Ref.

Set

ENCYCLOPAEDIA

of

FOOD SCIENCE
FOOD TECHNOLOGY

and

NUTRITION

ENCYCLOPAEDIA

of

FOOD SCIENCE
FOOD TECHNOLOGY
and
NUTRITION

Volume One

A–Cassava

Edited by

R. Macrae
University of Hull, Hull, UK

R. K. Robinson
University of Reading, Reading, UK

M. J. Sadler
Consultant Nutritionist, Ashford, UK

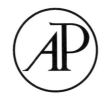

ACADEMIC PRESS

Harcourt Brace Jovanovich, Publishers
London   San Diego   New York
Boston   Sydney   Tokyo   Toronto

ACADEMIC PRESS LIMITED
24/28 Oval Road
LONDON NW1 7DX

United States Edition published by
ACADEMIC PRESS INC.
San Diego, CA 92101

A catalogue record for this book is available from the British Library

Library of Congress Cataloging-in-Publication Data
Encyclopaedia of food science, food technology, and nutrition/edited
    by R. Macrae, R. K. Robinson, M. J. Sadler.
        p.   cm.
      1. Food—Encyclopedias.   2. Food industry and trade—
    —Encyclopedias.   3. Nutrition—Encyclopedias.   I. Macrae, R.
    II. Robinson, R. K. (Richard Kenneth).   III. Sadler, M. J. (Michèle
    J.)
    TX349.E47   1993
    664′.003—dc20

ISBN   Volume 1 0-12-226851-2   Volume 5 0-12-226855-5
        Volume 2 0-12-226852-0   Volume 6 0-12-226856-3
        Volume 3 0-12-226853-9   Volume 7 0-12-226857-1
        Volume 4 0-12-226854-7   Volume 8 0-12-226858-X

ISBN Set 0-12-226850-4

EDITORIAL STAFF

Managing Editor
Gina Fullerlove

Assistant Editor
Sarah Robertson

Production Editors
David Atkins
Sara Hackwood

Production Controller
Anne Doris

Editorial Assistants
Jill Farrow
Lara King
Martina Tuohy

Copy Editors
Len Cegielka
Rich Cutler
Alison Walsh

Cross-referencer
Jane Wells

Proof Reader
Alison Woodhouse

Indexer
Merrall-Ross International

Editorial and Technical Support Manager
Christopher Gibson

Head of Book Production
Helen Whitehorn

Typeset by The Alden Press, Oxford
Printed in Great Britain by Butler and Tanner Ltd, Frome, Somerset, UK

D. B. Emmons
Food Research Centre, Ottawa,
Canada

O. R. Fennema
University of Wisconsin-Madison,
Madison, USA

D. L. Georgala
AFRC Institute of Food Research,
Reading, UK

M. J. Gibney
Trinity College Medical School,
Dublin, Eire

C. Gopalan
The Nutrition Foundation of India,
New Delhi, India

P. Gray
Commission of the European
Communities, Bruxelles, Belgium

M. S. Y. Hadaddin
University of Jordan, Amman,
Jordan

B. Hallgren
Swedish Nutrition Foundation,
Goteborg, Sweden

J. M. Hutchinson
FAO, Rome, Italy

B. Jarvis
HP Bulmer Ltd, Hereford, UK

M. E. Knowles
MAFF, London, UK

J. A. Kurmann
Institut Agricole de Fribourg,
Posieux, Switzerland

R. A. Lawrie
University of Nottingham, Lough-
borough, UK

F. A. Lee
Cornell University, New York, USA

D. X. Lin
Wuxi Institute of Light Industry,
Wuxi, People's Republic of China

V. Loureiro
Technical University of Lisbon,
Lisbon, Portugal

P. Lunven
FAO, Rome, Italy

E. J. Mann
International Dairy Federation,
Reading, UK

V. Marks
University of Surrey, Guildford, UK

H. E. Nursten
University of Reading, Reading, UK

R. Paoletti
Universita di Milano, Milan, Italy

K. L. Parkin
University of Wisconsin-Madison,
Madison, USA

G. T. Prance
Royal Botanic Gardens, Kew, UK

A. Reps
Institute of Food Biotechnology,
Kortowo, Poland

D. R. Richardson
Nestle, Croydon, UK

P. Richmond
AFRC Institute of Food Research,
Norwich, UK

A. Rougereau
Robert Debre Hospital, Amboise,
France

J. D. Schofield
Kings College, University of London,
UK

N. E. Schwartz
National Centre for Nutrition and
Dietetics, Chicago, USA

R. L. Sellars
Chr. Hansen's Laboratory Inc.,
Wisconsin, USA

J. Solms
Swiss Federal Institute of
Technology, Zurich, Switzerland

D. A. T. Southgate
AFRC Institute of Food Research,
Norwich, UK

K. R. Spurgeon
South Dakota State University,
South Dakota, USA

M. Stasse-Wolthuis
Netherlands Nutrition Foundation,
Wageningen, The Netherlands

P. S. Steyn
National Food Research Institute,
Pretoria, South Africa

P. Trayhurn
Rowett Research Institute,
Aberdeen, UK

A. S. Truswell
University of Sydney, Sydney, Australia

G. Varela
Universidad Complutense de
Madrid, Madrid, Spain

J. V. Wheelock
University of Bradford, Bradford, UK

E. M. Widdowson
Addenbrooke's Hospital, Cambridge,
UK

R. B. Wills
Food Industry Development Centre,
Kensington, Australia

BUCKINGHAM PALACE

Food is so vital for the survival and well-being of every society, that the provision of adequate supplies, and of the right quality, should be the central concern of Governments around the world. Thus, whether the problem is to ensure that the population of a less-developed country has sufficient food to avoid malnutrition, or to persuade sections of an industrialized society to have a properly balanced diet, the basic objectives are really the same, and it is sad to reflect upon the gap between intention and reality.

Half of the people of the world are still undernourished, and the problem increases daily as the world's population grows, apparently unabated. Yet each year, millions of tonnes of food are wasted as a result of inadequate processing and storage and, even more alarming, excesses of food produced in the West are being wasted. Recent decades have seen rapid progress in all aspects of the production, processing and distribution of nutritious foods. The knowledge and technical skills required to feed the world now exist and the extent of this expertise is vividly demonstrated by the range of topics covered in this Encyclopaedia.

Extending our knowledge of Food Science and Nutrition is similarly important to those of us who live under less arduous conditions. Changes in eating habits have resulted from the almost limitless choice of edible products. However, the increased consumption of processed and convenience foods need not lead to less nutritious diets, but it does demand our appreciation of all aspects of food handling. In the future we shall also see more emphasis placed on the correlation between diet and disease prevention, for example incidences of cancer or diabetes.

Choice of food is an individual choice, usually based on taste - not on Government recommendations. Choice can be and indeed should be - influenced by the best information available, but then it is up to the individuals to make their own choice.

For these reasons, I am extremely pleased to be associated with this remarkable informative publication, and it is particularly gratifying that so many scientists from around the world have been willing to make their expertise available. I wish the book every success.

Anne

HRH The Princess Royal

PREFACE

The food chain, in all its aspects, is an extremely diverse and complex subject. The starting point is food production and the end is the medical/nutritional implications of the food we eat. Along this tortuous route the food is subjected to all manner of chemical/biochemical and physical modifications which affect the quality, acceptability and nutritional value of the produce. This Encyclopaedia has been designed to provide the most comprehensive coverage possible of all aspects of the science of food, at all stages along the food chain. However, at a very early stage it became clear that some criteria for the selection of material would have to be agreed and, with this in mind, the initial stages of food production (agriculture and horticulture) have not been covered to the same extent as the mainstream topics of food science, food technology and nutrition. The decision to include a thorough coverage of nutrition, and indeed the physiological basis of nutritional studies, was not taken without some debate. However, it is the Editors' and publisher's view that an integrated approach to the subject, including nutrition, greatly enhances our understanding of what is happening to our food during processing, storage and cooking, and consequently how this affects our well being. It is believed that this is the first Encyclopaedic work to take this stance and we hope the balance of material will prove of interest to many readers.

Nevertheless, even with the selective criteria applied by the Editors, it has not been possible to cover every aspect of the subject in minute detail. The practical necessity of limiting the work to approximately 1000 articles, each of around 3000 words, was an essential restraint, and the failure of a few contracted authors to deliver their manuscripts to agreed deadlines has also resulted in some reduction in coverage. Even so, detailed information concerning the handling, composition and nutritional value of most important foodstuffs has been included, along with guidance for further reading, and hence there is little doubt that the work will meet the demands of most readers with ease.

The articles as far as possible, have been written with an international readership in mind and it is hoped that the entries with a local bias, e.g. Kefir, Sake and Samna, will, in fact, enhance the worldwide appeal of the Encyclopaedia rather than detract from it.

Robert Macrae
Richard Robinson
Michèle Sadler

INTRODUCTION

Food plays a central role in all of our lives, indeed it is the essential requirement for existence. In the developed world it is now taken for granted that there will always be a wide range of nutritious food available for consumption. Under these conditions of plenty, food, its preparation and its consumption, takes on additional roles at the very centre of culture, as a focus for family life, entertainment and even as a lubricant for the wheels of business. Furthermore as an area of employment, the food sector is crucial. However, while the developed world can ponder on the enormous choice of foods available a substantial proportion of the world population remains undernourished, and many millions are on the point of starvation. Whether as food scientists, technologists, or nutritionists, the problems facing those of us working in the food sector are truly staggering.

In the developed world the role of the food scientist is multifaceted and its importance to the 'health of a country' cannot be doubted. Yet it is also true that most people would survive, albeit with a greatly reduced standard and variety of diet, if the intervention of the food industry was to be scaled down. In less well developed countries the food scientist plays a critical role in ensuring survival. The reasons for malnutrition in parts of Asia, Africa, South America and other areas of the world are complex; nutritional status is inevitably conditioned by underlying environmental, social and cultural factors. In some areas the provision of adequate, uncontaminated water supplies poses the major difficulty. In other parts of the world malnutrition occurs not because of the actual lack of food *per se* but from inadequate supplies of the correct foods, in good condition, at the required places. In populations predominantly dependent on locally produced foods, deficiencies in specific micronutrients can cause disease, as in the occurrence of endemic goitre and cretinism in parts of the Himalayas and Andes where the soil has been leached of iodine through glaciation. In this respect the food scientist has a major role to play in the formulation and production of nutritious foods which are appropriate for their intended end use.

The problem of infant malnutrition is especially prominent in areas where infectious diseases are rife; together they are responsible for high infant mortality levels in many parts of the world. The nutritionist plays a crucial role in helping to solve such problems, for example through preventative programmes to promote the benefits of long term breast-feeding and informed weaning practices. The development and promotion of specialized weaning foods in centralized processing plants is also a major component of programmes in the developing countries. The food technologist can make an important contribution in this specific respect as well as in the general area of long-term preservation of nutritious foods under adverse conditions. The role of the nutritionist and the food scientist is also crucial in identifying the nutrients required and in ensuring that foods formulated are organoleptically acceptable.

In Europe, North America and other developed areas of the world changes in society have dictated significant shifts in the way that food is prepared. There is now demand for convenience foods which can be easily cooked and presented with the minimum of effort. This has extended to the feeding of infants, with very little weaning food being prepared in the home. The implications for the food industry are enormous, as foods must now be stable for long periods of time, whether dried, frozen, canned or preserved in some other way. Developments in technology have kept apace with this demand and the use of food additives such as antioxidants, stabilizers and preservatives have further increased the range of products available. However, further developments in food processing technologies, such as food irradiation, may reduce the need for preservatives. The urge to make foods attractive in appearance also leads to the use of added colours both synthetic and natural. Similarly the food industry has endeavoured to maintain the nutritive value of foods by replacement of nutrients lost during processing, and the fortification of some foods with nutrients above their natural levels, as for example in breakfast cereals. There is no doubt that the food industry has achieved remarkable success in presenting an ever increasing range of nutritious foods to the public. Nevertheless, in recent years there has been a move against the excessive use of food additives and this is most clearly illustrated by the reduced use of synthetic food colours and the increased market share of organically grown foods which have not been exposed to any 'added chemicals' during their growth and processing. Consumers are beginning to develop a greater interest in their diets and the resultant implications for health. The public increasingly look to nutritionists to provide firm guidelines on the optimum daily intake of both micronutrients (vitamins and trace metals) and macronutrients (proteins, lipids and carbohydrates). In some areas the recommendations are clear and unambiguous, for example the reduction in intake of saturated fats and the proportional increase of fruit, vegetables and cereals in the diet. Problems of obesity should be addressed with some urgency. In other areas the advice is less clear and the recommendations may depend on the sensitivity of the person concerned, an example that comes to mind is the rationale for drinking decaffeinated coffee. There is very little evidence to suggest that caffeine is toxic, but some individuals clearly react adversely to large intakes of coffee, which has been associated with caffeine. Other areas of concern are even more controversial with a wide range of conflicting views among the scientific community. The recent suggestion that vitamin supplementation in the diet of children may improve academic performance is a case in point and the debate will continue.

The increased proportion of factory prepared foods in diets should reduce the occurrence of food poisoning, and indeed it is true that overall the safety record of the industry in this respect is first class. However, increased incidences of outbreaks of disease such as salmonellosis and listeriosis are being reported. In some instances these can be attributed to undesirable agricultural practices, as in the feeding of untreated animal waste to chickens, although a significant cause can also be found in the poor understanding of potential hazards by those who prepare foods in institutions and in the home. Many pathogenic organisms are endogenous to our foods, and the risks to consumers can only be eliminated by correct and adequate processing coupled with detailed quality control of products.

A complete study of all of the aspects of food covers a very wide range of scientific disciplines. These subjects as applied to foods have traditionally been separated into food science, food technology and nutrition, but an appreciation of all branches of the science will be required if we are to solve the many problems the world faces on issues ranging from excess dietary intakes to food poisoning and malnutrition.

Robert Macrae
Richard Robinson
Michèle Sadler

GUIDE TO USE OF THE ENCYCLOPAEDIA

Structure of the Encyclopaedia

The material in the Encyclopaedia is arranged as a series of entries in alphabetical order. Some entries comprise a single article, whilst entries on more diverse subjects consist of several articles that deal with various aspects of the topic. In the latter case the articles are arranged in a logical sequence within an entry.

To help you realize the full potential of the material in the Encyclopaedia we have provided three features to help you find the topic of your choice.

Contents Lists

Your first point of reference will probably be the contents list. The complete contents list appearing in Volume 8 will provide you with both the volume number and the page number of the entry. Additionally each volume has a list of entries and articles to be found within that particular volume, which allows you to locate material within the volume without having to return to the complete contents list each time a new topic is required. On the opening page of an entry a contents list is provided so that the full details of the articles within the entry are immediately available.

Alternatively you may choose to browse through a volume using the alphabetical order of the entries as your guide. To assist you in identifying your location within the Encyclopaedia a running headline indicates the current entry and a running footer indicates the current article within that entry.

You will find 'Dummy Entries' where obvious synonyms exist for entries or where we have grouped together related analytical techniques or commodities. Dummy entries appear in both the contents list and the body of the text. For example, a Dummy Entry appears for Vitamin C which directs you to Ascorbic Acid, where the material is located.

Example

If you were attempting to locate material on Oranges via the Contents List.

Volume 5

Then once you have been directed to the correct location in the contents list this would then provide the page number.

If you were trying to locate the material by browsing through the text and you looked up Oranges then the following is the information you would be provided.

ORANGES

See Citrus Fruits

Alternatively, if you were looking up Citrus Fruits the following information would be provided.

CITRUS FRUITS

Contents

Types on the Market
Composition and Characterization
Oranges
Processed and Derived Products
* of Oranges*

Lemons
Grapefruits
Limes

Cross References

All of the articles in the Encyclopaedia have been extensively cross referenced.

The cross references, which appear at the end of a paragraph, have been provided at three levels:

1.   To indicate if a topic is discussed in greater detail elsewhere.

> **Groups at Risk of Vitamin C Deficiency (Scurvy)**
> The major determinant of vitamin C intake is the consumption of fruit and vegetables, and the range of intakes in healthy adults in Britain reflects this. The 2·5 percentile intake is 19 mg per day (men) and 14 mg per day (women), while the 97·5 percentile intake is 170 mg per day (men) and 160 mg per day (women). Deficiency is likely in people whose habitual intake of fruit and vegetables is very low. Smokers may be more at risk of deficiency; there is some evidence that the rate of ascorbate catabolism is two-fold higher in smokers than

in non-smokers. Clinical signs of deficiency are rarely seen in developed countries. *See* Scurvy

2. To draw the reader's attention to parallel discussions in other articles.

Fruit Morphology

Grapefruit is composed of three distinctly different morphological parts. The epicarp consists of the coloured portion of the peel and is known as the flavedo. In the flavedo are cells containing the carotenoids which give the characteristic colour to the fruit. The oil glands, also found in the flavedo, are the raised structures in the skin of the fruit that contain the essential oil, naringin, characteristics of the grapefruit. *See* Citrus Fruits, Oranges; Citrus Fruits, Lemons

3. To indicate material that broadens the discussion.

Plasma Concentration of Ascorbate

At intakes below 30 mg per day the plasma concentration of ascorbate is extremely low, and does not reflect increasing intake to any significant extent. As the intake rises, so the plasma concentration begins to increase sharply, reaching a plateau of 55–85 μmol l^{-1} at intakes between 70 and 100 mg per day, when the renal threshold is reached and the vitamin is excreted quantitatively with increasing intake. *See* Dietary Reference Values

Index

The index will provide you with the volume number and page number of where the material is to be located, and the index entries differentiate between material that is a whole article, is part of an article or is data presented in a table. On the opening page of the index detailed notes are provided.

Colour Plates

The colour figures for each volume have been grouped together in a plate section. The location of this section is cited both in the contents list and on the opening page of the pertinent articles.

Contributors and Referees

A full list of contributors and a full list of referees appears in Volume 8.

CONTENTS

Colour Plate Section appears between pages 556 and 557

ACCEPTABILITY OF FOOD

See Food Acceptability

ACESULPHAME

Acesulphame K (potassium salt of 6-methyl-1,2,3-oxathiazine-4 (3H)-one-2,2-dioxide; see Fig. 1) is a high-intensity artificial sweetener which is about 200 times as sweet as sucrose (compared to a 3% aqueous sucrose solution). It was accidentally discovered in 1967 by Dr Karl Clauss, a researcher with Hoechst AG in Frankfurt, FRG, during his experiments on new materials research. The sweetener is not metabolized by the human body and thus contributes no energy to the diet. It is now approved for use in more than 20 countries.

Sweetness

The sweetness properties of acesulphame K are similar to saccharin. It has a clean, sharp, sweet taste with a rapid onset of sweetness and no lingering aftertaste at normal use levels. However, at high concentrations, equivalent to 5% or 6% sucrose solutions, acesulphame K does possess a bitter, chemical aftertaste. The intensity of sweetness of acesulphame K, in common with other artificial sweeteners, varies depending upon its concentration and the type of food application. For example, it is 90 times sweeter than a 6% sucrose solution, 160 times sweeter than a 4% sucrose solution and 250 times sweeter than a 2% sucrose solution. *See* Carbohydrates, Sensory Properties; Saccharin; Sweeteners – Intense

Mixtures of acesulphame K with other intense sweeteners, such as aspartame or cyclamate, result in some synergistic increases in sweetness. Mixtures with saccharin are somewhat less synergistic.

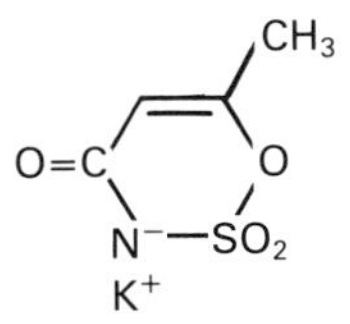

Fig. 1 Structure of acesulphame K.

Production and Physical and Chemical Properties

Acesulphame K (see Fig. 1) is structurally related to saccharin. It also has many of the same physical and chemical properties.

Acesulphame was one of a series of sweet-tasting substances synthesized by Hoescht AG in the late 1960s. All of these had in common the oxathiazinone dioxide ring structure. The synthesis involved reaction of fluorosulphonyl isocyanate with either acetylene derivatives or with active methylene compounds such as β-diketones, β-keto acids or esters. The latter reaction is used for commercial production of acesulphame K. A generalized reaction scheme for production of oxathiazinone dioxide ring is shown in Fig. 2. Many analogues have been prepared and evaluated for taste properties. The potassium salt of the 6-methyl derivative, acesulphame K, displayed the best sensory and physical properties and thus it has received extensive testing aimed at obtaining approval for its use in diet foods.

Acesulphame K is a white crystalline material which is stable up to 250°C at which temperature it decomposes. The free acid form of the sweetener has a distinct melting point of 123·5°C. Acesulphame K has a specific density of 1·83. When dissolved in water it produces a nearly

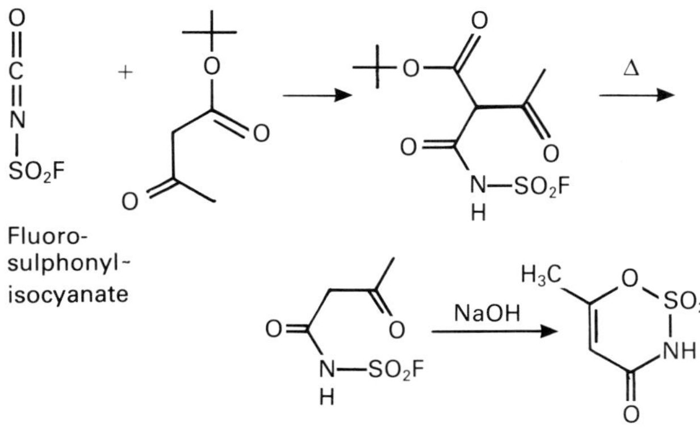

Fig. 2 Synthesis of the acesulphame ring structure using fluorosulphonyl isocyanate and *tert*-butylacetoacetate as starting materials.

Table 1. Typical use levels of acesulphame K in diet foods

Food product	Concentration (mg kg^{-1})
Soft drinks	1000
Coffee and tea	267
Jams and marmalades	3000
Ready-to-eat desserts	1000
Chewing gum	2000

neutral solution while the free acid is strongly acidic (pH of a 0.1 mol l^{-1} aqueous solution being 1.15). The sweetener is very soluble in water; a 27% solution can be prepared at 20°C. The solubility of acesulphame K increases significantly with temperature. At 80°C, 50% solutions can be prepared; because of this, greater than 99% purity can be obtained by crystallization. It is substantially less soluble in common solvents such as ethanol, methanol or acetone.

The stability of acesulphame K in the solid state is very good. It can be stored at ambient temperature for 10 years without decomposition. Aqueous solutions at pH 3 or greater may also be stored for extended periods without detectable decomposition or loss of sweetness. However, below pH 3, significant hydrolysis may occur at elevated temperatures. For example, at pH 2.5 an aqueous buffered solution of acesulphame K would decompose by about 30% after 4 months of storage at 40°C, whereas no decomposition occurs under the same conditions within the pH range of 3–8. At 20°C, less than 10% decomposition of acesulphame K occurs after 4 months' storage at pH 2.5, indicating that under normal storage conditions aqueous solutions of the sweetener are very stable.

Acesulphame K is stable under most food processing conditions, including the elevated temperature treatments encountered in pasteurization and baking.

Food Uses

Because of its stability, acesulphame K has been evaluated in a wide variety of diet food products, including table-top sweeteners, soft drinks, fruit preparations, desserts, breakfast cereals and chewing gum. Table 1 lists approximate concentration levels of acesulfame K typically used in several types of foods.

Safety and Regulatory Status

Acesulphame K has been subjected to extensive feeding studies in mice, rats and dogs. The substance is not considered to be carcinogenic, mutagenic nor teratogenic. It is excreted unmetabolized in test animals or humans. The current maximum acceptable daily intake (ADI) (the maximum amount that can be consumed daily for a lifetime without appreciable risk) established by the FAO/WHO (Food and Agriculture Organization, World Health Organization) Joint Expert Committee on Food Additives in 1990 is 5 mg per kg bodyweight. This value is based on the highest amount fed to animals for which there was no effect.

The first regulatory approval for acesulphame K was by the UK in 1983. Since then it has received approval for specific uses in more than 20 countries. *See* Legislation, Additives

Analysis

Thin-layer chromatography, isotachophoresis and high-performance liquid chromatography (HPLC) have been evaluated for the determination of acesulphame K in a variety of matrices, including liquid and solid food products, animal feed and biological fluids. Of the three, HPLC is perhaps the most useful since the efficiency of the chromatography coupled with selective detection (ultraviolet absorbance) enable quantitative measurements to be made in rather complex food samples. In addition, the sample preparation is minimal, usually involving a water extraction for solid samples or a filtration and dilution of liquid samples before direct HPLC analysis. Acesulphame K has been incorporated into a multisweetener analytical method employing HPLC. *See* Chromatography, High-performance Liquid Chromatography; Chromatography, Gas Chromatography

Bibliography

Franta R and Beck B (1986) Alternatives to cane and beet sugar. *Food Technology* 40: 116–128.

Hough CAM, Parker KJ and Vlitos AJ (1981) *Developments in Sweeteners* – 1. Essex: Elsevier Science Publishers.

Lawrence JF and Charbonneau CF (1988) Determination of seven artificial sweeteners in diet food preparations by reverse-phase liquid chromatography with absorbance detection. *Journal Association of Official Analytical Chemists* 71: 934–937.

James F. Lawrence
Sir FG Banting Research Centre, Ottawa, Canada

ACIDOPHILUS MILK

Acidophilus milk is a cultured dairy product which is known for its therapeutic properties. *Lactobacillus acidophilus* is the starter culture for this product. This microorganism is a normal inhabitant of the gut and a member of the intestinal microflora of humans and animals. It has been used as a beneficial dietary adjunct for the treatment of intestinal disorders. *See* Lactic Acid Bacteria; Starter Cultures

Definition

The absence of a unified world charter for the definition of fermented milk products makes a precise definition of acidophilus milk a difficult task. In broad terms, acidophilus milk, as it is traditionally known, is milk which has been nearly sterilized and inoculated with a pure culture of one or more strains of the bacterium *L. acidophilus*. It has been fermented under optimal conditions which favour growth and development of large numbers of this microorganism. The final product has acid taste and slightly viscous consistency. *See* Fermented Milks, Types of Fermented Milks

Historical Background

Nearly every civilization has known fermented milks. It has been claimed that they originated in the Near East and spread throughout eastern and central Europe. Traditional acidophilus milk and related products are widely recognized in southeastern Europe as well as central Europe and southwest Asia. In some of these countries, they occupy an important place in the diet of the population and form the staple ingredient for a variety of food products. Acidophilus milk products are also known to be associated with a long life, good nutrition and excellent health. *See* Fermented Milks, Products from Northern Europe; Fermented Milks, Kefir

Related Acidophilus Products

Acidophilus milk is one of several products containing *L. acidophilus* as the sole organism or in combination with other cultures (Table 1). Some of these products have been available to consumers as traditional fermented dairy products. Acidophilus milk and acidophilus-yeast preparations are examples of such products. Other products can be classified as fermented but nontraditional,

e.g. Bioghurt, Biogarde and acidophilus-bifidus yoghurt. More recently, new nonconventional and nonfermented products have been introduced, e.g. sweet acidophilus milk and concentrated acidophilus tablets.

Acidophilus products vary widely in their manufacturing methods. Their sensory, nutritional and therapeutic properties can be significantly influenced by the manufacturing method, as well as the type, number and viability of their culture.

Lactobacillus acidophilus

The importance of using a dietary adjunct to maintain balanced intestinal microflora has focused attention on *L. acidophilus*. This organism, along with *Bifidobacterium bifidum* and *L. casei*, have been most frequently

Table 1. Commercial preparations of acidophilus products

Product	Microorganism(s)
Acidophilus milk	*Lactobacillus acidophilus*
Acidophilus-yeast milk	*L. acidophilus, Saccharomyces fragilis, S. cerevisiae*
Acidophilus buttermilk	*L. acidophilus, Lactococcus lactis, Lac. lactis* subsp. *cremoris, Lac. lactis* biovar. *diacetylactis, Leuconostoc mesenteroides* subsp. *cremoris*
Acidophilus tablets	*L. acidophilus, Bifidobacterium bifidum*
Acidophilus paste	*L. acidophilus*
Acidophilus yoghurt	*L. acidophilus, L. delbrueckii* subsp. *bulgaricus, Streptococcus thermophilus*
Acidophilus-bifidus yoghurt	*L. acidophilus, Bif. bifidum, L. delbrueckii* subsp. *bulgaricus, St. thermophilus*
Biogarde	*L. acidophilus, Bif. bifidum, St. thermophilus*
Bioghurt	*L. acidophilus, St. thermophilus*
Biokys	*L. acidophilus, Bif. bifidum, Pediococcus acidilactici*
Cultura	*L. acidophilus, Bif. bifidum*
Sweet acidophilus	*L. acidophilus*
Yakult	*L. acidophilus, Bif. bifidum, Bf. breve, L. casei*

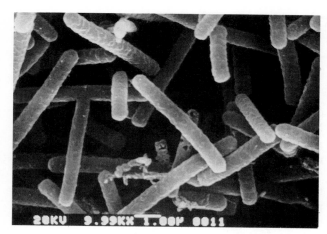

Fig. 1 A scanning electron micrograph of *Lactobacillus acidophilus*. The micrograph was obtained at magnification ×9990, 20 kV accelerating voltage. Scalebar, 1·00 μm. (Authorship and courtesy of Dr. Miloslav Kalab, Food Research Centre, Agriculture Canada, Ottawa, Ontario, Canada.)

described as intestinal lactobacilli. These bacteria are characterized by their ability to survive and grow in the intestinal tract. They can also produce substances that are antagonistic towards enteric pathogens.

Lactobacillus acidophilus, an acid-loving bacterium, is a homofermentative lactobacillus producing mainly DL-lactic acid. It is a Gram-positive rod with rounded ends (Fig. 1). It occurs singly, in pairs or in short chains. It is nonflagellated, nonmotile, nonspore-former, and is intolerant to salt. The size is 0·6–0·9 by 1·5–6·0 μm. It was originally isolated from the faeces of infants, but is also found in the mouth and vagina of human young and adults. *L. acidophilus* is described as a 'thermobacterium intestinale' which does not grow at 15°C, and some strains may not grow at 22°C. Growth can occur at 45°C but the optimum temperature is 35–38°C. Its acid tolerance varies from 0·3% to 1·9% titratable acidity, with an optimum pH of 5·5–6·0.

Although *L. acidophilus* is widely distributed in nature, it is a fastidious microorganism and has complex nutritional requirements. It grows slowly in milk, and some of its nutritional needs include acetate, nicotinic acid, riboflavin, and calcium pentathonate.

Manufacturing Methods

Acidophilus Milk

As a result of its fastidious nature, *L. acidophilus* does not grow rapidly in milk, and acid is produced rather slowly. This slow process of growth and acid production limits the ability of the organism to overcome contamination with other bacteria. Sterilizing the milk during propagation of the culture is therefore essential for

preservation of the purity and viability of this culture. Another limitation of this organism, during manufacture, is its sensitivity to acidity levels beyond the narrow range of its optimal pH of 5·5–6·0. Below pH 5, the numbers of this bacterium decline and, depending on the strain used, this decline can be significant and rapid.

Pure commercial cultures of *L. acidophilus* are obtained in a freeze-dried form or as a highly concentrated, wet biomass containing about 50×10^{12} viable organisms per ml of substrate. These cultures may require several propagations into mother or bulk cultures if they are to be suitable for direct inoculation of the process milk. Sterilized milk is used for the propagation of the mother cultures. After sterilization, this milk is cooled to 37°C, inoculated with the commercial culture using the manufacturer's specifications, and incubated to a titratable acidity of 0·6–1·0% lactic acid. Similarly, bulk cultures are prepared with 1% of the active mother culture.

Whole or partially skimmed milk is usually used in the preparation of acidophilus milk. This milk is nearly sterilized at 95°C for 1 h and cooled to 37°C. It is a good manufacturing practice to hold the milk at this temperature for a period of 3–4 h to promote germination of existing spores which survive the initial heat treatment. The milk is then reheated to destroy the vegetative cells, cooled down again to 37°C and inoculated with 2–5% of an active bulk culture. The milk is left to ferment. During this fermentation, it is essential that acidity is very closely monitored, so that after the cooling process a final product is obtained with a pH of 5·5–6·0 and a desirable bacterial count of $2–3 \times 10^9$ (colony-forming units) per ml of milk. After fermentation, the product is cooled to 5–10°C, stored at this range of temperature and rapidly distributed.

The production of a high number of viable bacteria in the product, and the maintenance of this number up to consumption time are both difficult tasks to accomplish in practice. It is therefore inevitable that the viability of the organisms will suffer, and a decline in number will be observed, especially after a week of storage.

Acidophilus Products

Acidophilus products have a wide range of compositions and methods of manufacture. Acidophilus-yeast milk, an old and traditional fermented milk, is a national sour milk beverage in the Soviet Union. It is prepared by inoculating 3–5% of acidophilus-yeast starter into nearly sterilized milk (90–95°C for 10 min) which has been cooled to 35–40°C. After inoculation, the milk is mixed, bottled and stored at 30°C until it is coagulated. The acidophilus bacteria and lactose-fermenting yeasts are prepared separately and mixed prior to inoculation of the milk. These cultures are selected for their ability to produce a desirable taste in the product, and also for their alcohol-forming properties and antibacterial action against a variety of pathogens, in particular against *Mycobacterium tuberculosis*. The final product is described as slightly viscous, ropy, effervescent due to liberation of carbon dioxide, and sourish in taste with a distinctive 'yeasty' aroma.

Acidophilus yoghurt products, such as acidophilus yoghurt, acidophilus-bifidus yoghurt, Biogarde and Bioghurt, are well known in Europe. They are presented by adding *L. acidophilus* and *Bifidobacterium bifidum* to the yoghurt culture during the process of yoghurt making. In some of these products, milk is fortified with growth stimulants to accommodate for the multiple culture and provide the desirable number of bacteria in the final product. *See* Yoghurt, Yoghurt-based Products

Sweet acidophilus milk and acidophilus tablets are relatively new acidophilus products, and more common to the USA. Sweet acidophilus milk is made by adding a highly concentrated cell mass of *L. acidophilus* to cold pasteurized milk (5×10^6 per ml of milk) and the product is stored below 5°C. Since *L. acidophilus* does not grow at this temperature, no fermentation will take place and the product remains sweet. Sweet acidophilus milk has stimilar organoleptic properties to pasteurized fresh milk and is appealing to the Western palate.

Acidophilus tablets are freeze-dried preparations of *L. acidophilus* and contain about 2×10^9 of this organism per tablet. These preparations are usually made with skim milk powder and lactose. It is also possible to use nondairy ingredients in such preparations. *Lactobacillus acidophilus* could be used either alone or in combination with other bacteria, such as *Bif. bifidum*.

In Japan, products bearing the name 'Yakult' have been developed with *L. acidophilus*, *L. casei* and bifidus bacteria. Beneficial effects have been attributed to these products.

Quality Aspects

Organoleptic Properties

Acidophilus milk can be described as a fermented milk with an acquired taste. In spite of its popularity in eastern Europe, it has a limited organoleptic appeal in the Western world because of its undesirable sour milk flavour. The main attraction of this product is in its therapeutic values rather than its sensory qualities. Attempts have been made to utilize the beneficial therapeutic effects of *L. acidophilus* by channelling the organism into products which are more palatable and appealing to consumers. Sweet acidophilus milk is an example of such a product. It permits the consumer to enjoy the familiar pleasant taste of pasteurized milk and, at the same time, to ingest large quantities of the acidophilus culture.

Nutritional Value

The nutrient composition of acidophilus milk is basically similar to milk, but some differences exist as a result of the addition of the microbial culture with all its inherent enzyme systems. Proteins, fats and carbohydrates (lactose) are exposed to hydrolytic breakdown and are favourably altered during this lactic acid fermentation. Although the total amino acid content is not different from milk, the free amino acids are significantly higher in acidophilus milk. The partial digestion of proteins in the product can be beneficial to individuals with impaired digestion. Protein quality and biological value, on the other hand, are similar in acidophilus milk and non-fermented milk. *See* Amino Acids, Properties and Occurrence

The carbohydrate, lactose, is partially broken down and converted into lactic acid. As a result, the lower level of lactose remaining in the product, in addition to the availability of lactase (β-galactosidase) enzyme from *L. acidophilus* for further breakdown of lactose in the digestive tract, makes acidophilus milk a better product for lactose-intolerant individuals. *See* Food Intolerance, Lactose Intolerances

The concentration of vitamins is usually lower in acidophilus milk and other fermented acidophilus products. Folic acid is an exception; it increases during the fermentation process. The vitamin content can be affected by the type, amount and method of manufacture of the product. Some strains of *L. acidophilus* were found to be capable of synthesizing nicotinic acid, ascorbic acid, vitamin B_{12} and folic acid. *See* Ascorbic Acid, Properties and Determination; Folic Acid, Properties and Determination; Nicotinic Acid, Properties and Determination

Absorption of minerals such as calcium and iron is enhanced in fermented milks. Minerals have to be ionized before absorption, and lactic acid facilitates this process. In evaluating the nutritional value of foods, concentration as well as bioavailability of nutrients should be recognized. Fermented dairy foods, in particular acidophilus milk and yoghurt, are excellent dietary sources of calcium because of the high concentration as well as the bioavailability of this mineral in these products. *See* Bioavailability of Nutrients; Calcium, Physiology; Iron, Physiology

Therapeutic Properties

In addition to their refreshing taste and high nutritional value, acidophilus milk products possess considerable therapeutic properties. The close association between intestinal lactobacilli and health was first advocated by Ilya Metchnikoff, a bacteriologist who shared a Nobel Prize in 1908. From his pioneering studies, he concluded that putrefaction in the large intestine produces dege-

Table 2. Therapeutic properties of acidophilus milk products

Therapeutic properties	Possible causes and mechanisms
Improved digestibility	Partial breakdown of proteins, fats and carbohydrates
Enhanced growth	Improved bioavailability of nutrients
Lactose tolerance	Reduced lactose in product and further availability of lactase enzyme
Antimicrobial action	Acidity and microbial inhibitors
Anticarcinogenic effect	Inhibit formation of carcinogens; reduce carcinogen-promoting enzymes; stimulate host immune system
Anticholesterolaemic effect	Production of inhibitors of cholesterol synthesis
Colonization in the gut	Survive gastric acid; resist lysozyme and low surface tension of intestine; adhere to intestinal mucosa and grow
Stimulation of the host immunological system	Enhancement of macrophage formation; stimulation of suppressor cells production and γ-interferon
Prolongation of life?	Reduce intestinal putrefaction and autointoxication

nerative factors, and he described this process as 'autointoxication'. This process, he claimed, was the main cause of old age, senility and natural death. In his book, *The Prolongation of Life*, he suggested the elimination of putrefactive bacteria by ingestion of large amounts of Bulgarian sour milk, which contained the bacterium he isolated and named *Bacillus bulgaricus*. Further investigations identified the organism he actually used as *B. acidophilus*. Metchnikoff postulated that after ingestion, these lactic acid bacteria will colonize the gastrointestinal tract and suppress toxin formation by producing an unfavourable acidic environment for the putrefactive bacteria.

However, Metchnikoff was unable to prove the colonization of these bacteria in the intestinal tract. Rettger and Chaplin (1921) succeeded in providing the first scientific evidence that some strains of *L. acidophilus* were able to implant themselves in the gastrointestinal tract.

The therapeutic properties of acidophilus products and their possible causes and mechanisms are summarized in Table 2. The subjects of the colonization by *L. acidophilus* and the therapeutic properties attributed to acidophilus milk products are both complex and contro-

versial. Most of the accumulated evidence concerning these issues has been accumulated *in vitro* or from *in vivo* studies on experimental animals. However, clinical evidence from studies of humans is insufficient at present to show conclusively a direct comparison between consumption of acidophilus bacteria and their therapeutic effects, particularly those properties related to anticarcinogenic effects and stimulation of the host immunological system. Manifestations of therapeutic properties, for example, will not be exhibited if the nutritional needs and growth requirements for *L. acidophilus* are lacking. Selection of specific strains, host specificity and viability of the culture organism are all critical parameters to be considered. Furthermore, uncertainties related to the chemical identity of the microbial inhibitors produced by these lactic bacteria continue to prevail. Several inhibitors, such as lactolin, lactocidin, acidolin, acidophilin and other unidentified compounds, have been isolated from *L. acidophilus*. Their chemical identity is still unknown. It is also unclear whether these inhibitors are separate compounds or merely the same substance with different names.

In spite of the prevailing uncertainties and controversies which necessitate further research, it is still widely accepted that acidophilus products possess exceptional nutritional and therapeutic properties.

Future Trends

As a result of the beneficial role they play in health and general well-being, acidophilus milk products could offer exciting potential for the future. Genetic engineering of microorganisms used in fermented milk products can improve the economics of processing of these products. It can also enhance flavour, texture, shelf life and nutritional qualities of such products. In providing tools for genetic engineering, bio-technology would be instrumental in engineering healthier organisms. Metabolic capabilities of *L. acidophilus* could be altered to produce more resilient and competitive strains with less complex nutritional requirements. New strains could be structured with powerful implantation capabilities, increased stability and enhanced therapeutic effects. In addition, new starter technology would provide highly concentrated cultures which are phage-resistant and ready for direct inoculation of milk without prior propagations.

What is needed in the future is an acidophilus milk product which is easy to manufacture and has attractive organoleptic properties. It should possess distinctive therapeutic values, and have sustained the viability of the culture during manufacture and storage.

Bibliography

Buchanan RE and Gibbons NE (eds) (1975) *Bergey's Manual of Determinative Bacteriology* 8th edn. Baltimore: Williams and Wilkins.

Chandan RC (ed.) (1989) *Yogurt: Nutritional and Health Properties*. Virginia: National Yogurt Association.

Gilliland SE (1979) Beneficial interrelationships between certain microorganisms and humans: candidate microorganisms for use as dietary adjuncts. *Journal of Food Protection* 42(2): 164–167.

Kosikowski FV (1977) *Cheese and Fermented Milk Foods* 2nd edn. New York: Kosikowski and Associates.

Metchnikoff I (1908) *The Prolongation of Life*. New York: GP Putnams and Sons.

Puhan Z (1990) Developments in the technology of fermented milk products. *Cultured Dairy Products Journal* 25(2): 4–9.

Rettger LF and Chaplin HA (1921) *A Treatise on the Transformation of the Intestinal Flora with Special Reference to the Implantation of* Bacillus acidophilus. Connecticut: Yale University Press.

Shahani KM and Chandan RC (1979) Nutritional and health aspects of cultured and culture-containing foods. *Journal of Dairy Science* 62: 1685–1694.

Speck ML (1975) Acidophilus food products. *Journal of Dairy Science* 58: 783–784.

Tamime AY and Robinson RK (1988) Fermented milks and their future trends. *Journal of Dairy Research* 55: 281–307.

Joseph P. Salji
Bedford, UK

ACIDS

Contents

Properties and Determination

In very general terms, an acid is a compound which contains or produces hydrogen ions in aqueous solutions, has a sour taste, and turns blue litmus paper red. A more comprehensive definition, given by the US chemist G. N. Lewis, states that acids are substances which can accept an electron pair or pairs, and bases are substances which can donate an electron pair or pairs. This definition, applicable to both nonaqueous and aqueous systems, requires that an acid be either a positive ion or a molecule with one or more electron-deficient sites with respect to a corresponding base.

The definition most widely used to describe acid–base reactions in dilute solution is one that was proposed independently by two scientists in 1923—the Danish chemist J. N. Brønsted and the US chemist T. M. Lowry. The Brønsted–Lowry theory defines an acid as a proton donor; that is, any substance (charged or uncharged) which can release a hydrogen ion or proton. A base is defined as a proton acceptor or any substance which can accept a hydrogen ion or proton.

This article discusses the physicochemical properties of acids and describes several methods for their analysis.

Strong versus Weak Acids

The strength of a Brønsted–Lowry acid depends on how easily it releases a proton or protons. In strong acids, owing to their weaker internal hydrogen bonds, the protons are loosely held. As a result, in aqueous solutions almost all of the acid reacts with water, leaving only a few unionized acid molecules in the equilibrium mixture. The reaction takes place according to eqn [1].

$$HA + H_2O \rightleftharpoons H_3O^+ + A^- \qquad (1)$$

In this equation, HA represents the undissociated acid; H_3O^+ the hydronium ion formed when a proton combines with one molecule of water and A^- the conjugate base of HA.

Unlike strong acids, weak acids exist largely in the undissociated state when mixed with water since only a small percentage of their molecules interact with water and dissociate. Most acids found in foods, including acetic, adipic, citric, fumaric, malic, phosphoric and tartaric acids and glucono-δ-lactone, are classified as weak acids.

Physicochemical Properties

Physicochemical properties, including the ionization constant, pH, pK_a and buffering capacity are discussed below.

Ionization Constant

The tendency for an acid or acid group to dissociate is defined by its ionization constant, also called the apparent dissociation constant (K_a). The ionization constant, given at a specified temperature, is expressed as

$$K_a = \frac{[H_3O^+][A^-]}{[HA]},\qquad (2)$$

where the brackets designate concentration in moles per litre. The ionization constant is a measure of acid strength: the higher the K_a value, the greater the number the hydrogen ions liberated per mole of acid in solution and the stronger the acid.

Acids having more than one transferable hydrogen ion per molecule are termed 'polyprotic' acids. Mono-protic or monobasic acids are those which can liberate one hydrogen ion, such as acetic acid and lactic acid. Those containing two transferable hydrogens ions are called diprotic or dibasic acids and include, for example, adipic acid and fumaric acid. Acids such as citric acid and phosphoric acid, which have three transferable hydrogens, are called triprotic or tribasic acids. Ionization of polyprotic acids occurs in a stepwise manner with the transfer of one hydrogen ion at a time. Each step is characterized by a different ionization constant.

pH

Measurement of acidity is an important aspect of ascertaining the safety and quality of foods. Such measurements are given in terms of pH which is defined as the negative logarithm of the hydronium ion concentration (strictly, activity):

$$pH = \log_{10}\frac{1}{[H_3O^+]} = -\log_{10}[H_3O^+].\qquad (3)$$

The lower the pH value, the higher the hydrogen ion concentration associated with it. A pH value of less than 7 indicates a hydrogen ion concentration greater than 10^{-7} M and an acidic solution; a pH value of more than 7 indicates a hydrogen ion concentration of less than 10^{-7} M and a basic solution. When the hydronium and hydroxide ions are equal in concentration, the solution is described as neutral. *See* pH – Principles and Measurement

It is also important to point out that because the pH scale is logarithmic, a difference of one pH unit represents a 10-fold difference in hydrogen ion concentration.

pK_a

The term pK_a is defined as the negative logarithm of the dissociation constant:

$$pK_a = \log_{10}\frac{1}{K_a} = -\log_{10}K_a.\qquad (4)$$

The pK_a corresponds to the pH value at the midpoint of a titration curve developed when one equivalent of weak acid is titrated with base and the pH resulting from each incremental addition of base is plotted against the equivalents of hydroxide ions added.

The pH of a system is at the pK_a when the concentrations of acid (HA) and conjugate base (A^-) are equal. At the pK_a and to a lesser extent in the area extending to within one pH unit on either side of the pK_a, the system resists changes in pH resulting from addition of small increments of acid or base. In other words, at the pK_a, acids and their salts function as buffers.

The number of pK_as an acid has depends on the number of hydrogen ions it can liberate. Monoprotic acids have a single pK_a, while di- and triprotic acid have two and three pK_as, respectively.

Strong acids have low pK_a values, and strong bases high pK_a values.

Buffering Capacity

A solution of a weak acid (or a weak base) and its corresponding salt is called a buffer solution. In these systems the hydronium ion content is not significantly changed when a small amount of acid or base is added to that solution. The reason buffer solutions resist appreciable changes in pH can be best illustrated by an example. If a small amount of hydrochloric acid is added to a buffer solution composed of acetic acid and sodium acetate, the protons from the hydrochloric acid would associate with the acetate ions to form unionized molecules of acetic acid. As the newly formed acid molecules ionize, the equilibrium would shift towards forming more hydronium ions (eqn [1]). This would result in only a very slight increase in pH.

Similarly, addition of a small amount of sodium hydroxide to the same buffer solution would have little effect on pH. Hydroxide ions from the sodium hydroxide would combine with hydronium ions in the equilibrium mixture, forming undissociated molecules of sodium hydroxide. More of the acid molecules would then dissociate to replace the hydronium ions lost; though a new equilibrium system would be created, it would produce only a minimal effect on pH.

The quantity of acid or base that a buffer solution is capable of consuming before a change in pH is realized is termed the 'buffering capacity'. The buffering capacity is defined as the number of moles of strong acid or base required to increase the pH by one unit in 1 litre of buffer solution. The buffering capacity of a solution is greatest at its pK_a value where the concentrations of acid and conjugate base are equal.

Analytical Methods

Quantitative determinations of acidity play an important role in ensuring food product quality and stability.

Information obtained on acid levels can help in detecting cases of food adulteration, monitoring fermentation processes, and evaluating the organoleptic properties of fermented foods. pH determination, titratable acidity, chromatographic methods, and capillary electrophoresis are procedures commonly employed by the food industry to determine food acids. *See* Adulteration of Foods, Detection

pH Determination

The measurement of pH can be undertaken by two techniques: colorimetric and potentiometric. The colorimetric method involves adding a suitable indicator to a solution and matching the colour of the solution to a standard solution containing the same indicator. This method can estimate pH to the nearest 0·1 pH unit.

A more accurate technique and the one most frequently employed, the potentiometric method, uses a pH meter to determine hydrogen ion concentration. The two electrodes of the meter—a calomel reference electrode and a glass indicator electrode—are immersed in the solution, of known temperature, whose pH is to be measured. The electrode potential of the indicator electrode is linearly related to changes in hydrogen ion concentration and therefore pH.

Titratable Acidity

The total concentration of acid in a solution can be determined by titration. The titration process is performed by placing in a flask a known volume of acid solution whose concentration is unknown. To the flask a few drops of indicator—e.g. phenolphthalein, which is colourless in acid solutions and pink in basic solutions—is introduced. A base solution of known concentration is then gradually added until the acid is completely neutralized. This point is indicated when the solution permanently changes colour. The concentration of acid can then be calculated from the volume of base solution used.

The value obtained, called titratable acidity, is an estimate of the total acid in the solution. It accounts for both the free hydronium ions present in the equilibrium mixture and the hydrogen ions released from undissociated acid molecules. For weak acids, the titratable acidity is different from the actual acidity (hydrogen ion concentration) since these compounds exist largely in the undissociated state in solution. For strong acids, however, titratable acidity and actual acidity are virtually the same, since strong acids and their salts are completely ionized in solution.

Chromatographic Methods

Gas chromatography (GC) and high-performance liquid chromatography (HPLC) have almost entirely replaced paper and thin-layer chromatography as methods for identifying and quantifying food acids.

Gas Chromatography

GC has been used to analyse organic acids in fruit and fruit juice. Analysis involves preparing volatile derivatives such as methyl esters of the organic acids, prior to their injection into the gas chromatograph. Derivatives are chromatographed on a nonpolar stationary phase column and detected by a flame ionization detector.

By use of GC, malic acid has been shown to be a major constituent of many fruits, including apples, pears, grapes, peaches and nectarines, while significant levels of citric acid were found in citrus fruits such as orange, lemon and grapefruit, and in noncitrus fruits, including pears, nectarines, cherries and strawberries. *See* Chromatography, Gas Chromatography

High-Performance Liquid Chromatography

HPLC is used more extensively than GC to determine organic acids because the technique requires little or no chemical modification to separate these nonvolatile compounds. Separation is usually done on either a reversed phase C8 or C18 column or a cation exchange resin column operated in the hydrogen mode. Acids are detected by either refractive index (RI) or ultraviolet (UV) detectors. RI detection requires prior removal of any sugars present which can potentially interfere with quantification; sugar removal is not required for UV detection at 220–230 nm.

Adulteration of a commercial cranberry juice drink was detected by use of HPLC when the test yielded different results for organic acids, sugars and anthocyanin pigments than those obtained for a standard juice drink. Atypical citric and/or malic acid contents and presence of a natural colourant, probably grape skin extract, confirmed the drink was adulterated.

In wine-making, HPLC is used to monitor concentrations of tartaric, malic, succinic, citric, lactic and acetic acids, which contribute tartness and stability to the finished product. A common approach involves using a column containing a strong cation exchange resin and eluting the sample with dilute sulphuric acid; the eluant is then analysed for acids by RI detection. This column has the additional advantage of permitting the simultaneous detection and quantification of ethanol and the monitoring of wine for adulteration with methanol. Organic acids in wine can also be separated using ion chromatography with a conductivity detector. *See* Chromatography, High-performance Liquid Chromatography

Capillary Electrophoresis

A relatively new technique, capillary electrophoresis is also useful for separating and quantifying organic acids in food systems. This technique utilizes an electrical field to separate molecules on the basis of their charge and size. Small volumes of sample, usually a few nanolitres, are injected onto a fused silica capillary tube which is usually less than 100 cm in length and 50 μm in internal diameter. The ends of the tube are placed in electrolyte reservoirs containing electrodes. A voltage in the range 20–30 kV is delivered to the electrodes by a power supply and causes the charged molecules to move. Because organic acids are negatively charged, they migrate away from more neutral or positively charged molecules, such as sugars and phenols, respectively. Acids are detected by a UV detector, and the signal is sent to a data collector. The resulting separation is graphically represented as a electropherogram. *See* Electrophoresis

Bibliography

Fennema OR (ed.) (1979) *Food Chemistry. Principles of Food Science*, part 1. New York: Marcel Dekker.
Lehninger AL (1975) *Biochemistry*, 2nd edn. New York: Worth.
Macrae R (1988) *HPLC in Food Analysis*. London: Academic Press.
Pomeranz Y and Meloan CE (1978) *Food Analysis: Theory and Practice*. Westport: AVI.

J. D. Dziezak
Institute of Food Technologists, Chicago, USA

Natural Acids and Acidulants

Acids, or acidulants as they are also called, are commonly used in food processing as flavour intensifiers, preservatives, buffers, meat-curing agents, viscosity modifiers and leavening agents. This article discusses the functions that acidulants have in food systems and reviews the more commonly used food acidulants.

Functions of Acidulants

The reasons for using acidulants in foods are numerous and depend on what the food processor hopes to accomplish. As outlined above, the principal reasons for incorporating an acidulant into a food system are for flavour modification, microbial inhibition and chelation.

Flavour Modification

Sourness or tartness is one of the five major taste sensations: sour, salty, sweet, bitter and umami (the most recently determined). Unlike the sensations of sweetness and bitterness which can be developed by a variety of molecular structures, sourness is evoked only by the hydronium ion of acidic compounds.

Each acid has a particular set of taste characteristics which include the time of perceived onset of sourness, the intensity of sourness, and any lingering of aftertaste. Some acids impart a stronger sour note than others at the same pH. As a general rule, weak acids have a stronger sour taste than strong acids at the same pH because they exist primarily in the undissociated state. As the small amount of hydronium ions is neutralized in the mouth, more undissociated acid (HA) molecules ionize to replace the hydronium ions lost from equilibrium (eqn [1]). The newly released hydronium ions are then neutralized until no acid remains. Taste characteristics of the acid are an important factor in the development of flavour systems.

$$HA + H_2O \rightleftharpoons H_3O^+ + A^- \qquad (1)$$

Acids also have the ability to modify or intensify the taste sensations of other flavour compounds, to blend unrelated taste characteristics, and to mask undesirable aftertastes by prolonging a tartness sensation. For example, in fruit drinks formulated with low-caloric sweeteners, acids mask the aftertaste of the sweetener and impart the tartness that is characteristic of the natural juice. *See* Flavour Compounds, Structures and Characteristics; Sensory Evaluation, Taste

Microbial Inhibition

Acidulants act as preservatives by retarding the growth of microorganisms and the germination of microbial spores which lead to food spoilage. The effect is attributed to both the pH and the concentration of the acid in its undissociated state. It is primarily the undissociated form of the acid which carries the antimicrobial activity: as the pH is lowered, this helps shift the equilibrium in favour of the undissociated form of the acid, thereby leading to more effective antimicrobial activity. The nature of the acid is also an important factor in microbial inhibition: weak acids are more effective at the same pH in controlling microbial growth. Acids affect primarily bacteria because many of these organisms do not grow well below about pH 5; yeasts and moulds, in comparison, are usually acid-tolerant. *See* Spoilage, Bacterial Spoilage; Spoilage, Moulds in Food Spoilage; Spoilage, Yeasts in Food Spoilage

In fruit- and vegetable-canning operations, the combined use of heat and acidity permits sterilization and spore inactivation to be achieved at lower temperatures; this minimizes the degradation of flavour and structure that generally results from processing. *See* Canning, Principles

Acidification also improves the effectiveness of antimicrobial agents such as benzoates, sorbates, and propionates. For example, sodium benzoate – an effective inhibitor of bacteria and yeasts – does not exert its antimicrobial activity until the pH is reduced to about 4·5. *See* Preservation of Food

Chelation

Oxidative reactions occur naturally in foods. They are responsible for many undesirable effects in the product, including discoloration, rancidity, turbidity and degradation of flavour and nutrients. As catalysts to these reactions, metal ions such as copper, iron, manganese, nickel, tin and zinc need to be present in only trace quantities in the product or on the processing machinery. *See* Oxidation of Food Components

Many acids chelate the metal ions so as to render them unavailable; the unshared pair of electrons in the molecular structure of acids promotes the complexing action. When used in combination with antioxidants such as butylated hydroxyanisole (BHA), butylated hydroxytoluene (BHT) or tertiary butylhydroquinone (TBHQ), acids have a synergistic effect on product stability. Citric acid and its salts are the most widely used chelating agents. *See* Antioxidants, Natural Antioxidants; Antioxidants, Synthetic Antioxidants

Other Functions

One of the most common reasons for adding acids is to control pH. This is usually done as a means to retard enzymatic reactions, to control the gelation of certain hydrocolloids and proteins, and to standardize pH in fermentation processes. In the first example, the lowering of pH inactivates many natural enzymes which promote product discoloration and development of off-flavours. Polyphenol oxidase, for example, oxidizes phenols to quinones which subsequently polymerize, forming brown melanin pigments that discolour the cut surfaces of fruits and vegetables. The enzyme is active between pH 5 and 7 and is irreversibly inactivated at a pH of 3 or lower. In the second example, acidification to 2·5–3 is required for high-methoxyl pectins to form gels. Because pH influences the gel-setting properties and the gel strength obtained, proper pH control is critical in the production of pectin- and gelatin-based desserts, jams, jellies, preserves and other products. In the final example, standardization of pH is done routinely in fermentation processes, such as wine-making, to ensure optimum microbial activity and to discourage growth of undesirable microbes. Acids are also added postfermentation to stabilize the finished wine. *See* Beers, Ales and Stouts, Biochemistry of Fermentation; Colloids and Emulsions; Enzymes, Functions and Characteristics; Phenolic Compounds

Acids are a major component of chemical leavening systems where they remain nonreactive until the proper temperature and moisture conditions are attained. The gas evolved by reaction of the acid with bicarbonate produces the aerated texture that is characteristic of baked products such as cakes, biscuits, doughnuts, pancakes and waffles. The onset and the rate of reaction of these compounds are controlled by such factors as the solubility of the acid, the mixing conditions for preparing the batter, and the temperature and the moisture of the batter. Many chemical leavening systems are based on salts of phosphoric and tartaric acids. *See* Leavening Agents

Commonly Used Acidulants

Among the most widely used acids are acetic, adipic, citric, fumaric, lactic, malic, phosphoric and tartaric acids. Glucono-δ-lactone, though not itself an acid, is regarded as an acidulant because it converts to gluconic acid under high temperatures. Table 1 shows the structures of these compounds and summarizes several of their physical and chemical properties.

Acetic Acid

Acetic acid is the major characterizing component of vinegar. Its concentration determines the strength of the vinegar – a value termed 'grain strength', which is equal to 10 times the acetic acid concentration. Vinegar containing, for example, 6% acetic acid has a grain strength of 60 and is called 60-grain. Distillation can be used to concentrate vinegar to the desired strength. *See* Vinegar

Fermentation conducted under controlled conditions is the commercial method for vinegar production. Bacterial strains of the genera *Acetobacter* and *Acetomonas* produce acetic acid from alcohol which has been obtained from a previous fermentation involving a variety of substrates such as grain and apples.

Vinegar functions in pH reduction, control of microbial growth, and enhancement of flavour. It has found use in a variety of products, including condiments such as ketchup, mustard, mayonnaise and relish; salad dressings; marinades for meat, poultry, and fish; bakery products; soups; and cheeses.

Pure (100%) acetic acid is called glacial acetic acid because it freezes to an ice-like solid at 16·6°C. Though not widely used in food, glacial acetic acid provides acidification and flavouring in sliced, canned fruits and vegetables, sausage, and salad dressings.

Natural Acids and Acidulants

Table 1. Structure, ionization constant, pK_a, and key physical and chemical properties of acidulants[a]

Acid	Structure	Ionization constant(s)	pK_a	Physical form	Melting point (°C)	Solubility (g per 100 ml water)	Hygroscopicity	Taste characteristics
Acetic acid	CH_3COOH	$1\cdot76 \times 10^{-5}$ at 25°C	$4\cdot76$	Clear colourless liquid	$-8\cdot5$	Soluble	—[b]	Tart and sour
Adipic acid	COOH—CH$_2$—CH$_2$—CH$_2$—CH$_2$—COOH	$K_1 = 3\cdot71 \times 10^{-5}$ $K_2 = 3\cdot87 \times 10^{-6}$ at 25°C	$4\cdot43$ $5\cdot41$	Crystalline powder	152	$1\cdot9$ g at 20°C 83 g at 90°C	Low level of hygroscopicity	Smooth lingering tartness; complements grape flavours
Citric acid	COOH—CH$_2$—HO—C—COOH—CH$_2$—COOH	$K_1 = 7\cdot10 \times 10^{-4}$ $K_2 = 1\cdot68 \times 10^{-5}$ $K_3 = 6\cdot4 \times 10^{-7}$ at 25°C	$3\cdot14$ $4\cdot77$ $6\cdot39$	Crystalline powder			Moderately hygroscopic	Tart; delivers a 'burst' of flavour
Anhydrous					153	181 g at 25°C		
Hydrous					135–153	208 g at 25°C		
Fumaric acid	COOH—CH=HC—COOH	$K_1 = 9\cdot30 \times 10^{-4}$ $K_2 = 3\cdot62 \times 10^{-5}$ at 18°C	$3\cdot03$ $4\cdot44$	White granules or crystalline powder	286	$0\cdot5$ g at 20°C $9\cdot8$ g at 100°C	Nonhygroscopic	Tart; has an affinity for grape flavours

continued

Table 1. *continued.*

Acid	Structure	Ionization constant(s)	pK_a	Physical form	Melting point (°C)	Solubility (g per 100 ml water)	Hygroscopicity	Taste characteristics
Glucono-δ-lactone	[structure: C=O; HC–OH; HO–CH; HC–OH; HC; O; CH$_2$OH]	$1·99 \times 10^{-4}$ (for gluconic acid)	3·7	White crystalline powder	153	59 g at 25°C	Nonhygroscopic	Neutral taste with acidic aftertaste, when hydrolysed
Lactic acid	CH$_3$; HC–OH; COOH	$1·37 \times 10^{-4}$ at 25°C	3·86	Liquid; also available in dry form	16·8	Very soluble	—	Acrid
Malic acid	COOH; HO–CH; CH$_2$; COOH	$K_1 = 3·9 \times 10^{-4}$; $K_2 = 7·8 \times 10^{-6}$ at 25°C	3·40 5·11	Crystalline powder	132	62 g at 25°C	Nonhygroscopic	Smooth tartness
Phosphoric acid		$K_1 = 7·52 \times 10^{-3}$; $K_2 = 6·23 \times 10^{-8}$; $K_3 = 2·2 \times 10^{-13}$; K_1 and K_2 at 25°C; K_3 at 18°C	2·12 7·21 12·67	Liquid		Very soluble in hot water	—	Acrid
Tartaric acid	COOH; HO–CH; HC–OH; COOH	$K_1 = 1·04 \times 10^{-3}$; $K_2 = 4·55 \times 10^{-5}$ at 25°C	2·98 4·34	Crystalline powder	168–170	147 g at 25°C	Nonhygroscopic	Extremely tart; augments fruit flavours, especially grape and lime

[a] Adapted with permission from *Food Technology*, Institute of Food Technologists.
[b] Not applicable.

Adipic Acid

Adipic acid, a white, crystalline powder, is characterized by low hygroscopicity and a lingering, high tartness that complements grape-flavoured products and those with delicate flavours. The acid is slightly more tart than citric acid at any pH. Aqueous solutions of the acid are the least acidic of all food acidulants, and have a strong buffering capacity in the pH range 2·5–3·0.

Adipic acid functions primarily as an acidifier, buffer, gelling aid, and sequestrant. It is used in confectionery, cheese analogues, fats, and flavouring extracts. Because of its low rate of moisture absorption, it is especially useful in dry products such as powdered fruit-flavoured beverage mixes, leavening systems of cake mixes, gelatin desserts, evaporated milk and instant puddings.

Citric Acid

The most widely used organic acid in the food industry, citric acid accounts for more than 60% of all acidulants consumed. It is the standard for evaluating the effects of other acidulants. Its major advantages include its high solubility in water; appealing effects on flavour, particularly its ability to deliver a 'burst' of tartness; and strong metal chelation properties.

Citric acid is naturally present in animal and plant tissues, and is most abundantly found in citrus fruits including the lemon (4–8%), grapefruit (1·2–2·1%), tangerine (0·9–1·2%) and orange (0·6–1·0%). *See* Citrus Fruits, Composition and Characterization

The principal method for commercial production of the acid is fermentation of corn. Formerly, the acid had been obtained by extraction from citrus and pineapple juices.

Citric acid has numerous applications. It is commonly added to nonalcoholic beverages where it complements fruit flavours, contributes tartness, chelates metal ions, acts as a preservative and controls pH so that the desired sweetness characteristics can be achieved. Sodium citrate subdues the sharp acid notes in highly acidified carbonated beverages; in club soda it imparts a cool, saline taste and helps retain carbonation. The acid is also used in wine production both prior to and after fermentation for adjustment of pH; in addition, because of its metal-chelating action, the acid prevents haze or turbidity caused by the binding of metals with tannin or phosphate.

Citric acid has also found use in confectionery and desserts. In hard confectionery, buffered citric acid imparts a pleasant tart taste; it is added to the molten mass after cooking, as this prevents sucrose inversion and browning. Citric acid is used in gelatin desserts because it imparts tartness, acts as a buffering agent, and increases pH for optimum gel strength.

Low levels of the acid, ranging from 0·001 to 0·01%, work with antioxidants to retard oxidative rancidity in dry sausage, fresh pork sausage and dried meats. Citric acid is also used in the production of frankfurters: 3–5% solutions are sprayed on the casings after stuffing and prior to smoking to aid in their removal from the finished product. Used at 0·2% in livestock blood, sodium citrate and citric acid act as anticoagulants, sequestering the calcium required for clot formation so that the blood may be used as a binder in pet foods.

In processed cheese and cheese foods, citric acid and sodium citrate function in emulsification, buffering, flavour enhancement and texture development.

Fumaric Acid

The extremely low rate of moisture absorption of this acid makes it an important ingredient for extending the shelf life of powdered food products such as gelatin desserts and pie fillings. Fumaric acid can be used in smaller quantities than citric, malic and lactic acids to achieve similar taste effects.

Fermentation of glucose or molasses by certain *Rhizopus* spp. is the method used to produce fumaric acid commercially. The acid is also made by isomerization of maleic acid with heat or a catalyst, and is a by-product of the production of phthalic and maleic anhydrides.

Applications of fumaric acid include rye bread, jellies, jams and juice drinks. In refrigerated biscuit doughs, the acid eliminates crystal formations that may occur in all-purpose leavening systems. In wine, it functions as both an acidulant and a clarifying aid although it does not chelate copper or iron.

Glucono-δ-lactone (GDL)

A natural constituent of fruits and honey, GDL is an inner ester of D-gluconic acid. Unlike other acidulants, it is neutral and gives a slow rate of acidification. When added to water, it hydrolyses to form an equilibrium mixture of gluconic acid and its δ- and γ-lactones. The acid formation takes place slowly when cold and accelerates when heated. As GDL converts to gluconic acid, its taste characteristics change from sweet to neutral with a slight acidic aftertaste.

GDL is produced commercially from glucose by a fermentation process that uses enzymes or pure cultures of microorganisms such as *Aspergillus niger* or *Aceto-bacter suboxydans* to oxidize glucose to gluconic acid. GDL is extracted by crystallization from the fermentation product, an aqueous solution of gluconic acid and GDL.

Because of its gradual acidification, bland taste and

metal-chelating action, GDL has found application in mild-flavoured products such as chocolate products, tofu, milk puddings and creamy salad dressings. In cottage cheese prepared by the direct-set method, GDL ensures development of a finer-textured finished product, void of localized denaturation. It also shortens production time and increases yields. In cured meat products, GDL reduces cure time, inhibits growth of undesirable microorganisms, promotes colour development and reduces nitrate and nitrite requirements. *See* Curing

Lactic Acid

Lactic acid is one of the earliest acids to be used in foods. It was first commercially produced about 60 years ago and only within the past two decades has it become an important ingredient. The mild taste characteristics of the acid will not mask weaker aromatic flavours. Lactic acid functions in pH reduction, flavour enhancement and microbial inhibition.

Two methods are used commercially to produce the acid: fermentation and chemical synthesis. Most manufacturers using fermentation are in Europe.

Confectionery, bakery products, beer, wine, beverages, dairy products and meat products are examples of the types of products in which lactic acid is used. The acid is used in packaged Spanish olives where it inhibits spoilage and further fermentation. In cheese production, it is added to adjust pH and as a flavouring agent.

Malic Acid

This general-purpose acidulant imparts a smooth, tart taste which lingers in the mouth, helping to mask the aftertastes of low- or noncaloric sweeteners. It has taste-blending and flavour-fixative characteristics and a relatively low melting point with respect to other solid acidulants. Compared with citric acid, malic acid has a much stronger apparent acidic taste.

Malic acid occurs naturally in many fruits and vegetables, and is the second most predominant acid in citrus fruits, many berries and figs. Unlike the natural acid which is laevorotatory, the commercial product is a racemic mixture of D- and L-isomers. It is manufactured during catalytic hydration of maleic and fumaric acids, and is recovered from the equilibrium product mixture.

The acid has been used in carbonated beverages, powdered juice drinks, jams and jellies, canned fruits and vegetables, and confectionery.

Phosphoric Acid

The second most widely used acidulant in food, phosphoric acid is the only inorganic acid to be used extensively for food purposes. It produces the lowest pH of all food acidulants. Phosphoric acid is produced from elemental phosphorus recovered from phosphate rock.

The primary use of the acid is in cola, root beer and other similar-flavoured carbonated beverages. The acid and its salts are also used during production of natural cheese for adjustment of pH; phosphates chelate the calcium required by bacteriophages which can destroy bacteria responsible for ripening. As chemical leavening agents, phosphates release gas upon neutralizing alkaline sodium bicarbonate; this creates a porous, cellular structure in baked products. The main reason for incorporating phosphates into cured meats such as hams and corned beef is to increase retention of natural juices; the salts are dissolved in the brine and incorporated into the meat by injection of brine, massaging or tumbling. When used in jams and jellies, phosphoric acid acts as a buffering agent to ensure a strong gel strength; it also prevents dulling of the gel colour by sequestering pro-oxidative metal ions.

Tartaric Acid

Tartaric acid is the most water soluble of the solid acidulants. It contributes a strong tart taste which enhances fruit flavours, particularly grape and lime.

This dibasic acid is produced from potassium acid tartrate which has been recovered from various by-products of the wine industry, including press cakes from fermented and partially fermented grape juice, lees (the dried, slimy sediments in wine fermentation vats) and argols (the crystalline crusts formed in vats during the second fermentation step of wine-making). The major European wine-producing countries, Spain, the FRG, Italy and France, have a higher consumption of the acid than the USA.

Tartaric acid is often used as an acidulant in grape- and lime-flavoured beverages, gelatin desserts, jams, jellies and hard sour confectionery. The acidic monopotassium salt, more commonly known as 'cream of tartar', is used in baking powders and leavening systems. Because it has limited solubility at lower temperatures, cream of tartar does not react with bicarbonate until baking temperatures are reached; this ensures maximum development of volume in the finished product.

Bibliography

Arnold MHM (1975) *Acidulants for Foods and Beverages.* London: Food Trade Press.
Bouchard EF and Merritt EG (1979) Citric acid. In: Grayson M (ed.) *Kirk-Othmer Encyclopedia of Chemical Technology*, 3rd edn, vol. 6. p. 150. New York: Wiley.

Dziezak JD (1990) Acidulants: Ingredients that do more than meet the acid test. *Food Technology* 44(1): 76–83.

Gardner WH (1972) Acidulants in food processing. In: Furia TE (ed.) *CRC Handbook of Food Additives*, 2nd edn, vol. 1, p. 225. Cleveland: CRC Press.

International Commission of Microbiological Specifications for Foods (1980) *Microbial Ecology of Foods*, vol. 1. New York: Academic Press.

J. D. Dziezak
Institute of Food Technologists, Chicago, USA

ADAPTATION – NUTRITIONAL ASPECTS

What is Adaptation?

Adaptation means to become, or have become, 'apt', and aptness in biology generally refers to the morphological or physiological equilibrium (or health) of an organism in relation to its environment. Of the many theories of adaptation that have emerged over the last 150 years, the best known are the purposeful adaptationism of Lamarck, Darwin's biological determinism, and the contemporary critiques of genetic determinism which postulate an interactive or reciprocal model of adaptation.

Theories of Adaptation

The French biologist Jean-Baptiste Lamarck (1744–1829) was the first to propose that species are not fixed, as had been previously believed, but evolve in response to organisms' changing needs in the face of a changing environment. Thus, for example, a bear, in its lifetime, might adapt to the seasonality of food supply with a range of heritable adaptations – hibernation, changes in body fat, eating certain foods, etc. New characteristics acquired in this way could, in Lamarck's view, be passed on to subsequent generations. Although inheritance of acquired characteristics has been rejected in evolutionary theory, Lamarck's belief in purposeful physiological processes is still widely accepted as a model for understanding adaptation in nutritional physiology.

For Charles Darwin (1809–1882), adaptation was the process whereby organisms endowed with advantageous characteristics survived through 'natural selection' to reproduce. However, Darwin did not know how new characteristics arose or were transmitted to subsequent generations, and it was not until the development of genetics, half a century later, that mechanisms were identified. These provided the basis for the neo-Darwinian synthesis: morphological variability within species was said to be the result of chance genetic mutation, while natural selection fashioned local evolutionary improvement and, through geographic isolation, facilitated divergence into new species.

Since the 1970s, numerous critiques of evolutionary determinism have emerged, based on the following observations: that many organisms are active in the process of environmental change; that genes, far from being 'fixed' and dominant players in physiology, constantly interact with their environment; and that the unit of survival in evolution is probably not an individual or species but the organism- or species-in-its-environment. As described by Gregory Bateson, Richard Lewontin and others, adaptation is now regarded as an ongoing process of interaction, reciprocity or mutual constitution, in which genes, physiological processes and the environment cannot be separated. This approach, which embodies elements of Lamarckian and Darwinian adaptation, is helpful in understanding how adaptation occurs in nutritional physiology. *See* Gene Expression and Nutrition

Adaptation at the Individual Level

While nutritional adaptation can clearly occur at a population level, through the ability of species and subpopulations to survive over generations in all sorts of ecological niches, most concern has been at the individual physiological level, in the ability of humans to maintain health in the presence of dietary changes.

Homeostasis and Adaptation

A major question which often arises is the difference between adaptation and homeostasis. Adaptation, at the individual level, is generally regarded as the purposeful process by which an organism responds to changes in its external or internal environment, so as to maintain, restore or improve its health or integrity.

Homeostasis, by contrast, is that dynamic state of

metabolic equilibrium, maintained within narrow parameters, by which organisms maintain health and functional integrity. Thus the stability of glycaemia, body temperature, acid–base balance, blood mineral values, etc., are maintained within a narrow fluctuating range.

Both of these concepts imply limits and regulation. If homeostatic limits are exceeded through environmental or endogenous change, an adaptive shift to a new homeostatic range may occur. For example, in humans, a move to increased altitude is accompanied within days by a higher level of haemoglobin, which is then maintained within a new homeostatic range. Another example is pregnancy, in which a lower than normal haemoglobin range is established. Adaptations of this kind are clearly reversible.

The Limits of Adaptation

The capacity of any organism to adapt to environmental change is limited. Beyond the limits, dysfunction occurs. For example, height in several species shows maximum limits, beyond which disproportionate growth occurs. The limits of adaptation are expressed as an interaction of genes and environmental conditions. *See* Growth and Development

Many argue that achieving the upper limits of adaptation, e.g. the maximum possible height for any individual, represents an ideal, a fulfilment of 'genetic potential'. Anything less than this is assumed to have adverse effects, i.e. to represent a 'cost'. However, what this upper limit might be for any individual cannot be predicted. Nor is it clear whether, under some circumstances, there may be 'benefits' associated with less than the maximum. The situation is even more complex if examined over time. Adaptive changes in response to one factor at a certain time may become disadvantageous at a later time; for example, bottle-fed babies with maximal weight-for-height may be at long-term risk of obesity.

Adaptation to Low Energy intake

Millions of infants and children in the developing world eat less and tend to grow smaller than their counterparts from developed countries. Tens of thousands die every day from undernutrition and infection. However, many appear to adapt to low energy intake by growing 'smaller'. A critical question here is as follows: at what point in the adaptive range is 'smallness' accompanied by functional impairment? *See* Malnutrition, Malnutrition in Developing Countries

Most of the research on this topic has examined the relationship between low energy intake and either the 'mental level' or 'work performance' of subjects, and the results are extremely difficult to interpret. Mental activity is heavily determined by social conditions, and its measurement is determined by cultural values. Although malnutrition and disease cause physical impairment of the nervous system, and would be expected to impair mental development, physical nutritional causes are extremely difficult to separate out from social causes, i.e. the effects of socio-economic and educational deprivation. 'Work performance' is equally problematic. Bigger individuals can do more muscle work per unit time than smaller ones, but smaller individuals may be biologically more efficient for their weight than larger ones. In addition, as with mental performance, associations with diet are confounded by other variables, such as motivation, gender and social support. Similar problems occur for any type of functional impairment one wishes to examine.

Changes in Energy Efficiency

Possible mechanisms for nutritional adaptation are also problematic: for example, there is little agreement on the processes of energy regulation, or even on whether such regulation occurs. The classic nutritional view of energy balance is based on the Second Law of Thermodynamics, which states that the energy (E) within a system can be transformed, but not lost or gained. This is generally translated as follows:

E intake (joules) =
$$E \text{ output (metabolism + heat + work + storage)} \qquad (1)$$

When heat is expressed as dietary-induced thermogenesis (DIT), and storage as fat storage (S_f), eqn [1] is expressed as follows:

$$E_i = E_o (E_M + DIT + W + S_f) \qquad (2)$$

The question involved in examining energy adaptation is this: under what circumstances do the factors on the right-hand side of the equation change in response to changes in energy intake (E_i)? The answer is that in spite of many years of investigation, we still do not know. The reasons for this are complex. One is the number of variables in energy output (E_o) and our lack of understanding of the many processes underlying these. Another is that relationships between the variables change over time. Yet another is the difficulty in accurate measurement of any of the variables. *See* Energy, Energy Expenditure and Energy Balance; Thermogenesis

One way to examine the problem is in terms of energy efficiency, i.e. the amount of work performed for the amount of energy put into each of the variables associated with E_o. If we define energy efficiency in terms of work (E_F), with W_E as the energy equivalent of work performed, and E_W as the energy input for the particular work performed, the equation is simple: $E_F = W_E/E_W$.

It has generally been assumed that E_F is *unchanged*, even when W_E or E_W change; if this assumption is correct, adaptation cannot occur in terms of human energy efficiency. However, there is increasing evidence, not yet accepted by all investigators, that E_F can vary for each of the variables contributing to F_o in eqn [1], and that adaptation can thereby occur.

Adaptation to Low Protein Intake

The lower limits of protein adaptation are usually defined as the 'adequate' or 'minimal adequate' protein intake, in terms of quality and quantity, that will provide for the growth of children and the maintenance of nitrogen balance in adults. Defining 'normal' or 'healthy' growth rates in children is problematic, but the adaptative range of nitrogen intake in adults is believed to be quite straightforward. *See* Protein, Requirements

Until recently it was assumed that the 'adaptation' of changes in protein intake could occur very rapidly over a period of 7–14 days, and that a suitable method for predicting requirements (minimal intake, plus a small protective increment) would be to alter protein intake over a range of three to five levels, feed at each level for about 10–14 days, measure nitrogen balance at each level, and plot the two. The point of interception of nitrogen intake and nitrogen balance was defined as the level of protein requirements (slope intercept method). The prior nutritional status of the individual was assumed to be 'normal'. However, this technique and its assumptions have now been questioned. Population studies suggest that people can exist for long periods of time on low intakes. Recent long-term balance studies in normal young men demonstrate that 'adaptation without any obvious cost' can occur at protein intakes of 0·5 g per kg of bodyweight per day or less.

As with energy balance, the nature of protein regulation is complex and controversial; it is difficult to estimate dietary intakes and expenditures in free-living populations, and long-term controlled studies are needed. Recent data suggest that the best available model to explain protein regulation is the stochastic process, in which the major variations can be explained by a first-order autoregression.

Summary

Organisms evolve as part of their 'environment', and humans are clearly able to maintain good health within a range of environments. The limits of any adaptation, however, cannot be easily determined. In nutrition, this has important ethical and political consequences. Millions of children in the developing world eat less than recommended intakes, and grow smaller than international standards. To the extent that their low food intake and 'smallness' are within the limits of adaptation, these children may be said to be adapted. However, the closer to the limits, the greater the risk; for marginally fed children, a relatively small change in just one of the factors that determine health (e.g. exposure to infection) may have disproportionately destructive effects. This is the conceptual basis for the well-known malnutrition–infection interaction. The unpredictability of the limits of adaptation, and of the adaptive process, reinforce the need for *all* children to be fed adequately, to be protected from disease, and to have access to the other elements of a decent life.

Bibliography

Bateson G (1972) *Steps to an Ecology of Mind.* New York: Ballantine Books.

Blaxter K and Waterlow JC (1984) *Nutritional Adaptation in Man.* Proceedings of a Symposium. April 1984. London: John Libbey.

Darwin C (1859) *The Origin of the Species by Means of Natural Selection; or the Preservation of Favoured Races in the Struggle for Life.* New York: Al Burt.

Lamarck J-R (1809) *Philosophie Zoologique.* Translated by Elliot H. (1963) as *Zoological Philosophy: An Exposition with regard to the Natural History of Animals.* New York: Hafner Press.

Levins R and Lewontin R (1985) *The Dialectical Biologist.* Cambridge: Harvard University Press.

Sukhatme PV and Margen S (1978) Models for protein deficiency. *American Journal of Clinical Nutrition* 31: 1237–1256.

Sheldon Margen and Michael G. Schwab
University of California at Berkeley, USA

ADIPOSE TISSUE

Contents

Structure and Function of White Adipose Tissue

Distribution and Physiological Roles of Adipose Tissue

White adipose tissue is quantitatively the most variable component of the body, ranging from a few per cent of bodyweight to over 50% in obese animals. In mammals, adipose tissue is found within the abdominal cavity, under the skin, within the musculature where it is found between muscles (intermuscular) and within muscles (intramuscular) (e.g. marbling of meat) and in a few highly specialized locations such as the eye socket. Within these locations the tissue occurs in discrete depots (e.g. perirenal, epididymal, omental, popliteal); there are about 16 in most species. Comparative studies have revealed that the distribution of adipose tissue depots evolved early in mammalian evolution and has been retained in most species. In some species (e.g. pigs, whales) subcutaneous depots have become enlarged and have fused to form a continuous layer; this also occurs in obese individuals. Adipose tissue depots are also found in birds, reptiles and amphibians.

The major function of white adipose tissue is the storage of energy as triacylglycerol (fat, lipid). Fat is a highly efficient form of energy storage, not only because of its high energy content per unit weight, but also because it is hydrophobic. Hence 1 g of adipose tissue may contain about 800 mg of triacylglycerol and about 100 mg of water. In contrast, protein and glycogen are much more hydrated. The development of copious stores of fat was probably very important for the evolution of homoiothermy in birds and mammals (these species have much higher basal metabolic rates than other vertebrates and so have a much greater requirement for nutrients). The ability to accrue copious amounts of adipose tissue was also essential for exploitation of northern regions; bears, reindeer and, to a lesser extent, sheep, build up substantial deposits of fat during the summer to provide reserves of nutrients during the winter. Such species thus have substantial seasonal fluctuations in the amount of adipose tissue in their bodies. *See* Energy, Energy Expenditure and Energy Balance; Energy, Measurement of Food Energy

It is now apparent that adipose tissues are not solely a store of fat. Subcutaneous adipose tissue will act as insulation; adipose depots in the eye socket may have a protective function. Adipose tissue produces a number of biologically active substances, e.g. prostaglandins, insulin-like growth factors, adipsin, oestrogens (adipose tissue is the major source of oestrogens in postmenopausal women). These substances are probably important for adipose tissue function but may also have other roles. The mammary gland grows in a bed of adipose tissue, and is thought to require factors secreted by adipose tissue for its development. Adipose tissue may also have a role in the immune system as it produces several components of the alternative pathway of complement formation.

In addition to white adipose tissue, there is also another form, brown adipose tissue, which differs morphologically and biochemically, and has an important role in thermogenesis. *See* Thermogenesis

Structure of Adipose Tissue

White adipose tissue is a soft, floppy tissue devoid of rigidity. The tissue is well supplied with capillaries and nerve endings from the sympathetic nervous system.

In mature animals, adipocytes (fat cells) comprise about 90% of the mass of the tissue but only 25% or less of the total cell population. The 75% or so nonadipocytes are often termed the stromal-vascular fraction and comprise mainly endothelial cells of blood vessels and adipocyte precursor cells. Adipocytes vary enormously in size from several picolitres to about 3 nl in volume, depending on the amount of lipid present. The mature fat cell is essentially a lipid droplet surrounded by a film of cytoplasm (containing mitochondria, endoplasmic reticulum, etc.) and bounded by a plasma membrane. Instead of lurking in the centre of the cell, the nucleus is pushed to the periphery and appears as a blip on the surface of the cell. Within a depot there will be fat cells of various sizes, so that it is usual to refer to the mean fat cell volume of a tissue. This varies amongst adipose tissue depots in an individual; in general, adipocyte mean cell volumes can be ranked by size, in descending order, as abdominal, subcutaneous, intermuscular, and intramuscular. Adipocyte mean cell volume also varies

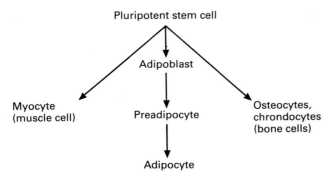

Fig. 1 Adipocyte development.

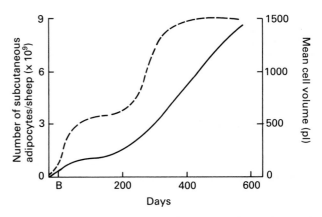

Fig. 2 Pattern of changes in the mean volume (———) and number (– – – – –) of subcutaneous adipocytes in sheep from 25 days before birth (B) until 600 days after birth.

with size of the animal, larger animals having larger fat cells; this occurs both within and between species. *See* Cells

Development of Adipose Tissue

Adipose tissue develops both by accretion of lipid in adipocytes and by increases in the number of adipocytes. Mature adipocytes are thought to be unable to divide; rather they are produced from a pool of precursor cells within the tissue. The sequence of events in the formation of mature adipocytes (Fig. 1) is still partly speculative and much has been gleaned from studies of certain cell lines which will differentiate and develop into adipocytes in cell culture. Current thinking envisages a pluripotent stem cell which can give rise to muscle and bone cells as well as adipocytes. Once commited to adipocyte formation, this cell is termed an adipoblast. This is envisaged (it has not been isolated) as an undifferentiated cell, devoid of lipid droplets but able to proliferate. At some point these cells begin to differentiate, acquiring in stages the enzymes and other proteins characteristic of adipocytes. Once differentiated, these cells can begin to accumulate lipid, which appears at first as a series of small droplets within the cell. As these become larger, they fuse to form the single lipid droplet characteristic of mature adipocytes. Both differentiating cells and cells with several small lipid droplets (multilocular phase) are often referred to as preadipocytes, the term adipocyte being used to describe cells with a single lipid droplet. Multilocular adipocytes are very similar in appearance to mature brown adipocytes and it was once thought that the brown adipocyte was a stage in the development of the white adipocyte. It is now recognized that this view is incorrect except possibly for a few special cases (e.g. the perirenal adipose tissue depot of newborn lambs, but this is a special adaptation to meet the need for heat production in the neonatal period).

In vivo, adipocytes begin to appear in the fetus about half-way through gestation, developing in small clumps around blood vessels. Within a depot both number and size of adipocytes increase in phases (Fig. 2). In addition, it is now clear that development is not synchronized in all depots; abdominal depots develop earlier than those associated with the musculature. In general, however, the fetal stage is an active period of proliferation but little hypertrophy, so that cells are small at birth. The suckling period usually results in rapid hypertrophy as well as hyperplasia; this is followed by a relatively quiescent period when muscle growth predominates; as the rate of muscle growth begins to slacken, nutrients are diverted into adipose tissue and the fattening phase begins. This phase is associated with a large increase in cell size and some further hyperplasia. Adipocytes do not increase in size indefinitely; once a maximum is reached (around 1–3 nl, depending on species) this seems to trigger the formation of new adipocytes from the precursor pool. The view prevalent in the 1970s that all hyperplasia occurred in young animals, including humans, is now thought to be invalid.

A great deal of research has gone into determining the hormones which promote the proliferation and differentiation of adipocyte precursor cells. At present the picture is far from clear, in part because of probable species differences and also because much of the work has involved the use of cell lines which do not all appear to have identical hormonal requirements for development. A variety of peptide growth factors (e.g. insulin-like growth factor 1, fibroblast growth factor, platelet-derived growth factor), growth hormone, thyroid hormones, sex steroids and glucocorticoids may be involved, but their precise roles are not known and for some (e.g. growth hormone) a role is still controversial. In addition to positive effectors, transforming growth factor β appears to inhibit differentiation, while epidermal growth factor may promote precursor cell proliferation but inhibit their differentiation. In contrast to hyperplasia, much more is known about the control of

Structure and Function of White Adipose Tissue

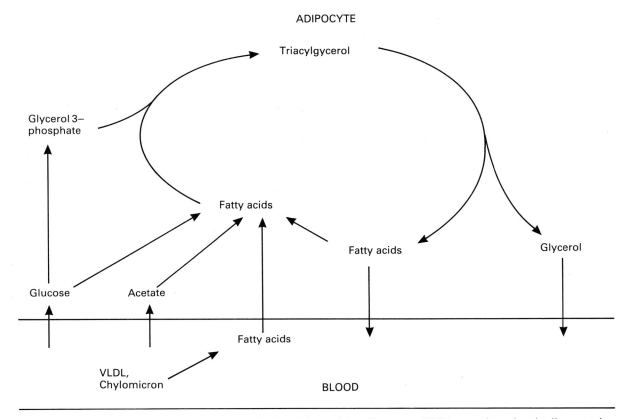

ADIPOCYTE

Fig. 3 Pathways for synthesis and hydrolysis of triacylglycerol in adipocytes. VLDL, very low density lipoprotein.

hypertrophy for this is dependent on the metabolic rates of the pathways of lipid synthesis and degradation. *See* Growth and Development

Deposition and Mobilization of Fat

The synthesis of triacylglycerol (esterification) requires a supply of fatty acids and glycerol 3-phosphate (Fig. 3). The latter is mostly synthesized from glucose. Fatty acids, however, may be synthesized *de novo* within the cell or obtained from blood triacylglycerols. Fatty acids can be synthesized in adipocytes from a variety of precursors, including glucose, acetate, lactate and some amino acids. Glucose is quantitatively the most important in man and some laboratory species (e.g. rats, mice), whereas acetate is most important in ruminants. In contrast to mammals, birds have essentially no capacity to synthesize fatty acids in adipocytes (liver is the major site of synthesis) and so obtain all their fatty acids from blood triacylglycerols. Liver is also an important site of fatty acid synthesis in many mammals, including humans; some of these fatty acids are incorporated into very-low-density lipoprotein (VLDL) triacylglycerols for transport to adipocytes and other tissues. Dietary fatty acids are also incorporated into triacylglycerols in the intestinal cells and secreted as

another form of lipoprotein called chylomicrons. Triacylglycerols are essentially insoluble in water and so cannot be taken up directly by adipocytes from blood lipoproteins; thus the fatty acids are released by the action of the enzyme, lipoprotein lipase. This enzyme is synthesized in adipocytes and then secreted, after which it migrates to the inner surface of the cells lining the blood capillaries. The relative importance of *de novo* synthesis and lipoprotein lipase activity as a source of fatty acids for fat synthesis depends on the diet and the species. When animals are fed high-fat diets, chylomicron lipids are the major source. When fed diets rich in carbohydrates, the major source becomes VLDL lipids or *de novo* fatty acid synthesis in adipocytes, depending on whether adipocytes or the liver are the major site of fatty acid synthesis in the species. *See* Fatty Acids, Metabolism; Glucose, Function and Metabolism

Once synthesized within the adipocyte, triacylglycerols are stored in the lipid droplet. Fatty acids are released from them when required by the action of the enzyme, hormone-sensitive lipase (distinct from lipoprotein lipase). This enzyme cleaves two molecules of fatty acids to yield a monoacylglycerol which is then hydrolysed to glycerol and fatty acid by a separate enzyme. Essentially all the glycerol is released from the cell as it cannot be metabolized by adipocytes. Some fatty acids, however, are usually re-esterified; hence the

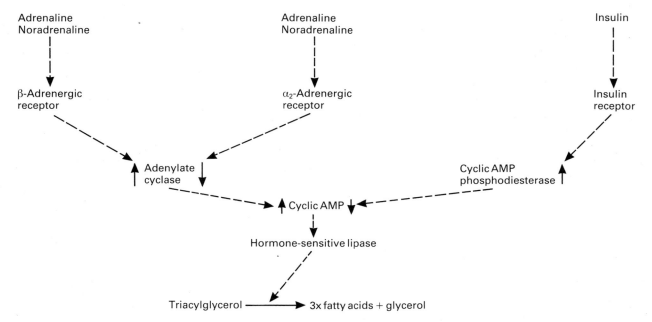

Fig. 4   Control of triacylglycerol hydrolysis (lipolysis) by the catecholamines (adrenaline and noradrenaline) and insulin. AMP, adenosine monophosphate; ↑, ↓ activity/concentration increased or decreased by stimulus respectively.

ratio of fatty acid to glycerol leaving the cell is normally less than the theoretical 3:1. Released fatty acid is bound to albumin in the blood, and transported to the liver and other tissues. Fatty acid esterification and triacylglycerol hydrolysis (lipolysis) occur continuously, i.e. there is a continual turnover of adipocyte triacyglycerol. Net accretion or loss of lipid thus depends on the relative rates of these two processes.

Regulation of Adipose Tissue Metabolism

Both lipid synthesis and hydrolysis are under complex hormonal control. Hormones regulate the amounts of key enzymes and other proteins involved, as well as their activities. In addition, the 'signal transduction' systems, (a series of reactions transmitting hormone-induced signals to targets in the cell) through which hormones achieve their effects, are also subject to endocrine control themselves. Control of fatty acid synthesis and lipolysis have been studied in greatest detail (Fig. 4).

Regulation of fatty acid synthesis depends on the precursor. For glucose, control begins at the point of entry into the cell where its transport is dependent on a specific carrier protein (transporter). Insulin stimulates glucose transport both by promoting recruitment of transporters into the plasma membrane and by increasing their activity. Within the cell, glucose is initially phosphorylated and then metabolized by a long series of reactions, some in the cytosol, some in the mitochondria, to produce acetyl coenzyme A (CoA) in the cytosol. Several enzymes, in particular phosphofructokinase and pyruvate dehydrogenase, have key roles in

controlling this flux. Insulin, for example, activates pyruvate dehydrogenase. For acetate, the control is much simpler as its initial reaction results in the production of acetyl CoA. The conversion of acetyl CoA to fatty acid is catalysed by two enzymes, acetyl CoA carboxylase and fatty acid synthetase. The former is thought to be the most important enzyme controlling flux. Both the amount of acetyl CoA carboxylase and its activation status (it is an enzyme which exists in active and inactive forms in the cell) change markedly with physiological, nutritional and pathological condition. The amount and activity, for example, are decreased by fasting, high-fat diets, diabetes and lactation. Insulin again increases both the amount and activity of the enzyme. These effects of insulin are antagonized by growth hormone. Catecholamines and glucagon also cause inactivation of the enzyme and hence a fall in the rate of fatty acid synthesis. In some species (e.g. ruminants, pigs) glucocorticoids act synergistically with insulin to increase acetyl CoA carboxylase activity and hence fatty acid synthesis. The gut hormones gastric inhibitory peptide and glucagon-like peptide 1 also increase fatty acid synthesis. *See* Hormones, Gut Hormones; Hormones, Steroid Hormones

Insulin increases the synthesis and secretion of lipoprotein lipase; this effect is accentuated by glucocorticoids. Gastric inhibitory polypeptide also increases lipoprotein lipase activity; this effect is likely to be important for promoting fat deposition in animals eating high-fat diets as such diets stimulate secretion of this hormone. Thus insulin and certain gut hormones increase fat synthesis by increasing the supply of fatty acids for esterification. Insulin also promotes glycerol 3-phosphate formation, in part at least, by increasing glucose uptake by adipocytes. The rate of fatty acid esterification itself may not be stimulated directly by hormones but varies directly with fatty acid availability.

The enzyme controlling lipolysis, hormone-sensitive lipase, exists in active and inactive states in the fat cell. A number of hormones, e.g. glucagon, adrenaline, adrenocorticotrophin, and also noradrenaline (which is released from nerve-endings of the sympathetic nervous system within the tissue itself), interact with specific receptor proteins in the plasma membrane. This causes activation of a key enzyme, adenylate cyclase, which synthesizes cyclic adenosine monophosphate (cAMP). Increased concentrations of cAMP both activate hormone-sensitive lipase and promote its movement from the cytosol to the surface of the lipid droplet, resulting in increased lipolysis. This stimulatory mechanism is attenuated by two inhibitory systems. Adenosine and prostaglandin E_2, which are both produced within adipose tissue, interact with their own receptors, leading to inhibition of adenylate cyclase. Curiously, adrenaline and noradrenaline can both activate and inhibit adenylate cyclase. They activate adenylate cyclase by interacting with the β-adrenergic receptor and inhibit by interacting with the α_2-adrenergic receptor. The effect of adrenaline and noradrenaline on lipolysis will thus depend in part on the relative number of β and α_2-adrenergic receptors in the adipocyte. One cause of the difficulty that some women experience when trying to lose fat from the thigh fat depots is a preponderance of α_2-adrenergic receptors in the fat cells. In addition to the above, insulin activates the enzyme, cAMP-phosphodiesterase, which catalyses the degradation of cAMP and so reduces its concentration. The rate of lipolysis then will depend on the concentration of a whole range of hormones, locally produced factors, and neurohumoral transmitters (substances, such as noradrenaline, which are released by nerve endings and act on cells). In addition, the ability of the 'signal transduction' system to transmit signals varies with age and with physiological state. For example, during lactation when fat is often mobilized to support milk production, the system can become more responsive to agents which promote lipolysis. Thyroid hormones, glucocorticoids, sex steroids, and growth hormone all act on one or more components of the signal transduction system, altering its ability to respond to stimulatory and/or inhibitory agents. *See* Hormones, Adrenal Hormones; Hormones, Thyroid Hormones

Adipose tissue metabolism is thus under complex control. In general, insulin promotes fat synthesis and inhibits lipolysis, whereas catecholamines and glucagon inhibit synthesis and promote lipolysis. In addition, steroid hormones, thyroid hormones, and growth hormone act to modulate the effects of insulin and catechol-

Table 1. Fatty acid composition of adipose tissue triacylglycerols

Fatty acid	Fatty acids (g per 100 g total fatty acids)			
	Humans	Pig	Sheep	Chicken
Myristic	4·1	1·3	6·3	0·6
Palmitic	23·3	24·2	20·4	31·7
Palmitoleic	9·0	3·1	2·2	5·3
Stearic	5·0	14·7	15·7	6·2
Oleic	49·4	45·6	38·0	45·2
Linoleic	3·0	7·7	1·7	10·2
Linolenic	0·8	2·2	4·1	0·6
Other	5·4	1·2	11·6	0·2

Data from Body DR (1988).

amines, in part at least, by modifying the ability of the signal transduction systems to transmit signals.

Composition of Stored Fat

Triacylglycerols comprise about 95% of adipose tissue lipid; the remainder includes diacylglycerols, phospholipids, unesterified fatty acids and cholesterol. The fatty acid composition of the triacylglycerols shows species variation (Table 1) but oleic and palmitic acids are the major components in all species. The proportions of polyunsaturated fatty acids (linoleic and linolenic) are usually low in adipose tissue from ruminant animals and higher in chicken and pig adipose tissue. This reflects the dietary supply; as described above, fatty acids are derived both from dietary lipid (via chylomicrons) and from *de novo* synthesis (which produces palmitic acid). There is some capacity for chain elongation of palmitic acid to produce stearic acid, and for desaturation which converts palmitic to palmitoleic and stearic to oleic acids, but the tissue cannot synthesize linoleic or linolenic acids. In simple-stomached species, such as humans and pigs, varying the fatty acid composition of the diet will alter the fatty acid composition of adipose tissue lipids. For ruminant animals, however, polyunsaturated fatty acids are mostly hydrogenated in the rumen to produce oleic and stearic acids. The small amount of linoleic and linolenic acids escaping this fate are conserved for essential functions (membrane synthesis, prostaglandin production), so that adipose tissue lipids (and milk fat) normally contain little linoleic or linolenic acids. This is ironic, for linolenic acids are the major fatty acids of the ruminant diet. If hydrogenation in the rumen is avoided (e.g. by coating dietary lipid with formaldehyde-treated casein), then large quantities of these polyunsaturated fatty acids are absorbed, producing adipose tissue rich in linoleic and linolenic acids. *See* Fatty Acids, Gamma Linolenic Acid

Structure and Function of White Adipose Tissue

Minor changes in the fatty acid composition occur during development and there are minor differences between adipose tissue depots, but these are small compared with the changes which can be elicited by dietary manipulation.

Manipulation of Adiposity

The current desire for leaner meat and the sheer economics of excess adipose tissue production in food animals (millions of pounds worth of excess fat are disposed of each year) have led to much interest in producing leaner animals and birds. There has been success in breeding leaner pigs and chickens but in addition a number of substances have been described which will decrease adiposity. Recombinant bovine and porcine somatotrophins (growth hormone) are very effective in this respect. Treatment of pigs in the USA (American pigs tend to be fatter than their European counterparts) decreased adipose tissue mass by over 50%. The molecular mechanism of this effect has not been fully resolved but, as indicated above, growth hormone antagonizes insulin stimulation of fatty acid synthesis and accentuates catecholamine stimulation of lipolysis. β-Agonists also decrease adiposity; again, the mechanism has not been fully resolved but it is at least partly based on their ability to stimulate cAMP formation via the β-adrenergic receptor, and thus to stimulate lipolysis. Sex steroids can also decrease adiposity. Use of such agents for reducing adiposity is controversial and is not allowed at present in the European Economic Community (EEC). Recombinant somatotrophin is licensed for use for increasing milk production in some countries (e.g. Czechoslovakia, Mexico, South Africa). Another approach has been to produce transgenic animals carrying extra copies of the growth hormone gene. While such animals have been produced which secrete additional growth hormone, many problems remain to be resolved (e.g. avoiding undesirable side-effects such as skeletal deformities).

Immunology offers a further option. Antibodies to adipocyte plasma membranes have been raised which, when injected, destroy adipocytes. This has been achieved in rats, pigs and sheep. The approach is attractive because it destroys adipocytes and also avoids problems of residues which arise with agents such as β-agonists and steroids. It has also been possible to produce anti-idiotypic antibodies which resemble growth hormone, providing a potential alternative to the use of recombinant somatotrophin. *See* Immunity and Nutrition

Bibliography

Body DR (1988) Lipid composition of adipose tissue. *Progress in Lipid Research* 27: 39–60.

Cryer A and Van RLR (1985) *New Perspectives in Adipose Tissue: Structure, Function and Development*. Oxford: Butterworth–Heinemann.
Flint DJ and Vernon RG (1992) Hormones and adipose tissue growth. In: Pang PKT and Schreibman MP (eds) *Vertebrate Endocrinology: Fundamentals and Biomedical Implications* (in press). Orlando: Academic Press.
Forbes JM and Hervey GR (1990) The control of body fat content. *International Monographs in Nutrition, Metabolism and Obesity* 1.
Pond CM and Mattacks CA (1985) Anatomical organisation of mammalian adipose tissue. In: Dunker HR and Fleischer G (eds) *Functional Morphology of Vertebrates*, pp 485–489. Stuttgart: Springer.
Vernon RG (1992) Control of lipogenesis and lipolysis. In: Buttery PJ, Boorman KN and Lindsay DB (eds) *The Control of Fat and Lean Deposition* (in press). Oxford: Butterworth–Heinemann.
Wood JD and Fisher AV (1990) *Reducing Fat in Meat Animals*. Essex: Elsevier Science Publishers.

Richard G. Vernon and David J. Flint
Hannah Research Institute, Ayr, UK

Structure and Function of Brown Adipose Tissue

Brown adipose tissue (BAT), or brown fat, is a small but highly specialized tissue, the main function of which is to produce heat (thermogenesis). This function requires a good blood supply and a dense population of mitochondria – two features which account for its reddish-brown colour. It is found in most mammals, particularly in the neonate, and plays an important role in the control of body temperature during exposure to the cold. There is evidence indicating that it is also involved in the regulation of energy balance. The tissue was first described some 300 years ago, but its thermogenic function was not recognized until the early 1960s, and only during the 1980s did its capacity for thermogenesis and its unique metabolism come to be fully appreciated. *See* Thermogenesis

Location

BAT is most obvious in small mammals, hibernators and neonates, and is usually found around the kidneys, heart and aorta, along the intercostal muscles and sternum, in the axilla, in the subcutaneous inter- and subscapular regions and deep within the neck, around the main arteries and veins. This distribution suggests that the tissue acts as a jacket to heat the major organs and warm the blood passing from the periphery into the trunk. The distribution varies considerably between species and some (e.g. dog, human) have little or no interscapular BAT, whereas in others (e.g. rodents) the interscapular depot may account for 20–30% of the total. BAT rarely exceeds 2–3% of body mass, and is present in such small quantities in large, adult mammals that it is often impossible to detect visually. In spite of this, BAT has been identified histologically in human adults up to the age of 80 or more years, and biochemical tests suggest that it might still retain its thermogenic activity.

Histology and Development

Brown adipocytes appear polygonal under the microscope, with a diameter of 10–15 μm, compared to 20–150 μm for white adipocytes. The adipocytes are organized in discrete lobules, surrounded by connective tissue, extensive blood vessels and numerous sympathetic nerves terminating on the adipocytes and blood vessels. Unlike white adipocytes, the nuclei are spherical and located centrally, and the lipid is stored in small, multilocular droplets. Between the droplets and packing the cytoplasm are numerous, well-developed mitochondria which possess distinctive and regular cristae, often traversing the width of the mitochondrion. The endoplasmic reticulum (particularly the rough reticulum) and Golgi apparatus are relatively small, but high densities of lysosomes, peroxisomes and clusters of glycogen granules are often present; adjacent cells are usually connected by gap junctions.

Cytogenetic studies indicate that brown adipocytes are derived from fibroblast-like stem cells closely associated with vascular structures, and it is now generally agreed that these are distinct from the stem cells that give rise to white adipocytes. Mature brown adipocytes cannot undergo mitosis, and the recruitment (hyperplasia) seen during cold-adaptation occurs by cytogenesis and mitosis of newly differentiated brown adipocytes. The first appearance of differentiated BAT cells varies between species, and in some neonates (e.g. guinea pig, rabbit, puppy, lamb) the tissue is well developed and functional at birth. In other species (e.g. rats, mice) the tissue is not fully functional at birth, but becomes thermogenically active within a few days. By contrast, the Syrian hamster is born without BAT, and it takes about 2 weeks for the tissue to develop, during which time the animal is essentially poikilothermic.

Innervation

The innervation of BAT is another feature that distinguishes it from white adipose tissue, since the metabolic activity of the tissue is almost entirely determined by the release of noradrenaline at sympathetic nerve terminals on the brown adipocytes. In some depots (e.g.

rodent interscapular BAT) the sympathetic nerves enter as obvious bundles. This makes experimental techniques such as surgical sympathectomy and nerve stimulation and recordings relatively easy to undertake, although there can be problems in distinguishing between effects on adipocytes and those on the vascular supply. The tissue content and turnover of noradrenaline is high, and the turnover is a good index of sympathetic activation in response to various environmental and dietary stimuli. Apart from noradrenaline, histamine, adenosine and various peptides may modulate the sympathetic activation of BAT. Neuropeptide Y (NPY) is found co-localized with noradrenaline in sympathetic nerve endings, and the depletion of sensory peptides – CGRP (calcitonin-gene-related peptide) and substance P – by capsaicin suggests that the tissue contains sympathetic afferents.

Blood Supply

The high oxygen supply required to support thermogenesis is provided by an extensive network of vessels, estimated to be four to six times denser than in white adipose tissue. The vascular supply can support a blood flow in excess of 20 ml per g of tissue per min; during maximal stimulation in cold-adapted rodents this relatively small mass of tissue can receive over 30% of cardiac output. Blood flow increases result partly from the vasomotor activity of the sympathetic nerves, but also from autoregulatory increases caused by sympathetic activation of metabolism and the release of metabolites. Aerobic heat production can be so intense that the oxygen supplied in arterial blood is almost completely extracted and the venous blood appears desaturated. The small amounts of oxygen remaining probably represent blood that bypassed the capillary network via arteriovenous anastomoses (i.e. vascular shunts). These vascular shunts, of which there are many, probably act to convect the heat generated away from the tissue, thereby avoiding thermal damage (BAT temperatures can rise to over 44°C). The thermogenic capacity of BAT can be determined from measurements of blood flow and oxygen extraction, and estimates of up to 500 W kg^{-1} can be compared with values of only 60 W kg^{-1} for the maximal aerobic power of skeletal muscle. *See* Exercise, Muscle

Metabolism

The exceptional heat-producing capacity of BAT is due to its mitochondria, which possess a 32 000 Da polypeptide known as uncoupling protein (UCP), or 'thermogenin'. The presence of this protein is unique to BAT mitochondria, and is responsible for the only known physiological example of uncoupled oxidative phosphorylation in mammalian metabolism. UCP forms a proton conductance channel in the mitochondrial inner membrane, and dissipates the proton electrochemical gradient generated by oxidation of substrates via the electron transport system. This has the effect of uncoupling oxidation from the phosphorylation of ADP (adenosine diphosphate) to ATP (adenosine triphosphate) thereby dissipating the energy released as heat, as well as increasing the rate of oxidation due to the loss of respiratory control.

The proton conductance pathway is under inhibitory control by purine nucleotides (e.g. ADP, ATP, GDP) which bind to UCP, and is activated by the free fatty acids released by lipolysis following sympathetic activation of the adipocyte β-adrenergic receptors. These fatty acids also provide the principal fuel for thermogenesis, and therefore act to uncouple their own oxidation. The rapid activation of the proton conductance pathway following sympathetic stimulation can be detected by measuring the mitochondrial binding of purine nucleotides – usually GDP (guanosine diphosphate) – in vitro, whereas chronic, adaptive changes in thermogenic capacity depend on immunoassay of mitochondrial UCP concentrations.

High rates of oxidation in any tissue require adequate levels of all the enzyme systems of intermediary metabolism, and BAT is particularly well endowed with those required for glycolysis, the tricarboxylic acid cycle and the mitochondrial electron transport chain. Since fatty acids are the main fuel for thermogenesis, adenyl cyclase activity and the subsequent cascade that leads to the intracellular release of fatty acids from stored triglyceride are prominent features of BAT metabolism. However, the lipid stored in the multilocular droplets is not sufficient to sustain thermogenesis for long periods, and brown adipocytes then rely on their remarkable capacity for lipogenesis. In cold-adapted rats and mice the lipogenic capacity of BAT is high enough to account for a major fraction of the amount of dietary carbohydrate that the animal converts to lipid. As well as the fatty acids supplied by de novo lipogenesis, the high level of lipoprotein lipase allows BAT to take up fatty acids released by the hydrolysis of circulating triglycerides.

In addition to the normal complement of respiratory enzyme systems, brown fat cells also contain peroxisomes, and these proliferate during chronic stimulation of the tissue. Peroxisomal oxidation of substrates is not linked to phosphorylation, and could therefore make a contribution to cellular thermogenesis. However, the contribution is probably very small, and their function may be more to do with the cytosolic metabolism of fatty acids that are not preferentially metabolized by mitochondria. Another interesting feature of BAT metabolism is the presence of an enzyme, 5-deiodinase, that converts thyroxine (T_4) to the physiologically active

hormone, triiodothyronine (T_3). The enzyme is under sympathetic control, and its activity can increase several-hundred-fold in cold-adapted animals. The T_3 produced is more than sufficient to saturate the nuclear receptors, and it is possible that much of the T_3 is exported and exerts effects on other tissues. *See* Hormones, Thyroid Hormones

Functions of BAT

Thermoregulation

Shivering is an acute response to cold exposure, and not a particularly effective mechanism for protecting the body against hypothermia. As a consequence, many animals resort to a form of heat production called nonshivering thermogenesis (NST) which, unlike shivering, can be sustained without fatigue and disruption of locomotor activity or sleeping behaviour. NST appears as an adaptive response to chronic cold-exposure in many mammals, but particularly in small animals where heat losses are greater due to their large surface area relative to body mass. High surface heat loss and immature neuromuscular development also explain why the neonates of most mammalian species (including humans) depend on NST to maintain body temperature until shivering, locomotor activity and other behavioural thermoregulatory responses develop. A third group are the hibernators, who rely on NST for the rapid rewarming that occurs during arousal.

Depending on the species, NST can raise heat production by 100–300% above that in a warm, thermoneutral environment, and is associated with large increases in the activity of the sympathetic nervous system. Pharmacological blockade (particularly with β-adrenergic antagonists) can inhibit completely the cold-induced rise in heat production, and demonstrates the dominant role of the sympathetic nervous system in mediating NST. The effector tissue is BAT, and a considerable body of evidence now exists to link BAT function to NST. For example, the capacity for NST is inversely proportional to age, bodyweight, and acclimation temperature, and this coincides with histological, physiological and biochemical indices of BAT activity. Conversely, deacclimation and decreased NST is associated with a parallel decline in BAT activity. Perhaps the most convincing evidence comes from in vivo measurements of BAT oxygen consumption which, in spite of enormous technical difficulties, have shown that the tissue can account for well over 60% of NST. Even this may be an underestimate, since it is not possible to measure the contribution of all the numerous, small and diffuse BAT depots.

Structure and Function of Brown Adipose Tissue

Energy Balance Regulation

Evidence linking BAT to energy balance regulation comes mainly from studies on laboratory rodents that represent examples of two extremes of metabolic efficiency. At one extreme there are normal, young rats and mice that fail to become obese in spite of an excessive energy intake, and at the other extreme there are examples of obesity developing in rats and mice (e.g. genetic and hypothalamic obesities) even when energy intake is normal. The explanation for these differences appears to depend on an adaptive form of heat production called diet-induced thermogenesis (DIT), which is absent or defective in obese animals, but provides a mechanism whereby normal animals can adjust energy expenditure to compensate for energy consumed in excess of requirements. DIT can produce increases in total heat production of 60–70%, and account for up to 90% of the excess energy consumed by hyperphagic rats. In rats feeding normally, the level of DIT is low, but sufficient to control energy balance by compensating for errors in the control of energy intake.

The control and metabolic origins of DIT are identical in almost every respect to NST, although cold is a more potent stimulus and produces more dramatic changes than dietary stimuli. As a consequence, the changes in sympathetic activity, BAT hypertrophy and hyperplasia, mitochondrial proliferation, GDP-binding and UCP concentration in rats exhibiting DIT are smaller than those seen in cold-adapted rats. However, these changes in BAT function are sufficient to account for up to 80% of the diet-induced changes in thermogenic capacity seen in hyperphagic rats. By contrast, BAT is usually atrophied and relatively inactive in obese rodents, although it will still respond to exogenous noradrenaline, and the animals retain the capacity to adapt to the cold and exhibit NST. This suggests that the defective DIT in these obese rodents is due to a failure of the sympathetic activation of BAT, rather than a defect in BAT itself.

Other Functions

In addition to cold- and diet-induced thermogenesis, there are several pathological conditions in which BAT has been implicated as the source of increased heat production. Fever, sepsis and cancer cachexia are three examples where increased sympathetic activation of BAT is thought to be at least partly responsible for the hypermetabolic response seen in animal models of these conditions. Patients with phaeochromocytoma (adrenomedullary tumour) have very high circulating levels of adrenaline and noradrenaline, and it is thought that the elevated heat production in this condition is due to the stimulatory effect of these catecholamines on BAT; the best examples of active BAT in human adults have been seen in patients with phaeochromocytoma.

In spite of increased energy intakes, pregnant rats and mice show little or no change in BAT activity, but during lactation the tissue atrophies and its sympathetic activity and thermogenic capacity declines to levels seen after sympathectomy or fasting. Similar reductions can be seen in warm-adapted nonlactating animals, which suggests that BAT thermogenesis declines to compensate for the elevated heat production associated with milk synthesis in the lactating mammary glands. Increased heat production during exercise could also account for the lower BAT activity seen in exercise-trained animals. This is particularly noticeable in cold environments, where exercise can prevent many of the changes in BAT function associated with NST.

Control of BAT

Neural

The control over the sympathetic supply to the various BAT depots originates from the hypothalamus, which receives afferent information on thermal and nutrient status from the periphery, as well as having its own receptor mechanisms and pathways. One of the main thermosensitive and thermoregulatory areas is the preoptic/anterior hypothalamus (POAH), but this is thought to modulate BAT thermogenesis via inhibitory pathways that descend to the lower brain stem. The area that appears to exert a major influence over BAT is one that has been classically associated with the control of energy intake – the ventromedial hypothalamus (VMH); often loosely referred to as the 'satiety centre'. Electrical stimulation of the VMH increases BAT thermogenesis, whereas lesions cause the tissue to atrophy, and the latter observation helps explain why VMH-lesioned animals can become obese without overeating. There are connections between the VMH and other hypothalamic areas concerned with feeding behaviour (e.g. lateral hypothalamus, paraventricular nucleus), and with the POAH, which provide a neural basis for integrating information on energy intake and body temperature, and modulate the level of NST and DIT accordingly.

Hormonal

Adrenaline stimulates BAT thermogenesis, but it is not as potent as noradrenaline, and in most physiological situations the circulating levels of adrenaline are probably not sufficient to activate the tissue's β-adrenoceptors. However, views may change on this in the light of recent, more sensitive measurements which show that circulating levels of adrenaline may have been previously underestimated. Although thyroid hormones (T_4 and T_3) are necessary to maintain BAT function, and T_3 is itself produced by the tissue, hyperthyroidism suppresses BAT activity. This is probably due to reduced sympathetic activation compensating for high levels of heat production in other, thyroid-sensitive tissues.

Glucocorticoids exert little or no direct effects on BAT, even though the tissue has glucocorticoid receptors. However, these adrenocorticoids have central inhibitory actions on the sympathetic outflow to BAT which are particularly noticeable in genetically obese rodents. Adrenalectomy in these rodents completely restores sympathetic activity, BAT thermogenesis and DIT to levels seen in lean animals. Only very low replacement doses of glucocorticoids are required to reverse the effects of adrenalectomy, suggesting that these obese animals are hypersensitive to the inhibitory actions of glucocorticoids. The glucocorticoids are thought to inhibit thermogenesis via feedback inhibition of hypothalamic corticotrophin-releasing factor (CRF). In addition to its effects on the pituitary, CRF is a potent stimulus for the sympathetic activation of BAT. Insulin exerts direct, metabolic effects on BAT that are essentially similar to those it exerts on white adipose tissue, but it also influences the tissue indirectly via its actions on the glucoreceptors of the VMH.

Pharmacological

For many years the β-adrenergic receptor subtype responsible for activation of BAT lipolysis and thermogenesis was thought to be the β_1-adrenoceptor. However, there is much recent evidence to suggest that the receptor is atypical (neither β_1 nor β_2), and it is now classified as the β_3-adrenoceptor. Much of this evidence came from experiments using novel thermogenic drugs developed for the treatment of obesity, and which were designed to be highly selective agonists of BAT thermogenesis, with little or no effect on β_1- or β_2-mediated functions. Subsequent to the pharmacological identification, the gene sequence for the β_3-adrenoceptor was identified in the human genome. BAT also contains α-adrenergic receptors, which are known to be important for activating the conversion of T_4 to T_3 by the 5′-deiodinase and may also play a minor, facilitatory role in thermogenesis. *See* Obesity, Treatment

Bibliography

Himms-Hagen J (1990) Brown adipose tissue thermogenesis. In: Schonbaum E and Lomax P (eds) *Thermoregulation – Physiology and Biochemistry*, pp 327–414. New York: Pergamon Press.
Lardy H and Stratman F (eds) (1989) *Hormones, Thermogenesis and Obesity*. New York: Elsevier.
Rothwell NJ and Stock MJ (1984) Brown adipose tissue. In: Baker PF (ed.) *Recent Advances in Physiology*, vol. 10, pp 349–384. Edinburgh: Churchill Livingstone.
Trayhurn P and Nicholls DG (eds) (1986) *Brown Adipose Tissue*. London: Arnold.

Michael J. Stock
St George's Hospital Medical School, London, UK

ADOLESCENTS

Contents

Nutritional Requirements

Because of the continuing sequence of growth and development over a period of 5–10 years during adolescence accurate quantification of the nutrient requirements of adolescents is probably more difficult than at any stage of the human life cycle. Significant differences in developmental patterns exist between females and males, so that the two genders must be considered separately. In addition, the actual development sequence within a gender varies greatly, so that in reality requirements shift according to maturational age rather than chronological age. Tanner staging is frequently used for this purpose (Tanner, 1962). Furthermore, the nutrient needs of active adolescents will differ from those of inactive, sedentary individuals of the same sex. Genetic and ethnic factors also play significant roles in adolescent development and determine to an important degree the nutrient requirements. Anthropometric standards are available for assessment of growth and nutritional status of adolescents (Frisancho, 1990). *See* Growth and Development; Nutritional Status, Importance of Measuring Nutritional Status; Nutritional Status, Anthropometry and Clinical Examination

Nutrient Requirements

Hormone-dependent changes in body composition which occur during prepuberty, puberty and the postpubertal growth spurt, drive the demand for energy, protein and other nutrients. Nutrient recommendations should ideally be applied according to developmental phase, since this approach would be more accurate than the traditional chronological strategy. Estimated requirements serve as the basis for setting nutrient allowances (Recommended Dietary Allowances or RDAs) which for all nutrients exceed estimated requirements by approximately 30%, the so-called safety factor. The RDA for energy, however, is set to equal the mean requirement of a given age- and sex-class since no safety factor needs to be built into this allowance. (Table 1 lists the US RDAs for adolescents.) Adolescents have greater energy requirements than adults on acount of the growth spurt. Requirements for protein are the same for adolescents and adults. Adolescents need more of those nutrients with requirements related to energy metabolism (thiamin, nicotinic acid). Calcium and phosphorus requirements are also greater than for adults. For male adolescents iron requirements are greater than for adult males, although for females iron requirements are the same during these two life stages. *See* Dietary Requirements of Adults

The energy requirements of adolescents are determined by many variables, including hereditary and environmental factors. Energy intake is related to a given stage of physical development, and hence the energy requirement varies among individuals by almost twofold during the postpubertal period, independently of age. The coefficient of variance (CV; standard deviation divided by mean of a given nutrient) exceeds 50% for almost all nutrient variables among adolescents and it may be as high as 200%. Thus other nutrients indexed to energy tend to have similarly high CVs. *See* Energy, Measurement of Food Energy

The relatively high level of nutrition in the more affluent nations has contributed to improved secular growth trends, i.e. greater height and weight, since the end of World War II. With high nutritional standards, adolescents in the technologically advanced nations have a greater chance of becoming overweight or obese. Excessive energy consumption relative to physiological needs is a major nutritional problem facing much of the economically developed world today. *See* Obesity, Aetiology and Assessment

Fat

Appropriate guidelines for adolescents are to limit fat consumption to approximately 30–35% of total energy consumption. A few studies have identified high total fat consumption among adolescents in the range of 40–45% of total energy. Such individuals invariably have high intakes of saturated fats and this is a significant dietary risk factor for coronary heart disease, stroke and other cardiovascular diseases. The National Cholesterol Education Programme of the USA has targeted adolescents, among other age groups in the population, for reducing saturated fat and cholesterol intakes. Childhood and adolescence are clearly appropriate times to initiate health promotion and disease prevention programmes. *See* Fats, Requirements

A concern has arisen among some paediatricians that both the energy consumption and the percentage of energy derived from fat could be reduced too much by overzealous, health-conscious adolescents (or possibly their parents) to help avoid obesity and cardiovascular diseases. Energy restriction has been shown to contribute to a significant delay in puberty, and to growth retardation or, minimally, developmental delay, in a group of 14 American children. The percentage of energy from fat in the diets of these children, however, was not so low, i.e. in the range of 30–35%. The possibility of growth retardation is less likely during adolescence than during the prepubertal stage of late childhood.

Carbohydrate

When fat consumption is lowered, carbohydrate intake must be increased to provide the same total amount of energy (kJ), with protein remaining approximately constant. Approximately 55–60% of energy should be derived from carbohydrates, especially complex carbohydrates (starches). *See* Carbohydrates, Requirements and Dietary Importance

Protein

Approximately 15% of total energy should come from protein. This requirement is readily met by nearly all adolescents in the USA and similarly affluent nations because of the wide availability of high-quality protein foods. Basal protein requirements are easily obtained on a typical Western diet high in animal protein because of the much greater digestive and absorptive efficiencies of animal proteins compared to plant proteins, although modern food processing methods in industrialized countries improve the effective utilization of plant proteins. This situation, however, does not hold for

Table 1.   US Recommended Dietary Allowances for adolescents

(a) Recommended Dietary Allowances (RDAs) for adolescents aged 11–18 years

Age (years)	Energy (MJ)	Protein (g)	Fat-soluble vitamins			
			Vitamin A (μg RE)	Vitamin D (μg)	Vitamin E (mg α-tocopherol)	Vitamin K (μg)
Males						
11–14	10·50	45	1000	10	10	45
15–18	12·60	59	1000	10	10	65
Females						
11–14	9·24	46	800	10	8	45
15–18	9·24	44	800	10	8	55

Water-soluble vitamins

	Vitamin C (mg)	Thiamin (mg)	Riboflavin (mg)	Niacin (mg nicotinic acid equivalents)	Vitamin B_6 (mg)	Folate (μg)	Vitamin B_{12} (μg)
Males							
11–14	50	1·3	1·5	17	1·7	150	2·0
15–18	60	1·5	1·8	20	2·0	200	2·0
Females							
11–14	50	1·1	1·3	15	1·4	150	2·0
15–18	60	1·1	1·3	15	1·5	180	2·0

Minerals

	Calcium (mg)	Phosphorus (mg)	Magnesium (mg)	Iron (mg)	Zinc (mg)	Iodine (μg)	Selenium (μg)
Males							
11–14	1200	1200	270	12	15	150	40
15–18	1200	1200	400	12	15	150	50
Females							
11–14	1200	1200	280	15	12	150	45
15–18	1200	1200	300	15	12	150	50

(b) Estimated sodium chloride and potassium minimum requirements of healthy persons

Age (years)	Weight (kg[a])	Sodium (mg[a, b])	Chloride (mg[a, b])	Potassium (mg[c])
10–18	50.0	500	750	2000

(c) Estimated safe and adequate daily dietary intakes

Age (years)	Vitamins		Minerals				
	Biotin (μg)	Pantothenic acid (mg)	Copper (mg)	Manganese (mg)	Fluoride (mg)	Chromium (μg)	Molybdenum (μg)
Males							
11–18	30–100	4–7	1·5–2·5	2·0–5·0	1·5–2·5	50–200	75–250
Females							
11–18	30–100	4–7	1·5–2·5	2·0–5·0	1·5–2·5	50–200	75–250

[a] No allowance has been included for large, prolonged losses from the skin through sweat.
[b] There is no evidence that higher intakes confer any health benefits.
[c] Desirable intakes of potassium may considerably exceed these values (approximately 3500 mg for adults).
[d] Values for those below 18 years assume a growth rate at the 50th percentile reported by the National Center for Health Statistics and averaged for males and females.
Source: National Research Council (1989b).

Nutritional Requirements

adolescents in much of the developing world, where low-quality proteins in plant staples serve as the primary sources of protein. In addition, the plant sources have lower digestibility efficiencies compared to animal products. *See* Protein, Requirements

Adolescent vegetarians should be able to obtain sufficient amounts of all the essential amino acids from plant sources to meet the requirements of growth if they include diverse protein sources in each meal or over the course of the daily meals. Physical growth and development depend on a ready supply of both energy and protein. If dietary energy is inadequate, amino acids derived from proteins in the diet will be used in part to meet energy needs, diminishing the availability of a large fraction of the body's pool of amino acids required for the protein synthetic pathways of growth. Vegetarians generally have less difficulty in meeting their protein (or amino acid) needs than their energy requirements for growth. *See* Vegetarian Diets

Whether or not high, long-term intakes of animal proteins have adverse effects regarding disease development has not been clearly established. Some investigators suggest that such intake patterns do exert an important effect as part of the multifactorial aetiology of renal diseases. Some researchers have generated supporting data for a role of excessive animal protein intake as a factor in the development of osteoporosis, whereas others have speculated that excessive protein intakes also play a role in cardiovascular diseases and even certain cancers. *See* Osteoporosis

Minerals

Adequate intakes of all minerals and trace elements are essential during adolescence. Of particular importance as this time are calcium and iron.

Calcium

Calcium is an unusual nutrient in two ways. First, it is available in large amounts from a relatively small number of foods. Second, the requirements for calcium by nearly all tissues except for the skeleton are very low. Thus the needs for calcium in cellular functions and blood clotting are small, but needs in the the continually renewed skeletal structures can only be satisfied by a fairly high calcium intake each day. Low bone mass or osteopenia later in adult life is correlated with fractures, especially in postmenopausal women. Amenorrhoeic or oligomenorrhoeic adolescent females may also be placed at risk of suboptimal bone mass development, even if calcium intakes are adequate, because of depressed serum oestrogen concentrations. *See* Calcium, Physiology

Calcium intakes should be near 1000–1200 mg per day during adolescence (US RDAs). These estimated allowances are based on the amount of mineral accumulated in the skeleton during both the prepubertal growth, and postpubertal growth spurt, as well as during the consolidation of bone mineralization after growth in length has ceased. Calcium requirements for skeletal retention during the growth spurts of adolescent girls have been estimated to be as high as 350 mg per day and for adolescent boys up to 450 mg daily. If the intestinal absorptive efficiency at this stage of life is assumed to be 40%, then adolescent girls will need as a minimum to support optimal skeletal development a daily intake of almost 1000 mg and adolescent boys approximately 1200 mg per day. These values are close to the recommended allowances (National Research Council, 1989b) but no gender distinction is made in the US recommendations. Furthermore, calcium intakes which approximate the adolescent RDAs are considered to optimize peak bone mass development in females, and possibly also in males, but the bone consolidation period in males continues for several years longer than in females. *See* Bone

The wise selection of foods from the relatively few calcium-rich foods becomes important for adolescent females, who are more likely to have to inadequate intakes than boys. Some girls tend to avoid dairy products in the USA because of their concern for their high fat content, despite the wide availability of many low-fat dairy choices. The increased acceptance of yoghurts and low-fat ice creams, as well as several kinds of reduced fat cheeses, make it much easier for adolescent girls to meet their calcium requirements. Dark green vegetables also contain useful amounts of calcium per serving. Foods are always recommended first for providing the amount of calcium to meet the body's needs, but if this cannot be achieved, supplements of calcium should be ingested in sufficient amounts to make up the difference between the allowance and the actual amount of calcium obtained from foods in a typical meal pattern. A dietitian or nutritionist would normally be needed to analyse the usual dietary pattern of an adolescent female in order to make this determination.

Iron

Iron is the trace element which is most deficient in the diets of females around the world. The satisfactory incorporation of enough mineral-rich foods in the diets of adolescent girls is as difficult for iron as it is for calcium. Weight-conscious females need to take care in selecting iron-rich lean meats and to include in their meals the dark meat portions of turkey and chicken which provide more iron than the white breast meat. Legumes are also a relatively good source of iron. *See* Iron, Physiology

Iron deficiency in females, uncomplicated by anaemia but showing clear deficits in iron stores and other functional indices of iron status, has been demonstrated experimentally to contribute to lower oxygen capacity and related performance parameters in female athletes. Nonanaemic iron deficiency adversely affects several enzyme systems, including those related to energy production in muscle and other tissues and to the normal function of neurons. Thus, even when a full-blown iron deficiency anaemia does not exist, menstruating females are placed at a disadvantage when their iron status is low, whether or not they are athletes. The gender-difference in the iron allowances (Table 1) relates to the greater losses of iron by menstruating females over the period of approximately one month, but the iron needs during rapid skeletal muscle development by males may equal those of adolescent females with normal cycles. Males who have low iron intakes, though not common in the USA, are also likely to have less-than-optimal physical performance in various types of activities, including strength and running tests. *See* Anaemia, Iron Deficiency Anaemia

Vitamins

Deficiencies of vitamins among adolescents are not common in the USA. It appears from national surveys that only small numbers of individuals have intakes of any vitamin below 67% of the US RDAs. Part of the reason for adequate vitamin intakes is widespread fortification of foods in the USA with thiamin, ribo-flavin, nicotinic acid, vitamin C, vitamin A and vitamin D. Another reason is the fairly common use of combination vitamin supplements, such as those that are taken once a day at recommended safe levels. Although toxicities of vitamins are always possible from excessive supplement usage, they have not been reported with any significant frequency. Thus vitamin intakes from foods and, to a lesser degree, from supplements satisfy adolescent requirements, at least in the USA. *See* individual vitamins

Dietary Fibre

Dietary fibre consists of several kinds of complex molecules (mostly polysaccharide in nature) obtained from plant foods, i.e. vegetables, fruits, nuts, seeds, cereal grains, legumes and seaweeds. Although not truly nutrients according to any strict definition, the diverse components classified as dietary fibre appear to be essential to good health, including bowel function and the regulation of both serum cholesterol and serum glucose. Thus, a reasonable amount of a variety of sources of fibre should be consumed. In the USA no

allowance has been recommended for dietary fibre, although general dietary guidelines promulgated by authorities include the suggestion that 30 g of fibre (18 g of nonstarch polysaccharides in the UK literature) should be consumed per day by adults and, presumably, by adolescents. *See* Dietary Fibre, Properties and Sources; Dietary Fibre, Physiological Effects; Dietary Fibre, Fibre and Disease Prevention

Special Needs of Adolescents

Certain subgroups of adolescents have special nutritional needs.

Adolescent Athletes

Adolescent athletes who strive for high performance must assure themselves of adequate nutrition. They have high requirement for carbohydrates and water, and female athletes, including ballerinas, must consume calcium and iron at recommended amounts (Table 1). If underconsumption becomes a regular pattern, performance levels may be compromised, injuries may become more likely, and healing from injuries may be slower. Good nutrition of adolescent athletes is extremely important, but little attention has been given to this by supervisory personnel in athletic and dance programmes. *See* Exercise, Metabolic Requirements

Strict Vegetarians

Strict vegetarians or vegans benefit from knowledge about food composition and the wise selection of many different foods. The concern about veganism is that optimal growth and development may be compromised because of insufficient energy intake and inadequate consumption of calcium, iron, and possibly other micronutrients, especially vitamin B_{12}. These concerns largely disappear as one or more animal products, particularly dairy products and eggs, are regularly included in the typical dietary pattern. Thus lacto-ovo-vegetarian patterns provide nearly all nutrients in satisfactory amounts to meet the allowances of adolescents, but iron may remain low or deficient if insufficient legumes and other plant sources of dietary iron are consumed. *See* Vegan Diets

Pregnant Adolescents

Pregnant adolescents have special nutrition-related problems imposed upon their incompletely developed bodies, depending on their stage of growth. Their bodies are sufficiently developed to allow egg fertilization and pregnancy to occur, but skeletal maturation, i.e. peak bone mass development and consolidation, clearly has not been completed. Much remains to be learned, however, about the skeletal development of early-maturing adolescent females, who are much more likely to become pregnant during adolescence than are late maturers, but the resultant low peak bone mass may be a significant outcome which places such females at increased risk of postmentopausal fractures. In addition, adolescent females who become pregnant almost invariably have poor nutritional habits and knowledge about wise food selection for themselves, let alone meeting the nutrient needs of a fetus as well. Adolescents who become pregnant require additional support to ensure nutritional adequacy of themselves and their fetuses. The nutritional demands of lactation are greater than those of pregnancy and an adequate diet is also essential for this period. The issue of adolescent pregnancy is nearly always further complicated by many other socioeconomic factors that nutritional matters become submerged, despite their critical importance to the health of the mother-to-be and the baby. Most nations, especially the USA, have not developed satisfactory programmes to deal with the nutritional needs of pregnant adolescents. *See* Lactation

Nutritional Education

Females are much more likely to have nutritional deficits, both of macro- and micronutrients, than males because they consume less food each day. In addition, females more frequently suffer from the eating disorders, anorexia nervosa and bulimia, because of major concerns about body image. Thus much greater emphasis on nutritional education among adolescent females would appear to be warranted in economically developed countries as well as in less developed nations. Males can also benefit from nutrition education, but they are generally more resistant to such an approach. *See* Anorexia Nervosa; Bulimia Nervosa; Nutrition Education

Bibliography

Anderson JJB (issue ed.) (1991) Adolescent nutrition – growth and body composition. *Nutrition Today* 26(No. 2): 7–39.
Falkner F and Tanner JM (eds) (1986) *Human Growth: A Comprehensive Treatise* 2nd edn. New York: Plenum Press.
Forbes GB (1987) *Human Body Composition: Growth, Aging, Nutrition and Activity*. New York: Springer-Verlag.
Frisancho AR (1990) *Anthropometric Standards for the Assessment of Growth and Nutritional Status*. Ann Arbor: University of Michigan Press.
Gong EJ and Heald FP (1988) Diet, nutrition, and adolescence. In: Shils ME and Young VR (eds) *Modern Nutrition in Health and Disease* 7th edn, pp 969–981. Philadelphia: Lea and Febiger.
Hetzel BS and Berenson GS (1987) *Cardiovascular Risk Factors in Childhood: Epidemiology and Prevention*. Amsterdam: Elsevier Science Publishers BV.
Institute of Medicine (1990) *Nutrition During Pregnancy: I. Weight Gain. II. Nutrient Supplements*. Washington, CD: National Academy Press.
Mahan LK and Rees J (eds) (1984) *Nutrition in Adolescence*. St Louis, Missouri: Mosby.
Meredith CN and Dwyer JT (1991) Nutrition and exercise: effects on adolescent health. *Annual Review of Public Health* 12: 309–333.
National Research Council (1989a) *Diet and Health: Implications for Reducing Chronic Disease Risk*. Washington, DC: National Academy Press.
National Research Council (1989b) *Recommended Dietary Allowances* 10th edn. Washington, DC: National Academy Press.
Pollitzer WS and Anderson JJB (1989) Ethnic and genetic differences in bone mass: A review with an hereditary vs. environmental perspective. *American Journal of Clinical Nutrition* 50: 1244–1259.
Pugliese MT, Lifshitz F, Grad G, Fort P and Marks-Katz M (1983) Fear of obesity: a cause of short stature and delayed puberty. *New England Journal of Medicine* 309: 513–516.
Tanner JM (1962) *Growth at Adolescence* 2nd edn. Oxford: Blackwell Scientific Publications.
Tanner JM and Preece MA (eds) (1989) *The Physiology of Human Growth*. Cambridge: Cambridge University Press.
US Department of Health and Human Services (1988) *Surgeon General's Report on Nutrition and Health*. DHHS Publication No. 88-50210. Washington, DC: US Government Printing Office.
Van Wieringen JC (1986) Secular growth changes. In: Falkner F and Tanner JM (eds) *Human Growth: A Comprehensive Treatise* 2nd edn. New York: Plenum Press.

John J. B. Anderson
University of North Carolina, Chapel Hill, USA

Nutritional Problems

Nutritional problems arise in adolescence as a result of both physiological and psychological changes. Rapid increase in lean body mass in boys and fat mass in girls contribute to nutritional stress. Dietary chaos may develop with noncooperation in family meals as adolescents express their independence. The intensity of emotion typical of adolescence also leads to eccentric or restricted diets adopted either for ethical or religious reasons or from excessive concern with body image. These may precipitate deficiencies of specific nutrients.

Poor nutrition may cause reduced linear growth, delayed pubertal development, poor skeletal mineralization, poor neurological function, and inadequate nutrition of the fetus in adolescent pregnancy. Poor nutrition may entrench inappropriate dietary habits at a stage when the adolescent is developing dietary practices which will continue into adult life.

The main features of adolescent nutritional habits include the following: missing meals; snacking; high consumption of fast foods; unconventional meals; alcohol and cigarette consumption; high consumption of soft drinks. An enormous variation in daily nutrient intakes results from these practices. In general, however, intakes are high in sugar, refined carbohydrates and saturated fats, and low in calcium, iron and vitamins, especially riboflavin, thiamin, vitamin B_{12}, folate and vitamin A. Clinical evidence of deficiencies is nevertheless surprisingly rare.

Between the ages of 11 and 15 years, British girls increase their energy intakes but reduce their intakes of sweets, carbohydrate snack items and fizzy drinks. Over the same age range the older boys consume more milk, bread and chips than the younger boys. Boys and girls show increasing chip and declining milk and fruit juice intakes with lower social class. *See* Snack Foods, Dietary Importance

Obesity

The incidence of obesity in adolescence is high in most Western societies but the precise figure is not clear because it is dependent upon the definition of obesity used and the age group studied. Some surveys suggest that about 3% of boys and 4% of 16-year-old girls have relative weights over 130% expected, whilst others suggest that as many as 30% of postmenarcheal girls and 12% of boys just prior to their pubertal growth spurt are obese. The true incidence is probably between these figures.

Obesity in adolescence is important since the proximity to adulthood makes obesity at this age likely to continue as obesity into adult life. Obesity occurs when energy intakes exceed energy expenditures. The frequently chaotic diets of adolescents, with high proportions of energy-dense snack foods and sweetened drinks, readily lead to excessive energy intakes. However, the low energy expenditure levels of some adolescents constitute another contributing factor. Bursts of vigorous activity (in sport or at discos) alternate with periods of extreme sloth spent lounging in bedrooms, in front of videos or television, or over computer games. In the USA, and probably in the UK as well, the percentage of overweight teenage boys increases in proportion to the hours spent watching television. *See* Obesity, Aetiology and Assessment

Slimming involves loss of adipose tissue and is dependent upon reduced energy intakes and increased energy output in activity. In those who are still growing, slimming is not necessarily the same as weight loss. In rapidly growing boys the changes of puberty with increasing lean body mass and reduction in percentage body fat may allow obese boys to slim in their teens

without weight loss. In postmenarcheal girls, where growth is slowing, slimming is almost certain to necessitate weight loss since the changes of puberty lead to increasing fat deposition with time.

Removal of snack items from the diet is critically important for slimming. Snack items feature highly in many obese adolescents' diets and they are almost always high in refined carbohydrates and fats and of low satiety value. Cooperation by obese adolescents is essential for successful dieting and this may be difficult to achieve since conformity with peers is important to the adolescent lifestyle. Parental desires for adolescents to slim provide an area of conflict between parents and children. Adolescents revolt by using diet as a means of demonstrating their noncooperation with parental wishes. The more the obese adolescent takes responsibility for the slimming regimen, the more likely he or she is to slim successfully. *See* Anorexia Nervosa; Bulimia Nervosa; Obesity, Treatment

Mineral Deficiencies

Calcium

Provided that adolescents have reasonable intakes of milk (e.g. 420 ml) of full, skimmed or semiskimmed per day), calcium intakes are likely to be adequate. Without substantial milk intakes it may be difficult to achieve recommended dietary requirements (15–17·5 mmol; 600–700 mg per day). Although there is little evidence that low calcium intakes in adolescence have significant effects on bone mineralization, the prevalence of osteoporosis in adult life may result from inadequate bone mineralization during rapid adolescent growth since it is suggested that osteoporosis is related to the amount of bone mineral present at the onset of bone mineral loss in the fourth decade. Bone mineralization is also influenced by exercise. Vigorous sport, or other physical activity during growth, may thus be important in achieving maximum lean body mass deposition in muscle and bone. *See* Calcium, Physiology; Osteoporosis

Iron

By adolescence, normal haemoglobin levels should be in the adult range for both girls and boys (11·5–14·5 g dl^{-1}). In girls, the onset of menstruation may be accompanied by irregular heavy periods, and iron requirements are high. Iron deficiency with or without anaemia is common in postmenarcheal girls but boys undergoing their growth spurt have requirements as high as girls for a short while. Low meat intakes, low vegetable intakes, and low intakes of vitamin C (which facilitates iron absorption), all contribute to iron deficiency. Vegetarian children and fussy children who tend to snack rather than eat meals, are likely to be iron deficient. The popularity of iron-fortified breakfast cereals may be important in preventing iron deficiency in many children. *See* Anaemia, Iron Deficiency Anaemia; Iron, Physiology; Vegetarian Diets

Iron deficiency in young children is associated with poor growth and poor intellectual development. In adolescence it may also be associated with poor learning, lethargy, lack of concentration and exacerbation of noncompliant behaviour since irritability, depression and apathy are psychological accompaniments of iron deficiency. Children with iron deficiency show low haemoglobin, hypochromia and microcytosis. Blood biochemistry, even when haemoglobin levels are in the normal range, shows low circulating iron, low ferritin which is a circulating indicator of iron stores, and high iron-binding capacity of proteins in the blood.

Iodine: Goitre

Goitre, i.e. enlargement of the thyroid gland, is a relatively common finding in adolescence. The gland is usually soft and diffusely enlarged. Adolescent goitre has been thought a normal association of the increased needs for thyroid hormone with vigorous growth and maturation at puberty. Girls are affected about six times more often than boys and there is a tendency for the finding to occur in families, making mild inborn errors of metabolism or asymptomatic autoimmune thyroiditis other possible explanations. Whatever the cause, most asymptomatic thyroid enlargements at puberty are not associated with clinically important abnormalities of thyroid function and resolve spontaneously. A few individuals with autoimmune thyroid antibodies develop hypothyroidism later. *See* Iodine, Physiology

In areas of iodine deficiency, previously borderline iodine intakes may become deficient during adolescent growth. The deficiency of iodine may be exacerbated by ingestion of goitrogens, particularly from high intakes of *Brassica* spp. Under these circumstances the thyroid enlarges secondary to increased thyroid-stimulating hormone production. Thyroid hormone production may be deficient despite the hypertrophy. The deficiency of iodine or the effect of goitrogens is variable, so that the thyroid goes through periods of enlargement and involution and these glands are usually nodular in consistency. In boys, adolescent enlargement secondary to low iodine intakes resolves as growth ceases. In girls, the enlargement may remain or increase with pregnancy and lactation. Treatment is to increase dietary iodine, usually by the use of iodized salt. *See* Goitrogens and Antithyroid Compounds; Thyroid Diseases

Vitamins

Vitamin D

Vitamin D intakes are commonly low in adolescence but circulating D metabolites are largely derived from conversion of 7-dehydrocholesterol in the skin to cholecalciferol during exposure to ultraviolet radiation around 300 nm in the summer months. Children with dark skins or those who remain indoors even in summer (often girls from the Indian subcontinent) are at risk of rickets in adolescence. This risk is exacerbated in those from the Indian subcontinent by the low-vitamin-D, low-calcium, high-fibre traditional diets, which tend to bind fat-soluble vitamins in the gut, leading to reduced absorption of the small quantities of dietary vitamin D. *See* Cholecalciferol, Physiology

Vitamins and Intelligence

There have been several studies of the effects of vitamin supplementation on intelligence of adolescent school children who are not considered vitamin-deficient by conventional terms. A review of adolescent children's intakes of vitamins showed many children had intakes below recommended levels. A trial of multivitamin preparations was instituted. Children receiving multivitamin preparations for 4 months showed improvement in intelligence quotient compared with children who received either no supplement or placebo, although the latter group showed some increase in intelligence quotient over the period of study. The original study was fiercely criticized and subsequent studies have not succeeded in proving the effect of vitamins on intelligence to critics' satisfaction. In one study the dose of vitamins given seemed very critical to whether or not a response was achieved, suggesting that factors in the study design may have been responsible for the changes rather than the vitamin supplements. High vitamin doses did not produce the same improvements as more moderate doses. It seems unlikely that blunderbuss vitamin supplementation will influence childrens' intellectual progress except amongst those few children who are suffering from inadequate intakes whose deficiencies deserve to be treated more specifically. *See* Mental Development and Nutrition

Pregnancy

Whilst relative youth is important for successful trouble-free pregnancy, the complications of pregnancy in immature girls are considerable. Low birthweight, resulting from prematurity or from intrauterine growth retardation, is common. Reductions in mean birthweights of just over 100 g can be expected in girls under 15. Several studies suggest that intakes do not meet recommendations for any of the main nutrients but pregnant teenagers are often very sedentary, so that energy requirements are greatly reduced. Intakes of iron, vitamin A and calcium are particularly likely to be below requirements.

In the USA, the neonatal mortality rate for infants born to mothers under 15 years of age was 41·2 per 1000 compared with 17·3 per 1000 livebirths overall in 1982. It is suggested that adolescent girls who become pregnant are at particular nutritional risk because linear growth is incomplete before conception and ultimate height is curtailed since the hormonal changes of pregnancy lead to epiphyseal fusion. Girls who have not yet completed linear growth are unlikely to become pregnant since the early years of menstruation are usually characterized by anovulatory cycles. Thus linear growth impairment is probably minimal.

Girls who become pregnant soon after menarche are more likely to have small-for-dates infants than those who become pregnant some years after menarche. Linear growth may have ceased but the nutritional demands of pregnancy compete with the physiological demands for energy for the storage of the fat so characteristic of female puberty. The fat store is an important reserve of utilizable energy which, once developed, protects fetal nutrition either in the first trimester, when vomiting causes low energy intakes, or in the last trimester, when fetal demands on maternal nutrition may exceed energy intakes.

In young adolescents still accruing lean and fat mass, deviation of calcium to the fetus may have a significant effect on their own calcium deposition, although the calcium deposited in fetal tissues is only about 2·5% of the maternal skeleton. Lactation creates greater nutritional demands, most notably for calcium, than pregnancy and this could be seen as a disadvantage for pregnant adolescents. The close bonding essential for successful breast-feeding, and the protective effects of maternal milk on fetuses at risk because of maternal emotional immaturity, outweigh any nutritional disadvantages to the mothers from breast-feeding. *See* Infants, Breast- and Bottle-feeding; Lactation

There is some evidence from long-term studies in the USA that women who consume higher protein intakes in early adolescence are more likely to have uncomplicated pregnancies later. This appears to be another indication for providing adolescents with good, balanced diets.

Acne

Acne is a common misery of adolescence. It develops as a result of increased sebum production by the sebaceous glands of the skin. Androgenic activity infuences the increase in sebaceous gland activity, which is why the problem only develops at adolescence.

Acne is characterized by the formation of comedones. Intrafollicular hyperkeratosis takes place in the sebum-forming hair follicles. The follicles fill with desquamated cells and sebum. Sebum itself is highly irritant and comedogenic. Open comedones form unsightly 'blackheads'. Closed comedones encourage inflammation and secondary infection, particularly with *Proprionobacter acnes* and coagulase-negative *Staphylococci*.

The role of diet in the development or persistence of acne is not clear. Many adolescents are sure their acne is influenced by their diet. The foods most commonly blamed are chocolate, fried foods, milk, cheese, and caffeine-containing drinks. There is little hard scientific evidence to support the effects of these foods on acne and it may be that there is tremendous variation in responses to individual foods. However, the irritant factors in sebum include free fatty acids and triglycerides. Increasing comedogenic effects are seen in rabbits with increasing saturation of fatty acids and chain length between C_{12} and C_{20}. Bacterial colonization of the follicles also converts triglycerides in sebum to free fatty acids and glycerol between secretion and reaching the skin surface. Thus it would seem possible for dietary fats to influence the type of fats excreted in the sebaceous glands. It would also seem logical for adolescents who feel that their diet is influencing their acne to exclude those nonessential dietary items which appear to exacerbate the condition. This is especially advisable for foods such as chocolate, fried foods and crisps.

Dental Caries

Perhaps 80% of an individual's incidence of dental caries occurs in the adolescent years. There is good evidence that dietary carbohydrates play a major role in the aetiology of dental caries. In adolescence, the demands of rapid growth directs minerals, particularly calcium, from tooth formation and enamel deposition to lean body mass, making teeth more susceptible to dental caries. All children should be encouraged to clean their teeth, especially before bed at night. Prebedtime snacks of carbohydrates or of the acid carbonated drinks so popular in adolescence, without teeth cleansing, encourage multiplication of cariogenic organisms in the mouth overnight when masticatory movements and the flow of saliva are at low levels. *See* Dental Disease, Aetiology of Dental Caries; Dental Disease, Role of Diet

There is little evidence that children have reduced their carbohydrate intakes over recent years or even that more children brush their teeth at night. Nevertheless, dental health in the UK has improved. This may be the result of widespread use of fluoride in toothpaste and the fluoridation of many water supplies. It may also be attributed to generally better health and nutrition leading to fewer interruptions in enamel deposition. Adolescents living in areas where water supplies are not fluoridated should be advised to take fluoride tablets equivalent to 1 mg per day to protect against dental caries. *See* Dental Disease, Fluoride in the Prevention of Dental Decay

Bibliography

Buckler J (1987) *The Adolescent Years*. Ware, Dorset: Castlemead Publications.

Department of Health (1989) *The Diets of British Schoolchildren*. Report on Health and Social Subjects 36. London: Her Majesty's Stationery Office.

Hetzel BS (1989) *The Story of Iodine Deficiency*. Oxford: Oxford University Press.

Lifshitz F and Moses N (1991) Nutrition for school child and adolescent. In: McLaren DS, Burman D, Belton NR, Williams AF (eds) *Textbook of Paediatric Nutrition* 3rd edn, pp 59–71. Edinburgh: Churchill Livingstone.

Mahan LK and Rees JM (1984) *Nutrition in Adolescence*. St Louis: Times Mirror/Mosby.

Poskitt EME (1987) Management of obesity. *Archives of Disease in Childhood* 62: 305–310.

Truswell AS and Darnton-Hill I (1981) Food habits of adolescents. *Nutrition Reviews* 39: 73–88.

E. M. E. Poskitt
University of Liverpool, Liverpool, UK

ADRENAL HORMONES

See Hormones

ADULTERATION OF FOODS

Contents

History and Occurrence
Detection

History and Occurrence

History

Food is a basic prerequisite for human survival and also for social and economic welfare and progress. Problems related to food have varied from one period of history to another, from continent to continent, and from country to country. The problem of food adulteration has been a major one and the protection of the consumer has occupied the attention of civil authorities from ancient times.

Food is considered adulterated in the following instances:

1. If the food contains poisons or other substances which may render it injurious to the health of the consumer.

2. If the food contains filth or is decomposed.

3. If the food contains a colouring agent or other food additive that is not approved, or contains materials that disguise inferior quality.

4. If any important constituent has been wholly or in part abstracted, or any specified ingredient has been substituted by a nonspecified ingredient.

5. If the food contains any substance that increases its weight and bulk or changes its strength, making it appear better than it is. *See* Contamination, Types and Causes

In US legislation, the term 'misbranding' is used as well as the term 'adulteration'. A food is misbranded if it is wrongly labelled or if it is a food for which standards of identity have been written and it fails to comply with these standards.

Food has been liable to adulteration to a greater or lesser extent since very early times. Mosaic and Egyptian laws made provision for preventing contamination of meat, while several centuries before the time of Christ India had regulations prohibiting the adulteration of grain and edible fats. Adulteration was also common during the Roman period. Evidence for this is given in Apicius' famous cookbook (*De Re Coquinaria*). During the Middle Ages in the UK, pepper and other costly spices imported from the East were adulterated by mixing with ground nutshells, local seeds and olive pits.

Between the thirteenth and sixteenth centuries, bread, wine, beer, spices, and valuable natural colouring materials were often adulterated. In the UK in 1319, a meat-market overseer succeeded in putting a butcher in the pillory for selling unsound beef. Wines were 'sophisticated' (adulterated) with burnt sugar, juices, starch and gums, and other substances. Such practices may have reduced the quality of the wine but they were not injurious to health. After the eighteenth century, however, food adulteration became dangerous. Vinegar was often adulterated with sulphuric acid, wine with preservatives containing lead salts, green vegetables in vinegar with copper (to improve colour), essential oils with oil of turpentine, confectionery products with colourings containing lead and arsenic, chocolate with Venetian red (ferric oxide), and red pepper with vermillion (mercury sulphide). 'Black extract', obtained by boiling poisonous berries of *Cocculus indicus* in water and concentrating the fluid, was used in beer. This extract imparted flavour, but also narcotic properties and intoxicating qualities to the beverage.

Bread was not only the basic item of diet for many centuries but also the one most subjected to adulteration. The incorporation of sieved boiled potatoes in the flour was a common fraudulent practice, but the most serious example was the addition of alum which whitened flour of inferior quality.

Recipe books of the eighteenth century contain instructions which today would cause alarm. The recipe for preserving green colour in pickles is characteristic: 'To render pickles green, boil them with a halfpenny or allow them to stand for 24 hours in copper or brass pans'. It is not surprising that records of that period list a number of deaths from copper poisoning.

Frederic Accum, writing from London in 1820, gives a vivid description of the adulteration of bread, alcoholic drinks, tea, coffee, and many other foods. Accum claimed that 'Indeed, it would be difficult to mention a single article of food which is not to be met with in an adulterated state; and there are some substances which are scarcely ever to be genuine'. Even if these accusations are somewhat overstated, the seriousness of

intentional adulteration of food which prevailed between 1800 and early 1900s is undisputed.

The second decade of the nineteenth century marks the beginning of the second period in the history of food adulteration. In the first period (ancient times to about 1820) food was procured from small enterprises and individuals who were, to a certain extent, responsible for their own transactions. In the second period (early 1800s to 1900s), the methods of food production changed significantly. Large-scale food production became necessary because of the industrial revolution which led to a move of population from country to city. This created conditions that were conducive to large-scale adulteration of food. Intentional adulteration of food remained a serious problem until the beginning of the twentieth century. At this point, regulatory pressures and the effectiveness of analytical methods reduced the frequency and magnitude of food adulteration. Further improvements have been achieved up to the present time and, owing to the strict legal standards and also to the growth of an increasingly critical public, deliberate adulteration in the industrialized countries has become less serious. Of course, fraudulent practices still continue in countries which lack adequate means to ensure that laws and regulations are enforced.

Food Additives

Modern food law in the developed countries has brought the more dangerous and fraudulent practices under control. However, the excessive use of additives and the use of additives that have not been approved present a serious threat to food safety. It could be argued that a fourth phase of food adulteration began some 40 years ago, when foods containing chemicals became prevalent in the diet.

In spite of being under legal control for more than three decades, food additives have assumed prominence as a source of consumer concern. Thus we have moved gradually from an outrage over fraud, sometimes practised with dangerous substances, to a growing concern over the more subtle toxic effects of common chemicals added to food to assist manufacture and storage. As a result, there has been a shift in focus from *food adulteration* to *safety of food*, and to a different approach which emphasizes not only evaluation of the food in its entirety, but also evaluation of individual components. Current legislation relating to food additives provides statutory lists of all permitted additives which may be used and, where appropriate, the maximum levels for their use. Nevertheless, as the food industry becomes increasingly sophisticated and relies more and more on the use of additives, many consumers believe that governments are unable to control the situation completely and that preservatives, antioxidants, colourings, flavour or texture modifiers, and other chemicals are and will always remain a potential hazard. *See* Food Additives, Safety

Food Legislation

The use of the regulatory powers of government to control the purity and safety of foods is very old but the first serious efforts to regulate malpractices took place only in the nineteenth century. The first general food laws were passed in the UK in 1860. Accum's book, *A Treatise on Adulteration of Food and Culinary Poisons* (1820), aroused the indignation of the British public. In 1850, Thomas Wakley, editor of the *Lancet*, established a Sanitary Commission under the direction of Arthur Hill Hassal, the first man to investigate food adulteration from a scientific point of view. The Commission's reports, published in the *Lancet* from 1851 to 1854, led to the formation of a parliamentary committee to investigate food adulteration and, in 1860, to the passage of the world's first Food and Drink Act. *See* Legislation, History

The law made it a criminal offence to sell adulterated food and drink. It also established the appointment of public analysts to examine foodstuffs produced throughout the country. In 1866, a second country, New Zealand, passed pure food legislation and, in 1874, Canada passed the Food and Drug Law.

In the twentieth century, new regulations were developed in the industrialized countries, and old regulations were repeatedly updated, taking into account the advice of governmental and international committees. Modern food law establishes and maintains standards for the composition of food, controls the use of additives and extent of contamination, controls packaging materials and unsanitary practices in the production of food and restrains unwarranted and misleading claims and advertisements. Effective food surveillance systems have also been developed which ensure that there is a constant supply of the right kind of food to keep people properly fed and that the food we eat is wholesome as a result of strict adherence to national and international law. *See* Legislation, International Standards; Legislation, Additives; Legislation, Contaminants and Adulterants; Legislation, Labelling Legislation; Legislation, Packaging Legislation

Food Legislation and Surveillance in the UK

The Food and Drink Act in 1860 and subsequent acts in 1875, 1928 and 1938 were succeeded by the 1955 Food and Drugs Act and the Food Act 1984. These continuous revisions and amendments have created a modern legislative framework, providing legal controls of food production and marketing.

Legislation in the UK is initiated by the Ministry of Agriculture, Fisheries and Food (MAFF) in conjunction with the Department of Health, the Department of the Environment and the Department of Trade and Industry. The ministry is advised by four advisory committees. The Food Advisory Committee advises the Government on the composition, labelling and advertising of food and on additives, contaminants and other substances, that are, or may be, present in food, or used in its preparation. The Committee on Toxicity of Chemicals in Food, Consumer Products and the Environment advises on the toxic risk to humans of chemicals in food, consumer products and the environment. The Veterinary Products Committee advises the licensing authority on the licensing of veterinary medicines. Finally, the Advisory Committee on Pesticides keeps under review all risks that may arise from the use of pesticides and other potentially toxic chemicals. *See* Ministry of Agriculture, Fisheries and Food

Monitoring the safety in the UK food supply is the responsibility of the Steering Group of Food Surveillance, a committee of senior government advisors which is linked to the above committees. The MAFF Surveillance Programme has now been running successfully for more than 10 years and the information provided by the steering group and its working parties is often used as a basis for discussions about the need for changes in UK or international regulations.

Regulating the Safety of Food in USA

In the USA there were no food regulation laws prior to the 1900s. At that time food companies could add anything to their products. In 1902, the Director of the Bureau of Chemistry in the US Department of Agriculture (USDA), Harvey Wiley, who was the leader of a campaign against adulteration of food, set up a group of male volunteers to evaluate the safety of common food preservatives and ingredients. This group became known as the 'Poison Squad'. At about the same time that the Poison Squad was formed, Upton Sinclair wrote a book, *The Jungle*, dealing with the unsanitary conditions of the Chicago meat-packing industry. This crusade resulted, in 1906, in the passage of the Pure Food and Drug Act, which defined food adulteration and made the distribution and sale of adulterated foods and drugs illegal. These early efforts of the Poison Squad marked the beginning of food toxicology and provided impetus for the regulation of substances added to foods.

In 1931, the Food and Drug Administration (FDA) was formed as a separate unit of the USDA to administer the law. This agency regulates food under two general criteria, adulteration and misbranding. The

FDA was ineffective until 1938, at which time the passage of the Federal Food, Drug and Cosmetic Act of 1938 updated and tightened the definition of adulteration. This gave the agency the power to fine violators of the laws.

After 20 years of application, interpretation and enforcement of this act, a significant revision took place in 1958, the Food Additives Amendment of 1958, which led to a major change in the FDA's approach to its activities. Congress applied the term 'safe' as the criterion for action, supplementing in this way the term 'adulteration'.

Over the years, with advances in science and analytical methods, the FDA has become more confident in its evaluation of food safety and the courts in the USA have given general endorsement to the agency's decisions.

The FDA has major responsibilities for food supply in the USA, but other agencies also exert significant regulatory control over foods and beverages. The major agencies are the Department of Health and Human Services, the US Department of Agriculture Inspection Services, the US Department of Commerce, and the Environmental Protection Agency.

International Standards

The Food and Agriculture Organization (FAO), the World Health Organization (WHO) and the Joint Codex Alimentarius Commission are concerned with the safety of food and food ingredients. The aims of the Codex Alimentarius include protecting the health of the consumer and ensuring fair practices in the food trade, co-ordination of all food standards work, determining priorities and initiating, guiding and finalizing the preparation of food standards. There are published recommended international standards for the individual foods (sugars, edible oils, canned fruits and vegetables, processed meat, fish products, cocoa products, etc.), as well as provisions with respect to food hygiene, food additives, contaminants, and labelling. *See* World Health Organization

All of the standards are detailed specifications, most of which require analytical methods for their realization. This task is backed by other standardizing organizations such as the International Union of Pure and Applied Chemistry (IUPAC), the International Standards Organization (ISO), and the Association of Official Analytical Chemists (AOAC) which are involved in the development of methods of sampling and analysis. These organizations consult with the the various international bodies representing individual commodity interests such as the International Dairy Federation (IDF), the International Association for Cereal Chemistry (ICC), the International Olive Oil Council (IOOC), the International Office of Cocoa and Chocolate (IOCC), and others.

European Economic Community Laws

In the European Economic Community (EEC), a huge market with a population of 320 million, a programme of food law measures is designed to create a single European Market in Foodstuffs by 1 January 1993. The laws of the community are expressed in the form of regulations and directives. Regulations, made under Article 43 of the Treaty of Rome, are binding on all member states and are directly applicable. The directive has no force of law in a member state until it is incorporated into the legislation of that country. Dates are prescribed in directives to ensure compliance within the time stated. Some of the rules and specifications of the EEC directives rely on Codex Alimentarius or other international guidelines. *See* European Economic Community, International Developments in Food Law

The community is also laying down tougher rules for food analysis which laboratories must adopt in time for the Single Market in 1992. The criteria to which EEC methods of analysis of foodstuffs should conform are as stringent as those recommended by any international organization.

Bringing a multitude of national laws into line with a common objective is a difficult task but food legislation at Community level is expected to deal successfully with questions such as protection of public health, consumer information and fair trading. The member states of the EEC are now speeding up harmonization, since their governments are aware that outdated legislation can no longer act as a basis for competition in this large market.

Toxicological Implications

In the past, deliberate adulteration of food with untested chemicals or poisonous substances was widespread. In this century, developments in the analytical field and improvement of legislation have brought many of these illegal and unethical practices under control, but cases of food adulteration with toxicological consequences have not disappeared completely.

One serious case of malpractice in the food industry is the use of denatured rapeseed oil for edible purposes, which caused the outbreak referred to as 'Spanish toxic oil syndrome'. In 1981, a disease broke out in Spain which rapidly took on epidemic proportions. The reported symptoms were respiratory distress, nausea, fever, vomiting, headaches, myalgias, abdominal pain and skin eruptions. Approximately 20 000 people were affected and more than 400 deaths were recorded.

For many years, scientists all over the world tried very hard to find an explanation and identify the toxic compounds which caused the illness. The situation was confused for many years. Today, toxicologists and chemists are convinced that the toxic oil syndrome should be attributed to aniline used for denaturation. The rapeseed oil was subjected to a refining process in an effort to remove the aniline and put the oil back on the market as an edible product in admixture with other vegetable oils. This treatment at high temperature caused the formation of compounds some of which have been shown to be acutely toxic.

1-Phenyl-5-vinyl imidazolidine-2-thione, which is presumably formed from aniline and the degradation products of glucosinolates (present in rapeseed oil), was initially reported to be one of the main causative agents. Very recent studies showed that the correct structure of the compound which is now believed to be the aetiological agent in Spanish toxic oil syndrome is N-(5-vinyl-1,3-thiazolidin-2-ylidene) phenylamine.

Examples of Current Practice of Food Adulteration

Cases of adulteration frequently reported in the literature concern oils and fats, fruit juices, alcoholic beverages, essential oils and flavourings, honey, dairy products, meat, chocolate, coffee and spices.

Some cases of the last decade with serious economic and other implications are briefly discussed below.

Wines

Some Austrian, German and Italian wines were found in 1985 to have been illegally supplemented with diethylene glycol (DEG), not a permitted food additive, to improve body and sweetness. Soon after the scandal, a 30% drop in demand for wines was observed in Austria. In 1987 some Japanese wines were also reported to contain the same adulterant.

Apple Juice

One recent case which involved economic fraud and cover-up efforts is the 'adulterated apple juice for babies' scandal. For many years, Beech-nut Nutrition Corporation purchased and used concentrated apple juice which contained cheap ingredients such as the corn syrup, invert sugar, malic acid, caramel and imitation flavour. Although the director of research and development discovered the use of the adulterants, he was forced to resign. The FDA took action and in 1988 the company was heavily fined. The director of the company was sentenced to 5 years on probation, and the vice president to a year in jail. The total cost to the company, of fines and losses of sales, is estimated to be 25×10^6. It has been said that the Beech-nut scandal will serve as 'a case study in Food Law courses for years to come'.

Vanilla Extracts

The adulteration of vanilla extracts with inexpensive synthetic vanillin represents a loss of millions of dollars to the vanilla extract industry. To obtain equal strength of flavour, either 28 g of synthetic vanillin or 4·5 l of single-fold vanilla extract is required. The ratio of cost is approximately 1 : 120, and this significant difference is a strong stimulus for adulteration.

Nonvanilla vanillin can be prepared from lignin, eugenol or guaiacol. Synthetic products have a characteristic vanilla-like note but they are inferior in organoleptic properties because the quality of natural vanilla derives not only from the concentration of vanillin but also from the presence of other valuable volatile flavour compounds.

Olive Oil

Olive oil, a food staple in the warmer regions around the Mediterranean, is now becoming more popular throughout Europe and in the USA. Olive oil is often adulterated with seed oils and olive residue oil (olive pomace, olive kernel or olive husk oil). Esterified oil, which is prepared by re-esterifying low-grade olive oil or olive oil soapstock recovered from alkali refining, has also been used to adulterate olive oil products. A survey in 1982 in the USA demonstrated that many olive oil products (imported or locally produced) contained undeclared olive husk oil, esterified oils and seed oils. These findings led to an FDA regulatory programme to control the market. In 1988 FDA officials reported that tight control by exporting countries and continuous surveillance in the USA were required to eliminate adulteration of olive oil.

Bibliography

Fennema O (ed.) (1976) *Principles of Food Science*, Part I, pp 2–7. New York: Marcel Dekker.
Firestone D, Carsan KL and Reina RJ (1988) Update on control of olive oil adulteration and misbranding in the United States. *Journal of the American Oil Chemists' Society* 65: 788–792.
Kochar SP (1984) The Spanish toxic oil syndrome. *Nutrition and Food Science* 90(11/12): 14, 15, 20.
MAFF (1989) *Food Surveillance*, Booklet PB 0025. London: Ministry of Agriculture, Fisheries and Food.
Middlekauff R (1984) Regulating the safety of food. *Food Technology* 43: 296–307.
Stewart GF and Amerine MA (1982) *Food Science and Technology*, pp 15–20. New York: Academic Press.
Wrolstad RE (1991) Ethical issues concerning food adulteration. *Food Technology* 45: 108–114.

Maria Tsimidou and Dimitrios Boskou
Aristotle University of Thessaloniki, Thessaloniki, Greece

Detection

Methods of detecting food adulteration are based on physical, chemical, biochemical and microscopic techniques. All these methods, which have replaced the early organoleptic and other empirical tests, are continuously updated because food adulteration is unceasing and new problems are always arising.

Proximate analysis of a foodstuff indicates the extent of abstraction for the main compositional components – moisture, fat, protein, carbohydrates and ash. However, it cannot answer problems of authenticity or speciation.

Very often adulteration can be detected from the presence of minor components that occur in the adulterant and not in the food itself. In such cases trace chemical analysis is necessary to assess the purity. Today, substances can be detected at the nanogram or even picogram level.

In recent years major advances in chromatographic separation have been achieved. Due to these analytical improvements, characteristic profiles of mixtures of chemically related components may be obtained and used to assess the authenticity of a suspect sample.

This article outlines the main applications of analytical techniques which are routinely used in laboratories authorized to check the purity of foods and drinks.

Sensory Methods

Sensory methods have not yet been incorporated into legislation for the detection of food adulteration although routine analysis of a sample always includes the examination of its organoleptic characteristics. International organizations such as the International Standards Organization (ISO), American Society for Testing Materials (ASTM), Office International de la Vigne et du Vin (OIV) and others have developed and recommended sensory methods for foods in general and for particular commodities. Moreover, the US Food and Drug Administration (FDA) has accepted results of sensory panel tests as *prima facie* evidence of product efficacy and in some cases legal decisions in the USA have relied exclusively upon sensory evaluation data. *See* Legislation, Contaminants and Adulterants

The limitations concerning the application of sensory methods for the detection of adulteration are fewer now that multivariate statistical techniques are employed. With these methods sensory data are better evaluated and more reliable conclusions can be drawn. Generalized Procrustes Analysis seems to be very promising and has been applied to classify coffee, tea and alcoholic beverages.

Physicochemical Methods

Among physicochemical techniques, chromatographic procedures are preferred when separation of the components of a mixture is needed; spectroscopic techniques are mainly used for quantitative determinations or qualitative identifications, very often in conjuction with chromatographic systems.

Chromatographic Methods

Gas Chromatography (GC)

GC has proved to be essential for the analysis of lipids and, therefore, is widely used in the detection of adulteration of edible fats. Adulteration of fats is usually detected by GC analysis of fatty acid methyl esters (FAMEs), sterols and triglycerides. *See* Chromatography, Gas Chromatography

Fatty Acid Composition. Separation of FAMEs is based on different molecular weights and degrees of unsaturation; it is usually achieved isothermally at 180–200°C using columns packed with diethylene glycol polysuccinate or diethylene glycol adipate; more recently, capillary columns have been used. Edible fats have characteristic fatty acid compositions and can be grouped into various categories. The percentage values for each fatty acid are compared to those recommended by national and international organizations. *See* Fatty Acids, Analysis

Analysis of Sterols and Triterpenoid Alcohols. Identification and determination of sterols by GC is mainly used to reveal the presence of vegetable fats in animal fats. The opposite is also feasible, provided that account is taken of the small amount of cholesterol naturally present in some vegetable fats (eg palm oil). The principle of recommended procedures (International Union of Pure and Applied Chemistry, IUPAC; Association of Official Analytical Chemists, AOAC) involves saponification of the sample, isolation of the sterols from the unsaponifiable matter on thin-layer plates and GC analysis of sterols or their derivatives. The separation is usually with SE-30, OV-17 or JXR at elevated temperatures (230–240°C).

A minor component of olive residue oil, erythrodiol (homo-olestranol), a triterpenoid diol, is used as an indication of adulteration of genuine olive oil with olive residue oil. The detection is based on GC of the combined sterol and triterpenoid diol fraction after silanization.

Triglyceride Composition. Triglycerides are separated according to carbon number. This is important for the detection of cocoa butter equivalents (CBEs) in cocoa products. The addition of 5% non-cocoa butter fat (rich in symmetrical triglycerides), apart from milk fat, is permitted in many countries and it is a common practice in the industry. Fincke, and also Padley and Timms, proposed a methodology based on the well-documented linear relationship betweenn C_{50} and C_{54} triglycerides for all cocoa butters. All CBEs contain fewer C_{52} triglycerides compared to cocoa butter, and this difference causes a significant deviation from the above relationship. *See* Triglycerides, Characterization and Determination

Recent Applications. Recent instrumental improvements as well as the development of high-resolution capillary columns have revitalized GC. GC–mass spectroscopy (GC–MS) techniques have been proved unequivocal in identifying the presence of undesirable components and in revealing adulteration. For example, a GC–MS method was used to identify the illegal addition of diethylene glycol in wines and also to elucidate the identity of the compounds responsible for the 'Spanish toxic oil syndrome'. These improvements in equipment and methodology require new sampling techniques. A variety of injection modes compatible with capillary columns have emerged. Headspace sampling techniques are ideal for trapping very volatile components prior to GC analysis. They can also be employed to explore the volatiles of samples that contain large amounts of nonvolatile components. This is the case in fermented beverages such as wine, beer and distilled liquors. The profile of the aromatic compounds of fermented beverages chromatographed by headspace techniques is used to check misbranding of these heavily taxed commodities. The test involves comparative GC analysis of the suspected sample and a standard for the particular brand.

High-performance Liquid Chromatography (HPLC)

HPLC techniques are increasingly being used in routine analysis and are now incorporated into the legislation of many countries. Today, well-established procedures for many classes of organic compounds or individual food components are available; many of these procedures can be used to check food adulteration. *See* Chromatography, High-performance Liquid Chromatography

Carbohydrate Composition. Carbohydrate analysis by HPLC is usually performed on amino-bonded reversed-phase columns. A 70–80% aqueous acetonitrile solution is suitable to elute low-molecular-weight sugars isocratically within 20 min; for the detection of eluate, refractive index detectors are necessary. The sample injected (10–100 μl) must be free from particulate material; therefore, careful extraction and clean-up are essential.

Simultaneous determination of glucose, fructose and sucrose are useful to detect the illegal addition of invert sugar in manufactured products. Nutritional claims may also be checked by HPLC profiling of carbohydrates. For example, lactose content is used to extrapolate the fat level of skim milk powder; raffinose and stachyose determination is an indicator of the addition of texturized soya in meat products, etc.

Oligosaccharide analysis is carried out by similar elution systems to those used for low-molecular-weight sugars (40–60% aqueous acetonitrile, ~ 30 min). Molecular weight carbohydrate analysis is necessary for the control of the addition of undeclared starch syrups in honey and other valuable natural products.

Triglyceride Composition. The HPLC analysis of triglycerides is achieved on reversed-phase columns, isocratically or by gradient nonaqueous elution. The separation is based on the concept of equivalent carbon number (ECN):

$$ECN = CN - 2DB, \qquad (1)$$

where CN is the carbon number of the triglyceride molecule and DB is the double bond number.

Triglycerides having the same equivalent carbon number are referred to in the literature as 'critical pairs'. The complete resolution of critical pairs is not necessary for detection of adulterated oils and fats or fat speciation as long as the separation is characteristic and reproducible. IUPAC recommends a simple isocratic procedure using acetone–acetonitrile mixtures and refractive index detection to determine the nature and the relative percentages of individual triglycerides in fats. Based on such simple procedures, the EEC has proposed a maximum level of 0·5% trilinolein for olive oil.

Amino Acid Composition. Ion exchange chromatography (automated or not) is the best analytical procedure for the separation of the 20 natural amino acids. However, it encounters specific difficulties which restrict its application in routine analysis. The search for an equally powerful technique for amino acid analysis may explain the fact that the first reported application of HPLC to food and beverage analysis was the determination of free amino acids in cocoa beans, in 1980. Precolumn derivatization of amino acids with various reagents (phenyl isothiocyanate, dansyl chloride, 2,4-dinitrofluorobenzene or *o*-phthaldialdehyde), reversed-phase columns, gradient elution with mixtures of acetonitrile (or methanol) and a buffer and ultraviolet detection are the usual chromatographic parameters. *See* Amino Acids, Determination

Among the most important applications are the determination of authenticity and type of juices and also the detection of the origin of honeys.

Fruit juices, beverages and syrups. The concentration

and relative proportions of amino acids are two of the best criteria for identification of the type of juices and for estimation of the content of juice in a beverage or syrup. This evaluation of results is based on the small variability of relative quantities of L-amino acids in juices, which cannot be easily manipulated. Besides, commercial amino acid mixtures are expensive adulterants.

Stepwise regression analysis performed on amino acid data produced by HPLC is very useful in solving complex problems of adulteration such as the presence of more than one adulterant, or the addition of acidulants and colouring agents.

Other Applications. HPLC is a very promising technique for the determination of minor components and metabolites. For example, illegal addition of colouring matter in juices and wine can be detected by HPLC analysis of pigments; diacetyl determination in butter, flavonoids in apple and pear juice and naringin and prunin in grapefruit are also used to detect aroma supplementation or the type of fruit.

HPLC analysis of minor components usually involves careful extraction and clean-up of the determinant. The widespread application of solid phase extraction with commercial cartridges facilitates these steps.

Electrophoresis

In recent years electrophoretic techniques have been used to reveal adulteration of many food products rich in protein. Among the most important applications reported are the detection of: the addition of soya protein to meat products (polyacrylamide gel electrophoresis, PAGE); the substitution of cow's milk for goat's milk in goat dairy products (PAGE, isoelectric focusing, IEF); the origin (season, area and strain) of wheat flour (PAGE); the partial replacement of wheat flour by other cereal flours (PAGE). Electrophoretic techniques are used almost exclusively for the species identification of fishery products. Electrofocusing is the most suitable technique because an equilibrium technique is easily standardized. *See* Electrophoresis

Fishery Products. The large number of fish species consumed, the close relations among some of them and the removal of the external features due to processing are the major difficulties in the identification of fish species. The latter is achieved using, as determinants, sarcoplasmic and myofibrillar proteins under well-established standard procedures. Reference samples are considered necessary for identification. Today, preparations of dry sarcoplasmic protein to yield species-specific proteins are commercially available. There are also publications containing the characteristic electrophoretic protein patterns and other information for a great number of fish species.

Spectrophotometry

Ultraviolet–visible techniques are frequently used for the assessment of adulteration of citrus juices, coffee and tea, virgin olive oils and coloured food products. Infrared radiation is the basis of automated equipment for the quality control of milk, grains or fats. More sophisticated techniques are employed where necessary (nuclear magnetic resonance, NMR or MS). *See* Spectroscopy, Infrared and Raman; Mass Spectrometry, Principles and Instrumentation; Spectroscopy, Nuclear Magnetic Resonance

Citrus Products. The approximation of orange juice and pulpwash content in citrus products is based on equations derived from absorption data of the alcoholic extract in the visible region (465, 443 and 425 nm; carotenes) and the ultraviolet (325, 280 and 245 nm; polyphenols, flavonoids, ascorbic acid) regions.

The ratio A273 nm/A326 nm is found to be constant for lemon juice. Deviation from this constant value indicates the addition of grapefruit, orange or apple juices. Luminescence spectrophotometry is also useful for the characterization of mixtures of citrus fruit juices. *See* Citrus Fruits, Composition and Characterization

Tea and Coffee. The caffeine content of these highly priced commodities and their products is a significant quality criterion. The method, which is based on measurement of the absorbance at 276 nm, is sensitive enough to test decaffeinated green or roasted coffee samples. HPLC is also widely used.

Oils and Fats. The state of autoxidation is indicated by the specific extinction values at 232 nm (conjugated dienes) and 268 nm (conjugated trienes). The specific extinction at 268 nm is also suitable to check admixing of virgin olive oil with residue or refined olive oil because conjugated trienes are present in the processed oils. *See* Vegetable Oils, Analysis

Coloured Foods. Ultraviolet–visible spectra of permitted and nonpermitted pigments are important for the identification of added colouring matter in food. Careful extraction and isolation of the dyes are necessary prior to analysis. Lists for permitted colours (FDA, EEC) and spectra for food colours are available for comparison (German Research Society). *See* Colours, Properties and Determination of Synthetic Pigments

Microscopic Methods

Standard microscopic methods have been developed for the authentication of herbs, spices, flours and honey. These techniques are simple in principle but the evaluation of the results requires considerable experience on the part of the microscopist.

Herbs and Spices. The sample is ground and a slide is prepared which is examined under different power objectives. For comparison, ISO standards describing histological characteristics of 68 spices and condiments can be used. *See* Spices and Flavouring Crops, Properties and Analysis

Honey. The potential of microscopic examination of pollen for the recognition of geographical origin of honey has been extensively studied. The principle of the method is the identification of pollen from characteristic and preferably indigenous plant species of a region. *See* Honey

Biospecific Methods

Enzymatic Methods

Enzymatic methods are applied to check the purity of fruit juices and starch and to characterize various sugars in foodstuffs, and formulae. *See* Enzymes, Use in Analysis

Fruit Juices. Among the various parameters required in the evaluation of fruit juice quality the determination of sugars and organic acids is extremely important. Enzymatic determination of sucrose and invert sugars is more accurate and specific compared to chemical methods. By applying enzymatic techniques, more reliable sugar/invert sugar ratios can be calculated.

Determination of organic acids is also useful in detecting adulteration or checking the type of processing and the raw materials used. The addition of synthetic D,L-malic acid is revealed by a combination of enzymatic determination of L-malic acid (the natural existing isomer) and HPLC. Deviation from the narrow range of the citric/isocitric acid ratio in orange juice indicates adulteration with sugar solutions and citric acid. Other organic acids such as ascorbic, dehydroascorbic, lactic and formic acids are also easily determined enzymatically.

Starches. There is a need for a reliable and reproducible technique to determine starch purity. The latter, for example, is extremely important for the EEC refunds for food-grade starches. The EEC Starch Working Group is now considering the utilization of a multienzyme regime consisting of α-amylase, amyloglucosidase and a debranching enzyme, pullulanase, to overcome the problem of incomplete starch hydrolysis. *See* Starch, Structure, Properties and Determination

Other Applications. Enzymatic determination of glucose, sucrose and starch or glucose, maltose, sucrose and partially hydrolysed starch are recommended by various bodies for the characterization of sugars added to meat products, sausages, baby foods, etc. These determinations of complex mixtures are readily carried out with commercial multienzyme test kits.

Very sensitive enzymatic methods are also available for the determination of ethanol. Such methods are particularly useful in the quality control of wine, beer, other alcoholic beverages, alcohol-free products and alcohol-containing chocolate products.

Immunochemical Methods

Immunochemical procedures were initially developed for clinical analysis but today they find many applications in food quality control. Immunodiffusion and newer techniques such as the various forms of enzyme-linked immunosorbent assay (ELISA) and radioimmunoassay (RIA) are the techniques most widely used in food analysis. *See* Immunoassays, Radioimmunoassay and Enzyme Immunoassay

Speciation of Meat and Meat Products.

The speciation of fresh, unheated frozen or mildly cooked meat is carried out by immunodiffusion and ELISA tests. Immunodiffusion procedures are used as screening techniques because they are influenced by the antigen content which varies from sample to sample. ELISA tests are more suitable for quantification.

Identification of thoroughly cooked meat species involves tedious steps for both sample (extraction and protein recovery) and sera preparation. Double-diffusion techniques are capable of detecting 5–10% meat species in cooked beef sausages by employing antigens resistant to thermal denaturation (e.g. adrenal antigens). Recently, multiple species-specific thermostable antigens have been used to detect various species with ELISA systems. In these cases, cross-reactivity has been reported for very closely related systems (beef/lamb and turkey/chicken). Combinations of immunoassays and electrofocusing in order to increase sensitivity have also been used to solve similar problems.

Detection of 'Foreign' Protein in Food Products. Soya protein in various forms – milk, meal and texturized – is added illegally to dairy and meat products to increase the total protein to a predetermined or a standard level. An array of different immunochemical precipitation techniques has been applied to the detection of soya protein in food products. The main limitation for all the techniques is that the immunoreactivity of soya antigens is influenced by the soya variety and the types of thermal process, which, in practice, are unknown. Such techniques are suitable for screening. ELISA techniques are preferred for quantification whereas RIA techniques, which offer equally accurate results to the former, are expensive for routine use. Indirect haemagglutination and immunoelectrophoresis, though more sensitive and specific, are laborious and expensive procedures and require trained personnel.

Other Applications. Gliadin, the ethanol-soluble fraction of gluten, can be routinely determined by ELISA tests but some precautions have to be taken to eliminate the problem of nonspecific binding. These tests are valuable for monitoring the legal limit of cereal proteins, added to foods for economic or technological reasons or to ensure the absence of gluten in gluten-free products.

Substitution of barley wort for maize or rice as a cheaper source of starch in beer manufacturing is determined by double diffusion and immunoenzyme assays. This replacement is illegal in some countries.

Other Methods

Isotope Ratios

The isotopic composition of various constituents has been used since the late 1970s as a means of determining the authenticity of foods of plant origin. Stable isotope ratio analysis (SIRA) and ^{14}C activity analysis are the most used techniques.

Stable Isotope Ratio Analysis

Photosynthesis initiates isotopic fractionation of ^{13}C and ^{12}C. Most plants cultivated for food fix carbon dioxide by Calvin synthesis (or the C_3 photosynthetic mode). Exceptions to this rule are sugar cane and corn which follow the Hatch–Slack (C_4) pathway. C_4 plant material is more abundant in ^{13}C and thus $^{13}C/^{12}C$ ratios are higher than in C_3 plants. Therefore, the $^{13}C/^{12}C$ ratios are used to detect the low-cost sugar cane and high-fructose corn syrups (HFCS) in valuable natural products such as honey, apple juice and orange juice. No other analysis could identify the above adulterants in these products. The AOAC has adopted a method for honey which involves complete burning of a sample to carbon dioxide and water, purification of carbon dioxide and measurement of the $^{13}C/^{12}C$ ratio in an isotope ratio mass spectrometer.

A very important application of the $^{13}C/^{12}C$ ratio is the detection of synthetic vanillin in vanilla extract. Vanilla plants follow an intermediate biosynthetic path compared to C_3 and C_4 modes and the extracts have very characteristic $^{13}C/^{12}C$ ratio limits. In this way, natural vanillin can easily be differentiated from its synthetic counterpart.

Another very important application is the discrimination between natural citrus juices and reconstituted ones. Plant water compared to ground- or rainwater is richer in ^{18}O and ^2H due to isotopic fractionation during evapotranspiration.

^{14}C Activity Measurement

The use of ^{14}C analysis in the food industry for determining the origin of ethanol in wines and other fermented beverages dates back to 1952. Since then, ^{14}C activity measurement has been extended to other natural products, e.g. spices and flavours. Atmospheric carbon dioxide through photosynthesis provides plants with the unstable isotope ^{14}C. The age of a certain plant or plant material is approximated from the measurement of its ^{14}C content. Hence, inexpensive artificial flavourings from petrochemicals, materials free of ^{14}C activity, are easily detected. However, the method fails in detecting substances chemically synthesized from natural sources.

The technique is also used in the USA to check the purity of champagne from artificially carbonated drinks. In a similar way, the vintage of a wine can be effectively determined because the ^{14}C activity of agricultural products has been well documented for the last 4 decades.

Bibliography

AOAC (1984) In: Williams S (ed.) *Official Methods of Analysis*, 14th edn. Arlington: Association of Official Analytical Chemists.

Baltes W (ed.) (1987) *Schnellmethoden zur Beurteilung von Lebensmitteln und ihren Rohrstoffen.* Hamburg: B. Behrs.

Egan H, Kirk RS and Sawer R (eds) (1981) *Pearson's Chemical Analysis of Foods*, 8th edn. Edinburgh: Churchill Livingstone.

FAO (1986) *Food Analysis: Quality, Adulteration and Tests of Identity. Manuals of Food Quality*, No. 8. Rome: Food and Agriculture Organization.

Gordon MH (ed.) (1990) *Principles and applications of Gas Chromatography*. Chichester: Ellis Horwood.

Hummel-Liljegren H (ed.) (1990) *Lebensmittelrechts-Handbuch.* Munchen: C. H. Beck's Verlagsbuchhandlung.

King RD (ed.) (1980) *Development in Food Analysis Techniques*, vols 1–3. London: Elsevier.

Macrae R (ed.) (1988) *HPLC in Food Analysis*, 2nd edn. London: Academic Press.

Piggot JR (ed.) (1986) *Statistical Procedures in Food Research*. London: Elsevier.

Pomeranz Y and Meloan CE (1982) *Food Analysis – Theory and Practice*, revised edn. Westport, CT: AVI.

Maria Tsimidou and Dimitrios Boskou
Aristotle University of Thessaloniki, Thessaloniki, Greece

AERATION AND FOAMING

Nature of Foam Formation

There is a wide variety of aerated foodstuffs; some of them belong to foamy systems, others belong to spongy systems or even felty systems, not to speak of powders which from a fundamental point of view also belong to air-containing systems. With the exception of powders and felty systems, the other systems often pass through a foamy state during their production. For example, in baking bread, which has a spongy structure, the rising dough has a foamy structure. With respect to foaming and aeration the following definitions can be given:

(1) Foaming: foaming is the process of making a foam. A foam is a dispersion of gas bubbles in a condensed, solid or liquid, phase. In a foam the condensed phase is the continuous phase whereas the gas is the discontinuous phase.
(2) Aeration: aeration is the process of making an aerated system. An aerated system is a system that consists of a gas phase and a condensed phase (solid or liquid). In an aerated system both phases (gas and condensed phases) can be continuous.

Foam Formation

In general, some form of mechanical agitation is needed to make a foam. The mechanical agitation serves two purposes: (1) the introduction of gas into the liquid and (2) the reduction of the bubble size. Other techniques by which bubbles can be formed are bubble formation in a liquid (water) oversaturated with carbon dioxide (beer) or allowing bubbles to be formed on a porous plate by means of gas injection. Formation of aerated systems having a spongy structure, as in bread making, initially requires the production of a foam. Due to collapse of the thin films between the bubbles this foam passes over to a spongy structure. To prevent collapse of this sponge, the remaining parts of the spongy structure (the Plateau borders, see below) must be stiff enough to keep the whole system upright.

Role of Surface Active Agents in Foam Formation and Stability

It is a matter of general experience that a stable foam can only be produced when surface active components are present. The essential property of these components is that they lower the surface tension of water. (The same reasoning is valid for oil, but because most of the interesting aerated foodstuffs are made from aqueous solutions, only aqueous systems are discussed in this article.) Surface active agents in foodstuffs like proteins, fatty acids, monoglycerides, lecithin, phospholipids and others lower the surface tension of water at room temperature from 72 mN m^{-1} to about half this value. *See* Stabilizers, Types and Function

Apart from the lowering in surface tension, an important contribution of surface active compounds to the stability of foam is caused by the fact that surface active agents are able to create a surface tension gradient along the surface of the liquid. This surface tension gradient gives the surface a certain amount of stiffness which has an important effect on the liquid flow in a foam, slowing down the liquid flow out of a foam considerably.

Another important property of surfactant solutions is that, especially during the mechanical agitation of foam making, the surfaces of the bubbles are not in equilibrium, which means that the surface tension may deviate considerably from the equilibrium value. Bubble surfaces may be expanded or compressed during agitation and, consequently, the dynamic surface tension can be considerably higher or lower than the equilibrium value.

When gas bubbles are formed in a liquid, for instance by allowing gas to flow through an orifice, the size of the bubbles escaping from the orifice is determined by the balance between the buoyancy force and surface tension force acting over the perimeter of the orifice. This means that a lower surface tension causes a smaller bubble. Since this process takes place at an expanding bubble, the dynamic surface tension during expansion of the surface comes into play.

Analogous reasoning can be used for bubble formation by means of a porous plate or behind a wire whip.

Reduction of Bubble Size by Mechanical Agitation

Bubbles can be broken up in a liquid by mechanical agitation when the hydrodynamic forces exerted by the liquid exceed the Laplace pressure in the bubble. The Laplace pressure of the gas in a bubble equals the overpressure Δp resulting from the surface tension of the bubble γ and the curvature of the bubble surface $1/r$ according to

$$\Delta p = \frac{2\gamma}{r}, \tag{1}$$

where r is the bubble radius.

Hydrodynamic forces can originate from shear flow, elongational flow or from turbulence. In the case of shear flow the hydrodynamic stress acting on the bubble is proportional to the viscosity of the liquid η and the velocity gradient perpendicular to the direction of the flow dV_x/dz. As long as this shear stress is larger than the Laplace pressure the bubble will be broken up into smaller ones. The ultimate bubble size that can be reached is given by the relation

$$r = \frac{2\gamma}{dV_x/dz\ \eta}. \qquad (2)$$

In the case of elongational flow the bubble is stretched in one direction by the velocity gradient acting in the same direction as the liquid flow dV_x/dx. This kind of flow is, for instance, present when a liquid is forced through a small orifice or slit. The elongational stress exerted on a bubble is proportional to the elongational velocity gradient and the elongational viscosity η_E, which, for a Newtonian liquid, equals three times the shear viscosity. Consequently, by applying elongational flow the ultimate bubble size that can be obtained is given by the relation

$$r = \frac{2\gamma}{dV_x/dx\ \eta_E} = \frac{\gamma}{3\ dV_x/dx\ \eta}. \qquad (3)$$

Practical experience suggests that in general it is easier to get smaller bubbles by applying elongational flow than by shear flow. In the case of turbulent flow, inertia forces become predominant which cause pressure fluctuations Δp leading to break up of the bubbles when they exceed the Laplace pressure. Pressure fluctuations originating from velocity fluctuations ΔV obey Bernoulli's law: $\Delta p = \frac{1}{2}\rho(\Delta V)^2$. Therefore, the ultimate bubble size which can be obtained by this mechanism is given by

$$r = \frac{4\gamma}{\rho(\Delta V)^2}. \qquad (4)$$

Applying this to the whipping of cream by using a wire whip moving with a velocity of $1\ \text{m s}^{-1}$, the resulting bubble size is about 0.1 mm, which is of the right order of magnitude ($\gamma = 40 \times 10^{-3}\ \text{N m}^{-1}$, $\rho = 10^3\ \text{kg m}^{-3}$).

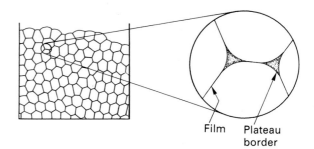

Fig. 1   Honey-comb like structure of a foam consisting of thin liquid films which meet each other in a plateau border under an angle of 120°.

Foam Stability

When a foam is made, three physical mechanisms can be distinguished which can contribute to the foam stability: drainage, coalescence and disproportion.

Drainage

Drainage is the flow of liquid out of a foam. Such a foam is built up by thin liquid films between the bubbles and Plateau borders, which are situated at the meeting point of three liquid films (Fig. 1). In a freshly made foam, liquid is flowing out of the thin films as a result of the force of gravity. This process proceeds in such a way that the film surfaces are almost motionless during the liquid flow. This is because the surface active agents present to stabilize the film generate a surface tension gradient along the film which keeps the surfaces motionless. This means that the amount of liquid flowing out of the film is small, especially when the film becomes thinner, because

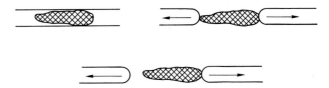

Fig. 2   Breaking of a thin aqueous film caused by the presence of a hydrophobic particle.

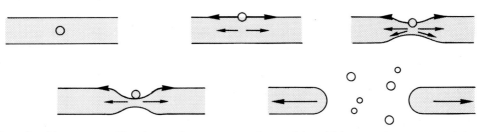

Fig. 3   Breaking of a thin aqueous film due to the presence of a particle which spreads over one of the film surfaces.

the flow rate is inversely proportional to the cube of the film thickness according to

$$Q = \frac{2}{3}\frac{\rho g}{\eta}d^3, \qquad (5)$$

where Q is the volume of liquid that flows out of the film per unit time (s) and per unit width of the film, g is the force of gravity and d is the film thickness.

The drainage of liquid out of the Plateau border continues until the curvature (the inverse of the radius of curvature) becomes so high that capillary suction compensates hydrostatic pressure according to

$$\rho g H = \frac{\gamma}{R} \qquad (6)$$

where H is the hydrostatic height of the Plateau border with respect to the liquid and R is the radius of curvature of the Plateau border. It may be expected that in most practical systems the drainage of liquid out of the Plateau borders also takes place when the surfaces are motionless.

Coalescence

When film drainage proceeds far enough, this process may slow down or even stop due to repulsive forces acting between the two approaching film surfaces. The reader is referred to a textbook on colloid chemistry for further details.

In practical systems, especially foodstuffs, it is often observed that before the film reaches its equilibrium thickness the film collapses, resulting in the coalescence of bubbles. Because these systems contain particles of various kinds such as emulsion droplets, crystals, fibres, cells and so on, it is to be expected that they play a role in the destabilization of thin films. Two mechanisms can be distinguished here: hydrophobic particles and spreading particles.

Hydrophobic Particles

When a hydrophobic particle makes contact with both surfaces of an aqueous film, due to a convex curvature of the film surface the film liquid flows away from the particle (Fig. 2). When the hydrophobicity is large enough (contact angle large enough) this results in collapse of the film.

Spreading Particles

When a particle is present in the film that is able to spread over the film surface, when it makes contact with one of the surfaces, the film may collapse. This is caused by the movement of the film surface away from the spreading particle. Due to this movement of the surface the film liquid also is squeezed away from the spreading particle (Fig. 3). When this process proceeds far enough the film becomes so thin that it collapses spontaneously.

Disproportionation

Disproportionation of gas bubbles is the growth of bigger bubbles at the expense of smaller ones. The driving force of this process is the higher gas pressure in the smaller bubbles according to Laplace's law. This causes a higher solubility of the gas in the liquid in the neighbourhood of the smaller bubbles. By means of diffusion the gas is transported to the bigger bubbles.

This process is in principle a self-accelerating process because when the smaller bubbles become smaller and smaller the driving force increases, leading to the implosion of those bubbles. In this way the number of bubbles decreases without breaking one film. The ultimate result of this process is a coarsening of the foam.

The rate of disproportionation increases with the solubility of the gas in the liquid. Because carbon dioxide is quite soluble in water, this process is one of the main causes of the foam instability of carbonated beverages such as beer.

Disproportionation, being a dynamic process, is very sensitive to dynamic surface properties. The surface of a disappearing bubble is continuously compressed which, when surface active compounds are present, causes a lowering of the surface tension and consequently a slowing down of the process. Under certain conditions the process of disproportionation can even be stopped.

Types of Aerated Foodstuffs

In aerated foodstuffs a distinction can be made between gas-discontinuous and gas-continuous systems. Foam is a gas-discontinuous system and whipped cream, whipped egg white and bread dough during rise are a few examples. Beer foam also belongs to this category but is an example of a creamed system as a result of the low viscosity of the continuous phase. In the other systems mentioned the rigidity of the whole system prevents creaming of the bubbles. Gas-continuous systems include sponges and other systems such as felty systems and powders. Sponges are usually made out of a foam: most bakery products such as bread and cake pass through a foamy state during their production. Sponges derive their typical structure from the foamy state in which the thin films between the bubbles are broken. These systems are only stable when the matrix is adequately stiff. An example of a felty system is a sugar spin consisting of thin threads of sugar which enclose a lot of air. *See* Bread, Breadmaking Processes; Cakes, Methods of Manufacture

Equipment Employed

Open or closed systems can be used for the production of aerated foodstuffs. Open systems operate in such a way that, in principle, the amount of gas (air) is infinite. Examples of this are a dough kneader, an open bowl for whipping cream or egg white and a high-speed pin stirrer such as an Ultra Turrax. Essential in this way of foam making is that both liquid and foam are subjected to the mechanical treatment of the moving parts of the equipment. The disadvantage of this method is that, in an attempt to make more foam and/or smaller bubbles by increasing the mechanical agitation, the result can be just the opposite. This is because mechanical agitation causes the break down of the thin films between the bubbles. So by increasing the mechanical agitation the amount of foam produced passes a maximum value whereas the bubble size passes a minimum value. The general characteristic of a closed system is that the gas/liquid volume ratio can be chosen at will by the setting of the apparatus. A further essential feature of a closed system is that the foam can be made under a pressure that is higher than 1 atm. This makes the foam less prone to the destabilizing action of the mechanical agitation. The required mechanical agitation in these apparatus can be achieved by means of a static mixer through which both phases are forced or by a rotating mixer such as a pin stirrer. Aerated foodstuffs can also be made by means of an extruder. In this apparatus the moist foodstuff is heated above 100 °C and kept under high pressure by means of a rotating screw. At the outlet of the apparatus the pressure drops suddenly to 1 atm and the resulting boiling of the water causes puffing of the foodstuff. A related process for producing foam is the expansion of a liquid which is oversaturated with a gas. Beer, fruit juices, soft drinks, sparkling wine and champagne are examples in which carbon dioxide is used. For the production of instant whipped cream, nitrous oxide is used because it has about the same solubility as carbon dioxide and is tasteless. *See* Extrusion Cooking, Principles and Practice

In all these cases the bubbles are formed by means of heterogeneous nucleation. The hydrodynamic conditions at the nucleation site, the dynamic surface properties of the liquid and the size and wetting behaviour of the nucleus determine, to a large extent, the size of the bubbles that are formed. The amount of foam is determined by the degree of oversaturation of the liquid.

Carbon dioxide can also be produced in foodstuffs by means of yeast (bread, champagne) or by baking powder (cakes), which produces this gas at higher temperatures.

Foam Control

For foam control it is essential that a given foam can be characterized in a quantitative way. Important physical parameters that characterize a foam are the bubble size distribution, the overrun and the foam stiffness. The bubble size distribution gives the number of bubbles present within a certain class width of bubble sizes per unit volume of the foam. This parameter can be measured by means of a newly developed glass fibre technique which measures the bubble size distribution of bubbles larger than 25 μm within a time of 1 min. From the bubble size distribution, various average bubble sizes can be calculated. Also, the overrun can be calculated, which is the ratio expressed as a percentage of the total volume of gas taken up in a foam and the volume of liquid in the foam. The overrun can also be measured in a simple way by weighing a known volume of foam. By measuring the bubble size distribution as a function of time, information can be obtained about the rate of drainage, coalescence and disproportionation. Information about coalescence and disproportionation can be obtained by using gases of different solubility in water: nitrogen, carbon dioxide or nitrous oxide. Information on these processes can also be obtained from the change in the bubble size distribution because, due to coalescence, the size distribution shifts only to larger sizes, whereas, as a result of disproportionation, the size distribution shifts to smaller sizes.

When the overrun of the foam is high enough, the foam has a certain yield value: it needs a certain minimum shear stress before it starts to flow. In this way, foam demonstrates a certain amount of stiffness which can be measured by using a couette-type apparatus. In using this technique, care must be taken that no slip of the foam along the walls of the cylinders takes place. Slip can be prevented by making the walls of the cylinders out of wire netting having a mesh size which matches the bubble size.

Hygiene

Foodstuffs have to be aerated under hygienic conditions. During production, contamination has to be prevented and after production the apparatus must be throughly cleaned.

Assuming that the product itself has been adequately decontaminated (time, temperature and heat exchanger configuration correct), important sources of contamination during aeration of foodstuffs may be the air as well as the equipment, in particular where there are moving parts (rotating and reciprocating shafts) and where there are dead ends and incorrectly designed seals.

A brief overview will be given of the main sources of contamination and how to ensure that aeration of foodstuffs is performed under hygienic conditions.

Air

Air usually contains between 500 and 10 000 viable microorganisms per cubic metre; hence, without a proper decontamination treatment, the air may recontaminate the product. It is relatively easy to reduce the number of microorganisms to an acceptably low level. HEPA (high-efficiency particulate air) filters reduce the number of particles of 0·3 μm diameter in air by a factor $\geq 3 \times 10^3$. In practice this means that microorganisms are retained by at least the same factor or better (many microorganisms are larger as they are often associated with larger dust particles). It is important that the filters are dry, as otherwise microorganisms may grow through filters. Self-evidently, it must be possible to free the filters from microorganisms. This may be done by either steam or by gaseous sterilants. The recommendations of the filter manufacturer should be followed.

Continuous Heat Treatment

The best way to ensure hygienic conditions during aeration of foodstuffs is to perform the operation at a high temperature. It may be helpful to combine the high temperature with a high pressure to improve the whipping behaviour of the foodstuff.

Temperature and Time

In order to control the above-mentioned process, the temperature and the holding time must be measured in a correct way. For the temperature measurement the thermometer must be present in the product stream as indicated in Fig. 4(a) and not in a dead leg as in Fig. 4(b), because in this case there is too much heat exchange with the surroundings. For the measurement of the holding time the pressure drop over the holding section can be used to indicate that, due to fouling or other causes, the flow rate is increased and consequently the holding time is decreased.

Flow Diversion

Flow diversion (see Fig. 5) is often applied in an aeration line. This arrangement facilitates the starting up of the process. Also in this case the diversion valve must be free from dead spaces. Figure 6(a) is an example of unsafe construction and Fig. 6(b) an example of a correct one.

Cleaning

Microorganisms in soil may have a water activity smaller than unity, reducing the effectivity of deconta-

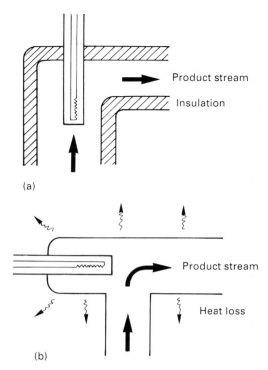

Fig. 4 Correct (a) and incorrect (b) methods of mounting a temperature probe in a process line.

mination with hot water or steam. In addition, soil residues will hamper heat transfer and in the case of chemical treatments may hamper the contact between microorganisms and chemicals. *See* Cleaning Procedures in the Factory, Types of Detergent, Cleaning Procedures in the Factory, Types of Disinfectant, Cleaning Procedures in the Factory, Overall Approach, Cleaning Procedures in the Factory, Modern Systems

Decontamination

Decontamination can be carried out with steam, hot water or a (hot or cold) aqueous chemical solution. To ensure a proper decontamination with hot water or steam the water activity must be unity. This means that no air or other gas must be entrapped in the equipment and that the temperature of the cleaning agent must not drop locally.

Especially when dead legs are present in the equipment, decontamination may be insufficient. When the dead leg is pointing upwards, hot water or a chemical solution may not contact the whole surface of the leg due to entrapped air (gas) (see Fig. 7). In addition, heat loss from the dead leg may cause too low a temperature. When the dead leg is pointing downwards, heat loss may cause condensation when steam is used. When hot water is used the temperature may be too low due to heat loss (see Fig. 8).

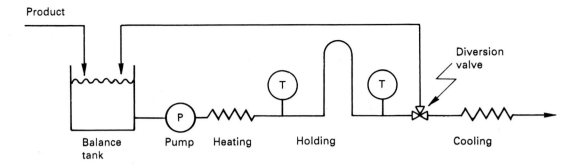

Fig. 5   Process line for heating and cooling of a liquid foodstuff provided with flow diversion.

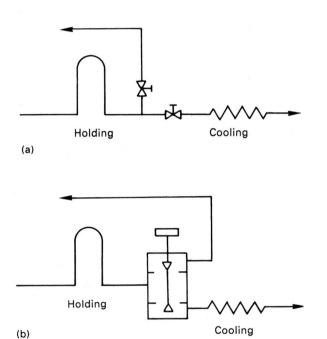

Fig. 6   Unsafe (a) and safe (b) constructions of a diversion valve. In (a) insufficient heated product may be trapped in the dead leg to the valve giving entry to the cooling section.

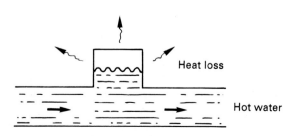

Fig. 7   Adverse effect of dead leg pointing upwards on decontamination of a process line, resulting in too low temperature and water activity.

Seals

Static Seals

When rubber O rings are used it should be remembered that the thermal expansion coefficient of rubber is about 20 times higher than that of steel. By heating the equipment the rubber O ring will cover an increasingly larger surface (see Fig. 9), protecting microorganisms from contact with steam or hot water. After cooling the equipment the survivors will be freed and infect the product.

If polytetrafluoroethylene or similar insufficiently resilient compounds are used for gaskets, after heating and cooling leaks are likely to occur (see Fig. 10). These leaks may be large enough to allow the passage of microorganisms but not large enough to cause leakage of the product.

The same is true when metal-to-metal couplings are

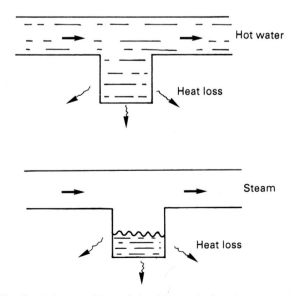

Fig. 8   Adverse effect of dead leg pointing downwards on decontamination of a process line with hot water or steam, resulting in too low temperature.

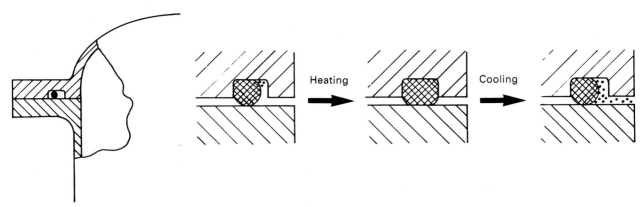

Fig. 9   Rubber O rings may protect microorganisms against contact with hot water or steam as a result of the difference in thermal expansion between rubber and steel.

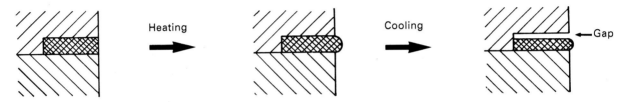

Fig. 10   Effect of heating and cooling on sealing with polytetrafluoroethylene. Due to lack in resilience a gap is formed after cooling of the system.

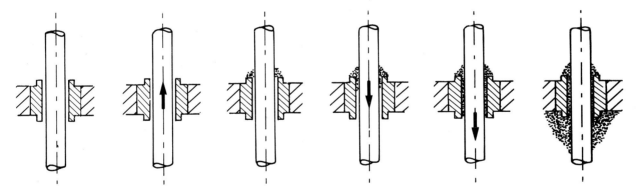

Fig. 11   Penetration of microorganisms through the seal of a reciprocating shaft.

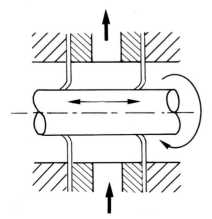

Fig. 12   Double-shaft seal. The vertical solid arrow indicates the flow of bacteriocidal agent.

used. Upon assembly for the first time tightening of the seal is accompanied by damage to the contact surfaces. After disconnection and reassembling, the damage may cause leakage, allowing ingress of microorganisms.

Dynamic Seals

Shaft passages will allow ingress of microorganisms, especially during axial movements (see Fig. 11). It should be realized that rotating shafts always exhibit some axial mobility and hence assist penetration by microorganisms. This problem can be solved by using a double-shaft seal (see Fig. 12) where a liquid – bacteriocidal or not – is used to flush the space between the seals.

In the case of shafts that just reciprocate, diaphragm

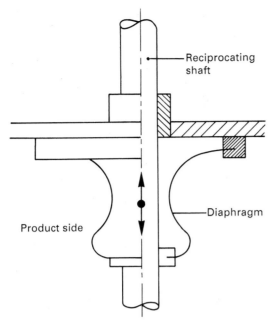

Fig. 13 Example of a diaphragm seal for a reciprocating shaft moving over a small distance.

seals may be more efficient than double-shaft seals (Fig. 13).

Corrosion

Hidden microbial leaks may occur as a result of corrosion. Corrosion may be initiated by mechanical damage of the chromium dioxide surface of the stainless steel. Once damaged, chloride ions will attack the steel underneath. Chloride ions may originate from the product itself, cleaning agents, sanitizer, water, insulation, gasket cements or refrigeration liquids. The result will be pitting and, eventually, microscopic leaks, allowing infection of the product by microorganisms. The chromium dioxide layer can be restored by a treatment with diluted nitric acid. **See** Corrosion Chemistry

Another cause of corrosion is incorrect welding. Proper welding of stainless steel requires that the connecting materials, such as pipes and welding rod, are of the same composition. In addition, welding has to be performed under a blanket of inert gas (argon). When these precautions are disregarded, corrosion may occur at those places where the foodstuff or other liquids make contact with the welded part of the production line.

Bibliography

Lelieveld HLM (1990) Processing equipment and hygienic design. *Microbiological and Environmental Health Issues Relevant to the Food and Catering Industries. Symposium Proceedings, Campden Food & Drink Research Association, Chipping Campden, 6–8 February*, p. 1–8.

Lucassen J (1981) Dynamic properties of free liquid films and foams. In: Lucassen Reynders ER (ed.) *Anionic Surfactants, Physical Chemistry of Surfactant Action*, chap. 6. *Surfactant Science Series*, vol 11. New York: Marcel Dekker.

Lucassen Reynders ER (1981) Surface elasticity and viscosity in compression and dilatation. In: Lucassen Reynders ER (ed.) *Anionic Surfactants, Physical Chemistry of Surfactant Action*, chap. 5. *Surfactant Science Series*, vol 11. New York: Marcel Dekker.

Prins A (1976) Dynamic surface properties band foaming behaviour of aqueous surfactant solutions. In: Akers RJ (ed.) *Foams*, pp. 51–60. London: Academic Press.

Prins A (1988) Principles of foam stability. In: Dickinson E and Stainsby G (eds) *Advances in Food Emulsions and Foams*, pp. 91–122. London: Elsevier.

Prins A (1989) Foam stability as affected by the presence of small spreading particles. In: Mittal KL (ed.) *Surfactants in Solution*, pp. 361–380. New York: Plenum Press.

Ronteltap AD and Prins A (1989) Contribution of drainage, coalescence and disproportionation to the stability of aerated foodstuffs and the consequences for the bubble-size distribution as measured by a newly developed optical glass-fibre technique. In: Bee RD, Richmond P and Mingins J (eds) *Food Colloids*, pp. 39–47. *Special Publication*, N. 75. London: Royal Society of Chemistry.

Ronteltap AD and Prins A (1990) The role of surface viscosity in gas diffusion in aqueous foams, II Experimental. *Colloids and Surfaces* 47: 285–298.

Ronteltap AD, Damsté BR, Gee M de and Prins A (1990) The role of surface viscosity in gas diffusion in aqueous foams, I Theoretical. *Colloids and Surfaces* 47: 269–283.

A. Prins
Agricultural University, Wageningen, The Netherlands

AEROMONAS

The genus *Aeromonas* belongs to the bacterial family Vibrionaceae and it has been suggested that this genus should be considered to contain some bacterial pathogens for humans, which may cause food poisoning. Other closely related genera within the family are *Vibrio* and *Plesiomonas* species. Both *Pl. shigelloides* and some *Vibrio* species are known to cause human gastroenteritis. With *Aeromonas* species, however, this pathogenic ability is not yet proven. These bacteria have traditionally been considered to be waterborne, although they may be isolated from a wide range of environments. *See* Vibrios, *Vibrio Cholerae*; Vibrios, *Vibrio Parahaemolyticus*; Vibrios, *Vibrio Vulnificus*

Aeromonas Species

Historically, the taxonomy of this genus has been confused, but the genus may be divided into two main groups. The first is the nonmotile species *A. salmonicida*. This microorganism is a pathogen for many species of fish and particularly the salmonids, but is not considered to be of significance in food safety or spoilage. Therefore, this species will not be considered further. The second group is the motile species of which the best known are *A. hydrophila*, *A. sobria* and *A. caviae*. Less well-recognized species include *A. veronii* and *A. schubertii*. It is claimed that all five species may cause human gastroenteritis. Much of the published literature on *Aeromonas* has not distinguished the motile species or has used out-of-date nomenclature. Consequently, the name *A. hydrophila* will be used as a general name for the motile species in this article. The name is derived from Greek, i.e. *Aeromonas* (a gas-producing unit), *hydrophila* (water-loving). Individual species may be distinguished by simple biochemical tests.

A. hydrophila as a Pathogen?

The significance of *A. hydrophila* as a direct cause of human gastroenteritis is a matter of debate. Although recognized as an opportunistic pathogen, it is only since the 1980s that there has been increased attention to its clinical significance in healthy individuals. To date (1990) there has been no fully confirmed outbreak of food poisoning caused by this bacterium.

Many studies have found that the incidence of *A. hydrophila* in diarrhoeal stools is significantly greater than in those from control groups (e.g. 10·6% positive compared with 0·6%, respectively), and it may often be obtained in high numbers. These observations are most pronounced in infants and young children. The presence of a bacterium in a diarrhoeal stool, however, does not confirm its role as the causative agent of the syndrome. Other pathogens (including bacteria, viruses or parasites) may initiate disease and alter the gut environment, and only then may *A. hydrophila* become prominent in the bacterial faecal flora. Much clinical data are of limited use as, in many cases, *A. hydrophila* was not looked for specifically, whilst, in other incidents, the presence of other pathogens could not be ruled out. The confusion in taxonomy and methodology for *A. hydrophila* may also have impaired the abilities of clinical microbiologists to isolate this bacterium from stool samples.

Many strains of *A. hydrophila* possess a wide range of potential virulence factors (i.e. strategies which may aid pathogenicity). These include the production of cytotonic and cytotoxic enterotoxins (which lead to fluid secretion in the gut), haemolysins (which attack cell membranes), haemagglutinin (which aid attachment to the gut) and protease enzymes (which cause tissue damage and enhance invasion). Similar virulence factors are present in many recognized foodborne bacterial pathogens. The virulence factors of *A. hydrophila* produce typical responses in both *in vitro* and *in vivo* model systems for pathogenicity. Human feeding studies with *A. hydrophila*, however, have been inconclusive, with only two of 57 volunteers getting diarrhoea after consuming high levels of enterotoxin-producing strains. The validity of this study has been challenged as the strains used may not have possessed all the other virulence factors necessary for gut colonization and so disease.

Consequently, in spite of the abundance of circumstantial evidence for pathogenicity, the case to include *A. hydrophila* as a foodborne pathogen resulting in gastroenteritis has not been conclusively proven.

Symptoms

Human infection with *A. hydrophila* may produce a wide range of localized and systemic illnesses. The symptoms are dependent on the bacterium, host, inoculum size and infection site. All the motile *Aeromonas* species have been implicated in human illness and it is likely that *A. sobria* and *A. caviae* have been mistakenly reported as *A. hydrophila* in the past.

The most common type of infection involves the

gastrointestinal tract and this is the illness of most concern to the food industry. Gastroenteritis may occur at all ages and in both sexes, although it is most commonly reported in young children. Symptoms are generally more pronounced in the very young, elderly and immunocompromised. The most common symptom is an acute profusely watery diarrhoea which may last for several days. Other associated symptoms include fever and vomiting. Generally, the disease is self-limiting and symptoms subside within 1 week. In a few cases, the disease may persist for more than 10 days and is classified as chronic. This results in weight loss and may require hospitalization. Chronic disease may last for several months. A second manifestation of gastroenteritis is a 'dysentery-like' illness characterized by diarrhoea containing blood and/or mucus and cramping abdominal pain. Hospitalization and antimicrobial therapy are often required. More rarely, a 'cholera-like' illness may occur when the diarrhoeal stool is turbid and contains white grains ('rice water stools'). This results in rapid and extensive dehydration, usually requiring hospitalization and aggressive antimicrobial therapy.

Other types of *A. hydrophila* illness include wound infection, septicaemia and localized infections. Wound infections are most common after traumatic injury and in many cases the injury has been associated with water or soil. Infection is most common in the hands, arms and legs. In most cases with healthy adults, the infection remains localized but, in the immunocompromised, it may become more serious and result in amputation, septicaemia or even death. Septicaemia and the infection of a variety of bodily sites occur most commonly, but not exclusively, with immuncompromised individuals. The symptoms of *A. hydrophila* septicaemia are similar to those produced by other Gram-negative bacterial pathogens and the mortality level in the immunocompromised is approximately 50%. Both septicaemia and localized infections generally require antibiotic therapy and often hospitalization.

Incidents of Foodborne Disease

Although there has not yet been a fully confirmed outbreak of *A. hydrophila* gastroenteritis, a number of suspected incidents have been reported. Three outbreaks affecting between three and 472 individuals have implicated oysters as the vector of transmission. Levels of the bacterium isolated ranged from 9 per 100 g to 2×10^4 per gram of food, although in the former case the value obtained was after frozen storage for 1 year.

Cooked prawns have been implicated in three small incidents (1–20 cases) in the UK. Levels obtained in one outbreak were approximately 5×10^6 cells of *A. hydrophila* per gram of food. The consumption of edible land snails in Nigeria, containing a level of 1×10^9 cells of *A.*

hydrophila per gram of food, resulted in a suspected incident of gastroenteritis. Several incidents implicating both treated and untreated water have also been reported.

A number of the incidents involving *A. hydrophila* cannot be fully confirmed as the faeces of individuals were not specifically tested for this bacterium. Confirmed outbreaks are more likely to be reported with the increased awareness of this bacterium. *See* Food Poisoning, Tracing Origins and Testing

Ecology

A. hydrophila may be isolated from a wide range of environmental sources, but has traditionally been considered to be an aquatic bacterium. It has been isolated from fresh waters, estuaries, coastal waters and, occasionally, open ocean waters. The incidence, numbers present and survival of the bacterium are affected by the pH, temperature, salt content and dissolved oxygen in the water. In the USA, levels up to 3600 cells of *A. hydrophila* per millilitre of water have been reported. Furthermore, *A. hydrophila* may be isolated (at low levels) from chlorinated and unchlorinated potable water supplies. A statistical relationship between *A. hydrophila* in water supplies and health risks has been suggested, but there is no firm evidence of serious health effects to humans after exposure to such drinking water. The presence of *A. hydrophila* in potable water supplies may be of concern to food-processing operations, as it may lead to product and/or equipment contamination. Adequate chlorination of the water will ensure destruction of the bacterium.

The presence of *A. hydrophila* in water undoubtedly contributes to its common occurrence in fish and seafood. The bacterium is a common component of the intestinal microflora of healthy fish. It is likely that poor processing techniques and poor hygienic practices may result in the contamination of fish flesh and seafood products. *See* Fish, Spoilage; Shellfish, Contamination and Spoilage of Molluscs and Crustacea

In addition to fish, *A. hydrophila* may be obtained from the faeces of a large range of both wild and domestic animals. In these studies the animals were considered to be healthy. As with fish, poor processing techniques and poor hygienic practices during slaughter, butchery, dressing and processing of meat and poultry products may contribute to the incidence of this bacterium in raw flesh foods. *See* Poultry, Chicken; Poultry, Ducks and Geese; Poultry, Turkey

A. hydrophila is not considered to be a normal inhabitant of the microbial flora of the human gut and its presence is usually transient. The faecal carriage rate for healthy individuals is usually 0–5%. Although asymptomatic carriers could serve as vectors for

Table 1. Incidence of motile *Aeromonas* in foods

Food type	Samples positive (%)
Seafood (including shellfish)	53–100
Poultry (raw)	69–98
Offal	84
Red meats (raw)	25–60
Milk (raw)	20–50
Vegetables (raw)	5–40
Cooked meat products	5–35
Drinking water	28
Preprepared salads	21
Mayonnaise salads	10
Milk (pasteurized)	0–10

transmission of this bacterium (e.g. food handlers), no documented evidence of this is available.

As a consequence of this bacterium in human and animal faeces, *A. hydrophila* can be commonly isolated from sewage samples and drainage from animal lairages. These may also contribute to the incidence in water samples.

Occurrence in Foods

A. hydrophila may be isolated from a very wide range of foodstuffs (Table 1). It is not surprising that it is common in a wide range of seafood including fish (both wild and farmed), shrimps (raw and cooked), oysters, crabs and scallops. The bacterium is also common in raw meats and may be isolated from a high proportion (50–100%) of red meat and poultry samples. Cooked meats may occasionally contain *A. hydrophila*, indicating that postprocess contamination has occurred. In fresh (and cooked) meats and poultry this bacterium is generally present in low numbers (less than 100 per gram) but may greatly increase during storage at chill temperatures, particularly when vacuum or modified-atmosphere packaging is used. In the past, *A. hydrophila* has been considered as a spoilage bacterium in these foods. Up to 50% of raw milk samples may contain *A. hydrophila* and it has also been isolated from pasteurized milk, cream and some dairy products. The incidence in pasteurized products is much lower than in raw milk and represents postprocess contamination. A wide variety of vegetable products (including parsely, spinach, celery, alfalfa, beansprouts, broccoli, lettuce and root vegetables) may contain *A. hydrophila* and the incidence is usually between 5 and 40% of samples positive. *See* Dairy Products – Dietary Importance

In addition to the above foods, *A. hydrophila* has been isolated from up to 28% of drinking water samples and also from bottled mineral waters, although levels are low (less than 10 per millilitre).

Factors Affecting Growth

Of particular concern with the incidence of *A. hydrophila* in foods is the ability of the bacterium to grow at refrigeration temperatures. This bacterium may grow at temperatures as low as 0°C. Consequently, refrigerated storage alone cannot be relied upon to inhibit the growth of *A. hydrophila* completely. On occasions, high levels of the bacterium have been isolated from chilled foods which had been stored for prolonged periods. Reducing the storage temperature, however, will reduce the rate of growth of *A. hydrophila* and refrigeration may act in combination with other preservation factors to inhibit growth. The optimum and maximum temperatures for growth are 28–30 and 42°C, respectively.

A. hydrophila is not heat-resistant and has a decimal reduction time (D value) of between 2·2 and 6·6 min at 48°C. Consequently, this bacterium will be readily destroyed by processes such as milk pasteurization and frankfurter processing. It is important to ensure that heat processes are carefully controlled to ensure microbial destruction.

This bacterium is not a good competitor with many other bacteria present in raw foods, but may reach high levels if the competing bacterial flora has been removed by heating or its growth is retarded. For example, vacuum packaging may prevent the growth of the main spoilage bacteria of raw meats (i.e. *Pseudomonas* species), but *A. hydrophila* may continue to grow and even dominate the bacterial flora. The use of modified atmospheres containing 100% carbon dioxide will inhibit growth of *A. hydrophila*, but a small decrease in this level may permit growth. *See* Chilled Storage, Effect of Modified Atmosphere Packaging on Food Quality; Chilled Storage, Packaging Under Vacuum

A. hydrophila is not an acid-tolerant bacterium and at chill temperatures (less than 5°C) it will grow only poorly, if at all, at pH values less than 6·0. Therefore, growth would not be expected in even mildly acidic refrigerated products. At lower pH values, the bacterium will slowly die, although this may require in excess of 20 days. When stored at 30°C the minimum pH value for growth has been variously reported to be between 4·0 and 5·0. As with other bacteria, organic acids (e.g. acetic, lactic and citric acids) which occur in foods are more effective in inhibiting growth than are mineral acids (e.g. hydrochloric acid).

The maximum level of salt permitting growth depends on the other conditions, but is 6% (w/v) when other conditions are optimal. With refrigerated samples (less than 5°C), growth is poor when the salt concentration exceeds 2% (w/v).

Irradiation, at the doses proposed for foods (i.e. 10 kGy), would successfully eliminate *A. hydrophila* from foods. The decimal reduction value is reported as 0·14–0·22 kGy. *See* Irradiation of Foods, Basic Principles

Little is known about the effect of freezing on *A. hydrophila*, but this process cannot be relied upon to ensure the destruction of the bacterium and it has been isolated from a wide variety of frozen foods.

The presence of *A. hydrophila* in chlorinated water suggests that the bacterium is resistant to this biocide. Chlorination can be a very effective means of controlling *A. hydrophila*, but the levels used must be carefully controlled. Other disinfectants, including those commonly used in the food industry, may also be effectively used to control *A. hydrophila*.

Overall, *A. hydrophila* is not a hardy bacterium and is readily controlled by many of the processes used in the food industry. Care is needed to ensure that postprocess contamination is minimized.

Detection Methods

A. hydrophila is not difficult to grow and produces good growth on many laboratory media. A wide variety of methods are used for this bacterium. Most of the media used have been developed from those used for the detection of Enterobacteriaceae or *Vibrio* species. In the past, it is likely that *A. hydrophila* has been misidentified as an enteric bacterium and so its incidence and clinical significance will have been underestimated.

The bacterium may be isolated using quantitative or qualitative procedures. With quantitative methods, the sample is inoculated directly on a solid selective agar medium, or a statistical most probable number (MPN) technique is used. With qualitative methods, the sample is usually placed in a liquid selective enrichment medium (to allow multiplication of *A. hydrophila*) prior to inoculation of the agar medium. Incubation temperatures used for both liquid and solid media range between 25 and 37°C, although 30°C is being increasingly accepted.

The solid selective agar media which are most widely used for food samples are starch–ampicillin, selective bile salts–irgasan–brilliant green and Ryan's *Aeromonas* agar media. With liquid media, alkaline peptone water and ampicillin broths are most widely used. Both liquid and solid media containing ampicillin have been shown to be very useful, although a few strains are sensitive to this antibiotic.

It is likely that the use of multiple solid and/or liquid media will be required for optimal recovery of this bacterium. The individual motile *Aeromonas* species can be separated using conventional biochemical tests. Additional tests to further identify biotypes and serotypes are not widely used for food isolates.

Bibliography

Abeyta C and Wekell MM (1988) Potential sources of *Aeromonas hydrophila*. *Journal of Food Safety* 9: 11–22.

Cahill MM (1990) Virulence factors in motile *Aeromonas* species. *Journal of Applied Bacteriology* 69: 1–16.

Janda JM and Duffey PS (1988) Mesophilic aeromonads in human disease: current taxonomy, laboratory identification, and infectious disease spectrum. *Reviews of Infectious Diseases* 10: 980–997.

Joseph SW, Janda M and Carnahan A (1988) Isolation, enumeration and identification of *Aeromonas* sp. *Journal of Food Safety* 9: 23–35.

Palumbo SA and Buchanan RL (1988) Factors affecting growth or survival of *Aeromonas hydrophila* in foods. *Journal of Food Safety* 9: 37–51.

Stelma JR (1989) *Aeromonas hydrophila*. In: Doyle MP (ed.) *Foodborne Bacterial Pathogens*, pp. 1–19. New York: Marcel Dekker.

S. J. Walker
Campden Food and Drink Research Association, Chipping Campden, UK

AFLATOXINS

See Mycotoxins

AGEING – NUTRITIONAL ASPECTS

The aim of this article is to give a brief introduction to the field of ageing and to discuss the role of nutrition in modifying the rate of age-associated change.

Ageing

The accepted definition of ageing is as follows: that period of the lifespan characterized by a failure to maintain homeostasis under conditions of physiological stress; this failure is associated with a decrease in viability and an increase in vulnerability of the individual. Most of the recognizable features of ageing occur after the period of reproductive activity has ceased. It has been proposed that ageing changes should satisfy four criteria: universal in the species, degenerative, progressive and intrinsic. These prerequisites separate ageing from the other time-related changes of development, maturation and age-associated disease. Clearly, this 'definition' requires considerable refinement before it can be used to separate ageing from other age-associated events in the adult organism. We have only one certainty, which is that lifespan is defined by a specific end-point – death – which enables us to determine longevity with accuracy. Unfortunately, the terms 'lifespan' and 'ageing' are frequently used interchangeably, and this can be misleading.

Particular emphasis is placed upon the failure to maintain homeostasis because it is in the integration of complex physiological functions that the greatest age-associated changes are observed. A successful theory of ageing should be able to explain the decline in the functional ability of older organisms. It must therefore explain the cellular and molecular events that result in the breakdown of cellular function and subsequent physiological deterioration.

Mechanisms or Theories of Ageing

The ideas about how and why we age can be conveniently divided into two groups. The first concerns possible genetic mechanisms that could bring about ageing. The second group deal with a series of random events which could explain age effects (stochastic mechanisms).

The Evolution of Ageing

It has been argued that ageing is an adaptive mechanism for the removal of individuals after the reproductive stage of the life-span. The implication is that encoded in the genome is a special mechanism, the purpose of which is to terminate life. In this case, ageing is considered a step in a programmed sequence of events. The study of survival indicates that there are characteristic species-specific lifespans, and survival curves are more or less constant within species, but this does not necessarily mean that lifespan is an inherited character. Furthermore, survival data do not support the idea of programmed ageing; there is no sharp increase in deaths at any particular stage of the lifespan. It is also difficult to envisage how a programme would be selected for during evolution because of the high, random mortality in the early part of the natural lifespan. In addition, natural selection is least effective in manipulating characters expressed late in life.

Disposable Soma Theory

A better explanation of the evolution of ageing is found in the disposable soma theory, which stems from attempts to explain senescence from a physiological viewpoint. Organisms must allocate the environmental resources available to them into various metabolic tasks. The disposable soma theory addresses the question of the optimal investment of these resources in maintenance of the soma. Senescence may be understood by focusing on the resources allocated to maintaining the somatic, or nonreproductive, parts of the body.

It is argued that senescence is caused by the accumulation of defects in macromolecules. The accuracy of synthesis of these molecules depends on the specificity of the transcription and translation system, and protective processes that remove defective products. Each organism would evolve an optimum level of accuracy for its macromolecular products. The frequency of errors would not be high enough to jeopardize normal function and not low enough to prevent the possibility of further evolutionary change. Since organisms occupy very different environments they might be expected to evolve different error levels, which would be directly related to the survival time prior to successful reproduction.

If an organism does not age (e.g. some prokaryotic cells), individuals will be in a physiologically identical state, irrespective of chronological age. In this case, the synthesis of macromolecules must be sufficiently accurate to prevent the development of any 'error catastrophes' (see below). This would involve a high energy expenditure with the cell using sophisticated 'proofreading' systems to enable the continuous production of accurate macromolecules. Other organisms may have found it selectively advantageous to reduce the energy expenditure associated with 'quality control' in somatic cells, and increase the rate of development and reproduction. The consequence would be degeneration and death of the soma. However, the 'disposable soma' requires a high level of macromolecular 'quality control' in the immortal germ cell line, or else an effective method for eliminating defective gametes.

Genome-based Theories

Damage to deoxyribonucleic acid (DNA) has been considered the prime target for the cause of ageing. Special attention has been given to the idea of accumulated damage because of a putative age-associated failure of repair. It is possible for DNA to be altered by a variety of endogenous or exogenous events. Free radicals (see below) and other reactive metabolites of normal cellular metabolism may cause 'cross-linkage' of DNA to DNA, or of DNA to intranuclear proteins. In mammals, the high body temperature (37°C) has been implicated in the loss of bases from the DNA polymer and the subsequent development of 'single-strand' breaks. Ultraviolet (UV) radiation, γ rays and X rays cause specific types of damage, ranging from the distortion of the helix to either base removal or damage from free radicals. Chemical mutagens and carcinogens also damage DNA, and viral DNA that has been inserted into the genome of the host will alter the information content of the cell. Mutations may also be a significant cause of age-associated dysfunction. *See* Nucleic Acids, Physiology

If damage of the kind described above accumulated unchecked it has been estimated that 10% of the bases in the DNA of the average cell of an old human would be altered, and this is not compatible with life. Any alteration of the information content of the DNA could have substantial effects on cellular function. However, the effect of the lesions would depend on several factors, including whether the cell was mitotic or nonmitotic.

There has been a search for evidence of damaged DNA or chromatin in older organisms. There are contradictory reports of the incidence of age-associated damage to DNA isolated from senescent cells and tissues (both *in vitro* and *in vivo*). Similarly, studies of DNA repair in old cells have not provided conclusive evidence of a decline in function. The outcome is that there is no clear relationship between DNA damage and ageing, and there is no convincing evidence of a decline in DNA repair with age.

Unprogrammed Events as a Cause of Ageing – Nongenomic Theories

Several theories seek to explain ageing as random chemical damage to cells. In the waste product theory it is argued that since most of the cells of ageing organisms contain increasing concentrations of age pigment (lipofuscin), this material must be accumulating to the detriment of cell function. However, it is now agreed that lipofuscin is associated with intracellular autophagy and is probably an indicator, rather than a cause, of intracellular damage. The occurrence of lipofuscin is increasingly linked to free-radical reactions. We know very little about the effect of lipofuscin on cell function, although the idea that it physically disrupts cellular activity is probably naive.

The rate of living theory has a similar theme. Lifespan is related to the rate of accumulation of random chemical damage, which is related to the metabolic rate. The metabolic rate of poikilotherms can be reduced by low temperature and increased by high temperature, and the lifespan increased or reduced respectively. However, the relationship between temperature and metabolic rate is not linear, and physical activity is also affected by temperature in these animals.

Free-radical Theory

Free radicals are formed by the splitting of a covalent bond in a molecule so that each atom joined by the bond retains an electron from the shared pair. These reactions are common in normal cell physiology, although they are thought to be rigidly controlled. However, uncontrolled free-radical reactions have been proposed as an important cause of cellular pathology, and as the primary event in ageing. Free-radical damage is thought to take place throughout the lifespan, causing a progressive deterioration of both nuclear and cytoplasmic components.

Free radicals can cause lipid peroxidation. Membrane lipids contain polyunsaturated fatty acid side-chains that undergo lipid peroxidation, producing carbon radicals and, finally, lipid hydroperoxides. The latter decompose into cytotoxic molecules, including malondialdehyde. Lipoproteins and DNA, particularly mitochondrial DNA, are thought to be the main targets for degradation.

The cell is protected against free-radical damage by several mechanisms. Glutathione protects against the toxic effects of oxygen. The catalases and peroxidases can remove hydrogen peroxide, and superoxide dismutase acts specifically to remove the superoxide radical. Several 'scavenging' systems are also present to protect the cell from lipid peroxides. Vitamin E is incorporated into membrane structure and may trap free radicals.

There are age-associated reductions in glutathione, glutathione reductase and superoxide dismutase in some tissues, but there is no correlation between the maximum lifespan potential and levels of superoxide dismutase in primates.

Attempts to extend animal survival by feeding antioxidants throughout the lifespan have been inconclusive. There is usually an increase of 10–15% on the mean lifespan, but the maximum lifespan remains altered. These experiments are difficult to interpret because only small numbers of animals have been studied, and most of these treatments result in a reduction in bodyweight. These animals may be restricting their food intake, which is recognized to modify the rate of ageing and extend survival (see below). *See* Antioxidants, Role of Antioxidant Nutrients in Defence Systems

Errors in Protein Synthesis

Orgel proposed that cell ageing would occur if old cells were more likely to insert incorrect amino acids into proteins, causing errors in protein synthesis. In proteins undergoing rapid turnover the ensuing changes may have little effect. However, errors in the DNA and RNA polymerases involved in processing genetic information would be more damaging. These polymerases have long half-lives and catalyse many reactions before they are degraded; any alteration in their function could introduce many copies of error-containing proteins that would accumulate within the cell. Orgel suggested that once a critical level of damaged proteins occurred in the cell there would be an 'error catastrophe', followed by cell death. Various approaches have been adopted to evaluate this proposal. Amino acid analogues have been fed to intact animals and cultured cells in attempts to induce errors in proteins. The thermal inactivation kinetics of enzyme proteins, and immunoprecipitation techniques, have been used to determine the presence of abnormal protein molecules in aged tissues. Frequently, the results have been contradictory. *See* Protein, Synthesis and Turnover

One ingenious and elegant test of Orgel's hypothesis employed the ability of viruses to use the protein-synthesizing machinery of host cells to make new viral protein. If senescent cells contain a transcription and translation apparatus prone to errors then this should result in either a reduction in the numbers of viruses produced, or abnormalities in the viral proteins. This in turn may make the assembly of the new viral particle less efficient, possibly altering the infectivity of new virus. Senescent cultures of cells supported infections by three different viruses as well as did young cultures, and the yields of new virus were equal in each case. The infectivity of the viruses was also identical; in addition, there was no evidence of an increased mutation rate.

It is now doubted that errors in protein synthesis are a primary mechanism in ageing. Recent studies of protein synthesis in cell-free systems suggest that the accuracy of the process is maintained in tissues derived from old animals. Inactive enzymes accumulate in the cells and tissues of ageing organisms but this is not a universal finding. Mechanisms have been suggested by which some proteins might accumulate in altered forms, while others might not, but further studies are required before this hypothesis can be properly evaluated.

Post-translational Protein Modifications

During ageing *in vivo* of human and rabbit erythrocytes several enzymes have been shown to accumulate in inactive or abnormal forms. Since protein synthesis does not occur in erythrocytes at the time of this accumulation, the production of these abnormal proteins must result from postsynthetic modifications. Altered proteins also accumulate in the fibre cells of the lens during ageing, even though protein synthesis has ceased at this site, again indicating that post-translational modifications must be occurring. Various postsynthetic changes have been recorded, including deamidation at asparagine or glutamine residues, cleavage of peptide bonds, acetylation of amino-terminal residues, and glycosylation of free amino groups. Other possible reactions include phosphorylation at serine residues, sulphydryl-disulphide bond interchange, changes involving cross-linking and oxidation. There are clear conformation changes in certain enzymes from aged animals.

The presence of aberrant proteins in old cells may be the direct result of a decrease in the degradation of these molecules. There are several pathways for the removal of proteins within the cell. Short-lived proteins, in either normal or abnormal form, are degraded in proteolytic pathways in the cytosol. The ubiquitin system is well known, and the cytosolic proteases, the calpains, also have a role in protein degradation. The balance of evidence suggests that protein degradation in the intact animal decreases with age. It is intriguing to speculate on the possible effects of age-associated changes in proteolysis, and the effects they may have on cellular senescence.

'Pacemaker' Theories

The theories described above are directed at the explanation of molecular and cellular changes that may cause ageing in multicellular organisms. If any of the events described above took place then cellular dysfunction would be observed. If the deterioration occurred in many cells, in many organs, there would be system inefficiency and, ultimately, 'ageing'. However, several theories have implicated 'organ systems' as a cause of ageing, the most notable involving the immune and neuroendocrine systems.

We know there are certain fundamental changes in molecules that take place with time, e.g. thermodynamic alterations. However, while these modifications take place at a given rate they may be modified by other external factors, including alterations in the *interne milieu* regulated by the endocrine system. It is possible that the endocrine system acts as a 'pace-maker' for ageing in multicellular organisms. For example, the rate of accumulation of DNA damage could be influenced by hormonal events that accelerate or retard repair.

Nutritional Modification of Ageing

Our understanding of ageing has been hampered by our inability to manipulate the lifespan effectively. It is easy to shorten lifespan but it is difficult to equate acute toxic effects and ageing. The development of strategies to retard the rate of ageing has proved difficult, particularly so for mammalian species. Only the restriction of energy intake is recognized as retarding physiological and actuarial rates of ageing in mammals. These dietary regimes are successful in delaying the onset of chronic age-related pathology, and slow the rate of physiological ageing. The diets are designed to avoid malnutrition, including vitamin and mineral deficiencies, while restricting energy intake to 30–70% of control levels. *See* Energy, Energy Expenditure and Energy Balance

Such diets increase mean, maximum and last decile survival by 30–60% in laboratory rodents. No one particular time within the post-weaning period of the lifespan is especially sensitive to the energy restriction effect. The survival of early-onset (1–1·5 months) and adult-onset (6–14 months) energy-restricted rodents has been compared. Adult-onset treatment results in average and maximum lifespans that are 89–95% as great as those animals experiencing early-onset restricted feeding. Returning energy-restricted animals to full feeding is detrimental to subsequent survival and is associated with the rapid onset of age-related pathology.

Mechanism of Action of Energy Restriction on Ageing

The extension in survival in chronic energy-restricted animals is achieved by retarding physiological ageing and delaying the appearance of several age-associated diseases. Chronic energy restriction has been shown to retard the development of genetically determined pathology and increase survival in animal models of human pathology, e.g. nephronophthisis in the KdKd mouse and hypertension-associated pathology in the sponta-

neously hypertensive rat. It is unknown whether these two effects result from the modification of a single basic mechanism, or are separate but interlinked processes.

Protein Turnover

It has been a general observation that the rate of protein turnover decreases with age as both the rate of protein synthesis and degradation fall. This increase in protein half-life in tissues from old animals leads to an increase in the proportion of labile or damaged proteins. Energy restriction retards the age-dependent accumulation of heat-labile proteins, thought to be the result of post-translational modification (see above). Several studies have shown that energy restriction results in an increase in the rate of protein turnover. The turnover of proteins and other cellular components is envisaged to provide not only for the removal of damaged molecules, but to endow the cell with metabolic flexibility. This effect can be shown in mice even after short periods of energy restriction (70 days), imposed as late as 24·5 months of age. A significant decrease in the proportion of heat-labile aminoacyl-tRNA (transfer ribonucleic acid) synthetases in liver and brain tissue is observed. Age changes in enzymes that are important in maintaining translation fidelity during protein synthesis are therefore susceptible to the effect of energy restriction.

Free Radicals

The heat-inactivation curves of aminoacyl-tRNA synthetases observed in fully fed, aged animals can be reproduced in an *in vitro* system by oxidative damage. The inactivation can be prevented by free-radical scavengers such as mannitol and benzoate. Free-radical generation has not been directly quantified in energy-restricted animals but some studies have attempted to assess rates of free-radical-induced damage. Such studies have shown a suppression of the age-related increase in lipid hydroperoxide formation in liver mitochondrial and microsomal membranes associated with an increase in the activities of several antioxidant enzymes. The increase in the activity of the antioxidant enzymes in energy-restricted rats appeared to arise from an increase in the transcription of the genes encoding for these proteins. Increased nuclear transcription rates have been shown in 18-month-old energy-restricted rats for the α_{2u}-globulin gene. This correlated with both increased synthesis of the α_{2u}-protein and its messenger RNA (mRNA). The expression of α_{2u}-globulin gene is under multihormone control and its enhanced expression in older energy-restricted rats is secondary to delayed ageing in the endocrine system. The control pathway by which increased transcription of the superoxide dismutase and catalase genes is induced by energy restriction is unknown. Similarly, the mechanism by which restricted-energy diets increase rates of protein synthesis and degradation have still to be determined. Preliminary data indicate that in older energy-restricted rodents, the elongation step in the translation process proceeds at a faster rate than in age-matched control animals. This aspect of protein synthesis is under direct thyroid hormone control but the details of the mechanism are unknown.

Conclusion

Ageing in mammals is typically manifest in a decreased ability to maintain homeostatic control. Several current theories about ageing have been critically discussed but clearly no single theory explains all the known facts about ageing; on the other hand, none of the proposed mechanisms can be completely excluded. This is evident from studies with the energy-restricted animal model of retarded ageing. Data exists to support the hypothesis that ageing results from an increase in labile or damaged proteins. Such proteins appear to accumulate as a result of free-radical and other metabolic actions inducing post-translational modifications. It is proposed that chronic energy restriction retards the rate of accumulation of damaged or labile protein by inducing an increase in the rate of protein turnover and enhanced expression of the genes coding free-radical scavenger enzymes. Although our knowledge of the interaction of diet on the rate of ageing is still rudimentary, the complexity of the ageing process may be such that single unitary theories will prove inadequate. *See* Elderly, Nutritional Status; Elderly, Nutritionally Related Problems

Bibliography

Fishbein L (ed.) (1991) *Biological Effects of Dietary Restriction.* International Life Sciences Institute Monograph. New York: Springer-Verlag.

Harding JJ, Beswick HT, Ajiboye R *et al.* (1989) Non-enzymatic post-translational modification of proteins in aging. A review. *Mechanisms of Ageing and Development* 50: 7–16.

Holliday R (1988) Toward a biological understanding of the aging process. *Perspectives in Biology and Medicine* 32: 109–123.

Ingram DK, Baker GT and Shock NW (1991) *The Potential for Nutritional Modulation of Aging Processes.* Trumbull Connecticut: Food and Nutrition Press.

Kirkwood TBL and Rose MR (1991) Evolution of senescence: late survival sacrificed for reproduction. *Philosophical Transactions of the Royal Society of London Series B: Biological Sciences* 332: 15–24.

Rothstein M (1982) *Biochemical Approaches to Aging.* New York: Academic Press.

Sohal RS (ed.) (1981) *Age Pigments.* Amsterdam: Elsevier/ North Holland Biomedical Press.

Sohal RS, Birnbaum LS and Cutler RG (eds) (1985) Molecular biology of aging: gene stability and gene expression. *Aging* 29: 49–65.

Warner HR, Butler RN, Sprott RL and Schneider EL (eds) (1987) Modern biological theories of aging. *Aging* 31: 177–182.

Weindruch R and Walford RL (1988) *The Retardation of Aging and Disease by Dietary Restriction.* Springfield, Illinois: Charles C Thomas.

Ioan Davies
University Hospital of South Manchester, Manchester, UK
Brian Merry
University of Liverpool, Liverpool, UK

AGGLOMERATION

Definitions, History and Scope

Agglomeration is a powder size enlargement process, where small particles combine to form large, relatively permanent masses in which the original particles are still identifiable. These agglomerates have a coarse, open structure and a mean particle size ranging from 0.1 to a few millimetres. The process uses mechanical agitation in the presence of the required proportion of a liquid phase and perhaps other binding agents and is normally followed by evaporative drying. Agglomeration is sometimes confused with granulation. The latter is, in fact, a term describing all size enlargement processes; compaction, extrusion, prilling, nodulization, sintering and agglomeration.

Agglomeration as a size enlargement process is not confined in its application to the food industry. The mineral-processing, chemical, surfactant and pharmaceutical industries use several methods of granulation, including agglomeration, to solve their powder handling problems. The advantages of agglomeration when compared with other granulation techniques such as compaction are lighter granules with large open pores and superior reconstitution properties.

Agglomeration started to be applied to food powders in the 1960s in the USA. Several processes were developed for dairy products, sugars, flour and cake mixes, chocolate drinks, instant coffee and tea and other special drinks. Some of these processes are still used today although the majority have been superseded by continuous straight-through fluid bed processes, which are more economical and have less down-time or product outside specification.

Agglomeration is employed to improve the handling properties of fine food powder materials when these are used either as intermediate raw materials or as final consumer goods. There are two distinct areas where agglomeration has a beneficial effect for both the consumer and the industrial user: dry handling and reconstitution of fine powders.

Dry Handling

Fine powders are used extensively in the food industry. They are produced from a variety of drying and crystallization processes such as oven drying, spray drying, vacuum or freeze drying, drum drying, etc., which may, when appropriate, be followed by a crushing and milling process. Fine powders invariably exhibit cohesive flow properties, which results in poor or no flowability in silos and hoppers, excessive dust formation, segregation and loss of control of bulk density. Agglomeration eliminates these problems. *See* Drying, Theory of Air Drying; Drying, Spray Drying

Agglomerated products exhibit:

(1) Improved flowability resulting from their having larger particles and a more uniform particle size distribution; for the consumer this means instantly and completely emptying packets with no material clinging to corners.
(2) Elimination of dust formation, owing to a substantial decrease in the proportion of fines.
(3) Uniform bulk density, which is usually a function of particle size and porosity, and less segregation in retail packages.

Reconstitution

The reconstitution of fine powders presents problems for the industrial user and the consumer. In industrial use long mixing times must be used with intensive mixing equipment interspersed with screening operations and settling tanks. For the consumer who is only equipped with a spoon and a cup, reconstitution of a soup mix or a chocolate drink needs to be convenient and quick, even in cold water and without the formation of partly hydrated lumps on the surface of the cup that may be mistaken for substandard product. Agglomerated powders are attractive because they have:

(1) greatly improved dispersion and rehydration characteristics because of their open porous structure, which allows water to penetrate and disperse the granule with minimum stirring;
(2) improved sensory properties, i.e. intense colour and an attractive appearance.

Instant Powders

An agglomerated powder with greatly improved dry handling and reconstitution properties is termed an 'instant' powder. The properties and standards for testing the quality of an instant powder differ according to the type of powder. Apart from microbiological requirements that have always had to be fulfilled, the properties for testing the quality of an instant powder can be divided into three groups:

(1) appearance, structure, size and handling properties of the powder;
(2) easiness and completeness of reconstitution;
(3) appearance and lack of defaults of the reconstituted solution.

Fat-containing powders such as whole milk, spray-dried fats, some chocolate drinks and soup or gravy mixes are difficult to reconstitute in cold water even if they are agglomerated. Such powders are usually covered by a thin layer of surface fat that makes them water-repellent. Coating these powders with small amounts of wetting agents such as lecithin dispersed in fat makes them wettable and cold-water-soluble. This operation has in some instances been termed 'instantization'. In fact, instantization is the production of an instant powder that fulfils certain predetermined standards and may be achieved either by agglomeration or some other form of granulation, lecithination or both.

The Agglomeration Process: Molecular Bonding and Growth

Knowledge of the types of bonds generated between agglomerating particles and the mechanisms of granule growth is of paramount importance in understanding the agglomeration process. Primarily, the bonds formed between solid particles are due to electrostatic and intermolecular attraction forces. In the presence of a liquid, though, the distance between centres of attraction is reduced and stronger bonds are formed. Their manifestation is termed 'liquid bridges'.

Liquid Bridges

As the name indicates, these are bonds formed between the liquid and the particles. They are strongly dependent on the wetting angle, the adsorption characteristics of the powder, and the amount and viscosity of the binding liquid. When the particles are held together by a low-viscosity liquid, owing to surface tension forces and depending on the liquid saturation, four different states are possible:

(1) Pendular state – the liquid is held in discrete lens-like rings at the point of contact between the particles. The air forms a continuous phase throughout the agglomerate.
(2) Funicular state – at higher liquid saturations the liquid rings coalesce to give a continuous liquid phase throughout the agglomerate, in which discrete pockets of air are entrapped.
(3) Capillary state – the pore space is completely saturated with liquid but the liquid does not cover the external agglomerate surfaces. A negative capillary pressure is built up within the agglomerate, which gives it a degree of tensile strength.
(4) In addition to the above, if the liquid covers the external surfaces of the agglomerate, the particles become completely encapsulated within the liquid.

Use of liquids with a high viscosity usually results in agglomerates of higher strength than is achieved using low-viscosity liquids, depending on the fluid cohesion strength and the fluid–solid adhesion force.

Solid Bridges

Liquid bridges hold the particles together during granule growth. Upon drying, these usually result in solid bridges through phase transformation, i.e. recrystallization of the dissolved material, hardening of binder liquid or chemical reaction. In this way the agglomerate comprises particles connected by solid bridges, in which capillary pores are present. The tensile strength of solid bridges is of the same order of magnitude as that of the constituent particles.

Mechanisms of Growth

The overall mechanisms of granule growth determine not only the rate of agglomeration but also the final properties of the agglomerate. Although these mechanisms are very strong functions of the process equipment used, the following steps are generally accepted:

(1) nucleation of primary particles by random coalescence;
(2) transition stage growth;
(3) final 'ball' growth.

In the initial nucleation period, the feed particles grow by rapid random coalescence. During the transition period, particles grow by preferred coalescence between large and small granules (in the case of wide particle size distributions) or by crushing and layering (in the case of a narrow particle size distribution). The growth rate passes through a maximum, which can be perceived as the rate at which the diameter of the granule increases to a size such that any further increase is accompanied by a corresponding increase in attrition crushing.

The principal variable used to control agglomeration is the liquid saturation necessary to achieve the surface tackiness, which leads to a greater propensity of particle coalescence. Research has shown that in many cases this critical moisture content is around 70–90% of that needed to saturate the voidage in the powder being agglomerated.

The choice of equipment and process parameters, such as fluidization velocity and speed of rotation, determine to a large extent the growth mechanism, which for the same moisture content can be based on coalescence or crushing and layering, or a combination of both. This explains the different densities of agglomerated products obtained from the same material and the same volume ratio of liquid to solids but made on different equipment or of products manufactured on the same equipment but at different agitation motions.

Characteristics of Agglomerated Powders in Contrast with the Starting Materials

It is the physical properties of fine powders that are the source of problems in power handling. Agglomeration is essential in order to modify these and improve the usefulness of fine powders. There follows a brief description of these properties and how they are modified by agglomeration.

Shape

The shape and surface roughness of particles dictate the number of contact points between adjacent particles and the minimum proximity. The shape has a pronounced effect on the flowability; for example, particles that have a fibrous, highly asymmetric shape can interlock and inhibit free flow. Agglomeration changes the shapes of the particles dramatically and, in general, creates more symmetrical particles with fewer 'cooking points' and therefore improved flowability.

Particle Size

Particle size is a contentious property, because most particulate matter has an irregular shape and its size differs according to the method used to measure it. It is usually defined as the 'dimension of an imaginary

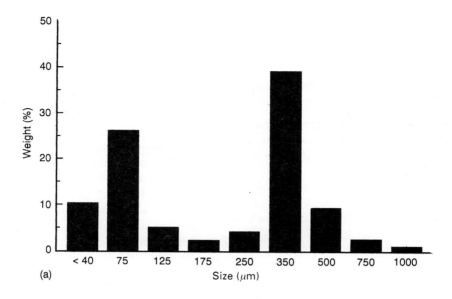

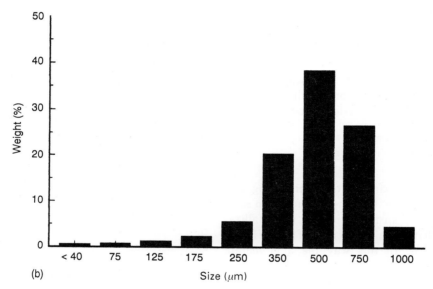

Fig. 1 Particle size distributions of (a) a fine powder showing a bimodal particle size range and (b) an agglomerate with a narrow range of particle sizes.

spherical particle having the same value in the physical property measured as the irregularly shaped particle'. Not all of the particles of a powder are the same size, and a particle size distribution is usually employed to characterize a powder. The particle size distribution correlates well with many other material properties and bulk characteristics.

Figure 1(a) and (b) show two particle size distributions. The first is typical of a powder resulting from a milling process. It contains a large proportion of very fine material, causing dust formation in dry handling and wet lump formation during reconstitution. Furthermore, the vast range of particle sizes will lead to acute flowability problems, time consolidation behaviour, variable density due to nonuniformity of packing and, finally, segregation or compaction during transportation. Thus, the effects of a wide particle size distribution are spread across the whole range of uses of powdered material. Agglomeration changes the particle size distribution in two ways (see Fig. 1(b)). First, it shifts the mean to a larger particle size, thus eliminating all problems arising from the presence of a very fine material. Secondly, it gives a product with more uniform size, thus narrowing the width of the particle size distribution curve, which eliminates all the other problems outlined above.

Density, Porosity, Surface Area, Pore Size Distribution

In the case of particulate matter, there are four types of density used – true, particle, pouring and tap density. True density is the density of the material when it does not include any interstitial pores; particle density is the density of the material when it is in particle form and includes interstitial pores; pouring density is the bulk density of the powder when it is poured into a container; and tapped density is the density measured after the container has been shaken and the powder has consolidated. Both of the latter include interparticle porosity. The difference between the poured and tapped densities determines the degree of consolidation and how much empty space will be left on top of a jar filled with product at the factory after it has been shaken through transportation. Density is also important during reconstitution. After wetting, the density of particles determines how fast they sink and whether they have time to dissolve or be stabilized in suspension.

The knowledge of surface area and pore size distribution provides insight into the structure and adsorption potential of particulate matter. This is often calculated from the particle size distribution and by use of the mercury porosimetry method.

In general, agglomerated granules are of larger size with a lower particle or bulk density. Such granules sink slowly into water and therefore can disperse and enter solution before reaching the bottom of the container. Agglomeration also increases the porosity and, particularly, the formation of large numbers of interconnecting micropores, which have potentially large capillary pressures during wetting, i.e. liquid is sucked into them by capillary action. It has been shown that the total wetting time is a decreasing function of porosity. Also, the presence of micropores is instrumental in the spontaneous deagglomeration process, which is essential for instant powders.

It is of interest to contrast the reconstitution of agglomerates with that of aggregates of fine powders. Agglomeration produces an increase in the amount of air between particles. During reconstitution air is replaced by water. In fine powders the surface area is large and the interstitial space small and usually not interconnected. As a result, water penetrates slowly and, after a short time, the space between particles is filled with high-concentration dissolution products, resulting in a sticky jelly with islands of unwetted powder and residual air. Furthermore, lumps form, which are wet and swollen outside, while dry inside. These hamper further reconstitution (even under strong agitation) because their structure is impervious to water. In an agglomerate the large amount of interstitial air results in the particles being dispersed in the liquid before the highly viscous solution is formed.

Cohesiveness

To ensure easy and successful handling during processing, powders must be sufficiently 'flowable'. The factors that influence flowability include surface properties, shape and size distribution, and the geometry of the processing equipment. The forces that are involved are gravitational, cohesive (between particles) and adhesive (between particles and walls).

Agglomeration produces granules that show a marked improvement in the flowability properties, which is qualified by a significant decrease in their angle of repose. This occurs because, in general, there is an increase of the mean particle size coupled with a narrowing of the width of the particle size distribution curve.

Hygroscopicity

Hygroscopicity is the quantity that expresses the propensity of the material to pick up moisture, which occurs when the equilibrium relative humidity of the product is below atmospheric humidity. Therefore, when nonagglomerated hygroscopic powders are used in containers open to the atmosphere, the powders tend to pick up moisture and form lumps that are hard on the outside and enclose dry material. These problems of caking and lumping are often encountered in the discharge of powders both in hoppers and in vending machines, particularly since in the latter the atmospheric humidity is high. Anti-caking agents are often included in hygroscopic powders and their function is to act as moisture scavengers and thus prevent moisture pick-up by the powder. The equilibrium relative humidity is a function of product moisture; thus, if water is used as an agglomerating medium it will at the same time increase product moisture content and product equilibrium relative humidity, decreasing the likelihood of moisture pick-up and caking.

Wettability

The wettability of a material is a property of the chemical composition of the surface of the material. Changes in the surface structure of a powder can be affected by the adsorption of a surfactant. The term 'instantizing' is often loosely used to describe a process whereby agglomeration is followed by coating with a surfactant, resulting in granules that are easily wettable. Fat-containing powders such as ordinary spray-dried whole-milk powder, chocolate drink powder or dried soup mix have poor wettability and the object of the instantizing process is to improve it. In the case of powder products, however, the effective contact angle of the material in powder form controls the wetting process. The effective contact angle is a function of particle size, porosity and moisture content as well as material wettability. The behaviour of complex powders cannot therefore be predicted by simple static contact angle measurements. By measuring the height of wetted beds of powders against time, however, it has been shown that agglomeration decreases the effective contact angle and the time required for bulk wetting provided that the agglomerate size lies within certain limits (0·4–1 mm for some powders).

Sensory Qualities

A final consequence of agglomeration is the change of the colour and appearance of the product. These are important qualities from the consumer's point of view and their change might improve or diminish consumer appeal. For example, the colour of an agglomerated product may be denser and richer than that of the original fine powder. Alternatively, a composite powder may be agglomerated to give a product of improved speckled appearance, which will also have minimum separation problems and enhanced reconstitution characteristics influenced by the most soluble of its individual components. *See* Sensory Evaluation, Sensory Characteristics of Human Foods

Equipment and Processes used for Agglomeration

There are two main types of process used to agglomerate powders – the re-wet process and the straight-through process.

The principle of the re-wet process is the addition of water, or water containing a binding agent, to a dry powder, and then mixing of the particles in such a way as to cause interparticle collisions to occur and agglomerates to form. The particles of the powder can occur either by addition of the liquid as a spray (droplet agglomeration) or by condensation of water from steam or humid air on to the surface of the powder (surface agglomeration). The liquid may act on the powder material in several different ways:

(1) It may dissolve part of it or transform it in such a way as to make the surface of the particles sticky or tacky and therefore make them adhere to each other in clusters.
(2) If the fluid contains a binder in solution or in suspension, this binder may be responsible for the bonding function between the particles either on contact with the particles or as the agglomerate is redried and the binder crystallizes or precipitates. This process is commonly used to agglomerate inert materials.
(3) It may be a material with a relatively high melting

point, used as (1) or (2) above, but which on cooling solidifies to form the interparticle bond.

The straight-through process uses liquid feed as the raw material. In the first stage, this is dried into a powder, usually by spray drying, allowing a moisture content a few per cent higher than that anticipated for the finished product. The particles thus formed show an increased tendency to adhere to each other. In the next stages of the straight-through process, the particles are agitated in ways similar to the re-wet process.

In the next sections some of the types of plant used in the re-wet or straight-through process will be described according to the mechanism used to promote interparticle collisions.

Agitation Tumbling Equipment

This category includes plant that provides agitation by the rotation of a container around its central axis. It can comprise either batch or continuous units and these are mainly variations on the inclined dish agglomerator or the rolling drum.

The essential element of the inclined dish agglomerator is a dish, which is rotated on an inclined axis. The feed or recycled particles enter the dish and are sprayed with water whilst undergoing rolling motion. The relative positions of the input of feed material and sprays influence the size and structure of the agglomerates formed. Other features include a side or bottom scraper. An important aspect of the dish agglomerator is the pronounced size segregation that occurs as a result of the centrifugal forces (Fig. 2). During continuous operation this allows the largest particles to be discharged first while the smaller particles have more time to grow. Therefore, a product of narrow particle size distribution is obtained and subsequent screening is unnecessary. Drying the product evaporates the moisture, leaving a granular product.

The rolling drum comprises a cylinder rotating around its longitudinal axis, which is slightly inclined to the horizontal so as to assist the continuous circulation of materials through the drum. It normally incorporates dam rings at either end in order to prevent spillback and increase the bed depth in the drum. The geometry of the drum makes it more suitable than the dish for handling dusty materials with minimum loss of fines although most industrial dishes are covered to prevent fines from escaping in the atmosphere. The solids are wetted near the inlet end of the drum and the wet powder cascades on to the tumbling bed. Build-up of moist material is prevented by incorporating a stationary scraping bar, knockers that rap the walls, and reciprocating scrapers, and by roughening the inner surface of the drum.

An important design parameter affecting the performance of the drum is the critical rotational speed at

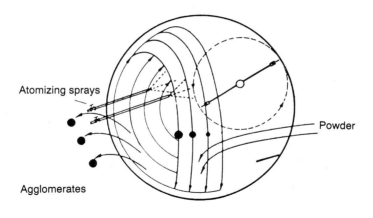

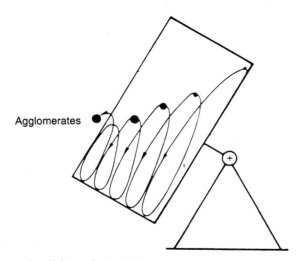

Fig. 2 Particle size segregation in the dish agglomerator.

which the material is carried completely around by centrifugal action. At low speeds the material forms a static bed and slides along the bottom with very little relative motion between the particles. Cascading takes place at around half the critical speed.

With all agitation and tumbling equipment the growth rate and final size depend on the residence time, binder saturation and bulk loading. The speed of rotation, the angle of inclination and the residence time can be varied to affect the density and strength of the granules produced. Sometimes mixers are incorporated inside the dishes to promote further particle collisions and break clusters in the case of very sticky materials. Agitation tumbling equipment has been used extensively in the chemical and mineral-processing industries but its use in the food sector is not so widespread. Maintaining a clean, contamination-free environment can be a problem as most available units are open to the atmosphere. Drying of the granules can be done using rotary drum driers or fluid beds. The large throughput and low cost of these units should make their appli-

cation financially attractive in the future for food applications provided that the contamination problems are solved.

Mixers/Agglomerators

In this type of equipment water is sprayed on to a powder while the latter is in a turbulent state or in the form of a falling curtain. Shear processing leading to the formation of granules can be carried out in batch equipment including planetary mixers, ribbon blenders, Z-blade units and high-speed intensive mixers. They rely on time and energy to effect the necessary contact between powder and liquid phases. All have their advantages for specific applications, although final granule properties may be adversely affected by excessive compression during prolonged mixing and the batch-mixed material requires sieving before drying in order to remove lumps.

In the NICA turbine mixer/granulator, the powder phase, accurately metered, enters the inner section of a turbine, which deagglomerates the material and throws it outwards as primary particles. A gear pump feeds liquid binder to the underside of the inner turbine, at the periphery of which it is atomized into a mist. Mixing under high shear conditions takes place in the outer turbine, the degree of work and properties of the granule being controlled by varying the area of the exit port. Contact time is thus reduced to a fraction of a second. The resulting agglomerate is fed directly into a close-coupled fluidized bed and drying commences immediately. In this way, time-dependent problems such as solubility of the binder or lumping are eliminated.

The Schugi mixer/agglomerator (Fig. 3) is a continuous device for blending small amounts of liquid with solids so that the product remains free-flowing. The mixing chamber consists of a 10 cm diameter, hollow, vertical, cylindrical tube with a shaft running through its centre. To the shaft are attached three sets of six knife-edged blades, the relative positions of which can be varied throughout the whole length of the mixing chamber. The shaft belt is driven at 3000 rpm. Liquids are introduced into the mixer through the jets, which are positioned above the top set of blades. The Schugi mixer is mounted vertically and solids are fed into the top. On entering, the solids are caught into contraflow turbulence created by the high peripheral velocity of the mixer blades. Liquids are pumped into the mixer under pressure and enter the mixing area as continuous threads of liquid. In the mixer the liquids are atomized by the combined action of the top set of blades, which act in a similar fashion to a disc atomizer, and also by the solids themselves, which because of their high speed have a high energy potential. The atomized liquid is dispersed through the powder and the two adhere together to form agglomerates, which leave by spiralling around the walls of the mixer. The residence time is very short, of the order of 0·5 s, and that limits the temperature increase of the product to 2°C.

The structure of the product formed depends both on the relative sizes of the liquid droplets and the powder particles and on the feed ratio of the two. Apart from the physical properties of the materials being mixed, the equipment control variables include the rotational speed, the position of the blades, the direction of rotation and the size of the liquid injection jets. The agglomerated product is dried in a fluid bed.

A third type of mixer agglomerator is referred to as the 'agglomerating tube'. In this device agitation is ensured by dropping the powder into a high-velocity stream of humidified air along the length of a tube. The resulting powder clusters are separated in a cyclone and then picked up by a hot air stream and blown through a second tube for drying. A considerable amount of impact between particles takes place inside the agglomerating tube, which makes it suitable for 'difficult' powders that tend to form sticky deposits easily.

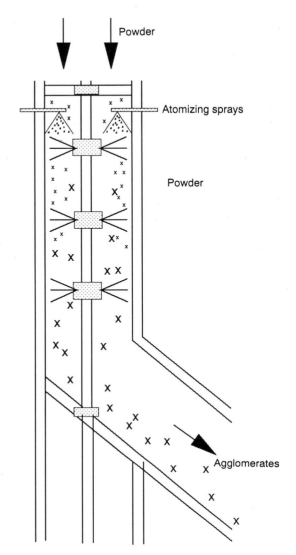

Fig. 3 The Schugi mixer.

In another process the powder is passed through a series of vibrating hoppers or conveyor belts and falls in the form of a thin continuous curtain inside the agglomerating vessel. Steam or atomized water is then injected on to the curtain, which has the force to redirect the travelling plane of the particles. The induced turbulence makes the particles collide and, because they are wet, adhere to each other. The powder clusters formed are carried on to a drying section.

It is evident that some of these units like the 'falling curtain agglomerator' are 'in-house' types of equipment developed and modified to suit the particular needs of specific products. Recently, they have been superseded by the fluidized bed agglomerators, which together with the straight-through process are the 'state of the art' agglomerators of the 1980s. It is, however, worth considering the use of mixing as the first stage in an agglomerating process, especially in cases where the nonwetting character of the powder requires high shear to effect the initial moistening of the material surface.

Fluid Bed Agglomerators – The Straight-through Process

Fluid bed operations are characterized by:

(1) good random mixing;
(2) stable, uniform temperature profile leading to effective interphase contact and controlled high rates of heat and mass transfer;
(3) high thermal efficiency, which allows use of low exhaust air temperatures and therefore avoids degradation of thermally sensitive food powder components.

These exceptional properties of fluidized beds are the cause of their almost universal use in agglomeration processes – batch, continuous, spouted beds, vibrofluidizers – or in straight-through combinations.

The continuous re-wet agglomerator usually consists of three sections that may or may not be separated by weirs. Powder is fed from the feed hopper into the first section of the fluid bed. Here it is re-wetted by means of steam, atomized water or binder solution delivered from jets positioned on top of the fluid-bed layer. The powder particles increase in size either by surface layering or random coalescence. Surface layering is more likely to happen with low-viscosity wetting agents which allow the moisture to distribute evenly around the particles. 'Blackberry'-type agglomerates form when particle surfaces are made just wet enough for collision of particles to lead to capture. Typical moisture contents of the re-wetted powder in the first section are 6–10%. Too high wetting will result in deposits in the bed and a blocked distributor plate. Too low wetting will reduce the level of agglomeration and produce less stable agglomerates. Vibration is used to reduce channelling and break powder clusters. The agglomerated material passes into the second section, where it is dried in a hot air stream. After drying it moves to the third section for cooling. Feed particle sizes range between 30 and 300 μm. Agglomerates of 0·5–1·5 mm in size are typically produced.

Straight-through combination systems consist of a spray drier in which liquid feed material is dried to produce a powder at a moisture content slightly higher than would be expected for a final stable product (6–9%). The partially dried powder is then fed to a number of static and/or vibrating fluid beds, where final drying and cooling take place. Fine unagglomerated material is removed pneumatically and taken back to the atomization zone in the spray drier, where it is mixed with the atomized droplets. Agglomeration occurs through contact of fine powder and liquid feed in the atomization zone as well as through interparticle collisions of the damp particles in the fluid beds. The remainder of the operation consists of final drying to 2–5% moisture and cooling and is similar to that in re-wet fluid bed agglomeration. If a lecithination (instantization) stage is required to be included to further improve the instant properties of the powder, this is usually carried out by spraying a lecithin-in-oil solution on the agglomerates after the drying stage. Lecithination may be carried out either by direct spraying on the fluidized powder or in a powder trap between two fluid beds. A conditioning fluid bed stage is then usually added to the process in order to distribute the lecithin uniformly on the surface of the particles.

A number of such straight-through systems differing in geometry and number of stages have been produced by companies such as APV, NIRO, STORK, DEC and others. Powders produced from the straight-through process are nondusty, free flowing and with a particle size ranging between 250 and 500 μm. The process has been applied successfully to a wide range of products where a liquid raw material needs to be dried and transformed into an instant powder. Its almost universal application is, however, offset by the high investment cost.

Microbiological Hazards of Agglomeration

Few outbreaks of foodborne diseases have been reported due to dried powders. Microbiological hazards are usually associated with the liquid raw materials and the emphasis of any manufacturer should be to ensure that adequate heat treatment is given to any liquid product that is going to be spray dried and agglomerated. Tests for *Salmonella*, Enterobacteriaceae (*Escherichia coli*, coliforms) and *Staphylococcus aureus* should be carried out routinely. There are, however, occasions where the product may be contaminated after drying through contact or handling. *See* Food Poisoning, Tracing Origins and Testing

Bibliography

James M, Brault M and Coucoulas L (1991) *Lecithination – Instant Character Dependence and Shelf-life Tests. LFRA Research Report No. 689.* Leatherhead: Leatherhead Food Research Association.
Pisecky J (1980) Instant whole milk powder. *Australian Journal of Dairy Technology*, Sept.: 95–99.
Pisecky J (1990) 20 years of instant whole milk powder. *Scandinavian Dairy Information* 2: 74–78.
Retsina T and Coucoulas L (1988) *Agglomeration of Powders. LFRA Scientific and Technical Survey*, No. 164. Leatherhead: Leatherhead Food Research Association.
Silliker JH, Baird-Parker AC, Bryan FL *et al.* (eds) (1988) Application of the hazard analysis critical control approach (HACCP) to ensure microbiological safety and quality. *Microorganisms in Foods*, vol. 4. Oxford: Blackwell Scientific

Leonidas Coucoulas
Leatherhead Food Research Association, Leatherhead, UK

AGITATION AND AGITATOR DESIGN

Food materials – whether individual or prepared meals – are invariably 'multi-component' systems. Agitation is both a means of rendering food systems more homogeneous and a means of dispersing further components into existing food systems. Agitation can be used to bring about physical and chemical changes in the system. Under the influence of shear and extensional forces generated by agitation, the rates of heat and mass transfer can be improved during processing. Agitation also enhances the rates of biochemical reactions by ensuring that reactants and enzymes are brought into intimate contact. Typical applications of agitation in food processing are (1) blending of soluble solids and liquids, (2) dispersing flavourings, preservatives, colourings and dressings, (3) disintegrating and comminuting animal and vegetable matter, (4) hydrolysing and reconstituting dried substances, (5) reducing agglomerates, (6) emulsification, and (7) aeration or de-aeration.

The principles of agitation as applied to food processes, as well as associated problems, are discussed here. In addition, the common types of agitation systems used for different applications are illustrated.

The *characteristic features* of food agitation and associated problems are as follows:

1.   Food systems cover a whole spectrum of materials, from dry free-flowing materials through thin and viscous liquids to slurries, pastes and doughs. Agitation of these materials involves many complex interfaces and free surfaces.
2.   Flow properties of the components and those of the mixture at any stage during mixing are both very complex and time-dependent. This is further complicated in situations which involve simultaneous chemical reactions.
3.   The shear stress generated by an agitator is very important in a food system: processes for making fine dispersions and emulsions need very high shear, while others, such as mixing nuts and chocolates or whole fruit into yoghurt, need low shear.
4.   Many food products contain particles of different sizes, some of which are fragile, and these particles may have to be dispersed into viscous liquids such as sauce. Agitation of such systems, to produce uniform product composition, is very difficult.
5.   Segregation of particles often occurs when blended products are discharged from mixing vessels. During the production of chilli con carne, for example, beans which have been dispersed uniformly by the agitator aggregate during discharge. This can cause valve blockage, as well as inconsistencies in the packaged product. It is not uncommon to observe significantly higher coefficients of variation between packs than between samples taken from the mixer.
6.   Mixing of food materials can involve the addition of high-value components, in very small amounts, into bulk materials. This process is particularly difficult when mixing into dry solids, as well as in the production of dough and batters.
7.   It is also difficult to monitor and control the extent of mixing in many food systems, since the end-point of agitation occurs some time after agitation has ceased. This is typical of processes involving gas inclusion, crystallization and texturization.
8.   A wide variety of agitating systems is available for use in food materials. Regardless of the size or shape of the mixer, its design features must ensure hygiene, as well as provide for in-place cleaning and, possibly, sterile operation. Most equipment is therefore available in crevice-free, polished stainless steel. *See* Plant Design, Designing for Hygienic Operation

The principles of agitation can be best illustrated by considering mixing phenomena in a single liquid phase.

Agitation of Liquids

Agitation of liquids can be discussed using stirred-tank agitators as examples, since these devices are not only fairly well understood, but are also widely used. A stirred-tank system consists of an impeller mounted on a shaft; the impeller rotates, immersed in a liquid contained in the tank. Mixing and dispersion are accomplished by dissipating mechanical energy through the impeller. Figure 1 shows the configuration of a typical stirred-tank system: the dimensions given in the figure are often considered to be 'standard', since most design information is available only for this geometric configuration; however, this configuration is not necessarily the best one for any given application. When the height of liquid in a vessel is greater than 1·5 times its diameter, it is advisable to use more than one impeller, generally fitted on the same shaft. Most mixing vessels used for low-viscosity liquids (less than 1 Pa s) are fitted with baffles which prevent the formation of a vortex*. Baffles also help to establish top-to-bottom circulation of fluid,

---

*Vortex is a swirling motion produced when an axially mounted agitator, regardless of type, is used to stir a low-viscosity liquid in an unbaffled vessel. The centrifugal force acting on the rotating liquid raises the level of liquid at the wall and lowers it at the shaft. Since the resulting liquid flow is predominantly tangential, mixing is very poor.

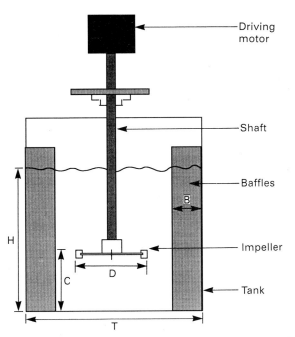

Fig. 1 Configuration of a standard agitated, cylindrical stirred tank of diameter T, fited with four baffles, each of width B. (Two baffles fitted diametrically opposite each other are shown in the figure; the remaining are fitted along the perpendicular diameter.) Standard ratios: $H=T$; $D/T=1/3$; $B/T=1/10$; and $C/T=1/3$.

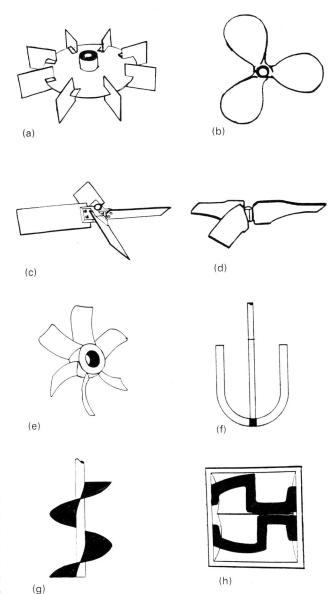

Fig. 2 Types of impeller: (a) disk, or Rushton, turbine; (b) propeller; (c) pitched-bladed; (d) hydrofoil; (e) convex-bladed mixed-flow; (f) anchor; (g) helical ribbon; (h) Sigma blade.

which moves the fluid to all parts of the vessel. In viscous liquids, unbaffled tanks can be used, since gross vortices are not readily formed.

Mechanically agitated devices are useful for mixing liquids of any viscosity up to 750 Pa s, depending on the size and shape of the impeller. Impellers are often classified according to the direction in which they discharge liquid. The disc turbine, shown in Fig. 2a, is a *radial-flow* impeller, since it discharges liquid in the radial direction as it rotates (see Fig. 3a). On the other hand, a propeller (Fig. 2b) is an *axial-flow* impeller (see Fig. 3b). Pitched-bladed turbine (Fig. 2c) and most of the recently developed impellers, such as the hydrofoil (Fig. 2d) and the convex-bladed mixed-flow impeller (Fig. 2e), are known as *mixed-flow* impellers, since they develop flows which have components of significant strengths in radial as well as axial directions. Figure 3c shows the flow pattern generated by a mixed-flow impeller.

The above mentioned impellers are often used in vessels conforming to the standard geometry described in Fig. 1. While dealing with viscous Newtonian liquids, or with non-Newtonian systems, which are more prevalent in the food industry, the impeller sizes are much larger, and stirrers that have a close clearance between the impeller body and the vessel walls are used. In pseudoplastic systems (fluids exhibiting lower viscosity at higher shear rate), anchor impellers (Fig. 2f) are often

used. Helical ribbons (Fig. 2g) are also used for high viscosity liquids, as well as for suspensions. These impellers sweep through a larger volume of the mixing vessel and facilitate heat transfer between the liquid and the vessel walls. For mixing applications involving paste-like materials (effective viscosity > 1000 Pa s), Z or Sigma blade agitators (Fig. 2h) are used. Figure 4 shows an agitator selection chart which is based on the effective viscosity of the material to be mixed.

Flow Pattern in Mixing Vessels

The liquid flow pattern generated by a rotating impeller can either be laminar (streamline) or turbulent, depend-

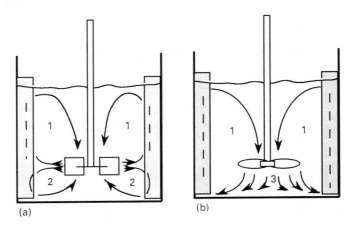

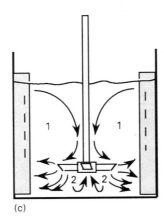

Fig. 3 Flow patterns with different impellers: (a) radial-flow; (b) axial-flow; (c) mixed-flow. (1) Upper loop; (2) lower loop; (3) discharged liquid jet.

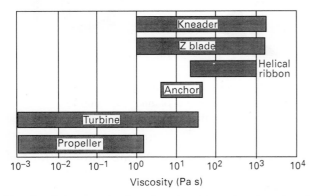

Fig. 4 Agitator selection chart based on the viscosity of the material to be stirred.

ing on the value of the Reynolds number, defined for Newtonian liquids as follows:

$$N_{Re} = (D^2 N \rho)/\mu \qquad (1)$$

Here D is the impeller diameter (m); N is the rotational speed (Hz); ρ is the liquid density (kg m^{-3}) and μ is its viscosity (Pa s). Flow is laminar when N_{Re} is < 10 and it

is fully turbulent when N_{Re} is $> 10\,000$. In between these two values, the flow is considered to be in the transition regime. For non-Newtonian fluids, the same definition of N_{Re} is valid, except that the denominator is replaced by an 'effective viscosity'. For example, in the case of pseudoplastic liquids following the power law constitutive equation $\tau = k\,\dot{\gamma}^n$ (where τ is the shear stress, $\dot{\gamma}$ is the shear rate, k is known as the consistency index, and n is known as the power law exponent), the effective viscosity is given by $\mu_{eff} = k\,\dot{\gamma}^{n-1}$. It is customary to express $\dot{\gamma}$ in terms of an 'average shear rate' in the agitated vessel, which is known to be proportional to the rotational speed. Thus $\dot{\gamma} = \beta N$, where β is a constant depending on the type of the impeller (β usually takes a value around 10 for most common impellers; see Uhl and Gray 1966). Therefore the effective viscosity of pseudoplastic fluids in an agitated vessel can be expressed as $\mu_{eff} = k(\beta N)^{n-1}$. With this value of μ_{eff}, the Reynolds number for pseudoplastic fluids can be defined as

$$N_{Re} = D^2 N \rho / k(\beta N)^{n-1} \qquad (2)$$

Just as in the case of Newtonian liquids, it is now possible to determine whether the flow pattern in a

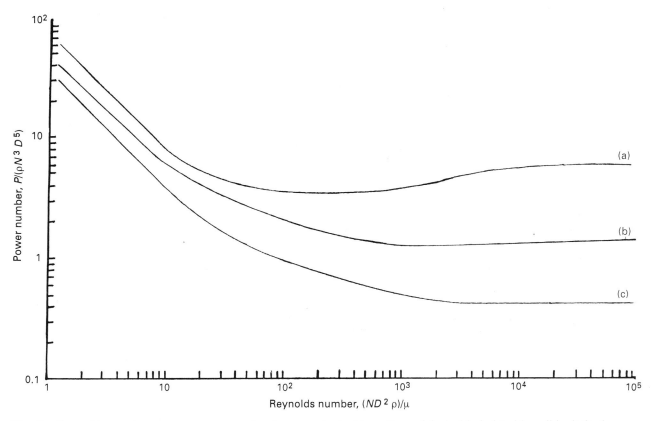

Fig. 5 Reynolds number versus power number for some typical impellers – (a) six-bladed turbine, (b) pitched-bladed turbine, (c) propeller – in standard baffle tanks.

pseudoplastic fluid is laminar or turbulent or in the transition regime during agitation.

Power Consumption of Impellers

The power consumed by impellers is a very important parameter because it determines the operating cost of running the mixer. For Newtonian liquids, it is related to fluid density and viscosity, rotational speed and impeller diameter. The relationship is graphically expressed by plotting power number (given by $N_{Po} = P/(\rho N^3 D^5)$), where P is the power drawn by the impeller) against the Reynolds number, N_{Re} (see Fig. 5). For any given impeller, the power number decreases with Reynolds number for low values of N_{Re}; for higher values, it is independent of N_{Re}. It may also be noted that, for a given impeller and for low values of N_{Re}, there is no difference in the N_{Po} versus N_{Re} relationship between baffled and unbaffled vessels. However, for high N_{Re} values, baffled vessels consume significantly higher power. Similar relationships between N_{Po} and N_{Re} are also valid for non-Newtonian fluids, provided that the effective viscosity is appropriately defined. Details of impeller power consumption in non-Newtonian fluids are given by Uhl and Gray (1966). Typically, to blend two low-viscosity liquids ($\mu < 0.1$ Pa s), a power dissipa-

tion of 0.2 kW m^{-3} is required; for high-viscosity liquids, the specific power dissipation could be 10 times higher.

Blending of Miscible Substances into Liquids

The *degree of mixing* is a very important indicator of the extent of homogeneity achieved during blending operations. The performance of an agitator is often characterized by the time and energy required to attain a given degree of mixing. The time required to attain 95% homogeneity is known as the *mixing time*. Allowable limits are often placed on the composition variances of blended products. Other statistical methods are also available to describe product uniformity, which can be used for controlling the operation, as well as for testing mixing equipment.

Blending of solute with non-Newtonian liquids (or to result in the formation of non-Newtonian solutions) could pose special problems. *Bingham plastic* fluids (fluids exhibiting shear only when the applied stress exceeds a threshold value known as *yield stress*), when agitated by small impellers, tend to form a cavern around the impeller, where the shear stress is high; there is little or no agitation in the regions remote from the impeller. A different kind of problem can be encoun-

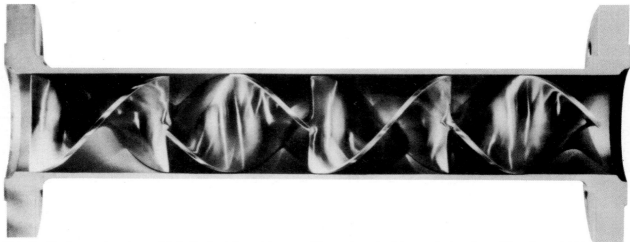

Fig. 6   Kenics static mixer with helical mixing elements. (Reproduced with permission from Chemineer Ltd.)

tered with certain *viscoelastic* substances, such as those having consistency similar to a thick sauce or jelly: these substances develop 'normal forces' as a result of elastic properties, in addition to the usual shear forces caused by viscous effects. The normal forces oppose the formation of vortices, and, instead of the liquid level falling around the rotating shaft as described earlier, it rises and climbs up the shaft. The phenomenon is known as the *Weissenberg effect*.

Agitation Equipment for Single-phase Systems

Apart from the impeller-agitated systems described above, various other types of agitating devices are also available. Most of these devices can be operated either batchwise or continuously.

When a blending operation demands or needs only low specific power dissipation levels (e.g. the blending of miscible liquids), a jet mixer can be used. In this device, a continuous recycle of the contents of a vessel is established by an external pump. The stream discharged by the pump re-enters the vessel with sufficient kinetic energy to cause mixing.

Motionless mixers or *static mixers* (Fig. 6) are a relatively recent development for continuous mixing, especially of viscous liquids. In this type of device, liquid is continuously pumped through conduits which are fitted with stationary mixing elements. These elements, which are available in various shapes, continuously interchange fluid elements between the walls and the centre of the conduits. The power consumption for agitating action in such devices is simply the power delivered by the pump to the fluid, in order to transport it across the length of the conduit.

Multiphase Agitation

Most practical situations relevant to the food industry involve agitation of several phases, e.g. dispersion of an immiscible liquid into another to form an emulsion, dispersion of air into liquids and pastes, and the mixing of powders (which always involves air and solid phases), pastes and suspensions. The mechanisms of multiphase mixing, as well as the equipment used, are complex, and these areas ought to be the focus of present and future research.

Liquid–Liquid Agitation

Immiscible liquids are agitated for either of the following purposes:

1.   To produce a uniform droplet dispersion of one phase (known as the *dispersed* phase) into another (referred to as the *continuous* phase), which would be stable over a period of time, sufficient to allow, for example, mass transfer to occur (as in the case of liquid–liquid extraction); the dispersion is subsequently separated by coalescence.
2.   Alternatively, and more often, to produce dispersions which are stable over a very long period of time. Such dispersions, known as emulsions, are the most common end products of many agitated liquid–liquid systems. Mayonnaise, salad creams, can greasing emulsions and confectionery fillings are all examples of this type of product.

Principles

The properties of liquid–liquid dispersions (including emulsions) are related to droplet size distribution, volume fraction of dispersed phase, interfacial tension, and attractive and repulsive forces between droplets. In the production of emulsions, coalescence suppressing agents known as emulsifiers are invariably added; they act by lowering the interfacial tension. Liquid–liquid dispersions are primarily produced by turbulent eddies

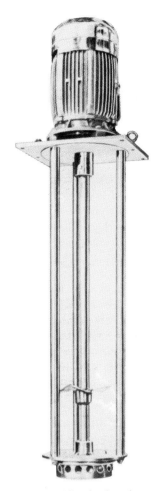

Fig. 7 Immersion emulsifier for batch operations. (Reproduced with permission from Silverson Machines Ltd.)

in the continuous phase, which shear the other phase into droplets. The power dissipated through the agitating device is responsible for the creation of turbulent eddies in the continuous phase. The maximum droplet diameter produced is known to be proportional to the following term:

$$d_{max} \propto \frac{\sigma^{0\cdot6}}{\rho_c^{0\cdot2}(P/V)^{0\cdot4}}$$

where σ is the interfacial tension; ρ_c is the density of the continuous phase and P/V is the power dissipated per unit volume of the dispersion.

Practice

Mass transfer operations such as liquid–liquid extractions are usually carried out in impeller-agitated vessels; a disc turbine is often the preferred choice for this purpose. Alternatively, spray and packed columns can also be used.

Emulsification is probably the most complicated mixing operation, since the nature of the final product varies greatly in character depending on the method of preparation. The order of addition of the components, as well as the rate at which they are added, can significantly affect emulsion quality. In a typical batch process, an immersion emulsifier (shown in Fig. 7) is lowered into the aqueous phase (in the case of oil–water emulsions). The various components are drawn into the working head, subjected to very high shear to form the dispersion, and finally the emulsion is expelled. Such devices are described as 'dispersion units'. Different designs of working heads are available and these can simply be fitted to the end of the frame; care must be taken to select the most appropriate one for any given operation. Emulsification can also be accomplished using in-line static mixers of the type already shown in Fig. 6. *See* Emulsifiers, Organic Emulsifiers

Liquid–Solid Agitation

The agitation of liquid–solid mixtures is carried out in a variety of situations. Dissolving solids into liquids is generally not difficult when the solids are readily soluble, e.g. salt and sugar in water. On the other hand, the role of agitation is crucial in dissolving substances such as carboxymethylcellulose, alginates and gums. In such cases, the rate of dissolution is slow, due to low solubility of these substances. The kinetics of this process is further complicated by variations in suspension rheological properties occurring as dissolution progresses. Care must be taken, especially in continuous processes, to provide adequate residence time for dissolution as well as for chemical reactions (e.g. hydrolysis) to occur. In all such situations, it is important to ensure that liquids are in a well-agitated state before commencing solid addition. When reconstituting substances such as milk and dried egg powder, the rate of powder addition is important: if the powder is added too quickly, it tends to agglomerate, thus prolonging process times.

The main difficulty with operations such as dispersing flavourings, spices, colouring, or preservatives, is that the quantities to be dispersed are very small in relation to the bulk. In such situations, it is advisable, where possible, to prepare a concentrated dispersion first, and then to mix it with the bulk.

Agitation accompanied by disintegration and comminution of substances such as meat, fruits and vegetables may be necessary in the manufacture of sauces, ketchups and infant foods. For each process a dispersion unit, as described in Fig. 7 and fitted with an appropriate working head, may be used.

In addition to the aforementioned situations, solid–liquid agitation may also be encountered during fermentations (e.g. suspensions of cell cultures and growth media), in holding vessels used as premixers, and in crystallizers. In these situations, the main objectives of agitation are to keep solids in suspension, and to disperse them uniformly so that any draw-off would have an identical solid concentration. Impeller-agitated devices, described earlier, are generally useful for these purposes; propellers, in particular, are known to be efficient for suspending solids in low-viscosity liquids. For a given impeller and solid–liquid system, there is a minimum rotational speed below which the impeller does not produce sufficient 'lift force' to suspend the solids. The threshold rotational speed, in general, depends on the size, shape and density of the solid particles, the solid concentration, the density and viscosity of the liquid, and the geometry of the mixing vessel. In food systems, the density difference between the particles to be suspended and the liquid phase is generally not high. It follows that the minimum rotational speed for solid suspension is not high. Nevertheless, it is quite problematic to ensure homogeneity after the particles have been suspended, especially when the particles are sensitive to collision and high shear. While information on threshold suspension speeds is readily available, the number of studies on the homogeneity of such dispersions in mixing vessels is very limited.

Air–Liquid Agitation

During the agitation of food products it is generally desirable to exclude air, since entrained air can cause spoilage during storage. However, there are certain situations where aeration is desirable: aerobic fermentations generally demand a continuous supply of air; processes such as cream whipping and ice-cream preparation involve air inclusion. Both aeration and de-aeration are therefore important to food processing.

Aeration, whether desirable or not, can occur from the surface of an impeller-agitated vessel. The action of the impeller induces circulation and turbulence in the liquid. When strong eddies are generated at the surface, air is entrained from the head-space to form bubbles, which are then dragged into the bulk by circulation currents. These bubbles are stabilized by surface-active agents which are invariably present in food systems, and the two phases co-exist. It has been noted that surface aeration occurs above a minimum impeller speed, and it is possible to estimate its value for a variety of systems. If aeration is detrimental to product storage, then either the impeller speed should be less than the minimum speed for surface aeration, or agitation should be followed by de-aeration. *See* Aeration and Foaming

Aerobic fermenters invariably need a continuous supply of air to sustain microbial growth. The main effect of sparging air into an impeller-agitated tank is to lower its power consumption. The reduction in power is a consequence of the formation of stable air cavities behind the impeller blades; the extent of the reduction depends on the size and shape of the cavities. At a given impeller speed, increase in air flow rate results in an increase in cavity size. However, the cavity size cannot increase indefinitely: once the cavities have grown to their maximum size at a given flow rate, further increase in air flow rate causes some of the excess air to bypass the cavities and hence the impeller blades. The cavities, in certain cases, may also coalesce. As a consequence, the impeller virtually stops pumping, and the phenomenon is described as 'impeller flooding'. An impeller-agitated fermenter operates well away from the flooding point. In practice, the disc turbine of Fig. 2a is the preferred impeller used in aerobic fermentation, mainly due to dispersion ability. This impeller, however, suffers from certain drawbacks: it is a high-shear impeller, and therefore causes shear damage to certain substances, its power consumption is very high, and, more importantly, a large fraction of the supplied power is dissipated in a relatively low volume fraction of the vessel. These disadvantages have been found to be critical to several processes, and there is an attempt to use alternative devices, such as the hydrofoil impeller of Fig. 2d.

Agitation of Particulate Material

Particle mixing is an extensive food processing operation used for mixing materials that include flour, sugar, dried milk, salt, flavouring materials, cereal flakes, etc. Wide differences among properties such as particle-size, shape, density, and surface characteristics (e.g. frictional and electrostatic), make particle mixing a difficult and a complex operation. The process can be further complicated in food systems by high moisture content, friability, complex flow properties and agglomeration or segregation. The desired end-point of solid-phase mixing is the attainment of a truly random distribution.

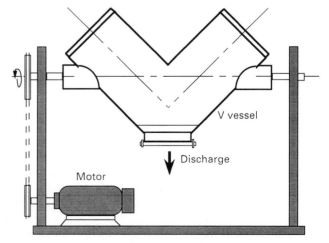

Fig. 8 V-shaped tumbler mixer for solid–solid mixing.

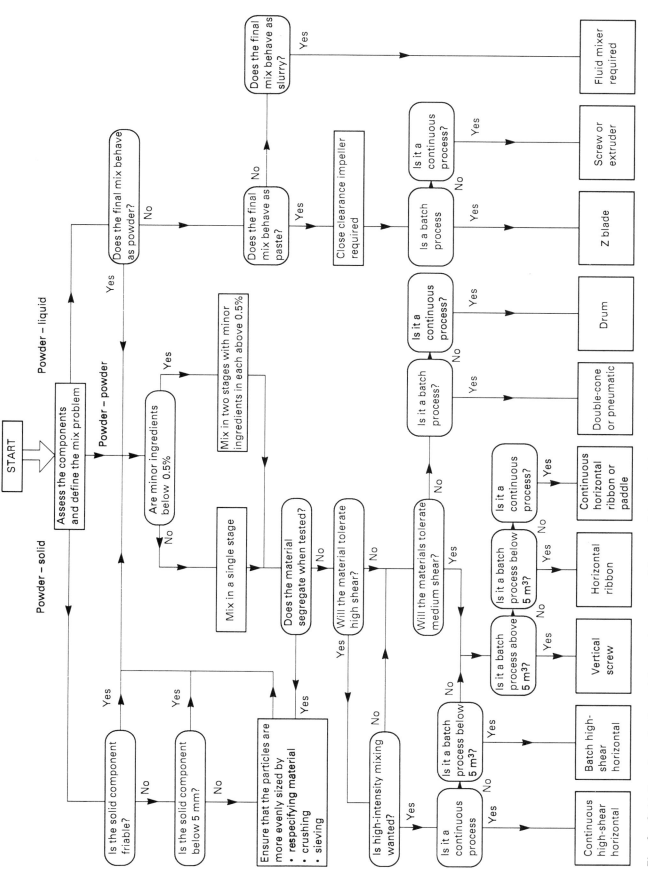

Fig. 9 Guidelines for selecting mixing equipment used for materials containing particles (Jones, 1985).

The following differences between mixing in particulate systems and fluid systems have been recognized:

1. There is no particulate motion equivalent to molecular diffusive transport in liquids and gases. Thus, when two miscible liquids or gases are in contact with each other, complete mixing eventually occurs. However, blending of particulate materials cannot occur without input of external energy.

2. Unlike fluids, mixing of particles is reversible. i.e. mixed solids, on storage, tend to segregate, primarily because of size differences; even marginal differences of 15–20% can cause 'unmixing'. Differences in other properties, such as density and shape, can only accelerate the process of unmixing. It has been recognized that, in general, heavier, smaller, or smoother and rounder particles tend to percolate and sink through lighter, larger or jagged ones.

3. Mixing in liquids and gases is far more intimate than in solids. The ultimate mixing elements of a particulate mixture have a coarser texture, and are of poorer quality.

Particulate materials may be broadly classified into two groups: (1) free-flowing or cohesionless powders and (2) cohesive powders. Cohesionless powders are mixed by convective transport, surface mixing and/or interparticle percolation; mixing and segregation occur simultaneously. Particles in cohesive powders move in clusters.

Mixers used for solids are normally batch type. Solid mixers can be broadly classified as (1) tumbler mixers, (2) convective mixers, and (3) hopper mixers. A V-shaped tumbler mixer is shown in Fig. 8. The vessel is typically filled to about half its volumetric capacity and is rotated on an axis between bearings, thus causing the particles to tumble and roll over each other. In the case of convective mixers, the mixing vessels are stationary and the solids are agitated by impeller blades, usually of ribbon or screw type. Cohesionless powders can also be mixed by discharging a mixture of the components through hoppers. Radial and axial mixing is achieved by returning the discharged material to the top of the hopper, and repeating the process till the solids are completely homogeneous.

Mixing of Doughs and Batters

Dough and batter, used in the making of bakery products, are formed by a series of agitation-induced interactions of such diverse components as water, flour, lipids, enzymes, salt, sweeteners, yeast, air, and oxidizing and reducing agents. When classified on the basis of the desired agitating action, most bakery products fall into two broad categories, *extensible doughs*, such as those used to make bread or puff pastry, and *flowable* or *friable mixtures*, used in the preparation of cake batters,

icings, etc. *See* Bread, Dough Mixing and Testing Operations

Mixing of doughs is more complex and energy-intensive. Although continuous processes are now being developed, mixing of doughs is invariably carried out batchwise in one or many stages. Single-stage mixing is mainly adopted by smaller bakeries, and it aims to complete dough development within its duration. On the other hand, in a two-stage process, the initial stage has a shorter duration, and it accomplishes blending and flour hydration (or hydration of the gluten proteins). Dough development and strengthening of the gluten network occurs more gradually during the second stage, promoted by repeated folding and stretching action caused by the mixer. An undesirable effect of the intense shearing action, especially in high-speed mixers, is the rapid increase in dough temperature. Provision for simultaneous cooling therefore exists in most mixers. Careful control of the process is necessary to obtain a dough structure optimum for baking purposes: at the right end-point, the dough has maximum consistency or minimum mobility; it appears smooth with a dry surface, and its elastic character is optimized. The end-point is reached when the dough starts to pull away from the mixer walls. Overmixed dough, on the other hand, is sticky and difficult to handle and its surface possesses a characteristic sheen.

The agitator in a dough mixer is mounted either on a horizontal shaft or on a vertical shaft. Vertical shafts generally rotate about a fixed axis; in some cases, planetary motion is also superimposed. In either case, there is a close clearance between the agitating blades and the mixing vessel, in order to eliminate stagnant regions and build-up of sticky material on the wall.

A general selection chart for solid mixing equipment is given in Fig. 9.

Bibliography

Aarons BL and Hepnor L (1975) Mixing and blending in the food processing industries. *Food Trade Review* 45(1): 7–11.

Harnby N, Edwards MF and Nienow AW (1985) *Mixing in the Process Industries.* Oxford: Butterworth.

Jones RL (1985) Mixing equipment for powders and pastes. *The Chemical Engineer* 419: 41, 43.

Matz SA (1972) *Bakery Technology and Engineering*, pp 307–327. Westport, Connecticut: AVI Publishing Company.

Nagata S (1975) *Mixing. Principles and Applications.* Tokyo: Halstead Press.

Uhl VW and Gray JB (eds) (1966) *Mixing Theory and Practice*, Vol. 1. New York: Academic Press.

Uhl VW and Gray JB (eds) (1967) *Mixing Theory and Practice*, Vol. 2. New York: Academic Press.

K. Niranjan and A. A. P. de Alwis
University of Reading, Reading, UK

AIDS

See HIV Disease and Nutrition

AIR CLASSIFICATION

Contents

Principles of Operation

In simplistic terms, air classification is a means of using air to effect a dry separation of objects having certain characteristics. These characteristics include physical properties such as size, shape, density and physicochemical nature. Air classification is an operation which applies the technology to fractionation of nonhomogeneous particles, suspended in an airstream, into classes of fairly uniform size, based on a common criterion of density or mass. Some segregation of light and heavy particles can be achieved by aspiration where airflow patterns are generated by a vacuum only, but true air classification makes use of airflow patterns induced through centrifugal motion with the assistance of vacuum. In general, air classifiers will segregate a heterogeneous particulate into two subclasses, one primarily below a targeted particle size and the remainder above this size. Air classification becomes a possible alternative when ordinary sieving fails to effect separation below 40 μm. Applications of air classification in the food industry are in the range of 2–60 μm, seldom exceeding 100 μm.

Principles of Method

If a predetermined particle size were selected (e.g. 15 μm), an ideal classification would permit a subdivision of a mixed-particle feedstock into two fractions: a fine fraction below the predetermined size and a coarse fraction above it. Figure 1a depicts a segregation of fine (shaded) and coarse (clear) fractions.

Under practical conditions, such a sharp separation cannot be achieved, and the separation is more realistically observed as the curves in Fig. 1b. A single 'cut size' is not achieved; instead, there is a range of particle sizes

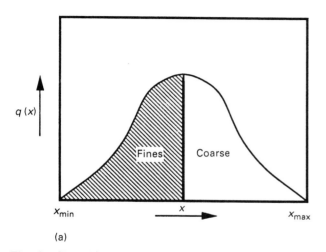

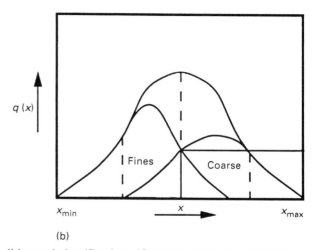

(a)

(b)

Fig. 1 Classification phenomena: (a) an ideal classification; (b) a real classification. (Courtesy of de Silva, 1983.)

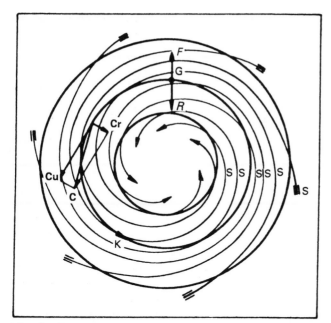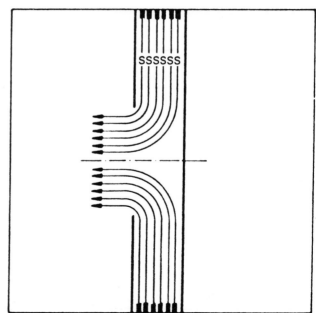

Fig. 2   Forces interacting in the spiral flow of an air classifier. *F*, centrifugal force; *R*, frictional force; *G*, cut size particle; *K*, circular path; *S*, spiral flow line; **C**, air velocity; **Cu**, peripheral component; **Cr**, radial component. (Courtesy of Alpine Aktiengesellschaft, Augsburg, FRG.)

present in both fine and coarse fractions, and these overlap in the region of a nominal cut size. The smaller the overlap, the better the separation efficiency.

The two major forces affecting air classification are the drag or frictional force exerted on the particle by the airflow, and an inertial force exerted by the accelerated motion of the particles. The latter is generally achieved by a centrifugal field or rotational airflow. A typical example of forces acting within a classifier are shown diagrammatically in Fig. 2. A particle ('G') of a certain diameter and density is exposed to two opposing forces: the centrifugal force (*F*) is produced by a rotating assembly, and frictional force (*R*) is produced by an airflow. Additional mathematics can be found in articles by Vose (1978) and de Silva (1983). As the air flows inwards in a spiral path, particles entrained in the flow are subjected to the opposing forces, *F* and *R*. Larger particles are dominated by the mass-dependent centrifugal force, small particles by the frictional force. When the forces are equal, a cut point or particle of a definite size can be established. Adjusting cut size can be achieved by manipulating the forces within the classifier.

Air classifiers are subdivided into types based on their principles of operation.

Free Vortex Principle

Air classification is achieved by adjusting a set of louvres, located at the periphery of the classifying zone, which allows the superimposed radial airflow to enter the zone at an angle. Typical of this group are designs

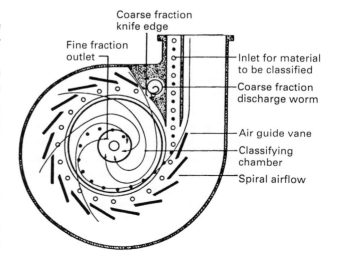

Fig. 3   Frontal cross-section view of a Mikroplex MP spiral air classifier. ○ Coarse particles; ● fine particles. (Courtesy of Alpine Aktiengesellschaft, Augsburg, FRG.)

such as Pallmann Galaxy and Alpine Mikroplex. The latter (Fig. 3) has been used in a large number of research studies and significant data have been published. This design uses a rotor on a horizontal axis, resulting in a vertical plane of centrifugal force, whereas most others use a horizontal plane which favours greater throughput but less precision in cut size. It is understood that the Mikroplex MPS model is being phased out of serial production in favour of equipment using the forced vortex principle.

Principles of Operation

Forced Vortex Principle

The force is provided by means of a turbine or rotor which disperses the particles into an airstream applied by a suction fan. Variations in equipment design then use airstreams to select fine or coarse particles. The Bauer Centri-Sonic was typical of this design, but its precision honeycomb rotor is costly to manufacture and the equipment is being discontinued. A new breed of classifiers, often referred to as turbine classifiers, are now being utilized for fine powder separation. The ABB Raymond 'Jet Stream' line illustrates this concept (Fig. 4). Other classifiers using this principle are Hosokawa Micron, Mikropul Acucut and Alpine ATP series classifiers, as well as those manufactured by Nisshin and Sturtevant.

Additional classifier designs use mixed vortex, countercurrent, co-current or cross-flow principles. Some are experimental, others have not been applied to the food industry. More comprehensive treatments of classifier types and their operating principles have been reviewed by de Silva (1983) and Klumpar *et al.* (1986).

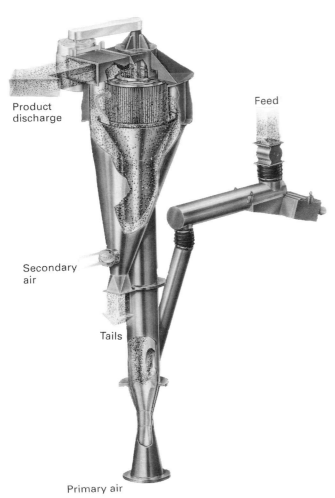

Fig. 4 Typical illustration of turbine-type air classifier (Raymond® High Performance Jet Stream™ Classifier). (Courtesy of ABB Raymond, Lisle, Illinois, USA.)

Factors Affecting Separation

The cell structure of food materials is most important for the mechanical separation or dry processing. Application has been primarily in protein and starch separations in legumes and cereals. Within the cell, the protein forms a matrix in which the starch granules are embedded. During comminution, the breakdown of this matrix into wedge protein or granular protein (and its size or homogeneity) is important and will affect the efficiency of classification (Fig. 5). The cell matrix must shatter easily, and the protein matrix must disintegrate readily. If compound starch granules are present, they must remain intact. A significant number of particles (e.g. starch granules) must be above the selected cut point. Typically, impact milling is the comminution of choice.

Three factors are of primary importance in achieving separation: particle density, shape and size. The difference between density of starch (1.5 g ml^{-1}) and protein (1.3 g ml^{-1}) are too small for density to have a significant role. Shape plays some role, in particular starch granules flattened by impact milling exhibit increased air drag and may concentrate in the fine fraction. Experience has shown that particle size is the predominating influence on quality of air classification.

Particle size of the starting material is an important factor in that, in general, the particles must be less than 100 μm and preferably lower, with a significant number being below the selected cut size. For example, if the granular and wedge protein can be pulverized into aggregates of 2–10 μm in size while the starch particles remain intact and are in the range of 15–45 μm, a separation is probably possible (Fig. 5). Some wedge protein of larger size will spill over into the coarse particle cut and some small starch granules will spill into the protein or fine fraction. Products that do not have a significant difference in the sizes of components are not suitable candidates for air classification.

Moisture content of grains and legumes affects the ability to disintegrate the cell contents and dislodge the protein from the starch. Practice suggests that the moisture content for satisfactory comminution preceding air classification should be in the range of 8%. Moisture contents above that do not lead to ideal size reduction but, on the other hand, moisture below 6% can lead to starch granule fragmentation and subsequent spillover into the fine fraction.

No well-documented research has been carried out on the influence of fat content of the starting material on air classification but, in general, fat contents have to be kept low in order to achieve dispersion in the centrifugal zone

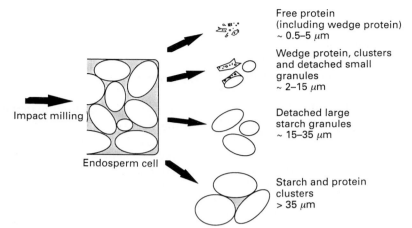

Free protein
(including wedge protein)
~ 0.5–5 μm

Wedge protein, clusters
and detached small
granules
~ 2–15 μm

Detached large
starch granules
~ 15–35 μm

Starch and protein
clusters
> 35 μm

Impact milling

Endosperm cell

Fig. 5 Conceptualized presentation of endosperm cells subjected to milling and subsequent fragmentation.

and minimize bridging in and around rotors, vanes and passageways. In general, a 1–2% fat content is the limit, although some results have indicated that flours containing up to 7% fat were separable but prolonged operating times were not established.

Sharpness of classification is affected by the feed rate and, as rates are elevated above optimal, the sharpness generally decreases.

Plant Design

The typical installation consists of a centrifugal fan generating a vacuum draw to a baghouse collector. An additional scrubber for fine particulate may be included after the baghouse filter, and some designs use an optional cyclone ahead of the baghouse collector. The fines that are separated by the classifier are drawn into the collector; the coarse particles are usually rejected by one of several ways – in an auger system, in an airstream to a cyclone, or within a cyclone built into the classifier. The classifier may be fed from a silo of premilled material or may be directly coupled to a fine grinding mill. Some criticism has been noted in this direct coupling method because changes in material composition or particle size affect the classifier cut fraction and thereby the final product composition, especially if it is being packaged directly from the line.

Some operating facilities, in particular for legumes, have used a double-milling, double-classification design sequence in which the initial mill is followed by a classifier, the coarse fraction remilled and reclassified, thereby yielding a final coarse fraction and two fine fractions that are generally pooled. This plan strives to increase the quantity recovered as fines, although there may be a sacrifice in quality, and to improve the purity of the coarse fraction.

Operating Conditions

In addition to the features of the feed material as given by composition, nature of particles, product uniformity and premilling influences, the variation of cut point and, subsequently, the quality and content of the separated fractions can be manipulated by classifier variables such as rotational speed of the rotor or disintegrator, the amount of airflow through the classifying chamber and the velocity of the airflow (both can be altered by adjusting either air intake or external booster fan), degree or angle of vane setting which deflects flow and, finally, the rate of feed delivered to the classifier. These options vary in both availability and degree of adjustment, depending on the manufacturer of the equipment. Some classifiers allow for easy adjustment of fineness from an external position while the unit is operating; others can only be adjusted after partial disassembly (such as alteration or adjustment of numbers or sizes of selection plates). However, by proper manipulation of these parameters, the classifier can produce a quality separation of high efficiency and yield.

Supplemental options are available for special applications whereby water cooling may be applied to the outside cone of certain separators to answer the need to cool product (prior to packaging) that has developed a temperature rise during the milling and classification sequence.

Bibliography

ABB Raymond (1991) *Raymond High Performance (HP) Jet Stream Classifier*. Data Sheet 911. Lisle, Illinois: ABB Raymond (Combustion Engineering Inc.).

Alpine Aktiengesellschaft (1978) *Alpine Mikoplex Spiral Air Classifiers MP, MPS*. Alpine Bulletin 31/6e. Augsburg, FRG: Alpine Aktiengesellschaft.

Jones CR (1960) New developments in milling processes. Protein displacement. *Milling* 135: 494–498.

Klumpar IV, Currier FN and Ring TA (1986) Air classifiers. *Chemical Engineering* 93: 77–92.

Lauer O and Prem H (1978) Protein enrichment in vegetable products by air classification. *Zeitschrift für Lebensmittel Technologie und Verfahrenstechnik* 29: 212–215.

Schubert H and Heideker HT (1986) Protein separation from vegetable sources by selective comminution and air classification. In: Le Maguer M and Jelen P (eds) *Food Engineering and Process Applications II, Unit Operations*, pp 293–303. London: Elsevier Applied Science Publishers.

de Silva SR (1983) Developments in air classifier theory and practice. *Institution of Chemical Engineers Symposium Series* 69: 387–410.

Vose JR (1978) Separating grain components by air classification. *Separation and Purification Methods* 7: 1–29.

Paul Fedec
POS Pilot Plant Corporation, Saskatoon, Canada

Uses in the Food Industry

Air classification is a technology which is based on physical principles. The use of chemicals is therefore precluded, and protein denaturation is avoided, as is the formation of artefacts. This dry treatment also avoids the production of polluting effluents and minimizes or obviates drying costs. Two of its negative aspects are (1) there may be a retention of antinutritional or undesireable components in one or both fractions, and (2) neither of the fractions produced are 'pure' when compared to those obtained through conventional wet processing, so that applications for products produced often need to be developed.

Application to Legumes

Considerable research work on the milling and classification of non-oleaginous, starchy legume seeds has been carried out in Canada at the National Research Council Prairie Regional Laboratory and the University of Saskatchewan, both in Saskatoon. Although a wide number of species were studied for their potential for commercialization, the focus on field peas led to the adoption of this dry separation process by industry. Similar procedures were adopted in France for the production of fababean protein concentrate. Other centres that have also explored fine grinding and air classification in legumes include the Agricultural and Food Research Council (AFRC) Food Research Centre and the University of Reading in the UK, the Technical University of Denmark and the Michigan State University in the USA. Most researchers have employed pin mills for fine grinding of the seed and a majority have focused on using the Alpine Mikroplex MPS series classifiers, although Alpine Zig Zag and Bauer Centri-Sonic series were also used. *See* Legumes, Legumes in the Diet

A flow diagram for the process developed at the Canadian Prairie Regional Laboratory and applied to legumes is shown in Fig. 1. Researchers have found that the milling of the seed is of overriding importance to the air classification process. Efficient size reduction in the initial milled flour should lead to improved separation of the protein and starch components. Whole or dehulled seeds are finely ground in a pin mill, and the resulting flour is classified in a spiral air stream classifier, set to a predetermined cut-point. This produces a fine (protein) fraction (F) and a coarse (starch) fraction (C). After the first pass, some protein bodies still remain attached to the starch granule surface and some agglomerates remain with starch granules embedded in a protein matrix. A second milling of the starch fraction disrupts these complexes further and a second classification generates additional protein (G), albeit at reduced yield and protein content, and a final starch fraction (E) which has low levels of protein. *See* Milling, Characteristics of Milled Products

In a typical example, the two-run process on field peas generated a combined protein fraction of 34·1% yield and a protein content of 56·6% (Fig. 1). For fababeans, a protein fraction of 37·2% yield and a protein content of 68·1% was produced. Starch fractions contained 6–7% residual protein. Repeated pin milling and air classification studies show that the starch fraction can be further purified, but even after four runs, the residual protein is still around 3% for field peas. It follows that a process based on more than two runs is unnecessary

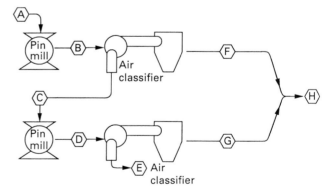

Fig. 1 Double-pass milling and air classification sequence for legumes. Field peas: A Dehulled seed; B 100 kg Pea flour (23% protein); C 77·7 kg Starch I (12·4% protein); D Remilled starch I; E 65·9 kg Pea starch (6·2% protein); F 22·3 kg Protein I (59·2% protein); G 11·8 kg Protein II (51·8% protein); H 34·1 kg Pea protein (56·6% protein). Fababeans: A Dehulled seed; B 100 kg Bean Flour (30·4% protein); C 78·9 kg Starch I (19·6% protein); D Remilled starch I; E 62·8 kg Bean starch (7·2% protein); F 21·1 kg Protein I (71·3% protein); G 16·1 kg Protein II (63·8% protein); H 37·2 kg Bean protein (68·1% protein). Adapted from Tyler, Youngs and Sosulski (1981).

Table 1. Yield, compositional data[a] and separation efficiency of fine and coarse fractions from air classification of milled legume flours[b]

Legume species	Protein content of starting flour (%)	Fraction yield		Protein content		Starch content		Protein recovery in fines	Starch recovery in coarse
		Fine	Coarse	Fine	Coarse	Fine	Coarse		
Field pea	20·4–25·3	22·3–53·0	77·7–47·0	62·5–42·6	14·5–6·5	1·4–24·7	60·0–86·2	58·1–88·8	99·8–75·3
Fababean	29·8–33·0	21·1–45·8	78·9–54·2	71·8–60·6	19·6–4·2	0–9·5	57·5–91·1	61·3–92·6	100–95·0
Navy bean	24·5–30·4	19·4–44·6	80·6–55·4	63·8–46·2	21·9–5·7	0·1–6·9	58·0–84·9	49·1–87·1	100–96·7
Lima bean	22·7–22·8	17·7–32·0	82·3–68·0	49·6–39·3	18·7–14·1	0–5·9	56·9–69·6	32·0–55·4	99·1–96·1
Great Northern bean	22·6–24·0	22·5–42·2	77·5–57·8	53·5–45·6	15·6–6·1	0–4·2	51·5–92·3	50·0–87·0	100–96·6
Lentil	22·6–27·1	21·9–44·6	78·1–55·4	64·6–46·5	14·5–3·3	0·2–19·3	65·8–89·7	63·0–91·9	99·2–84·3
Cowpea	23·6–24·4	24·1–33·5	75·9–66·5	51·6–41·8	17·2–14·2	3·2–14·6	67·8–73·7	48·7–60·0	97·0–89·2
Mung bean	25·8–26·5	27·1–29·0	72·9–71·0	61·4–60·4	12·3–11·7	2·0–6·1	67·7–74·0	66·1	96·4–96·3
Chickpea	17·7–19·5	8·5–29·0	91·5–71·0	40·0–28·9	15·5–11·4	3·7–30·3	53·1–62·7	19·2–50·2	94·5–81·4
Soybean	52·5	72·0	28·0	54·2	50·5	—	—	74·1	—

[a] Percentage on a dry-weight basis.
[b] Data are shown as a range of reported values from assorted classifier types and settings.

and, depending on economics, it may be sufficient to use only a single-run procedure.

A comprehensive review of the published data would be beyond this article. However, a summary table (Table 1) gives an overview of what may be achieved or expected from various legume flours. By way of caution, it should be noted that the data are drawn from a range of classifier types and operating parameters on starting flours that have varying protein levels, prepared by an assortment of mills from seed of varying moisture contents. The data are presented as in the form of minimum–maximum ranges recorded in the literature. All data are based on a single-impact milling followed by a single air classification, generally using dehulled seeds.

Low fine yields generally have a correspondingly higher level of protein content, as well as a higher protein level in the coarse (starch) fraction. As the yield of fines increases, the protein content of the fine fraction decreases and the quantity of the coarse fraction will show a decrease. The protein content in the coarse fraction will decrease and the starch proportion will increase correspondingly. In all cases the recovery of protein into the fine fraction is not as efficient as the recovery of the starch into the coarse fraction. *See* Protein, Food Sources; Starch, Sources and Processing

The initial protein content of the starting legume flour has an influence on the classification result. At the same yield or split ratio, higher protein levels in the starting flour will result in a higher protein content in the fines fraction. Alternatively, if the protein content in the fines fraction is kept constant, a higher yield of that fraction can be expected. Finely milled soybean meal has been added to Table 1 for comparative purposes and serves to

indicate that unless there is a high proportion of relatively large and uniform starch granules, a shift of protein cannot be accomplished, in spite of achieving a separation into two fractions.

Comparing the legumes, good separation may be expected with faba, lima, mung, navy and Great Northern beans, lentils and peas. Chickpeas are a poor candidate for air classification, presumably because of higher oil content in the flour and a high proportion of small starch granules. *See* Peas and Lentils

The separation efficiency (i.e. the percentage of total protein recovered in the fine fraction or the percentage of total starch recovered in the coarse fraction) is dependent upon moisture at the time the legumes are milled. In peas, an increase in moisture to 14% from 10% reduced the separation efficiency by 20%. As the seed moisture decreases, there is a decrease in the starch yield, in the protein content of the starch fraction and in the protein content of the protein fraction. On the other hand, there is an increase in the yield of the protein fraction as well as the protein separation efficiency. It has been suggested that a moisture range of 8–10% is ideal for an impact milling, air classification process operation in legumes.

The effect of seed maturity on air classification suggests that presence of immature seeds, even at high levels, has little effect on subsequent milling and classification. There is concern that green and shrunken seeds may make dehulling difficult and translate to high fibre levels in the starch fraction.

Protein content of the starting flour and, initially, of the seed supply prior to milling has a significant effect on fractionation. In a study of pea flours of widely varying protein content, it was noted that the percentage of protein in all classified fractions was positively correlated to the percentage of protein in the flour, whereas lipid and cell wall material was negatively correlated. Starch and protein separating efficiencies generally increase with an increased protein content. An unpublished rule of thumb has been applied to evaluating the potential of legume seed for air classification. If the flour is finely milled and a 33% fines fraction yield is sought, the protein content of that fraction is apt to be 2–2·25 times the initial protein value of the flour. To ensure uniform products by air classification technology, it is suggested that in any particular legume being processed, the seeds fall within a narrow range of protein content.

Shifting of other components also occurs as a result of air classification. In terms of fibre present in the flour, the hull fibre tends to segregate into the coarse fraction and the cell wall fibre into the fine fraction. Dehulling may somewhat enhance the efficiency of the process and may be a prerequisite if coloured hulls are present. If the coarse (starch) fraction is of lesser importance, dehulling need not be practised as it only has a small effect on the crude fibre content of the protein fraction.

Legume flours containing α-galactosides – especially raffinose, manninotriose, stachyose and verbascose – generally show the protein fraction to be 40–90% higher in these components than the initial flour, while the starch fractions become depleted. Legumes that contain trypsin inhibitors, haemagglutinating factors, saponins, phytic acid, vicine and convicine will exhibit elevated concentrations of these components in the protein fractions.

The protein fraction from legumes also tends to be enriched in ash and lipid, the latter having ramifications for storage of the concentrate. The lipid presence probably results from a lipid-rich coating on the protein bodies.

Protein concentrates prepared by air classification may be used as emulsifiers or supplements in meat products and patties, beverages, bread, noodles and spaghetti. There may be a requirement to inactivate some of the antinutritional factors. The starch fractions are being utilized in the paper industry and in ore refining. Peas have shown the greatest potential for commercial application of the technology. There are few major nutritional or technological problems except for the 'pea flavour' and in some cases a darker green colour of some end products. The main problems are agronomic, the quest for a year round supply at competitive price and of high quality, and establishment of markets for the products. *See* Emulsifiers, Uses in Processed Foods

Application to Cereal Grains

Although the early work in application of air classification techniques to food products began in several USDA (US Department of Agriculture) laboratories with protein shifting in wheat flours, classification is less efficient than in legume flours because of the high proportion of small starch granules that cannot be readily separated from the fine protein particles. Approximately 81% of the granules fall below 7·5 μm, 6% between 7·5 and 15 μm and 13% between 15 and 30 μm, but the quantities by weight represented in those fractions are 4%, 3% and 93%, respectively. *See* Flour, Analysis of Wheat Flours; Wheat

To obtain a protein-rich flour, a separation cut-point of 15 μm is usually sufficient, especially in soft wheat. Two separations may, however, be required to obtain a low protein–starch fraction. As an example, soft wheat flour containing 10·8% protein can be fractionated into three cuts: <15 μm, 15–35 μm and >35 μm, with yields of 12%, 43% and 45%, having 19·5%, 7·1% and 12·0% protein content, respectively. In a single operation, a 20% yield of 21–22% protein fine fraction and an 80% yield of a coarse fraction having 7·5–8% protein can be achieved from soft wheat flour of around 10·5% initial protein.

The protein-rich fractions generated from wheat can be used as the basis for preparation of protein isolates, or the high-protein fraction can be added to low-protein base flours to improve dough and baking characteristics. This enhancement is due to the nature of the protein components present and the alteration of starch and ash components during air classification. As in legumes, the soluble sugars are also concentrated into the high-protein fraction.

To improve the efficiency of fine grinding and subsequent air classification it has been suggested that a treatment of 0·1–1·0% sulphurous acid be applied for several hours as an aid in loosening the starch–protein complex. Sorghum subjected to such treatment gave increased yields of protein-rich and starch-rich fractions. *See* Sorghum

Barley – especially dehulled malted barley – lends itself to successful separation by air classification. Dehulled malted seed containing 11·5% protein can be impact milled and classified into a high-protein, low-fibre fraction with 26–27% protein content and a starch portion having about 9·5% protein. The split ratio was in the region of 16:84. Regular dehulled barley containing 15% protein showed up to 40% protein in the fine fraction with a 17·5% yield. The benefits of such application may be in a defibred, starchy malt or barley flour or a high-starch malt flour which may be used in rapidly brewed malt drinks. *See* Barley

Nonconventional use of the air classification technique has been applied to oats. Instead of classifying finely ground flour, the groats were coarsely milled and then subjected to air classification in order to produce a high-bran coarse fraction and a fine flour fraction. The bran fraction can serve as an enriched fibre source for cereal applications or as a starting material for the preparation of β-glucans. Inactivation of enzymes would be a prerequisite. *See* Oats

Other Minor Uses

Cottonseed proteins are rarely used in edible foods because of pigment glands containing gossypol. Air classification has been shown to produce an edible protein fraction if there is minimal pigment gland damage during the milling of extracted flakes. Yields of 35–40% protein-rich fractions, containing up to 65% protein and meeting food and drug directorate standards, are possible.

Utilization of rapeseed and canola meals could be enhanced if crude fibre levels could be reduced by 50% or less. Small protein shifts of 11–17% have been achieved in roughly 50:50 splits but in spite of the fibre being shifted into the coarse fraction, the two end products are not sufficiently improved to warrant commercialization.

Although rice protein has high nutritional value, attempts at recovery of this protein by air classification have failed to demonstrate significant protein shifting. Air classification of defatted, finely ground rice bran provided a high protein–bran fraction with 50% yield and 23% protein content from an initial 19·4% protein level in the flour. Unfortunately, the ash content of the protein-enriched fraction also increased, rendering the product unsuitable for direct food use. *See* Rice

Potato granules produced by spray drying from a wet milling process have been successfully classified. Granules having about 10% protein were classified into a 15:85 ratio of fine to coarse, containing 38% and 3·1% protein respectively. Assuming the economics of spray drying is favourable, the protein fraction can provide a source of undenatured protein concentrate for food applications.

Air classification techniques applied to finely ground flours have produced a wide range of protein- and starch-rich fractions, with variable degrees of success. The process is advantageous in that drying and effluent disposal costs for wet plants are reduced or excluded. There is also some flexibility for the processor to vary the resulting flours to suit the end-user. Increases in capital and operating costs for the operation must be considered in the light of these benefits.

Bibliography

Gueguen J (1983) Legume seed protein extraction, processing and end product characteristics. *Qualitas Plantarum, Plant Foods and Human Nutrition* 32: 267–303.

Kadan RS, Freeman DW, Ziegler Jr GM and Spadaro JJ (1979) Air classification of defatted, glanded cottonseed flours to produce edible protein product. *Journal of Food Science* 44: 1522–1524.

King RD and Dietz HM (1987) Air classification of rapeseed meal. *Cereal Chemistry* 64: 411–413.

Kohnhorst AL, Uebersax MA and Zabik ME (1990) Production and functional characteristics of protein concentrates. *Journal of the American Oil Chemists' Society* 67: 285–292.

Reichert RD (1982) Air classification of Peas (*Pisum sativum*) varying widely in protein content. *Journal of Food Science* 47: 263–1271.

Sosulski F and Youngs CG (1979) Yield and functional properties of air-classified protein and starch fractions from eight legume flours. *Journal of the American Oil Chemists' Society* 56: 292–295.

Sosulski FW, Walker AF, Fedec P and Tyler RT (1987) Comparison of air classifiers for separation of protein and starch in pin-milled legume flours. *Lebensmittel wissenschaft und Technologie* 20: 221–225.

Tyler RT, Youngs CG and Sosulski FW (1981) Air classification of legumes. I. Separation efficiency, yield and composition of the starch and protein fractions. *Cereal Chemistry* 58: 144–148.

Vose JR, Basterrechea MJ, Gorin PAJ, Finlayson AJ and Youngs CG (1976) Air classification of field peas and horsebean flours: chemical studies of starch and protein fractions. *Cereal Chemistry* 53: 928–936.

Wu YV and Stringfellow AC (1980) Protein isolate from alkaline extraction of air-classified high-protein soft wheat. *Journal of Food Science* 45: 1383–1386.

Paul Fedec
POS Pilot Plant Corporation, Saskatoon, Canada

AIR DRYING

See Drying

ALCOHOL

Contents

See also Cirrhosis and Disorders of High Alcohol Consumption

Properties and Determination

The earliest written records indicate that alcohol (ethanol or ethyl alcohol) has been enjoyed in the human diet for thousands of years. In spite of past and present prohibitions among some groups, an impressive number and variety of alcoholic beverages have been developed, refined, and extolled in an extensive and rich literature. While the discovery of alcohol was undoubtedly accidental, its microbial origin was only established some 120 years ago through the work of Louis Pasteur. Microbial physiologists have since shown that alcohol formed through different fermentative pathways in various microbial species always serves the same purpose: regeneration of an oxidized cofactor, usually the oxidized form of nicotinamide adenine dinucleotide (NAD^+).

Major classes of alcoholic beverages include primary products of alcoholic fermentations (beer and wine), products of mixed alcoholic–lactic acid fermentations, and since the discovery of distillation—known to the Chinese at least 3000 years ago and to the ancient Egyptians even earlier—distilled and fortified beverages. Because alcohol is an excellent extractant, exhibits low toxicity, and possesses antimicrobial activity, it also enjoys wide use as a solvent for food ingredients such as spices and flavours. *See* Lactic Acid Bacteria

Physical and Sensory Properties

Ethanol is a clear, colourless, flammable liquid miscible with water and many organic solvents in all ratios. It is hygroscopic and relatively nontoxic, exhibiting an oral LD_{50} in rats of 13.7 g kg^{-1} (grams of ethanol per kilogram of body weight required to kill 50% of the animals). When ethanol is added to water, a rise in temperature due to the heat of solvation occurs with a consequent increase in volume. When the mixture cools to the original temperature, the volume decreases, becoming slightly less than the sum of the initial water and ethanol volumes. Maximum contraction occurs at a molar ratio of eight parts of water to one part of ethanol. At a pressure of 1 atm, a mixture of 95·6% ethanol and 4·4% water on a mass basis forms a constant boiling-point mixture called an azeotrope. In practice, this means that the concentra-

Table 1. Physical properties of ethanol

Formula	CH_3CH_2OH
Molecular weight (Da)	46·07
Boiling point (°C)	78·32
Freezing point (°C)	−114·1
Density, d_4^{20} (g ml^{-1})	0·7893
Refractive index, n_D^{20}	1·361
Viscosity at 20°C (cP)	1·17
Dielectric constant at 20°C	25·7
Heat of fusion (J g^{-1})	104·6
Heat of vaporization at 78·32°C (J g^{-1})	839·31

tion of ethanol cannot be increased beyond 95·6%, by simple distillation. Some important physical properties of ethanol are listed in Table 1.

Ethanol has a slightly sweet taste and a characteristic aroma. The aroma threshold determined in one study ranged from 4 to 5 mg of ethanol per 100 ml of total aqueous solution. At high concentrations, it causes a burning sensation in the mouth. It moderates the taste of acids, as shown by the greater tartness of dealcoholized wines relative to the same untreated wines. It is said to impart 'body', which may be due to the fact that at room temperature it is more viscous than water. Addition of sugar to an ethanol–water solution increases the threshold for ethanol, indicating that sugar masks its taste and/or aroma.

Sources of Alcohol

The natural source of alcohol is fermentation which has been defined as the oxidation of organic compounds (generally carbohydrates) in the absence of external electron acceptors. Pasteur called it 'life without air'. Microorganisms ferment in order to obtain the energy necessary for growth and reproduction and alcohol is one of several possible fermentation products. In most countries, use of alcohol in beverages is restricted to that made by fermentation. The vast amount of alcohol used industrially as a solvent and substrate in various chemical syntheses is made synthetically from ethylene. The amount derived from the fermentation of agricultural products is largely dependent on economic con-

Table 2. Major classes of alcoholic beverages

1.	Fermented	
	A. Beer	
	B. Wine	
	C. Sake	
2.	Mixed alcoholic–lactic acid fermentation	
	A. Kefir	
	B. Koumiss	
3.	Distilled	
	A. Whiskies, vodka	
	B. Rum	
	C. Brandy	
	D. Tequila	
	E. Liqueurs	
4.	Fortified	
	A. Port	
	B. Vermouth	

siderations, e.g. alcohol produced by fermentation is used as a substitute for petrol in Brazil.

Alcoholic Beverages

All alcoholic beverages are derived either directly or indirectly from fermented products. As indicated in Table 2, the major groups are fermented beverages, products of mixed alcoholic–lactic acid fermentations, beverages made by distillation, and by fortification. Fruits containing high sugar concentrations at maturity and nutrients at levels sufficient to support growth of fermenting yeasts, primarily *Saccharomyces cerevisiae*, have traditionally been the raw materials from which wines are made. Grapes are unusual in that they contain sufficiently high levels of sugars, nutrients, and acids to produce wines that are microbiologically stable.

Beer and sake are produced from barley (other grains are possible sources) and rice, respectively. Unlike wines, these beverages are derived from carbohydrates that are not initially fermentable. Conversion of carbohydrates into fermentable sugars requires the action of amylases produced by barley in the case of beer, and by the fungus *Aspergillus oryzae* during sake production. Kefir and koumiss are examples of beverages produced by the fermentation of cow's and mare's milk, respectively, by a mixture of lactic acid bacteria and lactose-fermenting yeasts. Although almost unknown in some Western countries, kefir and koumiss continue to enjoy great popularity in Eastern Europe. *See* Beers, Ales and Stouts, Fermentation Systems; Fermented Milks, Kefir; Sake

Distilled beverages are derived from fermented grains and potatoes (whiskies and vodka), sugar cane by-products (rum), fruits (brandies), and other plants such as mezcal (tequila). Liqueurs are distilled beverages that have been flavoured and sweetened. Fortified beverages require the addition of alcohol during production, generally in the form of brandy. Special fruit preserves are fortified to assure preservation. The intact fruits, usually cherries, are steeped in brandy for a period of months prior to consumption. *See* Brandy and Cognac, Brandy and its Manufacture; Rum; Whisky, Whiskey and Bourbon, Products and Manufacture

Use as a Preservative

Ethanol is not particularly toxic. As a sole agent of preservation in beverages, minimum concentrations ranging from 18 to 21% by volume are required to assure microbiological stability. Table wines which contain significantly less alcohol are stable because of additional factors: their natural high acidity, low pH, high content of phenolic compounds, and lack of sugar. The toxicity of ethanol towards microorganisms is due to a number of effects. At very high concentrations, as in flavour extracts, ethanol acts as a dessicant and protein denaturant. At lower concentrations, 10–20% by volume, the toxicity is believed to result primarily from interactions with cell membranes. In the yeast *S. cerevisae*, ethanol has been shown to inhibit several solute transport systems. In the presence of sugar, the toxicity of ethanol is enhanced. This explains the stability of a class of sweet dessert wines which contain several per cent sugar and only 7–10% ethanol.

Analysis

Several methods are available for quantitative measurement of ethanol. Some are based on ethanol-specific chemical reactions, such as dichromate and enzyme-catalysed oxidation. Others are based on selected physical properties of the product or sample which are functions of its ethanol content, such as boiling point or relative density. Often, separation of the ethanol from other compounds by chromatography, distillation, or other means is required prior to quantification. The choice of method depends on the need for accuracy and precision, analysis time, potential for interfering substances, and expense. *See* Chromatography, Principles

Boiling Point Determinations (Ebulliometry)

Boiling point depression is probably the most commonly used measure of ethanol in liquid systems. The method is based on Raoult's law of partial pressures. Under ideal conditions, the law states that the total pressure above a mixture of two miscible liquids is equal to the sum of their partial pressures, and that the partial pressure of each component is directly proportional to its mole fraction in the mixture. Stated mathematically,

$$P_T = P_A + P_B = P^0_A X_A + P^0_B X_B, \qquad (1)$$

where P_T is the total pressure above a solution of liquids A and B, P_A is the partial pressure of component A, P_B is the partial pressure of component B, P^0_A is the vapour pressure of component A above pure liquid A, X_A is the mole fraction of component A in the mixture, P^0_B is the vapour pressure of component B above pure liquid B and X_B is the mole fraction of component B in the mixture. Ethanol–water mixtures have boiling points ranging from slightly less than 78·32°C (100% ethanol) to 100°C (0% ethanol) at 1 atm pressure. The ethanol–water azeotropic mixture (95·6% ethanol) boils at 78·2°C. Deviations from Raoult's law are exhibited by mixtures of nonideal liquids, in which significant molecular interactions occur between components. Ethanol–water mixtures are examples of nonideal systems because ethanol exhibits significant hydrophilic character. Generally, the boiling point of pure water is measured in addition to that of the sample and tabulated ethanol content–boiling point data are adjusted accordingly, to account for variations in atmospheric pressure. To prevent significant evaporative loss of ethanol during boiling and measurement, ebulliometers are fitted with a small condenser, and readings are taken shortly after a constant temperature is attained.

Boiling point measurements require relatively large samples, up to 50 ml, which limits their utility. Their accuracy is reduced in the presence of high concentrations of other dissolved solutes. Since ebulliometers are simple devices, relatively inexpensive, and sufficiently accurate for production purposes, small wineries have used them extensively.

Relative Density Measurements (Hydrometry)

Relative density (specific gravity) is the ratio of the density of a solution to the density of a reference solution (usually water at 4°C). Relative densities of aqueous solutions are dependent on the concentration of dissolved solutes. Two general approaches are used to obtain relative densities.

The first is to measure the mass of known volumes of sample and standard reference solutions. This is accomplished by use of a pycnometer, a small, relatively lightweight flask of known volume. Since specific volume is temperature-dependent, the pycnometer is immersed in a water-bath maintained at a standard temperature. The mass of the sample and reference solutions is then determined on an analytical balance and compared to tabulated standard values. The relative density of aqueous ethanol solutions reflects the concentration of ethanol, assuming it is the only (or major) dissolved solute.

The second general approach is based on Archimedes' principle which holds that an object immersed in a liquid appears to lose an amount of mass equivalent to the mass of liquid it displaces. The Westphal balance illustrates this principle. Its design is similar to that of an equal-arm, two-pan balance. At one end, a tube of known volume and weight is immersed in a reference solution and the beam is balanced by addition of weights to compensate for the buoyancy of the liquid. The procedure is repeated by immersion in the unknown liquid sample. In this manner, a relative density is determined. A more commonly used device, based on the same principle, is the hydrometer. Hydrometers are glass instruments with narrow, calibrated stems much like a thermometer at the top, but with much expanded bottom halves that are weighted with lead to ensure that they float upright. When the hydrometer is placed in a liquid sample, it sinks to a depth that results in displacement of a volume of liquid equal to its weight. The alcohol content is read from the calibrated stem at the point where it intersects the liquid surface. Hydrometers designed for alcohol measurement are standardized for use at a specific temperature and calibrated either in per cent alcohol, or °proof (°proof = 2 × % ethanol by volume). Correction tables are available for measurements taken at nonstandard temperatures. Hydrometers are accurate over a limited range of alcohol concentrations. Consequently, a set of instruments may be required to cover the range of interest.

Since the relative density of a solution depends on the concentration of all dissolved solutes, it is often necessary to separate the ethanol from the other solutes. To accomplish this, the ethanol contained in a specified volume of product is separated by distillation. The distillate is diluted to a known volume with water, and the relative density of the resulting solution is measured. In fermented beverages, the concentration of other volatiles that codistill is significant from a sensory perspective, but is very low compared to that of ethanol and does not significantly affect the relative density. In some beverages, such as Bourbon whiskey, the concentration of soluble solids other than ethanol is sufficiently low to permit direct measurement of relative density without need for distillation.

The International Association of Official Analytical Chemists (AOAC) has approved methods based on specific gravity for determination of ethanol in distilled beverages, beers, and wines. The methods require relatively large samples, and are somewhat tedious due to the need for distillation and strict temperature control. However, the equipment is relatively inexpensive and readily available, and precise results can be expected from a skilled technician.

Enzymatic Determination

The enzymatic analysis of ethanol is generally based on the reaction catalysed by alcohol dehydrogenase. As shown in eqn [2], the oxidation of ethanol by NAD^+ yields acetaldehyde and NADH.

$$CH_3CH_2OH + NAD^+ \rightarrow CH_3CHO + NADH + H^+ \quad (2)$$
$$\text{Ethanol} \qquad\qquad\qquad \text{Acetaldehyde}$$

The reaction is monitored photometrically at 340 nm since NAD has no significant absorbance at this wavelength in the oxidized form (NAD^+), but has a molar extinction coefficient of 6.23×10^3 l mol^{-1} cm^{-1} when reduced (NADH). Primary alcohols other than ethanol can interfere, but this is rarely a problem in foods. Determination of ethanol concentration requires that conditions be adjusted such that the equilibrium is shifted toward acetaldehyde formation. One approach is to trap the aldehyde as it forms by reaction with semicarbazide. Another is to carry out the reaction at alkaline pH. A third is to couple the reaction with a second enzyme, aldehyde dehydrogenase, which converts the acetaldehyde to acetic acid. In the latter case, 2 mol of NADH are formed per mole of ethanol. *See* Enzymes, Use in Analysis

Enzyme assays have high sensitivity relative to other methods and good accuracy due to the specificity of the reaction. Often, samples require treatment such as dilution, pH adjustment or decolorization prior to analysis. Material needs for this type of assay are simple: volumetric glassware, a photometer and reasonable temperature control. A recurring expense is the enzyme itself, which must be stored and handled appropriately.

Dichromate Oxidation

Chemical oxidation may be used to quantify the amount of ethanol in a sample. In the dichromate procedure, the quantity of dichromate required to oxidize ethanol to acetic acid is measured. In complex beverages, the ethanol is usually separated from potentially interfering compounds by distillation. The ethanol in the ethanol–water distillate is then oxidized with a known excess of dichromate in the presence of sulphuric acid. Residual dichromate is then reduced by ferrous ammonium sulphate in a standard oxidation–reduction titration. A useful end-point indicator is 1,10-*o*-phenanthroline-ferrous sulphate, which turns brownish purple from blue-green. Potassium dichromate is available in sufficient purity to be used as a primary standard. Ferrous ammonium sulphate may be used as an approximate standard, but solutions that are not fresh must be standardized against dichromate.

The dichromate oxidation method for the measurement of alcohol in wines has been approved by the AOAC. The method is appropriate for routine analyses only when the reagents are standardized regularly.

Refractive Index

The refractive index (RI) of a medium is dependent on its chemical composition, since under controlled conditions composition dictates its electrical and magnetic properties. The RI of a sample is defined as the ratio of the speed of light in a vacuum to its speed in the sample medium. Consequently, RI values are always greater than one. The RI of aqueous ethanol solutions can be measured directly to indicate ethanol concentration. When interfering compounds are present, the RI of a distillate can be measured. Since the RI of a liquid is temperature-sensitive, measurements taken at nonstandard temperatures must be corrected by use of conversion tables.

The AOAC has approved RI-based methods for determining ethanol in beers and wines. For wines, the measurement is made on the distillate. Measured RI values for beer are used in conjunction with specific gravity measurements to calculate ethanol content.

Chromatography

Chromatography is based on the separation of sample components due to their differing affinities within a stationary–mobile phase system. A successful chromatographic run results in separation of the analyte of interest from all sample components that would otherwise interfere with its analysis. The separated analyte may then be quantified by one of several detectors. The ethanol in most samples can be readily separated by chromatography. Since ethanol is volatile, direct measurement by gas chromatography (GC) is possible. Several commercial vendors have columns specifically designed for determining the ethanol content of beverages. Simple, 2 m packed columns are commonly used. Depending on the sample, it is often beneficial to carry out a simple pretreatment to extend the life of the column by removing nonvolatile components. Ethanol exiting a GC column is commonly quantified with a flame ionization detector or by thermal conductivity. Ethanol separations using high-pressure liquid chromatography (HPLC) are also possible. An advantage of HPLC over GC is the possibility of simultaneous determination of certain nonvolatile sample components. Commercial HPLC columns for ethanol analysis are available. Chromatographic methods, which are expensive, are widely used in analytical laboratories because of their specificity, increasingly simple operation, and potential for automation. *See* Chromatography, High-performance Liquid Chromatography; Chromatography, Gas Chromatography

Bibliography

Amerine MA and Ough CS (1980) *Methods for Analysis of Musts and Wines.* New York: Wiley.

Amerine MA and Roessler EB (1983) *Wines. Their Sensory Evaluation*. New York: W.H. Freeman.

Amerine MA, Berg HW, Kunkee RE, Ough CS, Singleton VL and Webb AD (1980) *The Technology of Wine Making*, 4th edn. Westport, Conn.: AVI Publishing.

Association of Official Analytical Chemists (1990) *Official Methods of Analysis*, 15th edn. Arlington, Virginia: Association of Official Analytical Chemists.

Heath HB and Reineccius G (1986) *Flavor Chemistry and Technology*. New York: Van Nostrand Reinhold.

Pederson CS (1979) *Microbiology of Food Fermentations*, 2nd edn. Westport, Conn.: AVI Publishing.

Sherman PD and Kavasmaneck PR (1980) Ethanol. *Encyclopedia of Chemical Technology*, 3rd edn, vol. 9. New York.

Sommer AE and Bücker R (1983) Ethanol. *Encyclopedia of Chemical Processing and Design*, vol. 19. New York: Marcel Dekker.

Zoecklein BW, Fugelsang KC, Gump BH and Nury FS (1990) *Production Wine Analysis*. New York: Van Nostrand Reinhold.

A. T. Bakalinsky and M. H. Penner
Oregon State University, Corvallis, USA

Metabolism, Toxicology and Beneficial Effects

In the context of this article, 'alcohol' is taken to mean ethyl alcohol, with the molecular formula of C_2H_5OH, although the term is generally applied collectively to the potable liquors produced by fermentation from a carbohydrate substrate, with or without subsequent distillation. The ethanol content ranges from about 2% to 6% in beers, 10% to 20% in wines, and 40% and 50% in spirits such as gin, whisky and brandy. In addition, other agents, which either arise naturally from the manufacturing and storing process, or are deliberately added, give the distinctive scent and flavour to the final product.

Among human communities the predilection for alcoholic drinks can be traced back to early history, with the votaries of Dionysus and Bacchus bearing impressive witness to the effects. History, too, is replete with accounts of over-indulgence influencing not only modest folk, but also dynasties, civilizations and the destiny of nations.

Physics and Chemistry

Pure ethanol is a clear, colourless, freely flowing liquid, with a somewhat fiery odour. Among the beverages, vodka is the one that most closely resembles it in character, being an aqueous solution at a concentration of 40–50% without any perceptible, extraneous ingredients.

Absorption, Distribution, Metabolism and Excretion

The fate of ethanol in the body has been intensively studied, probably more than any other chemical. The pattern which emerges in relation to pure ethanol is similar to that for alcoholic drinks as consumed.

Absorption and Distribution

Depending on the alcohol concentration in the ingested drink the subject is aware of a sharp or even stinging sensation upon the tongue and buccal mucosa, followed by a similar, if milder, feeling as the drink is swallowed. This may partly explain the attractions of an alcoholic drink as an aperitif. In the stomach the presence of alcohol is not so apparent to the drinker, although it impinges directly upon the gastric mucosa and tends to dilate the blood vessels. Occasionally, it may predispose to eructation, especially if it is swallowed as a liqueur. Uptake is rapid, both from the stomach itself and from the small intestine. In the presence of ingested food, absorption may be delayed. Peak blood levels of alcohol are normally attained within 30–60 min after ingestion.

Metabolism and Excretion

Reaching the body systemically, ethanol is not compartmentalized, but is dispersed throughout the body water, crossing the blood–brain barrier as well. Part of the total dose is excreted unchanged via the kidneys, while another portion is exhaled, also unchanged, in the breath, to an extent that depends upon the dose and upon the systemic blood level. Ethanol undergoes biotransformation, almost entirely within the liver. Alcohol dehydrogenase, with the coenzyme nicotine adenine dinucleotide (NAD), produces acetaldehyde (CH_3CHO):

$$CH_3CH_2OH + NAD^+ \xrightleftharpoons[\quad]{\text{Alcohol dehydrogenase}} CH_3CHO + NADH$$

To a much lesser extent, ethanol is also converted to acetaldehyde by peroxidation, by the enzyme catalase, in conjunction with any hydrogen peroxide that may be present:

$$CH_3CH_2OH + H_2O_2 \xrightarrow{\text{Catalase}} CH_3CHO + 2H_2O$$

Furthermore, it is postulated that other enzyme systems, notably those depending on mixed-function oxidases, may also make some contribution to the metabolism of ethanol. Controversy persists over the extent to which these other routes account for the metabolism of ethanol in humans because the alcohol dehydrogenase mechanism seems to predominate.

The resulting acetaldelyde is converted to acetate by its corresponding dehydrogenase, which is found in the cytosol of human liver cells, again in conjunction with NAD:

$$CH_3CHO + NAD^+ + H_2O \xrightarrow[\text{dehydrogenase}]{\text{Acetaldehyde}} CH_3COOH + NADH + H^+$$

The acetate becomes distributed generally to the tissues of the body, where it is probably oxidized to water and carbon dioxide.

The rate at which ethanol is metabolized by the human body is remarkably constant between one individual and another, of the order of 15–20 mg per 100 ml of blood per hour, in a linear fashion. In children the rate is rather less. For an adult with an initial blood level of 100 mg of alcohol per 100 ml, it would take little more than an hour for this to fall to 80 mg per 100 ml and 5–6 h for it to reach zero, provided that no further alcohol is ingested.

Biological and Biochemical Effects

These require consideration under two headings – acute and chronic – for the consequences are quite distinct.

Acute Overdose

In the acute situation the dominating response is seen in the central nervous sytem, where ethanol acts fundamentally as a neuronal depressant. Contrary to public belief there is no central stimulation. Instead, as the dose increases – in a manner similar to a volatile anaesthetic – suppression of the activity proceeds successively in the brain from the higher centres subserving intellect, mood and the like, then to the motor centres and, ultimately, to those parts of the medulla regulating respiration and the cardiovascular system.

To begin with, the inhibitions emanating from the cerebral cortex may be obtunded, so that the mood is less withdrawn and diffident, with the release, in some instances, of what is almost primitive conduct. Cheerfulness and elation are common, frequently with volubility and enhanced gregariousness. The senses of discrimination, memory and mental concentration become blunted. Integrated control over neuromuscular movements, especially those of a finer nature, may deteriorate.

As the dose is increased, the individual may become assertive, arrogant and aggressive. At the same time the motor actions of the musculature are overtly incoordinated, speech becomes dysarthric, and arm and leg movements lack steadiness and precision, with a loss of balance. Simultaneously, the reflexes are slowed.

With the body level of ethanol rising still further, stupor may overtake the subject and, finally, coma may supervene, with respiratory depression and death.

The impact of ethanol on other parts of the body may be less obvious. The peripheral blood vessels may dilate, falsely creating a sense of bodily warmth when, instead, this increases heat loss from the body. Some compensating tachycardia may be noted, but it is doubtful whether the coronary arteries dilate to any meaningful degree. The salivary and gastric secretions may be increased, but the reputation of certain alcoholic liqueurs as aperitifs is more likely to be attributable to their taste, for they contain complementary and somewhat bitter ingredients.

Renally, ethanol is a diuretic, possibly by a direct effect on tubular reabsorption, although most likely with a reduction in the output of the antidiuretic hormone from the posterior pituitary gland. *See* Hormones, Pituitary Hormones

The mechanism by which ethanol interferes with the activity of the central nervous system is still not clearly understood. A plausible explanation is that modifications take place in the membrane surrounding the brain cells, or neurons. These are said to be deranged, becoming more fluid, so that the enzymes they contain no longer function normally. Neuronal function is consequently inhibited, with a corresponding effect upon the brain as a whole, albeit selectively in the different regions, as already described. The higher centres of the cerebral cortex are the first to be subdued, followed by the lower centres, with the vital centres in the medulla, subserving respiration and cardiovascular performance, being spared until the ethanol concentration in which they are bathed becomes overwhelming.

With an acute surfeit, as long as the vital centres are not suppressed, total recovery can follow, as the body load of ethanol decreases, in the same way as with a general anaesthetic.

Levels of Alcohol in the Body

What is so remarkable about ethanol, by contrast to the majority of drugs, including the recognized psychotherapeutic agents, is the close parallel between the blood concentrations and the manifest conduct of the individual, both mentally and physically. Whilst seasoned drinkers may exhibit some apparent compensation for what would otherwise be a departure from normality, the intensity of intoxication may be graded, generally speaking, as follows:

1. 50–150 mg alcohol per 100 ml blood: mild intoxication; delighted and devilish.
2. 150–300 mg alcohol per 100 ml blood: moderate intoxication; dizzy and delirious.
3. 300–500 mg alcohol per 100 ml blood: severe intoxication; dazed, dejected and drunk.
4. Over 500 mg alcohol per 100 ml blood: coma and death.

In some people, possibly of certain ethnic groups, there may be some variation but, overall, the figures are reliably indicative.

There is an almost constant correlation between levels of alcohol in the blood and those on the breath. Measurements of the ethanol in an expired sample of the air have found legal application in the laws promulgated in many countries for judging whether someone is fit to drive. Thus, in the UK, under the Road Traffic Act 1988 and its regulations, it is a statutory offence for anyone to have, on testing, a blood alcohol level in excess of 80 mg per 100 ml, or a level in an expired sample of air shown by an 'intoxi-meter' to be above 35 μg per 100 ml.

Chronic Ingestion of Alcohol

The effects of chronic alcoholism on the body differ from those of acute overdose.

The effects of chronic ingestion of alcohol on the brain are attributed to interference with the nutrient supply, particularly of vitamins, to the brain cells. Thus the effects tend to be accentuated whenever malnourishment concurrently exists. Changes are seen in behaviour, mood, sociability and judgement, coupled with muscular tremors and dysarthria. These may lead to Wernicke–Korsakoff syndrome, showing gross loss of memory with relatively little disruption of intellect. The peripheral nerves may exhibit damage recognizable as clinical polyneuritis. This may progress to Wernicke's encephalopathy, with ocular palsies interfering with vision, together with spasticity of the skeletal musculature and ataxia. The cerebellum may be involved, with gross changes in gait and speech.

Not infrequently, dementia may be a predominant feature, with euphoria and/or paranoia, either alone or in association with the other abnormal presentations already listed as being caused by brain damage.

Clinically the picture is often polymorphic, rather than pathognomonic, and diagnosis must rest on other features, including the patient's history.

Acute infection or sudden withdrawal of alcohol may lead to delirium tremens (DTs), which is associated with epileptiform convulsions, disorientation and vivid hallucinations. The hazards of long-term alcohol misuse are not confined to the brain; other organs may also be at risk.

Despite the magnitude of these mental and physical aberrations induced by habituation to alcohol, they can be reversible. Complete withdrawal, coupled with counselling, support and active management, can lead to complete rehabilitation, even if this may demand a closed environment at the outset, unrelenting professional surveillance and a patience to withstand the often long delay before recovery is achieved.

Liver

It is axiomatic that heavy drinkers suffer from liver disease. This belief is far from inaccurate, but such a fate is not universal. In this respect individual variation is common and, inexplicably, some alcoholics seem to escape completely from this complication. Whether there is a genetic explanation for this is not yet established. *See* Liver, Nutritional Management of Liver and Biliary Disorders

Liver complications may become apparent when anorexia, morning nausea and, perhaps, some diarrhoea and abdominal discomfort are noted. By this stage, biochemical tests of liver function, usually but not invariably, reveal damage to the liver cells. Even when such criteria are negative, direct liver biopsy may still demonstrate histologically the pathological appearance of swelling of the parenchymatous cells, with fatty infiltration.

As cirrhosis develops, the liver may become enlarged and, microscopically, may show widespread fibrosis, either portal in its distribution, or centrilobular. This may lead to obliteration of the bile ducts and, at the same time, obstruction of the portal vein. Allied to this, varices may develop at the lower end of the oesophagus, where the venous blood flow is shunted from the portal to the systemic route. Disruption of these distended vessels may be the cause of bleeding into the oesophagus and the vomiting of blood.

Jaundice of the skin, mucosae and eyes may be apparent, together with the presence in the skin, chiefly of the face, head, neck, shoulders and upper arms, of curious abnormalities of the veins which, being of arachnoid shape, are described as 'spider naevi'.

Gross liver failure may ensue, with all its devastating accompaniments – ascites (free fluid in the abdomen), a predisposition to uncontrollable infection and encephalopathy.

Heart

Ethanol acts as a direct toxin to the heart muscles, weakening their performance and bringing about cardiac failure. This may be quite independent of the other adverse effects of alcohol, as on the brain and liver.

Once the drinking is discontinued, cardiac decompensation may resolve. On the other hand, it may prove fatal, sometimes by sudden cardiac arrest.

It is clear that excessive alcohol consumption increases the risk of coronary artery disease. However, epidemiological studies point significantly to a lower incidence of this condition among moderate drinkers in comparison with teetotallers, indicating a protective effect of moderate levels of alcohol.

Pancreas

Pancreatic failure, which is often of uncertain aetiology, commonly features in conjunction with alcoholism. In the chronic form the alliance of the two conditions is well documented, but the sudden emergence of pancreatitis as an acute event is not so convincingly explained against an alcoholic background.

Gastrointestinal Tract

Although acute gastritis is widely accepted from an immoderate bout of drinking, the mucosa of the stomach soon returns to normal – as long as further alcohol is avoided. Habitual drinkers, however, are prone to chronic gastritis, without this necessarily predisposing to peptic ulceration.

There is some suggestion that alcohol disturbs the transport mechanisms of the small intestine, but the clinical relevance of this is dubious.

Effects in the Male

That a resort to drinking may incapacitate man's sexual prowess has been noted for centuries. Shakespeare, indeed, must have been minded of this when his porter in *Macbeth* declared '. . . it provokes the desire, but it takes away the performance'. Today these misgivings have been verified scientifically, for male alcoholics have been shown to suffer hypogonadism, with loss of libido and potency, testicular atrophy, lowered fertility, feeble beard growth, gynaecomastia and atypical distribution of body fat and hair.

Effects in the Female

In the female, the effects may be less obvious. However, besides raising the risk of spontaneous abortion, drinking alcohol during pregnancy can distort fetal development, bringing about, in its severe form, 'fetal alcohol syndrome'. The infant has a reduced birthweight, small head size, peculiar facial changes, mental deficiency, muscular incoordination and odd behavioural patterns. Lesser degrees of these defects may go unrecognized. *See* Pregnancy, Safe Diet

Endocrine System

Investigations have revealed hormonal changes in alcoholics, apart from those implicated in reproduction, but they are of uncertain clinical significance.

Nutrition

Chronic drinking is frequently attended by malnutrition, although the aetiology of this is complex. *See* Malnutrition, Malnutrition in Developed Countries

Cancer

There is support for a relationship between alcohol intake and cancer of the upper alimentary and respiratory tracts, in addition to cancer known to affect the liver.

Social Effects

With such a forbidding catalogue of calamities that can overtake anyone given to more than moderate drinking, in both body and mind, it is perhaps astonishing that alcohol consumption remains so popular. Health authorities inveigh against the practice with resounding intensity, yet, according to recent statistics, the consumption of such beverages, rather than falling, is rising both nationally and internationally.

As part of the World Health Organization (WHO) 'Health for All by the Year 2000' project, the UK is committed to make 'significant decreases in health damaging behaviour such as the use of alcohol'. How this is going to be achieved is unclear. Raising the price by swingeing additions to the excise duty has been vigorously advocated but, despite some limited benefit, it is doubtful whether this would deter other than small sections of the community. Meanwhile, the drinks industry continues to mount the most powerful and persuasive sales campaigns, and an increasing number of sports organizations are grateful for the sponsorship offered by drinks manufacturers. While the public at large remains relatively unperturbed, the explanation for such an attitude may be that, whereas nearly everyone has seen, or known, individuals whose lives have been disrupted personally, occupationally and domestically by licentious drinking, the vast majority of people imbibe socially without coming to any overt harm. Alcohol, it must be remembered, is pharmacologically a psychotropic (psychoactive) drug. If we are to rely on what the psychologists and psychiatrists tell us, a very large proportion of the population is beset by minor mental problems – from which alcohol may offer some relief.

Furthermore, so many of the favoured beverages are endowed with their own, characteristic flavours which can delight the palate – hence their role as aperitifs, accompaniments to the meal, digestifs and the like. Indeed, there are those people who drink discriminatingly more for the gustatory than for the psychotropic responses.

Well intentioned as the more zealous of the anti-alcohol campaigners may be, it is possible that total abstinence within the community is, after all, a chimera. The failure of the prohibition era in the USA is not to be forgotten. As with so many of the pleasurable diversions in life, it is possible that moderation in drinking will prove to be the desirable '*modus vivendi*', rather than total rejection.

Safe Level for Drinking

The consensus of various medical authorities is to set the maxima for alcohol intake at 21 'units' per week for men and 14 'units' for women, i.e. two to three standard drinks per head per day.

R. Goulding
London, UK

Alcohol Consumption

Trends and Levels of Alcohol Consumption in Different Countries

While the terms 'alcohol' and 'alcoholic beverages' tend to be used interchangeably to designate the product consumed, a distinction must be made between alcohol and ethanol. Alcohol consumption is usually expressed in grams of ethanol, which is a convenient standard to express the consumption of alcoholic beverages as varied as wine, beer or spirits. Personal interviews on alcohol intake tend to underestimate true intake, especially when subjects are only asked about drinking habits. Large-sample surveys provide distribution graphics for daily alcohol consumption in populations over their lifetime. In the USA, in 1981, alcohol dependence was most prevalent among men aged 21–34, and women in the reproductive years (ages 21–49) drank more heavily than older women. In France, the proportion of habitual drinkers increases with age, the heaviest alcohol drinkers belonging to the 45–54-year age group. *See* Dietary Surveys, Measurement of Food Intake

Household budget surveys contribute to national statistics by providing the share spent on alcoholic beverages. Caution must be exercised when using these figures as they do not take into account expenditure on alcohol outside the home. Furthermore, the choice of reference years may also imply some distortion when assessing time trends. In France, a country of high alcohol consumption, alcoholic beverages contributed 2% of the total household budget in 1985, whereas food products contributed 18%.

Although individual-based assessments of alcohol consumption are of benefit, time-trends and inter-country comparisons are also collated, along with information such as national statistics of production and trade in alcoholic beverages (Table 1). These statistics are calculated as the difference between the quantities produced and imported, and the quantities exported and in stock. They can also be calculated on the basis of sales statistics collected for taxation purposes. *See* Dietary Surveys, Surveys of National Food Intake; Dietary Surveys, Surveys of Food Intakes in Groups and Individuals

The regional disparities in alcohol consumption within a country must be considered, along with disparities in different population groups. For example, in Ireland, one third of the adult population is totally abstinent.

In order to take into account the variety of alcoholic beverages and their ethanol content, three groups have been determined: beer, wine and distilled spirits. These groupings are not clear-cut: for example, fortified wines are referred to as wines despite being richer in ethanol than table wines. The ethanol content of each class (beer, spirits and wine) is respectively approximated to 5%, 40% and 12% by volume.

International statistics show that since World War II alcohol consumption has dramatically increased in most developed countries, some having doubled or tripled

Table 1. Alcohol consumption in major consumer countries

Country	Consumption (litres per head per year)
France	13·0
Luxemburg	13·0
Spain	12·7
Switzerland	11·0
Hungary	10·7
Belgium	10·7
FRG	10·6
Portugal	10·5
GDR	10·5
Italy	10·0
Austria	9·9
Denmark	9·6
Bulgaria	8·9
Argentina	8·9
Australia	8·8
Czechoslovakia	8·6
The Netherlands	8·3
New Zealand	8·3
Romania	7·6
USA	7·6
Yugoslavia	7·6
UK	7·3
Poland	7·1
Finland	7·1
Japan	6·3
Uruguay	5·5
Sweden	5·4
Ireland	5·4
Greece	5·4
Chile	5·2
South Africa	4·4
USSR	3·2

Produktschap voor gedistilleerde dranken schiedam, Netherlands (1988). From: Statistiques, édition 1989. Paris: Association Nationale de Prévention de l'Alcoolisme.

Table 2. Percentage change in consumption of commercial alcoholic beverages (as ethanol) per head by type of beverage in six WHO regions, 1970–1977

Beverage	Africa	The Americas	Eastern Mediterranean	Europe	Southeast Asia	Pacific
Wine	−16·7	6·9	0·0	−4·2	0·0	200·0
Beer	9·1	17·1	8·3	15·6	100·0	20·7
Spirits	11·1	8·8	71·4	4·3	20·0	−24·3
All	7·3	11·3	12·5	3·0	25·0	−4·4

From Moser J (ed) (1985). *Alcohol policies in National Health and Development Planning.* WHO Offset Publication No. 89. Geneva: World Health Organization.

their consumption. Actually by the middle of the nineteenth century, the intake of alcoholic beverages was higher in most countries in Europe and North America than it is today. Alcohol intake in the USA peaked in 1830, at a rate twice that estimated for 1970. In the UK, alcoholic drinks were consumed in larger quantities in the eighteenth and nineteenth centuries than in the twentieth century, although there has been an increase from the historical low of 1930–1960. Beer, spirits and wines once provided at least 2 MJ per person per day compared with 0·67 MJ in 1975.

The world drinking pattern has been modified during the last 10 years. While in some countries, such as Finland and The Netherlands, alcohol consumption has recently become stable, or has even decreased, as in France, Portugal and Italy, it has increased in other countries, such as Japan, Korea, and some developing countries. In the latter, except in Muslim countries, European-style beverages have partly replaced traditional beverages, and an increasing trend is observed. Alcohol intake figures, which generally do not take into account consumption of locally produced beverages, are scarce in developing countries. However, available statistics show that some countries which experienced low consumption (about 1 l per head per year) have seen that figure double in 10 years. Some African countries, such as Burundi and Uganda, experience alcohol intakes as high as 13·8 and 11·7 l per head per year. Between 1970 and 1977 alcohol drinking has doubled in some islands, such as Barbados (16·2 l per capita per year in 1977), Trinidad, Tobago, Netherlands Antilles and Cyprus. An overview of percentage changes between 1970 and 1977 in the consumption of commercial alcoholic beverages (ethanol-equivalent) per head in six World Health Organization (WHO) regions shows the steady increase in consumption in Southeast Asia, the eastern Mediterranean and the Americas; Europe has experienced the lowest increase. Beer consumption has increased by 100% in Southeast Asia and spirits by 71% in the eastern Mediterranean region (Table 2).

National trends based on average consumption levels are only one aspect of the situation for it is clear that the pattern of beverages consumed has changed over the last 40 years. Generally, in countries such as France, where wine is the major alcohol drink and may represent 60% of the total consumption, beer consumption tends to increase, whereas in countries where beer is the preferred drink there is a shift to wine and spirits.

Some surveys of drinking habits, undertaken in Europe and North America, indicate that the consumption of alcoholic beverages is skewed, so that the relatively small group of heavier drinkers accounts for a large proportion of the country's alcohol consumption (1–10%). The general tendency in developed countries is to consume episodically a high quantity of alcoholic beverages. While a decreased intake is noticed in older age groups, abstention seems to be declining globally among teenagers in many countries. However, in the 1980s in some countries, such as the USA and Sweden, there has been a decline in alcohol use by teenagers. Although statistical data about developing countries is less frequent and not always reliable, it is likely that alcohol use follows in some way the pattern in developed countries.

Factors Influencing Alcohol Intakes

Because the influential factors vary between regions and countries, between groups within a country, between individuals belonging to the same social and ethnic groups, and between different times in the life of an individual, it is not a straightforward matter to portray precisely the factors that influence alcohol consumption. Nearly as far back as human beings have been traced on Earth, alcohol consumption has been identified. Initially consumed by religious leaders and ritualized during religious feasts, alcohol consumption extended to the general population in most ancient civilizations. In Egypt, 3500 years BC, wine and beer were consumed during ritual libations, funeral meals and feasts. Wine was often deified, and Osiris was widely considered as the homologue of Bacchus, the god of wine. Indo-European, Greek and Roman civilizations produced alcoholic beverages, and references to wine are found in the Old and the New Testament. Alcoholic beverages are mentioned in rituals of all the civilizations, although they can be forbidden by some religions such as Buddhism and Islam. The mythical and symbolic aspects of alcohol, and, more generally, the social aspects have continued through the centuries, even if certain restrictions appeared at an early stage. For example, pregnant women were advised against wine, and priests were not allowed to drink wine before entering the sacred tent.

With time, alcoholic beverages have become the trade commodities. Although alcohol drinking has become more a matter of individual taste in most societies, the social aspects of alcohol consumption are important. Positive and negative images of alcohol are numerous. Alcohol is known to remove inhibitions, yet it can be synonymous with depravity. These images and representations are strongly influenced by historical and sociological schools of thinking. At the beginning of the century, alcohol was considered to be a cause of degeneration and, reciprocally, degeneration and heredity were thought as responsible for alcoholism. Nowadays, owing to the profusion and the multiplicity of information from the mass media, the representations of alcohol are not straightforward. Advertising may influence alcohol consumption, especially in some sensitive social groups such as young adults, but its effectiveness remains an open question. Indeed, econometric studies based on correlations between the level of advertising and aggregate alcohol consumption have produced relatively weak and contradictory results.

Genetic predisposition to the utilization of particular substances has been shown in animal experiments and there is now some evidence that hereditary factors may predispose to harmful consequences of alcohol. Both features of an individual's personality and environmental factors play a major role in determining alcohol dependence. Education is important as these can be acted upon. For example, many studies have shown that alcoholics often mention family dismantling, scholastic problems or episodes of stress. Although poverty, unemployment and belonging to the unfavoured social classes may be considered risk factors, they are not systematically the major ones.

Historically, social controls on alcohol consumption have been stricter for women than for men. Differences in alcohol use between men and women, once dramatic, are narrowing. In France, 67% of men against 39% of women regularly drink one or more alcoholic beverages per day. Men are still at greater risk than women, but evidence shows that women with professional occupations consume more alcoholic drinks on average than men. Data collected in some developing countries show that the percentage of drinkers among young women is close to that observed in men of the same age.

Modifications in social habits and in the way of life can influence drinking patterns. Thus, in France, as meals tend to be taken out of the home, wine which traditionally accompanies meals tends to be substituted with beer and spirits. As migration, uncertainty of life conditions and social change have been direct or participative causal factors in high alcohol consumption reported in the USA in the eighteenth and the nineteenth centuries, these same factors are now met both in developing and developed countries. Investigations of social factors that influence drinking patterns have focused their concern on heavy drinkers, and our knowledge about the spread of alcohol use throughout society as a whole is not satisfactory.

A much as social factors, the economical factors influence alcohol intake. Over the centuries, the fluctuations in the consumption of alcohol closely follow the rise and fall in the national general trade. By replacing traditional techniques of processing alcohol beverages, industrial techniques have allowed increased production of alcoholic beverages, which has decreased market prices. In this respect, beer and distilled spirits have benefited more from these improvements than wines. Alcohol consumption has been shown to be sensitive to purchase price. For example, alcohol consumption has dramatically increased between 1950 and 1970 in the UK and at the same time the number of working minutes required for a manual worker to pay for a large loaf, a pint of beer and a bottle of whisky has changed from 9, 23 and 659 respectively in 1950 to 11, 12 and 209 in 1976.

As there is not one single and unique factor that influences alcohol drinking pattern, there is not one unique strategy to prevent alcohol abuse and its consequences. It is recognized that to be effective in the long term, national alcohol policies must emphasize information, prevention of alcohol dependency and control of alcohol availability. In fact, very few countries have fixed national objectives, e.g. to limit alcohol consumption at less than 5% of the total energy intake. It is generally agreed that education plays a major role in preventing alcoholism. Some authors claim that education has not yet shown its complete efficacy and that educational programmes seriously need to be directed at target groups and evaluated. It has been argued that a better knowledge of the consequences of alcohol abuse is unlikely to prevent the genesis of alcohol drinking unless it is associated with an active participation of concerned subjects, thereby leading to changes in attitudes and behaviour. Some education programmes have even been accused of reinforcing alcohol consumption. The prevention of alcoholism recidivism has shown little effect and primary prevention of alcohol abuse now seems preferable. The main objective is not to eradicate alcohol consumption but to prevent abuse of alcohol, and overall to encourage future generations, if they drink alcohol, to do so in moderation. To achieve that

Alcohol Consumption

aim, education must be initiated as soon as possible and the family is a favoured target area. To support this argument, one must be conscious that 61% of young Europeans between 11 and 15 years old have already taken alcohol at least once and that one child in four has had his or her first alcoholic drink before the age of 11, notably in Greece, the UK and Denmark.

Disorders Caused by Alcohol Intake

Alcoholism on its own has been recognized by the WHO as a disease: 'Alcoholics are excessive drinkers whose dependance on alcohol is such that they present either a discernible mental disorder or their physical and mental health, their relationships with others and their social and economic behaviour are affected'. Although that definition is a good reflection of the evidence that the effects of alcohol on public health are multiple and varied, alcohol-related problems cannot be limited to alcoholism. The impact of alcohol drinking is both specific in developing diseases and nonspecific in maintaining some morbidity states and giving rise to sociodemographic disorders. It is very difficult to quantify this in terms of public health and there is a general tendency to underestimate the related morbidity and mortality. Recent advances in medicine and biology have shown that the detrimental effects of alcohol are wider than previously thought and it is very likely that further advances are going to bring more evidence of those effects. *See* Diseases, Diseases of Affluence

Mortality resulting from alcohol use is very often roughly assessed from deaths classified as caused by alcoholism, alcoholic psychosis and liver cirrhosis. The cirrhosis death rate has long been considered as an indicator of alcohol use. In Europe, male mortality rates from liver cirrhosis and chronic diseases ranged from 3·5 per 100 000 in Ireland to 49·1 per 100 000 in Italy in 1980–1983; the female mortality rates ranged from 2·9 per 100 000 in Ireland to 20·2 per 100 000 in Hungary. A small and very recent decline in cirrhosis has been monitored; this is partly a result of decreased alcohol consumption but also a result of increased treatment of alcohol abuse, changes in diet and nutrition. Data collected in several countries show that the mortality rates are two to four times higher in excessive drinkers than in the general population. In France, 50 000 deaths are estimated to be attributed to alcohol, i.e. about 8% of the total mortality rate. It is quite obvious that mortality rates do not take account of moderate drinkers and the other deaths which could be explained by alcohol intake. Alcohol may partly contribute to death in accidents (traffic, occupation), deaths from suicides, homicides, bronchial diseases (e.g. tuberculosis) or unspecified causes, but the proportions are difficult to assess. *See* Liver, Nutritional Management of Liver and Biliary Disorders

There is now a body of evidence that alcoholic beverages are causally related to some cancers: oral cavity and pharynx, larynx and oesophagus. People with a daily consumption above 36 g ethanol have a two- to six-fold increased risk for oral cavity and pharyngeal cancer compared with nondrinkers. Heavy drinkers who are also heavy smokers, have a risk 15 times higher when compared with people who neither smoke nor drink. The risk for oesophageal cancer is 10- to 18-fold higher in people who drink more than 80 g ethanol per day when compared with non-drinkers. This risk is even higher (44-fold) in people who smoke more than 20 cigarettes per day. Suggestive but inconclusive data exists for a causal role of alcohol drinking in other cancers: rectum, liver and breast. *See* Cancer, Epidemiology; Oesophageal Cancer

Alcohol may contribute to many varied disorders such as gastritis, gastric ulcer, chronic pancreatitis, hepatitis and liver steatosis. Alcohol can lead to nutritional disorders such as deficiencies of vitamins B and A, folates and selenium, as well as energy–protein malnutrition. Alcohol and nutrition may interact in the genesis of liver cirrhosis. Obesity is also often present in alcohol users before they experience nutritional deficiencies. Metabolic disorders such as hypertriglyceridaemia and hyperuricaemia (gout) can be provoked or made worse by alcohol drinking. *See* Folic Acid, Physiology; Malnutrition, The Problem of Malnutrition; Obesity, Aetiology and Assessment; Selenium, Physiology *See also* individual vitamins

Effects of alcohol abuse on the central and peripheral nervous systems are numerous and abundantly described. They are as banal as inebriety and slower reflexes and as severe as delirium tremens, peripheral polyneuritis, paralysis, encephalopathy of Gayet-Wernicke (vitamin B deficiency) and Korsakoff's syndrome. In France, about one-third of male admissions to psychiatric hospitals are related to alcoholism.

Excessive consumption of alcoholic beverages during pregnancy is associated with the development of a syndrome of physical and mental manifestations – fetal alcohol syndrome – and of mental retardation in the offspring. Effects of moderate consumption have been associated with reduced birthweight, and behavioural deficits deserve further investigations.

Dependence on alcohol dramatically increases the incidence of cardiovascular diseases and the death rate peaks in 50-year-old men. A higher blood pressure is very often reported in heavy drinkers, and cerebral haemorrhage becomes less frequent as intemperance breaks off. Effects of low doses of alcohol on cardiovascular diseases are currently and extensively debated. Some authors argue that moderate intakes reduce the risk of coronary diseases, but more conclusive evidence is awaited. *See* Coronary Heart Disease, Intervention Studies; Wines, Dietary Importance

As scientific knowledge increases, a major problem in identifying the effects of alcohol on health is that alcohol intake is often associated with other behaviours and habits (tobacco, drugs, nutrition) which also affect health. It is not always straightforward to disentangle these effects from alcohol intake.

Finally, social and psychological disorders due to alcohol (rape, assaults, disabilities, lower productivity) must not be neglected even if they are not easy to assess quantitatively. When not taking account of human sufferings, the annual cost of alcohol-related disorders, both biomedical and psychosocial, was assessed at about $43 in 1979 by the US Department of Health, Education and Welfare. *See also* individual beverages

Bibliography

Barrucand D (1988) *Alcoologie*. France: Riom Laboratoires-CERM.
IARC (1988) *Evaluation of Carcinogenic Risks to Humans; Alcohol Drinking*, vol. 44. Lyon, France: International Agency for Research on Cancer.
Partanen J and Montonen M (1988) *Alcohol and the Mass Media*. EURO Reports and Studies 108. Copenhagen: World Health Organization, Regional Office for Europe.
Plant M (1990) *Alcohol-Related Problems in High-Risk Groups*. Report on a WHO Study. EURO Reports and Studies 109. Copenhagen: World Health Organization, Regional Office for Europe.
Regan TJ (1990) Alcohol and the cardiovascular system. *Journal of the American Medical Association* 264: 377–381.
Rotily M, Durbec JP, Berthezene P and Sarles H (1990) Diet, alcohol and liver cirrhosis: a case control study. *European Journal of Clinical Nutrition* 44: 595–603.
Spring JA and Buss DH (1977) Three centuries of alcohol in the British diet. *Nature* 270: 567–572.
Walsh B and Grant M (1985) Public health implications of alcohol production and trade. WHO Offset Publication No. 88. Geneva: World Health Organization.
WHO (1980) Alcohol-related problems. *World Health Organization Technical Report Series* 650.

M. Rotily
CAREPS Centre Hospitals, Grenoble, France

ALES

See Beers, Ales and Stouts

ALGAE

See Single-cell Protein and Marine Foods

ALKALOIDS

Contents

Properties and Determination

The alkaloids comprise a large group of basic nitrogenous compounds distributed widely, though in quantitatively minor amounts, in plant material. Their significance is due to the wide variety of marked physiological effects that result from their ingestion. Some of them, in attacking the central nervous system, can be rapidly fatal. Others, or the same ones in smaller doses, can cause narcotic, stimulatory or hallucinogenic effects. Addiction and dependence can frequently ensue. Yet others may be carcinogenic, or their toxicity may be manifest through effects on specific organs, e.g. the liver.

The function of alkaloids, from the point of view of the plant, has been widely debated. It has been established that they are not essential to the growth of plants, whether by serving as sources of soluble nitrogen or contributing to the preservation of ionic balance during growth. They may therefore be 'useless' metabolic end products. However, they may have a more positive role, having developed specifically as defence mechanisms against predators to ensure the plant's survival.

The term 'alkaloid' has not been precisely defined. Here it is confined to heterocyclic nitrogen bases derived biosynthetically directly from amino acids, involving oxidations, reductions, *trans*-alkylations or intra- or intermolecular condensations. It excludes the caffeine group of bases and favism factors, which, though physiologically active purines or pyrimidines, originate from nucleic acids. It also excludes linear bases such as ephedrine and mescaline, in which the basic nitrogen is not part of a ring. *See* Caffeine

Alkaloids are best known as drugs or poisons. However, several occur in foods, potential foods or food contaminants. Appropriate screening of certain common food commodities and of foods under development from new sources is important in quality assurance so that risks may be evaluated or eliminated.

Classification and Evaluation Problems

Alkaloids can be grouped in at least four different ways, in accordance with the discipline under consideration. Chemists, biochemists, botanists and physiologists will see them in terms, respectively, of chemical structure,

biogenetic origins, plant taxonomy and physiological response.

From a taxonomic viewpoint, though alkaloids are to be found in only a minority of plant species, these are widely, almost randomly, distributed throughout the plant kingdom. However, specific chemical classes tend to concentrate in defined plant families; for example, the isoquinoline alkaloids in the Papaveraceae, the quinolizidines in the Leguminosae and the carboline alkaloids in the Eleagnaceae. Many members of the same families will, however, be alkaloid-free.

In a single species, alkaloid levels will vary markedly in different parts of the plant. Thus, the solanine content of potatoes is high in the leaves, less in the sprouts, very low in the skins and negligible in the tissues of the tubers. Quantities vary considerably with variety, plant maturity and environmental conditions of growth.

A further complication is that one is dealing usually not with a single alkaloid but with two or more chemically distinct, if related, compounds in a single plant. These may well vary in relative amounts and in physiological response. Thus, though the group of lupin alkaloids includes at least five chemically individual compounds, one of them, lupanine (Fig. 1), is by far the most toxic.

Food Relevance

Major Crops

In terms of production volumes, plant material from three of the top-ranking world food crops, potatoes (sixth), tomatoes (15th) and rye (19th) may contain significant quantities of alkaloids. *See* Potatoes and Related Crops, Fruits of the *Solanaceae*; Rye; Tomatoes

Plant material from potatoes (*Solanum tuberosum*) may contain solanine (Fig. 2). The highest proportions of alkaloid are to be found in the leaves, though portions of the tubers exposed during growth, and consequently green, also contain appreciable levels. However, significant amounts do not normally occur in edible material. In the tomato (*Lycopersicon esculentum*) the closely related tomatine, also a glycoside of a steroid alkaloid, is to be found almost exclusively in the leaves of the plant or in the green unripe fruit. It should be remembered that other members of this family (the Solanaceae) contain highly toxic alkaloids (e.g. atropine, Fig. 2).

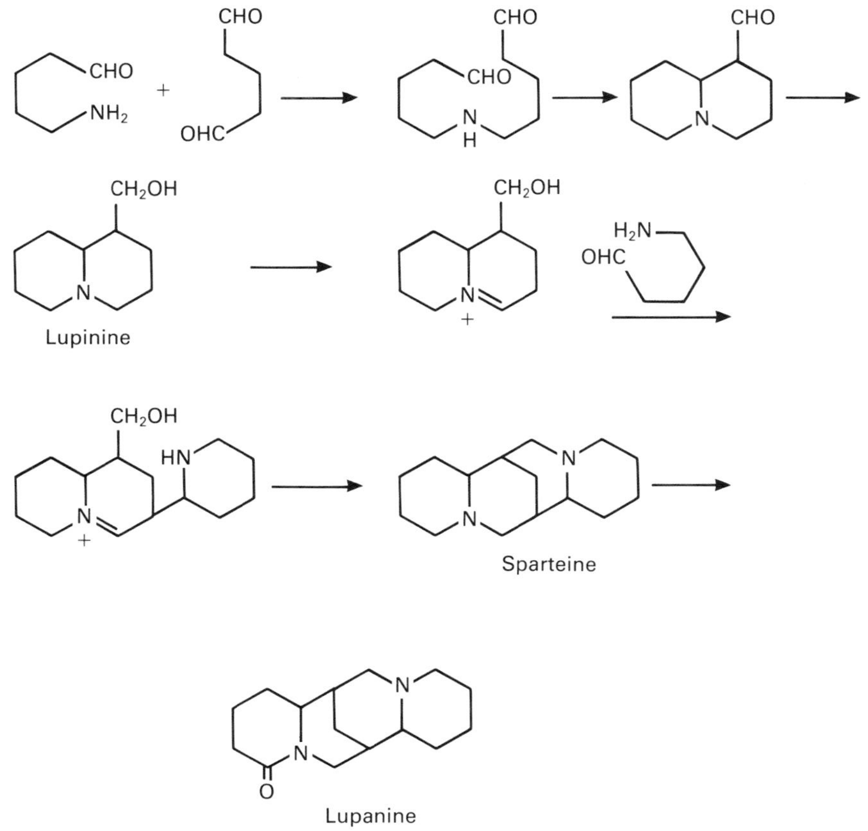

Fig. 1. Biosynthesis of some *Lupinus* alkaloids.

The case of rye (*Secale cereale*) is different. The crop as such is alkaloid-free but it may harbour the fungus *Claviceps purpurea* (ergot), which contains the highly toxic ergot alkaloids, such as ergonovine (Fig. 2).

Minor Crops and Crops under Development

Alkaloids are known to be present in several of these. For example, species of lupins (genus *Lupinus*) are important indigenous food plants in many countries, and under development in others. The beans may contain quite high proportions (up to 2%) of quinolizidine alkaloids. With a view to encouraging the use of such crops for food, selective breeding programmes have been undertaken to reduce the alkaloid contents. It has proved possible to develop alkaloid-free varieties in several species without deleterious effects on growth, maturation or yield. Other methods of removing alkaloids, such as prolonged soaking of beans in water and discarding the extract, are also practised. *See* Lupin

Weeds and Contaminants

Standard food raw material may occasionally be contaminated with alkaloid-bearing weeds. It is important that growers undertake seed analysis checks from time to time. Thus, though weed seeds can often be easily eliminated from main crop material by classification, if their seed sizes and ripening dates are similar they may escape detection. Thus, seeds of *Solanum nigrum* (black nightshade) may occasionally be found in those of poppyseed or rapeseed ('oilseed rape'), both of which are small-seeded crops.

Unconventional or locally traditionally foods, depending on domestic gathering of wild plants, are particularly at risk from adventitious contamination. Thus, the widespread occurrence of liver poisoning in several parts of the world has been attributed to the consumption of pyrrolizidine alkaloids (e.g. retronecine, Fig. 2) in foods varying from cereal products to herbal teas. Potent, but not exclusive, sources of these alkaloids are *Senecio* species (e.g. groundsel and ragwort). Stock pastured on land on which these are endemic are well known to avoid them meticulously when grazing.

Fungi

Though they are not plants, fungi should not be overlooked in the context of alkaloids in food. Mush-

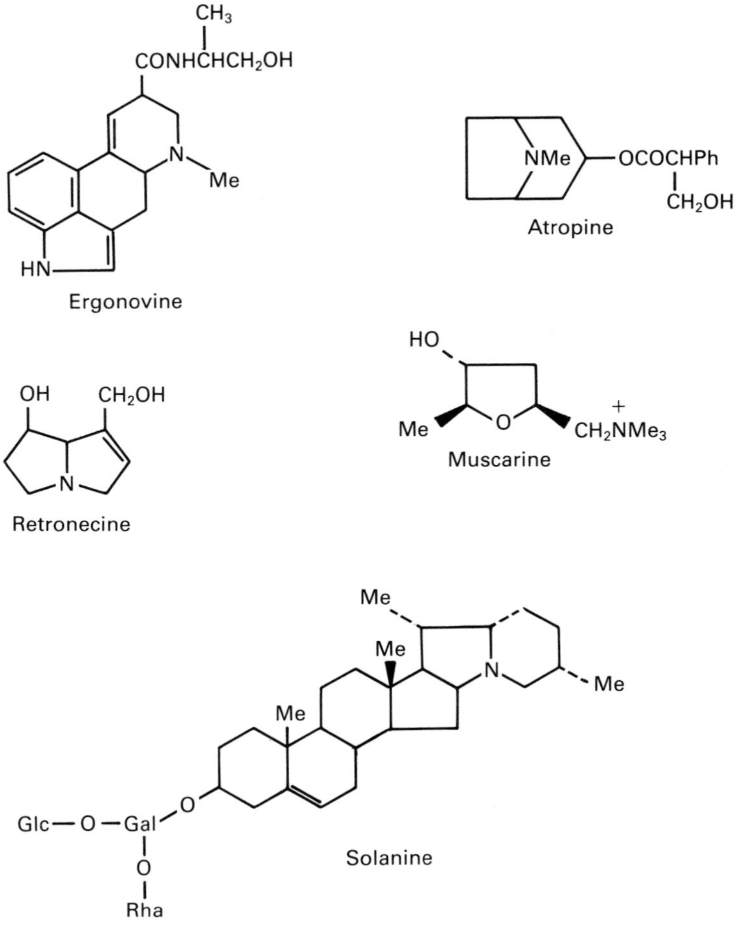

Fig. 2. Some alkaloids of possible relevance to food.

rooms, both cultivated and wild, are consumed in large quantities. Most of them are safe, but a few, especially those belonging to the genus *Amanita*, contain highly toxic 'alkaloids' such as muscarine (Fig. 2). Examples are *Amanita muscaria* (fly agaric) and *Amanita phalloides* (death cap). *See* Mushrooms and Truffles, Classification and Morphology

Biosynthesis, Chemical Structures and Properties

Details of biosynthetic pathways leading to specific alkaloids have still, in the main, not been fully elucidated. However, they are known to originate from amino acids. In the case of the lupin alkaloids (Fig. 1), lysine is decarboxylated to cadaverine, which, following oxidative deamination, affords lupinine. Intermolecular condensation leads to sparteine and this, finally, is oxidized to lupanine, the most predominant and toxic of the lupin alkaloids.

From Figs 1 and 2 some idea can be obtained of the diversity of structures to be found in the plant alkaloids.

Though they are usually tertiary bases they may contain various additional functional groups and they encompass a very wide range of molecular weights. Further, as tertiary bases, some of them are prone to facile oxidation to *N*-oxides, distinctively different from their parent bases. These features contribute to their widely disparate physical properties, and this in turn emphasizes the difficulty of recommending a general method of isolation from plant material and of subsequent identification. Suitable specific techniques are therefore applied to defined chemical groups (e.g. the quinolizidines) or botanical classes (e.g. the Compositae). A few key structures have been outlined in Fig. 2.

Alkaloid Analysis in Food Material

The presence of alkaloids in plant material can sometimes be detected immediately, e.g. from the characteristic bitter taste, as in leaves of *Lupinus* species, or the bright yellow colour in root tissue, due to the presence of berberine, in *Berberis* species. Normally, however, the investigation of plant material in which alkaloids are

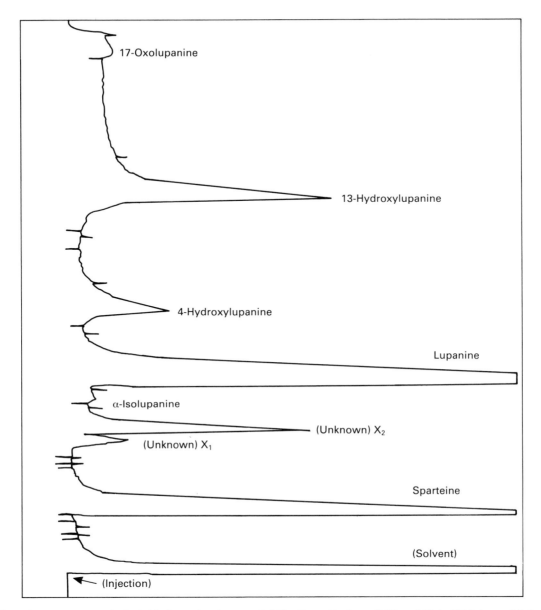

Fig. 3. Gas chromatogram of alkaloids from *Lupinus mutabilis*. From Hudson BJF and Gale MM (unpublished).

known or suspected to be present involves the extraction of finely powdered, dried plant tissue, which may be leaves, roots, flowers, fruit or seeds.

Extraction and Isolation

Dried plant tissue is extracted thoroughly with dilute hydrochloric acid or acetic acid and the solution clarified, concentrated and basified with ammonia. Alkaloids are liberated as solids, gums or (occasionally) liquids. Some are slightly water-soluble and necessitate extraction with chloroform. The dried alkaloid fraction, in the form of a standard solution in chloroform, is then subjected to a series of qualitative tests to establish its class and obtain some idea of individual components.

Qualitative Analysis

Paper chromatography was originally a favoured technique for preliminary investigation, but this has now been largely replaced by thin-layer chromatography (TLC), usually on silica gel, which is more sensitive and reproducible. Standards, most of which are commercially available, are run alongside test material. Elution is with a solvent system appropriate to the class of alkaloid under study. A good general system is methanol/concentrated ammonia (200:3, v/v). An acidic medium, in which ammonia is replaced by acetic acid, sometimes provides a useful contrast. *See* Chromatography, Thin-layer Chromatography

Spots are detected and identified either directly (colour, fluorescence under ultraviolet light, or fluores-

Properties and Determination

cence quenching on plates incorporating a fluorescent background) and/or after using specific spray reagents. Three of these, Dragendorff, Iodoplatinate and Marquis reagents, are used universally. Full details are to be found in the literature (see the Bibliography).

Quantitative Analysis

TLC, especially after the destructive application of spray reagents, is not suitable for quantification. It is therefore sometimes accompanied by ultraviolet spectrophotometry, particularly when a single alkaloid is involved and absorption maxima are in the region 250–350 nm. The many alkaloids incorporating aromatic systems, e.g. those based on pyridine, quinoline, isoquinoline and indole, are readily amenable to this form of quantification. However, others, such as the steroid alkaloids, and the pyrrolizidine and quinolizidine groups, do not respond usefully.

Alkaloids with some degree of volatility can be quantified by gas chromatography (GC). The lupin alkaloids may be analysed successfully by GC, using a 10% SE-30 column programmed to operate at 220–260°C. All individual components are clearly differentiated by this method (Fig. 3). *See* Chromatography, Gas Chromatography

The steroid glycoalkaloids are not determined by the foregoing methods. They, as well as several other classes of alkaloids, can be analysed, however, by high-performance liquid chromatography (HPLC). A Zorbax SIL column with hexane/methanol/acetone (18:1:1, v/v/v) as the solvent is used, detection depending on the ultraviolet absorption maximum at 213 nm. For food specialists this is an important group of alkaloids. A new method of analysis relies on enzyme-linked immunosorbent assay (ELISA), involving an antiserum raised against a solanine–bovine serum albumen conjugate. Potato crops can be rapidly screened by this technique. *See* Chromatography, High-performance Liquid Chromatography; Immunoassays, Radioimmunoassay and Enzyme Immunoassay

Bibliography

Clarke EGC (1970) The forensic chemistry of alkaloids. In: Manske HF (ed.) *The Alkaloids*, vol. XII, pp 514–590. New York: Academic Press.

Harborne JB (1984) *Phytochemical Methods*, 2nd edn pp, 192–202, 218–221. London: Chapman and Hall.

Hudson BJF, Fleetwood JG and Zand Moghaddam A (1976) Lupin: an arable food crop for temperate climates. *Plant Foods for Man* 2: 81–90.

Hill GD (1977) The composition and nutritive value of lupin seed. *Nutrition Abstracts and Reviews Series B* 47: 511–527.

Huxtable RJ (1980) Herbal teas and toxins: novel aspects of pyrrolizidine poisoning in the United States. *Perspectives in Biology and Medicine* 24: 1–13.

Mattocks AR (1967) Detection of pyrrolizidine alkaloids on thin-layer chromatograms. *Journal of Chromatography* 27: 505–508.

Morgan MRA, McNerney R, Matthew JA, Coxon DT and Chan HW-S (1983) An enzyme-linked immunosorbent assay for total glycoalkaloids in potato tubers. *Journal of the Science of Food and Agriculture* 34: 593–598.

Rehacek Z and Sajdi P (1990) *Ergot Alkaloids–Chemistry, Biological Effects, Biotechnology*. Amsterdam: Elsevier.

Siegler DS (1977) *Alkaloids*, vol. 16, pp 1–82. New York: Academic Press.

Stumpf PK and Conn EE (1981) *Secondary Plant Products. The Biochemistry of Plants*, vol. 7. New York: Academic Press.

B. J. F. Hudson
University of Reading, Reading, UK

Toxicology

Alkaloids are widely distributed in the plant kingdom and many are highly toxic to animals and man. It is unsurprising, therefore, that in general these compounds do not feature widely amongst plants grown as human foods or animal feedstuffs. There are exceptions, notably the glycoalkaloids in the potato and other members of the family Solanaceae, and the quinolizidine alkaloids of range and grain lupins. Mention must also be made of the isoquinuclidine alkaloids of yams (*Dioscores* spp.), a staple food in many tropical countries, and the pyrrolizidine alkaloids, which may enter the food chain through a number of channels, including contamination of grain, use of herbal medicines or 'health' products. This article briefly reviews the nature, occurrence and toxic effects of these structurally diverse compounds.

Solanum Glycoalkaloids

Solanum glycoalkaloids are found primarily in the common potato (*Solanum tuberosum* L), and also occur in the tomato (*Lycopersicon esculentum*), aubergine, and red and green peppers. Since the beginning of the last century it was thought that the cultivated potato contained only one alkaloid, 'solanine', but this is now known to be a mixture of solanines and chaconines. A number of other, minor alkaloids, such as α- and β-solamarine, and demissidine, have now been isolated from *S. tuberosum*. These were introduced as a result of the use of 'wild' (noncultivated and nonedible) varieties, such as *S. chacoense* and *S. demissum*, in breeding programmes; other alkaloids, such as leptinines, leptines, demissine and commersonine, may be introduced in a similar manner. Whilst tomatines are found together with other steroidal alkaloids in the genus

Solanum, they occur alone in *Lycopersicon* species. *See* Potatoes and Related Crops, Fruits of the *Solanaceae*; Tomatoes

Structure

Potato glycoalkaloids comprise a nitrogen-containing steroidal aglycone attached to a sugar chain at the C3 position. α-Chaconine (Fig. 1a) and α-solanine (Fig. 1a) both contain a common aglycone, solanidine (solanid-5-en-3β-ol) linked to the trisaccharides, β-chacotriose and β-solatriose, respectively. The β- and γ-chaconines and solanines possess di- and monosaccharide chains, respectively. Tomatine (Fig. 1b) contains the tetrasaccharide, β-lycotetraose, linked to the aglycone, tomatidine. Partial hydrolysis yields β(1)- and β(2)-tomatines (loss of xylose and glucose, respectively) and γ-tomatine (loss of both xylose and glucose).

Occurrence and Levels

In the potato, glycoalkaloids occur in all parts of the plant, with highest levels being found in sprouts (2–4 g per kg fresh weight), flowers (3–5 g kg^{-1}) and leaves (0·4–1 g kg^{-1}). In the tubers the alkaloids are located mainly in the skin and peel. Typical figures for commercial varieties are shown in Table 1.

α-Tomatine had been isolated from all parts of the tomato plant (Table 2). The alkaloid is readily metabolized to allopregnenolone (3β-hydroxy-5α-pregn-16-en-20-one) during ripening; red-ripe tomatoes lose almost all of their α-tomatine content if left on the plant for 2–3 days.

Factors Affecting Levels

The levels of glycoalkaloids, like those of other secondary metabolites, are affected by a number of factors.

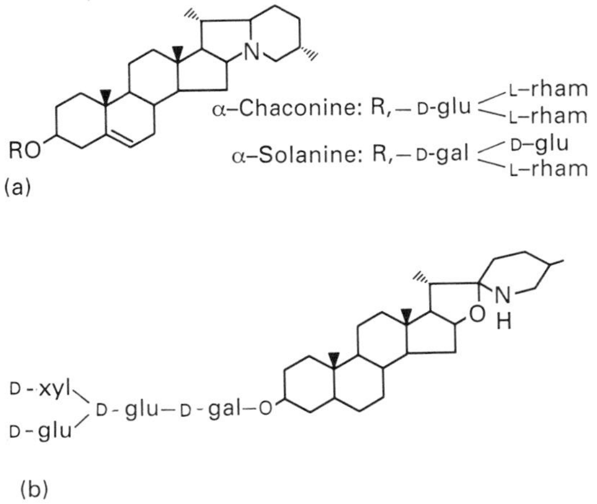

Fig. 1   (a) α-Chaconine and α-solanine; (b) tomatine.

Table 1.   Total glycoalkaloid contents of flesh and peels of commercial potato tubers

Variety	Fresh flesh (mg kg^{-1})	Peel (mg kg^{-1})
Russet Burbank	16–45	380–700
Kennebec	13–42	830–1070
Katahdin	3–6	310–730
Green Mountain	1–5	220–260
Superior	1–3	210–260
Russet	0·4–2	40–70

From Bushway RJ *et al.* (1983) *Journal of Food Science* 48: 84, with permission.

Table 2.   α-Tomatine content of tomato plant and fruit

Plant part	α-Tomatine content (mg kg^{-1})
Leaves	8600–19 000
Flowers	9300–22 000
Fruit	
Green	870
Yellow	450
Red (ripe)	360

From Jadhav *et al.* (1981), with permission.

Cultivar type, agronomy, environment and climate can all significantly affect levels. When field or harvested potatoes are exposed to light, chlorophyll will accumulate and 'greening' occurs. Increased synthesis of glycoalkaloids will occur under these conditions, giving rise to the warning against consuming green potatoes. Since high levels of glycoalkaloids will also be found in potato sprouts and around damaged and blighted areas, quality control is vital when selecting potatoes for cooking and processing. This is particularly important since most domestic and industrial potato processing conditions, including frying, have little effect on glycoalkaloid levels. Since the synthesis of chlorophyll and glycoalkaloids are stimulated by light of different wavelengths, the absence of greening cannot be taken necessarily as an indication of low glycoalkaloid content. Tomato plants will accumulate α-tomatine in response to fungal infection. Any process which encourages the ripening of the fruit would be expected to reduce alkaloid levels.

Mechanical damage (including bruising, slicing and cutting, as well as cellular disruption caused by infection or infestation) will result in accumulation of glycoalkaloids, the extent of which will depend upon the variety, the degree of damage, and the nature and length of subsequent storage. Since this effect will be enhanced at higher temperatures it is important that cut potato products be stored at low temperatures, and out of high light intensity, prior to further processing and cooking.

Bitterness

Potatoes containing more than 140 mg of glycoalkaloids per kg possess a bitter taste, with higher levels causing a burning sensation in the mouth and throat. Whilst such undesirable characteristics are certainly an indication of toxic levels, it must be realized that in strongly flavoured or spiced dishes, the taste sensations may be partly or wholly masked.

Toxicity

Potato glycoalkaloids are effective cholinesterase inhibitors; losses of poultry and livestock following ingestion of potato vines, sprouted and culled potatoes and potato peel have been recorded. In humans, severe illness and even deaths have followed the accidental consumption of damaged, green, sprouted or otherwise poor-quality potatoes. Poisoning is characterized by abdominal pain, vomiting and diarrhoea, with additional neurological symptoms of apathy, drowsiness, mental confusion, hallucinations, dizziness, trembling and visual disturbance also being common. Acute poisonings have been linked to the ingestion of potatoes containing over 300 mg of glycoalkaloids per kg. The suggestion that potato glycoalkaloids might also be responsible for the incidence of two severe birth defects, anencephaly and spina bifida, is no longer credited. Glycoalkaloids have caused illness and death in pigs consuming green tomato plants. Bearing in mind the reduction in levels in ripe fruit, it is unlikely that there is a danger to human health from this source, but the risk that small children may eat green tomatoes, and potato 'apples' is real. The latter, and *S. nigrum* berries, have been occasionally reported in processed (canned, frozen) beans.

Mean daily intake of glycoalkaloids in the UK is approximately 25 mg. Of more interest will be the intakes of those individuals consuming large amounts of potato daily; recent dietary trends, in particular the regular consumption of potato peel (in the form of jacket potatoes, or whole potato snack products), will also increase glycoalkaloid intakes. Some people currently consume potato peel in the mistaken belief that it is rich in fibre and nutrients; neither of these claims is true and the excessive consumption of potato peel in any form should be discouraged. Recent findings indicate that glycoalkaloids have a potent permeabilizing effect on the intestine. Further research is needed to ascertain

the extent of this effect in humans, and to determine the nature of any chronic toxicity.

Lupin Quinolizidine Alkaloids

The genus *Lupinus* contains both poisonous species, and others which have been widely cultivated as grain crops and forages. The potential of lupin as a source of animal feed and human food has been limited by problems of bitterness and toxicity which are associated with the presence of a number of alkaloids possessing the di-, tri- and tetracyclic quinolizidine skeletons. Considerable efforts to reduce the levels of these compounds in domesticated lupins have been made by plant breeders, whilst the possibility of their post-harvest removal has also been investigated.

Structure

Approximately 70 quinolizidine alkaloids have been reported in wild and cultivated lupins. The bicyclic quinolizidines are based on lupinine (Fig. 2a), whilst angustifoline (Fig. 2b) is typical of the tricyclic alkaloids. The largest group are the tetracyclic compounds, which may be further sub-divided to groups based on sparteine (Fig. 2c), lupanine (Fig. 2d), anagyrine (Fig. 2e) and multiflorine (Fig. 2f).

Occurrence and Levels

Factors Affecting Levels

There is very considerable variation in alkaloid content amongst different lupin species. Within a given species, considerable fluctuations have been reported for both the levels and occurrence of individual compounds. This clearly makes overreliance on literature values, or data gathered from previous seasons, dangerous. 'Sweet' cultivars of lupin species containing as little as 0·1% of the initial levels (equivalent to 20–30 mg per kg of seed) have been developed, and corresponding improvements might be expected in other species following the application of the newer techniques of plant biotechnology. Environmental, developmental and cultural factors are all known to affect the profiles and contents of lupin alkaloids, and hence the toxicity of the plant. There is considerable variation in alkaloid levels between different parts of the same plant. Alkaloids accumulate in the upper, green parts during vegetative growth and are translocated to the pods and seed after flowering; levels in the latter may be 10–15 times greater than in the green tissue.

Traditionally, lupins have been processed to reduce toxic alkaloids by washing the seed. This process, as

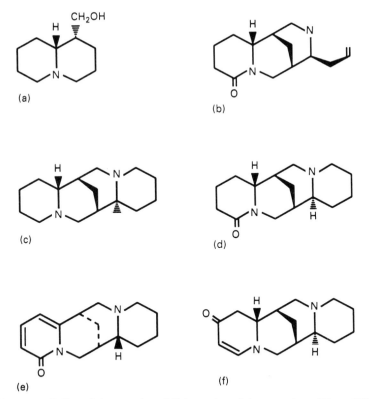

Fig. 2 (a) Lupinine; (b) angustifoline; (c) sparteine; (d) lupanine; (e) anagyrine; (f) multiflorine.

carried out by Andean families may reduce levels to less than 1 g kg^{-1}, but has the disadvantage of considerable loss of protein. Improved washing processes may reduce the original alkaloid content to 20 mg kg^{-1}, with 90% of the protein retained. Other techniques have utilized solvent extraction, both on the seed itself (whereby an important oil fraction is also produced) or after an initial defatting process. As with all such processes, the introduction of these or other methods will be determined by economic judgements.

Toxicity

In grazing animals, lupin toxicity may be characterized by a number of symptoms, including laboured breathing, lethargy, trembling and convulsions, with death resulting from respiratory paralysis. A congenital deformation of cattle, 'crooked calf' disease, is a result of maternal consumption of lupin species containing the teratogenic alkaloid, anagyrine. There is considerable species sensitivity to lupin alkaloids; for guinea pigs the most toxic alkaloid is lupanine and for mice, sparteine. In general, the minimum lethal doses (intraperitoneal; ip) range between 20 and 200 mg per kg bodyweight.

Symptoms of lupin poisoning in humans include lethargy, nausea, respiratory arrest, visual disturbance, ataxia, progressive weakness and coma. Human fatalities have followed the ingestion of doses of 11–46 mg total alkaloids per kg, whilst an oral dose of 30 mg of sparteine per kg caused death. In a pregnant woman, ip injection of 2 mg of sparteine per kg proved fatal. On the basis of such data it may be concluded that 25 g of bitter (alkaloid content 30 g kg^{-1}) lupin would cause severe illness, if not death. In contrast, over 20 kg of a sweet cultivar would need to be consumed to cause an equivalent effect. Although no anagyrine was found in a limited survey of lupin selections used as human food, the fact that it has been found in the milk of a goat fed lupin seeds emphasizes the importance of vigilance in this area.

Isoquinuclidine Alkaloids

Tubers of wild Dioscorea yams, although toxic, are commonly used as an emergency food in West Africa (*Dioscorea dumetorum*) and Southeast Asia (*D. hispada*). If the plants are not properly processed prior to consumption, serious illness and death may result. Highly toxic yams are sometimes planted amongst cultivated yams to protect against thieves.

Structure

Many species of yam contain dioscorine (Fig. 3) and its dihydro derivative, possessing the isoquinuclidine skele-

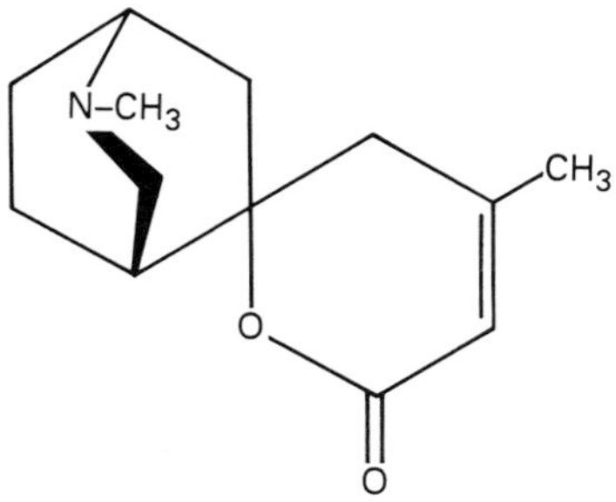

Fig. 3 Dioscorine.

ton, but the opening of the lactone ring may lead to the formation of a number of other alkaloids.

Toxicity

The symptoms of Dioscorea poisoning include speech disturbance, abdominal pain, vomiting and diarrhoea, vertigo and delirium; in acute cases, death occurs between 3 h and 7 days. Even small quantities of toxic yams may cause death, whilst ingestion of sublethal quantities of dioscorine and its analogues are associated with anorexia and distension. Detoxification is usually achieved by thorough washing and leaching of the water-soluble alkaloids.

Pyrrolizidine Alkaloids

It has been estimated that 3% of the world's flowering plants, some 6000 species, contain pyrrolizidine alkaloids, and their possible entry into the human food chain is considerably more diverse than for the other alkaloids considered above. Major losses of livestock around the world have resulted from ingestion of *Senecio* species (including *S. jacobaea*, tansy ragwort), *Echium* species, *Crotolaria spectabilis*, *Cynoglossum officinale* and *Heliotropium europaeum*. Human intoxications have followed the consumption of grains (contaminated with *Heliotropium*, *Senecio* and *Crotolaria* spp.), of *Symphytum* or *Petasites* as green vegetables, and the use of a variety of pyrrolizidine-alkaloid-containing 'health' products, herbal remedies and tonics. Additional, secondary exposure routes, via milk and honey, are also possible but only in extreme cases are these judged likely to represent a serious health hazard to humans. *See* Health Foods, Definition and Dietary Importance; Health Foods, Dietary Supplements; Herbs, Herbs and their Uses

Structure

Not all pyrrolizidine alkaloids are toxic; the requirements for toxicity appear to be unsaturation at the C1

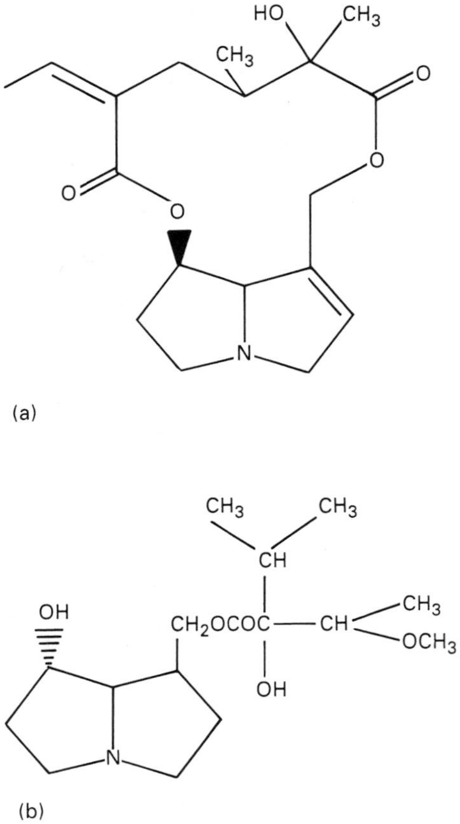

(a)

(b)

Fig. 4 (a) Senecionine; (b) heliotrine.

position of the bicyclic nucleus, and branching of the ester grouping. Typical examples are senecionine (Fig. 4a) and heliotrine (Fig. 4b); cyclic diesters, such as the former, are most toxic. The toxicity of the pyrrolizidine alkaloids is caused by the formation of pyrrole metabolites.

Occurrence and Levels

Pyrrolizidine alkaloids, and their corresponding N-oxides are found in all parts of the plant. In Russian comfrey (a hybrid of comfrey, *Symphytum officinale*, and *S. asperum*) mixtures are found at levels ranging from 30 to 1150 mg kg^{-1}, whilst roots of *S. asperum* contain over 5 g kg^{-1}. Alkaloid contents of 0·3–3·9 and 0·3–0·95 ppm have been found in honeys from bees feeding on *Senecio* and *Echium*, respectively. Tissue levels of pyrrolizidine alkaloids and their metabolites are metabolized very rapidly after exposure and are almost completely removed after 24 h; hence only in the unlikely situation of animals being killed and eaten immediately after a large intake would there be any likelihood of human exposure from this source. The contents of pyrrolizidine alkaloids in certain herbal teas will vary according to the nature of the plant, its origin and the presence of contaminating species. The method of preparation is also important. For example, a cup of tea prepared from a comfrey root preparation contained 8·5 mg of alkaloids, but when the gelatinous residue was consumed, the exposure increased to 26 mg. Alkaloid contents of comfrey-containing digestive aids vary from 270–2900 mg kg^{-1}, implying a likely daily dose of up to 2 mg.

Factors Affecting Levels

Alkaloid levels vary with the plant part examined, climate, soil conditions and plant maturity. In comfrey, for example, they are highest in the early stages (preflower and early bud stage) of vegetative growth and decline with maturity. The roots contain higher levels than the leaves, and drying of the latter further concentrates the toxic principles. Storage of dried *Senecio* plants for 22 months had no effect on alkaloid levels. Pyrrolizidine alkaloids in hay are not decomposed by curing, and although some decomposition will occur during ensilage, the amounts consumed by animals and the toxicity of the alkaloids have resulted in numerous cases of poisonings. Since there is variation in the natures of the alkaloids found in different parts of the plant, toxicities will also vary; thus ragwort flowers and leaves (containing sneciphylline and jacobine, respectively) were more toxic to rats than to the roots, whilst the stems were apparently nontoxic.

Toxicity

In animals, typical symptoms of pyrrolizidine alkaloid poisoning include enlargement of the hepatocytes, liver fibrosis, biliary hyperplasia and consequent signs of liver dysfunction, such as hyperbilirubinaemia, hypoalbuminuria, jaundice and ascites. Once again there is considerable species sensitivity, with cattle and horses much more susceptible than sheep and goats.

In humans, poisonings usually involve liver damage and in particular, veno-occlusive disease. This latter condition, which may be considered characteristic of pyrrolizidine alkaloid poisoning, is characterized by a dull ache in the right upper abdomen, which is rapidly filled with ascites and consequently distended. Mortality is high, from liver failure or, in chronic cases, the consequences of cirrhosis. Liver diseases caused by the contamination of cereal grains has been reported in rural areas of India, USSR, South Africa and Afghanistan. In the largest outbreak in Afghanistan 8000 people were affected, and an incidence of mortality of 20–25% was recorded. Human poisonings resulting from the use of pyrrolizidine-alkaloid-containing herbal products have been reported in all parts of the world, with the main species involved being *Crotolaria*, *Heliotropum*, *Senecio*, *Symphytum* and *Gynura*. *Symphytum*-containing preparations (including those based on comfrey or Russian comfrey) are considered to pose a particular hazard through their widespread use, variable composition and generally high exposure. In view of the published data, it is appropriate to echo the recommendations of RJ Huxtable (in Cheeke, 1990) concerning ways of reducing the risk of pyrrolizidine-alkaloid poisoning:

1. Do not give herbs to babies.
2. Do not take a large quantity of any one preparation.
3. Do not take anything containing comfrey.

See Plant Toxins, Detoxification of Naturally Occurring Toxicants of Plant Origin

Bibliography

Cheeke PR (ed.) (1990) *Toxicants of Plant Origin*. Boca Raton, Florida: CRC Press.
Cheeke PR and Shull LR (1985) *Natural Toxicants in Feeds and Poisonous Plants*. Westport, Connecticut: AVI Publishing.
Jadhav SJ, Sharma RP and Salunkhe DK (1981) Naturally-occurring toxic alkaloids in food. *CRC Critical Reviews in Toxicology* 5: 21.
Kinghorn AD and Balandrin MF (1984) In: Pelletier SW (ed.) *Alkaloids, Chemical and Biological Perspectives*, vol. 2. New York: John Wiley.
Kuc J (1975) In: Runeckles VC (ed.) *Recent Advances in Phytochemistry*. New York: Plenum Press.
Maga JA (1980) Potato alkaloids. *CRC Critical Reviews in Food Science and Nutrition* 12: 371.
Mattocks AR (1986) *Chemistry and Toxicology of Pyrrolizidine Alkaloids*. London: Academic Press.
WHO (1988) *Pyrrolizidine Alkaloids*. Environmental Health Criteria 80. Geneva: World Health Organization.

R. Fenwick
Food Research Institute, Norwich, UK

ALLERGENS

Substances that give rise to allergic symptoms are called allergens. Usually the term is restricted to antigens that induce specific immunoglobulin E (IgE) production in susceptible individuals leading to a type I allergic or immediate hypersensitivity reaction following a second or subsequent contact with the same antigen. Although, in principle, any antigen or hapten may act as an allergen, it is not understood what makes an antigen an allergen. There are no known common structural or physicochemical properties of allergens distinctive from nonallergenic antigens. Most known allergens are proteins or glycoproteins, whilst a few have been found to be polysaccharides. Most isolated protein or glycoprotein allergens are globular proteins with molecular weights in the range of 10 000–40 000 Da and isoelectric points in the range pH 4–6. Amino acid sequencing and molecular cloning of allergens reveal no structural homologies that discriminate allergens from other antigens.

So far there is little known about the biological function of most allergens. Some have been shown to be enzymes such as the insect venom allergens phospholipase A_2 and hyaluronidase, some are transport proteins like mammalian serum albumin and some have digestive functions such as the major allergen Der p I of the house dust mite *Dermatophagoides pteronyssinus*, which was recently shown to have significant amino acid sequence homology with a cysteine protease.

Allergens may enter the body by inhalation, ingestion or injection. Inhalent allergens enter the body through the mucosa of the nose and lung. Many are derived from environmental sources such as pollens of trees, weeds and grasses. These allergens are seasonal because their occurrence depends on blossom periods in defined seasons. Further important sources of inhalent allergens are mould spores and mycelia, proteins derived from animal dander, serum, saliva and urine, and the perennial indoor allergens derived from arthropods like house dust mites, storage mites and cockroaches. Ingested allergens are those present in certain foods and drugs. Adverse reactions to food are most common during infancy and childhood. IgE antibodies to food allergens frequently occur in atopic children and at low titres also in some nonatopic children. Symptoms may occur if food allergens penetrate the gut barrier and interact with their corresponding IgE antibodies on the mast cells in the gut wall, skin or respiratory tract. The most important allergens in food-induced allergic reactions are derived from eggs, milk, nuts, seafood, legumes and cereals. Recently proteins of potatoes have been characterized as another cause of food allergy. Since food allergens are often affected by degradation during digestion, the diagnosis of food allergic reactions can be very difficult. Allergenic drugs as well as food additives like dyes can act as haptens that induce IgE responses after combining with human protein. Injected allergens are mainly venom components of stinging insects like bees, vespids or ants.

Allergen Extracts

Allergens are responsible for IgE-mediated allergic reactions in humans like hay fever, rhinitis, asthma, etc. Since 1911, extracts prepared from different allergen sources have been used continuously and systematically in human medicine for diagnosis and therapy of IgE-mediated allergic diseases. The success of diagnosis and therapy is strongly influenced by the quality of the extracts. A prerequisite for good allergen extract is the quality of the source material as well as use of a standardized production process. It is essential that each raw material is as pure as possible. The source material should be described in a very detailed manner. This description must include particulars concerning collection, preparation and storage. Today most raw materials are produced by specialized companies on an industrial scale. From such raw materials produced under controlled conditions allergen extracts are prepared.

High-quality raw materials are available for most important allergens, e.g. pollens, animal epithelia, moulds, mites (Fig. 1) and venoms. At present, some companies are also starting to produce high-quality raw materials of different foods such as pesticide-free apples or antibiotic-free milk.

Pharmaceutical allergen preparations must be manufactured in compliance with the principles of good manufacturing practices (GMP) as established by the World Health Organization and in the near future according to the EEC guide to GMP.

Figure 2 shows a flow diagram for the preparation of an extract starting with the raw material and ending with the bulk material. Prior to extraction the quality of the raw material will be checked by microscopic analysis. Most raw materials are defatted with petroleum ether (boiling point 40–60°C) and then extracted with a physiological salt solution. Extraction is performed by stirring the raw material with the salt solution at 4–6°C overnight (if the extract is to be freeze dried, a 'volatile buffer' must be used). Then it is clarified by centrifuga-

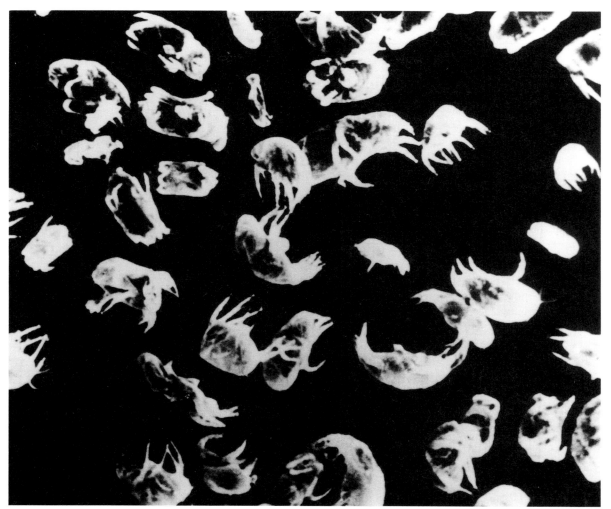

Fig. 1 Scanning electron micrograph of house dust mite (*D. pteronyssinus*) bodies. Only mite bodies can be seen and no contamination with culture medium on which the mites are grown.

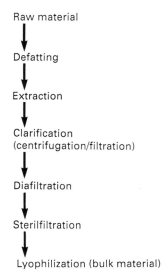

Raw material
↓
Defatting
↓
Extraction
↓
Clarification
(centrifugation/filtration)
↓
Diafiltration
↓
Sterilfiltration
↓
Lyophilization (bulk material)

Fig. 2 Flow diagram for the preparation of an allergen extract.

tion and filtration. To exclude low-molecular-weight substances, like histamine and histamine-related substances, which may cause irritation when used for diagnosis and therapy, the extracts are dialysed or diafiltered, respectively. This is also of special importance for food allergens since some foods, like fish, etc., can contain free histamine. After diafiltration the extracts are sterile filtered and freeze dried. From this freeze-dried bulk material the medical products used for diagnosis and therapy are prepared. *See* Histamine

Allergen extracts are complex mixtures that can be composed of five or even more than 50 individual antigenic components. In general, all proteins can be regarded as potential allergens. As most of the allergens are proteins or glycoproteins, chemical, biochemical and immunochemical methods are used for characterization of allergen extracts. Since there are numerous procedures reported for allergen extracts, many different guidelines have been prepared. The methods shown in Table 1 are the most frequently used *in vitro* methods

Table 1. Methods frequently used in allergen extract characterization and standardization

Protein determination
Carbohydrate determination
High-performance thin-layer chromatography (HPTLC)
High-performance liquid chromatography (HPLC)
Isoelectric focusing (IEF)
Sodium dodecyl sulphate polyacrylamide gel–electrophoresis (SDS–PAGE)
Crossed immunoelectrophoresis (CIE)
Crossed radioimmunoelectrophoresis (CRIE)
Immunoblot: immunoprint (IP), Western blot (WB)
Radioallergosorbent test (RAST) inhibition
Enzyme-linked immunosorbent assay (ELISA) using monoclonal antibodies

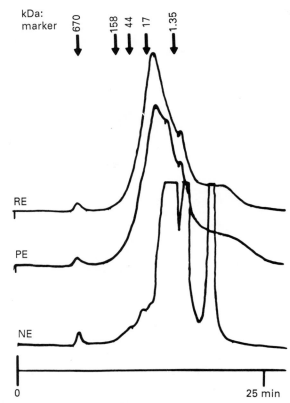

Fig. 3 Size exclusion HPLC traces of three timothy pollen allergen extracts: PE, production extract; RE, reference extract; NE, nondiafiltered extract.

in allergen extract characterization and standardization. As allergens are mostly proteins, protein determinations are often carried out. Molecular weight distributions can be determined by size exclusion high-performance liquid chromatography (HPLC) and sodium dodecyl sulphate–polyacrylamide gel electrophoresis (SDS–PAGE). HPLC can be used both analytically and preparatively. Figure 3 shows size exclusion HPLC traces of three timothy pollen allergen extracts. The traces of the production lot and of the in-house reference extract look similar, whereas the third trace exhibits a quite different pattern. This is due to the high amount of low-molecular-weight substances present in this sample because it did not undergo diafiltration. Figure 4 shows the preparative HPLC trace of a *D. pteronyssinus* allergen extract and Fig. 5 the isolated fractions analysed by crossed radioimmunoelectrophoresis (CRIE). *See* Chromatography, High-performance Liquid Chromatography; Immunoassays, Radioimmunoassay and Enzyme Immunoassay

Although most of the major allergens have molecular weights between 10 000 and 40 000 Da, preparative investigations of a *D. pteronyssinus* extract (purified mite bodies) showed that high-molecular-weight fractions (> 100 000 Da) also exhibit allergenic activity. One major allergen, namely D.pt.4, had a molecular weight of 244 000 Da (see CRIE of fraction 4). Therefore, for purification, extracts should only be diafiltered to exclude low-molecular-weight substances (≤ 5000 Da). This will ensure that extracts contain all the allergens which are relevant for the patients, including major as well as intermediate and minor allergens which can be of higher molecular weights. It must be remembered that in nature the allergic patient is not only in contact with allergen fractions but with the whole spectrum of allergens.

Figure 3 shows the HPLC trace of a nondiafiltered extract. The degree of diafiltration effect can also be investigated by high-performance thin-layer chromato-

graphy (HPTLC). Figure 6 shows chromatograms from HPTLC analysis of diafiltered and nondiafiltered extracts. Only the nondiafiltered extracts contain ninhydrin-positive low-molecular-weight substances with free amino groups. In the diafiltered extracts these were excluded. *See* Protein, Determination and Characterization

Since proteins/allergens have different isoelectric points and molecular weights, isoelectric focusing and SDS–PAGE provide useful methods of analysis. IgE-binding components in the extract can be determined by immunoblotting methods like immunoprint and Western blot. Figure 7 shows the Western blot of three timothy pollen allergen extracts. Nearly comparable allergen patterns appear from lot to lot.

Antigen and allergen pattern can also be determined by crossed immunoelectrophoresis (CIE) and crossed radioimmunoelectrophoresis (CRIE). A limitation of CIE and CRIE is that antisera are used which are obtained by immunization of animals – mostly rabbits – with the respective allergen extract. The quality of these antisera strongly influences the quality of the CIE and CRIE results. Figure 8 shows CIE of a cat epithelium allergen extract. Three different antisera produced by three different companies were used for the investigation. Although these results suggest that three different

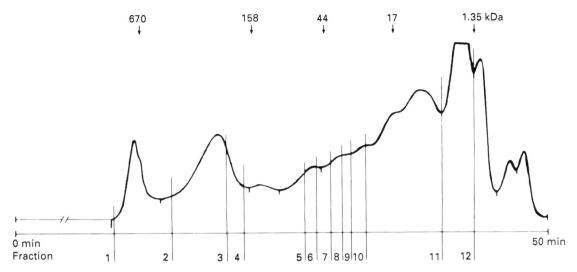

Fig. 4 Preparative HPLC trace of a *D. pteronyssinus* allergen extract. 1–12 isolated fractions.

extracts were examined, the differences are only due to different qualities of the antisera used. To overcome those limitations, immunoblot should be performed. For immunoblot no animal antisera but sera of the allergic patients are used directly to identify allergens. Furthermore, in contrast to CRIE, immunoblot can demonstrate the isoelectric points and molecular weights of single allergens in allergen extracts. This is very important for the characterization of allergen extracts to obtain information on their molecular structure. *See* Electrophoresis

Total allergenic activity of allergen extracts are determined by radioallergosorbent test (RAST) inhibition, which is one of the most important methods in allergen extract standardization. For RAST inhibition, allergen discs, pool serum, allergen extracts and labelled anti-IgE (enzyme or radio labelled) are needed. For RAST inhibition it is only necessary to know the species of the allergen extract which should be measured. Information about the protein content of the extract or the allergenic composition, etc. are not necessary. However, it is not possible to quantify single allergens by RAST inhibition, which is nowadays more often requested. This can be done by monospecific radio rocket immunoelectrophoresis or by using monoclonal antibodies in an enzyme-linked immunosorbent assay (ELISA) system (Fig. 9). For the determination of single allergens in crude extract a reference curve (Fig. 10) must be prepared. Using this reference curve the amount of single allergens in samples can be determined.

Since raw materials used for the extract preparation can differ in their composition, the previously mentioned methods can also be used for the investigation of raw materials. Using these methods, differences were found for ragweed pollen extracts when the raw materials were purchased from different suppliers. However, when raw material from the same supplier was tested a

high conformity of extracts was found. To ensure that the extracts prepared from different manufacturers are comparable, international standards (ISs) were created. The ISs are not intended to be used as templates; that is, commercially available extracts need not demonstrate the identical allergenic composition and activity as the IS. The ISs should rather be used as yardsticks for preparing in-house reference extracts or national reference preparations. Sometimes the IS does not reflect absolutely the composition of all in-house references and this is the case for *D. pteronyssinus*. Different results were obtained with different extracts; this was caused by variability of the raw materials used for extract preparation. For timothy pollen extracts a high conformity was shown between extracts prepared from commercially prepared extracts and the ISs.

The activity of allergen extracts must also be investigated *in vivo*. This can be done by biological standardization. The aim is to express the allergenic activity of the extracts in biological, allergy or other related units which are obtained by testing the extracts in humans. By using the sera of patients who have taken part in the biological standardization process, allergens in the tested extracts can be classified as major, intermediate and minor. Major allergens are those that appear by CRIE after 3 days of autoradiography on an X ray film in more than 50% of the patients and in more than 90% of the patients after a time of autoradiography of 2 weeks. If allergens appear on the X ray film in 25% of the patients they are defined as intermediate, and in less than 25% of the patients they are defined as minor allergens. The determination of major, intermediate and minor allergens is only a statistical definition and is obtained by *in vitro* investigations. To check whether the same range of importance of single allergens would be detected *in vivo*, each single allergen has to be isolated and tested. This is not generally feasible. Figure 11

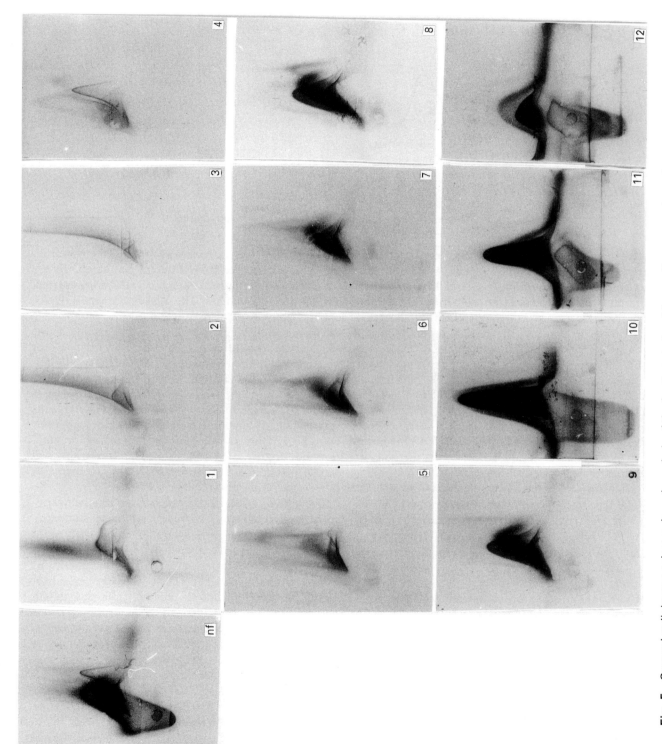

Fig. 5 Crossed radioimmunoelectrophoresis analysis of the fractions isolated from a *D. pteronyssinus* allergen extract (see Fig. 4).

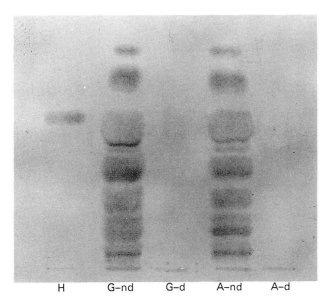

Fig. 6 HPTLC analysis of diafiltered (d) and nondiafiltered (nd) allergen extracts: H, histamine control solution; G, grasspollen extract; A, alternarratenuis (mould) extract.

shows the allergogram of a *D. pteronyssinus* allergen extract. Some allergens were classified as major, some as intermediate and some as minor allergens. Allergen extracts should contain major as well as intermediate and minor allergens, which for some patients can be as important as the statistically defined major allergens.

When keeping in mind all the conditions mentioned above, allergen extracts can be prepared with a high reproducibility. Fifteen production lots of *D. pteronyssinus* extracts prepared from 26 different lots of rat material – harvested during a period of 4 years – were investigated. The coefficients of variation of the data obtained when using the several methods were between 14 and 23% (Table 2). By immunoblot, all extracts showed nearly similar allergen patterns (Fig. 12) and Der p I content, as can be seen by similar peak height of the Der p I rockets (Fig. 13).

Allergen extracts used in diagnosis and therapy must be stable. Lyophilized allergen extracts stored at $-20°C$ are stable for more than 10 years. Aqueous (containing 0·4% phenol) and glycerol-based extracts (e.g. *D. pteronyssinus* allergen extracts) showed a stability of 3–5 years when stored at 5°C.

Current Status of Allergen Research

Rapid progress in protein chemistry as well as in immunological methodology during the past few years has provided powerful tools for allergen research on a molecular basis. These tools are used for different strategies, e.g. to improve our understanding of allergic diseases, or for a more sophisticated standardization of allergen extracts, or for developing new therapeutic pathways. Molecular protein chemistry can characterize protein molecules to obtain information about primary, secondary and tertiary structural features. The first step towards a detailed picture of a protein is to identify its physicochemical and immunological properties, followed by purification and analysis of its amino acid sequence. Allergenic properties of such a well-defined protein can be investigated using epitope mapping, leading to the determination of B and T cell epitopes. Another approach towards a definition of proteins as allergens has come from comparative studies of genetically determined properties of allergic patients.

A very important immunological method that improved allergen research was the development of hybridoma technology for raising monoclonal antibodies (mabs). As shown in Fig. 14 mabs are used for many different applications. Meanwhile, mabs have been raised against allergens from many species, including house dust mites, cat, horse, insects and pollens of grass and birch. Mabs are very useful as reagents in immunoassays for quantification of single allergens in crude allergen extracts or in the environment. Even

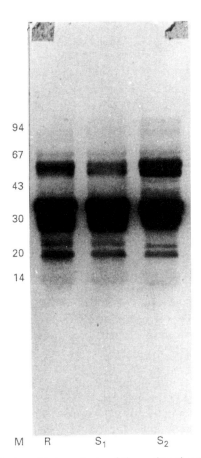

Fig. 7 Western blot analysis of three timothy pollen allergen extracts: R, reference extract; S$_1$, sample 1; S$_2$ sample 2; M, kDa of the marker proteins.

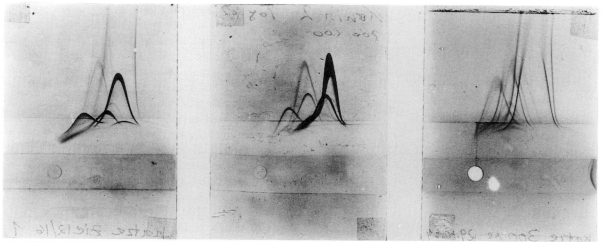

Fig. 8   CIE analysis of a cat epithelium allergen extract using antisera purchased from three different companies.

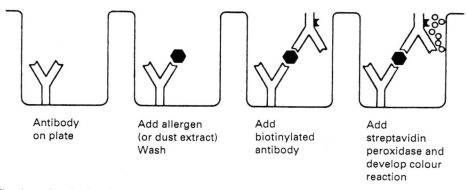

Antibody on plate

Add allergen (or dust extract) Wash

Add biotinylated antibody

Add streptavidin peroxidase and develop colour reaction

Fig. 9   Quantification of a single allergen using monoclonal antibodies in an ELISA system.

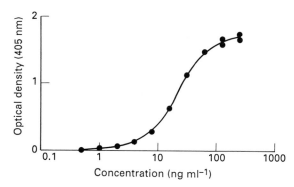

Fig. 10   A typical reference curve for the determination of a single allergen in a crude extract.

allergens which are closely related (showing a high degree of homology) like house dust mite group I allergens Der p I and Der f I were distinguishable in immunoassays by mabs. Another application of mabs is the purification of allergens from crude allergen extracts by affinity chromatography, thus leading to one-step purification procedures instead of complex purification schemes based on classical chromatographic methods. Thus, the purification of allergens that are difficult to separate because of their heterogeneity can be achieved with high yields of nearly pure protein, without any loss of IgE reactivity. Supplied with such a large stock of pure proteins, studies of molecular structures have become possible.

Purified allergens have been subjected to epitope mapping in order to develop two side immunoassays as well as to find antigenic or even IgE reactive binding sites. By competitive inhibition assay, overlapping and nonoverlapping epitopes have been identified. When performing inhibition assays involving IgE antibodies it is also possible to define IgE-binding sites.

In recombinant techniques mabs can be useful tools in screening procedures. Isolation of messenger RNA from different allergens, e.g. house dust mite, birch pollen and different grass species, and transcription of these messenger RNAs into complementary DNA (cDNA) by an enzyme called reverse transcriptase has provided material for two different subsequent pathways. First, cDNA can be brought into *Escherichia coli* and then, after multiplying, a screening procedure using appropriate labelled oligonucleotides is applied. Secondly, when using another vector for infection of *E. coli*, not only is cDNA synthesized, but also the protein for which the

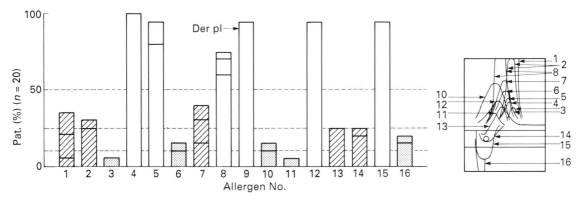

Fig. 11   The allergogram of a *D. pteronyssinus* allergen extract (right). Graphical presentation of the allergens (*N*=16) that could be detected in the sum of the CRIEs of 20 mite *D. pteronyssinus* allergic patients.

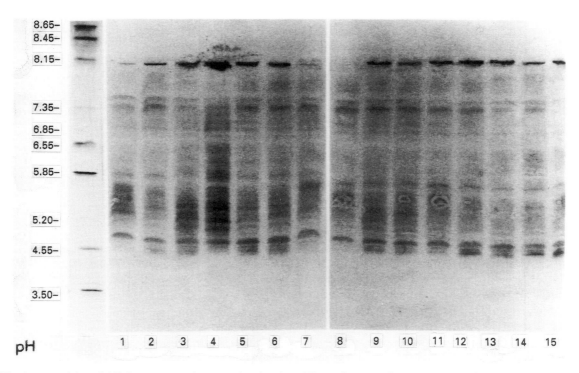

Fig. 12   Immunoblot of 15 *D. pteronyssinus* production lots. Time of autoradiography 14 d. On the left, pH of the marker proteins.

Table 2.   Mean values and coefficients of variation for data from *D. pteronyssinus* allergen extracts

Property	Coefficient of variation (%)
Extract (*N* = 15): 2% w/v	
PNU per mg of lyophilisate: 12 705	14
Protein: 0·542 mg ml^{-1}	19
Allergenic activity: 369 693 BU ml^{-1}	23
Specific activity: 683 BU (μg protein)$^{-1}$	23

PNU, protein nitrogen units; BU, biological units.

cDNA is coding. These recombinant proteins can be detected by mabs, thus identifying the *E. coli* clones bearing well-defined chromosomal DNA. For this procedure sera from allergic patients are also used.

Sequencing the appropriate DNA nucleotide sequences of allergens and deduced amino acid sequences have been reported. Today sequences of several allergens are known: Lol p II, Bet v I, Poa p IX, Amb a I, Amb a III, Der p I, Der p II, Der f I and Der f II.

From these data, it became possible to synthesize peptide fragments of allergens and analyse a set of such peptides for antigenic or allergenic epitopes of an allergenic protein. Based on this methodology, five allergenic epitopes were translated in house dust mite

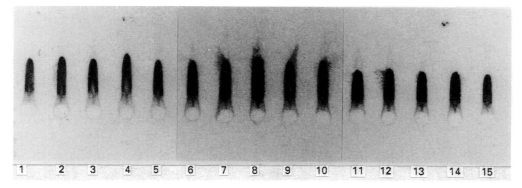

Fig. 13 Radio rocket immunoelectrophoresis analysis of the same 15 *D. pteronyssinus* extracts as in Fig. 12. Fusing a monospecific Der p 1 patient serum.

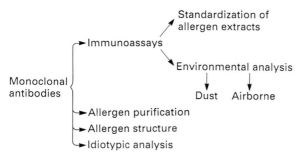

Fig. 14 Importance of monoclonal antibodies in allergen research.

group I allergens of *D. pteronyssinus* Der p I. When testing extracts of the closely related *D. farinae*, containing Der f I, in inhibition experiments, only three of the five epitopes were found to be cross-reactive; the remaining two peptides did not remove reactivity. Furthermore, peptides bearing allergenic protein sequences were used to localize T as well as B cell epitopes.

When assessing amino acid homologies of allergens and other known proteins no general principle became evident in defining or specifying proteins as allergens. For example, homologies were found when comparing the amino acid sequence of the major allergen of birch pollen, Bet v I, with alder, hazel and hornbeam, thus confirming cross-reactivity of these allergens with human IgE. On the other hand, no homologies exist between birch pollen and house dust mite or house dust mite and grass pollen allergens. So it is obvious that amino acid sequence data alone cannot serve as an answer to the problem of what makes a protein an allergen. Structural aspects other than epitopes have to be considered, e.g. secondary or tertiary structure, size, charge and other properties.

Another approach in this field based on comparison of genetically derived sequence data came from investigations of *HLA-D* genes, which code for certain cell marker proteins. Analysis of genomic DNA from Lol p

III (grass pollen allergen) responder and nonresponder subjects revealed an association of responsiveness with a specific *HLA-D* sequence. However, as stated by the authors, these findings do not demonstrate a cause–effect relationship. This has to be confirmed by investigations of antigen-specific T cell clones and antigen-presenting cells of various *HLA-D* phenotypes.

Bibliography

Anderson MC, Baer H and Ohman JL (1985) A comparative study of the allergens in cat urine, serum, saliva and pelt. *Journal of Allergy and Clinical Immunology* 74: 563.

Kurth R (ed) (1985) Regulatory control and standardization of allergenic extracts. *Fourth International Paul-Ehrlich Seminar*, 16–17 October 1985. Stuttgart: Gustav Fischer.

Kurth R (ed) (1985) Regulatory control and standardization of allergen extracts. *Fifth International Paul Ehrlich Seminar*, 2–4 September 1986, 41–44. Stuttgart: Gustav Fischer.

Ansari AA, Shinomiya N, Zwollo P and Marsh DG (1991) *HLA-D* gene studies in relation to immune responsiveness to a grass allergen Lol p III. *Immunogenetics* 33: 24–32.

Baldo BA (1987) Standardization of allergens. Examination of existing procedures and the likely impact of new techniques on the quality control of extracts. *Allergy* 38: 535–548.

Chapman MD (1988) Allergen specific monoclonal antibodies: new tools for the management of allergic disease. *Allergy* 43(suppl. 5): 7–14.

Chapman MD (1989) Monoclonal antibodies as structural probes for mite, cat and cockroach allergens. *Advances in the Biosciences*, vol 74, pp 281–295. Oxford: Pergamon Press.

Dreborg S, Einarsson R and Longbottom L (1986) The chemistry and standardization of allergens. In: Weir DM (ed.) *Immunochemistry. Handbook of Experimental Immunology*, 4th edn, vol. 1, chap. 10. Oxford: Blackwell.

Frandsen PF and Bachman A (1989) Registration of allergen preparations. *Nordic Guidelines*, 2nd edn, *NLN Publication*, No. 23, Uppsala: Nordiska Lakemedelsnamnden (Nordic Council on Medicines).

Greene WK, Chua KY, Stewart GH and Thomas WR (1990) Antigenic analysis of group I house dust mite allergens using random fragments of Der p I expressed by recombinant DNA libraries. *International Archives of Allergy and Applied Immunology* 92: 30–88.

King TP (1990) Insect venom allergens. In: Baldo BA (ed.)

Molecular Approaches to the Study of Allergens. Monographs in Allergy, vol. 28, pp 84–100. Basel: Karger.

Malling HJ (1988) Immunotherapy position paper. *Allergy* 43(suppl. 6): 13–15.

Ohman Jr JL (1985) Selection of source materials for reference preparations, mammalian allergens. *Proceedings of the 4th International Paul Ehrlich Seminar on the Regulatory Control and Standardization of Allergenic Extracts*, Bethesda, pp 58–78.

Tovey ER, Chapman MD and Platts-Mills TAE (1981) Mite faeces are the major source of house dust allergens. *Nature* 289: 592–593.

Wahl R and Franke D (1992) State of the art of allergen extract standardization. Regulatory control and standardization of allergenic extracts. *Sixth International Paul-Ehrlich Seminar*, 5–7 September 1990. 197–205. Stuttgart: Gustav Fischer.

Wahl R, Meineke D, Oliver J, Schultze-Werninghaus G and Hauck P (1989) Comparison of in-house allergen extracts of *Phleum pratense* (timothy grass) pollen with the international standard and investigation of IgE specificities of a grass pollen serum pool from West Germany and of the one recommended by the World Health Organization. *Journal of Allergy and Clinical Immunology* 84(4): 448–456.

Wahl R, Lau S, Maasch HJ and Wahn U (1990) IgE-mediated allergic reactions to potatoes. *International Archives of Allergy and Applied Immunology* 92: 168–174.

Wahl R, Oliver JD, Hauck P, Schultze-Werninghaus G and Paap A (1991) Comparison of fifteen production batches of house dust mite extract (*Dermatophagoides pteronyssinus*). *Annals of Allergy* 66(4): 348–353.

R. Wahl, B. Weber and D. Franke
Allergopharma Joachim Ganzer, K.G., Reinbek, FRG

ALLERGY

See Food Intolerance

ALMONDS

The almond is the major commercial tree nut crop of the world. This importance has been achieved by the very large increase in acreage and production in California during the past 20 years. This article reviews the areas of production, principal cultivars, important uses, and methods of handling and storage.

The Crop and its Importance

Global Distribution

The cultivated sweet almond (*Prunus dulcis* Miller (D. A. Webb) syn. *P. amygdalus* Batsch) originated from within the wild species known originally as *Amygdalus communis* L. which grew on the lower slopes of mountains in central Asia. About 30 related almond species have been described occupying specific ecological niches in the arid steppes, mountains and deserts of central and southwestern Asia and southern Europe.

The geographical range of the cultivated almond corresponds to the three stages of cultural evolution: (1) *Asiatic* (southwest and central Asia), (2) *Mediterranean* (countries bordering both sides of the Mediterranean sea), and (3) *Californian* (central valleys of California, parts of Australia, central Chile and areas of South Africa).

Almonds are adapted to Mediterranean, steppe and desert climates characterized by mild, rainy winters and hot dry summers. Although they have traditionally been grown with other arid tree and vine crops, such as olive, pistachio and grape, almond trees respond so well to supplementary irrigation, fertilizers, good soil, disease and insect control and other intensive culture methods that yields can be increased 5- to 10-fold over the traditional culture practised for centuries.

Commercial Importance

Since 1950, almonds have become the most important world tree nut crop, with present annual production of approximately $350–400 \times 10^6$ kg ($800–900 \times 10^6$ lb). In any given year, California produces about 70% of the world's supply of almonds (Figs 1 and 2), with most of the balance coming from Mediterranean countries

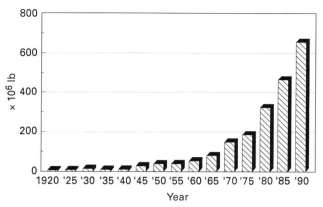

Fig. 1   California almond production.

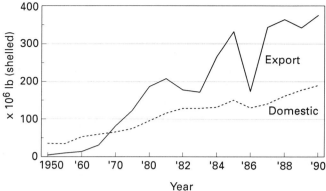

Fig. 2   Changes in the export and domestic distribution of almond production since 1950.

(Spain, Italy, Greece, Portugal, Morocco, Tunisia, Canary Islands, France). Almonds are also grown, often in primitive culture, as local crops in Iran, Israel, Afghanistan, Pakistan, southeastern USSR, northwest India, Syria, Turkey, and Iraq.

Cultivars

Older botanical literature described two botanical varieties as *Prunus amygdalus* var. *dulcis*, the sweet almond, and *P. amygdalus* var. *amara*, the bitter almond. In reality, bitter and sweet kerneled trees exist side by side in seedling populations with the same parents, the difference apparently due to a single dominant gene. Some of the more primitive almond growing areas (e.g. in Asia and Morocco) still grow almond trees as seedling populations (wild or cultivated).

Modern orchards grow selected cultivars, which are clones that are vegetatively propagated by budding or grafting upon specific rootstocks. Rootstocks include almond and peach seedlings, as well as certain plums and peach × almond hybrids. Historically, many cultivars were apparently identified when superior individual trees were selected to replace 'bitter' trees within seedling orchards. In recent years, controlled breeding has created cultivars with special qualities. Use of genetic engineering methods will augment genetic improvement.

Although many cultivars exist in the world, a limited number have dominated industrial and local use within specific production areas. Cultivars are selected for performance in the orchard. Flowers on most current cultivars are self-incompatible, so that two or more cultivars that bloom at nearly the same time need to be planted together, preferably in adjoining rows. Hives of honey bees are placed within the orchard to effect cross-pollination. Combinations of cultivars are also chosen to facilitate an economical harvest. Other cultivar characteristics of importance include yield, tree habit, disease and insect resistance, ease of harvest and

processing, and other specific characteristics. Nuts of different cultivars vary from very hard-shelled to soft- and paper-shelled. Cultivars are also chosen for their marketing potential, and specific marketing classes have evolved.

California

Nonpareil accounts for around 50% of the production. Kernels are uniform in shape, relatively flat, smooth, attractive in appearance, easy to blanch and are versatile in processing and utilization. The nut has a thin, papery shell and is easy to remove without damaging the kernel. This shell is subject to worm and bird damage. The cultivar is subject to a genetic variant referred to as 'noninfectious bud-failure' which can be controlled primarily through proper selection of propagation sources.

Mission (Texas) is an old cultivar which produces small, round, plump nuts. Kernels have a relatively strong 'almond' flavour owing to higher levels of amygdalin. The pellicle is difficult to remove during blanching. The shell is hard and protective of worm damage. Padre is a similar cultivar, the kernels of which can be combined with Mission. Peerless is grown to a limited amount as a pollinator of Nonpareil. The shell is hard and the nuts are sold primarily in the shell.

Ne Plus Ultra has a large, elongated kernel, blooms early and cross-pollinates Nonpareil. The cultivar is gradually becoming obsolete in California, but orchards still exist and represents 3% of the total crop.

In the mid-1960s, Merced and Thompson were planted to replace Ne Plus Ultra, Peerless and Mission. Similarly shaped and blanchable kernels of these and later introduced cultivars have been mixed and marketed under the name 'California'. Other cultivars of this group include Price, Fritz, Monterey, and others.

Carmel became popular in the mid-1970s and is the second most important cultivar in new plantings. Sonora was introduced in the mid-1970s and is becoming popular as an early blooming pollinator for Non-pareil and has large, elongated nuts sometimes marketed with Carmel.

Additional cultivars that have recently been planted in California include Butte, Livingston, LeGrand, Mono and Ruby. Their nuts are grouped either as 'Mission' or 'California' marketing classes.

Spain

Marcona and Desmayo are the most important cultivars in Spain, each accounting for about 25% of Spanish production. Marcona has large, heart-shaped, flat, high-quality kernels which blanch easily. Desmayo produces large, elongated, flat kernels, the pellicle of which is thin and can be readily removed after roasting by rubbing between the fingers. Many other cultivars exist in specific production areas of Spain but their kernels are usually mixed together for marketing.

Italy

Most of the older areas, (Puglia, Sicily and Sardinia) are reducing production. Kernels of the many cultivars are mixed together for marketing. The main cultivars in newer orchards include Tuono, Felipo Ceo, and Genco, which are self-fertile.

France

New, late-blooming, high-yielding, vigorous cultivars derived from breeding programmes are being planted not only in France but other countries of the Mediterranean area. These cultivars include Ferragnes and Ferraduel, kernels of which are marketed together with those from other cultivars.

Morphology and Anatomy

Fruit

The almond fruit is known botanically as a *drupe*, which is composed of three basic parts: (1) exocarp (skin), which in almond is pubescent; (2) mesocarp, which is fleshy and becomes the hull; (3) endocarp (shell). This overall structure is the same as stone fruits, such as peaches, plums and apricots, but differs in that the almond mesocarp does not enlarge into fruit, but dehisces (splits) at maturity and dries. The hull is an important feed for livestock.

Seed

The almond *kernel* is the seed which develops from the ovule. Although two ovules are present in the flower,

only one normally develops to produce the single kernel. The seed is edible because it lacks amygdalin, the bitter compound in many seeds. The seed consists of the embryo (also referred to as the 'meat'), surrounded by seed coats or testae (also referred to as the 'pellicle' and sometimes the 'skin'). The embryo consists of the hypocotyl–root axis with growing points for roots and shoots which appear upon germination, and two massive cotyledons, which are storage organs and contain the high-energy compounds characteristic of almond.

Almond kernels of different cultivars have characteristic sizes, shapes, appearances, thickness of pellicle and, to some extent, flavour. 'Double' kernels result when two kernels develop within the same nut shell. 'Twin' kernels result when two or more embryos develop within the same pellicle.

Harvesting, Handling and Storage

Harvesting

Almond nuts should be harvested as soon as possible after maturation to avoid quality losses and to minimize problems with fungal attack and insect infestation. Indices used to determine maturity stage and optimum harvest dates for almonds include hull dehiscence (splitting), separation of the hull from the shell, decrease of the fruit removal force and drying of hulls and kernels. Almond harvesting in California is by machines. Almonds are shaken from the tree to the ground by various kinds of shakers. After about a week of drying, the nuts are raked into rows and the nuts picked up by mechanical harvesters. They are then transported in bulk to hulling machines which separate the hull from the in-shell product.

Post-harvest Handling

Dehydration of the kernel begins while the nut is still on the tree. Further drying takes place after the nuts are knocked to the ground. Under rainy and/or cool weather conditions, heated air dehydrators may be used to reduce moisture content to 7% or less. Most almonds sold commercially range from 4% to 5% in moisture. Dried almonds are transported in bulk to processing plants where they are stored in bins, silos, or other bulk-storage containers for a few weeks to several months before final processing and preparation for market.

In-shell almonds are fumigated with methyl bromide or aluminium or magnesium phosphide, which are lethal to all insect life stages. Residues are monitored to ensure that levels in finished products are below legal limits. *See* Fumigants

Alternatively, almonds can be kept in a controlled

atmosphere of 0·5% oxygen and about 10% carbon dioxide (balance nitrogen) to control insects. Freezing the nuts can be used for insect control at home, or for small-scale operations. *See* Controlled Atmosphere Storage, Applications for Bulk Storage of Foodstuffs

Storage

Compared to other nuts, almonds and almond products have a long life. This is attributable in part to their low moisture, the presence of relatively low levels of polyunsaturated fatty acids, and high tocopherol levels.

Raw almonds should be stored at 0–5°C, 65–70% relative humidity (RH), to minimize deterioration during storage. Prolonged exposure to direct sunlight causes the skins to darken and reduces shelf life. Since almonds readily absorb odours, they should never be exposed to pungent odours from onions, fresh fruits, fish, cheeses, paint, chemicals or other compounds.

Both the maintenance of quality and safety of almond and the extension of storage life depend upon the initial moisture content, the RH and temperature of storage, and the exclusion of oxygen and insect pests. *See* Storage Stability, Parameters Affecting Storage Stability

The Food and Drug Administration (FDA) regulations for tree nuts define a 'safe moisture level', (i.e. the moisture content which will not support fungal growth) as a water activity level that does not exceed 0·70 at 25°C. This is equal to a moisture content of about 7%. The optimum range for unroasted almonds is 4–6% moisture.

The relationship between moisture content and equilibrium relative humidity (ERH) is temperature-dependent. From 20% to 80% ERH (for any given moisture content), ERH rises approximately 3% for every rise in temperature of 10°C. At a given RH, air will contain more water vapour at a high temperature than at a low temperature. Temperatures between 0°C and 5°C are recommended for almonds, the lower temperatures allowing longer storage life (up to a year).

Low oxygen (0·5% or lower) atmospheres are beneficial for keeping flavour quality, delaying rancidity, and controlling stored products insects. Exclusion of oxygen is usually achieved by vacuum packaging or replacement with nitrogen in storage facilities and transport vehicles. The storage life of raw almonds can be extended up to 2 years under low-oxygen atmosphere at 0°C. *See* Chilled Storage, Packaging Under Vacuum

Quality and Safety Factors

Important appearance factors for almonds marketed in the shell include shell integrity, suture opening, and shell colour. Kernel defects include damage from insects, mould and mechanical injury, gum, callus growth, shrivelling and doubling. Kernels are graded for size. Quality criteria used in the grade standards include freedom from dust particles and other foreign materials, and uniformity of shape and colour.

Textural factors, including crispness and firmness, are influenced by moisture content. Thus roasted almonds are usually more crisp than raw almonds.

Flavour quality depends upon sweetness, oiliness, intensity of almond flavour, and absence of off-flavours resulting from rancidity, staleness or other causes. A problem called 'concealed damage', which appears as internal darkening and poor flavour after roasting, is related to wet conditions and high temperatures during temporary storage following harvest.

Safety factors relate primarily to the potential contamination of almonds with mycotoxins, especially aflatoxin produced by the fungus, *Aspergillus flavus*. Contamination can occur in the orchard or during postharvest handling if recommended handling and storage procedures are not followed. Elimination of nuts exhibiting any symptoms of fungal contamination is an integral part of market preparation. *See* Mycotoxins, Occurrence and Determination

Residues of pesticides used to control the major insect pest, navelorange worm (*Anyelois transitella* Walk), have been reduced by 40% during the last 10 years. This reduction was made possible through such integrated pest management procedures as orchard sanitation, maintaining natural predator balance, and prompt harvest. *See* Pesticides and Herbicides, Residue Determination

Propylene oxide, the only sterilant approved for nuts, is generally effective against bacteria, but less effective against yeasts and moulds. The nuts are treated in a specially designed vacuum chamber. After treatment, a series of air washes under vacuum removes traces of the remaining gas. Each chamber load then enters a post-conditioning staging area until cleared for both residue level and microbial load. Propylene-oxide-treated products are recommended when raw almonds are incorporated into dairy products, such as cheese or yoghurt, or in high moisture foods, or used for other microbially sensitive applications.

Composition

The chemical composition and nutritive value of almond are summarized in Table 1. *See* individual nutrients

Market Forms

Almonds are eaten alone as snacks and are included in many processed foods to enhance their appeal. The wide

Table 1. Chemical composition and nutritive value of almonds (per 100 g edible part)

Component	Mean
Water (%)	4·4
Proteins (%)	19·9
Fats (%)	52·2
Carbohydrates (%)	20·4
Fibre (%)	2·7
Ash (%)	3·0
Sugars (%)	4·4
Food energy (MJ)	2·47
Fatty acids	
Saturated (g)	4·9
Monounsaturated (g)	33·9
Polyunsaturated (g)	11·0
Vitamins	
Vitamin A (IU)	0
Thiamin (mg)	0·2
Riboflavin (mg)	0·8
Nicotinic acid (mg)	3·4
Pantothenic acid	0·5
Vitamin C (mg)	0·6
Minerals (mg)	
Calcium	266
Phosphorus	520
Iron	3·7
Sodium	11·0
Potassium	732
Magnesium	296

Source: USDA Agricultural Handbook (1984) Composition of foods: Nuts and seed products – raw, processed and prepared. 8–12: 137.

variety of foods includes sweets, health foods, baked goods, cereals, ice cream, dry mixes, garnishes for food entrées and packaged snacks.

Almonds may be used directly as a whole nut, or it may be appropriate for them to be chopped, diced, sliced, split, halved, slivered or cube-cut. They are available in an array of kernel sizes as segregated by round and slot-holed screens which separate according to kernel width and thickness. There is also a wide range of smaller-sized products, such as flakes, slivers and meals. The variety of shapes, sizes and colours available makes almonds appropriate for many different food applications.

The largest usage category is confectionery. Many premium confectionery products are enhanced by the combination of chocolate and almonds. Almonds enhance the flavour and acceptability of confections by lowering the sweetness of the finished piece, by adding crunch, enhancing the nutritional value and adding sales appeal.

Manufacturing

Roasting

The flavour of most almond varieties is quite mild before they are roasted. The strong flavour and crunchy texture desired in most applications are developed by roasting. Most almonds added to chocolate are roasted almonds. Almonds may be roasted by hot air or in hot oil. Almonds roasted in oil may pick up some of the flavour of the roasting oil. Dry-roasted almonds usually possess the same roasted flavour, a somewhat harder texture and slightly lower moisture (below 2%).

The amount of oil absorbed by almonds in oil roasting is minimal, usually 3–4%, roughly equal to the amount of moisture driven off by roasting. This small amount of oil has a minimal impact on the fat content of the final product. The degree of roast in a given application is determined by experimentation and/or sensory testing.

Blanching

Blanching is the process of soaking the almonds briefly in hot water, then slipping the skins from the kernels using rollers.

Blanched almonds have a milder flavour and softer texture than unblanched almonds. The only cultivar which is not blanchable is Mission. Blanched almonds are preferred in applications where the brown skin may come loose upon cooking, or a light nut is desired.

Almond Butter

Almond butter is made by grinding (dry) roasted almonds with other ingredients, such as salt, sugar and stabilizer. The predominant flavour of almond butter is that of roasted almonds. Almond butter is similar to peanut butter in appearance with a slighly oilier texture. It is used in a wide variety of food applications.

Almond Paste and Marzipan

Almond paste and marzipan have long been used in baked goods, pastries and confections, particularly in Europe. Marzipan is traditionally shaped into figures for holidays and, in some countries and, in some countries, is enrobed in chocolate. Almond paste is among the oldest of confections and is made by grinding raw blanched almonds with sugar.

Extending Shelf Life

The package as well as the moisture, temperature and water activity of the surrounding environment must be considered in predicting shelf life of products using almonds. With higher moistures and water activities in the surrounding environment, the shelf life is usually shorter.

As a general rule, blanching reduces shelf stability by about 25–50%. Any cutting, such as slicing and dicing, has a similar effect. Roasting accelerates deterioration, and roasted nuts should be packaged to exclude oxygen. When properly packaged in cans, foil or glass under vacuum or nitrogen flushed, both dry-roasted and oil-roasted almonds can last a year or longer at room temperature. Dry-roasted almonds tend to have a longer shelf life than oil roasted. The quality and stability of oil-roasted almonds depends upon the type and quality of roasting oil. Finely ground products, such as almond paste and almond butter, have a long shelf life (> 1 year) because the particles pack tightly together, excluding oxygen.

Roasted almonds in oxygen-free packaging have a shelf life of 1–2 years at room temperature. If longer storage is desired, or if harsh storage conditions exist, antioxidants should be considered. A variety of natural and artificial antioxidants will contribute to a two- to threefold improvement in shelf life. The ideal package for almonds excludes both moisture and oxygen. Shelf life in some packages may be improved by addition of oxygen and/or moisture scavenger packets. *See* Antioxidants, Natural Antioxidants; Antioxidants, Synthetic Antioxidants

Bibliography

IPM Manual Group (1985) *Integrated Pest Management for almonds*. Publication No. 3308. Oakland: University of California Division of Agricultural and Natural Resources.

Kester DE and Gradziel TH (1993) Almond breeding. In: Janick J and Moore JS (eds) *Advances in Fruit Breeding* 2nd edn. Indiana: Purdue University Press (in press).

Kester DE, Gradziel T and Grasselly C (1991) Almonds. *Germplasm Resources in Fruit and Nut Species*. Wageningen, The Netherlands: International Society for Horticultural Science.

Micke WC (1993) *Almond Production Manual* 2nd edn. Oakland: University of California Division of Agricultural and Natural Resources.

Rosengarten Jr F (1984) *The Book of Edible Nuts*. New York: Walker and Co.

Ryall AL and Pentzer WT (1982) *Fruits and Tree Nuts* 2nd edn., vol. 2, chap. 10. Westport, Connecticut: AVI Publshing.

Soderstrom EL and Brandl DG (1990) Controlled atmospheres for preservation of tree nuts and dried fruits. In: Calderon M and Barkai-Golan R (eds) *Food Preservation by Modified Atmospheres*, pp 83–92. Boca Raton, Florida: CRC Press.

Woodruff JG (1979) *Tree Nuts: Production, Processing, Products*. Westport, Connecticut: AVI Publishing.

Dale E. Kester and A. A. Kader
University of California, Davis, USA
Sam Cunningham
Blue Diamond Almond Growers, Sacramento, USA

ALUMINIUM

Contents

Properties and Determination

Aluminium metal has been commercially produced for just over 100 years; a relatively short period of time compared to other metals. The potential for adverse biological effects on human health, postulated to be associated with elevated environmental and food aluminium levels, has resulted in its in-depth investigation in recent years. This article will review the physical and chemical properties of aluminium, its speciation in water, occurrence in foods, uses in utensils and packaging and determination in simple and complex matrices.

Physical and Chemical Properties

In pure form, aluminium is a silvery-white, light-weight, malleable, ductile metal with a melting point of 660°C and boiling point of 2327°C. It is also a good conductor of both heat and electricity. Aluminium is located in group IIIA of the periodic table and has an atomic number of 13 with an atomic weight of 26·9815.

Aluminium is the earth's most abundant metal. Preceded by oxygen and silicon, aluminium is the third most abundant element, accounting for approximately 8% by weight of the earth's crust. It is indeed ubiquitous, being prevalent in soils, clays, minerals, air and water. The extremely reactive nature of aluminium accounts for the fact that aluminium does not exist in the 'free' or metallic state but, rather, is always found as chemically bound species, predominantly with silicon or oxygen, often in ionic forms as aluminosilicate and aluminohydroxyl ions.

An invisible, protective outer layer of aluminium oxide forms immediately metallic aluminium is exposed to moist air. It is this dramatic affinity for oxygen, and the ability of the oxide so formed to bind firmly to the exposed metal, which affords aluminium its many diverse applications. Not only does this coating of oxide protect the surface of aluminium against further oxidation, it also protects the metal from reaction with many other chemicals. The oxide exhibits excellent resistance to corrosion by many inorganic and organic chemicals within a pH range of 4·5–9, but is susceptible to reaction with both acids and bases outside of this range. *See* Corrosion Chemistry

Bauxite is a mixture of alumina (aluminium oxide), silica and iron oxides and is the chief ore from which aluminium is extracted and subsequently purified. Following extraction, the aluminium oxide is electrolytically reduced to the free metal for the production of a variety of products.

Aluminium is trivalent in all of its stable combinations and exhibits a normal electrode potential in aqueous solution (E^0(aq) $Al^{3+} \rightarrow Al^0$) of -1.66 V.

Speciation and Soluble Forms

In aqueous solution the speciation of aluminium is influenced by several factors, including pH, temperature, ionic strength and the presence of complexing ligands such as F^-, SO_4^{2-} and organic anions.

The ionic radius of Al^{3+} closely resembles that of Fe^{3+}. In addition, the hydrolysis behaviour of Al^{3+} in aqueous solution is also quite similar to that exhibited by Fe^{3+}. An understanding of the speciation of aluminium in aqueous solution is critical to the study of its biological activity.

The octahedral hexahydrate $Al(H_2O)_6^{3+}$ cation is stable only in solutions at pH < 5 and, for convenience, is written as Al^{3+}. As the pH of the solution increases, deprotonation of the Al^{3+}-bound water occurs, with the formation of $Al(H_2O)_5(OH)^{2+}$ and $Al(H_2O)_4(OH)_2^+$. The formation of a trihydroxide precipitate $Al(OH)_3$ in neutral solutions at approximately pH 6·5 is the limiting factor for aluminium solubility. As the solution becomes basic, the $Al(OH)_3$ precipitate redissolves, forming $Al(OH)_4^-$, the tetrahedral aluminate anion, which is the predominant species at pH 7·4.

The mononuclear speciation of aluminium in aqueous solution may thus be summarized by eqns [1]–[4].

$$Al(H_2O)_6^{3+} + H_2O \rightleftharpoons Al(H_2O)_5(OH)^{2+} + H_3O^+ \qquad (1)$$

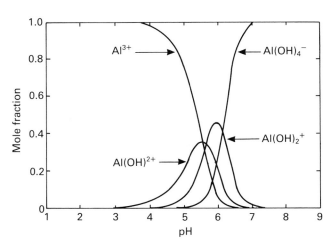

Fig. 1. Distribution of soluble, mononuclear aluminium ion species in aqueous solutions. The ordinate scale is the mole fraction of aluminium ions occurring as each designated species. At any given pH the individual mole fractions sum to unity. Reproduced by permission from Martin RB (1988).

Equation [1] is more conveniently written as eqn [2].

$$Al^{3+} + H_2O \rightleftharpoons AlOH^{2+} + H^+ \qquad (2)$$

Similarly, the sequential hydrolysis steps are represented by eqns [3] and [4].

$$AlOH^{2+} + H_2O \rightleftharpoons Al(OH)_2^+ + H^+ \qquad (3)$$

$$Al(OH)_2^+ + H_2O \rightleftharpoons Al(OH)_4^- + 2H^+ \qquad (4)$$

At pH < 5, the octahedral hexahydrate $Al(H_2O)_6^{3+}$ cation predominates, whereas at pH > 6·2 the tetrahedral aluminate anion $Al(OH)_4^-$ predominates. As indicated in Fig. 1, a mixture of the species is observed between pH 5 and 7. *See* pH – Principles and Measurement

Entry into the Food Chain

Although its concentration and speciation may vary widely, aluminium is present in all soils. It is, therefore, not surprising that, as a result of natural leaching, most foods as well as water and air samples exhibit detectable quantities of aluminium.

This natural dissolution of soil-bound aluminium is highly favoured under acidic conditions but is also dependent upon geological factors, soil pH, temperature and proximity to sources of pollution. The aluminium cycle of pathways through which aluminium gains direct, natural entry into the human food chain has been effectively illustrated by Epstein and is depicted in Fig. 2.

Occurrence in Food

As indicated, the ubiquitous nature of aluminium implies that most foods naturally contain some alumi-

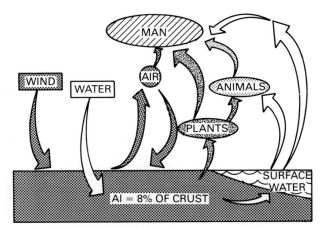

Fig. 2. The aluminium cycle. Reproduced by permission from Epstein SG (1990).

nium. However, the concentration of aluminium within similar types of food can vary immensely as a result of large variations in the aluminium levels of soil and water as well as from that attributed to processing aids and processing methods. In general, the aluminium concentrations in commonly consumed foods are less than 10 mg kg^{-1}.

Natural Sources

The natural sources of aluminium entry into the food chain are depicted in Fig. 2.

Nonnatural Sources

The amounts of aluminium that can be added to a food during its preparation is dependent upon the type of food, its processing requirements, such as pH and cooking time, as well as the type of container in which it is processed and/or stored prior to consumption. Obviously, aluminium containers, whether processing vessels or final packaging, have the potential to contribute greater levels of aluminium to the food than do nonaluminium ones.

Processsing Aids as a Source

Clarifying agents such as bentonite, leavening agents such as sodium aluminium phosphate (acidic), emulsifiers such as sodium aluminium phosphate (basic), anticaking agents such as sodium aluminium silicate, colouring agents such as aluminium lakes of various food dyes and colours, and firming agents such as aluminium sulphate are some of the processing aids that

are commonly used within the food industry and which may contribute to residual aluminium levels. It must be noted that such processing aids are only used with the approval of government regulatory bodies. *See* Colours, Properties and Determination of Synthetic Pigments; Emulsifiers; Phosphates as Meat Emulsion Stabilizers; Leavening Agents

Although water is considered a natural source of aluminium, some of the aluminium occurring in municipal water supplies may result from the aluminium flocculants used by many water treatment plants to clarify the water. *See* Water Supplies, Water Treatment

Pharmaceutical Sources

Although in North America the current trend for antacids is shifting towards the substitution of aluminium by calcium-based compounds, many antacids still contain significant quantities of aluminium. Similarly, most antacids, buffered analgesics, antidiarrhoeals and certain antiulcer drugs contain significant quantities of aluminium-based compounds.

Aluminium compounds are also prevalent in many vaccines as adjuvants and carriers. Many antiperspirants contain significant quantities of aluminium-based compounds.

Cooking Utensils as a Source

Foods cooked in aluminium containers generally exhibit elevated levels of aluminium. The nature of the food in question and the method of preparation will obviously have a dramatic effect on the level of aluminium accumulated in food during preparation. This is especially accentuated when acidic foods are cooked in plain or unconverted vessels and concentrations of up to 10 mg l^{-1} can be realized under such conditions. On the other hand, the invisible outer protective layer of aluminium oxide normally found on the surface of metallic aluminium is not susceptible to attack by neutral foods, especially those low in salt content. These foods exhibit virtually no increase in aluminium content during cooking. The contribution to dietary aluminium resulting from the use of aluminium cookware is, however, relatively small, even under the worst case scenario, when compared with that found naturally in foods as a result of differing soil, water and growing conditions.

In recent years, an increasing portion of aluminium cookware has been manufactured with a protective coating of either sintered fluorocarbon (e.g. Teflon) or stainless steel. No accumulation of aluminium is observed in foods cooked in these converted utensils.

Packaging Materials as a Source

In common with tin and steel, aluminium is impervious to oxygen, moisture, light, odours and grease. These attributes, but more particularly its relative light weight for required strength, account for the widespread use of aluminium by the food-packaging industry. For packaging purposes, aluminium is used in either plain or converted forms.

Plain aluminium packaging involves those materials in which the aluminium surface is untreated. The only barrier between the packaged product and the metallic aluminium is the protective layer of aluminium oxide. Converted aluminium packaging refers to those materials which have been coated with an additional protective layer of lacquer, plastic, paper or cardboard and within which the packaged goods do not intimately contact the metal. Converted packaging materials are used for both liquid and solid foodstuffs and may be fabricated into flexible, semirigid and rigid types of packages.

Plain aluminium packaging applications are mainly household foils, foil trays and foil wrappings which have been laminated with paper or plastic coated to ensure closure of the package (such as for chocolate and deliquescent/effervescent tablets). Household foils are used extensively in a variety of applications, whereas foil containers, in general, are used for chilled and frozen foods, bakery products such as meat pies and fast food products. The amount of aluminium which migrates into such foodstuffs is negligible.

For converted packaging materials, aluminium may be treated with various epoxyphenolic, vinyl, polyolefin or polyurethane resin protective coatings. The packaging applications for these materials are almost limitless. In most countries regulatory agencies strictly regulate the materials which can be used in direct contact with foods and beverages. Migration of aluminium into foods or beverages packaged in converted aluminium materials is observed to be minimal provided that the integrity of the coating is assured throughout the fabrication and packaging processes. In instances where that integrity is compromised, the risk to the food or beverage is clearly dependent on its properties (e.g. pH) and the conditions of storage until consumption.

Aluminium Determination

The determination of aluminium in complex food and biological matrices has proven to be a formidable challenge. In recent years, analytical chemists have successfully overcome interferences and contamination difficulties, two major hurdles which have continually plagued aluminium analyses. For example, the currently accepted level of aluminium in human serum is approximately 100 times less than that first reported. This apparent dramatic decrease has been achieved, over many years, by the elimination of contamination errors and matrix interferences. Significant improvements in both instrumentation and methodology have also contributed to increased sensitivity of the methods. The erroneous inflated results now known to have been reported for blood plasma have also cast a shadow over the validity of levels previously reported for food, water and beverages.

Accurate and precise methods to monitor aluminium levels in human biological samples are clearly essential to assess accurately any health and disease implications of aluminium, particularly with the seemingly increasing number of people suspected of having elevated levels of blood aluminium. Accurate and precise analytical methods for aluminium in complex food and beverage matrices are also required to determine the dietary contributions of aluminium from these sources.

Numerous classical analytical methods employing gravimetric, titrimetric, photometric, fluorometric and polarographic techniques are available for the analysis of aluminium. Most of these methods, which were originally developed for the analysis of water or aqueous metal alloy samples, are subject to interferences from other metals and reagent contamination. In general, they also lack the sensitivity required and cannot be used for complex matrices.

Other techniques which have proven to be more accurate and reliable for the analysis of complex matrices are X ray fluorescence, neutron activation analysis (NAA), atomic emission spectrometry using either flame (FAES) or inductively coupled argon plasma combined with either emission (ICAPES) or mass spectrometry (ICAPMS) detection and atomic absorption spectrometry using flame (FAAS) or flameless, electrothermal (EAAS) atomization. The operating principles and sensitivity for each of these methods are readily available in the literature. The best of these methods for the analysis of aluminium in complex biological and food matrices, at this time, appear to be those based on EAAS, NAA and ICAPES or ICAPMS. EAAS has been the method most frequently used and is the recommended method for biological samples. Currently, EAAS methods are also being adapted to the analysis of aluminium in food and beverage matrices. *See* Spectroscopy, Fluorescence; Mass Spectrometry, Principles and Instrumentation

Sample Preparation

The three most sensitive methods, NAA, ICAP and EAAS, all require dissolution of the sample prior to analysis. As already mentioned, the acquisition of accurate and precise data requires the elimination of all matrix interferences.

In EAAS, reagents or modifiers are incorporated to reduce, as far as possible, the effects of matrix components on the atomization of the analyte. Choice of the appropriate matrix modifier eliminates the need for sample pretreatment and, therefore, many samples can be analysed directly. Contamination errors are minimized by the choice of appropriate modifiers, which are low in aluminium content, and by the incorporation of blank samples into the analysis protocol.

Acid digestion is required with some liquid and all solid samples for analysis. In many cases, concentrated nitric acid is sufficient to oxidize all the organic material present and provide a clear sample which can be analysed directly by EAAS. More difficult matrices, such as those high in fat content, may require stronger acids (e.g. sulphuric acid/peroxide mixtures or perchloric acid) for digestion. Microwave heating may also be used to assist the digestion process. In general, the more complex the sample pretreatment, the greater is the potential for contamination errors and consequently the greater is the care which must be exercised to ensure the accuracy and precision of the results.

Bibliography

Browning E (1969) *Toxicity of Industrial Metals*, 2nd edn, pp 3–22. London: Butterworths.

Epstein SG (1990) *Human Exposure to Aluminium. Environmental Geochemistry and Health*, No. 12 (1/2), pp 65–70. Washington, DC: American Chemical Society.

Greger JL (1988) Trace minerals in foods. In: Smith KT (ed.) *Tin and Aluminium*, pp 291–323, New York: Marcel Dekker.

Lucier GW and Hook GER (eds) (1974) *Aluminium in the Environment and Human Health. Environmental Health Perspectives*, vol. 8, pp 3–95. Washington DC: National Institute of Environmental Health Sciences.

Martin RB (1988) Metal ions in biological systems. In: Sigel H and Sigel A (eds) *Bioinorganic Chemistry of Aluminium*, pp 1–57. New York: Marcel Dekker.

Massey R and Taylor D (eds) (1988) *Aluminium in Food and the Environment. Special Publication*, No. 73. Cambridge: The Royal Society of Chemistry.

Savory J and Wills MR (1988) Metal ions in biological systems. In: Sigel H and Sigel A (eds) *Analysis of Aluminium in Biological Materials*, pp 348–372. New York: Marcel Dekker.

Savory J and Wills MR (1989) Aluminium and health, a critical review. In: Gitelman HJ (ed.) *Analytical Techniques for the Analysis of Aluminium*, pp 1–26. New York: Marcel Dekker.

Tikhonov VN (1973) Analytical chemistry of aluminium. In: Vinogradov AP (ed.) *Physiochemical and Analytical Description of Aluminium and its Compounds*, pp 1–23. New York: Wiley.

Herbert P. Wagner
John Labatt Limited, London, Ontario, Canada

Toxicology

Toxicology

Essentiality of Aluminium

Although aluminium is ubiquitous in nature, and biological systems have probably evolved in the presence of high concentrations of this element, no essential role has been established for aluminium in living systems. Nutritional research has been unable to define a deficiency state associated with minimal aluminium intake.

Intakes and Requirements of Aluminium

A number of authors have accepted 20 mg as a representative figure of a typical daily intake of aluminium. However, there are some indications that this estimate may be too high and 2–3 mg of aluminium per day will probably be more accurate. Nevertheless, amounts as different as 3·5–51·6, 3–100, 7–50 or 20–40 mg have also been reported as mean daily aluminium intakes by various authors.

Sources of Aluminium Exposure

Sodium aluminium phosphate is the main aluminium compound used in foods. The acidic forms of this compound are commonly added to cake mixes, frozen doughs, pancake mixes and self-raising flours to react with sodium bicarbonate and leaven these products when they are moistened. Moreover, the alkaline forms of sodium aluminium phosphate are widely used as additives in processed cheeses and cheese foods. These salts function as emulsifying agents, giving the cheese products a soft texture and easy melting characteristics. Alum (aluminium potassium sulphate) is an additive used to clarify sugar as a firming agent, and as a vehicle for bleaching agents. Although considered safe, in larger quantities alum and other aluminium compounds can interfere with the body's retention of phosphorous. Lastly, the aluminium silicates are commonly used as anticaking agents in salt, non-dairy creamers and other dry, powdered products. *See* Emulsifiers, Uses in Processed Foods; Leavening Agents

Aluminium compounds are also widely used in various non-prescription drugs. They include some antacids, buffered aspirins, antidiarrhoeal products, douches and haemorrhoidal medications. Of the aluminium compounds currently used in non-prescription antacids, aluminium hydroxide is by far the most common. Aluminium hydroxide is also used as a leavening agent in baked goods. Aluminium hydroxide is considered safe, but its use should be restricted in those with kidney disease. The aluminium content per dose of the antacids that contain aluminium hydroxide ranges from 35 to 208 mg. Moreover, other solutions currently used therapeutically can permanently or intermittently contain large amounts of aluminium which may be transferred from the fluid to the patients.

Aluminium cooking utensils such as pans, pots, kettles, trays, and foil are widely used in homes, restaurants, cafeterias and the food industry. Although the amount of aluminium ingested as a result of preparing food in aluminium cookware appears to be of no significance in comparison with the amount consumed from other sources, in some cases release of aluminium from aluminium untensils has been reported to constitute more than 20% of the daily intake of this element. Thus, for example, the intake of one pack of Chinese noodles was reported to cause ingestion of 3·3 mg of aluminium, including 2·6 mg of aluminium released from an aluminium pan.

Air emissions of aluminium due to human activities are much lower than the natural release. Aluminium is one of the most abundant elements in soil. Natural acidification processes result in increasing solubility of aluminium and, as soils become moderately acidic (pH < 5·5), aluminium begins to appear as the exchangeable cation which dominates in the lower mineral horizons. Concentrations of soluble and exchangeable aluminium in acid soils may reach many micrograms per gram of soil and can be toxic to plants, with reduced productivity of crops. In particular, the combination of low phosphorus, low pH and high aluminium – stress conditions characteristic of many tropical and subtropical soils – has been reported to be detrimental to soya bean yields and can be expected to reduce the yield of all leguminous crops. Several mechanisms have been proposed to explain the aluminium toxicity in plants: (1) disturbance of the metabolism of mineral nutrition, (2) binding of aluminium to plasma membrane and calmodulin, thereby inhibiting their functions, and (3) inhibition of cell division. The disturbance of nuclear activity by aluminium seems to be the main cause of aluminium toxicity.

Absorption, Distribution and Excretion of Aluminium

Absorption

The average body burden of aluminium in most tissues is less than $4\,mg\,kg^{-1}$ dry weight and the total body burden is less than 50 mg. Normally, very little aluminium is absorbed from the gastrointestinal tract. Balance studies indicate <2% of oral load is absorbed with no aluminium retention on a dietary intake of

<5 mg of aluminium per day. However, when the amount of ingested aluminium is markedly increased, some of this excess aluminium is absorbed, with an aluminium retention rate of 0·3–10%. Moreover, studies in perfusates of rat gut have shown that the reaction of gastric acid with various aluminium organic chelators – frequently present in the diet as food additives (citric, ascorbic, gluconic, lactic, malic, oxalic or tartaric acids) – solubilizes aluminium cations, resulting in the equilibrium formation of a soluble complex of aluminium, which by preventing reprecipitation, may result in aluminium absorption and elevated plasma aluminium levels. Recently, it has also been demonstrated that oral intake of citric or ascorbic acids, combined with prolonged high ingestion of aluminium hydroxide, results in significant absorption and retention of the metal in the brain and bone tissues of rats. Because of the propensity of uraemic patients to retain aluminium, even if not given oral aluminium compounds, in order to prevent the potential aluminium accumulation and toxicity, it is important to carry out a careful surveillance of the diet of chronic renal failure patients. *See* Ascorbic Acid, Physiology

Another modulator of aluminium absorption may be the fluoride content of the ingested diet and water, since aluminium has been shown to form tight complexes with fluoride. Aluminium and fluoride are both present in variable concentrations in the water supply. Aluminium sulphate has been frequently added as a coagulant agent to flocculate the organic matter and so clarify the water. The benefits of systemic fluoride for children are well established, whereas different studies have also shown that elderly persons are less susceptible to root caries if they have been lifelong residents of communities where water is fluoridated. The recommended optimal level of fluoride set by the Environmental Protection Agency (USA) for municipal water systems is 0·7–1·2 ppm, with a maximal acceptable level of 4 ppm. Since it has been demonstrated that aluminium does decrease fluoride absorption from the gastrointestinal tract, this might suggest that fluoride may also decrease aluminium absorption, although this has not been directly studied. On the other hand, a 1000-fold enhancement of aluminium leaching from cooking utensils has been reported when 1 ppm fluoride was present in the cooking water. Notwithstanding, subsequent studies demonstrated minimal enhancement by fluoride of aluminium leaching from aluminium cooking utensils. These observations are of considerable concern to both proponents and opponents of water fluoridation, especially because the question of toxicity of ingested aluminium in individuals with normal renal function is unresolved. Finally, there are certain plants, including the Theaicae (tea family), that are aluminium accumulators. Thus it seems possible that individuals who drink large amounts of tea may have additional aluminium loads.

Distribution

In subjects without aluminium accumulation, the highest levels of aluminium are found in the lungs (35 mg kg^{-1} wet weight) followed by the skeleton (12 mg kg^{-1}) and the skeletal muscle (4 mg kg^{-1}). Consequently, bone and muscle account for about 40% of total body aluminium and the lungs for 12%. In patients with aluminium overload, e.g. chronic dialysis patients, although brain, bone and muscle aluminium levels all increase with increased duration of dialysis, the bone largely overruns the skeletal muscle as the major storage organ in severe renal failure. It has been suggested that the bone sequesters aluminium, thus protecting the brain from aluminium toxicity.

Excretion

Despite large variations in aluminium intake in people with normal renal function, most absorbed aluminium has been reported to be excreted in urine. In adults receiving a diet with < 5 mg of aluminium per day, the urinary aluminium excretion is very low, accounting for < 6% of the oral load and usually in the range of 1–2% or less. Urinary aluminium excretion increases with increased aluminium loading whether it is from increased intestinal absorption, or intravenous loading in adults or infants.

Although it appears that biliary aluminium excretion may be of little importance after parenteral administration, biliary aluminium concentration has been shown to exceed urinary concentration in liver transplantation candidates who have normal renal function and who ingested aluminium-containing antacids. Even though excretion rates of aluminium via both routes were not compared, this observation raises the possibility that aluminium absorbed after oral intake may be handled differently by the liver to aluminium administered intravenously.

Toxicity of Aluminium

Experimental

The intraperitoneal median lethal dose (ip LD_{50}) for aluminium nitrate nonahydrate was reported to be between 327 and 901 mg kg^{-1} in rats, and between 320 and 1587 mg kg^{-1} in mice, whereas the reported oral LD_{50} values in rats ranged from 260 to 4280 mg kg^{-1} depending on rat strain, sex, age, period of observation, etc. The LD_{50} of aluminium sulphate in mice is 1400 mg kg^{-1} injected intraperitoneally compared to 6200 mg kg^{-1} when given orally. The LD_{50} of aluminium chloride following oral administration is

380 mg kg^{-1} in mice, 400 mg kg^{-1} in guinea pigs, and 400 mg kg^{-1} in rabbits. Decreased locomotor activity, piloerection, weight loss, and decreased food and water consumption are the most remarkable physical signs appearing after acute aluminium intoxication.

No significant toxic effects have been observed when aluminium nitrate nonahydrate was given orally to rats at doses of 375, 750 or 1500 mg per kg of bodyweight per day for one month or over a period of 100 days at 360, 720 and 3600 mg per kg of bodyweight per day, whereas dietary administration of sodium aluminium phosphate for six months at concentrations of 3% or lower caused no toxicological effects in beagle dogs. Chronic oral administration of aluminium sulphate induces cognitive impairments in the rat without producing major changes in the cholinergic system, and aluminium chloride administration in the diet of rats produces varying deficits on shuttle-box avoidance behaviour depending on rat strain, sex, and whether or not parathyroid hormone was administered.

Neurofibrillary degeneration has been induced in widespread regions of the central nervous systems of experimental animals by intracranial injection of aluminium compounds.

Carcinogenicity and Mutagenicity

Animal studies have failed to demonstrate carcinogenicity attributable to aluminium metal powder, aluminium hydroxide, aluminium oxide or aluminium phosphate administered by various routes to rats, rabbits, mice and guinea pigs. Aluminium fibres were not carcinogenic following ip injection to rats, whereas sarcomas were produced at the site of injection of aluminium-dextran in mice. In contrast, aluminium nitrate nonahydrate given at doses of 50–400 mg kg^{-1} reduced growth of intraperitoneally transplanted Walker 256 carcinosarcoma in rats. However, this compound had little activity against P388 leukaemia cells and none against L1210 leukaemia, K1964 leukaemia, plasma cell YPC-1, or Erlich ascites carcinoma. *See* Carcinogens, Carcinogenic Substances in Food

With regard to the mutagenic effects of aluminium, it has been described that aluminium chloride causes chromosome aberrations. Nevertheless, aluminium chloride did not give positive effects when tested by the rec assay with two strains of *Bacillus subtilis* (H17 and M45). When inhibition of cellular growth by a chemical is more pronounced with recombination-repair-deficient (rec^-) than with wild bacteria (rec^+), it is supposed that this chemical is damaging cellular DNA. Negative responses were also obtained when aluminium chloride was examined for its potential to induce forward mutations at the thymidine locus in L5178Y mouse lymphoma cells. This compound failed to induce reverse mutations in the *Salmonella typhimurium* TA102 strain at doses ranging from 10 mmol per plate to 1000 mmol per plate. Aluminium sulphate, aluminium chloride, aluminium oxide and aluminium phosphate also gave negative results in the rec assay with the same two strains of *Bacillus subtilis*: H17 and M45. *See* Mutagens

Reproductive Toxicity

When aluminium sulphate was administered to rats by intratesticular injection at 0·08 mmol per kg of bodyweight, the testes were focally necrosed within two days after aluminium injection. All the spermatozoa were also destroyed by this dose within seven days after aluminium administration. In contrast, a single subcutaneous (sc) injection of aluminium sulphate (0·08 mmol kg^{-1}) had no effect on the testes weight in rats, but daily administration of the salt reduced this weight in mice. In addition, aluminium sulphate caused shrinkage of the tubules and spermatogenic arrest without affecting the interstitium.

Developmental Toxicity

In recent years, the developmental toxicity of aluminium has been investigated by a number of authors. The incidence of fetal deaths and resorptions was significantly increased when aluminium chloride was administered by ip injection to pregnant rats and mice at different dose levels and different stages of gestation. Nevertheless, aluminium chloride given orally to rats during the period of organogenesis, or intravenously to mice before implantation or in early organogenesis had no significant effect on resorption rates or on fetal weights. Developmental alterations in fetuses and offspring of rats and mice have been observed after oral administration of aluminium nitrate or aluminium lactate during gestation. However, no evidence of maternal toxicity, embryo/fetal toxicity or teratogenicity has been observed with aluminium hydroxide in mice or rats at doses as high as 266 or 768 mg per kg of bodyweight per day, on gestation days 6 through 15. These doses would be equivalent to those consumed by people of 60 kg weight who ingest 5·5 or 16 g of aluminium per day respectively. Moreover, the maternal-placental aluminium concentrations are not significantly different between control and aluminium-treated rats, whereas the metal was not detected in the fetuses. However, recent investigations have shown that the concurrent administration of citric acid and aluminium hydroxide presents some signs of maternal toxicity and fetotoxicity in rats.

No adverse effects on fertility or reproductive parameters were evident when aluminium nitrate nonahyd-

rate (180, 360 and 720 mg per kg of bodyweight per day) was given to male rats for 60 days prior to mating with female rats treated for 14 days prior to mating and also during the periods of gestation and lactation. Notwithstanding, the survival rates were higher for the controls, and a dose-dependent delay in the growth of the offspring could be observed in the aluminium-treated groups. No overt fetotoxic effects were noted when the same doses of aluminium nitrate were given orally to pregnant rats from the 14th day of gestation through 21 days of lactation, but the growth of the offspring was also significantly less from birth for the aluminium-treated groups.

Aluminium Toxicity in Humans

The spectrum of clinical aluminium toxicity has expanded gradually since its initial description as the cause of dialysis dementia. In 1976, Alfrey *et al.* suggested that dialysis encephalopathy, previously a uniformly fatal neurological syndrome, resulted from aluminium intoxication. Based on additional biochemical and epidemiological data, this supposition was confirmed and now it is generally accepted that aluminium is indeed the cause of this syndrome.

During the last two decades, it has been clearly established that aluminium accumulates in serum and tissues of patients receiving long-term haemodialysis against aluminium-containing dialysis fluids. Although aluminium has been implicated in the aetiology of several neurological disorders, such as Alzheimer's disease, amyotrophic lateral sclerosis and parkinsonian dementia of Guam, the dialysis encephalopathy syndrome is the main neurotoxic condition of aluminium. This syndrome includes a mild or severe speech disorder, hallucinations, twitching, myoclonus, seizures, mental changes and typical EEG (electroencephalogram) abnormalities. Aluminium accumulation has also been reported to be the cause of vitamin-D-resistant osteomalacia in some dialysis patients. The lines of evidence include epidemiological associations, bone biopsy correlations, animal models of osteomalacia produced by aluminium loading, and the favourable clinical response to the removal of aluminium by chelation therapy. Patients with dialysis osteomalacia typically present with severe symptoms of axial skeletal pain, and proximal muscular weakness, fractures of the ribs, vertebral bodies, pelvis and hips are common. These sometimes lead to severe disability, skeletal deformities and even death. Serum calcium levels are usually normal or modestly increased, serum phosphorus levels are normal or increased, and the serum levels of immunoreactive parathyroid hormone (iPTH) are generally lower than those usually noted in dialysis patients.

Aluminium has also been implicated as the cause of a microcytic, hypochromic anaemia in patients with

Table 1. Aluminium toxicity in humans

Source of aluminium	Clinical disorder
General population	
Occupational exposure	Chronic pulmonary disease
	Progressive encephalopathy
Parenteral nutrition	Osteomalacia
Antacids	Phosphate deficiency syndrome
Vaccines, medications, antiperspirants	Granuloma
Dietary aluminium	Neurological disorders: Alzheimer's disease (controversial)
Patients with chronic renal insufficiency	
Diffusate	Dialysis osteodystrophy
	Dialysis encephalopathy
Phosphate binder	Microcytic hypochromic anaemia (non-iron-deficient)

chronic renal failure, but other ions, trace metals in excess or deficiency and potentially toxic substances cannot be excluded yet. A summary of the clinical disorders associated with aluminium toxicity is presented in Table 1.

With the exception of premature infants who receive prolonged infusions of hyperalimentation products that contain substantial quantities of the metal, aluminium toxicity has been almost exclusively a disease of those with renal failure on dialysis who had a lengthy history of ingesting aluminium-containing phosphate binders and/or had been dialysing with water that had a high aluminium concentration. The health threat from diffusate fluids has been reduced by the recommendation that the diffusate contains less than 10 μg of aluminium per litre. However, although phosphate binders that do not contain aluminium, such as calcium carbonate, are being used more frequently, for some patients these do not provide satisfactory phosphate control at well-tolerated dosages.

On the other hand, aluminium-containing antacids are also widely used non-prescription medications for dyspepsia. Until recently, it was thought that the gastrointestinal tract was an impervious barrier to the passage of aluminium, but in 1977 it was clearly demonstrated that although the gastrointestinal tract is a formidable barrier to the entry of aluminium, it is not impervious. Furthermore, normal renal function is necessary to eliminate aluminium from the body. Thus both decreased urinary excretion and increased gastrointestinal absorption of aluminium are thought to explain why this treatment occasionally leads to symptomatic disease due to aluminium toxicity in patients with chronic renal failure.

Prevention and Treatment of Aluminium Overload

Because of the propensity of uraemic patients to retain aluminium, even if not given oral aluminium compounds, in order to prevent the potential aluminium accumulation and toxicity, a careful surveillance of the diet of these patients (citric, ascorbic, etc) should be carried out. Moreover, sodium bicarbonate and calcium carbonate or calcium acetate would appear to be adequate substitutes for Shohl's solution and calcium citrate respectively.

Despite these preventive measures, aluminium removal is essential to treat patients with aluminium overload. Currently, the most effective method is the chelation of aluminium with desferrioxamine (or deferoxamine, DFO), a chelator traditionally used in the treatment of iron overload. Desferrioxamine administration results in decreases of tissue aluminium levels and regression of aluminium-associated pathology. However, because of the serious toxic side-effects of DFO therapy, other chelators which may be therapeutically efficacious but with lower toxicity than DFO are being investigated.

Aluminium and Alzheimer's Disease

Aluminium is a proposed risk factor in the aetiology of Alzheimer's disease (AD), but it remains a controversial topic of cause versus effect. The fundamental disagreement among researchers concerning aluminium in AD revolves around the issue of timing and causality – whether aluminium is deposited in the brain as a result or a cause of AD. Four principal sites of aluminium accumulation in grey matter have been identified in AD: DNA-containing structures of the nucleus, the protein moieties of neurofibrillary tangles, the amyloid cores of senile plaques and cerebral ferritin. Whereas in some studies elevated concentrations of aluminium have been found in the brains of AD patients compared to age-matched controls, other studies have been unable to substantiate these findings.

In summary, outside the dialysis dementia syndrome, to date there is no evidence that aluminium has a role in the observed pathological changes, signs and symptoms in AD, amyotrophic lateral sclerosis and parkinsonian dementia.

Bibliography

Alfrey AC, LeGendre GR and Kaehny WD (1976) The dialysis encephalopathy syndrome. Possible aluminium intoxication. *New England Journal of Medicine* 294: 184–188.

Cannata JB and Domingo JL (1989) Aluminium toxicity in mammals: a minireview. *Veterinary and Human Toxicology* 31: 577–583.

Domingo JL (1989) The use of chelating agents in the treatment of aluminium overload. *Clinical Toxicology* 21: 103–109.

Elinder CG and Sjögren B (1986) Aluminium. In: Friberg L, Nordberg GF, Vouk VB and Kessler E (eds) *Handbook on the Toxicology of Metals* 2nd edn, pp 1–25. Elsevier: Amsterdam.

Koo WWK and Kaplan LA (1988) Aluminium and bone disorders: with specific reference to aluminium contamina-

tion of infant nutrients. *Journal of the American College of Nutrition* 7: 199–214.

Krueger GL, Morris TK, Suskind RR and Widner EM (1984) The health effects of aluminium compounds in mammals. *CRC Critical Reviews in Toxicology* 13: 1–24.

Jose L. Domingo
University of Barcelona, Barcelona, Spain

AMARANTH*

Amaranth, a legacy of the Aztecs, Mayas and Incas, continues to be an underexploited plant with a promising economic value due to the variety of uses it can have and the benefits it can provide to producers, processors and consumers. Present interests have developed because the plant offers leaves of high nutritional quality when used as a vegetable, because the grains, and because the whole plant offers a highly acceptable forage. The amaranth plant is also attractive since it adapts itself to a large number of environments, grows with vigour, produces large amounts of biomass, and resists drought, heat and pests. Less attractive features of the plant include leaves which tend to accumulate nitrate and oxalates, and a very small grain size which necessitates a large labour force when harvesting. With only a relatively small research effort, a strong knowledge base is being constructed and is beginning to reveal the economic value and nutritional benefits of this ancient legacy crop.

Origin and Distribution

The Amaranthacea comprise over 60 genera which include around 800 species of dicotyledonous, herbaceous plants, of either annual or perennial growth. There are three species of the genus *Amaranthus* which produce relatively large inflorescences with often more than 50 000 edible seeds per plant. These are *A. hypochondriacus* from Mexico, *A. cruentus* from Guatemala and *A. caudatus* from Peru and other Andean countries. Vegetable amaranths grow very well in the hot, humid regions of Africa, Southeast Asia, Southern China and India; they are represented by various amaranth species, such as *A. tricolor*, *A. dubius*, *A. cruentus*, *A. edulis*, *A. retroflexus*, *A. viridis* and *A. hybridus*.

---

* The colour plate section for this article appears between p. 556 and p. 557.

Grain amaranth was an important crop for the pre-Hispanic, New World civilizations. Its presence goes back some 4000 years BC in the Tehuacan Valley in Mexico, also the most likely site for the origin of maize. It is said that its use was highly associated with religious festivities, which were forbidden by the Spanish conquerors and which resulted in the elimination of the crop. Its production declined to small and insignificant levels, but it did not disappear. From Mesoamerica and the Andean region, grain amaranth was apparently carried as a weed, ornamental, or grain to other parts of the world.

Classification

Amaranth is a dicotyledonous plant, not a grass like most cereals which are monocotyledonous; rather it is a pseudocereal. Amaranth shows an extreme botanical plasticity in adaptation, which contributes to difficulties and confusion in its taxonomy. It is classified by means of flower structure, the form and proportion of leaves and inflorescence. These highly variable characters also allow for a high hybridization frequency, and assure the availability of a large germ plasm reserve. *See* Cereals, Contribution to the Diet

Plant Description

Amaranths are broad-leafed plants, which can grow from about 1·5 to 3·0 m high. The plant has a variable growth pattern in the type and number of branches, all of which end with a small seed head, sometimes maturing at the same time as the main seed head. Leaf shape varies from lanceolate to ovate to elliptic. Leaf number and size show great variability within and between species. The leaves, stems and flowers of amaranth can be green, gold, reddish-purple or of

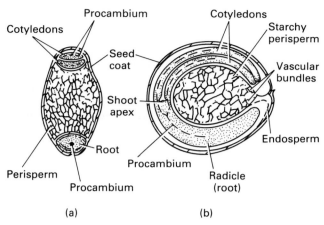

Fig. 1   *A. cruentus* seed in (a) cross- and (b) longitudinal sections as viewed in a light microscope. Source: Irving DW, Betschart AA and Saunders RM (1981) Morphological studies on *Amaranthus cruentus*. *Journal of Food Science* 46(4): 1170–1174.

various shades. The seed head, some 50–60 cm high, varies from pendulous to spiked and seed colour is usually black, gold, or cream.

Amaranths, like many cereals and grasses, carry on photosynthesis by the C_4 pathway, which uses carbon dioxide very efficiently by fixing it in the chloroplasts of specialized cells surrounding the leaf vascular bundles. This characteristic is also responsible for lower water losses by transpiration in association with the stomata. C_4 plants also have the capacity to photosynthesize at high rates at high temperatures and, through osmotic adjustment, the amaranth plants can tolerate some lack of water without wilting.

Grain Description

It has been found that the main amaranth inflorescence may produce from 49 to 89 g of grain (50 000–100 000 seeds). The grain is very small, lenticularly shaped, 1–1·5 mm in diameter, and weighs from 0·6 to 1·3 mg per seed, with the structure shown in Fig. 1. The germ, which is circular in shape, encircles the perisperm in one plane, and represents, together with the seed coat, around 25–26% of the weight of the seed as obtained by milling techniques. This fraction is relatively rich in fat and protein. In cereal grains, such as maize, the seed coat plus germ represent around 16–18% of the weight of the kernel, with the germ representing about 65%. *See* Wheat, Grain Structure of Wheat and Wheat-based Products

Production

Grain

Production depends on many variables, such as agronomic practices, plant density per ha, method of harvest in which seed shattering is important, uniformity of grain maturation, and the type of seed head. Yields in some localities have ranged from 1·1 to 1·5 t ha^{-1}, but in Mexico some reports indicate yields of 3·0–5·9 t ha^{-1}. Annual production has been estimated at 470×10^6 t per year worldwide. High yields can be obtained through high plant population densities (320 000–360 000 plants per ha), as well as from the appropriate application of organic and inorganic fertilizers.

Whole Plant

With respect to vegetable production, yields between 1·4 and 11 t of dry matter per ha at 4 weeks have been reported. In one study, dry matter yield at 25, 40 and 60 days after emergence was 66·6, 681·8 and 3452·0 kg ha^{-1}, yielding 19·7, 154·3 and 514·7 kg of protein per ha. Yields of edible leaves are obviously much lower, with values varying from 0·30 to 0·70 t ha^{-1} of dry matter. From a study on 14 varieties, the average dry weight of the whole plant, prior to seed harvest, was 208·5 g, of which 40% was represented by the weight of the stems, 26% by the inflorescence, and 34% by the seed.

Vegetable Amaranth

The use of amaranth leaves as a vegetable has been well established in a number of countries. *A. tricolor* is the main vegetable species in Asia, while *A. hybridus* and *A. cruentus* predominate in Africa and Latin America. Today, there is probably more amaranth consumed as a vegetable than as grain. The young leaves and the softest sections of the plant are boiled, sometimes in several changes of water, and consumed often mixed with cooked tomatoes, and other condiments. Usual forms of consumption include soups, salads, boiled, made into a purée with tomatoes and consumed with cooked root crops or with lime-cooked tortillas. The flavour of cooked amaranth leaves and young stems is pleasantly mild and not much different from that of similar greens.

Chemical Composition

The chemical composition of the vegetative part of amaranth is quite variable, since the content of organic and inorganic compounds changes as a result of climate, plant nutrition, agricultural practices, physiological stage, species and cultivar type and position of the leaves taken for analysis (Table 1). The moisture content for all species varies from about 70% to 94%, or from 6% to 30% dry matter. On a dry-weight basis (dwb), protein varies from 18% to 38% and total crude lipids from

Table 1. Chemical composition of amaranth[a]

	Vegetable	Grain	Forage
Moisture (g per 100 g)	85.0 ± 4.4	9.9 ± 2.0	87.8 ± 0.76^b
Dry matter (g per 100 g)	15.0 ± 4.4	90.1 ± 2.0	12.2 ± 0.76
Protein (N × 6·25)	24.1 ± 4.2	15.2 ± 1.7	19.2 ± 5.6
Total lipids (g per 100 g)	3.8 ± 0.68	7.0 ± 1.6	2.9 ± 1.3
Crude fibre (g per 100 g)	14.9 ± 3.7	6.2 ± 3.2	16.6 ± 6.2
Dietary fibre (g per 100 g)	—	13.6 ± 4.8	—
Ash (g per 100 g)	17.7 ± 1.6	3.3 ± 0.5	19.0 ± 3.9
Carbohydrate (g per 100 g)	42.9 ± 4.6	62.1 ± 7.6	43.8 ± 8.6
Amylose (g per 100 g)	—	6.1 ± 1.2	—
Energy (g per 100 g)	284	366	337
Metabolic energy ($kJ\ g^{-1}$)	—	12·2	—
Nitrate (g per 100 g)	0.55 ± 0.19	—	—
Oxalate (g per 100 g)	4.5 ± 1.8	—	5.86 ± 1.89
Phytate (g per 100 g)	—	1.03 ± 1.16	—
Tannins (g per 100 g)	—	0.18 ± 0.14	—
Cell walls (g per 100 g)	—	—	63.5 ± 7.7
Neutral detergent fibre (g per 100 g)	—	—	43.4 ± 10.9
Acid detergent fibre (g per 100 g)	—	—	34.6 ± 15.0
Acid detergent lignin (g per 100 g)	—	—	5·2
Cellulose (g per 100 g)	—	—	23·4
In vitro digestion (%)	—	—	60.0 ± 4.1

[a] Data, except moisture are given on dwb
[b] Moisture content varies widely depending on processing

Table 2. Mineral content of amaranth

Mineral	Vegetable (g per 100 g, dwb)	Grain (mg per 100 g, dwb)	Forage (g per 100 g, dwb)
Phosphorus	0.66 ± 0.22	578 ± 38.9	0.70 ± 0.28
Potassium	0.19 ± 0.02	541 ± 80.7	—
Calcium	2.57 ± 0.62	212 ± 66.0	2.45 ± 0.76
Magnesium	1.10 ± 0.30	327 ± 42.8	—
Sodium	—	22.5 ± 6.9	—
Iron	0.19 ± 0.15	35.6 ± 32.9	—
Copper	—	1.81 ± 1.06	—
Manganese	—	3.42 ± 0.90	—
Zinc	—	3.83 ± 0.38	—
Sulphur	—	150	—
Aluminium	0·015	1·0	—
Selenium	0·003	—	—

Table 3. Vitamin content of amaranth

Vitamin (mg per 100 g, dwb)	Vegetable	Grain
Thiamin	0.68 ± 0.32	0.136 ± 0.076
Riboflavin	2.24 ± 0.43	0.223 ± 0.056
Nicotinic acid	7.47 ± 1.66	1.153 ± 0.161
Biotin	—	42.5 ± 1.5
Folic acid	—	43.8 ± 1.5
Vitamin C	570.7 ± 89.6	4·47
Carotene	33.3 ± 16.68	4·6

1·3% to 10·6%. The lipid fraction contains 53·6% nonpolar lipids, 33·8% glycolipids and 12·6% phospholipids. The main fatty acids include linolenic (30–70%) and palmitic (13–14%) as well as oleic and stearic acid (see Table 5). *See* Fatty Acids, Properties; Lipids, Classification

The variability in crude fibre is also quite large, from 5·4% to 24·6% (dwb). This variability can be explained on the basis of the age of the plant, with young leaves and shoots showing the highest values. Finally, the ash content ranges from 7·6% to 22·2%. *See* Dietary Fibre, Properties and Sources

Minerals and Vitamins

The levels of calcium, potassium and magnesium are quite high, with calcium in the largest amount (2–3 g%; Table 2). Large quantities of phosphorus are also found, with values ranging from 0·49 to 0·79 g%. There is a relatively high concentration of iron, varying from 0·08 to 0·50 g% (dwb). Other minerals have been reported in smaller amounts.

The amounts of vitamins B_1 and B_2, nicotinic acid and ascorbic acid are similar to those found in other greens,

but the content of β-carotene is as high or higher than that reported for other green vegetables (Table 3). *See* individual minerals and vitamins.

Other Compounds

Amaranth, like many other fast-growing plants, has a tendency to accumulate nitrates. Reported values range from 0·27% to 0·74% nitrate (dwb) (0·046–0·104% fresh weight; Table 1). There is significant variation among cultivars, also due to environmental factors, since the same cultivar grown over different years had different values. The stems contain about twice as much nitrate as the leaves on a fresh-weight basis (fwb). The levels of nitrate in amaranth leaves are similar to those found in spinach and chard. Nitrogen fertilizer increases nitrate accumulation in green vegetables, including amaranth. Nitrates seldom cause problems to consumers because of their relatively low concentration and because, upon cooking, they leach out of the vegetable.

Another compound of greater concern is oxalate, which accumulates in leafy vegetables such as amaranths, particularly during dry weather. Oxalate levels are nutritionally important because they can bind

Table 4. Essential amino acid content of amaranth

Essential amino acid (mg per 100 g N)	Vegetable	Grain
Leucine	421 ± 76·5	356 ± 17·6
Isoleucine	327 ± 38·7	226 ± 15·9
Lysine	300 ± 34·9	351 ± 21·4
Methionine	78 ± 43·6	124 ± 17·7
Cysteine	24 ± 8·1	124 ± 6·4
Phenylalanine	314 ± 78·0	270 ± 40·1
Tyrosine	232 ± 48·7	220 ± 32·6
Threonine	356 ± 75·9	238 ± 21·3
Tryptophan	80	76 ± 12·3
Valine	355 ± 31·4	256 ± 14·1

essential divalent minerals, particularly calcium, making it nutritionally unavailable. On a dry weight basis, the oxalate in amaranth ranges from 1·1% to 7·9% (0·20–1·02% fwb); the stems contain significantly lower amounts than the leaves. The variability is as a result of both genetic makeup of the plant, and environmental factors. The oxalate in amaranth is bound to sodium, potassium, calcium and magnesium, but about 40% is free and therefore capable of binding other minerals. During processing in boiling water, oxalates are removed when water is changed, so that an intake of 100 g of cooked amaranth would provide approximately 0·2–1·0 g of oxalic acid. Assuming that 40% of oxalate is free and lost during cooking, the level will drop to 0·12–0·6 g which is nontoxic. Toxic levels for humans have been indicated to be 2–5 g per day. For populations consuming low levels of calcium, some of this mineral would become unavailable because of its complexing affinity to oxalic acid.

Other Uses

Amaranth leaves have been used in the preparation of leaf protein concentrates. These represent 24–36% of the leaf protein and contain 61–80% protein, which is of a light colour, almost odourless and nonbitter. Their essential amino acid content is attractive and high in lysine, but the sulphur amino acid content is low (Table 4).

Nutritional Value

The chemical composition of amaranth leaves shows that they provide relatively good nutritional value. The iron and β-carotene contents are highly available. Not much information is available on the quality of the protein in amaranth leaves, but they make a very good

supplement to maize and rice, either alone or with common beans at levels of up to 5% (dwb), because of their relatively high content of lysine, an amino acid which is deficient in both cereal grains.

Grain Amaranth

Chemical Composition

The gross chemical composition of amaranth grain is shown in Table 1. The crude protein content ranges from 11·8% to 17·6%. The reasons for the large variation amongst the different species is not known. While it may be of a genetic nature, it may also be due to environmental conditions and cultural practices. Nitrogen fertilization of amaranth has not consistently increased the crude protein in the grain. *See* Cereals, Dietary Importance

The variability in total lipid content for all species is 4·8–8·1%. Nutritionally, a high lipid content is of interest for the high energy that grain amaranth can provide in comparisons with cereal grains and food legumes.

Dietary fibre data for grain amaranth are not abundant. Values for *A. caudatus* have been reported to vary from 7·6% to 16·4%.

The ash concentration is relatively constant among species, and the variability for each element is also small.

Vitamin contents appear to be relatively constant among species. Some of the vitamins, e.g. nicotinic acid, are low in comparison with the nicotinic acid content in cereal grains, which show values about two to three times higher.

Starch is the most abundant chemical component in amaranth grain; the content varies from 48% to 69%. It occurs as very small polygonal or spheric granules (1–3 μm in diameter), and is readily digested by α-amylases. The starch is present mainly as highly branched amylopectin, but some varieties of amaranth grain contain from 4·8% to 7·22% of amylose, a linear starch. Other carbohydrates include sucrose, raffinose, stachyose and maltose in small but variable amounts. Microgranule starches, like those in amaranth, are being studied for paper coatings, fat substitutes, and biodegradable applications. *See* Carbohydrates, Classification and Properties; Starch, Structure, Properties and Determination

Fatty Acids

Amaranth seed oil is rich in the essential fatty acid, linoleic acid, with values ranging from 43·4% in *A. cruentus* to 51·4% in *A. hypochondriacus*. Oleic acid content is second in concentration, with values of 21·3% for *A. hybridus* and 31·9% for *A. cruentus*. Amaranth oil

Table 5. Fatty acid content of amaranth

Fatty acid (g per 100 g)	Vegetable	Grain
Myristic acid 14:0	1·1	0·53 ± 0·3
Palmitic acid 16:0	13·3	20·4 ± 2·0
Stearic acid 18:0	4·6	3·5 ± 1·5
Oleic acid 18:1	4·7	26·1 ± 5·6
Linoleic acid 18:2	6·4	48·0 ± 7·3
Linolenic acid 18:3	34·4	1·43 ± 0·8
Arachidonic acid 20:0	0·5	1·6 ± 0·9

contains 18·6–21·3% palmitic acid. The reported variability suggests differences between species and also differences between varieties of the same species. Other lipid classes include sterols, of which spinasterol is found at around 0·20% of the crude oil. In the unsaponifiable fraction, the isoprenoid, squalene, is found in relatively large amounts, around 6·8%. The total unsaturated fatty acid content is around 77% for amaranth oil (Table 5). *See* Essential Fatty Acids, Physiology

Protein

Protein distribution in the grain The endosperm of the grain contains 35·0% of the total grain protein, while the remainder is in the seed coat and germ or embryo. This distribution is quite different from that found in maize, sorghum and rice, wherein the germ contributes between 12·5% and 18·5%, and the endosperm from 81·5% to 87·5% of the total protein of the grain. The physical distribution of the protein in amaranth is responsible for its higher total protein content, as compared to common cereal grains, since the protein concentration in the germ is higher than the concentration in the endospores.

Protein Fractions in Amaranth

A few studies have been carried out on amaranth protein fractions. The quantity of albumin was found to vary between 19% and 23%, while that of the globulins from 18% to 21%. The alcohol-soluble prolamines varied from 2% to 3%, and alkali-soluble glutelin-like proteins ranged from 42% to 46%. Values of around 5–14 g per 100 g of protein have been reported for nonprotein nitrogen. The data available suggest that no great differences are found in the quantity of protein fractions among species or among cultivars.

Amino Acids

Table 4 presents average values for all species. Comparison of the essential amino acid content in grain amaranth with the FAO/WHO (Food and Agriculture Organization/World Health Organization) 1973 refer-

ence pattern reveals that the most deficient amino acid is leucine. Nevertheless, other amino acids, such as valine, isoleucine and threonine, could be limiting. Biological tests, however, revealed that threonine rather than leucine was the most limiting essential amino acid. Amaranth protein is a good source of lysine, tryptophan and sulphur amino acids. In contrast, cereal grains are deficient in lysine. The essential amino acid balance of grain amaranth protein is significantly better than that of many other proteins of vegetable origin. Since germ proteins are richer sources of essential amino acids (as compared to the storage proteins of the endosperm), the higher proportion of germ proteins in amaranth may explain the higher concentration of lysine in amaranth grain than that in cereal grains. *See* Protein, Quality

Nutritive Value

Oil

The digestibility of amaranth crude oil varies between 91·7% and 94·1% at the 5% level of addition and between 91·1% and 93·8% at the 10% level. These results are significantly lower than those from refined cottonseed oil at both levels of addition. The lower digestibility is probably caused by the presence of sterols (0·37% total) and unsaponifiable matter (1·4%) in crude amaranth oil; however, no deleterious effects from its consumption have been reported.

Metabolizable Energy of Amaranth Grain

The two main sources of energy in amaranth grain are the carbohydrate fraction and the oil content. The metabolizable energy (ME) of light- and dark-coloured. *A. cruentus* grain was 11·8 and 11·72 kJ g^{-1} (2·81 and 2·79 kcal g^{-1}), respectively. Heat processing increased the value for both seed colours, with extrusion cooking giving the highest values of 17·72 and 14·11 kJ g^{-1} (4·22 and 3·36 kcal g^{-1}), respectively.

Protein

A number of researchers have uncovered an important conclusion: the protein value (protein efficiency ratio) of the raw amaranth grain does not reflect the amino acid pattern of the protein. Furthermore, amaranth grain processed by wet cooking gives a higher protein quality value than that of the raw grain in all amaranth species. When processed under conditions which do not damage the availability of essential amino acids, its protein quality is very close to that of casein or milk protein. The effect of processing is evident in both the consumption of the diet and the weight gains of test animals. This effect is still unexplained and deserves some research. It has been suggested that the presence of antiphysiological factors which are inactivated by heat may be responsible; well-known antigrowth factors such as trypsin inhibitors, tannins and lectins are present at low levels in amaranth grain.

Some processes, such as expansion, flaking and wet cooking, apparently do not affect protein digestibility. However, the product from toasting gives equal or lower protein digestibility than the raw grain.

Although human studies on grain amaranth protein quality have been conducted, the data are not readily available. Some results with adult human subjects indicate that extrusion-cooked grain amaranth had a protein value of 89% relative to the value of cheese, while the popped material gave a value of 81% of the value of cheese. Digestibility values followed the same order.

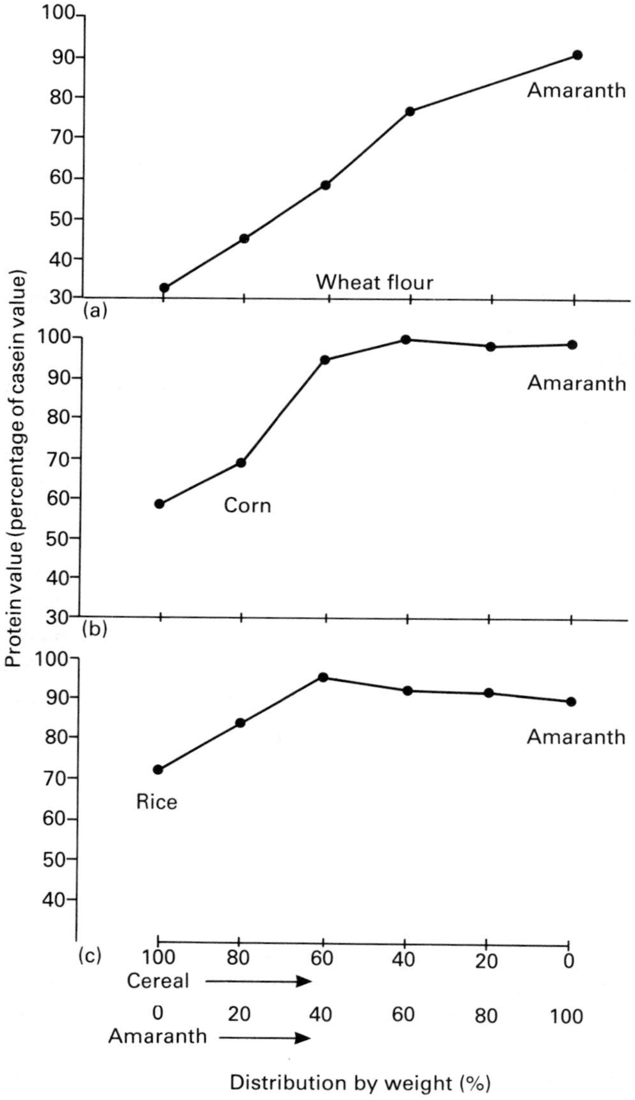

Supplementary Value

As a result of its high lysine content, the addition of amaranth grain to cereal flours improves the quality of the mixture (Fig. 2). The available data show an increase in protein quality of 62% for wheat flour, 40% for maize and 25% for rice, from the addition of 30% amaranth flour to 70% of each cereal grain. The high protein quality of amaranth means that it can be used alone or as a fortifier in cereal grain mixtures.

Grain Uses

Popped or parched amaranth are time-honoured edible forms of whole amaranth. The methods of preparation have persisted for centuries in Mexico, Peru and India. In recent research, grain amaranth flour has been tested as a supplement to wheat, maize and rice flours to be used in pastries, tortillas and similar products. Likewise, amaranth grain flour has been tested as a component of high-quality protein foods and as a drink in blends with milk. Product possibilities are numerous, but very few have been commercialized. A total of 60 cereal grain foods containing small amounts of amaranth are marketed in the Americas. In Mexico eight different amaranth grain flours are marketed, with the most popular product being alegría, a mixture of popped amaranth with sugar. Product and market development will be crucial to amaranth's growth in the food chain.

Fig. 2 Complementation between amaranth and cereal protein. (a) Wheat flour plus processed amaranth, 10% protein in diet; (b) corn flour plus processed amaranth, 9·0% protein in diet; (c) rice flour plus processed amaranth, 8% protein in diet. Source: Bressani R (1989).

Bibliography

Bressani R (1989) The proteins of grain amaranth. *Food Reviews International* 5: 13–38.

Saunders RM and Becker R (1984) Amaranthus: a potential food and feed resource. In: Pomeranz Y (ed.) *Advances in Cereal Science and Technology*, vol. 6, p 357. St Paul, Minnesota: American Association of Cereal Chemists.

Teutonico RA and Knorr D (1985) Amaranth: composition, properties and applications of a rediscovered food crop. *Food Technology* 39: 49–60.

Paredes-López O, Barba de la Rosa AP, Hernández-López D and Carabéz-Trejo A *Amaranto. Características Alimentarias y Aprovechamiento Agroindustrial.* Irapuato, México: Laboratorio de Biotecnología de alimentos, Centro de Investigación y de Estudios Avanzados, Instituto Politécnico Nacional.

Ricardo Bressani
Instituto de Nutrición de Centro América y Panamá, Guatemala

AMINES

Amines are aliphatic, aromatic or heterocyclic organic bases of low molecular weight, which arise as a consequence of metabolic processes in animals, plants and microorganisms.

Biogenic amines may be defined as aliphatic mono-, di- and polyamines, aromatic amines and related compounds which are biologically active (Figs 1 and 2). They are usually formed by enzymatic decarboxylation of the corresponding amino acids (Table 1). *See* Amino Acids, Properties and Occurrence; Enzymes, Uses in Food Processing

Biologically active amines are generally either psychoactive or vasoactive. Psychoactive amines act on the neural transmitters in the central nervous system, while vasoactive amines act, either directly or indirectly, on the vascular system. Pressure amines are vasoactive amines that cause a rise in blood pressure.

Biologically active amines are normal constituents of many foods and have been mainly found in several natural fruits (e.g. bananas and citrus fruits), in microbiologically processed foods (e.g. cheese, meat products, wine, beer and fermented vegetables) and especially in spoiled foods (e.g. fish, meat and cheese).

Biogenic amines do not represent any hazard to individuals, unless large quantities are ingested or the natural mechanisms for their catabolism are inhibited or are genetically deficient.

Formation

Amino acid decarboxylation takes place by the removal of the α-carboxyl group to give the corresponding

Methylamine	CH_3-NH_2
Dimethylamine	$(CH_3)_2-NH$
Trimethylamine	$(CH_3)_3-N$
Ethylamine	$CH_3-CH_2-NH_2$
Diethylamine	$(CH_3-CH_2)_2-NH$
Propylamine	$CH_3-(CH_2)_2-NH_2$
Butylamine	$CH_3-(CH_2)_3-NH_2$
Amylamine	$CH_3-(CH_2)_4-NH_2$
Hexylamine	$CH_3-(CH_2)_5-NH_2$
Ethanolamine	$HO-(CH_2)_2-NH_2$
Propanolamine	$HO-(CH_2)_3-NH_2$
Cysteamine	$HS-(CH_2)_2-NH_2$
Taurine	$HO_3S-(CH_2)_2-NH_2$
Methylthiopropylamine	$CH_3-S-(CH_2)_3-NH_2$
Putrescine	$H_2N-(CH_2)_4-NH_2$
Cadaverine	$H_2N-(CH_2)_5-NH_2$
Spermidine	$H_2N-(CH_2)_3-HN-(CH_2)_4-NH_2$
Spermine	$H_2N-(CH_2)_3-HN-(CH_2)_4-HN-(CH_2)_3-NH_2$
Agmatine	$H_2N-\underset{\underset{NH}{\parallel}}{C}-HN-(CH_2)_4-NH_2$

Fig. 1 Structures of some aliphatic amines.

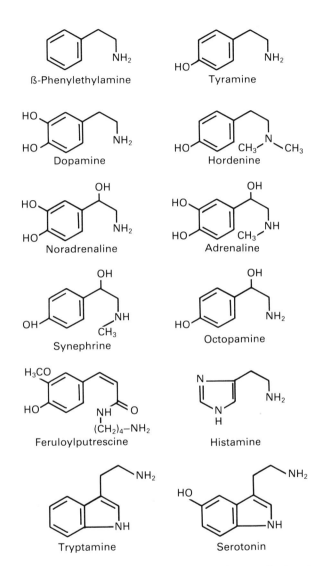

Fig. 2 Structures of some aromatic amines and related compounds.

amine. Decarboxylases are specific for each amino acid and are widely distributed in plants and animals, including microorganisms, but mainly in bacteria. Amine build-up in foods is mainly the result of the growth of decarboxylase-positive bacteria (especially histidine and tyrosine decarboxylases) under conditions favourable to enzyme synthesis and activity. Decarboxylation is a part of protein degradation and may also be a protective mechanism used by bacteria against an acid environment. *See* Amino Acids, Metabolism

The factors that govern the formation of amines in foods include:

Table 1. Some biogenic amines and their precursors

Amines	Precursors
Agmatine	Arginine
n-Amylamine	Norleucine
Isoamylamine	Leucine
n-Butylamine	Norvaline
Isobutylamine	Valine
Cadaverine	Lysine
Cysteamine	Cysteine
Dopamine	Dihydroxyphenylalanine
Ethanolamine	Serine
Ethylamine	α- and β-Alanine
Histamine	Histidine
Methylamine	Glycine
2-Methylbutylamine	Isoleucine
3-Methylthiopropylamine	Methionine
Noradrenaline	Dihyroxyphenylserine
β-Phenylethylamine	Phenylalanine
Propanolamine	Threonine
n-Propylamine	α- and β-Aminobutyric acid
i-Propylamine	α-Aminoisobutyric acid
Putrescine	Ornithine
Serotonin	5-Hydroxytryptophan
Taurine	Cysteinic acid
Tryptamine	Tryptophan
Tyramine	Tyrosine

From Askar A and Treptow H (1986).

- The presence of particular substrate amino acids. Autolytic and microbial proteolysis play a role in the release of such amino acids.
- The presence of microorganisms that have the genetic potential to synthesize decarboxylase enzymes.
- Favourable conditions for the growth of microorganisms and for the production of the enzymes (e.g. temperature, pH, water activity, absence of preservatives, etc.).
- The presence and activity of microbial monoamine oxidases (MAOs) and diamine oxidases (DAOs) which are responsible for the oxidative desamination of amines and which play a major role in their degradation. *See* Enzymes, Functions and Characteristics

Importance

The presence of amines in foods is of interest for several reasons. Secondary amines, such as dimethylamine, can react with nitrite added to meat products to form carcinogenic nitrosamines. The highly volatile alkylamine trimethylamine (TMA) has highly undesirable sensory properties and is an index for fish quality. Di- and polyamines, such as putrescine, spermidine and spermine, stimulate the growth of animal and plant

systems. Histamine is a capillary dilator, can produce hypotensive effects and is responsible for scombrotoxin fish poisoning. Tyramine is the most active of pressor amines and causes a rise in blood pressure. All phenethylamine derivatives appear to be triggers of dietary migraine.

During the last few years, the possibility of using histamine, putrescine and cadaverine concentrations in food as indices of microbial quality and spoilage of meat, fish, cheese, wine and fermented vegetables has received much attention. *See* Fish, Spoilage; Nitrosamines; Histamine; Cheeses, Dietary Importance; Migraine and Diet

Histamine Poisoning

Among the many food hazards which have been implicated in a number of outbreaks of food poisoning is histamine. At the present time a histamine concentration of 1000 ppm in food is considered to be the critical level for histamine poisoning, although 500 ppm is often considered as a hazard action level.

Histamine in food results from the microbial decarboxylation of histidine. Consequently, those foods which originally contained large amounts of histidine and which have been exposed to microbial degradation or fermentation may contain sufficient histamine to cause occasional food poisoning episodes.

The food most often implicated in such outbreaks has been fish. Histamine toxicity from fish, often called 'scombroid poisoning', generally involves the ingestion of scombroid fish from the families Scomberesocidae and Scombridae. Scombroid fish include various species of tuna, mackerel, bonito and skipjack which normally contain large amounts of free histidine in their muscle tissue. From the 'nonscombroid' fish, dolphin fish (or mahi-mahi), herrings, sardines and anchovies have been most commonly implicated in histamine poisoning.

However, histamine poisoning can also occur with aged cheese that has undergone spoilage, e.g. Swiss cheese, Cheddar, Emmental, Gruyère, blue cheese and Camembert. Such cheeses may have histamine levels over 1000 ppm.

Symptomatology

Many foods contain small amounts of histamine which can be easily tolerated and are not necessarily hazardous. Intestinal bacteria also produce histamine. A fairly efficient detoxification system exists in the intestinal tract to metabolize histamine. The system has two distinct enzymes: DAO and histamine *N*-methyltransferase (HMT). The enzymes convert histamine into nontoxic products.

The detoxification system is adequate for handling normal dietary intakes of histamine. However, it apparently fails to detoxify the large amounts of histamine that can be ingested with spoiled fish or cheese (usually over 500 ppm).

Since it is an intoxication, the incubation period is short (less than 1 h to a few hours) following ingestion, with wide variation from individual to individual. It is usually a mild illness of short duration (about 8 h). The most consistently noted symptoms are nausea, cramps and an oral burning sensation. Diarrhoea, flushing, headache, vomiting, urticaria and/or palpitations can also occur. Most individuals suffering from histamine poisoning experience only a few of these symptoms. The facial flush is principally caused by the dilating action of histamine on the small blood vessels, capillaries and venules. The flush is usually followed by a headache, which becomes a continuous dull ache deep inside.

Prevention of Histamine Poisoning

Good hygienic practices and storage at temperatures between 2 and 10°C can prevent the formation of large amounts of amines in food, including histamine. The microflora of fish or milk is a reflection of the microflora of their environment, of which histamine-producing bacteria are a part. Fresh fish and fresh milk are practically devoid of histamine. Postcatching and post-handling contamination with histamine-producing bacteria may occur in processing plants and in the distribution chain. The optimal temperature for histamine generation ranges from 15 to 35°C.

Tyramine and Hypertensive Crisis

Tyramine, an active pressor amine, occurs naturally in many foods. Tyramine is formed during cheesemaking and storage by microbial degradation of milk protein and subsequent decarboxylation of tyrosine. Tyramine generally does not represent any hazard to individuals unless large amounts are ingested or the normal routes of catabolism are inhibited or are genetically deficient.

Usually, tyramine is metabolized to *p*-hydroxyphenylacetic acid by MAO in the human intestine, liver and kidneys and excreted via the urine. However, tyramine can cause a hypertensive crisis in patients treated with MAO inhibitor (MAOI) drugs, which block the pathway for catabolism and inactivation of the amine after ingestion. Tyramine raises the blood pressure by releasing noradrenaline and norepinephrine. When MAOI drugs were first used in the treatment of tuberculosis and later for depressive illness (antidepressants), a number of patients developed severe hypertension after ingestion of cheese, mainly due to its content of tyramine. The symptoms of the 'cheese reaction' (or 'cheese effect') include high blood pressure, headache (a feeling of fullness in the head), fever and sometimes vomiting. A sudden increase in blood pressure can occur as a result of ingestion of 10–25 mg of tyramine, particularly in patients receiving MAOI treatment. Cheese (aged or spoiled) has been reported to contain tyramine at concentrations of up to 5000 ppm and was the food initially associated with hypertensive disturbances noted in patients undergoing treatment with MAOI drugs.

Quantitative studies have shown tyramine to be present at variable concentration in meat extracts, yeast extracts, pickled herring, chicken liver, beer, wine, coffee, chocolate, sauerkraut and fermented soya bean products. Some of these products were shown to induce a hypertensive crisis similar to that attributable to cheese.

Thus, patients taking MAOI drugs are routinely given dietary warning cards.

Phenethylamine and other catecholamines, which may be present in some foods, may have the same effect as tyramine.

Migraine-inducing Amines

Migraine can be defined as a symptom complex occurring periodically and characterized by pain in the head (usually unilateral), vertigo, nausea and vomiting, often with photophobia and scintillating appearance of light. Food may play a role in the migraines of some individuals, and a type of migraine is known as 'dietary migraine'. Food may serve as a migraine trigger through an allergic reaction to food proteins or through the amine content of the food.

Chocolate, cheese and citrus fruits are associated with dietary migraine. Phenethylamine, tyramine and related compounds has been widely studied as potential causes of migraine. About 3 mg of phenethylamine or 125 mg of tyramine induced headache in patients who suffer from dietary migraine.

Phenethylamine- and tyramine-containing foods can cause most dietary migraine patients to suffer a classical migraine attack. Phenethylamine occurs in varying concentrations in chocolate, wine, cheese and fish.

Di- and Polyamines

Putrescine, spermidine and spermine occur universally in plants and animals, including microorganisms. These amines are important in the regulation of nucleic acid function and protein syntheses in ribosomes, and play a role in the stabilization of membranes, control of cell pH, and cell proliferation. Polyamines are growth-promoting 'hormones' and occur, therefore, in high concentration in rapidly growing tissues. Polyamine levels are also increased in cancer cells, and an increased excretion of polyamine in urine is an index for cancer. *See* Cancer, Epidemiology; Nucleic Acids, Physiology; Protein, Synthesis and Turnover

In plants, arginine is decarboxylated to agmatine, and putrescine is formed from agmatine via *N*-carbamylputrescine. In conditions of potassium and magnesium deficiency, agmatine and putrescine accumulate in plants. Spermidine and spermine are formed from putrescine. Fertilization seems to increase the polyamine content of seeds. In the embryo of mature seeds the spermidine content can reach a level as high as 1 mg g^{-1}. These amines are responsible for seed development and germination.

Occurrence in Foods

Amines in Fish

Trimethylamine

TMA is one of the major components of the smell of spoiled marine fish, and its level is used as an objective index of fish quality. For most fish, the usual sensory borderline of acceptable quality is 15 mg of TMA nitrogen per 100 g of tissue. The international limits are between 5 and 15 mg per 100 g. Trimethylamine oxide (TMAO) is present in the muscle of marine fish and in some freshwater fish. The amount in marine fish ranges from 75 to 250 mg of nitrogen per 100 g. Non-bacterial enzymes present naturally in the flesh (endogenous enzymes) degrade TMAO into DMA and formaldehyde. Spoilage bacteria reduce TMAO to TMA. Thus, the amount of TMA present in fish can give an indication of the degree of bacterial spoilage.

Biogenic Amines

Histamine is formed in fish having a high content of free histidine, by bacterial action. A histamine concentration of over 1000 ppm in fish is poisonous even before spoilage can be detected by organoleptic examination. A concentration of over 500 ppm in fish is seen as the hazard action level of histamine. Most countries do not have firm regulations for permitted levels of histamine in fish; however, the provisional limit of 100–200 ppm has been established in some countries (e.g. the USA, the FRG). A histamine content of over 50 ppm indicates that the fish has been unnecessarily exposed to high temperatures.

Histamine formation in fish rich in free histidine (mainly scombroid fish) depends on the presence of microorganisms able to produce histidine decarboxylase and temperatures of over 0°C. Histamine-produc-

ing bacteria can be divided into two categories: those species capable of producing large quantities of histamine (> 1000 ppm) in tuna fish infusion broth (TFIB), during a short incubation period (< 24 h) at a temperature above 15°C; and those species capable of producing somewhat smaller quantities of histamine (< 25 ppm) in TFIB after a prolonged incubation (> 48 h) at a temperature of 30°C or above. *Proteus morganii, P. mirabilis, Klebsiella pneumoniae, Hafnia alvei, Clostridium perfringens* and *Enterobacter aerogenes* appear to belong to the category of prolific histamine producers. Most active are various strains of *P. morganii* (*Morganella morganii*), which has been identified as the main histamine-producing bacterium in fish. *See* Clostridium, Occurrence of *Clostridium Perfringens*

Putrescine and cadaverine increase markedly as the decomposition of fish progresses and are recommended as indices for quality. A concentration between 1 and 10 ppm is an indicator of initial decomposition, while a concentration of over 10 ppm indicates advanced decomposition.

In order to evaluate the degree of decomposition of fish, a chemical quality index (QI) has been defined (concentrations of amines in parts per million):

$$QI = \frac{\text{Histamine} + \text{Putrescine} + \text{Cadaverine}}{1 + \text{Spermidine} + \text{Spermine}}.$$

The QI classifies the quality of fish materials as acceptable, borderline (initial decomposition) and unacceptable) (advanced decomposition).

Amines in Milk Products

The biogenic amine concentration (tyramine, histamine, putrescine, cadaverine) in fresh milk, yoghurt, milk powder, cottage cheese, quark, cream cheese and butter milk is quite small (less than 1 ppm). The formation of large amounts of biogenic amines in cheese has been reported only in aged and spoiled cheeses. The major factors that govern the formation, concentration and type of amines are the availability of free amino acids, and hence the proteolysis of cheese, the presence of bacteria with decarboxylase activity and the existence of proper conditions for growth and activity (pH, temperature, salt, water activity). Biogenic amines found in cheese may be aromatic (tyramine, histamine, phenethylamine and tryptamine) or aliphatic (putrescine and cadaverine).

Tyramine

The tyramine content of cheese is known to be variable not only in different types of cheese but also in the same type (from 0 up to 5000 ppm, but usually less than 100 ppm). These levels of tyramine are only toxic for patients receiving MAOI drugs. As little as 6 mg of tyramine taken orally can cause a rise in blood pressure.

Microorganisms of the starter cultures seldom produce the enzymes which create the amines in question. The high concentration of tyramine found in some cheeses, such as cheddar, Emmental, Gouda, blue cheese, Gorgonzola, Mascarpone and Camembert, are associated with poorly controlled cheese production and storage at an elevated temperature for an abnormally long period. Microorganisms responsible for tyramine formation in some cheeses are *Streptococcus* spp. (e.g. *S. faecalis*), coliforms (e.g. *Escherichia coli*), *Clostridium* spp., *P. mirabilis* and *Pseudomonas reptilivoriae*. *See* Enterobacteriaceae, Occurrence of *Escherichia Coli*; Starter Cultures

Histamine

Reported incidents of histamine poisoning in relation to cheese consumption, usually involves products with more than 1000 ppm of histamine. In some cases, concentrations of more than 18 000 ppm have been determined. A histamine-producing strain of *Lactobacillus buchneri* isolated from Swiss cheese was responsible for an outbreak of histamine poisoning. *Lactobacillus delbrueckii* (L. 30a) and *Streptococcus lactis* are also histamine producers in cheeses such as Swiss cheese, Gouda, Gruyère, Cheddar, Emmental, blue cheese and Camembert. There is no clear relation between the quality of cheese and the amount of histamine. Most cheeses have a histamine concentration of less than 10 ppm.

Putrescine and Cadaverine

These amines usually occur in a concentration of less than 5 ppm. In aged and spoiled Tilsiter, Roquefort, Gorgonzola, Camembert and similar cheeses the concentration can be over 1000 ppm.

Amines in Meat

Recent investigations on biogenic amines in meat suggest the possibility of using the content of cadaverine and putrescine in meat and meat products as indicators of freshness and quality. In ground beef, pork and poultry the putrescine and cadaverine content is less than 1 ppm, and increases gradually during storage. Before spoilage occurs the concentration increases by a factor of 10, and at the initial stages of spoilage by a factor of 100. Typical spoilage bacteria, such as members of the Pseudomonadaceae and Enterobacteriaceae, produce such amines and correlate with the content of putrescine and cadaverine in meat. Cadaverine is the only amine that correlates significantly with

coliform bacteria in meat. Tyramine and histamine concentrations in meat products increase during the fermentation stage and during storage to reach levels of up to 500 ppm. *See* Meat, Slaughter

Amines in Wine

A wide range of histamine concentrations in wine has been reported (from 0 to 40 ppm). Tyramine may occur in some wines. Chianti wine may contain a high content of tyramine (up to 25 ppm). Red wines contain an average of about 3 ppm of histamine, which is higher than that in white wines (about 1·2 ppm). This may be because red wine vinification methods lead to much higher contamination with bacteria. An upper limit of about 2 ppm of histamine in wine has been proposed, since wine manufactured under optimum conditions from a hygienic viewpoint should contain practically no amines. *See* Wines, Production of Table Wines

Alcohol may potentiate the effects of biogenic amines in wine and other foods by the inhibition of MAO and DAO and by facilitating amine absorption through the intestinal mucein.

Intoxication due to a high content of histamine or tyramine in wine has not been described and it appears unlikely that normal consumption of wine could precipitate poisoning or hypertension.

Amines in Fermented Vegetables

Amines are normally present in small quantities in fermented vegetables and lactic acid-fermented vegetables are rarely involved in food poisoning caused by biogenic amines. The histamine content is usually less than 50 ppm in fermented cabbage in the production of sauerkraut; however, the level increases simultaneously with the appearance of *Pediococcus cerevisiae*.

Amines in Fruits

The presence of several biogenic amines in bananas was discovered by accident. In a study on the excretion of 5-hydroxyindoleacetic acid (5-HIAA) as an index for the clinical diagnosis of carcinoid tumours, in monkeys fed with bananas, the final estimate of 5-HIAA in the urine was increased about 25-fold. 5-HIAA is the metabolite of serotonin. Thus, bananas, (and also pineapples, figs, walnuts and tomatoes) due to their serotonin content (5–15 ppm), should be excluded from the diet before attempting to diagnose a carcinoid tumour. Serotonin inhibits gastric secretion and bananas have been recommended for the treatment of peptic ulcers. The amount of serotonin in banana pulp decreases and in banana peel increases during maturation. Tryptamine, noradrenaline and dopamine and a series of aliphatic monoamines have also been found in bananas. *See* Bananas and Plantains

Citrus fruits contain varying amounts of tyramine and its derivatives such as synephrine, octopamine and feruloylputrescin, which are vasoactive. *See* Citrus Fruits, Composition and Characterization

Analysis of Amines in Food

The current most sensitive, fast and accurate methods for the determination of biogenic amines in foods makes use of amino acid analysers or high-performance liquid chromatography. Both methods can be recommended. If these techniques are not available, thin-layer chromatography and gas chromatography can be used. *See* Amino Acids, Determination; Chromatography, Thin-layer Chromatography; Chromatography, Gas Chromatography; Chromatography, High-performance Liquid Chromatography

For the determination of histamine itself, fluorometry provides the basis for the most accurate and fastest method, after suitable fluorogenic labelling. *See* Spectroscopy, Fluorescence

There is a voluminous literature on the extraction, purification and determination of amines in food and the interested reader is referred to the Bibliography.

Bibliography

Arnold SH and Brown WD (1978) Histamine toxicity from fish products. *Advances in Food Research* 24: 113–154.
Askar A and Treptow H (1986) *Biogene Amine in Lebensmitteln*. Stuttgart: Ulmer.
Franzen F and Eyesell K (1969) *Biologically Active Amines Found in Man*. New York: Pergamon Press.
Mietz JL and Karmas E (1977) Chemical quality index of canned tuna as determined by high-pressure liquid chromatography. *Journal of Food Science* 42: 155–158.
Smith IA (1980) Amines in food. *Food Chemistry* 6: 169–200.
Tabor CW and Tabor H (1984) Polyamines. *Annual Review of Biochemistry* 63: 749–790.
Treptow H and Askar A (1990) Analytische Methoden für die Bestimmung von biogenen Aminen in Lebensmitteln. *Ernährung/Nutrition (Wien)* 14: 9–17.

A. Askar
University of Suez Canal, Ismailia, Egypt
H. Treptow
Technical University of Berlin, Berlin, FRG

AMINO ACIDS

Contents

Properties and Occurrence

Any molecule that contains both a carboxylic acid and an amino group can be called an amino acid. An α-amino acid has both the primary amino and carboxylic acid groups attached to the same carbon atom (the α-carbon; see Fig. 1). Also attached to the α-carbon is a hydrogen atom and a unique group of atoms (designated 'R'). R can be any of the groups listed in Table 1.

Amino acids will readily ionize in aqueous solution. By adjusting the pH of the solution it is possible to find a pH where both the α-amino and the α-carboxylic acid groups are equally ionized. At this pH (the isoelectric point pI) the amino acid is electrically neutral. This neutral form (shown in Fig. 1) is known as a zwitterion

(derived from the German word meaning 'hybrid ion'). Figure 2 shows the structure of the zwitterion form of the α-amino acid alanine. Note that the R group for alanine is a methyl group. *See* pH – Principles and Measurement

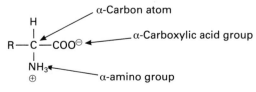

Zwitterion (dipolar)

Fig. 1 The structure of an α-amino acid shown as a zwitterion.

Table 1. The 20 amino acids commonly found in proteins showing the polarity of their R group at pH 7

Polarity of R group	Amino acid (abbreviations)	R group or side-chain
Nonpolar (hydrophobic)	L-Alanine (Ala or A)	$-CH_3$
	L-Valine (Val or V)	$-CH(CH_3)_2$
	L-Leucine (Leu or L)	$-CH_2-CH(CH_3)_2$
	L-Isoleucine (Ile or I)	$-CH(CH_2-CH_3)(CH_3)$
	L-Phenylalanine (Phe or F)	$-CH_2-$ (benzene ring)
	L-Proline (Pro or P)	(ring structure: $O=C(O^-)$, CH, CH_2, CH_2, CH_2, H_2N^+)
	L-Methionine (Met or M)	$-CH_2-CH_2-S-CH_3$
	L-Tryptophan (Try or W)	$-CH_2-$ (indole ring, NH)
Polar but uncharged	L-Glycine (Gly or G)	$-H$
	L-Serine (Ser or S)	$-CH_2-OH$
	L-Glutamine (Gln or Q)	$-CH_2-CH_2-C(=O)-NH_2$
	L-Threonine (Thr or T)	$-CH(CH_3)(OH)$
	L-Cysteine (Cys or C)	$-CH_2-SH$
	L-Asparagine (Asn or N)	$-CH_2-C(=O)-NH_2$
	L-Tyrosine (Tyr or Y)	$-CH_2-$ (benzene ring)$-OH$
Polar charged	L-Aspartic acid (Asp or D)	$-CH_2-COO^-$
	L-Glutamic acid (Glu or E)	$-CH_2-CH_2-COO^-$
	L-Lysine (Lys or K)	$-CH_2-CH_2-CH_2-CH_2-\,^+NH_3$
	L-Arginine (Arg or R)	$-CH_2-CH_2-CH_2-NH-C(=\,^+NH_2)-NH_2$
	L-Histidine (His or H)	$-CH_2-C=CH$ (imidazole ring: NH, $^+$NH, CH)

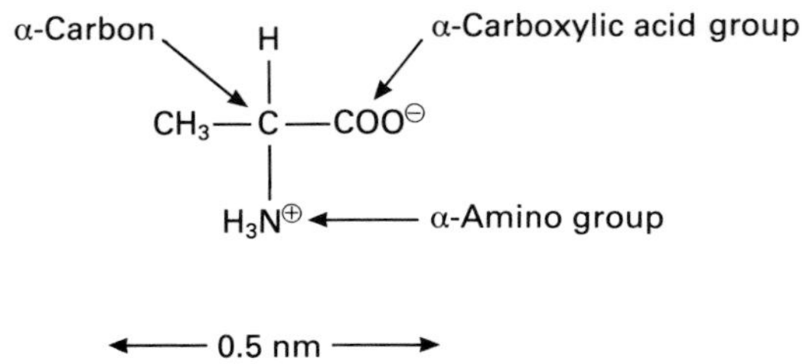

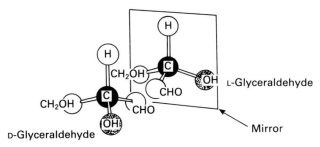

Fig. 2   Alanine – a typical α-amino acid.

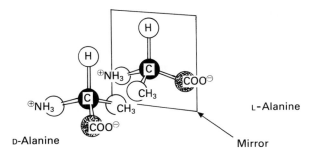

Fig. 4   The stereoisomers of alanine.

Fig. 3   The stereoisomers of glyceraldehyde.

Isomers

With the exception of glycine, all the commonly encountered α-amino acids contain at least one asymmetric carbon atom, i.e. their α-carbon atoms are bonded to four different substituent groups. Most amino acids therefore exist in two different arrangements or isomers. However, certain amino acids, i.e. isoleucine, threonine, hydroxylysine and hydroxyproline, have a second asymmetry centre and each one has, therefore, four stereoisomers. The stereoisomers of amino acids are mirror images of each other. They differ in their ability to rotate polarized light. These isomers are designated by either a $(+)$ or $(-)$ suffix (formerly *d* or *l*) to indicate that a pure solution of the stereoisomer would rotate polarized light clockwise (dextrorotatory) or anticlockwise (laevorotatory), respectively.

An amino acid is also designated as either the D or L isomer according to whether it can be prepared from or converted to D($+$)-glyceraldehyde or L($-$)-glyceraldehyde, respectively. This designation is the 'absolute configuration' of the amino acid. The relationship between the D and L isomers of glyceraldehyde and alanine can be seen in Figs 3 and 4.

Amino Acids and Proteins

Proteins are linear chains of L-α-amino acids linked together by peptide bonds. Different proteins have different sequences of amino acid residues along this

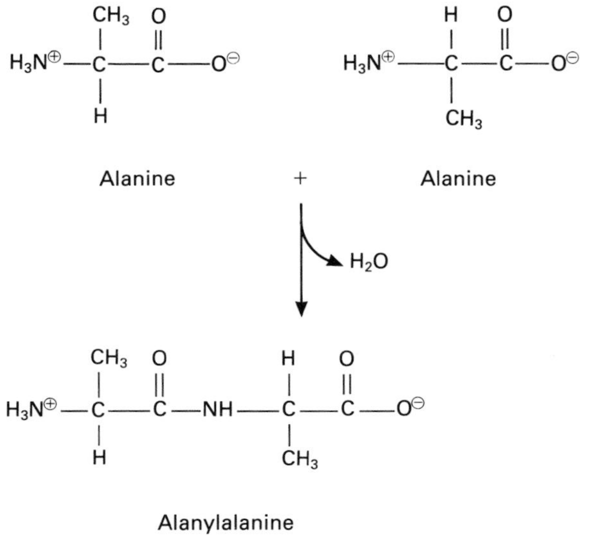

Fig. 5   The formation of a peptide bond between two molecules of alanine.

chain (the primary structure). Amino acids are often called 'the alphabet of proteins' because, when linked in a peptide chain, they are like letters in a word and spell out the 'name' of the protein. *See* Protein, Chemistry

Interestingly only the L forms of the α-amino acids are found in normal proteins. D-Amino acids are not involved in the metabolism of higher organisms. However, they can be part of the structural components of the cell walls of certain bacteria. They are included in some peptide antibiotics. L-Amino acids will slowly convert to mixtures containing equivalent amounts of D- and L-amino acids (racemization) with time or as a result of severe cooking or processing.

A peptide bond is formed between the α-amino and α-carboxylic acid groups of two amino acids. Figure 5 shows the formation of the dipeptide linkage between two alanine residues.

A peptide bond is a resonance hybrid between two configurations. One structure has a C=O double bond and a C—O single bond while the other has a C—O

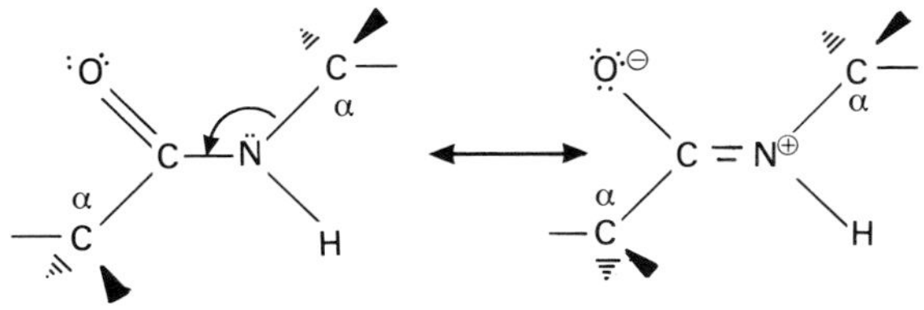

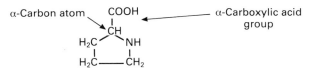

Fig. 8   Structure of proline.

Fig. 6 The two structures contributing to the resonance hybrid structure of the peptide bond.

cis   *trans*

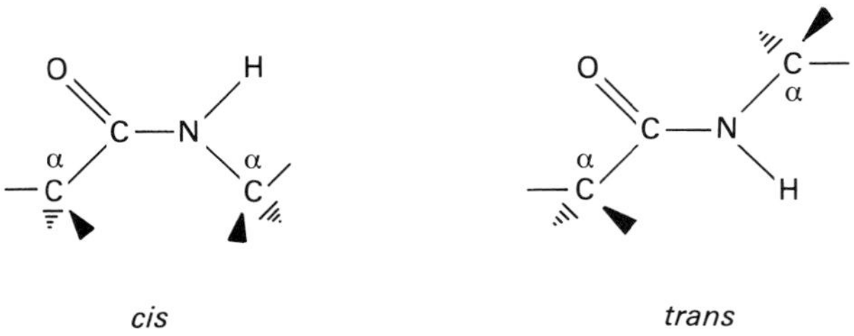

Fig. 7 The *cis* and *trans* configurations of the peptide bond.

Table 2.   The nonessential and essential amino acids required by humans

Nonessential	Essential
Alanine	Arginine[a]
Asparagine	Histidine
Aspartate	Isoleucine
Cysteine	Leucine
Glutamate	Lysine
Glutamine	Methionine
Glycine	Phenylalanine
Proline	Threonine
Serine	Tryptophan
Tyrosine	Valine

[a] Insufficient arginine is synthesized by a growing child.

single bond and a C=N double bond (see Fig. 6). The hybrid structure behaves as if it has a 'semi-double' bond, holding the four atoms of a peptide bond and the two α-carbon atoms in the same plane. The amino acid residues are not able to rotate freely due to the planar nature of the peptide bond, and the movement of the peptide chain is restricted. The peptide bond is limited to two configurations.

The peptide bond exists in nature in either the *cis* or *trans* configuration. The *cis* configuration is rare and is usually associated with proline residues. The *trans* configuration, holding the bulky atoms well apart, is by far the most common in nature (see Fig. 7).

The primary structure of a protein is very important as it contains all the information required for the protein to fold correctly. The effect exerted by the planar nature of the peptide bond and the amino acid composition and sequence in the peptide will determine the ultimate size and shape of a protein.

Amino Acids Commonly Found In Proteins

The same 20 α-amino acids (the standard amino acids) are commonly found in proteins. The combination of these 20 amino acids in any sequence, in any amount, can produce an almost infinite number of different proteins. The amino acids found in proteins are termed 'standard' (or occasionally 'primary' or 'normal'). This is to distinguish them from the large number of compounds that can be correctly classified as amino acids, but are not found in proteins. Within this last

group are a few amino acids that are important because they appear during protein metabolism or can be used as drugs.

Imino Acids Found in Proteins

Proteins often contain the imino acid L-proline (often abbreviated to 'Pro' or 'P') and, more rarely, L-4-hydroxyproline. Unlike α-amino acids (which have primary amines) the imino acids have secondary amines. The cyclic structure of proline is shown in Fig. 8. Notice that the nitrogen group attached to the α-carbon is also attached to the last carbon on the side-chain, making this a secondary amine.

A proline (or a hydroxyproline) residue in a polypeptide introduces a 'kink' or bend in the peptide chain. If the content of proline in a peptide is high then the peptide is likely to fold randomly. If the imino acid residues are positioned regularly along the peptide (as is true of collagen, the precursor of gelatin) then the protein is able to fold into a regular structure.

The Classification of Amino Acids

Amino acids can be usefully classified in many different ways. The two most common ways of classifying amino acids are by the polarity of the R group at pH 7 or whether they are essential or not in the diet of a healthy animal (see Table 2). As most proteins and amino acids function in aqueous environments at physiological pH, the first method is most helpful when considering the function of an amino acid in a protein *in vivo*. Hydrophobic R groups tend to be found in the interior of folded proteins. Table 1 shows the structure of the 20 amino acids commonly found in proteins classified according to their polarity in solution at pH 7.

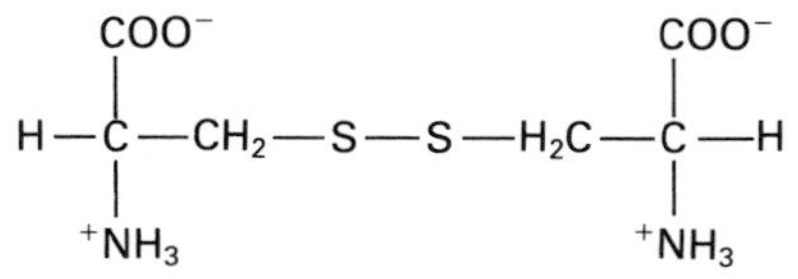

Physical, Chemical and Sensory Properties of Amino Acids (and Imino Acids) Found in Proteins

All amino acids are white crystalline solids that melt at high temperatures. Their molecular weights range from 75 to 204. The average molecular weight is estimated at 110 when calculating the number of amino acids in a protein (i.e. a protein with a molecular weight of 33 000 contains approximately 300 residues). Most of the amino acids are insoluble in organic solvents. They have varying solubilities in water.

Amino Acids Commonly Found in Proteins

Glycine (M_r 75.1). This amino acid has a sweet taste and its name is derived from the same Greek word as glucose ('glycos'). The R group is a single hydrogen atom, making it the smallest amino acid. Glycine is a small residue and will enable a protein to fold into a compact shape. Collagen is able to fold into a tight triple helix because every third amino acid is glycine. (The primary sequence of collagen is often abbreviated to Gly-Pro-X]$_n$ where X is often hydroxyproline.) The hydrogen atoms attached to the α-carbon atom are too small to influence the high degree of polarity of the α-amino and α-carboxylic acid groups.

Alanine (M_r 89.1). This is the next simplest amino acid. The R group of alanine is a methyl group (see Fig. 2). Like glycine this amino acid is found in high concentrations in tightly folded proteins such as keratin and collagen, including proteins in spiders' webs.

Serine (M_r 105.1). A hydroxyl group at the end of the side-chain makes serine polar but uncharged at pH 7. Like the other polar but uncharged amino acids (glycine, threonine, cysteine, tyrosine, asparagine and glutamine), serine is able to form hydrogen bonds with water, making it very soluble. Serine is an essential amino acid in the active sites of enzymes, especially the digestive enzymes trypsin and chymotrypsin. *See* Enzymes, Functions and Characteristics

Cystine (M_r 240.2) *and Cysteine* (M_r 121.1). These amino acids have R groups that contain sulphur either oxidized as a disulphide or reduced as a thiol. Cystine is two molecules of cysteine linked through a disulphide bond

Fig. 9 Disulphide bond in a cystine molecule linking two molecules of cysteine.

(see Fig. 9). When incorporated into proteins the disulphide bond between cysteine residues effectively 'pins' proteins together. It is interesting that nearly all proteins secreted by cells contain disulphide bonds. They help maintain the shape of the protein in what may be a hostile environment. The intracellular fluids are mildly reducing, a condition that favours cysteine; however, the extracellular environment is sufficiently oxidizing to favour cystine. The thiol of cysteine is essential for the catalytic activity of some enzymes.

Aspartic Acid (M_r 133.1). This amino acid is normally abbreviated to 'asp' but if, when it is determined, no distinction is made between aspartic acid and asparagine (the corresponding amide) it is abbreviated to 'Asx'. Aspartate has an acidic, net negatively charged R group at pH 7. It is electrically neutral at pH 2·98.

Asparagine (M_r 132.1). This was the first amino acid to be isolated (1806). It derives its name from asparagus, the plant from which it was first isolated.

Valine (M_r 117.1). Valine has a bulky, very hydrophobic R group. It is an essential amino acid for humans (the average person requires 1·5 g per day).

Leucine (M_r 131.2). The R group on leucine is aliphatic, nonpolar, bulky and very hydrophobic. It is an essential amino acid for humans (the average person requires 2·0 g per day).

Isoleucine (M_r 131.2). This amino acid is hydrophobic. It has two asymmetric carbon atoms and therefore can exist as any of four isomers. Only one isomer exists in proteins. It is an essential amino acid for humans (the average person requires 1·3 g per day).

Methionine (M_r 149.2). Like cysteine, methionine is a sulphur-containing amino acid. The sulphur in methionine, however, is unable to form disulphide bonds. The R group on methionine is nonpolar. Methionine plays an important role in protein synthesis. In eukaryotic cells all proteins translated from nuclear nucleic acid begin with a methionine residue. It is an essential amino acid for humans (the average person requires 2·02 g per day.

Threonine (M_r 119.1). This amino acid has a hydroxyl group as part of its R group, making it polar, but uncharged at physiological pH. It has two asymmetric carbon atoms and therefore can exist in any of four isomers. Only one form exists in proteins. This was the last amino acid to be identified (1938). It is an essential amino acid for humans (the average person requires 0·91 g per day).

Glutamine (M_r 146.1). The abbreviation for this amino acid is, 'Gln' (or 'Q') but 'Glx' (or 'Z') when no distinction is made between glutamic acid and the corresponding amide glutamine). Glutamine has a polar but uncharged R group. Glutamine is found in large amounts in the gliadin and glutenin fractions of wheat.

Glutamic Acid (M_r 147.1). This amino acid has an acidic, negatively charged R group. It therefore is found on the surface of proteins. It was first discovered in 1908 in edible seaweed when it was recognized as a flavour potentiator or enhancer. The salt monosodium glutamate (MSG) has a sweet and salty taste at very low concentrations. MSG increases sensitivity to sour and bitter tastes. Other amino acids such as ibotenic acid and tricholomic acid have been reported to have similar effects.

Lysine (M_r 146.2). A positively charged R group with a second amino group that can react with other residues to form covalent cross-links is found in this amino acid. These cross-links are very important in skin where they are involved in ageing effects. Lysine is very reactive with sugars and, through the Maillard reaction, can be responsible for an array of different flavour and colour compounds. Lysine is an essential amino acid for humans. Cereal protein is particularly low in lysine. The average person requires 1·5 g per day. *See* Browning, Nonenzymatic

Arginine (M_r 174.2). This amino acid has a positively charged guanidine group on the end of the R chain. This is a much stronger base than the amino group of lysine. Consequently, arginine is 100% protonated with a charge of +1 at physiological pH. Ammonia intoxication results in children (and cats) if this amino acid is absent from a fasting diet.

Histidine (M_r 155.2). A positively charged R group that contains a weakly ionized imidazole group is present in this amino acid. It is often found in the active sites of proteins and can be shown to be essential for the catalytic activity. For all practical purposes histidine is the only amino acid with significant buffering power near the pH of intracellular fluids and blood. Haemoglobin has a uniquely high content of histidine in order to buffer the effects of carbon dioxide.

Phenylalanine (M_r 165.2). This amino acid has an aromatic, nonpolar hydrophobic R group. Phenylketonuria is a disabling disease that is estimated to occur in 1% of mentally handicapped patients. It is caused by a failure to metabolize phenylalanine and sufferers must avoid eating foods containing phenylalanine.

Tryptophan (M_r 204.2). This amino acid has an aromatic, nonpolar hydrophobic R group. It is an essential amino acid for humans (the average person requires 0·5 g per day). Pellagra is a disease where victims develop skin rashes in response to sunlight. They also suffer diarrhoea, severe nervous depression and partial paralysis. The administration of tryptophan or the vitamin nicotinic acid reverses these symptoms. *See* Niacin Physiology

Tyrosine (M_r 181.2). This amino acid has an aromatic, polar but uncharged R group. Tyrosine is an important intermediate in the synthesis of adrenalin and thyroxin. Foods such as chocolate and cheese contain high levels of tyrosine and it has been suggested that tyrosine is responsible for some migraine-type headaches. *See* Migraine and Diet

Unusual Amino Acids

There are a number of unusual amino acids, derived from one of the 20 standard amino acids found in proteins.

Selenocystine. An analogue of cysteine where the sulphur atom has been replaced by selenium, this amino acid is found in the active site of selenium-dependent enzymes such as glutathione peroxidase. These enzymes are important for the removal of toxic hydrogen peroxide from cells. Generally, selenium salts are considered toxic when present in large amounts; however, small amounts are required for the synthesis of selenocystine. *See* Selenium, Physiology

Amino Acids Formed by the Posttranslational Modification of Proteins

Some amino acids found in proteins have been generated by modification of amino acids after they have been incorporated into a peptide.

Hydroxylation

Hydroxylation. Proline may be modified to 3-hydroxyproline or 4-hydroxyproline after it has been incorporated into a precursor peptide for collagen.

5-Hydroxylysine. Another unusual amino acid found in collagen. Hydroxylysine is a modification of lysine which occurs after lysine has been incorporated into a peptide.

Scurvy symptoms occur when these hydroxylations do not take place. *See* Scurvy

Phosphorylation

Phosphoserine residues bind calcium and consequently are found in proteins such as casein. The phosphorylated forms of threonine and tyrosine are also found in tissues. Phosphotyrosine is involved in the transformation of normal cells in cancer cells.

Carboxylation

γ-Carboxyglutamic acid. This amino acid is associated with calcium binding and is found in proteins such as prothrombin, the protein involved in blood clotting.

Methylation

ε-N-Methyllysine. This amino acid is found in the contractile muscle protein myosin and in cytochrome *c*. *See* Exercise, Muscle

Occurrence in Foods and Metabolism

Proteins are the most abundant macromolecules in living cells. All living tissues are able to synthesize protein and some amino acids, they therefore contain protein and amino acids. Higher plants are more versatile than animals. They can synthesize all the amino acids they require. Bacteria differ in their ability to make the amino acids they require. *Escherichia coli*, for instance, can make all the amino acids needed, but lactic acid bacteria must obtain certain amino acids from their environment. *See* Enterobacteriaceae, Occurrence of *Escherichia Coli*; Lactic Acid Bacteria

All animal foods such as meat, fish, milk and eggs contain protein. Most plant foods are poorer in protein. The exceptions are leguminous seeds and nuts. Their protein is, however, deficient in the sulphur-containing amino acids, particularly methionine. Leafy vegetables are somewhat richer in protein than root vegetables whereas fruits are very low in protein. Most plant foods are much poorer in protein than their seeds. The proteins found in cereal grain (seeds) are deficient in the essential amino acids lysine (maize grain is also low in tryptophan). *See* Protein, Food Sources

Glycosylation

Many proteins have carbohydrate side-chains. The sugars (often galactose and glucose) are attached to asparagine, serine or threonine residues, or through hydroxylated amino acid residues. Glycoproteins can form gel structures that control the water activity in foods and influence the texture of foods.

Covalent Cross-linking Amino Acids

Desmosine. The structure of desmosine is shown in Fig. 10. It is a derivative of lysine and forms a covalent cross-

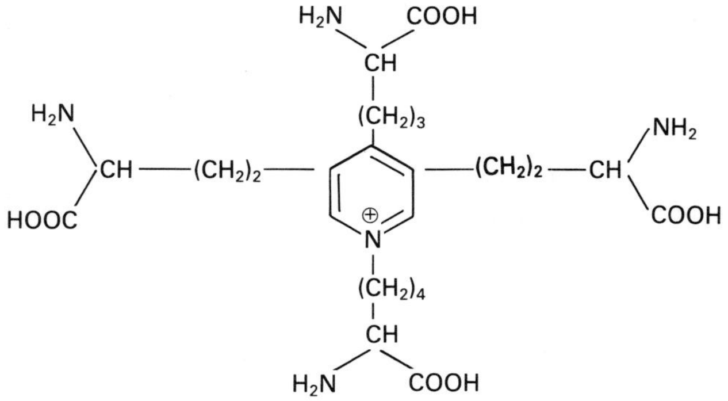

Fig. 10 The structure of desmosine.

link between proteins. It is found mainly in elastin and has been linked with the ageing effects seen in skin.

Animals can only synthesize some 20 amino acids. Those amino acids that cannot be synthesized by an organism (or cannot be synthesized in large enough amounts for metabolic requirements for synthesis) are called the essential amino acids. Humans can synthesize only 10 of the 20 amino acids required for their protein synthesis. The rest they must obtain from their diet if they are to remain healthy (see Table 2). *See* Protein, Synthesis and Turnover

Interestingly, the metabolism of children and adults is slightly different. The growing child has a greater requirement for arginine and histidine. Adults synthesize sufficient arginine for their daily requirement.

Protein rather than free amino acids are the main source of dietary amino acids. Some amino acids are recovered from damaged or degraded protein, but this process is less efficient in energy terms. About 75% of amino acid metabolism in a normal healthy adult is devoted to the synthesis of protein. This protein is essential for maintenance, repair and growth of tissue and also for the production of active enzymes, plasma protein, muscle creatine and, in females, the production of milk proteins. The remaining 25% of amino acid metabolism produces intermediates of the tricarboxylic acid (TCA) cycle, hormones and neurotransmitters.

Amino Acids in Physiological Fluids

Amino acids can be either metabolic intermediates or form parts of molecules that are biologically active. Ornithine and citrulline (Fig. 11) are just two examples of metabolic intermediates. They play an important part in the metabolic oxidation of amino acids carried out by the liver.

Amino Acid Neurotransmitters and Hormones

The amino acids glutamate, glutamine, aspartate, glycine and *γ*-aminobutyric acid (GABA) will act as

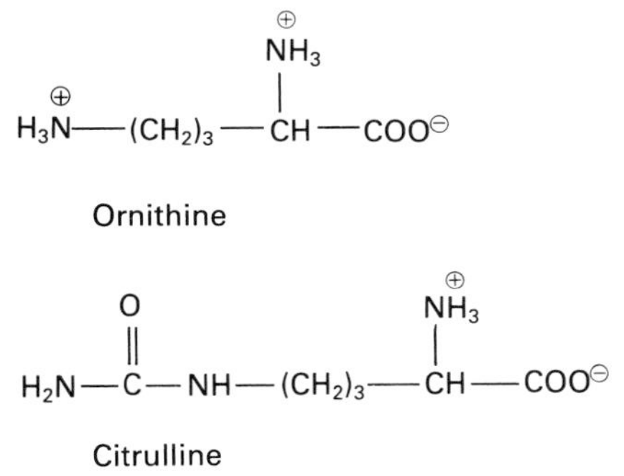

Fig. 11 The structures of ornithine and citrulline.

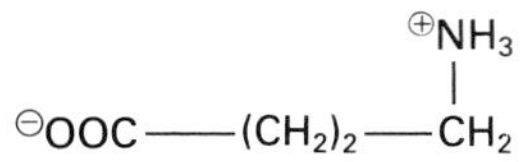

Fig. 12 The structure of γ-aminobutyric acid.

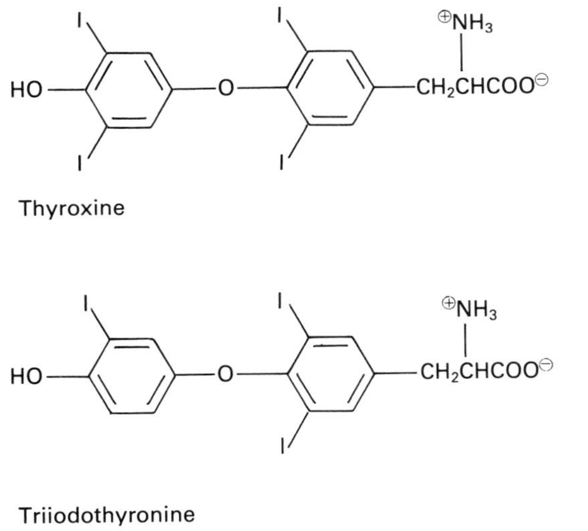

Fig. 13 The structures of thyroxine and triiodothyronine.

neurotransmitters for specific types of neurones or regions of the brain. Glutamate is one important excitory transmitter in the central nervous system of invertebrates and possibly in humans. GABA is found in relatively high concentrations (at around 0·8 mM), almost exclusively in brain tissue. It acts as an inhibitory transmitter by making it more difficult for a nerve to 'fire'. The structure of GABA is shown in Fig. 12.

Thyroxine and triiodothyronine (Fig. 13) are hormones derived from the amino acid tyrosine. Both these hormones stimulate metabolism in tissues. *See* Hormones, Thyroid Hormones

Chemical Properties Relevant to Foods

Deamination

Amino acids undergo deamination during fermentation. This is important in the production of flavour compounds in bread and beers. If deamination is allowed to go too far diamines may form, giving the food a fishy or spoiled odour. *See* Flavour Compounds, Structures and Characteristics

Maillard Browning

Under low-moisture and high-temperature conditions, amino acids undergo condensation reaction with carbonyl groups, i.e. aldehydes, ketones and reducing sugars. The products of these reactions are numerous. They are complex colour compounds referred to collectively as 'melanoids' that have a slightly bitter flavour. They are very important in the perception of food acceptability, especially of baked foods.

Processing Aids

L-Cysteine, L-glutamyl-L-cysteine, L-cysteinylglycine and glutathione (γ-L-glutamyl-L-cysteine-glycine) are naturally present in wheat flour. In certain dough processes flour can be enriched with these molecules or with mixtures of these molecules with oxidizers to produce desired properties in the dough or to reduce mixing times. *See* Flour, Dietary Importance

Amino Acids in Artificial Sweeteners

Aspartame is composed of two amino acids, aspartic acid and phenylalanine. This molecule is about 200 times as sweet as sucrose and has no aftertaste. It breaks down slowly at room temperature and rapidly at higher temperatures, making it unsuitable for baked foods. People with phenylketonuria cannot tolerate this sweetener because of the phenylalanine content. *See* Sweeteners – Intense

Bibliography

Bigwood EJ (ed.) (1972) Protein and amino acid functions. *International Encyclopaedia of Food and Nutrition*. Oxford: Pergamon Press.

Brown WH (1987) *Introduction to Organic and Biochemistry*, 4th edn. California: Wadsworth.

Lehninger AL (1987) *Lehninger – Principles of Biochemistry*, 5th edn. New York: Worth.

Barbara Brockway
University of Reading, Reading, UK

Determination

Analysis of foods to determine their amino acid composition has long been of importance nutritionally, but there are an increasing number of other applications, including detection of adulteration and potentially toxic amino acids produced by new food-processing technologies. This article will review current methods of the determination of amino acids.

Isolation of Free and Protein Amino Acids

Although determination of the total amino acid composition of foods, after protein hydrolysis, is the prime requirement it is sometimes necessary to determine free amino acids in foods, beverages, physiological fluids and tissues. To do this it is necessary to remove any protein before analysis. Methods of deproteinizing include precipitation with acids or alcohols, high-speed centrifugation, ultrafiltration, ion-exchange and equilibrium dialysis. None are perfect but precipitation with sulphosalicylic acid is the most popular method although not always suitable for all derivatization procedures.

It may be necessary to remove nonprotein substances from samples before hydrolysis since they can affect the accuracy of the analysis or damage stationary phases by irreversible adsorption. Since the extraction procedures are lengthy and can result in losses of protein they are normally only used when these substances are present in high concentrations, e.g. lipids in mechanically separated meat. Such samples are homogenized with 15 ml g^{-1} of an acetone/chloroform (3:1) mixture and filtered on a Buchner funnel until air dry. In addition to lipids it is claimed that this procedure removes nucleic acids and most of the carbohydrates. Nucleic acids may also be removed by heating the lipid-free sample with 10% NaCl at 85°C, removing the NaCl with water and drying with acetone. After hydrolysis or deproteinization, nonprotein substances can interfere with precolumn derivatization procedures used for reversed-phase chromatography (RPC) and gas–liquid chromatography (GLC). Lipids can be extracted with chloroform and salts, carbohydrates and acids by cation exchange followed by recovery of the amino acids with 2 M NH$_4$OH. The strength of the NH$_4$OH is critical since concentrations > 2 M can lead to degradation of amino acids. *See* Chromatography, Gas Chromatography; Chromatography, High-performance Liquid Chromatography

Hydrolysis Procedures

Acids, alkalis or enzymes may be used for protein hydrolysis. Alkaline hydrolysis is generally only used in the determination of tryptophan since other amino acids are degraded.

Enzymatic Hydrolysis

Enzymatic hydrolysis is rarely used except for the determination of glutamine and asparagine which are converted to aspartic and glutamic acids together with ammonia by acid hydrolysis. Since no single protease will hydrolyse all the peptide bonds in proteins the procedure is lengthy and there is evidence of contamination by amino acids derived from the enzymes. A better method is to analyse the sample before and after treatment with bis(1,1-trifluoroacetoxy)iodobenzene which converts the carboxamide residues to their corresponding amines. *See* Enzymes, Use in Analysis

Acid Hydrolysis

The most favoured procedure involves heating the protein with excess 6 M HCl under reflux or in a sealed tube *in vacuo* or under nitrogen at 110°C for 24 h. After filtration the HCl must be removed, usually by rotary evaporation or neutralization with NaOH, before analysis. However, this procedure is a compromise, since no one method can provide satisfactory values for all amino acids. The problem of tryptophan has already been mentioned, but cystine, cysteine and methionine undergo variable degradation through oxidation during acid hydrolysis, and an alternative procedure must be used. Tyrosine losses can also occur due to oxidation but this may be reduced by the addition of phenol to the HCl.

There are smaller, but progressive, losses of threonine and serine which may be compensated for by corrections of 5 and 10% respectively, or more precisely by hydrolysing for 24, 48 and 72 h and calculating to zero time. Since isoleucine and valine are difficult to liberate completely in 24 h, for the most accurate values it is again necessary to hydrolyse for 24, 48 and 72 h and then to calculate to infinite time. This is rarely carried out for foods.

To obtain the ideal amino acid analysis much time and care must be spent on the hydrolysis stage. Since analysis time has been reduced from 24 h to around 30 min there have been many efforts to automate and reduce the time of the hydrolysis. Commercial systems are available for 42 samples to be hydrolysed in 24 h at 110°C using standard liquid phase HCl. The same number can be hydrolysed in 1 h at 150°C using vapour phase hydrolysis. In liquid phase hydrolysis HCl is added directly to the sample. In vapour phase hydrolysis, tubes containing the sample are sealed into a larger vessel containing HCl. As the vessel is heated the HCl vaporizes so that only the vapour comes into contact with the sample. This has the advantage of avoiding contamination from amino acids present in all but the highest-purity HCl. A recent development is microwave irradiation in which samples can be hydrolysed in liquid phase HCl at $180 \pm 5°C$ in 5 min in a microwave oven. Special tubes that can resist high temperatures and pressures must be used. In common with most new innovations developed for use with pure proteins care should be taken in applying them to foods where the presence of carbohydrates often results in losses of amino acids during hydrolysis.

Chromatographic Methods

After hydrolysis or deproteinization it is necessary to separate the amino acids from each other and for this chromatography is the method of choice. Chromatographic separations may be of three types: column chromatography in which the stationary phase is packed into glass or metal columns; thin-layer chromatography (TLC) in which the stationary phase is coated onto inert plates; and paper chromatography in which the stationary phase is supported by the cellulose fibres of a paper sheet. Neither of the latter two methods are particularly quantitative and are little used, although TLC is used to monitor inborn errors of metabolism. Column chromatography consists of GLC and high-performance liquid chromatography (HPLC). *See* Chromatography, Principles; Chromatography, Thin-layer Chromatography

High-performance Liquid Chromatography

HPLC can be subdivided into methods involving post- or precolumn derivatization.

Postcolumn Derivatization

Postcolumn derivatization involves separating underivatized amino acids on a chromatographic column, mixing a derivatization reagent with the eluent from the column, passing the mixture through a reaction coil and then through a detection system (spectrophotometer or fluorometer). This type of HPLC is usually carried out using ion-exchange chromatography (IEC) with sulphonated polystyrene cation exchange resins as the stationary phase and aqueous sodium citrate (for hydrolysates) or lithium citrate (for physiological fluids) mobile phases. This, when coupled with derivatization with ninhydrin, is the traditional method and still considered to be the best. Other derivatizing reagents, o-phthalaldehyde (OPA), fluorescamine, dabsyl chloride (DABS-Cl) and 4-fluoro-7-nitro-2,1,3-benzoxadiazole (NBD-F), have been used to increase sensitivity, as the derivatives formed can be detected by fluorescence.

Precolumn Derivatization

In precolumn derivatization the mixture of amino acids is treated with a reagent to form derivatives which are highly fluorescent or ultraviolet-absorbing and can be separated by reversed-phase chromatography (RPC). RPC, a fairly recent innovation to amino acid analysis, is a partition system in which the mobile phase is more polar than the stationary phase. The most popular stationary phases are octadecyl-bonded silicas with acetate buffer as the mobile phase and a gradient of acetonitrile or methanol.

Many derivatizing reagents have been used, e.g. OPA, DABS-Cl, 1-fluoro-2,4-dinitrobenzene (FDNB), dansyl chloride (DNS-Cl), phenylisothiocyanate (PITC), 9-fluorenylmethyl chloroformate (FMOC), 4-N,N-dimethylaminoazobenzene-4′-isothiocyanate (DABITC), 1-fluoro-2,4-dinitrophenyl-5-L-alanine amide (FDAA) and 4-chloro-7-nitro-2,1,3-benzoxadiazole (NBD-Cl). Although giving high sensitivity, there are problems with all of these reagents (Table 1). Cleanup and derivatization are laborious but can be automated in commercial instruments, where DABS-Cl, PITC and FMOC are most commonly used.

Gas–Liquid Chromatography

In GLC the stationary phase is a liquid such as silicone grease supported on an inert granular solid and the mobile phase is an inert gas (N, He, Ar). Since amino acids are not volatile they must be converted to volatile derivatives before analysis. This is not difficult but there are even more derivatives than for RPC. However, the N-trifluoroacetyl (N-TFA) n-butyl and N-heptafluorobutyl (N-HFB) isobutyl esters appear to be the best. Derivatization is laborious although it has recently been automated. The major difference between these derivatives is their chromatographic separation. All the N-HFB isobutyl esters of protein hydrolysates can be readily separated on a single methylsilicone-packed column (e.g. OV 101, or 3% SE30 coated on 100–200 mesh Gaschrom Q) in 35 min or in less than 10 min with a capillary column (DB-1). Capillary columns are recommended for physiological fluids, analysis taking 1 h. With the popular N-TFA n-butyl esters it is impossible to separate all the amino acids on a single column. A column of 1% OV 7 + 0·75% SP2401 on 100–200 mesh Gaschrom Q is used for histidine, arginine and cystine and one of 0·65% EGA on 80–100 mesh Chromasorb W for the remainder. A major advantage of GLC is its sensitivity and specificity; since the mobile phase is gaseous, flame ionization, electron capture and nitrogen-specific detectors can be used. It is possible to detect femtomole levels of amino acids as their N-HFB isobutyl esters using capillary columns and electron capture detectors or mass spectrometry. Another

Table 1. Comparison IEC, RPC and GLC methods of amino acid analysis

	IEC	RPC	GLC[a]
Analysis time (min)			
Hydrolysates	30	30	10
Physiological fluids	90	50	35
Sensitivity (pmol)	50[b]	10	0·01
Disadvantages	Expensive instruments Complex mobile phases Low sensitivity	Some multiple or unstable derivatives Complex purification and derivatization Interference from salts, lipids and reagent contaminants Shorter column life Resolution poor for some amino acids	Complex purification and derivatization Interference from carbohydrates and lipids
Recommended applications	Protein hydrolysates Complex mixtures	Individual amino acids Peptide hydrolysates Screening metabolic disorders Enantiomeric analysis	Enantiomeric analysis Identification of amino acids

[a] N-HFB isobutyl esters, capillary column, electron capture detector.
[b] 5 pmol with OPA replacing ninhydrin.

advantage of GLC is that it can be linked with a mass spectrometer to provide confirmation of the identity and purity of peaks.

Comparison of IEC, RPC and GLC

Good agreement between these methods has often been claimed but usually in comparative studies with pure proteins. The choice of method is difficult and often depends on the applications, sensitivity and urgency required. Table 1 summarizes their main features. It is often suggested that a major advantage of RPC and GLC is that the instruments can be used for other analyses. If the requirement for amino acid analysis is small, and RPC and GLC instruments and expertise are already available, then these would be the methods of choice. The traditional, well-tried method is IEC followed by derivatization with ninhydrin. This is ideal for protein hydrolysates and complex mixtures where maximum accuracy and reproducibility are required and there is no shortage of sample. The sensitivity, analysis times and the cost of the instruments have improved considerably. Sample purification is rarely necessary since it is almost completely insensitive to sample matrix. The time taken for sample purification and derivatization for RPC and GLC should not be ignored and recent automation of these stages adds to the overall cost. The higher sensitivities of RPC and GLC are ideal where the amount of sample is limited, but care should

be taken to avoid contamination by amino acids from reagents and glassware.

A major problem with RPC is the choice of derivative, with little agreement on which is the best, since none are ideal. Ideally, it would be better if pre- and postcolumn derivatization could be avoided altogether. The separation of underivatized amino acids, at picomole levels, using anion exchange chromatography followed by pulsed amperometric detection has recently been proposed for protein hydrolysates. This uses complex aqueous mobile phases and would be difficult to apply to more complex mixtures. Whichever method is selected it should be stressed that the hydrolysis of proteins and the deproteinization of physiological fluids are still major problems.

Methods for Specific Amino Acids

Methionine and Cystine

These amino acids are difficult to estimate because they are present in low concentrations and undergo oxidation to multiple derivatives during acid hydrolysis. To overcome this problem, controlled oxidation of methionine to methionine sulphone and cystine to cysteic acid must be carried out with performic acid prior to acid hydrolysis. This consists of oxidizing the sample with performic acid–hydrogen peroxide for 16 h at 0°C. After removal of excess oxidizing reagents, acid hydrolysis is carried out as normal.

Tryptophan

Tryptophan is also present in low concentrations and extensively degraded during acid hydrolysis. However, there is no measurable end product and so it is normal to use alkaline hydrolysis specifically for tryptophan analysis. Sodium, barium or lithium hydroxides may be used at concentrations ranging from 4 to 6 M, with additives such as maltodextrin, starch or thiodigycol often recommended to reduce tryptophan losses. Hydrolysis may be for 8 h at 145°C or 20 h at 110°C using polypropylene vessels. Ideally the tryptophan should be separated from interfering compounds, e.g. lysinoalanine (LAL) by IEC or RPC. The latter takes only a few minutes and precolumn derivatization is unnecessary since tryptophan can be detected by its native fluorescence.

Tryptophan has also been estimated by acid hydrolysis of intact proteins in the presence of ninhydrin with which it reacts before it can be degraded. Corrections must be made for tyrosine.

Lysine and Available Lysine

There has been considerable interest in a specific method for lysine. However, even RPC methods take 15 min and would appear to have little advantage over complete analysis. However, available lysine is usually determined separately. If foods are subjected to heat during processing lysine can become nutritionally unavailable if its free ε-amino group reacts with, for example, carbohydrates, forming bonds which are resistant to digestive enzymes. Available lysine can be measured by treating proteins with FDNB or 2,4,6-trinitrobenzene sulphonic acid which reacts with the free ε-amino groups of lysine to form either ε-dinitrophenyllysine (DNP-lysine) or ε-trinitrophenyllysine (TNP-lysine). The lysine derivatives can be separated by RPC from other DNP or TNP amino acids in 15–20 min.

Lysinoalanine

Alkaline treatment of proteins is used extensively in food processing, e.g. in the preparation of textured proteins. This results in the formation of amino acids such as LAL, ornithinoalanine, lanthionine and β-aminoalanine. LAL is formed by reaction of the ε-amino group of lysine with the double bond of dehydroalanine which can result in the loss of available lysine and toxicity problems. LAL can be measured in 16 min by RPC after derivatization with DNS-Cl. Alternatively, LAL and all the common amino acids can be determined by IEC followed by ninhydrin derivatization in 110 min.

3-Methylhistidine

3-Methylhistidine is an analogue of histidine found mainly in skeletal muscle. Methylation of histidine occurs after its incorporation into the peptide chains of actin and myosin. Since after the catabolism of these proteins 3-methylhistidine is not recycled but quantitatively excreted in the urine, it has been proposed as an index of muscle protein turnover. It has also been used to determine the meat content of foods where vegetable or microbial protein have been added for economic or fraudulent reasons. 3-Methylhistidine may be estimated after derivatization with fluorescamine. Histidine and 3-methylhistidine give acid-stable fluorescent derivatives which can be separated by RPC in 20 min.

Hydroxyproline

If 3-methylhistidine is used as an index for meat protein, hydroxyproline must also be measured to correct for the collagen content. Collagen has a low content of essential amino acids, and excessive amounts in foods reduces their nutritive value. New technologies also make it possible to incorporate collagenous materials into meat products at high levels. There are histochemical, histological and immunological techniques available, but for routine purposes there is a British Standards method available. This involves oxidation of the hydroxyproline with chloramine T to pyrrole, followed by photometric determination of the reaction product of the pyrrole with p-dimethylaminobenzaldehyde. An RPC method taking 10 min also exists using NBD-Cl derivatization.

D- and L-Amino Acids

During alkali or heat treatment L-amino acids in proteins are racemized to their D-isomers. Since most D-amino acids cannot be utilized by humans and some are toxic their determination is of considerable interest. The D- and L- isomers have identical chemical properties and must first be converted to diastereomeric dipeptides by reaction with chiral (optically active) reagents before chromatography or separated by chiral stationary or mobile phases. The leucyl-DL-aspartic acid dipeptides are prepared by coupling aspartic acid with L-leucine N-carboxy anhydride (NCA). Basic amino acids are coupled with L-glutamine NCA. N-t-Butoxycarbonyl-L-cysteine and OPA are other chiral agents that have been used. Separation of 21 enantiomers in 40 min can be achieved by RPC and fluorescence detection. Precolumn derivatization can be avoided by using a chiral mobile phase, a copper–proline (Cu–Pro) complex, with IEC. Diastereomeric Cu–amino acid complexes are formed on the column and detected by postcolumn derivatization with OPA. Alternatively an RPC method using a chiral stationary phase, in which the Cu–Pro or Cu–hydroxyproline complex is bound to a silica stationary phase, can be used.

D- and L-amino acids can also be determined by GLC with the introduction of a second, optically pure, asymmetric centre into the molecule to make diastereoisomers which can be separated on conventional packed columns. The use of (+)-butan-2-ol to form (+)-2-butyl esters appears to be the best method. Alternatively the enantiomers, converted to normal derivatives, e.g. TFA isopropyl esters, can be separated on capillary columns coated with chiral stationary phases, e.g. *N*-TFA-L-valyl-L-valine cyclohexyl ester.

Bibliography

Bech-Anderson S, Mason VC and Dhanoa MS (1989) Hydrolysate preparation for amino acid determinations in feed constituents 9. Modifications to oxidation and hydrolysis conditions for streamlined procedures. *Zeitschrift für Tierphysiologie, Tierernährung und Futtermittelkunde* 63: 188–197.

Cohen SA and Strydom DJ (1988) Amino acid analysis utilizing phenylisothiocyanate derivatives. *Analytical Biochemistry* 174: 1–16.

Deyl Z, Hyanek J and Horakova M (1986) Profiling of amino acids in body fluids and tissues by means of liquid chromatography. *Journal of Chromatography* 379: 177–250.

Gehrke CW and Zumwalt RW (1987) Symposium on chromatography of amino acids. *Journal of the Association of Official Analytical Chemists* 70: 146–147.

Williams AP (1986) General problems associated with the analysis of amino acids by automated ion-exchange chromatography. *Journal of Chromatography* 373: 175–190.

Williams AP (1988) Determination of amino acids. In: Macrae R (ed.) *HPLC in Food Analysis*, 2nd edn. pp 441–470. London: Academic Press.

Alwyn P. Williams
AFRC Institute of Grassland and Environmental Research, Hurley, UK

Metabolism

Naturally occurring amino acids may be conveniently grouped into three categories: protein amino acids (sometimes known as 'standard', 'primary' and 'normal'), uncommon amino acids, and nonprotein amino acids. Protein amino acids are those that are coded for in the genes and incorporated directly into proteins. For some time it seemed well established that all proteins, whatever their origin, were constructed from the same set of 20 amino acids. Recent studies, however, have shaken the foundation of this classical dogma. It now seems that the genetic code may dictate the incorporation of more than 20 amino acids. Thus, for example, selenocysteine and phosphoserine, previously consid-

ered to be uncommon amino acids, can be directly incorporated into the polypeptide chain. All protein amino acids are α,L-amino acids. It is not clear why amino acids incorporated by organisms into proteins are of the L form, since L-amino acids have no obvious inherent superiority over their D isomers for biological function. Thus, in this article, unless otherwise stated, an L configuration is assumed.

The 20 classical protein amino acids may be grouped into several classes reflecting important characteristics of their side-chains: straight aliphatic amino acids (glycine, alanine), branched-chain amino acids (valine, leucine, isoleucine), hydroxy amino acids (serine, threonine), sulphur-containing amino acids (cysteine, methionine), aromatic amino acids (phenylalanine, tyrosine), heterocyclic amino acids (tryptophan, histidine), basic amino acids (lysine, arginine), acidic amino acids and their amides (aspartate, glutamate, asparagine, glutamine) and imino acid (proline). Amino acids can also be classified on the basis of the polarity of their side-chains. *See* Protein, Chemistry

Analyses of proteins have revealed that they contain well over 100 different amino acids. The occurrence of uncommon amino acids in proteins is the result of post-translational, covalent modification of protein amino acids. Cystine, for example, is formed by the post-translational cross-linking of two cysteine residues. Citrulline, *N*-formylmethionine, *O*-galactosylserine, and *N*-acetylthreonine constitute other examples of amino acids found in proteins.

The amino acids found in proteins are by no means the only ones to occur in living organisms. Thus the term 'nonprotein amino acids' is used to include those naturally occurring amino acids which are present in free or combined forms but not in proteins. Over 200 nonprotein amino acids are known, most of them occurring in plants and frequently limited, in each case, to certain taxonomic groups. Some, such as cystathionine and saccharopine, fulfil important roles in the primary metabolic pathways. However, the great majority of these compounds have obscure functions and are generally regarded as secondary products. Many of the nonprotein amino acids from plants are known to be toxic to animals, plants and microorganisms. Some accumulate to exceptionally high levels, as in the case of 5-hydroxytryptophan, canavanine or 3,4-dihydroxyphenylalanine, which may constitute up to 14% of the seed weight in some Leguminosae species. Storage and protection against predation are probably two of the many possible roles that these amino acids play in plants.

Essential and Nonessential Amino Acids

Organisms differ greatly in their abilities to synthesize the amino acids required for protein synthesis. Many microorganisms and plants are entirely self-sufficient in that they can synthesize the entire basic set of protein amino acids. However, the bacterium *Leuconostoc mesenteroides* can synthesize only four of the protein amino acids, whereas *Lactobacillus*, which flourishes in milk, must be provided with all amino acids required for protein synthesis. Mammals are intermediate, being able to synthesize about half of the protein amino acids. Amino acids which cannot be synthesized by an organism in adequate amounts are called essential or indispensable because they must be supplied by the diet. Those which can be synthesized by an organism from readily available precursors in sufficient amounts to meet its needs are not required in the diet and are referred to as nonessential or dispensable amino acids. A consensus of current nutritional opinion indicates that the L-isomers of 10 amino acids – arginine, histidine, isoleucine, leucine, lysine, methionine, phenylalanine, threonine, tryptophan and valine – are considered to be essential for mammals, including humans.

The designations of essential and nonessential amino acids refer to the needs of an organism under a particular set of conditions. Thus essential amino acids are often species specific, i.e. the set of amino acids that are essential for a particular organism is not necessarily the same for other organisms. The essential amino acids requirements depend on a variety of factors including age, sex, physiological conditions and diet. Arginine (see *Urea Cycle*, below) and histidine are synthesized by humans in quantities sufficient to meet the needs of an adult but not those of a growing child. These amino acids have been termed semi- or half-essential. Adults have proportionally lower demands for essential amino acids than infants and children because adults are able to efficiently recycle such amino acids, whereas infants need them for tissue growth. When the ratio of total essential amino acids required to total protein required is considered, it is 0·37 for infants and 0·15 for adults. Tyrosine and cysteine are considered nonessential amino acids for mammals only as long as the diet contains adequate amounts of, respectively, phenylalanine and methionine; this is because, in mammals, tyrosine is formed in one step directly from phenylalanine, and cysteine derives its sulphur uniquely from dietary methionine (see *Synthesis of Amino Acids* below). Hence the apparent quantitative phenylalanine requirement is actually a requirement for phenylalanine plus tyrosine, whereas that of methionine is for methionine plus cysteine.

The essential amino acids include those with complex structures, which are formed by complex routes, whereas the nonessential are those whose syntheses are the simplest and whose intermediate precursors are always present in all organisms. Indeed, 59 enzymes are required by prokaryotic cells to synthesize the essential amino acids for humans, but only 15 are required for the

non-essential. Essential amino acids other than lysine and threonine (the only amino acids that, in mammals, do not participate in transamination reactions; see *Transamination and Deamination*, below) can be replaced by their α-keto analogues in the diet. This indicates that the carbon skeleton of the essential amino acid is the fundamental part of the amino acid molecule.

A deficiency of even one essential amino acid in the diet of an organism results promptly in a negative nitrogen balance, i.e. total nitrogen excretion exceeding total nitrogen intake, indicating that tissue protein is being degraded and used to supply the missing amino acid for those 'high priority' proteins that need to be continually synthesized. The remaining amino acids then accumulate and are shunted into catabolic pathways – hence the loss of nitrogen. Under these conditions protein synthesis is severely inhibited because the ribosome – mRNA (messenger ribonucleic acid) – nascent polypeptide complex must suspend its operation at the point where the missing amino acid should be incorporated. Thus the degree of negative nitrogen balance is similar whether only one, several or all of the essential amino acids are missing. This is logical because nearly all body proteins contain all the essential amino acids.

Regardless of the organism or of the essential amino acids considered, the net result of its deficiency involves inevitably a decreased growth rate, increased susceptibility to disease and biochemical dysfunctions along with ultimate death. However, deficiencies of a specific essential amino acid may also result in disturbances characteristic of that particular amino acid. This is the case for tryptophan in nicotinic acid formation, and lysine in the formation of hydroxylysine in the biosynthesis of collagen. *See* Niacin, Physiology

Amino Acid Biosynthesis

Amino acid metabolism involves the dynamic occurrence of anabolic and catabolic pathways. It is sometimes difficult to distinguish between catabolic and anabolic reactions because the catabolism of one amino acid may be involved in the biosynthesis of another. Because of the complexity and multiplicity of these pathways only a simplified version of the major routes will be considered.

Nitrogen Assimilation

Inorganic nitrogen is incorporated into organic nitrogen compounds as ammonium. This process, called ammonium assimilation, leads to the formation of glutamate, glutamine and carbamoyl phosphate. Utilization of the nitrogen of carbamoyl phosphate is limited to the biosynthesis of arginine (see *Urea Cycle*, below) and pyrimidine nucleotides. Essentially, all other nitrogen atoms of amino acids and other nitrogenous compounds are derived directly or indirectly from glutamate or glutamine.

The reductive amination of 2-oxoglutarate by ammonium ions (NH_4^+), catalysed by glutamate dehydrogenase, is the simplest route to the formation of α-amino groups:

$$2\text{-Oxoglutarate} + NH_4^+ + NADPH + H^+ \longrightarrow$$
$$\text{glutamate} + H_2O + NADP^+$$

(NADPH, $NADP^+$ represent the reduced and oxidized forms of the nicotinamide adenine dinucleotides.) This reaction occurs in plants and bacteria only under situations of high NH_4^+ concentration, which is toxic to cells and does not happen frequently under natural conditions, implying that this enzyme does not play a significant role in primary ammonium assimilation. Under natural conditions, the glutamate synthase cycle constitutes the major pathway by which plants and microorganisms assimilate NH_4^+. This cycle involves the sequential action of two enzymes: glutamine synthetase, which catalyses the adenosine triphosphate (ATP)-dependent amidation of glutamate to produce glutamine, and glutamate synthase, which catalyses the reductive transfer of the δ-amino group of glutamine to 2-oxoglutarate, to produce two molecules of glutamate. The sum of these reactions is as follows:

$$2\text{-Oxoglutarate} + NH_4^+ + NADPH + ATP \longrightarrow$$
or
reduced
ferredoxin

$$\text{glutamate} + NADP^+ + ADP + P_i$$
or   (inorganic
oxidized   phosphate)
ferredoxin

Synthesis of Amino Acids

The biosyntheses of protein amino acids arise as branching pathways from a few key intermediates in the central metabolic routes that are common to all cells, namely glycolysis, the pentose phosphate pathway, and the tricarboxylic acid (TCA) cycle. It is convenient to divide the 20 classical protein amino acids into six biosynthetic families according to the central metabolites that serve as starting points for their syntheses. *See* Glucose, Function and Metabolism

The Glutamate Family

2-Oxoglutarate, a TCA cycle intermediate, serves as the starting point in the formation of glutamate and the

other members of the glutamate family, glutamine, proline, arginine and, in the fungi and *Euglena*, lysine:

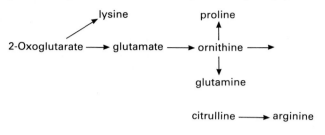

The Serine Family

3-Phosphoglycerate, an intermediate of the glycolytic pathway, serves as a precursor for the serine family of amino acids, comprising serine and its derivative amino acids, glycine and cysteine:

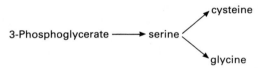

In common with carbon and nitrogen, environmental sulphur is available to organisms in the form of inorganic compounds. Sulphur assimilation is largely confined to plants and microorganisms since higher animals, unable to assimilate inorganic sulphur, must rely on ingested methionine and cysteine. Thus, whilst some microorganisms can reduce sulphate, thiosulphate or elemental sulphur, higher plants use sulphate for amino acids synthesis. Reductive assimilation of sulphate, i.e. incorporation of sulphate sulphur into thiol groups of amino acids and other organic compounds, requires the reduction of sulphate to sulphite and, subsequently, of sulphite to sulphide.

Two major pathways exist for the biosynthesis of cysteine in living organisms. Plants and microorganisms, which utilize H_2S as the source of sulphur, synthesize cysteine by the direct sulphhydrylation pathway. However, in mammals, which synthesize cysteine by the transsulphuration pathway, cysteine derives its carbon skeleton from serine but its sulphur atom is obtained uniquely from methionine.

The Aspartate Family

Oxaloacetate, an intermediate of the TCA cycle, provides the carbon skeleton for the synthesis of six different amino acids: aspartate, asparagine, lysine (in bacteria and plants but not in fungi), methionine, threonine and isoleucine, which constitute the aspartate family of amino acids:

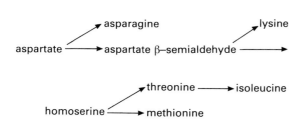

However, isoleucine is frequently included in the pyruvate family since four of its five biosynthetic enzymes are common to the valine pathway. Methionine derives its sulphur atom from cysteine.

The Pyruvate Family

The pyruvate family of amino acids includes alanine, valine and leucine:

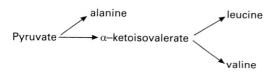

Pyruvate, a glycolytic intermediate, gives rise to the carbon skeletons of alanine and valine, and to 4 of the 6 carbons of leucine. In addition, pyruvate also donates 2 carbon atoms to the synthesis of isoleucine and, on average, 2·5 carbons to the synthesis of lysine in bacteria and plants. As mentioned earlier, isoleucine, a member of the aspartate family, is most conveniently considered along with valine, since the biosynthesis of both involves a common set of enzymes.

The Aromatic Family

Phenylalanine, tyrosine and tryptophan, which comprise the aromatic family of amino acids, are synthesized from phosphoenolpyruvate and erythrose 4-phosphate, intermediates of glycolysis and the pentose phosphate pathway, respectively:

Phosphoenolpyruvate + erythrose 4-phosphate⟶

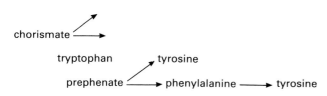

These amino acids are synthesized by a branched pathway in which chorismate is the major branch-point

metabolite. Chorismate is synthesized by a seven-step pathway, often referred to as the shikimate or common aromatic pathway, to build the benzene ring.

In some organisms, including humans, tyrosine can be synthesized by hydroxylation of phenylalanine in a reaction catalysed by phenylalanine hydroxylase. This reaction, the only known reaction of aromatic amino acid biosynthesis in animals, accounts for the nonessentiality of tyrosine in mammals, and is not reversible, which explains why tyrosine cannot replace the nutritional requirement for phenylalanine.

The Histidine Family

Histidine is synthesized from ribose 5-phosphate, a pentose phosphate pathway intermediate, by a pathway unrelated to those of the other amino acids.

Uncommon amino acids are synthesized by post-translational, covalent modification of protein amino acids. These modifications, which may either be enzyme-catalysed or occur spontaneously, involve a variety of chemical processes including glycosylation, phosphorylation, hydroxylation, methylation, acetylation and amidation. Hydroxyproline and hydroxylysine, for example, are two uncommon amino acids almost exclusively associated with collagen. The preformed amino acids, as they may occur in ingested food protein, are not incorporated into collagen since there are no tRNAs (transfer RNAs) capable of recognizing and inserting them into a nascent polypeptide chain. Rather, these amino acids are synthesized by hydroxylation of prolyl and lysyl residues, in reactions catalysed by prolyl hydroxylase and lysyl hydroxylase, respectively. 3-*N*-Methylhistidine constitutes another example of an uncommon amino acid. This amino acid, found in actin and myosin, is synthesized by methylation of an histidyl residue in an enzymatic reaction that utilizes *S*-adenosylmethionine as the methyl group donor. This process is clearly highly specific because only one histidine out of the 35 found in the heavy chain of myosin is methylated. Furthermore, the extent of methylation varies with a number of factors including age and diet and is generally not complete in that specific residues are found to be methylated in only a fraction of the myosin molecules.

Relatively little work has been done on the biosynthesis of non-protein amino acids. There are four different ways by which these amino acids may be formed: (1) as intermediates in protein amino acid synthesis; (2) modification of protein amino acids; (3) modification of pathways to protein amino acids; (4) novel pathways.

Regulation of Amino Acid Biosynthesis

Living cells contain a small pool of free protein amino acids resulting from a precise and coordinated control of the rates at which each amino acid is synthesized and degraded. The mechanisms that control amino acid synthesis vary widely in the various pathways and, for the same pathway, in different organisms. Most studies have been performed with microorganisms, in particular with *Escherichia coli*, *Bacillus subtilis* and *Salmonella typhimurium*. The regulation of amino acid biosynthesis occurs at two levels: regulation of enzyme activity or metabolite flow over a pathway and regulation of enzyme amount. *See* Enzymes, Functions and Characteristics

Control of Enzyme Activity

The control over the flow of metabolites into an amino acid biosynthetic pathway can be efficiently achieved by blocking the first, usually irreversible step which is specific for that amino acid. The inhibition of the committed step by the end product, i.e. the amino acid itself, constitutes the simplest kind of feedback inhibition. Some examples include the regulation of the biosynthesis of proline, arginine, histidine and of the branched-chain amino acids. Alanine, aspartate, glutamate and glycine are four amino acids for which no form of feedback inhibition is known. However, these amino acids are usually in equilibrium, by means of reversible reactions, with compounds that are key intermediates in the central metabolic routes. Metabolite flow into the biosynthetic pathways of the remaining 16 protein amino acids is controlled by several types of feedback inhibition.

Sequential feedback inhibition regulates the synthesis of aromatic amino acids in *B. subtilis*. The first divergent steps in the synthesis of these amino acids are inhibited by their final products. If all three are present in excess, the branch-point intermediates chorismate and prephenate will accumulate, inhibiting the first common enzyme in the overall pathway, i.e. the first reaction of the shikimate pathway.

Enzyme multiplicity regulates the synthesis of aromatic amino acids in *E. coli*, *S. typhimurium* and *Neurospora crassa* and the synthesis of the aspartate family of amino acids in *E. coli*. In the former, those organisms possess three isoenzymes which catalyse the first reaction of the shikimate pathway – one inhibited by phenylalanine, one by tyrosine, and one by tryptophan. In the latter, three forms of the enzyme catalysing the first reaction of the pathway leading from aspartate to aspartate β-semialdehyde exist – one inhibited by methionine, one by threonine, and one by lysine.

Bacillus polymyxa and *Rhodopseudomonas capsulata* possess a single enzyme catalysing the first reaction of the pathway leading from aspartate to aspartate β-semialdehyde, and its regulation is achieved by concerted feedback inhibition. Lysine and threonine alone

are only weak inhibitors, but when both present, a strong synergistic inhibition occurs.

The regulation of *E. coli* glutamine synthetase, a key enzyme in the flow of inorganic nitrogen to organic compounds, is an example of cumulative feedback inhibition. Eight inhibitors are either metabolic end products of glutamine (tryptophan, histidine, carbamoyl phosphate, glucosamine 6-phosphate, cytidine triphosphate and adenosine monophosphate, or AMP) or in some other way indicators of the general status of amino acid metabolism (alanine and glycine). Each of the eight compounds alone gives only partial inhibition, but in combination, with each acting independently of the others, the degree of inhibition is increased until the activity is almost completely switched off when all eight compounds are simultaneously present.

Other ways of controlling enzyme activity include the following: (1) activation of enzyme activity by metabolites; (2) modification of enzymes (e.g. adenylation of certain enzymes may render them more susceptible to feedback inhibition); (3) protein–protein interactions (e.g. activity of multienzyme complexes may change with the amounts of its components present).

Control of Enzyme Amount

The amount of an enzyme may be controlled by a number of different mechanisms: (1) end-product repression of enzyme synthesis (e.g. the coordinate repression of the synthesis of all the enzymes involved in histidine biosynthesis in *E. coli* by histidine); (2) substrate induction of enzyme synthesis (e.g. the induction of the synthesis of the first enzyme involved in cysteine biosynthesis in *E. coli* by the product of its reaction); (3) metabolite depression of enzyme synthesis (e.g. the synthesis of all amino acid biosynthetic enzymes is strongly reduced when *E. coli* is grown in a rich medium); (4) regulation of enzyme degradation. Very little is known on this last topic. Nevertheless, the protection of a given enzyme against proteolysis is probably an important regulatory process.

Amino Acid Catabolism

All living cells undergo intracellular protein degradation, with the resulting amino acids being recycled into proteins or degraded oxidatively to yield energy. In microorganisms and plants amino acids are not generally present in excessive amounts. In higher animals, however, where amino acids intake may largely exceed the metabolic needs, amino acids present in excess are not stored or excreted as such. Instead, they are used for energy production. It is estimated that amino acids supply about 15% of the total energy required by an average human adult. This value may be increased under conditions of energy insufficiency or nutritional pathologies. Amino acids can also constitute an important energy source in plants, during the germination of protein-storing seeds, and in microorganisms, when carbohydrates or fatty acids are not available. This is the case in many bacteria that can grow in media containing amino acids as the source of energy, carbon and nitrogen. These organisms utilize amino acids catabolic pathways analogous to those of higher animals.

The catabolic metabolism of amino acids is mainly concerned with the separation of the amino groups from the carbon skeletons and the subsequent fate of both the amino groups and the carbon chains. *See* Energy, Measurement of Food Energy

Transamination and Deamination

In general, one of the first steps in the degradation of amino acids involves the removal of the α-amino group to give the corresponding 2-oxo acid. Two distinct types of reactions are known to accomplish this task: transamination and deamination.

Transamination, the most common mechanism for deamination of amino acids, involves the transfer of an amino group from a donor amino acid to an acceptor 2-oxo acid, with the formation of a new amino acid and a new oxo acid. Transamination reactions are catalysed by pyridoxal phosphate-dependent enzymes termed transaminases or, more properly, aminotransferases. These enzymes have a twofold specificity in that they are specific for the acceptor 2-oxo acid but nonspecific for the donor amino acid. Most aminotransferases are specific for 2-oxoglutarate as the acceptor 2-oxo acid, although some may use either pyruvate or oxaloacetate. Accordingly, there are three classes of aminotransferases, which form glutamate, alanine and aspartate, respectively. More than 50 aminotransferases have been identified. With the exception of lysine and threonine, the α-amino groups of all the amino acids found in proteins can be removed by transamination. Moreover, transamination is not restricted to α-amino groups since, for example, the δ-amino group of ornithine is readily transaminated. Transaminases fulfil central catabolic as well as anabolic functions in the metabolism of several amino acids because they catalyse freely reversible reactions, having equilibrium constants close to unity.

Transamination does not result in a net removal of nitrogen from amino acids. It does, however, allow for the collection of amino groups in glutamate. Oxidative deamination of glutamate by glutamate dehydrogenase results in the liberation of ammonium. The 2-oxoglutarate thus produced can either be used as the acceptor 2-oxo acid in further transamination reactions or enter the TCA cycle. Glutamate is the only amino acid for which a specific and highly active dehydrogenase exists. This pathway, i.e. the concerted action of the aminotransferases and glutamate dehydrogenase, is responsible for most of the ammonium produced by the catabolism of amino acids.

Additional minor routes for the deamination of amino acids are provided by amino acid oxidases, capable of oxidizing most naturally occurring amino acids, and by dehydratases, capable of removing non-oxidatively the amino groups of some amino acids.

Urea Cycle

Plants and microorganisms commonly excrete very little nitrogen. Growth of these organisms is often restricted by a limited availability of nitrogen so that nitrogen liberated by catabolic pathways is usually reassimilated. However, because high concentrations of NH_4^+ are extremely toxic to cells, animals must get rid of the excess ammonium produced by the catabolism of amino acids, either by direct excretion or, when removal of NH_4^+ by simple diffusion is difficult, by conversion to less toxic excretory products. Most terrestrial vertebrates, including mammals, excrete ammonia in the form of urea. Urea is highly soluble in water but non-toxic to cells.

Urea is synthesized by the urea cycle, which is carried out almost exclusively in liver cells. This cycle, discovered by Hans Krebs and Kurt Henseleit in 1932, consists of five sequential enzymatic reactions:

1. $NH_4^+ + HCO_3^- + 2ATP \longrightarrow$
   $\qquad\qquad$ carbamoyl phosphate $+ 2ADP + P_i + H^+$
2. Carbamoyl phosphate $+$ ornithine $\longrightarrow$
   $\qquad\qquad$ citrulline $+ P_i$
3. Citrulline $+$ aspartate $+$ ATP $\longrightarrow$
   $\qquad\qquad$ argininosuccinate $+ AMP + PP_i$
4. Argininosuccinate $\longrightarrow$
   $\qquad\qquad$ arginine $+$ fumarate
5. Arginine $+ H_2O \longrightarrow$
   $\qquad\qquad$ ornithine $+$ urea

The sum of these reactions is as follows:

$$NH_4^+ + HCO_3^- + 3ATP + H_2O + aspartate \longrightarrow$$

$$urea + 2ADP + AMP + 2P_i + PP_i + H^+ + fumarate$$

Virtually all organisms synthesize arginine from ornithine by reactions 2–4. However, only ureotelic organisms are capable of catalysing the hydrolysis of arginine (reaction 5), the reaction responsible for the cyclic nature of the urea cycle. The synthesis of urea is energetically expensive, requiring the hydrolysis of 4 molecules of ATP per turn of the cycle (2 molecules of ATP are needed to convert AMP to ATP). The fumarate produced is hydrated to malate and oxidized to oxaloacetate by TCA cycle enzymes. Aspartate is then

Table 1. Metabolic fates of the carbon skeletons of amino acids

Amino acid	Product(s) of catabolism	Metabolic fate
Alanine	Pyruvate	Glycogenic
Arginine→glutamate	2-Oxoglutarate	Glycogenic
Asparagine→aspartate	Oxaloacetate	Glycogenic
Aspartate	Oxaloacetate, fumarate[a]	Glycogenic
Cysteine	Pyruvate	Glycogenic
Glutamate	2-Oxoglutarate	Glycogenic
Glutamine→glutamate	2-Oxoglutarate	Glycogenic
Glycine→serine	Pyruvate	Glycogenic
Histidine→glutamate	2-Oxoglutarate	Glycogenic
Methionine	Succinyl-CoA	Glycogenic
Proline→glutamate	2-Oxoglutarate	Glycogenic
Serine	Pyruvate	Glycogenic
Threonine	Pyruvate	Glycogenic
Valine	Succinyl-CoA	Glycogenic
Isoleucine	Succinyl-CoA, acetyl-CoA	Glycogenic and ketogenic
Phenylalanine→tyrosine	Fumarate, acetoacetate	Glycogenic and ketogenic
Tryptophan	Pyruvate, acetyl-CoA, acetoacetate	Glycogenic and ketogenic
Tyrosine	Fumarate, acetoacetate	Glycogenic and ketogenic
Leucine	Acetyl-CoA, acetoacetate	Ketogenic
Lysine	Acetoacetate	Ketogenic

[a] See text (*Urea Cycle*).

regenerated from oxaloacetate by transamination. Thus both amino groups of urea originate from amino acids: one is derived from ammonium produced by deamination (reaction 1) and the other is provided by aspartate (reaction 3). Bicarbonate (reaction 1) furnishes the carbon atom of urea. In this respect it is interesting to note that not all the urea produced in the human liver is excreted in the urine, a considerable fraction being hydrolysed in the colon by bacterial ureases. The mucosa of the human colon is relatively permeable to urea. However, the great majority of the urea molecules is rapidly hydrolysed within the lumen of the colon with a large proportion of the resulting ammonia nitrogen being absorbed into the portal system or metabolised by the intestinal flora. The ammonium absorbed from the colon may be available for transamination into amino acids in the liver or resynthesized to urea also in the liver, with some of this urea distributed back to the gastrointestinal tract for degradation to ammonia and consequent recycling.

Catabolic Pathways

Once the amino groups of amino acids have been removed, the remaining carbon skeletons are funnelled into seven major metabolic intermediates, namely pyruvate, acetyl coenzyme A (acetyl-CoA), acetoacetate, 2-oxoglutarate, succinyl-CoA, fumarate, and oxaloacetate (Table 1), which may be either directly oxidized into carbon dioxide and water by the TCA cycle or reincor-

porated into glucose or fatty acids. Glycogenic amino acids are those possessing carbon skeletons which generate pyruvate or TCA cycle intermediates and can, therefore, be converted to glucose via gluconeogenesis. In contrast, amino acids possessing carbon skeletons which are metabolized to acetyl-CoA or acetoacetate, precursors of fatty acids and ketone bodies, are termed ketogenic. Recall that, with the exception of some species of plants and microorganisms which possess the glyoxylate cycle, all other organisms lack a pathway for the net synthesis of glucose from acetyl-CoA or acetoacetate. A few amino acids are both glycogenic and ketogenic since portions of their carbon skeletons are converted into carbohydrate derivatives whereas other portions are converted into ketone bodies. Note that the classification presented in Table 1 is not universally accepted because several amino acids are glycogenic under some conditions but ketogenic under others.

Regulation of Amino Acid Catabolism

Microorganisms regulate the level of their amino acid degradative enzymes in different ways. (1) The enzymes are subjected to catabolite repression, i.e. repression of the amino acid catabolic pathway by a carbon and energy source, even in the simultaneous presence of that amino acid as the only source of nitrogen. Thus these enzymes are induced only when carbon and energy limit growth (e.g. the induction of tryptophanase – the enzyme which cleaves tryptophan to yield ammonium, pyruvate and indole – by tryptophan in *E. coli*). (2) The enzymes are induced when nitrogen limits growth (e.g. the induction of proline oxidase – the enzyme which catalyses the first step of proline degradation – by proline in *E. coli*, even in the presence of ample carbon supply). (3) The enzymes are induced independently of carbon and energy or nitrogen supply (e.g. the induction of threonine dehydrogenase – an enzyme involved in threonine catabolism – in *E. coli* by growth in leucine, even in the presence of other carbon and nitrogen sources). In some microorganisms, catabolite repression can be bypassed by a nitrogen limitation signal that allows the induction of a particular amino acid catabolic pathway. This nitrogen limitation signal is probably related to the complex regulation mechanisms of glutamine synthetase (see *Regulation of Amino Acid Biosynthesis*, above).

In animal cells, amino acid catabolism is also subjected to control mechanisms. Thus, for example, removal of amino groups from amino acids is regulated mainly by control of glutamate dehydrogenase. This enzyme is allosterically inhibited by ATP and guanosine triphosphate (GTP) and stimulated by ADP and GDP. Hence, when cellular energy charge is low the rate of amino acid oxidation increases. On the other hand, the urea cycle is controlled by *N*-acetylglutamate. This compound is a positive allosteric effector of carbamoyl phosphate synthetase, which catalyses the first and rate-limiting step in the pathway. *N*-acetylglutamate is also a precursor of arginine and its synthesis is inhibited by arginine. However, the amino acid catabolic enzymes of animal cells are much more often subjected to a hormonal control than are the microbial enzymes. Thus, for example, the synthesis of tryptophan oxygenase, regulated by adrenal activity, is developmentally controlled so that the enzyme is formed only in certain tissues and at certain times during development. A high-protein diet is also a factor that is known to stimulate the formation of a number of amino acid degradative enzymes in liver, namely urea cycle enzymes and tryptophan oxygenase.

Synthesis of Biologically Important Compounds

In addition to their role in protein synthesis, energy production, and gluconeogenesis, many amino acids serve as precursors for the synthesis of other amino acids and other biologically important compounds.

Many oligopeptides containing up to 20 residues, including hormones, antibiotics and antitumour agents, are synthesized in living organisms by mechanisms different from the usual ribosome-dependent processes of protein synthesis. The dipeptides carnosine (β-alanyl-histidine) and anserine (β-alanyl-1-*N*-methylhistidine)

are synthesized enzymatically from β-alanine and histidine, and from carnosine and *S*-adenosylmethionine, respectively.

Glutathione (γ-glutamylcysteinylglycine) plays a variety of roles in living organisms. This tripeptide is synthesized by a two-step enzymatic pathway: (1) the formation of a peptide linkage between the γ-carboxyl group of glutamate and the amino group of cysteine, to produce γ-glutamylcysteine; (2) the condensation of this dipeptide with glycine, to form glutathione. Thus the order of the amino acids in glutathione is specifically determined by the enzymes catalysing the formation of each peptide bond.

At least 90 different peptide antibiotics are produced by strains of *Bacillus subtilis* and *B. brevis*. Gramicidin S, for example, is a cyclic decapeptide composed of two identical pentapeptides (D-phenylalanine-L-proline-L-valine-L-ornithine-L-leucine). Gramicidin S is synthesized by a multienzyme complex, gramicidin synthetase, composed of two enzymes, one of which, serving as a template, specifies the amino acid sequence in the antibiotic.

S-Adenosylmethionine (SAM), the metabolically activated form of methionine, functions as an important source of methyl and propylamino groups for a wide variety of compounds, including alkaloids, choline, creatine, adrenaline, *N*-methylated amino acids, nucleotides, and polyamines, as well as for phospholipids, proteins, polysaccharides, and nucleic acids. It is synthesized from methionine and ATP, in a reaction catalysed by SAM synthase.

A wide variety of amines occurring in bacteria, plants and animals are derived directly or indirectly from amino acids by decarboxylation; these include ethylamine (from alanine), agmatine (from arginine), γ-aminobutyric acid (from glutamate), methylamine (from glycine), histamine (from histidine), cadaverine (from lysine), putrescine (from ornithine), phenylethylamine (from phenylalanine), ethanolamine (from serine), tryptamine and 5-hydroxytryptamine (from tryptophan), and tyramine and dopamine (from tyrosine). These amines and their derivatives often play a variety of physiologically important roles. For example, γ-aminobutyric acid, phenylethylamine, tryptamine, 5-hydroxytryptamine, or serotonin, tyramine, dopamine, noradrenaline, and adrenaline are all neurologically active compounds, whereas histamine, a powerful vasodilator, is involved in allergic reactions. *See* Amines

Tyrosine plays several important roles in animal metabolism as a precursor to melanins, thyroid hormones (thyroxine and triiodothyronine), and catecholamines (dopamine, noradrenaline and adrenaline). In the synthesis of melanins, tyrosinase catalyses first the hydroxylation of tyrosine to 3,4-dihydroxyphenylalanine (dopa), followed by the oxidation of dopa to phenylalanine-3,4-quinone (dopaquinone). Dopaquinone undergoes a sequence of reactions, including polymerization, to yield both red and black melanins. Another enzyme forming dopa is tyrosine hydroxylase, which catalyses the first reaction in the sequential enzymatic pathway leading to the biosynthesis of catecholamines. Dopa is then decarboxylated to yield 3,4-dihydroxyphenylethylamine (dopamine). Dopamine is hydroxylated to norepinephrine (noradrenaline), which in turn is methylated by SAM to give epinephrine (adrenaline). *See* Hormones, Adrenal Hormones; Hormones, Thyroid Hormones

Putrescine, or 1,4-diaminebutane, is synthesized by decarboxylation of ornithine, in a reaction catalysed by ornithine decarboxylase, a highly regulated enzyme. Another route to putrescine formation involves the conversion of arginine to agmatine by arginine decarboxylase, followed by cleavage of agmatine to putrescine and urea by agmatine ureohydrolase. Putrescine is an intermediate in the biosynthesis of two important polyamines, spermidine and spermine. Spermidine is synthesized enzymatically by the SAM-mediated transfer of a propylamino group to putrescine. The enzymatic transfer of an additional propylamino group from SAM to spermidine produces spermine. These polycations play multiple roles in stabilizing negatively charged intracellular components such as nucleic acids and membranes.

Creatine phosphate, which serves as a source of high-energy phosphate in mammalian muscle and brain, is synthesized in three steps from arginine, glycine, and methionine.

There are four classes of tetrapyrrole compounds, haems, chlorophylls, phicobilins and cobalamins, all of which are synthesized from a common precursor, δ-aminolevulinic acid (ALA). In bacteria and animals, ALA is synthesized by the condensation of glycine and succinyl-CoA, with loss of carbon dioxide, in a reaction catalysed by ALA synthase. In plants, however, ALA is formed from glutamate by a three-step pathway.

An enormous amount of carbon in the biosphere passes through the pathway leading to lignin biosynthesis, the major constituent of woody tissue. In the first reaction, phenylalanine ammonia lyase catalyses the cleavage of phenylalanine to *trans*-cinnamic acid and NH_4^+. Cinnamic acid is a precursor for the synthesis of a huge number of plant substances, including lignin, tannins, flavonoids, pigments, many of the flavour components of spices, and various alkaloids, such as morphine and colchicine. *See* Lignin

In addition, the synthesis of a variety of other important molecules utilizes various amino acids as precursors. Thus β-alanine is a component of CoA, asparagine is a major form of transport of organic nitrogenous compounds in plants, and aspartate is involved in purine and pyrimidine biosynthesis. Glutamate is a precursor of folic acid; glutamine contributes to the synthesis of a variety of substances, including purines, pyrimidines, ATP, cytidine triphosphate (CTP), NAD, amino sugars, and glycoproteins; cysteine is a precursor of taurine, isethionic acid, CoA, vasopressin, various types of pigments, including phaeomalins and trichochromes, and other sulphur-containing compounds. Glycine also plays multiple roles, including contributions to the one-carbon pool and as a precursor of purines, glyoxylate, and various conjugates such as hippurate and glycocholate. Histidine is involved in ergothionine and homocarnosine biosynthesis, and methionine, via SAM, is the precursor of the plant hormone ethylene, which influences plant growth and development and induces the ripening of fruits. Serine is involved in the biosynthesis of phospholipids, and tryptophan is the precursor of several important physiological substances, including NAD, NADP, and the plant hormone indole 3-acetic acid. *See* Niacin, Physiology; Ripening of Fruit

Bibliography

Fowden L, Lea PJ and Bell EA (1979) The non-protein amino acids of plants. *Advances in Enzymology* 50: 117–175.

Kulka HE and Schwarz RS (1988) A flexible genetic code, or why does selenocysteine have no unique codon? *Trends in Biochemical Sciences* 13: 419–421.

Miflin BJ and Lea PJ (1977) Amino acid metabolism. *Annual Review of Plant Physiology* 28: 299–329.

Murray RK, Granner DK, Mayes PA and Rodwell VW (1988) *Harper's Biochemistry.* East Norwalk, Connecticut: Appleton and Lange.

Orten JM and Neuhaus OW (1982) *Human Biochemistry.* St. Louis, Missouri: CV Mosby.

Rawn JD (1989) *Biochemistry.* Burlington, North Carolina: Neil Patterson Publishers.

Smith EL, Hill RL, Lehman IR *et al.* (1983) *Principles of Biochemistry: General Aspects.* Singapore: McGraw-Hill.

Umbarger HE (1978) Amino acid biosynthesis and its regulation. *Annual Review of Biochemistry* 47: 533–606.

Zapsalis C and Beck RA (1985) *Food Chemistry and Nutritional Biochemistry.* New York: John Wiley.

Zubay G (1983) *Biochemistry.* Reading, Massachusetts: Addison-Wesley.

Ricardo M. B. Ferreira and Artur R. N. Teixeira
Technical University of Lisbon, Lisbon, Portugal

ANAEMIA

Contents

Iron Deficiency Anaemia

Iron deficiency is both the commonest nutritional disorder in human beings and the commonest cause of anaemia. Anaemia occurs when body iron stores have been exhausted and the rate of delivery of iron to developing red blood cells in the bone marrow is insufficient to support the level of haem synthesis required to maintain a normal circulating red cell mass and haemoglobin concentration. It is estimated that more than 500 million people throughout the world suffer from iron deficiency anaemia. This article will review the causes, methods of detection, physiological consequences, as well as treatment and prevention of iron deficiency anaemia. *See* Iron, Physiology

Iron Balance

Iron balance in human beings is uniquely dependent on the body's ability to match the rate of iron absorption from the proximal small intestine to iron requirements. During childhood, iron absorption normally exceeds requirements, ensuring a positive balance and the gradual establishment of an iron store. In the adult, the level of absorption is approximately equal to a relatively fixed rate of loss which is governed by factors unrelated to iron balance. When requirements are increased, e.g. with pregnancy and lactation, absorption increases to replace the storage iron that is used up. *See* Children, Nutritional Requirements; Lactation

When iron stores are exhausted by increased demand, anaemia supervenes if adaptive changes in the rate of absorption are insufficient to restore iron balance. While dietary iron intake almost always exceeds the body's requirements by a large margin, the ability of absorptive mechanisms to extract the iron from food may be limited. Iron deficiency anaemia is therefore most commonly encountered when the relationship between requirement and dietary intake of bioavailable iron is least favourable. Periods of increased vulnerability are infancy, adolescence (particularly among girls after the onset of menstruation) and women of child-bearing age (Table 1). Chronic blood loss, either from the uterus or from the gastrointestinal tract, will further contribute to an unfavourable balance. For example, the monthly menstrual loss in 10% of healthy women is more than 80 ml (average for most women is 30 ml). This increases the daily iron requirement by about 0·8 mg or 6% of the dietary intake. It would be necessary for such an individual to absorb 16% of the iron present in her daily diet. Hookworm infestation, which is prevalent in many developing countries, may induce sufficient blood loss to increase iron requirements by 3–4 mg per day. Iron balance would only be maintained if percentage absorption from the diet were increased by 20–30%. Many of these individuals will become anaemic because maximal total absorption from a normal diet is usually only 3–

Table 1.   Relationship between iron requirements and dietary iron supply

	Aged 0–6 months[a]	Aged 6–12 months	Aged 1–2 years	Adolescent		Adult	
				Male	Female[b]	Male	Female[c]
Weight (kg)	3·3–7·8	7·8–9·8	9·8–12·3	60	50	70	60 (60)
Food intake (MJ)	3·6	4·2	5·1	12·6	10·5	13·4	9·7 (9·7)
Iron intake (mg)	3·3	6·0	7·4	18	15	19·2	13·8 (13·8)
Iron requirement (mg)	0·49	0·90	0·75	1·32	1·45	1·0	1·4 (2·2)
Absorption requirement (%)	15	15	10	7	10	5	10 (16)

[a] Caloric iron density 3·8 mg per 4200 kJ.
[b] Menstruating.
[c] Values in brackets are for women with monthly menstrual blood loss exceeding 80 ml (10% of women).

4 mg per day. *See* Menstrual Cycle and Premenstrual Syndrome – Nutritional Aspects

The diet of most Western adults contains large quantities of meat, which is rich in highly available haem iron, as well as fresh fruit and other sources of vitamin C, which increases the absorption of inorganic iron. This diet provides sufficient bioavailable iron to prevent anaemia even in the presence of higher requirements. For example, a recent study in which dietary iron absorption was measured over a 2-week period indicated that a menstruating woman eating a mixed diet containing meat would absorb about 10% of the iron and maintain an iron store of approximately 350 mg. The composite 10% absorption value is achieved by assimilation of about 30% of the haem iron and 6% of the nonhaem iron. Even a woman with relatively high menstrual losses (Table 1) would be expected to remain in iron balance by increasing her non-haem iron absorption to 12%, although her iron store would be estimated at only 200 mg. Supplementary iron will usually be necessary during pregnancy and may also be required by some women with high menstrual losses to ensure that iron deficiency does not occur. In infancy, relative iron requirements are highest in the first year. Even in Western countries it is unlikely that sufficient iron will be extracted from an unfortified infant diet to prevent iron deficiency when breast milk is no longer the major source of nutrition. *See* Ascorbic Acid, Physiology; Diseases, Diseases of Affluence; Meat, Dietary Importance; Offal, Dietary Importance

The situation is much less satisfactory in developing countries, where the composition of the diet is such that the iron bioavailability is usually low. Haem iron is often absent from the diet since meat is not eaten in significant quantities. Severely iron-deficient individuals may be able to absorb only 5–10% of the non-haem dietary iron. Under these circumstances even modestly increased requirements may not be met. Unfortunately, poor dietary iron availability is often accompanied by high requirements due to factors such as multiple pregnancies and hookworm infestation. As a result iron deficiency anaemia is widespread.

Prevalence

On the basis of data obtained in the USA during the Second National Health and Nutrition Examination Survey (NHANES II, 1976–1980), the highest prevalence rates for anaemia which was predominantly caused by iron deficiency occurred in infants (5·7%), teenage girls (5·9%), and menstruating women (2·6–5·8% depending on analytical method). Iron deficiency anaemia was rare in men and postmenopausal women. Among the elderly, inflammatory disease, not iron deficiency, was the commonest cause of anaemia. Iron

Table 2. Laboratory evaluation of iron deficiency anaemia

Purpose of test	Laboratory test
Confirm presence of anaemia	Haemoglobin
	Haematocrit
Evaluate iron status	
Iron stores	Bone marrow iron
	Serum ferritin
Iron supply	Transferrin saturation
	Free erythrocyte protoporphyrin
	Red blood cell indices

deficiency anaemia is much more commonly encountered in developing countries. Depending on the criteria used for identification, some prevalence estimates for pregnant women are as high as 80%.

Laboratory Diagnosis

Iron deficiency anaemia may be suspected on the basis of the clinical symptoms and the setting in which it occurs, but precise identification depends on the results of laboratory tests designed to confirm the presence of anaemia and evaluate iron status (Table 2).

Haemoglobin or Haematocrit

Anaemia is identified by the finding of a haemoglobin concentration or haematocrit below the normal range. This usually presents little difficulty in the clinical situation since symptoms only occur in individuals with moderate or severe anaemia. On the other hand, prevalence studies of nutritional anaemia depend on the identification of mild anaemia in an otherwise healthy population. The World Health Organization (WHO) criteria established in 1975 are the most widely accepted. Haemoglobin concentrations below 13 g dl^{-1} for adult males, 12 g dl^{-1} for menstruating women, and 11 g dl^{-1} in pregnancy are considered indicative of anaemia.

Unfortunately, the use of a single value for diagnosing mild iron deficiency anaemia is limited by the significant overlap in the frequency distribution curves for anaemic and normal populations. In one study using a single value criterion, 17% of women responded to oral iron despite the fact that they were classified as normal, while 35% of 'anaemic' women failed to show any change in haemoglobin after being treated. The problem is even more complex in children, where developmental changes affect the normal haemoglobin concentration. The use of percentile curves instead of single values is more satisfactory in childhood.

Iron Status

Specific laboratory tests of iron status are used both to distinguish iron deficiency from other causes of anaemia and to facilitate the recognition of mild iron deficiency anaemia in nutritional surveys. They supply specific information about iron stores and internal iron supply.

Iron Stores

Bone marrow iron Histological evaluation of storage iron by using the Prussian-blue method to stain macrophage haemosiderin in needle aspirate or biopsy specimens of bone marrow provides a semiquantitative estimate of storage iron. Iron deficiency anaemia is characterized by an absence of stainable bone marrow iron. This procedure remains the gold standard in patients suffering from complicated illnesses, but is rarely necessary under most other circumstances and impractical in nutritional surveys.

Serum ferritin Body iron not immediately required for haemoglobin synthesis or other metabolic processes is stored in cells as ferritin and haemosiderin. Ferritin is also present in very small amounts in the plasma. The development of sensitive immunological methods has made it possible to measure serum ferritin (SF) accurately. This has become the most useful indirect estimate of body iron stores since the SF concentration is directly proportional to the size of the storage pool in health and in uncomplicated iron deficiency or iron overload; $1 \mu g \, l^{-1}$ is equivalent to 8–10 mg storage iron in adults (SF $1 \mu g \, l^{-1}$ is equivalent to $140 \mu g \, kg^{-1}$ storage iron). Serum ferritin below $12 \mu g \, l^{-1}$ is diagnostic of iron deficiency. Unfortunately, higher SF levels do not exclude iron deficiency when disorders such as infection, chronic inflammatory diseases, malignant disorders and liver disease are present because they elevate SF values independently.

Internal Iron Supply

Transferrin saturation As body iron stores become depleted, the concentration of the iron transport protein, transferrin, in the plasma increases, leading to a rise in the total iron binding capacity (TIBC). Once iron stores are exhausted and the tissue demands exceed the rate of supply, the serum iron (SI) concentration falls. Since impaired iron supply is characterized by a rising TIBC and a fall in SI, a reduction in the transferrin saturation (TS = SI/TIBC) from the normal value of approximately 35% to less than 16% is the best single criterion of a suboptimal supply.

Free erythrocyte protoporphyrin Impaired iron supply can also be recognized by measuring the protoporphyrin IX (free erythrocyte protoporphyrin; FEP) in peripheral red blood cells. Insufficient iron limits the final step in haem synthesis, leading to the accumulation of FEP in red cell precursors. The cellular content remains unchanged throughout the lifespan of the red cell. Peripheral blood FEP values therefore reflect iron supply during red cell production. Modern instrumentation has made it possible to measure FEP directly on a single drop of venous or capillary blood. Unfortunately, FEP levels are also raised in lead poisoning. If exposure to lead can be excluded, a raised FEP provides the same information as a reduced TS, but it is more stable. FEP is raised only after several weeks of iron-deficient erythropoiesis and requires a similar period for normalization once an adequate supply of iron is re-established.

Red blood cell indices As the severity of iron deficiency progresses, morphological abnormalities (microcytosis and hypochromia), resulting from reduced haemoglobin synthesis, appear in the peripheral blood. The sensitivity with which these changes can be recognized has improved dramatically with the introduction of electronic counting and sizing equipment. Both the mean corpuscular volume (MCV) and the mean corpuscular haemoglobin (MCH) are reliable measures of impaired haemoglobin synthesis, although not specific for iron deficiency. The MCV is the more widely used.

The best approach to diagnosing iron deficiency anaemia depends on the setting in which it is being evaluated. The accuracy of prevalence studies of nutritional anaemia is improved by the concurrent measurement of haemoglobin or haematocrit and one or more specific tests for iron status, such as SF, FEP or TS. All of these measurements may be carried out on a single sample of venous or capillary blood. A similar approach or a therapeutic trial of oral iron may be satisfactory for clinic or office patients in whom iron deficiency is considered likely. In hospital patients, anaemia complicated by other illnesses may require the direct evaluation of bone marrow iron stores. *See* Nutritional Status, Anthropometry and Clinical Examination; Nutritional Status, Biochemical Tests for Vitamins and Minerals; Nutritional Status, Functional Tests

Physiological Consequences of Iron Deficiency Anaemia

Related to Anaemia

Mild anaemia usually causes few symptoms in individuals with sedentary occupations because of compensatory physiological adjustments, including increased cardiac output and a shift in the oxygen dissociation curve with improved oxygen delivery to tissues. However, aerobic work capacity in human beings is reduced when the haemoglobin concentration falls below $12 \, g \, dl^{-1}$.

Table 3. Causes of iron deficiency anaemia

Underlying disorder	Site of action	Causal factors
Nutritional deficiency		Low dietary bioavailability
		Unrefined cereal diet
Malabsorption		Gastric surgery
		Clay eating
		Gluten-induced enteropathy
Blood loss	Uterine	Menorrhagia
	Gastrointestinal	Hookworm, schistosomiasis
		Peptic ulcer disease, oesophagitis
		Stomach and colorectal cancer
		Angiodysplasia, hereditary telangiectasia
		Aspirin, NSAIDs
		Inflammatory bowel disease
		Diverticulosis, haemorrhoids
	Renal tract	Haemoglobinuria
		Severe haematuria
	Lung	Idiopathic pulmonary haemosiderosis

NSAIDs, nonsteroidal anti-inflammatory drugs.

The social consequences of the significant limitation that chronic iron deficiency anaemia places on sustained physical activity is most evident among agricultural labourers in developing countries. For example, a study carried out among Indonesian rubber plantation latex tappers, who were paid a daily wage based on the weight of latex they collected, demonstrated a direct correlation between haemoglobin concentration and income. Anaemic men were 18·7% less productive than their nonanaemic fellow workers; when they were given 100 mg elemental iron per day for 60 days their income increased by 37%.

Severe iron deficiency anaemia during pregnancy has been reported to be associated with a higher maternal mortality rate. Prenatal infant loss as well as prematurity and higher infant mortality rates have also been observed. However the evidence is not conclusive; it is possible that other factors including folate deficiency may have been equally important. *See* Folic Acid, Physiology

Unrelated to Anaemia

Many clinical symptoms and signs have been attributed to associated tissue iron deficiency in patients with iron deficiency anaemia. They include fatigue, malaise and mucosal or epithelial abnormalities such as angular stomatitis, glossitis, oesophageal webs, atrophic gastritis and koilonychia. The apparent decrease in the frequency of these findings in recent years and the marked geographic variation in their prevalence suggest that factors other than iron deficiency may have played an important role in their aetiology.

Other consequences of tissue iron deficiency do appear to be related specifically to iron lack and have been the subject of intense study recently. They include impaired exercise tolerance due to skeletal muscle dysfunction, impaired cell mediated immunity, behavioural, cognitive and neurological dysfunction, and abnormalities of temperature regulation.

Treatment and Prevention

Treatment

The recognition of iron deficiency anaemia is never a complete diagnosis. Iron administration may produce a rapid and gratifying correction of the anaemia, but a satisfactory long-term solution to the problem depends on a clear understanding of the reasons for increased requirements and/or reduced absorption. For example, iron deficiency anaemia in Western men is usually a symptom of unsuspected blood loss from the gastrointestinal tract. Identification of the underlying disorder is essential (Table 3).

Oral iron therapy using a soluble ferrous salt such as the sulphate, gluconate or fumarate, providing 60–120 mg kg^{-1} elemental iron per day in adults, or 2–3 mg kg^{-1} in children, is usually the most appropriate method to both repair the anaemia and restore a normal body iron store in patients with moderate or severe anaemia. Once this has been accomplished, continued iron balance can only be assured if the cause of excessive requirements is eliminated or if more available dietary iron is supplied.

Prevention

The prevalence of nutritional iron deficiency anaemia in Western societies has fallen markedly in recent years. The many factors that have been suggested to contribute to this improvement in adults include dietary fortification, a general improvement in income level and diet, a large increase in the sale of medicinal iron preparations, routine iron supplementation in pregnancy, and reduced menstrual blood loss as a result of the widespread use of oral contraceptives.

Similarly, increasing awareness of the importance of adequate iron nutrition in early infancy has reduced the prevalence of, although by no means eliminated, iron deficiency in young children. As with adults, improved iron nutrition reflects several different factors, including increased awareness of the importance of breast-feeding, the use of iron-fortified formulae, and the provision of medicinal iron when appropriate.

The situation in developing countries is far less satisfactory. Attempts to reduce iron losses or improve the intake of bioavailable iron have had only a limited success. Iron supplementaton (usually the provision of iron tablets) has been effective in pilot studies, but the inadequacy and cost of distribution systems, as well as poor compliance owing to gastrointestinal side-effects, have limited the value of this approach as a long-term solution. Nevertheless, supplementation is the preferred method of intervention in severely anaemic individuals and during pregnancy.

Increasing the population's intake of bioavailable dietary iron is the only feasible means of improving iron nutrition at the national level. Despite years of research and numerous field trials, this has proved to be extremely difficult to achieve. The traditional diet of people in most developing countries tends to inhibit iron absorption. Dietary customs are not easily modified. In addition, foods that promote iron bioavailability tend to be expensive. Iron fortification of the diet has also encountered several obstacles. The introduction of iron into the food chain in developing countries is complicated by the difficulty of identifying a suitable vehicle. Most foods are produced at the local level and not processed or distributed through a small number of centres where the fortificant could be introduced into the food. In addition, the inhibitory effect of vegetable diets on bioavailability tends to reduce the effectiveness of the fortificant. Finally, iron salts that do not affect the appearance or organoleptic and storage properties of foods tend to be poorly bioavailable. Despite these formidable obstacles, limited field fortification trials targeted to specific population groups in Chile

(children) and South Africa (adults) have been very successful. *See* Food Fortification

Bibliography

Bothwell TH, Charlton RW, Cook JD and Finch CA (1979) *Iron Metabolism in Man.* Oxford: Blackwell Scientific Publications.

Clydesdale FM and Wiemer KL (eds) (1985) *Iron Fortification of Foods.* New York: Academic Press.

Cook JD (1982) Clinical evaluation of iron deficiency. *Seminars in Hematology* 19: 6–18.

Cook JD (1990) Adaptation in iron metabolism. *American Journal of Clinical Nutrition* 51: 301–308.

Cook JD and Reusser ME (1983) Iron fortification: an update. *American Journal of Clinical Nutrition* 38: 648–659.

Expert Scientific Working Group (1985) Summary of a report on assessment of the iron nutritional status in the United States. *American Journal of Clinical Nutrition* 42: 1318–1338.

Sean R. Lynch
Eastern Virginia Medical School, Norfolk, USA

Megaloblastic Anaemias*

The word 'megaloblast' is derived from the Greek, *megas*, meaning large, and *blastos*, meaning germ or sprout. It was first used by the Austrian biologist Paul Ehrlich in the nineteenth century to describe the abnormal appearance of developing red cells (erythroblasts) in a condition known as pernicious anaemia. This appearance has subsequently been seen in other conditions and is the result of abnormal nuclear maturation caused by disturbed deoxyribonucleic acid (DNA) synthesis. Megaloblasts are larger than normal erythroblasts (normoblasts) at all stages of maturation. Their nuclei contain smaller quantities of condensed chromatin than the nuclei of normoblasts of similar cytoplasmic maturity and thus have an abnormal, open, lacy appearance (Fig. 1 and Plate 5). Circulating red cells derived from the maturation of megaloblasts are abnormally large (macrocytic). The defect in DNA synthesis leads to a variety of secondary disturbances and results in the destruction of many cells before they are mature, a process known as ineffective erythropoiesis.

Although B_{12} and folate deficiencies are the most common causes of megaloblastic erythropoiesis, there are others. These include the following: drugs such as azathioprine, cytarabine or hydroxyurea, which interfere with DNA synthesis; some acquired defects of the

---

* The colour plate section for this article appears between p. 556 and p. 557.

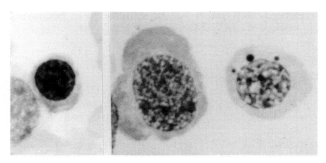

Fig. 1 An erythroblast from a normal bone marrow (left) compared with two megaloblasts from a patient with severe pernicious anaemia (right). The smaller megaloblast contains three cytoplasmic inclusions consisting of nuclear material (Howell–Jolly bodies).

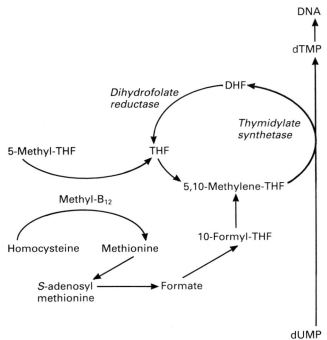

Fig. 2 Role of methyl-B_{12} and 5,10-methylenetetrahydrofolate (5,10-methylene-THF) in the formation of deoxythymidine monophosphate (dTMP). The dTMP is converted to dTTP and the deoxythymidine moiety then inserted into DNA.

dUMP, deoxyuridine monophosphate; DHF, dihydrofolate.

haemopoietic stem cell (certain myelodysplastic syndromes and leukaemias); and some inherited conditions, e.g. hereditary orotic aciduria. This article deals only with the nutritional causes, namely B_{12} and folate deficiency. *See* Cobalamins, Physiology; Folic Acid, Physiology

Vitamin B_{12} and Folate Deficiency

Biochemical Considerations

Vitamin B_{12} and folate deficiency cause megaloblastic changes by impairing DNA synthesis. The probable roles of B_{12} and folate in DNA synthesis are shown in Fig. 2. Folate deficiency appears to reduce intracellular levels of 5,10-methylenetetrahydrofolate (5,10-methylene-THF) and, consequently, impairs the synthesis of deoxythymidine triphosphate (dTTP), the source of one of the two pyrimidine bases of DNA. Deficiency of B_{12} also causes reduced intracellular levels of 5,10-methylene-THF but there is uncertainty as to the mechanism by which this happens. According to the methylfolate trap hypothesis, the reduction in 5,10-methylene-THF results from the known role of methyl B_{12} in the 5-methyltetrahydrofolate (5-methyl-THF)-dependent methylation of homocysteine to methionine. When B_{12} is deficient, there is impaired generation of THF from 5-methyl-THF and, consequently, impaired conversion of THF to 5,10-methylene-THF. However, there are more recent data suggesting that the failure of synthesis of methionine also leads to impaired formate synthesis and reduced synthesis of 10-formyl-THF, a precursor of 5,10-methylene-THF. According to some investigators, the impaired production of 5,10-methylene-THF in B_{12} deficiency may be related more to reduced formate synthesis than to reduced THF availability. *See* Nucleic Acids, Physiology

Demyelination, which is the characteristic early lesion in the neuropathy of B_{12} deficiency, may also be related to the impairment of the methyl-B_{12}-dependent conversion of homocysteine to methionine, referred to above. It has been suggested that this impairment may lead to a failure of synthesis of S-adenosylmethionine and, consequently, to impaired methylation of the constituents of myelin sheaths.

Since both B_{12} and folate are required for DNA synthesis, a deficiency of these vitamins will affect not only erythroblasts but also all other rapidly dividing cells. These include other haemopoietic cells and the epithelial cells lining the gastrointestinal, respiratory, urinary and female genital tracts. Microscopically, these cells too are characteristic, being enlarged with finely stippled nuclear chromatin. The gonads are also affected.

Clinical Features

Apart from the more pronounced neurological deficits seen in B_{12} deficiency, the clinical features of B_{12} and folate deficiency are similar. Initially, patients may be asymptomatic, picked up by chance from an examination of their blood. Later, patients may present with symptoms and signs of anaemia. As the anaemia develops slowly, there is time for the body to compensate for the effects of anaemia, and the haemoglobin may become very low before the patient seeks medical attention.

In severe B_{12} or folate deficiency, the concentrations of white cells and platelets in the blood are also often low and this may very occasionally lead to problems with infection and bruising or bleeding.

Impaired proliferation of epithelial cells may lead to other symptoms, such as a sore tongue (glossitis) and lips (cheilitis), and to altered bowel habit and weight loss. The increased cell breakdown associated with the gross ineffectiveness of haemopoiesis may cause jaundice and a mild fever. The combination of jaundice and anaemia gives rise to the characteristic lemon-yellow tinge which has been observed in these patients. Impotence is not uncommon, and infertility in both sexes is usual.

Vitamin B_{12} deficiency can cause marked neurological abnormalities, including peripheral neuropathy, degeneration of the dorsal columns and pyramidal tracts of the spinal cord (a condition known as subacute combined degeneration of the cord), and optic atrophy. It may also affect cerebral function, leading to altered cognition and even dementia and psychosis. Folate deficiency can cause mental changes, particularly mental slowing, and occasionally causes peripheral neuropathy.

Features of the Blood and Bone Marrow

The haemoglobin concentration in the blood is normal in a mild deficiency state but decreases when the deficiency is more marked. The mean corpuscular volume (MCV) of red cells is high and, in severe deficiency states, the white cell and platelet counts may be low. The appearance of the blood film in megaloblastic anaemia is characteristic. The red cells are large and often oval in shape. There are also some fragmented and irregularly shaped red cells. The neutrophils often have abnormal nuclei with an increase in the number of nuclear segments. This may not be seen in the presence of infection when neutrophils are released early into the circulation. Hypersegmented neutrophils are a valuable clue to the presence of megaloblastic anaemia when red cell changes are masked by a coexistent iron deficiency anaemia or the anaemia of chronic disease.

The bone marrow is commonly hypercellular, with a reduction in the ratio of myeloid to erythroid cells. Megaloblastic red cell precursors are seen, as described above, and there is often an excess of immature erythroblasts due to selective death of more mature forms. In the granulocyte series, giant and abnormally shaped metamyelocytes (a stage in the formation of white cells) are found. Megakaryocytes (large cells in the bone marrow which produce platelets) may also be enlarged, with increased numbers of nuclear lobes.

Vitamin B_{12} Deficiency

Mechanism of B_{12} Absorption

Vitamin B_{12} is synthesized solely by bacteria. Humans must absorb about 1–3 μg of B_{12} per day and this comes mainly from animal produce, meat and dairy foods. Since B_{12} is a large hydrophilic molecule, a specialized mechanism has evolved for its absorption. The steps involved are shown in Fig. 3. Almost all B_{12} is absorbed via a process which requires a glycoprotein known as intrinsic factor (IF) produced by parietal cells in the fundus and body of the stomach. The B_{12} in the B_{12}–protein complexes found in ingested food is released within the stomach by peptic digestion. About half of the released B_{12} immediately binds to IF; the remainder attaches to R-binder (a B_{12}-binding protein present in all body fluids, including gastric juice). The B_{12} attached to R-binder is released in the jejunum following digestion of the binder by pancreatic proteolytic enzymes, and the released B_{12} then binds to IF. The B_{12}–IF complex is resistant to digestion and travels to the distal ileum, where there are specific receptors on the ileal cells which bind the complex. From here the B_{12} molecules are transferred across the ileal cells, from which they enter the capillary circulation bound to transcobalamin II(TCII), the plasma transport protein which carries B_{12} to the liver and elsewhere for storage and use.

Vitamin B_{12} is not broken down within the body but is excreted unchanged in the urine and faeces. It also undergoes an enterohepatic circulation in which it is excreted in bile and largely reabsorbed in the terminal ileum. This circulation is important as it conserves B_{12} stores.

Causes of B_{12} Deficiency

Reduced entry of B_{12} into the circulation may be due to problems at each of the stages shown in Fig. 3. The main causes are reduced intake of B_{12}, impaired IF secretion, and absence or disease of the terminal ileum. Sometimes, B_{12} deficiency can result from utilization of B_{12} by organisms within the gut or, very rarely, from absence of TCII.

Dietary Deficiency

Worldwide, inadequate dietary intake of B_{12} is probably the most common cause of B_{12} deficiency. The average daily requirement of B_{12} (1–3 μg) is easily supplied by a normal Western diet. If the diet has been adequate, there is about 2–5 mg of stored B_{12} which is enough to last about 2–7 years if absorption ceases. The people who most commonly become B_{12}-deficient are vegans, who exclude meat, fish and dairy produce from their diet.

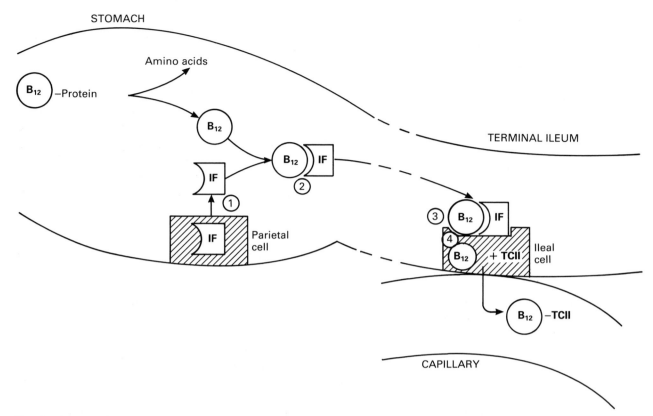

Fig. 3 Schematic diagram to illustrate the interaction of vitamin B_{12} and intrinsic factor (IF) in B_{12} absorption: (1) release of IF from gastric parietal cell; (2) binding of free B_{12} to IF (for the sake of simplicity, an intermediate step, involving the binding of some of the free B_{12} to R-binder in the gastric juice, has been omitted); (3) interaction of B_{12}–IF complex with ileal cell receptor; (4) binding of B_{12} to transport protein, transcobalamin II (TCII).

They do, however, receive a small amount of B_{12} from bacterial contamination of other foods and, because the enterohepatic circulation of B_{12} is intact, symptomatic B_{12} deficiency is infrequent. Nevertheless, subclinical B_{12} deficiency (i.e. low serum B_{12} level without macrocytosis or anaemia) is very common; for example, it affects about 50% of Hindu Indians living in London. The prevalence of megaloblastic anaemia in vegans is uncertain, but one hospital in the UK encountered 138 cases over a period of 14 years. *See* Vegan Diets

The other group of individuals who may develop megaloblastic anaemia are breast-fed infants of B_{12}-deficient mothers. The anaemia develops after the infant's meagre stores of B_{12} are depleted and is usually diagnosed at 3–6 months of age.

Impaired Secretion of Intrinsic Factor

The next most common cause of B_{12} deficiency is impaired absorption as a result of a lack of IF. This may arise in three ways: first, in a condition known as pernicious anaemia, autoimmune destruction of gastric parietal cells leads to a failure to secrete acid and IF; second, in rare inherited conditions, there is an isolated failure of IF secretion or the secretion of a functionally

inactive form of IF; third, gastric parietal cells are removed during surgical resection of part or all of the stomach.

Pernicious anaemia (PA) Although generally considered to be predominantly a disease of northern Europe, PA occurs in all other parts of the world. Its frequency in Africans and Asians has not yet been adequately determined but the estimated prevalence in Gujerati Indians living in London is the same as that in Caucasians. In the UK, the prevalence is about 1·2 per 1000 of the population, with a female to male ratio of about 1·6:1. About 90% of cases diagnosed are over the age of 40 years and the frequency of the condition increases with increasing age; as many as 1–2·5% of the population over the age of 65 are affected. It is rare under the age of 30, although a juvenile form can occur in children. There is a higher prevalence in close relatives of patients with PA and in people with other autoimmune conditions, and these groups tend to present earlier, at an average age of 51 years, compared to 66 years in those without such a history.

The symptoms and signs are mainly those described above for megaloblastic anaemia. Neurological symptoms, usually paraesthesiae, are common, occurring in up to 45% of cases in some studies. In addition, it has been noted that PA is associated with early greying and blue eyes. Evidence of other autoimmune disease such as vitiligo or hypothyroidism may be present.

Histologically, a gastric biopsy in PA shows a gastritis in which all layers of the body and fundus of the stomach are atrophied and there is infiltration by lymphocytes and plasma cells. Gastric parietal and chief cells are lost and replaced by mucus-secreting cells, and intestinal metaplasia may be present. With loss of acid secretion, very high serum gastrin levels are found in PA and lead to the proliferation of endocrine cells in the antral mucosa. The incidence of polyps and carcinoid tumours of the stomach is increased, as is that of carcinoma of the stomach, which in males with PA is about three times that in the general population.

The histological changes can be at least partially reversed by the administration of corticosteroids. This fact, in addition to the association of PA with other autoimmune conditions, makes it likely that PA itself is an autoimmune disease. This is further supported by the finding of abnormal circulating antibodies.

About 90% of people with PA have circulating anti-gastric-parietal-cell antibodies (GPA) and about 60% have anti-intrinsic-factor antibodies (IFA). Although GPA are common in PA they are by no means diagnostic. They are also found in about 16% of healthy females over the age of 60 and in a substantial proportion of both patients with other autoimmune conditions and relatives of PA patients. Anti-intrinsic-factor antibodies are more specific for PA.

Although the antibodies probably have a role in pathogenesis, it is likely that the autoimmune damage is largely cell-mediated. In support of this is the observation that the incidence of PA is increased in people with immunoglobulin A (IgA) deficiency or with complete hypogammaglobulinaemia who do not usually have GPA or IFA.

The prognosis of PA has changed dramatically since treatment with B_{12} became available. Without treatment, the disease was uniformly fatal, with a life expectancy of less than 3 years in most cases. With treatment, the life expectancy for women with PA equals that of the general population. For men it is slightly reduced, probably due to gastric neoplasms.

Loss or Abnormality of Epithelial Cells of the Terminal Ileum

Vitamin B_{12} deficiency can sometimes be caused by a lack or abnormality of the ileal cells which bear the receptors for the B_{12}–IF complexes. This may be due to surgical resection of the terminal ileum or to diseases such as Crohn's disease and chronic tropical sprue, which affect this part of the bowel. A few hundred patients have also been investigated who have congeni-

tal, isolated, cobalamin malabsorption and proteinuria, the so-called Imerslund–Gräsbeck syndrome. *See* Colon, Diseases and Disorders

Utilization of B_{12} by Organisms in the Gut

In normal circumstances the small bowel contains a very small bacterial load. Some conditions, however, may lead to bacterial overgrowth and since bacteria utilize and inactivate B_{12} they can give rise to B_{12} deficiency. The conditions which predispose to bacterial overgrowth are those which cause stagnation of intestinal contents, e.g. jejunal diverticulosis or the creation of a blind loop at surgery. *See* Microflora of the Intestine, Role and Effects

A species of fish tapeworm called *Diphyllobothrium latum* may live in the small intestine of man and can also absorb B_{12} from food. A single worm can cause B_{12} deficiency and give rise to megaloblastic anaemia. The condition is more or less confined to Finland, the Baltic states and the Soviet Union and humans become infected by eating raw or undercooked freshwater fish containing the larvae of the worm.

Other Causes of B_{12} Deficiency

Other causes of B_{12} deficiency are rare. Congenital lack of transcobalamin II leads to megaloblastic anaemia which presents within a few weeks of birth. Prolonged administration of the anaesthetic gas, nitrous oxide, may cause B_{12} deficiency by oxidizing and thereby inactivating methyl-B_{12}.

Folate Deficiency

The metabolism and function of folate have been described elsewhere. This section briefly reviews the source of and requirements for folate and goes on to discuss some of the causes of folate deficiency.

There are over 100 derivatives of folic acid (folates) in nature. Folates are found in all foods, especially in liver, kidney, green vegetables, yeast, nuts and fruit. Since folate is easily destroyed by cooking, the best sources are raw or lightly cooked food. The average daily requirement is about 50–100 μg, which may be increased several-fold at times of increased demand such as during pregnancy. The average stores are about 5–20 mg and deficiency can occur within a few months if intake ceases.

Causes of Folate Deficiency

Folate stores depend on the balance between the amount of folate ingested and absorbed on the one

Megaloblastic Anaemias

hand, and the amount utilized and excreted on the other. Deficiency can result from reduced ingestion or absorption, or from increased utilization or excretion. In addition, some drugs exert their effect by interfering with folate metabolism. *See* Drug–Nutrient Interactions

Reduced Ingestion

Dietary folate deficiency is common. It occurs in those who, for various reasons, eat little fruit or fresh vegetables. These include many elderly people living alone, alcoholics and those on very low incomes.

Reduced Absorption

The jejunum and proximal part of the ileum are the main sites of folate absorption. Folate polyglutamates in the diet are degraded enzymatically to monoglutamates prior to their absorption, and the monoglutamates are converted to 5-methyl-THF before release from the intestinal epithelial cells into the extracellular fluid and plasma. Diseases affecting the upper region of the small intestine, such as coeliac disease or tropical sprue, commonly cause folate deficiency. Others, such as Crohn's disease, amyloid or lymphoma or extensive jejunal resection, may also reduce folate absorption. Whereas stagnant loops of bowel may cause B_{12} deficiency, they tend to increase serum folate because of increased synthesis of folate by microorganisms within the gut. *See* Coeliac Disease

Increased Utilization

In conditions associated with increased cell turnover there is increased utilization of folate and, if the greater demand for folate cannot be met by the dietary intake, folate deficiency eventually develops. This is occasionally seen in haematological conditions in which there is shortened red cell survival, e.g. thalassaemia major and sickle cell disease. It can also occur, although to a lesser degree, in malignant conditions such as leukaemias and carcinoma and in some chronic diseases such as rheumatoid arthritis, tuberculosis and psoriasis. Folate deficiency developing in psoriasis is related both to increased utilization of folate for nucleic acid synthesis in the skin and to increased loss of folate due to excessive desquamation of skin cells.

The other situation in which folate requirements are increased is pregnancy. It is estimated that an extra 100–300 μg of folate are needed per day for transfer to the fetus. Many pregnant women who do not take folate supplements are in negative folate balance. The frequency of megaloblastic haemopoiesis in the latter part of pregnancy is high, varying from about 25% in the UK, Canada and the USA to over 50% in South India.

The prevalence of megaloblastic anaemia is lower, being around 0·5–5% in the UK and 24% in Malaysia. Megaloblastic anaemia usually presents after the 36th week of pregnancy or in the puerperium. It is especially common in twin pregnancies.

Newborn infants with their rapid growth rate can also become folate-deficient, especially those born prematurely whose stores are small.

Increased Excretion

Loss of folate can increase in certain circumstances, e.g. in patients with renal failure undergoing dialysis. Increased folate excretion may also occur in patients with liver disease or congestive heart failure in whom folate is released from damaged liver cells.

Disturbed Folate Metabolism

Some drugs exert their action by interfering with folate metabolism. Methotrexate, pyrimethamine and trimethoprim are, respectively, strong, weak and very weak inhibitors of human dihydrofolate reductase (Fig. 2). Methotrexate and high doses of pyrimethamine cause macrocytosis and megaloblastic changes in folate-replete individuals. By contrast, standard doses of pyrimethamine (used in chemoprophylaxis of malaria) and trimethoprim have no effect on folate-replete subjects but aggravate pre-existing mild folate or B_{12} deficiency. Other drugs, such as phenytoin sodium and barbiturates, have also been reported to cause folate deficiency, although the exact mechanisms are not fully understood.

Investigation of Megaloblastic Anaemia

In most suspected cases the blood count and film are abnormal, with some or all of the features described earlier. There are three stages in the diagnosis and investigation of a megaloblastic anaemia. The first is to demonstrate megaloblastic haemopoiesis, the second to establish whether the megaloblastic changes are due to vitamin B_{12} and/or folate deficiency, and the third to establish any underlying cause.

Some conditions that cause macrocytosis have normal-looking erythroblasts (normoblasts) in the bone marrow, e.g. chronic alcoholism (most cases), liver disease and hypothyroidism. To make a diagnosis of a megaloblastic anaemia, therefore, a bone marrow aspirate is required.

The concentration of B_{12} in serum and of folate in red cells can be measured using microbiological assays or competitive protein-binding radioassays. In B_{12} or folate deficiency one or both of these measurements are usually low. Low B_{12} or red cell folate levels are presumptive but not definitive evidence of B_{12} or folate deficiency, respectively, since low B_{12} levels may be seen in folate deficiency and vice versa. In addition, low B_{12} or folate levels may be found in conditions other than B_{12} or folate deficiency. An investigation which can be used to detect B_{12} or folate deficiency is called the deoxyuridine (dU) suppression test (see Wickramasinghe and Matthews, 1988). *See* Immunoassays, Radioimmunoassay and Enzyme Immunoassay

Once B_{12} or folate deficiency has been diagnosed, the next question is why is it present? A comprehensive history (including a dietary history) and examination of the patient may already have provided some clues. However, it is often necessary to perform further investigations, looking for underlying causes such as PA or malabsorption. The most important test in the diagnosis of PA is the Schilling test. This assesses B_{12} absorption, first without (part 1) and then with (part 2) IF. A low absorption in part 1 which increases in part 2 is highly suggestive of PA. If both parts show low absorption, it is likely that malabsorption or excessive utilization by gut bacteria is the cause. The latter can sometimes be detected by repeating the test a third time, this time after the administration of antibiotics which will reduce the gut flora of the small bowel.

Treatment of B_{12} or Folate Deficiency

Folate deficiency can usually be treated by large oral doses of folic acid, even when malabsorption is the cause. Parenteral treatment is usually only indicated when patients cannot swallow. It is important to ensure that B_{12} deficiency is not also present as the prolonged administration of folate to a B_{12}-deficient patient could precipitate vitamin B_{12} neuropathy. Folate supplements are sometimes administered prophylactically in situations in which there is increased demand for folate, such as during pregnancy or in people with sickle cell anaemia.

If the diet cannot be changed, nutritional B_{12} deficiency may be treated by the daily oral administration of B_{12} (cyanocobalamin). Other forms of B_{12} deficiency require intramuscular injections of hydroxocobalamin. These are usually given every 2–3 months once stores have been replenished and, in the case of PA, need to be continued throughout life. Oral preparations of B_{12} plus hog IF have been tried in the treatment of PA but rapidly become ineffective as antibodies develop against the IF.

Bibliography

Chanarin I (1990) *The Megaloblastic Anaemias* 3rd edn. Oxford: Blackwell Scientific Publications.
Lindenbaum J, Healton EB, Savage DG *et al.* (1988) Neuro-
psychiatric disorders caused by cobalamin deficiency in the absence of anemia or macrocytosis. *New England Journal of Medicine* 318: 1720–1728.
Shorvon SD, Carney MWP, Chanarin I and Reynolds EH (1980) The neuropsychiatry of megaloblastic anaemia. *British Medical Journal* 281: 1036–1038.
Wickramasinghe SN and Matthews JH (1988) Deoxyuridine suppression: biochemical basis and diagnostic applications. *Blood Reviews* 2: 168–177.
Wintrobe MM, Lee GR, Boggs DR *et al.* (1981) *Clinical Hematology* 8th edn. Philadelphia: Lea and Febiger.

C. Beatty and S. N. Wickramasinghe
St Mary's Hospital Medical School, Imperial College of Science, Technology and Medicine, University of London, London, UK

Other Nutritional Causes

The main dietary causes of anaemia are iron, B_{12} and folate deficiencies, which have been described in the preceding two articles. A number of other components of the diet can also cause anaemia through their absence or excess, or by an effect on susceptible individuals, e.g. fava beans in people deficient in the enzyme, glucose-6-phosphate dehydrogenase. The broad categories that are covered in this article are protein-energy malnutrition, deficiency or excess of minerals, vitamin deficiency, favism and alcohol toxicity.

The deficiency syndromes discussed below are rarely caused by the lack of a single nutrient. Instead, a number of substances required for erythropoiesis are usually missing from the diet. The resulting blood and bone marrow appearances vary and reflect the combination of factors that are deficient. The circulating red cells may be normal in size (normocytic) or abnormally large (macrocytic). Sometimes, the formation of haem is affected and when this occurs the red cells are pale (hypochromic) and small (microcytic). The developing red cells (erythroblasts) in the bone marrow may look normal (normoblastic) or, where deoxyribonucleic acid (DNA) synthesis is affected, may be megaloblastic, as described in the previous article. There are sometimes other morphological abnormalities in erythroblasts, indicating disordered erythropoiesis (dyserythropoiesis). Occasionally, iron-laden mitochondria are formed which, under the light microscope, are seen as a ring of iron-positive (siderotic) granules around the nucleus.

Protein–Energy Malnutrition

Severe protein–energy malnutrition (PEM) affects between 0·5% and 20% of children below the age of 5 years in the poorest communities of Asia, Africa and

South America, and it is almost always associated with anaemia. Infectious diseases, such as measles and parasitic infestations of the intestine, may aggravate the nutritional deficiency by causing an increased loss or enhanced breakdown of protein, or impaired absorption of amino acids. *See* Protein, Deficiency

The severity and characteristics of the anaemia depend on whether the nutritional deficiency of protein and energy is complicated by a deficiency of other nutrients, especially folate. The degree of anaemia and response to treatment can be difficult to assess since severe PEM is associated with a markedly reduced plasma volume, which concentrates the red cells and results in a falsely elevated haemoglobin concentration. *See* Folic Acid, Physiology

In the absence of folate or iron deficiency, the anaemia of PEM is generally mild or moderate, and the mean corpuscular volume (MCV) of erythrocytes is usually normal. The percentage of newly released red cells (reticulocytes) is inappropriately low in relation to the degree of anaemia, indicating that the production of red cells by the bone marrow is impaired. Levels of erythropoietin, the hormone produced by the kidney which stimulates erythropoiesis, are appropriately high. Red cell lifespan may be slightly reduced in kwashiorkor and marasmic kwashiorkor (^{51}Cr half-life values of 11·4–24 days; mean, 17 days) but not in marasmus. This reduction results from both a corpuscular and an extracorpuscular defect. *See* Iron, Physiology; Kwashiorkor; Marasmus

If the bone marrow is examined, there is often erythroid hypoplasia or even aplasia (a reduction or absence of red cell precursors). Sometimes, however, the percentage of erythroblasts may be either normal or increased. The marrow is usually normoblastic but, even in the absence of folate deficiency, may be mildly megaloblastic. In either case, giant forms of metamyelocytes (a stage of white cell development) may be seen. Occasionally, the erythroblasts show nonspecific morphological abnormalities indicative of dyserythropoiesis. Iron stores are variable: in some parts of the world they are often normal or increased, while in others they are usually absent. The number and size of siderotic granules within erythroblasts may be increased and there may occasionally be a few ring sideroblasts.

It seems, therefore, that the anaemia of PEM is due mainly to impaired erythropoiesis, sometimes together with a shortened red cell lifespan. Since a recent study showed no major abnormality in the ultrastructure or cell cycle distribution of the erythroblasts in the bone marrows of seven Nigerian children with PEM, it seems likely that, at least in some cases, impairment of erythropoiesis results mainly from an abnormality of the erythroid progenitor cells (i.e. the very earliest cells committed to erythropoiesis) rather than from abnormalities in, or death of, more mature red cell precursors.

While protein deficiency *per se* seems to cause the anaemia in many patients, other deficiencies may coexist and can aggravate the haematological picture. When folate deficiency is also present, the blood film shows macrocytosis and the bone marrow displays megaloblastic changes, often of a marked degree. Coexisting iron deficiency causes microcytosis. Even when iron stores are present at diagnosis, treatment with a high-protein diet may be followed by the emergence of an iron deficiency picture, presumably because the rate of supply of iron to erythropoietic cells is inadequate to cope with the rapid rise in red cell mass. This can be prevented by the administration of iron. However, in view of the possibility that early iron therapy may cause a flare-up of pre-existing subclinical infections by providing iron for the growth of microorganisms, some authorities advise that the institution of iron therapy be delayed until signs of iron deficiency emerge.

Minerals

Deficiencies

Of the 14 essential trace elements, three have an unequivocal role in haemopoiesis. These are cobalt, iron and copper. Deficiencies of other elements, such as zinc, selenium and nickel, have occasionally been reported to cause or exacerbate anaemia but, as yet, the evidence is inconclusive.

The effects of cobalt (in vitamin B$_{12}$) and iron deficiencies have been described in the preceding two articles. This section therefore covers only the anaemia of copper deficiency.

Copper Deficiency

Although it has been known for a long time that copper is an essential element, the number of reported cases of isolated copper deficiency is small. The reasons for this are that copper is found in most foods, is only required in minute amounts, and is easily absorbed. The main groups in which deficiency may occur are premature babies, malnourished infants, patients subjected to total parenteral nutrition and those in whom the enterohepatic circulation of copper is interrupted, e.g. after extensive small bowel resection. Some people have also become copper-deficient by ingesting excessive quantities of zinc which competitively inhibits copper absorption. *See* Copper, Physiology; Zinc, Physiology

Copper is required in a number of enzyme systems. These include cytochrome *c* oxidase, ascorbic acid oxidase, tyrosinase, monoamine oxidase and superoxide dismutase. About 90% of the copper in the blood is bound to caeruloplasmin, an α-globulin which acts as an oxidase on a variety of substrates, including ferrous iron (Fe^{2+}). Copper deficiency causes a reduction in the activities of these enzymes and leads to a number of abnormalities. There have been reports of malnourished, copper-deficient children in whom there is anaemia and neutropenia (a reduction in the number of circulating neutrophils) associated with skeletal abnormalities resembling those seen in scurvy. It is not clear how much of this picture is caused by the copper deficiency and how much by a lack of other dietary components. In adults, the first evidence of copper deficiency is usually neutropenia, which is followed by anaemia.

The anaemia of copper deficiency is usually characterized by hypochromic and macrocytic red cells, although microcytic red cells have also been reported, possibly in association with dietary iron deficiency. The blood film may also contain spherocytes (red cells with a spherical shape instead of the normal biconcave disc shape). The most consistent bone marrow findings are vacuolation of both erythroid and myeloid cell lines and a reduced number of granulocyte precursors. Several case reports have described mild megaloblastic erythropoiesis and increased siderotic granulation of erythroblasts, including the formation of ring sideroblasts. One case report described such changes which were reversed when copper sulphate was administered by mouth, reappeared on stopping the treatment and again resolved when copper sulphate was given intravenously.

The mechanisms underlying the anaemia of copper deficiency are not fully characterized. Iron metabolism is certainly affected. Iron is transported bound to apotransferrin, in the ferric form (Fe^{3+}). Reduced activity of copper-containing oxidant enzymes leads to trapping of iron in the ferrous form and consequent hypoferraemia, despite adequate iron stores. For entry into mitochondria to form haem, iron needs to be converted back to the ferrous state. This step also seems to be impaired, probably as a result of reduced cytochrome oxidase activity. Failure to incorporate iron to form haem accounts for the hypochromia of the red cells and the increased siderotic granulation of the erythroblasts. Iron uptake from the gut may also be impaired.

In addition to being hypochromic, red cells are often macrocytic, and megaloblastic changes are seen in the marrow. This may imply a defect in DNA or ribonucleic acid (RNA) synthesis, although the site of the defect is not known.

Animal work suggests that the anaemia of copper deficiency may be caused not only by reduced red cell production but also by shortened red cell survival. Superoxide dismutase catalyses the conversion of the superoxide anion, O_2^-, to molecular oxygen and peroxide. Reduced activity of this enzyme may render cells susceptible to oxidant damage, and studies in copper-deficient lambs have shown increased production of Heinz bodies (red cell inclusions formed of denatured haemoglobin).

Copper deficiency is treated by giving copper sulphate either orally or intravenously.

Toxicity

It is not only the deficiency of minerals which can cause anaemia but also their presence in excess. As mentioned above, ingestion of excessive quantities of zinc can impair copper absorption and lead to copper deficiency anaemia. High levels of two other metals, copper and lead, exert a direct toxic effect and are discussed below. *See* Heavy Metal Toxicology; Lead, Toxicology

Copper Toxicity

Copper toxicity can cause anaemia by haemolysis. Acute toxicity can occasionally occur as a result of excess copper ingestion or haemodialysis against fluid contaminated by copper. This produces symptoms of nausea, vomiting and diarrhoea, as well as causing haemolysis. Chronic copper toxicity can also occur, usually as a result of a rare inherited condition known as Wilson's disease. This is caused by a defect in copper excretion and is also characterized by episodes of haemolysis and by hepatic and/or cerebral damage.

The reason for the haemolysis is not well understood. It is known, however, that copper accumulates in the red cells, and this may interfere with intracellular metabolism, leading to membrane damage, Heinz body formation and shortened red cell survival.

Lead Toxicity

The metabolism of lead and the effects of lead toxicity have been described elsewhere. The following paragraphs, therefore, merely summarize the features of the anaemia caused by excess lead.

Chronic lead ingestion causes a mild to moderate anaemia. The red cells may be normochromic or mildly hypochromic and microcytic, and there is often a slight increase in reticulocytes. Basophilic stippling of some red cells is a characteristic, although not universal finding and is due to the clumping of polyribosomes, probably the result of inhibition of the enzyme pyrimidine-5-nucleotidase. The bone marrow shows erythroid hyperplasia and increased siderotic granulation of erythroblasts, often with ring sideroblasts.

The cause of the anaemia is multifactorial. There is a shortening of red cell survival, probably due to blocking of sulphydryl groups which causes damage to structural proteins. Haem synthesis is also impaired at several stages. The two key enzymes affected are δ-aminolaevulinic acid dehydratase (ALA-D), which catalyses the formation of porphobilinogen, and ferrochelatase, which is needed for the incorporation of ferrous iron into haem.

A fast-moving minor band may be found on haemoglobin electrophoresis, presumably due to postsynthetic modification of haemoglobin A.

Vitamin Deficiencies

Deficiency of a number of vitamins has been reported to cause anaemia. The effects of vitamin B_{12} and folate deficiency have already been discussed in the preceding two articles. This section therefore covers deficiencies of vitamin A, riboflavin, pantothenic acid, vitamin B_6, vitamin C and vitamin E.

Vitamin A

Deficiency of vitamin A can cause anaemia with a picture similar to that seen in iron deficiency. It is associated with a low serum iron in the face of normal iron stores. *See* Retinol, Physiology

Most of the studies correlating low vitamin A levels with anaemia have been carried out in malnourished children, often with other nutritional deficiencies. However, it has also been shown experimentally in otherwise healthy adults that vitamin A deficiency causes a mild anaemia which is reversed by giving vitamin A. The effects of vitamin A deficiency may be aggravated in the presence of protein deficiency since the latter causes a reduction in the serum levels of a specific retinol-binding transport protein.

The blood film usually shows microcytosis and hypochromia. At autopsy, the bone marrow of animals and infants with severe vitamin A deficiency may show hypoplasia and fibrosis.

Riboflavin (Vitamin B_2)

Naturally occurring deficiency of riboflavin in man is almost always associated with deficiencies of other nutrients. Experimentally, subjects fed on a riboflavin-deficient diet and given the antagonist, galactoflavin, develop a normocytic, normochromic anaemia. In these subjects, the bone marrow shows erythroid hypoplasia and may show vacuolation of normoblasts. The flavin-coenzyme-dependent reactions involved in these abnormalities of erythropoiesis have not yet been identified. The enzyme, glutathione reductase, requires flavin adenine dinucleotide for activation and in riboflavin deficiency its activity is low. Despite this, however, vitamin B_2 deficiency does not seem to cause a haemolytic anaemia or increased susceptibility to oxidant damage. *See* Riboflavin, Physiology

Pantothenic Acid

Pantothenic acid deficiency, when artificially induced in humans, is not associated with anaemia. Swine, however, do develop a mild normocytic, normochromic anaemia associated with other changes. *See* Pantothenic Acid, Physiology

Vitamin B_6

Vitamin B_6 compounds that are absorbed from food are converted *in vivo* to pyridoxal 5-phosphate, which acts as a coenzyme in the decarboxylation and transamination of amino acids and in the synthesis of haem. Vitamin B_6 deficiency has been reported rarely and may cause an hypochromic, microcytic anaemia. This picture may also be seen in patients receiving the drugs, isoniazid, pyrazinamide, cycloserine or penicillamine, which interfere with B_6 metabolism. Some patients with hereditary or acquired sideroblastic anaemia show a variable degree of response to high doses of pyridoxine, although they are not vitamin B_6-deficient. *See* Vitamin B_6, Physiology

Vitamin C

Experimentally induced, mild, isolated vitamin C deficiency does not cause haematological changes. By contrast, clinically severe scurvy is usually associated with mild to moderate anaemia. The blood and bone marrow appearances can be very variable. Red cells are usually normochromic and normocytic, but may be hypochromic and microcytic or macrocytic. The bone marrow shows normoblastic or megaloblastic erythropoiesis and a wide variation in cellularity. This diversity probably reflects the fact that scorbutic diets are very often deficient in other nutrients in addition to vitamin C. *See* Ascorbic Acid, Physiology; Scurvy

The anaemia is at least partly caused by the lack of vitamin C itself. Some patients with scurvy and anaemia have responded to the addition of ascorbic acid alone to their diet. More often, however, there are additional dietary deficiencies, especially of iron and folate. Furthermore, part of the effect of vitamin C deficiency may result from altered iron and folate metabolism.

Vitamin C depletion causes iron deficiency in two ways: it reduces iron absorption since ascorbic acid helps to convert iron to its ferrous form, in which it is best absorbed; it also promotes increased iron loss as scurvy impairs collagen formation, leading to an increased tendency to bleed, e.g. around the gums.

Vitamin C is also required in folate metabolism. Urinary excretion of 10-formylfolic acid is increased in scurvy and diminishes when ascorbic acid is given. It is postulated that vitamin C is required to prevent the irreversible oxidation of tetrahydrofolates to 10-formylfolic acid and, hence, their loss from the metabolic pool.

Thus there may be increased demand for iron and/or

folate in scurvy at a time when nutritional intake of these compounds is often reduced.

Vitamin E

Vitamin E deficiency has been most extensively studied in animals. In monkeys, prolonged vitamin E deficiency gives rise to a normochromic, normocytic anaemia. Erythrocyte life-span is reduced but the reticulocyte count is not appropriately increased. The anaemia is therefore caused by a combination of haemolysis and impaired erythropoiesis. Bone marrow examination reveals marked morphological abnormalities in the erythroblasts. Vitamin E is known to be an antioxidant, and the shortened red cell survival is the result of increased susceptibility to haemolysis, particularly when exposed to oxidant agents. *See* Tocopherols, Physiology

In humans, vitamin E deficiency is very rare. Adults have substantial stores of the vitamin and, following inadequate dietary intake, may take years to become deficient. Premature infants have low stores of the vitamin and are most at risk. Some cases of haemolytic anaemia caused by vitamin E deficiency have been reported in this group, although this condition is probably not as common as once thought, and recent studies have shown no clear benefit from routinely giving vitamin E supplements to premature, low-birth-weight babies. The haemolysis seems to be aggravated by the high oxygen tension to which such infants are exposed, and to the administration of iron or a diet rich in linoleic acid. Older children can also be affected and there have been reports of malnourished infants with a megaloblastic anaemia which responded to administration of vitamin E. In addition, children and adults with chronic fat malabsorption (e.g. due to cystic fibrosis) may become vitamin E deficient and consequently have a moderately shortened red-cell lifespan, usually without anaemia.

Favism

Fava beans are an important source of protein in the Middle and Far East and in North Africa, and are hazardous to those with a deficiency of the enzyme, glucose-6-phosphate dehydrogenase (G6PD). Such individuals are unable to generate enough reduced glutathione to reduce the oxidants formed from constituents in the fava beans (Fig. 1). These are assumed to be the glycosides, divicine and isouramil.

Over 400 variants of G6PD have been described and some show deficient enzyme activity. It is estimated that more than 200 million individuals worldwide suffer from G6PD deficiency. The inheritance is sex-linked and only hemizygous males and homozygous females are

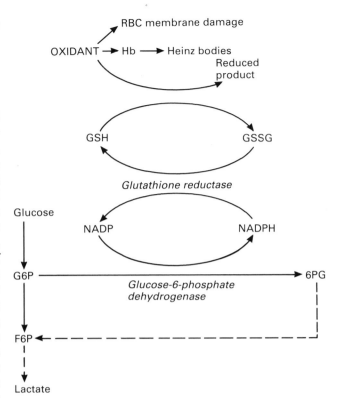

Fig. 1 Schematic diagram illustrating the biochemical pathways involved in favism. In glucose-6-phosphate dehydrogenase deficiency, NADPH synthesis is impaired, leading to reduced glutathione (GSH) formation and making the red blood cell (RBC) membrane and haemoglobin (Hb) vulnerable to oxidant damage.

G6P, glucose 6-phosphate; 6PG, phosphogluconate; F6P, fructose 6-phosphate; GSSG, oxidized glutathione; NADP, nicotinamide adenine dinucleotide phosphate; NADPH, reduced NADP.

usually clinically affected. In Blacks with G6PD deficiency, the level of G6PD in newly formed red cells is near normal and the level decreases markedly as the red cells age. As the proportion of young red cells increases during a haemolytic episode, the haemolysis is self-limited. In the Mediterranean type of deficiency even newly formed red cells may have very low levels of G6PD, and most reported cases of favism have had this variant. Favism does not affect Blacks.

The main feature of favism is an acute haemolytic anaemia developing 5–24 h after ingestion of the bean. The initial symptoms are of headache, nausea, vomiting, lumbar pain and fever. These may be followed by haemoglobulinuria and jaundice and, in some cases, death may ensue. Since only some G6PD-deficient members of one family may suffer from favism, it appears that factors other than the enzyme deficiency are involved in this condition. Favism accounts for 1–2% of paediatric hospital admissions in affected areas (e.g. Cairo).

Alcohol Toxicity

Chronic alcoholism is often associated with anaemia. The cause is multifactorial, with poor diet, gastrointestinal bleeding, liver dysfunction and a direct toxic effect of alcohol on the blood and bone marrow all playing a part. *See* Alcohol, Metabolism, Toxicology and Beneficial Effects

A number of haematological appearances are encountered in alcoholics. Acute alcoholism may cause stomatocytosis (the presence in the peripheral blood of stomatocytes, red blood cells with an elongated area of central pallor, shaped like a mouth). Chronic alcoholism often causes macrocytosis, which persists for several weeks after alcohol ingestion ceases. This may or may not be associated with anaemia and is often the result of a direct toxic effect of alcohol and/or its metabolite, acetaldehyde, on the bone marrow. The marrow usually shows normoblastic erythropoiesis but may occasionally show megaloblastic changes which are unrelated to folate deficiency. Megaloblastic changes are more often a result of concomitant folate deficiency, which is common in poorly nourished alcoholics, especially those who drink wine or spirits as opposed to beer which is rich in the vitamin. Erythroblasts often contain cytoplasmic vacuoles. Sometimes there is a small population of hypochromic microcytes in the blood, and the bone marrow contains ring sideroblasts. This alcohol-induced sideroblastic anaemia is more common in those whose diets are low in pyridoxine.

The anaemia of alcohol toxicity is often caused by impaired red cell production, as described above. It may also be due in part to increased red cell loss. Gastrointestinal haemorrhage resulting from peptic ulcers or bleeding oesophageal varices is common, and may lead to anaemia and iron deficiency. When alcohol-induced hepatic dysfunction is also present, alcohol may cause a haemolytic anaemia. In Zieve's syndrome, acute haemolytic anaemia is associated with spherocytosis, hyperlipidaemia, and either alcohol-induced fatty changes in the liver or early cirrhosis. In spur cell anaemia, there is marked haemolysis associated with acanthocytosis (the presence in the blood of acanthocytes, red cells with blunt projections from their cell membranes) and advanced liver disease.

Apart from the red cell changes, alcohol toxicity may also cause other haematological abnormalities. Acute alcohol toxicity may be associated with thrombocytopenia, and chronic ingestion may impair platelet aggregation. In chronic alcoholics, granulocyte precursors often show vacuolation of their cytoplasm, and the neutrophils produced may be defective in function. There are also functional abnormalities in mononuclear phagocytes and lymphocytes.

Bibliography

Beutler E (1991) Glucose-6-phosphate dehydrogenase deficiency – a review. *New England Journal of Medicine* 324: 169–173.

Blackfan KD and Wolbach SB (1933) Vitamin A deficiency in infants, a clinical and pathological study. *Journal of Paediatrics* 3: 679.

Crandon JH, Lund CC and Dill DB (1940) Experimental human scurvy. *New England Journal of Medicine* 223: 353.

Dunlap WM, James III GW and Hume DM (1974) Anaemia and neutropenia caused by copper deficiency. *Annals of Internal Medicine* 80: 470–476.

Edozien JC and Rahim-Khan MA (1968) Anaemia in protein malnutrition. *Clinical Science* 34: 315–326.

Herbert V (ed.) (1980) Haematological complications of alcoholism: over-view. *Seminars in Haematology* 17 (1 and 2).

Hodges RE, Sauberlick HE, Canham JE, *et al.* (1978) Haematopoietic studies in vitamin A deficiency. *American Journal of Clinical Nutrition* 31: 876.

Hodges RE, Bean WB, Chlson MA and Bleiler RE (1959) Human pantothenic acid deficiency produced by omega-methylpantothenic acid. *Journal of Clinical Investigation* 38: 1421.

Lane M and Alfrey CP (1963) The anaemia of human riboflavin deficiency. *Blood* 22: 811.

Snyderman SE, Holt Jr LE, Carretero R and Jacobs K (1953) Pyridoxine deficiency in the human infant. *Journal of Clinical Nutrition* 1: 200.

Stokes MB, Melikian V, Leeming RL *et al.* (1975) Folate metabolism in scurvy. *Americal Journal of Clinical Nutrition* 28: 126–129.

Wickramasinghe SN (1988) Nutritional anaemias. *Clinical and Laboratory Haematology* 10: 117–134.

Wickramasinghe SN, Akinyanju OO and Grange A (1988) Ultrastructure and cell cycle distribution of bone marrow cells in protein-energy malnutrition. *Clinical and Laboratory Haematology* 10: 135–147.

Wintrobe MM, Lee GR, Boggs DR *et al.* (1981) *Clinical Hematology* 8th edn. Philadelphia: Lea and Febiger.

Zipursky A, Brown EJ, Watts J *et al.* (1987) Oral vitamin E supplementation for the prevention of anaemia in premature infants: a controlled trial. *Pediatrics* 79: 61–68.

C. Beatty and S. N. Wickramasinghe
St Mary's Hospital Medical School, Imperial College of Science, Technology and Medicine,
University of London, London, UK

ANALYSIS OF FOOD*

See specific commodities for Analysis and specific analytes for Determination

Food analysis became a profession as a consequence of human urbanization. Although the quality of certain basic food commodities such as ale, bread and spices had been maintained in earlier centuries by trade guilds and specifically appointed officers, the gross adulteration of foods became more common following the movement of the population from the countryside to the towns in the last century as the industrial revolution expanded. An organized food industry hardly existed and the supply to the growing cities must have been an enormous problem, with ample scope for malpractice.

By the beginning of the 19th century, Berzelius and Liebig had established some of the fundamentals of quantitative organic chemistry; however, the microscope was clearly the first advanced analytical technique used by pioneer analysts such as Accum and Hassall to identify food components and to detect adulteration. The improving analytical capacity to determine the composition of foods, accelerated by the introduction in 1885 of Kjeldahl's method for nitrogen (thereby establishing the basis of nutritional analysis), together with the concern over adulteration, all aided the introduction of national statutory controls over the composition of important food products. These forms of control continued for about 100 years until the 1970s when rapid advances in food science and technology revolutionized food manufacture, retailing and eating habits in the advanced countries. Traditional meals started to give way to the plethora of prepared, convenience, novel and snack foods. Media attention focused on the possible hazards of food contaminants such as metals, toxins, agrochemical residues and on industrial chemicals used as food additives, and also on the 'un-naturalness' of many modern foods and food products. Media attention has also brought public awareness of the links and causations between diet and health. As a result, the cosmopolitan and sophisticated consumers of the present day have become more concerned over the quality and composition of their food purchases, the ingredients, additives and contaminants present and the nutritional value. Also, in the EEC these technological changes have resulted in a reduction of restrictive statutory compositional controls for food commodities

with more emphasis being given to informative labelling.

Fortunately, modern food analysis techniques have been able to meet the challenge of providing the information needed to monitor and control these advances. *See* Adulteration of Foods, Detection; Antioxidants, Natural Antioxidants; Antioxidants, Synthetic Antioxidants; Aspartame; Colours, Properties and Determination of Natural Pigments; Colours, Properties and Determination of Synthetic Pigments; Cyclamates; Saccharin

Basic Principles

Analysis of food is carried out essentially to find out what it contains, what are its physical properties and what condition it is in. These tasks are made difficult by the fact that foods are very complex mixtures of thousands of different chemical substances with widely differing chemical and physical properties. However, the great majority of the chemical constituents of food can be grouped together on the basis of their properties and behaviour when analysed by a few basic test methods. These groups of substances, known as the proximate components, are moisture, protein, fat and mineral matter. Moisture content is determined by drying, protein by determination of the nitrogen content of the food, fat by solvent extraction and mineral matter by ashing the foodstuffs to remove the organic matter. The remaining part of the food after the addition of moisture, protein, fat and mineral matter content was, prior to the relatively recent introduction of modern methods of analysis, deemed to be the 'carbohydrate-by-difference' content. *See* Carbohydrates, Determination; Protein, Determination and Characterization

Apart from the moisture content of foods, methods of analysis to determine the constituents of the other proximate components were, until recent years, strictly limited and of dubious accuracy and precision, relying on non-specific chemical reactions and physical measurements, and on spectroscopic techniques. However, since the 1960s, sensitive and selective techniques based on commercially available instruments, have made possible the detection and determination of a large proportion of the constituent chemical substances in the proximate components; for example, the amino acids and individual proteins making up the protein content,

---

* The colour plate section for this article appears between p. 556 and p. 557.

the fatty acids, sterols, phospholipids and oil-soluble vitamins within the fat content, the elemental composition of the mineral matter including the trace heavy metals, and the specific sugars, starch and dietary fibre constituents of the carbohydrate fraction of the food. *See* Amino Acids, Determination; Dietary Fibre, Determination; Fatty Acids, Analysis; Phospholipids, Determination; Starch, Structure, Properties and Determination; Vitamins, Determination

Food analysis is carried out for various reasons. In industry-related laboratories the main reasons are to support quality control and continuous monitoring of the composition of ingredients, raw materials and manufactured food products, dealing with complaints, examination of competitor's products, and in the development of new products. In official and enforcement laboratories the main reasons for food analysis include law enforcement, import/export trade regimes and compositional surveys.

Sampling

Not only is the analysis of foods difficult because of their complexity, but also the results of analysis are subject to considerable variability due to the heterogeneous nature of foods. For these reasons correct sampling of the food or food product is vitally important in order to obtain a representative sample for analysis. Sampling from bulk, from tankers or from trays or pallets of food commodities and products is a specialist and very broad subject in itself, but the value of the results of food analysis depend crucially on correct sampling. Moreover, the sample for analysis must be very thoroughly homogenized so that each sample portion for an analytical determination is as identical as possible in composition.

Techniques and Methods

The analytical techniques involved in food analysis can be categorized as chemical, physicochemical, physical and biological.

Chemical techniques include gravimetric and titrimetric methods, and many procedures involving an instrument to measure the results of a chemical reaction. Examples are the determination of the proximate components, sulphur dioxide, and anions and some metals (by colorimetry). *See* Spectroscopy, Visible Spectroscopy and Colorimetry

Physicochemical techniques are mainly instrumental techniques which utilize the different physical properties of atoms and molecules to effect their separation and often a physical property to detect the separated components. Examples are chromatographic techniques (gas–liquid chromatography, high-performance liquid chromatography, thin-layer chromatography, size exclusion chromatography and ion-exchange chromatography) and spectroanalytical methods. Substances determined by chromatography include fatty acids and other lipids, various additives, sugars, alcohols, colours, vitamins, and organic contaminants. Spectroanalytical methods include near-infrared reflectance spectroscopy, which allows rapid determination of major components, and flame photometry, atomic absorption spectrophotometry and plasma emission spectroscopy, all of which are invaluable for the determination of trace levels of metals and other elements. Electrophoresis relies on the separation of proteins under the influence of an electric field. *See* Electrophoresis

Physical techniques are based on the measurement of a physical property of a solid or liquid food substance or a solution. Procedures include refractometry, polarimetry, density, pH, viscosity and texture measurement.

Biological methods include microbiological analysis, enzymatic methods based on specific enzyme reactions, immunoassays to detect and identify proteins and microbiological assays for vitamins. Chromatographic and spectroscopic methods, immunoassays, microscopy and physical properties are discussed in other articles. *See* Immunoassays, Principles; Immunoassays, Radioimmunoassay and Enzyme Immunoassay; Microscopy, Image Analysis

Basically, methods of food analysis can be classified into two types, routine and reference. Routine methods include quantitative, semiquantitative and qualitative methods, as well as spot tests. Reference methods are those which have been prepared and issued by standards organizations, and have been thoroughly tested, e.g. by extensive use or by collaborative study, and found to be acceptably precise for both within-laboratory repeatability and between-laboratory reproducibility.

The Association of Public Analysts in the UK classifies initial routine or sorting methods as 'first action'. Where legal proceedings could develop, a reference method of analysis will then be carried out. The US Association of Official Analytical Chemists (AOAC) categorizes methods initially as 'interim official first action' when published in their journal. Once adopted by vote the method's status becomes 'official first action'. After a minimum of 2 years, if it has been reported to perform successfully by users, the method will achieve 'official final action' by affirmative vote at the annual meeting of the AOAC. Every 5 years, newly adopted or revised methods are published in a new edition of the compilation volume *Official Methods of Analysis*.

The Codex Alimentarius Commission of the Food and Agriculture Organization of the United Nations defines types of food analysis methods as follows:

Table 1.   Organizations which issue standard food analysis methods

Initials/acronym	Name	Area of concern
AACC	American Association of Cereal Chemists	Cereals
AFNOR	Association Française de Normalisation (French Standards Organization)	General
AIIBP	Association Internationale de l'Industrie des Bouillons et Potages (International Association of the Stock and Soup Industry)	Soups
AMC	Analytical Methods Committee of the Royal Society of Chemistry (UK)	Various
AOAC	Association of Official Analytical Chemists (USA)	Food, agriculture
APA	Association of Public Analysts (UK)	Various
BSI	British Standards Institution	General
CIRF	Corn Industries Research Foundation Inc.	Starch products
DGF	Deutsche Gesellschaft für Fettwissenschaft (German Society for the Science of Oils and Fats)	Oils and fats
EEC	European Economic Community	Various
FAO	Food and Agriculture Organization (UN)	Agriculture
FOSFA	Federation of Oils, Seeds and Fats Association	Oils and fats
IASC	International Association of Seed Crushers	Vegetable oils and fats
ICC	International Association for Cereal Chemistry	Cereals
ICMSF	International Commission on Microbiological Specification for Food	Food (general)
ICUMSA	International Commission for Uniform Methods of Sugar Analysis	Sugar
IDF	International Dairy Federation	Dairy products
IOB	Institute of Brewing (UK)	Beer
IOCCC	International Office of Cocoa, Chocolate and Sugar Confectionery	Cocoa, confectionery
IOFI	International Organization of the Flavour Industry	Flavour
ISO	International Organization for Standardization	General
IUPAC	International Union of Pure and Applied Chemistry	General
NMKL	Nordisk Metodik-Kommittee för Livsmedal (Nordic Committee on Food Analysis)	Food
NNI	Nederlands Normalisatie-Instituut (Standards Institution of the Netherlands)	General
OIV	Office Internationale de la Vigne et du Vin (International Office of Wine and Vine)	Wine

(1) Defining methods (type I). Methods, such as drying and other empirical methods and also those which interpret the results by use of a conversion factor, e.g. protein content, which determine a value defined entirely by the methodology, and are used for calibration purposes.

(2) Reference methods (type II). Methods which determine absolute chemical entities. Used for dispute and calibration purposes where type I methods do not apply.

(3) Alternative approved methods (type III). Methods suitable for regulatory or control purposes which are not reference methods.

(4) Tentative methods (type IV). Traditional or new methods for which performance criteria have not been established.

Standardization of Methods

As analytical techniques developed and analytical data accrued, it was recognized that the analysis of complex organic matrices, such as foods, was particularly subject to experimental and sampling errors. The earlier attempts before and between the two world wars to minimize error in chemical analysis were mainly the standardization and calibration of basic tools such as glassware, physical measuring instruments and balances, together with assay standards for the composition and purity of analytical reagents. These developments made it possible following interlaboratory collaboration to standardize analytical methods themselves as a means of improving the quality and validity of analytical measurement. The standardization of methods has gained pace since commencing in the 1930s, and particularly since about 1970. Table 1 lists organizations currently producing standard methods.

Statistical analysis techniques were introduced and applied, notably by the AOAC, to the results of interlaboratory collaborative studies of food methods, to measure their efficiency. For many years the standards organizations have pursued their own quite varied procedures for carrying out and reporting collaborative studies of methods. The different approaches made it difficult to compare a standard method and its performance from one organization with another standard method from another organization. In an attempt to overcome these difficulties, harmonized protocols have been developed by the IUPAC for the adoption of standardized food methods and for the presentation of their performance characteristics.

The general criteria for the selection of Codex Alimentarius methods of food analysis are:

(1) specificity;
(2) accuracy;
(3) precision, within and between laboratories;
(4) limit of detection;
(5) sensitivity;
(6) practicality and applicability.

Additional criteria which are now regarded as equally important are safety and cost.

Accreditation

Notwithstanding the standardization of food methods, in the early 1980s there was growing evidence from international interlaboratory studies of wide variations in results from different laboratories. This lack of reproducibility was illustrated in the results of a 1982 study by a working group of the UK Ministry of Agriculture, Fisheries and Food (MAFF), in which foodstuffs were monitored for heavy metals. Some 27 laboratories from universities, research institutes and associations, public analysts, hospitals and the food industry reported significantly different lead levels in dried cabbage compared to results from a subgroup of expert official laboratories. Such poor precision between laboratories, especially in trace analysis related to health and safety, raised many questions on the value of food analysis and gave impetus to the implementation of more effective quality control in analysis. Analytical quality control, however, cannot be treated in isolation, but only as part of a laboratory's wider quality assurance system of operation.

As a part of a quality assurance scheme or a manufacturer's total quality management system, the laboratory analytical work needs to be assessed by an independent authority. Various schemes and arrangements have developed over recent years, based on the recognized standards of competence to be expected in a laboratory claiming to produce valid and reliable measurements in mechanical, electrical and physical testing and in analytical chemistry. The National Measurement Accreditation Service (NAMAS), as a part of the UK National Measurement System developed by the National Physical Laboratory, became an accreditation service for food analysis laboratories carrying out chemical, physical and microbiological testing. The NAMAS accreditation standard is consistent with the provisions of ISO Guide 256 'General requirements for the technical competence of testing

laboratories' and EN 45001 'General criteria for the operation of testing laboratories'. Meeting the NAMAS standard also implies that laboratories conform to the appropriate requirements concerning adequacy of testing and calibration contained in the ISO 9000, EN 2900 and BS 5750 series of specifications relating to quality assurance in manufacture and similar activities. NAMAS accreditation approves a laboratory to carry out a schedule of test methods for any customer. Accreditation to meet the requirements of the BS 5750 series of standards is carried out by the British Standards Institution Quality Assurance Services or by Lloyds Register Quality Assurance Ltd (LRQA). Accreditation by these two organizations is for a company's food analysis facilities as part only of a total quality assurance system, and not for food analysis operations for external customers. Compliance with the principles of good laboratory practice (GLP), as laid down by the UK Department of Health, deals with those aspects of food and chemical analysis associated in a programme of toxicological testing of industrial and pharmaceutical chemicals and food additives. It does not cover contract food analysis.

All the above schemes for laboratory accreditation are quite similar in that they lean heavily on a fully documented and maintained quality assurance system in the form of manuals covering staff, their qualifications and training, instrument maintenance and calibration, quality control procedures, laboratory housekeeping and other operating procedures, report writing and audit and review procedures. There are agreed statements on their overlapping areas in the accreditation of testing laboratories and arrangements for mutual cooperation in carrying out assessments. There are also international mutual recognition agreements by participation with Western European Laboratory Accreditation Co-operation (WELAC), and national accreditation bodies around the world. The setting up of a laboratory quality assurance system to meet the requirements of one of the accreditation standards is a daunting task, particularly in the preparation of the quality assurance manuals. However, the experience of the author, as a consultant assessor for NAMAS, has shown that once the initial paper work has been completed and the laboratory operating procedures, especially audits, have been installed, the quality assurance system then requires only a modicum of attention. The additional quality control measures used, such as control charts, tend to increase the analyst's interest in their tasks.

The main reasons for accreditation include:

(1) The provision of a due-diligence defence in the event of civil, criminal or contractual actions against the laboratory.

(2) Compunction by the terms of contract with, for example, large retailers or suppliers.
(3) As a part of a company's total quality assurance system.
(4) As a means of increasing efficiency and confidence in analysis.
(5) For publicity and promotional purposes.

Post-1992 EEC legislation is expected to make it necessary for certain laboratories which carry out official or linked EEC work to be accredited. Such laboratories are also likely to be required to participate and show competence in organized sample check programmes.

Analytical Proficiency

A documented quality assurance system cannot by itself guarantee that the results of food analysis are correct. The system can only increase the degree of confidence in the result. Involvement in a proficiency testing/sample check scheme is essential to monitor continuous analytical competence. The MAFF introduced in 1990 their food analysis performance assessment scheme (FAPAS) to help provide the effective implementation and enforcement of the UK Food and Environmental Protection Act, the Food Safety Act and future EEC 'single market' legislation. Samples of prepared food types requiring analysis for proximate and nutritional components, fatty acids, preservatives, sweeteners, metals, aflatoxins, pesticide and veterinary residues are dispatched regularly to voluntary participating coded laboratories. The results are statistically appraised and reported to the coded laboratories, whom alone can monitor their performance in comparison with the other participating laboratories. By the end of 1991 over 140 laboratories were participating, approximately half of them from the food industry. More recently, a similar assessment scheme for assisting the performance of laboratories carrying out food microbiological analyses has been introduced by the Public Health Laboratory Service. *See* Ministry of Agriculture, Fisheries and Food; Pesticides and Herbicides, Types, Uses and Determination of Herbicides

Analytical Quality Control

Reliable and valid food analysis depends on efficient laboratory operations, trained staff, suitable reagents, fully calibrated and maintained equipment and instruments, and effective sampling and sample preparation. Furthermore, in order to have confidence in the results of a food analysis, the method used must have known and acceptable minimum performance characteristics, and it must be applied with all the calibrations, controls and checks necessary to make sure that the method operates to the degree of accuracy and precision expected. The calculated mean result from replicate analyses of the prepared sample, usually duplicate analysis, will minimize repeatability errors and provide confirmation that the repeatability performance of the method is being achieved. Duplicate analysis also provides evidence whether or not the laboratory sample has been thoroughly homogenized. If batches of the same sample type are being analysed, duplicate analysis with routine methods can with sufficient confidence be confined to, say, one in 10–20 samples, but more frequently for complex methods. In food industry quality control laboratories, where regular analysis of known products is most often the rule, samples are predominantly analysed singly alongside periodic in-house reference samples of the same sample type. Quality control charts of the results on the reference samples should be applied to monitor analytical variability or drift.

Where suitable and appropriate reference food materials with certified composition are obtainable, their use to monitor the accuracy of the analytical method is probably the best form of quality control available to the food analyst.

For methods which determine a chemical entity, e.g. a preservative, sweetener, trace metal or pesticide residue, and where no suitable certified reference material is available, the continued efficiency or relative accuracy of the method should be frequently checked by recovery analysis of a known quantity of the determinand added to the sample as early as possible in the methodology, commonly known as 'spiking'. Provided that the calculated percentage recovery of the added substance at the appropriate level of concentration is within the known or expected range for the method, the method can be regarded as correctly functioning. If the percentage recovery is outside the acceptable range, the analytical protocol or its operation is at fault and must be corrected until satisfactory recoveries are achieved. The percentage recovery of a spike is not intended to be used to correct a food analysis result to 100% recovery, except in very special circumstances, e.g. the determination of trace labile organic compounds. The results of an analysis to be valid must be subject to known limits of detection and determination, and, considering the sensitivity of the method, should only be reported to significant figures of concentration.

Summary

Food analysis is an important branch of food science and technology, aiding economy and efficiency in food production, manufacture and sale, and providing information on the quality, safety and nutritional value of

---

foods for the consumer. New techniques are providing greater insight into the nature and composition of foods, and developments in instrumentation are providing the means for rapid and economical analysis. Nevertheless since foods are such heterogeneous and chemically complex substances, food analysis remains a very broad and difficult subject, requiring great care in its execution if valid data are to be obtained. Quality assurance systems, standardized methods and analytical quality control are important features of an efficient food analysis laboratory, but motivated and well-trained staff are the prime factors for demonstrating and maintaining the value of food analysis.

Bibliography

Aurand LW, Woods E and Wells MR (1987) *Food Composition and Analysis*. New York: Van Nostrand Reinhold.

Dux JP (1986) *Handbook of Quality Assurance for the Analytical Laboratory*. New York: Van Nostrand Reinhold.

Garfield FM (1984) *Quality Assurance Principles for Analytical Laboratories*. Arlington, VA: Association of Official Analytical Chemists.

Keenan Taylor J (1987) *Quality Assurance of Chemical Measurements*. Michigan: Lewis.

Kirk RS and Sawyer R (1991) *Pearsons Composition and Analysis of Foods*, 9th edn. Harlow: Longman.

Pocklington WD (1990) *Guidelines for the Development of Standard Methods by Collaborative Study*, 5th edn. Teddington: Laboratory of the Government Chemist.

Pocklington WD (1990) Harmonized protocols for the adoption of standardized analytical methods and for the presentation of their performance characteristics. *Pure and Applied Chemistry* 62(1): 149–162.

Pomeranz Y and Meloan CE (1987) *Food Analysis*. New York: Van Nostrand Reinhold.

Williams S (ed.) (1990) *Official Methods of Analysis of the Association of Official Analytical Chemists*, 15th edn. Arlington, VA: Association of Official Analytical Chemists.

R. S. Kirk
Fanfare Consultants Ltd, Fleet, UK

ANALYTICAL TECHNIQUES

See Chromatography, Immunoassays, Spectroscopy and Mass Spectrometry

ANIMAL FATS

See Fats

ANIMAL MODELS OF HUMAN NUTRITION

Experimentation with animals has been fundamental to human nutrition knowledge. By using small animals, researchers can economically control experimental diets to determine the biological effects of dietary constituents. Studies with small animals fed controlled diets led to the discovery of most of the vitamins and essential trace minerals. Because of animal research, nutrient deficiency diseases of humans have been eradicated in many countries. Animals continue to contribute to our knowledge about diet and biological function. Animal research in the future should help us understand how diet affects disease, reproduction, brain function and longevity.

Advantages of using animals in nutrition research include: (1) large groups can be studied economically; (2) dietary consumption and living conditions can be carefully controlled; (3) short life-spans improve the feasibility and efficiency of developmental, longevity or multiple generation studies; and (4) controlled breeding reduces biological variability. The use of animals in food and nutrition research protects human safety. If dietary deficiencies or imbalances are suspected of causing disease in humans, these hypotheses should be tested in controlled studies with animals. Likewise, new dietary additives should be tested in animals to protect human safety. Although animal research is indispensable for our expanding knowledge about diet and health, investigators must weigh the benefits of such knowledge against the discomfort of animals in research. New knowledge for the health of our own and possibly other species should be obtained with an ethical responsibility for the humane treatment of experimental animals.

History

Since earliest times, human have recognized that they share with animals a basic need for food and water. Accordingly, the history of nutrition is replete with examples of animal experimentation. Erasistratus (310–250 BC), tested his ideas that *pneuma* in the atmosphere became spirit in the body. He placed fowls in a jar and weighed them and their excreta before and after food. Galen (130–200 AD) studied digestion in hogs and concluded that in the stomach foods were reduced to smaller particles that could later be absorbed.

In 1774, Joseph Priestley (1733–1804) exposed mercuric oxide to focused sunlight to produce 'pure dephlogisticated air' (oxygen). He demonstrated that this air caused a candle flame to burn brighter and that mice could live in it.

Guinea pigs were employed by Crawford, Lavoisier and Laplace, and by Despretz in the late eighteenth and early nineteenth centuries to study respiration and body heat production. Lavoisier and Laplace invented an ice calorimeter and compared the amount of ice melted by a guinea pig with the amount of carbon dioxide produced. In addition to using guinea pigs, Lavoisier measured his own respiratory exchanges and those of his friends and assistants. These studies led to the conclusion that respiration was a combustion of carbon and hydrogen which transformed oxygen into carbon dioxide, similar to the burning of a candle or an oil lamp.

Spallanzani (1729–1799) first obtained gastric juice from the stomach of a hawk by using a sponge and string. He demonstrated that it dissolved flesh, bones and bread without putrefaction.

Boussingault performed the first balance study in 1839 on a cow, by measuring carbon, hydrogen, oxygen, nitrogen and salts in the feed, urine, faeces and milk. Later, he performed similar experiments with a horse and a turtle dove.

In 1849, Regnault and Reiset used rabbits, dogs and fowl to determine the effect of various foods on the ratio of carbon dioxide produced to oxygen inspired, later

called the 'respiratory quotient'. The animals were in a 45-l bell jar which was part of a sealed, closed-circuit apparatus.

Dogs were used extensively in the last half of the nineteenth century by German investigators studying protein and energy metabolism. Voit (1831–1908) demonstrated 'nitrogen equilibrium', and an increase from negative to positive nitrogen balance as dogs were fed greater amounts of meat. He also discovered that muscular work by the dog did not increase protein metabolism. Rubner (1854–1932), a student of Voit, employed dogs to show that similar measurements of energy utilization could be obtained by direct and indirect calorimetry, and he measured the 'specific dynamic action' (increased heat production) associated with protein consumption by studying a dog fed meat. From his measurements of metabolic rates of various species, including humans, Rubner developed his surface area law, which stated that the basal metabolism is proportional to the surface area of the animal.

Animals played an indispensable role in the discovery of the vitamins. In 1897, Eijkman, a Dutch physician in Java, reported that chickens fed polished rice developed a paralysis. This paralysis was similar to that of the disease beriberi in humans. Unmilled rice or a water extract of rice polishings cured the chickens. Hölst, a Norwegian, repeated Eijkman's experiments, and obtained similar results with pigeons. However, he and Frölich reported in 1907 that guinea pigs fed a cereal diet developed scurvy, rather than the paralysis of beriberi. This fortunate discovery – of one of the few species in addition to humans that require ascorbic acid – soon led to a biological assay for the antiscorbutic potency of foodstuffs.

In 1906, Hopkins reported from the University of Cambridge, UK, that mice required the amino acid tryptophan. This initiated the concept of essential amino acids and differences in the biological value of proteins. Hopkins studied both mice and rats and reported in 1912 that animals could not live on purified protein, fat, carbohydrates, and minerals alone; other unknown nutrients were essential.

In 1907, at the University of Wisconsin, USA, McCollum set out to identify what was lacking in purified diets that did not nourish small animals. Frustrated by tedious studies with cows fed various grains, he recognized the advantages of studying animals which have a short lifespan and eat little. Smaller dietary volumes would make dietary control and analysis both practical and economical. McCollum decided to use rats because of their convenient size, omnivorous feeding habits, and lack of economic value. Within 5 years, McCollum and Davis reported a fat-soluble factor (later named vitamin A) in butterfat that was not present in lard or olive oil. Vitamin A deficiency was later found to be a major cause of human blindness.

In the UK, Mellanby used dogs, known to be susceptible to rickets, to show that the disease resulted from a dietary deficiency. Incidental to this research, Mellanby discovered that nitrogen trichloride bleaching of wheat flour caused canine hysteria, a nervous disorder that also occurred in ferrets, cats and rabbits. Rats, which had been used in safety testing, were less sensitive to the compound. Commercial use of nitrogen trichloride in flour for human consumption was discontinued after Mellanby's discovery.

McCollum used rats to differentiate between the effects of vitamins A and D. He developed the 'line test', a measure of the width of a line of new calcification in the bone of a deficient rat given vitamin D. This became a widespread biological assay for vitamin D in foods.

Rats were the principal animal used to discover most of the vitamins, the essential trace elements, and the essential amino acids. As a result, more is known about the nutritional requirements of the rat than about any other species. Dogs, chickens, pigeons, mice and guinea pigs have also made valuable contributions to our knowledge of nutrition.

Animals as Models of Human Nutrition in Research

Factors considered when selecting an animal model include anatomical, physiological and biochemical similarities to humans, similarities of disease processes, susceptibility to aetiological agents, availability, cost, breeding lines available, behaviour, size, genetic characteristics, lifespan, resistance to infections, suitability for experimental manipulation, and accumulated pathobiological information. Considerations particularly pertinent to nutrition research are as follows.

Natural Diet in Habitat

The omnivorous feeding patterns of the rat usually make it a better model for human nutrition questions than a strict herbivore such as the rabbit. The natural diets of nonhuman primates vary considerably. Primates include insectivores, herbivores, and omnivores, which makes some primate species poor models for human nutrition research. Strict carnivores such as cats have associated differences in nutrient metabolism and requirements. For instance, the cat requires arachidonic acid and preformed vitamin A from animal foods, as it cannot synthesize those from the respective plant-food precursors, linoleic acid and β-carotene.

Nutrient Requirements

The requirement for vitamin C is a striking example of qualitative differences between species; few species require it in the diet. Humans share this uncommon requirement with other primates, the guinea pig, the red-vented bulbul, and some Indian fruit-eating bats.

Dietary fibre may provide a more subtle example of species differences in nutrient requirements. Two herbivores, the guinea pig and the rabbit, require dietary fibre, according to the US National Research Council (NRC). Other laboratory animals are apparently not as vulnerable to a fibre deficit. However, fibre is routinely added to research diets for rodents, and continued research may reveal reduced gastrointestinal diseases associated with fibre in the diets of primates.

Quantitative comparison of nutrient requirements across species is difficult: limited research on some species has yielded knowledge of adequate intakes without determination of minimum requirements. Differences in vitamin requirements between species are influenced by differences in production by intestinal flora. The mineral requirements of most species are quite similar, with the possible exception of a higher iron requirement of primates.

Digestion and Absorption

The relative influence of gastrointestinal microorganisms on metabolism of digesta varies widely between species. Extensive fermentation in the pregastric chambers of ruminants and the hindgut of the horse makes these animals poor models for human nutrition. Dogs and pigs are similar to humans in many aspects of gastrointestinal morphology and physiology, including relative length of small and large bowels, ingesta transit times, influence of dietary factors on gastric emptying, glucose or xylose absorption, faecal fat excretion, activities of intestinal brush border and pancreatic enzymes at maturity, and colonic volatile fatty acid concentration. However, humans, dogs and pigs differ in the developmental patterns and primary structure of some digestive enzymes. The composition of bile and the structure of bile acids differs substantially between humans and pigs. Colonic volatile fatty acids may be an important energy source for the pig, but not for the dog; the importance of colonic fermentation for humans probably falls between these two species. Numerous strains of miniature pigs have been developed and used in experiments related to digestion and absorption.

Body Composition, Nutrient Metabolism, and Excretion

Species differences in chemical composition may influence the suitability of animals as models for human nutrition problems. As an example, differences in skeletal mass may reduce the usefulness of animal models for bone health and related nutrients. The skeleton comprises about 16% of the adult human body, as compared to 11% of the rat, 10% of the rabbit, and 7·7% of a 28-week-old pig. This probably accounts for considerably higher amounts of calcium and phosphorus per kilogram of fat-free body tissue in humans than in pigs, cats, rabbits, rats, or mice. Human cortical bones have greater nitrogen and lower calcium : nitrogen ratios than those of pigs, cats, rabbits, rats, and fowl. Differences in nutrient excretion may complicate animal modelling further. For example, the rat excretes less than 1% of dietary calcium in the urine, which is an important route for calcium excretion (and its hormonal control) in humans. These examples may help explain why there has not been a satisfactory animal model for human osteoporosis.

Coprophagy (the ingestion of faeces) by rabbits and rodents can confound dietary intake measurements in nutrition studies. By increasing the total nutrient intake, coprophagy can lower apparent requirements and reduce signs of deficiency for many nutrients. Particularly affected are those nutrients synthesized or made more bioavailable through colonic microbial flora, including the B-complex vitamins and essential fatty acids. To study signs of deficiency for such nutrients, steps must be taken to prevent coprophagy.

Reproduction

Animal studies have demonstrated vital roles for nutrition from oestrus to parturition and lactation. For example, animal studies have shown the essentiality of zinc for normal oestrus cycling and fertility, development of preimplantation eggs, normal development of organ systems (especially the skeletal and central nervous systems), fetal growth, and normal labour and delivery. Zinc deficiency during specific stages of gestation causes postnatal abnormalities in behaviour and immune function.

Special considerations when evaluating animals as models of human reproduction include the number of fetuses, the type of placentation, the tendency to abort or reabsorb fetuses under teratological conditions, the rate of development, and the maturity of the fetus at delivery. Maturity at birth can determine the suitability of an animal model for studies of late gestational development. For example, epiphyseal calcification of the femur is much greater in newborn piglets than in newborn humans, and pigs walk soon after birth. This would limit the usefulness of the pig in some studies of prenatal bone development. Maturation at birth is also a concern when selecting animals to study early infant development. Another difficulty is that newborn mammals often require maternal lactation, limiting the investigator's control of dietary variables in early life.

Animal Models of Nutrient Evaluation

Because living organisms are always used in research determining the essentiality of nutrients for life, they naturally provide the earliest means of evaluating foods as a source of nutrients. Biological assays for vitamins in foods were mentioned previously. Historically, animals were useful for food evaluation because chemical techniques were inadequate for direct analysis of foods. While chemical analysis difficulties have been largely overcome, difficulties predicting nutrient bioavailability have not.

Bioavailability is the proportion of a nutrient in food which is absorbed and utilized. It is affected by chemical form, interactions with other food components, and, probably, physiological responses to food. For example, the zinc bioavailability of foods fed to rats depends on the amount of food fed, even though the foods are compared in amounts providing similar quantities of zinc. Pancreatic secretion responds to quantitative and qualitative differences in foods. Zinc is a cofactor of pancreatic carboxypeptidase, and perhaps the reabsorption of endogenous zinc from pancreatic secretions competes with absorption of dietary zinc. Zinc absorption mechanisms may also involve coabsorption with ligands such as histidine which have separate facilitated pathways of absorption. *In vitro* measurements of zinc absorption are generally static, involving measurements of food composition or physicochemical properties in a gastrointestinal simulation. Until the dynamic nature of the gastrointestinal response to differing foods in varying quantities is understood, accurate *in vitro* simulation may not be possible. *See* Bioavailability of Nutrients

For investigating the bioavailability of some nutrients, even animal models may not be sufficient. For example, the haem form of iron present in foods of animal origin is much better absorbed by humans than ionic ferrous iron. This is not true for rats. Rats deficient in iron apparently absorb haem iron less efficiently than ferrous iron.

Food bioavailability is poorly understood for many nutrients, including the extensively researched macronutrient protein. The nutritional quality of dietary proteins has been evaluated since as early as 1917 by measures of animal growth or nitrogen retention. Despite attempts since the mid-1940s to replace the biological assays with a 'chemical score' of amino acid composition, the biological assays continue to be used extensively. Chemical scoring accounts for essential amino acid composition and requirements. However, scoring does not account for amino acid bioavailability, which can be reduced by chemical changes during heating, or by inhibitors of proteolytic digestion.

In vitro testing has progressed substantially and is often preferred by scientists for efficient use of resources. However, the complexity of living organisms remains incompletely understood, and the nutritional value of foods or diets is frequently more accurately evaluated by direct *in vivo* testing than by modern, highly technological *in vitro* testing.

Animal Models of Disease States

With the help of animal models, a major cause of human disease – overt nutrient deficiency – was largely solved as a scientific problem (it unfortunately remains as a political and economic problem). Scientific emphasis has turned to diet and chronic disease. Perhaps because they are as yet unresolved, the problems of chronic disease seem more complex. Dietary variables are likely to be slight deficiencies, excesses, or imbalances in a lifelong interaction with other genetic and environmental factors. Animal models can provide the advantage of controlled environmental and dietary factors over a short lifetime. However, genetic differences, although confirming inheritability, limit application to humans. The use of animals to study nutrition and major chronic diseases is considered briefly below.

Atherosclerotic Cardiovascular Disease

The responsiveness of serum cholesterol and atherosclerosis to dietary cholesterol and saturated fatty acids varies among animal species. Rabbits, guinea pigs, swine, rhesus and cynomolgus monkeys are more susceptible than humans. Rats and dogs are more resistant. Baboons and vervet monkeys are in the same moderate range of susceptibility as humans. Genetic differences in lipid metabolism are confirmed by the variation observed within and between species. *See* Atherosclerosis

Hypertension

Hypertension in response to dietary salt is not observed in all animal models but occurs in specific animal strains without sufficient renal capacity to excrete salt rapidly. The Dahl S and the Kyoto spontaneously hypertensive rat are susceptible to dietary salt, and the addition of potassium to high-salt diets reduces the incidence of stroke in these animals, and in the Sprague-Dawley rat. Research on animal models verifies an interaction between diet and genetic susceptibility to hypertension, and susceptible animals may be useful in identifying dietary variables that affect susceptible humans. *See* Hypertension, Physiology; Hypertension, Hypertension and Diet

Obesity

Genetically obese strains of rodents – obese (*ob/ob*) and diabetic (*db/db*) mice and obese (*fa/fa*) rats – confirm

that inheritance can contribute to obesity. Obesity in such models has been associated with hyperinsulinaemia and abnormal glucose tolerance. Hyperphagia also occurs, but pair-feeding studies indicate that genetically obese rodents have an unusually high body fat composition even with normal diets. Rats without genetic obesity increase their food intake and thermogenesis in response to a 'cafeteria' diet of mixed human food. The relationship between energy intake, physical activity, thermogenesis and bodyweight has been extensively studied in rodents. Results of these studies generally support the biological maintenance of a 'set-point' for bodyweight; this varies only slightly and controls energy balance. *See* Obesity, Aetiology and Assessment

Cancer

Approximately one third of human cancer mortality may be related to diet. Animal studies are useful in the investigation of specific dietary components and the mechanism of action. Animal studies, mostly using rats, have indicated that tumour development is enhanced in a variety of tissues by high-fat diets, especially diets rich in ω-6 (but not ω-3) polyunsaturated fatty acids. This effect of high-fat diets has not been completely differentiated from the effect of high energy consumption. Retinoids can prevent cancer at several sites in laboratory animals. However, research has focused on new synthetic retinoid compounds because the naturally occurring retinoids are commonly toxic at doses necessary to inhibit carcinogenesis. Animal models have shown that selenium inhibits both the initiation and proliferative phases of tumorigenesis. The effect of some dietary components may depend on the specific site, type and stage of carcinogenesis. The effects of specific nutrients may depend on the relative nutrient requirements of host and tumour. Zinc deficiency in animals increases the incidence of oesophageal carcinoma induced by methylbenzylnitrosamine, but decreases the incidence of tumours induced by 3-methylcholanthrene and 4-nitroquinoline-*N*-oxide. *See* Cancer, Epidemiology; Cancer, Diet in Cancer Prevention; Cancer, Diet in Cancer Treatment

Testing food additives for carcinogenicity requires animal models. Careful studies generally involve more than one species and exposure over an extended portion of the lifespan. However, the evaluation of research results must consider whether dietary characteristics have been experimentally exaggerated, and whether extrapolation to humans is realistic. A US food additive law, known as the Delancy Clause, prohibits the use of a food additive in any amount if it has been shown to produce cancer in animal studies or in other appropriate tests. This law has been controversial because it can be applied to prohibit any amount of a substance that may have been tested in high amounts. Carcinogenicity of dietary constituents should be evaluated with consideration of average and peak human exposures to the substance, the potency of the substance, and the quality of experimental data.

Osteoporosis

Diets low in calcium or high in phosphorus increase bone reabsorption and decrease bone mass in rats, mice, cats, dogs and nonhuman primates. In contrast with experimental animals, calcium balance in humans is relatively insensitive to high dietary phosphorus. Animal research related to bone health has too often involved animals that were young and growing or animals that were very old. There are few animals that experience the spontaneous ovarian failure in middle age that occurs in humans. Researchers have not identified an appropriate animal model of postmenopausal or age-related osteoporosis (see *Body Composition, Nutrient Metabolism, and Excretion*, above). *See* Osteoporosis

Diabetes Mellitus

Experimental diabetes can be induced in animals by pancreatectomy or injection of β-cell toxins such as streptozotocin or alloxan. There is a genetically obese strain of diabetic (*db/db*) mice. Unlike most rodents, the sand rat remains lean and nondiabetic in the wild, but becomes obese and diabetic under laboratory feeding conditions. In normal strains of animals, greatly inccreased food intake for an extended time leads to adiposity and an increased incidence of insulin resistance, which is reversible with weight reduction. This insulin resistance is confounded by both adiposity and ageing. It has not been possible with animal research to show that high energy consumption causes diabetes.

Interpretation and Extrapolation of Data

Animal studies are most appropriately applied to humans when they complement and are consistent with human studies. Highly controlled experimental trials in animals can confirm epidemiological associations between diet and health in humans. Short-term experimental results in humans can be compared for similarity to short-term results in animals, and then continued to determine longitudinal effects in animals. As with all scientific research, reliable conclusions should be reproducible in different laboratories and supported by various methods. Relevance of animal research to humans is more likely if the results are confirmed in several animal species.

The highly uniform experimental conditions charac-

teristic of animal models can provide disadvantages as well as advantages. For example, energy restriction reproducibly increases longevity in rodents. However, such studies were usually conducted under laboratory conditions in which the rodents spent their entire lives in a small space; they formed no social relationships, did not reproduce, experienced low exposure to hazardous biological or chemical substances and sunlight, and had little need for physical activity or development of self-preservation skills. Scientists must evaluate whether the food-restricted animals would have an improved *quality* or even *quantity* of life if tested under more realistic living conditions.

The control of experimental diets in animal nutrition studies can present similar problems in extrapolation to humans. To enhance experimental control and comparability between studies, animal diets for nutrition research are often standardized, purified, and fed *ad libitum*. Purified diets are commonly composed of a small number of refined ingredients, such as commercially refined proteins, carbohydrates and fat, with added vitamin and mineral mixtures. While such diets allow a controlled supply of specific nutritional variables, they also limit the context of the experiment. Unlike many animal research diets, human diets contain thousands of compounds and are usually scheduled in meals. Metabolic adaptation occurs in response to eating schedules and to specific dietary components, but this is not well defined for most dietary constituents. As nutrition research moves from single nutrient deficiencies to more complex dietary interactions that affect health, laboratory diets and other conditions may need to become more like human conditions to facilitate comparability to humans. An example is the 'cafeteria' diet of mixed human food used to attain overeating in rodents.

Animal studies are often most valuable for initial nutritional studies preparatory to human studies and for studies of basic biological mechanisms. Animal models are often helpful in evaluating dose–response relationships. Some biological responses to dietary variables are more credible when an increased exposure results in an increased response. Essential nutrients can often be characterized by biological responses that are linear below requirements and possibly above safe amounts, but stable at intermediate intakes that do not overpower homeostatic adaptation. Quantitative relationships between dietary amounts and biological responses should also be tested in humans to determine realistic exposures and outcomes.

Limitations of Animal Models in Nutrition Research

Nutritional knowledge has rapidly expanded in the nineteenth and twentieth centuries. During this time, an increasing share of biomedical advances depended on animal research. Some 67–75% of major biomedical advances in the 1900s required the use of animals. This trend was accompanied by an antivivisectionist movement in Victorian England in the late 1800s, which may be a predecessor of the current 'animal rights/liberation' movement. This movement has raised ethical questions about animal research. The movement appropriately emphasizes the value of humane treatment of animals but inappropriately harms humanity when it prevents animal research and the resulting knowledge about health. Most people recognize the inconsistency of vandalism and terrorism in the name of animal rights. A more insidious threat to research is the reduction of resources through excessive regulation and bureaucracy. High-quality animal care helps both research results – by improving reliability of experimental results – and the researcher – by engendering public trust.

The US NRC's Committee on the Use of Laboratory Animals in Biomedical and Behavioral Research concluded in 1988 that animals should be used when research with animals is the best available method to improve the human condition. The committee also recognized the ethical obligation of scientists to ensure animal wellbeing and minimize pain and suffering through humane treatment. Scientists realize that they must be involved in public policy influencing legal regulations that benefit humans through science, while treating animals humanely and without inefficient bureaucracy.

One suggested means of minimizing animal pain and suffering has been for researchers to consider possible alternative methods. This may include differentiation among species; public opinion prefers the experimental use of rodents over the use of dogs, cats, and monkeys. Most nutrition research has been conducted with rodents, especially rats. However, as societal preferences influence researchers to use nonmammalian vertebrates, invertebrates, and microorganisms, the valid extrapolation of results to human nutrition becomes more difficult. Some nutrition knowledge may be gained by using cell and tissue cultures, human tissues removed at surgery or at autopsy, *in vitro* systems and mathematical models. Such methods can be more efficient, controlled and economical than research with living animals. However, researchers must be cautious not to extrapolate to human nutrition without adequate validation of the simpler model.

A straightforward alternative to using animals is to study humans directly. Although the technology for safe study of humans continues to improve, many nutrition research topics require animal models. Such topics include the effects of nutrition on reproduction, growth and development, longevity, and behaviour. Animal experiments can verify observations in humans that often cannot be controlled sufficiently to be conclusive. Use of animals for initial experiments in nutrition research improves efficiency and the rate of progress in knowledge. Animal studies facilitate the investigation of physiological and molecular mechanisms. Animal research has been instrumental in identifying required nutrients and developing the science of nutrition. For the foreseeable future animal research will be necessary to answer questions about nutrition and health that can be learned only from living organisms.

Bibliography

Lusk G (1933) *Nutrition*. New York: Paul B Hoeber.

NRC (1988) *Use of Laboratory Animals in Biomedical and Behavioral Research*. Committee on the Use of Laboratory Animals in Biomedical and Behavioral Research, National Research Council. Washington, DC: National Academy Press.

NRC (1989) *Diet and Health. Implications for Reducing Chronic Disease Risk*. Committee on Diet and Health, National Research Council. Washington, DC: National Academy Press.

Phillips RW (ed.) (1984) *Animal Models for Nutrition Research*. Report of the Fifth Ross Conference on Medical Research, Ross Laboratories, Columbus, Ohio.

Widdowson EM (1986) Animals in the service of human nutrition. *Nutrition Reviews* 44: 221–227.

Janet R Hunt
US Department of Agriculture Human Nutrition Research Center, Grand Forks, USA

ANNONACEOUS FRUITS

The main commercial species of *Annona* grown throughout the world are the cherimoya (*A. cherimola*), the atemoya (*A. hybrids*) and the sugar apple (*A. squamosa*). Expansion of production of these three species in many subtropical countries is limited by several factors, including low yields of better-quality cultivars, unattractive external appearance of the fruit, a high susceptibility of the fruit to blemishing, poor and unreliable internal fruit quality, and a very short post-harvest shelf and storage life. In the short term, fruit quality can be improved by field management practices. In the longer term, selection and breeding of new varieties will be necessary.

Classification

The family, Annonaceae, comprises 50 genera. Three genera (*Annona*, *Rollinia* and *Asimina*) produce edible fruit, but only two genera are of commercial importance – *Annona*, comprising approximately 100 species, and *Rollinia*, comprising approximately 50 species. The four most commercially important species are the cherimoya, the sugar apple, the atemoya, and the soursop (*Annona muricata*). The cherimoya is native to the subtropical highlands of Peru and Ecuador, and is grown commercially in Chile, Spain, California and New Zealand. The atemoyas, most of which are hybrids between *A. cherimola* and *A. squamosa*, are grown commercially in Florida and Australia. Both the sugar apple and the soursop are widely distributed throughout the tropical regions of Southeast Asia and Central America, where they are found growing wild. The rollinia (*Rollinia mucosa*) and biriba (*R. deliciosa*) are native to the jungles of South America. A list of the edible species of *Annona* and *Rollinia* grown throughout the world is presented in Table 1. It should be noted that common names, such as custard apple, have been used with reference to many different species.

Climate

Most *Annona* species are tropical or subtropical in their growth requirements. Both the atemoya and the cherimoya are best grown in frost-free locations as the young trees are killed at $-1°C$ and mature trees at $-3°C$. The cherimoya is more cold-tolerant than the atemoya and is able to stand a longer duration of cold at $-3°C$. The sugar apple and the soursop, on the other hand, are very

frost-sensitive. Most cherimoya and atemoya cultivars are semideciduous and enter either a true rest or environmentally induced dormancy in the late winter or spring. This dormancy or rest period allows the plant to avoid the effects of late-winter frost and drought.

Different species exhibit varying climatic requirements for fruit development and maturation. Excessively low temperature during the fruit maturation period may retard the process, while excessively high temperatures during this period may cause premature ripening and fermentation of the fruit whilst still on the tree. For example, atemoya cultivars grown in cool subtropical regions of California or New Zealand may fail to mature properly. In these regions the main commercial species grown is the cherimoya. In contrast, cherimoya fruit grown in tropical climates often fails to develop full flavour, and post-harvest shelf life is short.

Besides the influence of temperature on fruit maturation, physiological disorders such as skin russetting are more prevalent under cool night temperatures, particularly when ambient temperatures fall below about $13°C$.

Fruit Morphology

The cherimoya, atemoya and sugar apple fruits are syncarpiums, made up of many individual carpels which are fused together with the receptacle to form a fleshy mass. Each carpel, if pollinated, contains an oval seed. Depending on species and cultivar the number of seeds per 100 g of flesh can vary from 5 to 15. The fruit ranges in shape from conical, through globular to ovoid, and the skin type may be smooth, finger-imprinted, or bumpy. The skin is relatively thick and contains numerous stomata. The mesocarp consists mainly of parenchyma, cholenchyma and sclerenchyma cells, the latter often being highly lignified, similar to those found in pears.

Varietal Selection and Breeding

The atemoya and the cherimoya produce fruit superior in quality to other *Annona* species. The fruit of some species, such as the bullock's hearts (*A. reticulata*) and ilama (*A. diversifolia*), are barely edible. The fruit of the sugar apple are highly seeded and are not grown commercially in regions where cherimoya or atemoya can be grown. The fruits of rollinia and biriba, although

Table 1.   Important species of the genera *Annona* and *Rollinia*

Species names	Common names	Chromosome number (2n)	Gene centre	Potential uses
Annona hybrids	Atemoya Cherimorinones Custard apple	16	Various	Fresh fruit Rootstock Processing with dairy products
A. cherimola Mill	Cherimuyu Cherimoyer Cherimoya Cherimola Custard apple	16	Andean valleys of Peru and Ecuador	Fresh fruit Rootstock Processing with dairy products
A. squamosa L.	Sugar apple Sweetsop Sitaphal Ata Custard apple	16	West Indies	Fresh fruit Rootstock Processing with dairy products
A. reticulata L.	Bullock's hearts Ramphala Custard apple (often considered the true custard apple)	16	West Indies, Mexico	Fresh fruit Rootstock
A. muricata L.	Soursop Guanabana Corossol Graviola	16	West Indies, Mexico	Fresh fruit Drinks and purées Processing with dairy products
A. glabra L.	Pond apple Alligator apple	28	Florida (USA)	Rootstock
A. senegalensis	Wild Transvaal apple		South Africa	Pollinator species Rootstock
A. diversifolia Safford	Ilama Cherimoyer of the lowlands		Mexico, Guatemala, El Salvador	Fresh fruit
A. montana Macf.	Mountain soursop	16	Cuba, West Indies	Fresh fruit Rootstock
A. purpurea Moc. & Sesse	Soncoya Manirote		Mexico	Fresh fruit Rootstock
A. longiflora	Wild cherimoya		Mexico	Rootstock
A. scleroderma Safford	Posh te		Mexico, Guatemala	Fresh fruit
Rollinia deliciosa Safford	Biriba	48	Brazil	Fresh fruit Rootstock
R. emarginata Schlecht			Brazil, Paraguay	Fresh fruit Rootstock
R. mucosa	Rollinia		Brazil, Paraguay	Fresh fruit Rootstock

edible, deteriorate rapidly within a few days after harvesting, thus limiting their commercial acceptabilty for local markets only.

The University of Puerto Rico's Agricultural Experiment Station at one time catalogued 14 different types of soursop. In El Salvador, two types of soursop are grown: guanaba azucaron (sweet), eaten raw and used for drinks, and guanaba acida (very sour), used only for drinks. A yellow, fibreless form of soursop has been selected in Cuba.

The most important commercially grown cultivars are as follows: of cherimoya, Bronceada (Chile), Fino de Jete (Spain), and Bays (California); of atemoya, African Pride (Australia) and Gefner (Israel, Florida and Hawaii); of soursop, Cuban Fibreless. Wide genetic variability exists between different species of cherimoya and atemoya. Selection of varieties with round, symmetrical shape, smooth skin, high ratios of flesh to seed, and long post-harvest storage life is highly desirable. Intensive varietal selection programmes for cherimoya are currently being undertaken in Spain, New Zealand and Chile. A small breeding programme, currently in progress in Queensland, Australia, has produced promising new interspecific and intraspecific hybrids.

Maturity and Quality

No reliable quantitative maturity indices for when to harvest *Annona* fruit have been developed. Individual trees are normally harvested up to 10 times, and fruits judged to be mature when the skin changes from a darker to a lighter green and becomes smoother. In some regions, fruits which develop during the colder winter months may fail to mature properly. Total soluble solids contents at full maturity can vary from 18% to 28%.

Physiological Disorders

Fruit Splitting

Fruit splitting may occur while fruits are still on the tree or after harvest. Splitting appears to be related to sudden changes in fruit moisture content or temperature. Some cultivars appear to be less susceptible than others.

Russetting

Superficial russetting of skin seems to be caused by low night temperatures (less than 13°C), accompanied by low humidity. Near-mature fruit appear to be particularly susceptible. Cherimoya cultivars are apparently less susceptible than atemoya cultivars.

Crocodile Skin

The extremely wavy and pointed carpels that are symptomatic of this disorder are particularly severe on highly vigorous trees, which may indicate some harmful effect of tree vigour on pollination processes. Based on fruit and leaf analyses, nutrition does not appear to be implicated.

Hard Seed Casing and Brown Lumps

Possible causes are boron deficiency or sudden changes in fruit water content.

Post-harvest Handling and Physiology

The skin of most *Annona* fruits, in particular those cultivars which produce fruit with protruding carpels, is easily damaged by rough handling. Fruits are usually size-graded by hand because of their irregular shape, and are packed into single-layer trays before shipment. The cherimoya and atemoya are classified as climacteric fruits which show two peaks in carbon dioxide production. The fruit softens, develops pleasant aroma and flavour and is considered ripe at the beginning of the second respiratory rise. Compared with other fruits the cherimoya and atemoya have high rates of ethylene production and respiration. With the exception of a few cultivars, post-harvest shelf life is short (between 7 and 10 days). *See* Ripening of Fruit

Storage

The optimum storage temperatures for atemoya and cherimoya fruit are between 13°C and 16°C. At these temperatures most atemoya and cherimoya cultivars can be stored for up to a maximum of 2 weeks with minimum loss of quality. One cultivar of cherimoya, Bronceada, has a reported cool storage life of 3 weeks. Storage at temperatures below 13°C for more than 1 week can cause severe chilling injury. Chilled fruit develops blackened skin, discoloration of the core, and watery patches in the fruit flesh; after removal from storage the fruit fails to ripen properly. However, fruit used for processing can be stored for 1 week at between 5°C and 10°C without loss of internal fruit quality. For short-distance transport precooling of fruit at 10°C for up to 18 h prior to shipment at ambient temperatures has been shown to be beneficial in extending shelf life by 3–4 days. Because of the presence of numerous stomata on the surface of the fruit, one of the main problems during storage is rapid water loss. Maintenance of relatively high humidity during storage should improve the appearance of fruit after the removal from storage. The main post-harvest disease is anthracnose, caused by a range of disease organisms (*Colletotrichum* spp., *Phomopsis* spp., *Rhizopus* spp.). Post-harvest fungicidal dips have successfully controlled fruit rots, provided that recommended dipping temperatures and concentrations are adhered to. Only limited studies have been conducted on controlled atmosphere storage of *Annona* species. Further studies are needed to evaluate the benefits of packaging fruit in polyethylene bags, which may help to prevent water loss and blackening of fruit during storage. *See* Controlled Atmosphere Storage, Applications for Bulk Storage of Foodstuffs; Fungicides; Storage Stability, Mechanisms of Degradation

Fresh Food Uses

The flesh of most *Annona* species is most commonly eaten out of hand. Because seeds of the fruit are

Table 2. Chemical and nutritional composition (per 100 g of ripe fruit) of the more important *Annona* spp. fruits

Parameter	Cherimoya	Atemoya	Sugar apple	Soursop
Water (g)	74·6–82·8	71·5–78·7	72·5–79·0	77·9–84·0
Fibre (g)	1·5–4·3	0·05–2·5	1·0–1·6	0·8–1·2
Starch (g)	NA	1·1	NA	NA
Sugar (g)	12·0–15·0	18·1	14·6	10·4–12·5
Ash (g)	0·6–1·0	0·4–0·75	0·4–1·4	0·6–0·9
Fat (g)	0·1–0·4	0·4–0·6	0·4–0·6	0·6–1·0
Protein (g)	1·0–2·4	1·1–1·4	1·3–2·4	0·7–1·7
Total acidity (citric acid equivalent)	0·17–0·50	0·2–0·6	NA	0·9–1·3
pH	3·9–4·8	4·4–5·1	3·9–4·8	3·6–4·8
Total energy (kJ)	NA	310–394	368–398	267–297
Ascorbic acid (mg)	4·3–16·8	50	10–51	13–32
Carotene (mg)	0·0–0·02	0·0–0·02	0·01	0·0–0·01
Thiamin (mg)	0·06–0·13	0·05	0·11–0·17	0·05–0·11
Riboflavin (mg)	0·11–0·15	0·07	0·08–0·16	0·03–0·05
Nicotinic acid (mg)	0·73–2·03	0·80	0·7–1·0	0·57–1·28
Calcium (mg)	8·0–32·0	17	19·4–44·7	8–26
Magnesium (mg)	27	32	NA	NA
Phosphorus (mg)	30·2–47·0	NA	23·6–55·3	27–29
Potassium (mg)	298–370	250	NA	179–265
Sodium (mg)	4–6	4·5	NA	9·0–14·0
Zinc (mg)	NA	0·2	NA	NA
Iron (mg)	0·8	0·3	0·28–0·36	0·5–0·8

NA, no data available.
Major sources: Morton (1987); Fruit and Vegetables (R.B. Duckworth); Tropical and Sub-tropical Fruits (S. Nagy and P.E.Shaw)

interspersed throughout the flesh, cultivars containing few seeds are the most desirable. Eating quality of atemoya and sugar apple fruit, which are particularly sweet, may be enhanced by adding a few drops of lime juice to the flesh. Soursops of least acid flavour and least fibre are the only ones suitable for eating fresh. The best eating quality is obtained from fruit that has been ripened at 17–20°C and then placed in the refrigerator to cool just before eating. In terms of appearance, colour, flavour and texture, the most acceptable pulp for both eating and processing is to be found 1 day after the first detectable softeniing. Softened fruit can be stored in the refrigerator (4°C) for about a week with a minimal loss in flavour, but some skin blackening will result. Segments of the pulp can be added to fruit salads, or used for making sherbets or ice cream.

Processed Products

Atemoya, cherimoya and soursop pulp has potential for mixing with dairy products such as ice cream and yoghurt, and sweetened soursop juice can be made into a canned beverage. Because of its higher acidity, soursop pulp is the most suitable of all the *Annona* species for processing. Cultivars with a low level of grit or fibre in

the flesh have been found to be more suitable for processing than others. Passing the flesh through fine screens (20 000–10 000 μm), and homogenization, as used for guava pulp, should eliminate this problem. The pulp can also be used to make semidried fruit 'leathers', and jams and jellies of fair flavour and quality. In Central America, sweet soursop pulp is sieved and squeezed, diluted with either milk or water, and sweetened, before canning to make a refreshing drink. When mixed with a little cream or ice cream the frozen soursop concentrate makes a delicious dessert.

Some species of *Annona* have been used in the production of soaps, domestic cooking oils, essential oils, herbal medicines, alcohol, fertility drugs, and insecticides. However, the commercial potential of these products at the present time appears limited.

Pulp Extraction

The production of pulp on a commercial scale does not appear to be easy because the skin of *Annona* fruits, at full ripeness, is soft and disintegrates easily if conventional processing techniques are used for skin removal. Other processed fruits, such as mango, passion fruit and guavas, have leathery skins which are brushed clean of pulp before being discarded. *Annona* fruit disintegrates and is brushed through the screens and mixed in with the pulp. The skins of most *Annona* fruits are high in polyphenols. This causes two problems when the skin is mixed with the flesh – a rapid browning of the pulp and a strong off-flavour. The Food Industry Development Centre of the University of New South Wales, Australia, has evaluated two methods for removing custard apple pulp – a screen pressing process and a reaming process. Although the reaming process offers yield advantages, it requires the use of skilled labour, and this would reduce its potential economic advantages. A prototype screen press extractor has been developed but this unit has yet to be tested commercially. *See* Phenolic Compounds

Pulp Storage

Heating or pasteurization impairs pulp flavour considerably, and often results in the development of a bitter character. However, unblanched frozen pulps treated with either ascorbic acid (1500–2000 mg per kg) or potassium metabisulphite (500 mg per kg) can be stored for up to 120 days with minimal loss of flavour. Upon thawing, pulp treated with ascorbic acid may develop a pinkish discoloration, whereas pulp treated with potassium metabisulphite retains a bright, fresh colour. *See* Ascorbic Acid, Properties and Determination

Nutritional Value

The fruit is rich in starch when firm but increases markedly in sugar as it softens. The main sugars are glucose and fructose (80–90%). There is some phenolic content associated with an increase in the activity of peroxidase, which causes oxidation of the pulp. The volatile fraction consists of alcohol, esters, carbonyls and hydrocarbons. The nutritional properties of the more important *Annona* species are presented in Table 2. Compared with other fruits, the *Annona* fruits contain significant quantities of vitamin C, thiamin, potassium, magnesium and dietary fibre content. The calorific value of the flesh is high (300 kJ per 100 g) and is almost double that of peach, orange and apple. *See* individual nutrients

Marketing Characteristics

Both the cherimoya and the atemoya are best eaten as fresh fruits. Both fruits are currently virtually unknown on world markets, and Chile is the only country which exports significant quantities. The major problem facing expansion of cherimoya and atemoya production throughout the world is the high perishability of the product. The transportation of atemoya and cherimoya to distant export markets, given current cultivars and post-harvest technology, is difficult. The processing potential of soursop and other *Annona* fruits is yet to be fully exploited. *See* Fruits of Tropical Climates, Commercial and Dietary Importance

Bibliography

Bueso CE (1980) Soursop, tamarind and chironja. In: Nagy S and Shaw PE (eds) *Tropical and Subtropical Fruits*, pp 357–407. AVI Westport, Connecticut: AVI Publishing.

Duckworth RB (1966) *The composition of fruits and vegetables*. Fruit and vegetables, Appendix A. London: Pergamon Press.

Edwards RA (1989) *The processing of custard apple and the development of pulp extraction equipment*. Report of the Food Industry Development Centre, University of New South Wales, Australia.

George AP and Nissen RJ (1985) The custard apple, Part 1. Species, variety and rootstock selection. *Australian Horticulture* 83 (10): 100–107.

George AP, Nissen RJ and Brown BI (1987) The custard apple. *Queensland Agricultural Journal* 113 (5): 287–296.

Morton JF (1987) *Fruits of Warm Climates*, pp 65–91. North Carolina: Media Incorporated, Greensboro.

Sanewski GM (1988) *Growing Custard Apple*, pp 86. Brisbane: Queensland Department of Primary Industries.

A. P. George and R. J. Nissen
Maroochy Horticultural Research Station, Nambour, Queensland, Australia

ANOREXIA NERVOSA

Definition

Anorexia nervosa (AN) is an eating disorder that is characterized by self-imposed starvation accompanied by an idealization of thinness and a morbid fear of becoming fat. The resultant emaciation leads to significant medical and psychiatric complications. Contrary to the literal meaning of its name, AN does not reflect a true loss of appetite except in the later stages of starvation; rather, it is a determined battle waged against sensations of hunger in order to achieve an illusory sense of control. Since its initial modern description by Sir William Gull in 1874, diagnostic criteria for AN have evolved to reflect the biological, behavioural, and psychological disturbances characteristic of the disorder. The formal criteria as defined by the American Psychiatric Association in 1987 are listed below:

1. Refusal to maintain bodyweight over a minimal normal weight for age and height, e.g. weight loss leading to maintenance of bodyweight 15% below that expected; or failure to make expected weight gain during period of growth, leading to bodyweight 15% below that expected.
2. Intense fear of gaining weight or becoming fat, even though underweight.
3. Disturbance in the way in which one's bodyweight, size, or shape is experienced, e.g. the person claims to 'feel fat' even when emaciated, believes that one area of the body is 'too fat' even when obviously underweight.
4. In females, absence of at least three consecutive menstrual cycles when otherwise expected to occur (primary or secondary amenorrhoea). (A woman is considered to have amenorrhoea if her periods occur only following hormone, e.g. oestrogen, administration.) *See* Menstrual Cycle and Premenstrual Syndrome – Nutritional Aspects

Prevalence

AN is, in about 90% of cases, a disorder of females, typically between the ages of 12 and 40. Studies of the age of onset of this disorder reveal bimodal peaks at 14 and 18 years of age; at these ages, the demands of secondary sexual development and autonomy in the context of leaving home may be related to the increased incidence. The current accepted prevalence rate for AN among Western adolescent and young adult women is approximately 1%. AN is, relatively speaking, a culture-bound disorder limited to industrialized societies with Western values. *See* Adolescents, Nutritional Requirements

Aetiology and Groups at Risk

The aetiology of this disorder is unknown; most clinicians and researchers endorse a multidimensional model of AN which acknowledges psychological, biological and social risk factors that exist at the level of the individual, the family and society. While dieting is an almost ubiquitous behaviour among women in Western society, the significant medical and psychiatric manifestations of AN and its characteristic psychological features argue for the definition of AN as a distinct disorder, and not a simple exaggeration of Western social values.

At the level of the individual, women who by career choice experience pressures to be thin, and to achieve, may be particularly vulnerable. This includes ballerinas, fashion models and gymnasts, in whom thinness and perfectionism are not only demanded but also equated. Conflicting pressures on women to nurture and to perform professionally may intensify concerns about control that are shifted onto weight regulation as a focus.

At the familial level, there may be a magnification of social idealization of thinness and denigration of obesity. Genetic influences through vulnerability to a variety of psychiatric disorders such as depression or alcoholism in other family members may also play a role. First-degree relatives also display a five-fold increase in the prevalence of eating disorders over control levels. Twin studies indicate a 56% concordance rate for AN in monozygotic (identical) twins versus 5–10% in dizygotic (nonidentical) twins.

At the level of society, the last 75 years have witnessed shifting models of the ideal female form toward thinness, in contrast to the increasing biologically ideal weights for women in the context of good nutrition. However, it must be remembered that the description of AN in 1874 long predates our cultural preoccupation with thinness and a broader understanding of the disorder must be sought.

Psychopathology

The focal point of AN is the individual's relentless pursuit of thinness and the associated conviction that her body is too large. This may emanate from a variety of sources, including a past history of obesity and the social humiliation and sense of failure associated with it. Alternatively, AN may reflect a symbolic focus in the search for personal mastery that in turn betrays a personal sense of ineffectiveness. It may also allow retreat from the maturational demands of adolescence, as expressed by the development of secondary sexual characteristics. Associated psychopathological features often include a fear of losing control in many spheres, self-esteem that is highly dependent on the opinions of others, an all-or-nothing thinking style that allows no middle ground between being thin and being fat, and a pervasive sense of helplessness.

Clinical Features

The initial manifestations of AN are deceptively benign; the disorder frequently commences with dieting behaviour. However, this particular form of dieting leads to increased criticism of one's appearance and greater social isolation than typical adolescent dieting behaviour; further, weight goals continue to drift downward as they are approached. Food aversion becomes more general than specific and, as emaciation progresses, the individual exhibits a marked denial of her thinness. A typical but not universal characteristic of AN is a distortion of body image in which the individual overestimates her body size substantially, believing herself to be fat even when thin. This perceptual disturbance is usually accompanied by feelings of loathing of one's appearance.

At the level of behaviour, routine dieting evolves into more elaborate food avoidance and other activities to counteract the effect of ingested calories. Individuals restrict their intake dramatically, skip meals, or secretly dispose of food. Elaborate rituals related to eating develop, and decreased consumption of food is paralleled by a heightened cognitive preoccupation with it. This translates into thinking, reading and dreaming about food, or working in food-related industries. Weighing oneself becomes not only a frequent ritual but also a regulator of subsequent eating, socialization and self-esteem. In addition to calorie restriction, individuals may exercise intensively for the express purpose of weight loss, or use purgative techniques such as diuretics, diet pills, laxatives, or self-induced vomiting.

Initially, because the consequences of the disorder are consistent with the individual's desire to be thin, there is seldom the motivation to seek help, or to acknowledge the evolving AN as a problem. Rather, the individual with AN may contact a nutritionist, physician or other health professional, seeking advice on dieting in the absence of obesity or help in dealing with the secondary medical and psychiatric effects of starvation.

Physiological Effects

Virtually no body system is spared the effects of nutritional deprivation in AN. The changes seen reflect not only loss but also homeostatic compensatory mechanisms to minimize energy expenditure in the context of decreased energy intake. Loss of menstrual function is the most classically recognized of these sequelae to the point that it is a diagnostic criterion thought to reflect disturbances in gonadotrophin function in the hypothalamus. Other common starvation effects include lowered body temperature and heart rate, dry skin and the development of a fine body hair, abdominal bloating and constipation, and oedema.

Psychological Effects

Starvation due to AN also produces distinct psychological effects such as depressed, irritable or anxious mood, cognitive preoccupation with food, and impairment of concentration. Individuals with AN may appear to suffer from a coexistent depressive illness and are vulnerable to the long-term development of such disorders. However, many of the psychological sequelae of the disorder – which are more troubling to the individual than the dieting itself – are reversible with adequate nutrition.

Nutritional Status

The food restriction of AN may be severe. Individuals may abstain from all solid foods for days at a time or subsist on as little as 200 to 500 calories per day. Typically, there is an avoidance of perceived high-calorie foods and foods become imbued with moral as well as nutritional value. Individuals may develop frank cachexia, with vigorous dieting and exercise behaviours persisting at weights as low as 30 kg. Fasting hypoglycaemia, abnormal glucose tolerance tests, and increased insulin sensitivity are among the metabolic responses to this form of starvation. Elevations of cholesterol and carotene may occur and plasma zinc levels have been variably reported as low. Low platelet, red blood cell and white blood cell counts, accompanied by a relative paucity of precursors in bone marrow, have been described as a consequence of the disorder. *See* Glucose, Glucose Tolerance and the Glycaemic Index; Hypoglycaemia for Nutrition

The nutritional status of AN patients may have implications for the chronicity of the disorder. Brain neurotransmitters such as serotonin and noradrenaline are integral in the hypothalamic regulation of appetitive behaviour. Serotonin synthesis is itself dependent on the dietary availability of its precursor, the essential amino acid tryptophan. Tryptophan availability may be decreased in AN, and both neuroendocrine provocation tests and cerebrospinal fluid metabolite assays indicate a decrease of serotonin activity in AN. This may be associated with disturbances in satiety, mood and sleep found in eating disorders. Delayed gastric emptying may occur in response to the decreased volume of food consumed. This further contributes to altered senses of satiety; an augmented sense of fullness may perpetuate food restriction.

Diagnosis

The diagnostic criteria of the American Psychiatric Association listed above reflect the confluence of biological, behavioural and psychological factors characteristic of AN. However, clinicians may perceive them as arbitrary, particularly with regard to the determination and degree of weight loss required. Epidemiological research demands strict criteria, while clinical practice requires recognition of disorders in evolution. The diagnosis of AN in a young woman with weight loss requires consideration of other psychiatric and medical illnesses with similar presentation. These include depression, schizophrenia and conversion disorder, as well as endocrine disorders, inflammatory bowel disease and malignancy. All of these differential diagnoses typically lack the central psychological preoccupation of AN – the relentless pursuit of thinness. The nonspecific sequelae of starvation and weight loss may be present in a variety of disorders other than AN.

Treatment

The goal of treatment of AN includes but is not limited to nutritional rehabilitation. Clearly, if weight gain is the only purpose of therapy for an individual dedicated to the attainment of weight loss, her commitment to treatment will be poor. At the same time, however, treating personnel cannot ignore the nutritional status of the individual while focusing on psychological issues; when this occurs, it results in collusion with the denial of the individual of her thinness and obscures the connection between food deprivation and psychological symptoms.

The initial phase of treatment is a careful diagnostic assessment, with emphasis on both the evolution of the disorder and its various sequelae. A family assessment is often relevant, particularly in younger patients, both to understand familial influences and to substitute education for guilt. A target weight range is established, allowing the minor fluctuations that are normal (1–2 kg). This range should be able to be maintained without dieting, should allow return of normal men-

strual function, and should reflect consideration of the individual's longitudinal weight history. Generally, a target weight range is above 90% of the average for the individual's weight and height or a body mass index (kg m^{-2}) greater than 20. Despite a seemingly encyclopaedic knowledge of nutrition, these individuals usually require directive counselling regarding meal frequency, portion size, and macronutrient selection. A daily diary of eating and associated thoughts, feelings and behaviours is helpful. An initial intake of 1500 calories per day is usually sufficient to promote weight gain without inducing the gastric dilatation that can complicate refeeding. A rate of weight gain of 0·5–1·0 kg per week is desirable; more rapid weight gain may induce its own complications, including hypophosphataemia and oedema, as well as mistrust in an individual reluctantly relinquishing weight control. Caloric intake is usually increased by 200 to 300 calories per week toward a goal of 2400 to 3000 calories per day. To date, controlled clinical trials indicate no role for drugs in the promotion of eating or weight gain in AN; food remains the drug of choice.

Psychotherapy is usually offered in conjunction with nutritional rehabilitation, and builds on the establishment of a trusting relationship. Issues include the recognition of feelings, self-trust, and disconnecting one's sense of self-worth from bodyweight. A variety of methodological approaches, from psychodynamic to cognitive-behavioural, may be employed. Family therapy may be particularly helpful with the younger AN patient.

Hospitalization is not necessary for the majority of individuals with AN; rather, it is reserved for cases where the weight loss has been either precipitously acute or impinging on basic function, where medical sequelae such as hypokalaemia pose an imminent risk, where suicidal tendency accompanies the AN, where AN coexists in a threatening fashion with another illness such as diabetes mellitus, or where other forms of treatment have been ineffective.

Prognosis

AN is usually a gradual, covert and sometimes chronic disorder. Long-term follow-up studies indicate that while two thirds of patients show eventual improvement or recovery, less than one third recover within three years. More disturbing, recent large-scale follow-up studies still indicate a mortality rate of 10–20% as a consequence of AN. In addition, these women are vulnerable over the long term to the development of mood and anxiety disorders, regardless of whether the AN is active or quiescent. They are also susceptible to such diverse medical conditions as osteoporosis with pathological bone fractures, and a form of atrophy of brain tissue. Beyond reversal of the nutritional deprivation and weight loss, there is no established method of tertiary prevention.

Bulimia

Up to 50% of individuals with AN will, in addition to calorie restriction, experience periods of binge eating. During these episodes, 3000 to 6000 calories may be consumed rapidly in a manner that is experienced as compulsive. This is usually followed by efforts to purge the ingested calories through a variety of techniques. When bulimia nervosa (BN) coexists with AN, it is often associated with impulsive behaviours, substance abuse and premorbid obesity. At other times, BN may emerge after resolution of an episode of AN; BN may also exist in the absence of a history of AN. *See* Bulimia Nervosa

Adolescents

Disordered eating behaviour is common among adolescents, whether it describes dieting, food cravings, or pleasurable eating binges; AN is relatively rare. Nevertheless, the adolescent period represents the peak incidence of AN, and health professionals need to be aware of the common clinical presentations of this potentially chronic and debilitating disorder.

Bibliography

American Psychiatric Association (1987) *Diagnostic and Statistical Manual of Mental Disorders*, 3rd edn. Washington, DC: American Psychiatric Association.
Brownell KD and Foreyt JP (eds) (1986) *Handbook of Eating Disorders*. New York: Basic Books.
Garfinkel PE and Garner DM (1982) *Anorexia Nervosa: A Multidimensional Perspective*. New York: Brunner/Mazel.
Garfinkel PE, Garner DM and Goldbloom DS (1987) Eating disorders: implications for the 1990s. *Canadian Journal of Psychiatry* 32: 624–631.

David S. Goldbloom and Paul E. Garfinkel
University of Toronto, Toronto, Canada

ANTHROPOMETRY

See Nutritional Status

ANTIBIOTICS AND DRUGS

Contents

Uses in Food Production

Veterinary medicines are used to improve or maintain the health of animal species regardless of whether these are intended for food production. They are designed and manufactured to cover a wide variety of prophylactic and therapeutic purposes and they are administered to household pets, exotic species and wild animals in addition to food-producing animals.

Most countries possess a governmental regulatory authority charged with assessing veterinary medicines and granting some form of marketing authorization before a product may be sold, and the UK's system is used here to exemplify this in practice. Veterinary medicines, like their human counterparts, are assessed against three basic criteria – efficacy, quality and safety – although the terms of these criteria differ from country to country. Efficacy is ability of the drug to accomplish the task claimed for it by its producer.

Quality refers to pharmaceutical quality; the levels of contaminants must meet acceptable criteria, the shelf life must be as claimed by the manufacturer, and the product must be produced to appropriate standards. Safety means that the product must not harm the animal patient, the environment, the users of veterinary medicines or the consumer of food of animal origin. This latter aspect is of paramount importance when assessing the safety of veterinary medicines. When a veterinary drug is given to an animal, most of the dose will be excreted in urine, faeces and expired air, but small amounts will remain in body tissues. These are known as residues and it is the responsibility of regulatory authorities to ensure that these do not pose a threat to the consumer when veterinary medicines are used in food-producing animals.

Uses of Veterinary Medicines

In general, veterinary medicines are available to treat most of the types of animal disease state which are encountered in humans. In practice, diseases such as cancer are not usually treated in food-producing species, largely for economic reasons, although they are frequently dealt with in companion animal medicine. The majority (but not by any means all) of the medicines used in food-producing animals are for the prevention or treatment of diseases caused by infectious agents. These fall into a number of categories and they are described briefly below.

Antibiotic and Antimicrobial Agents

Antibiotics are antibacterial agents derived from living organisms, but the term includes closely related synthetic analogues. The archetypal compound is penicillin, the structure of which has now formed the basis for a wide range of naturally occurring and semisynthetic analogues. Other major categories of antibiotics used in veterinary medicine are the tetracyclines, the aminoglycosides, the macrolides and the polymixins. Sulphonamides constitute the major class of antimicrobial agent, drugs which are unrelated to naturally occurring compounds. A number of sulphonamides have been prepared for fast, medium or long-acting functions. Sulphadimidine is one of the most widely used sulphonamide drugs in veterinary medicines, particularly in pig production where it is employed to combat respiratory disease.

Ectoparasiticides

Cattle and sheep are often subject to attack by ectoparasites. For example, in the UK and other parts of Europe

(and indeed elsewhere) cattle are susceptible to attack by the warble fly (*Hypoderma* spp.) which in addition to causing animal suffering results in considerable economic loss. Sheep scab is another disease which poses serious animal welfare and economic problems, and in several countries, including the USA and the UK, it is a notifiable disease. Both diseases are treated and prevented by the application of organophosphorus compounds. For warble fly, treatment is usually in the form of a relatively viscous formulation which is spread onto the back of the animal (a pour-on formulation); in the case of sheep scab, dipping and showering are the most therapeutically and economically effective methods currently available.

Fish too are susceptible to external parasites and as fish farming (aquaculture) becomes more important, so the effects of disease become more significant. Salmon farming is a fast-growing industry in many parts of the world, particularly in North America, Chile, Norway and Scotland. Salmon are vulnerable to infestation by the sea louse, an arthropod which attacks the external surface of the fish and in severe cases causes death. At the time of writing the only formulation authorized in the UK is a product containing the organophosphorus compound dichlorvos.

Anthelmintics

'Anthelmintics' is a term almost universally abused to describe agents used to treat internal parasite infestations and not merely those caused by helminth worms. Many of the diseases caused by internal parasites can be extremely distressing to affected animals and all can result in substantial economic losses. A number of drugs have been developed to combat these diseases, including the benzimidazoles, levamisole and ivermectin.

The first benzimidazole to achieve widespread use in veterinary medicine was thiabendazole, but newer compounds include albendazole, oxfendazole, fenbendazole and mebendazole. Levamisole is extremely efficacious in the treatment of gastrointestinal nematodes in cattle, sheep and pigs. Ivermectin is a mixture of two closely related compounds derived from abamectin, a metabolite of *Streptomyces avermitilis*, and it has found wide use as an antiparasitic agent in veterinary medicine (and in some areas of human medicine).

Antifungal Agents

In veterinary medicine, several drugs have found uses as antifungal agents for application to the external surfaces of the body. These include ketoconazole, thiabendazole, aliphatic acids and benzoic acid. Nystatin and griseofulvin are extensively used as systemic treatments for fungal infections in both food-producing and other species.

Steroid Hormones

It has long been known that testosterone exerts anabolic effects in both humans and animals, and testosterone and chemically related steroid hormones have been widely used for this purpose in beef production. However, the EEC has prohibited the growth-promoting uses of steroid hormones in animal production, although certain so-called zootechnical (e.g. synchronization of oestrous for mating) and therapeutic (e.g. treatment of recurrent abortion) uses are still permitted using naturally occurring compounds or closely related derivatives. In other countries, notably in the North and South Americas, the growth-promoting uses of steroid hormones are legally permitted.

Regulatory Control of Veterinary Medicines

Regulatory control of the uses of veterinary medicines is almost universal and, as described earlier, drugs must meet exacting standards of efficacy, quality and safety. In the UK, for example, human and veterinary medicines are controlled by the Medicines Act 1968 and by integrated EEC legislation. Product licences and other forms of marketing authorization are granted by a licensing authority established under the act. The Licensing Authority is defined in the act as the Health and Agriculture Ministers acting together and, in practice, responsibility is given over to civil servants working in the Department of Health for human medicines, and in the Veterinary Medicines Directorate (VMD) of the Ministry of Agriculture, Fisheries and Food (MAFF) for veterinary medicines. Applications for product licences are submitted to the VMD by companies together with the quality, efficacy and safety data. Staff of the VMD then vigorously assess these data and submit it with their appraisals to the independent Veterinary Products Committee appointed under the Medicines Act. This committee may then recommend licensing, require further information or refuse the application. When a product is not recommended for licensing, companies have recourse to an appeals procedure whereby they can submit their arguments. *See* European Economic Community, The Common Agricultural Policy; Legislation, Contaminants and Adulterants; Ministry of Agriculture, Fisheries and Food

Essentially similar systems exist in other countries including other member states of the EEC. For this latter group, national laws are amended from time to time to incorporate EEC legislation. Three European directives are worthy of note for the impact which these have had on national legislation within the EEC.

The two Veterinary Medicines Directives (81/851/ EEC and 81/852/EEC) provide a legislative framework for the European 'licensing' of conventional veterinary medicines. They establish an expert committee, the Committee for Veterinary Medicines Products, and offer a system of control, including a multistate authorization procedure within the EEC. Moreover, they provide comprehensive guidelines on safety, quality and efficacy. The so-called Feed Additives Directive (70/524/ EEC) covers both medicinal and nonmedicinal ingredients intended to be added to the animal feeds. Although conventional veterinary medicines and medicinal feed additives are therefore dealt with separately at community level, in the UK they are subject to the same treatment under the Medicines Act, once they have been accepted by the EEC.

On a worldwide basis, the marketing authorization of veterinary medicines and the steps preceding this can be summarized briefly as follows: development of a drug and its formulations; testing to fulfil the requirements of safety, quality and efficacy; submission of an application for marketing authorization with the data from safety, quality and efficacy tests to the appropriate national authorities; appraisal, assessment and consideration by those authorities; granting or refusal (or requirement for further studies) of marketing authorization.

Safety Data Requirements

Safety data with respect to consumer safety can be divided into two main categories: toxicity data and residues data. In recent years there has been an increasing demand for data on microbiological safety with respect to possible effects on the gastrointestinal flora of consumers.

Toxicology Studies

Toxicology data usually take the form of the results from a package of studies using laboratory species and *in vitro* tests. Pharmacokinetic and pharmacodynamic data are also used where relevant in the interpretation of the results of these endeavours. The precise requirements for toxicology testing differ from country to country but in general terms they are exemplified by those of the EEC, which include the following:

- Single-dose (acute) toxicity.
- Repeated-dose toxicity.
- Reproductive toxicity: effects on reproduction; effects on the embryo or fetus and teratogenicity (birth defects).
- Mutagenicity studies.
- Carcinogenicity (induction of tumours) studies.
- Pharmacodynamics.

- Pharmacokinetics.
- Observations in humans.

There are three basic aims in conducting toxicology studies: to identify a no-observed effect level (NOEL), to calculate an acceptable daily intake (ADI), and to determine a maximum residues limit (MRL).

The NOEL is the lowest dose level, usually quoted in mg per kg bodyweight, below which an effect or range of effects do not occur in the species being investigated (usually mice or rats). It is usually necessary to eliminate those effects thought to be irrelevant – usually because they are known to occur only in rodents or because they represent a phenomenon induced by excessive doses – and then select the study thought to be of most relevance, although in practice the lowest NOEL from the battery of tests is often used.

The ADI is calculated by dividing the NOEL by an arbitrary safety factor. This is usually 100 for minor toxic effects, but factors of up to 2000 may be used with severe effects or when the battery of tests is considered to be deficient in some relatively minor aspect; if deficient in some major area, e.g. if a carcinogenicity study has not been conducted, an ADI may not be set. The ADI is often expressed in terms of human weight by use of the additional factor of 65 kg, this being widely accepted as representing human adult weight. Hence, the ADI can be expressed (in mg per day) as follows:

$$ADI = (NOEL \times 65)/\text{safety factor}$$

The MRL is the maximum permitted level of the drug residue which regulatory authorities perceive as being acceptable in food of animal origin on the basis of the results of the safety studies described earlier. As such, it is often difficult to describe in purely arithmetical terms for although it is based primarily on the ADI, it must take into account other factors, not the least of which is the intake of the food commodity in question. Every consumer has a varied intake of most of the products of food of animal origin, such as muscle, fat, kidney and liver; some, for example, eat more liver or kidney than others. To try to cover the majority of possibilities, the FAO/WHO (Food and Agriculture Organization, World Health Organization) Joint Expert Committee on Food Additives (JECFA) has recommended standard daily intake values of 300 g of muscle, 100 g of liver, 50 g of fat, 50 g of kidney, 100 g of egg and 1·5 l of milk to be used in the elaboration of MRLs. The types of food-producing animals are shown in Fig. 1. In general terms, the ADI is 'spread' across the different types of food commodity, bearing in mind their relative standard intakes, so that MRLs, which will not result in the ADI being exceeded, can be elaborated.

When considering values for MRLs, a major factor which must be taken into account is the chemical nature of the residues and their resultant biological activity. This is an extremely complex area and one which is not

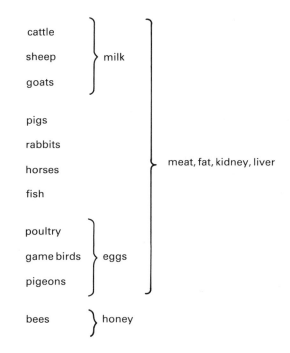

Fig. 1 Major food-producing species and their products important in considering maximum residues limits (MRLs) and residues studies.

devoid of controversy. Most chemicals, including veterinary medicines, when given to animals are converted to a range of metabolites, usually but not exclusively by the liver. Consequently, the residues present in tissue may be the parent compound or a mixture of metabolites or both. Moreover, either the parent drug or its metabolites may be highly reactive and may therefore combine with cellular constituents to give rise to so-called bound residues. In these circumstances it is desirable and sometimes essential to know to what extent these may be released to yield potentially harmful substances following consumption of products of animal origin. The most likely place for such a release to occur is in the gastrointestinal tract of the consumer and a number of animal as well as several chemical models have been developed in an attempt to provide information on this area of hazard assessment. One of these makes use of a technique known as relay toxicology, although in this context relay pharmacology might be more appropriate. The radiolabelled drug is administered to the food-producing animal which is later slaughtered, and its tissues, known to contain bound residues, are fed to laboratory animals such as rats. Detection of radioactivity in the plasma (for example) of these animals would indicate that the bound residues are bioavailable and, as a result of digestive processes, have been released for subsequent absorption. Chemical methods using solvent extraction and acid–base treatments investigate the ease with which bound residues can be released. These methods then determine whether or not the contribution from bound residues needs to be taken into account in the MRL setting procedure.

As indicated earlier, microbiological safety testing has been proposed for use in the hazard assessment process and indeed has been incorporated into some testing guidelines, including those of the EEC. The requirement for such testing is based on the premise that residues of some antibiotic and antimicrobial compounds may have the potential to affect adversely the gastrointestinal flora of the consumer, either by favouring the growth of resistant bacteria or by allowing the growth of organisms not normally found in any numbers in the gastrointestinal tract, by reducing the numbers of other organisms which normally suppress them. This is an extremely controversial area of safety assessments for two main reasons. First, despite the use of antibiotic and antimicrobial drugs in veterinary medicine for many years, there is no evidence to suggest that harmful effects have arisen in the human population as a result of biological changes in the gut flora. Second, the tests proposed to identify these effects have not been validated, so that even if the effects do exist, it is not known whether or not the proposed tests would actually detect them.

There are three tests currently available. Human volunteer studies involve the administration of the drug and subsequent examination of faeces and the oral cavity for changes in floral composition. The major alternative involves the use of germ-free rodents in which human gut flora have been seeded into the gastrointestinal tract. These are then given the drug under investigation and changes in the gut flora monitored. The third approach makes use of *in vitro* studies of the susceptibilities of various types of bacteria to antibacterial drugs, before and after exposure to low, sublethal levels of the drug. The numerical results in terms of dose can then be employed in the calculation of the ADI.

Residue Studies

Having determined an MRL value (or values) for a drug it is then essential to ensure that residues in the tissues or other products of food-producing animals do not exceed these. This is achieved by determining the withdrawal (or withholding) period for the drug in question. Small groups of animals are treated with the medicine, usually at the maximum dose recommended for its use in practice. The animals are then slaughtered in a serial manner after various intervals to determine when residue levels fall below the MRL. This time period for depletion of residues to below the MRL is then usually chosen as the withdrawal period; animals must be retained unmedicated during this time as the minimum interval between drug administration and slaughter.

Where appropriate, milk, eggs and honey must be discarded until this minimum time has elapsed.

Enforcement

There is little point in progressing through the various procedures detailed above if the withdrawal period is ignored and unacceptable levels of residues result. There is often pressure to ensure that animals are sent to slaughter at particular times, and this can lead to abuse.

To ensure that withdrawal periods are observed, most countries operate some form of residues surveillance scheme. In the UK, for example, over 40 000 samples are taken annually from slaughterhouses and these are tested for residues of various veterinary drugs in compliance with the requirements of the EEC Residues Directive (86/469/EEC). Other EEC member states carry out similar surveillance in order to comply with the requirements of this directive. The system allows enforcement officers to trace carcases back to farms to determine why the problem arose and where necessary to take legal proceedings against offenders.

The Codex Alimentarius Commission

The Codex Alimenatarius Commission is a joint WHO and FAO body and one of its objectives is to ensure that food of plant and animal origin worldwide is safe for human consumption. It has recently commenced work on establishing MRLs for veterinary drugs, having been involved for many years in setting these for pesticide residues. The Codex is advised on toxicological and residues issues by JECFA, the published scientific reports of which summarize the major conclusions and the proposed MRLs.

Given the international standing of the Codex system and of the JECFA, it seems likely that the MRL values which it promulgates will find their way eventually into various national regulations. In particular, it offers a basis for scientific assessment not currently available in some poorer and less developed nations.

Concluding Considerations

In most countries of the world, veterinary medicines are assessed for their ability to induce toxic effects and these effects and the doses which produce them are taken into account when calculating the ADI, which is in turn used to determine an MRL value or values. Residues studies are then used to determine when levels of the drug and its metabolites deplete to below the MRL in food-producing animals. Residues surveillance is essential to ensure that withdrawal periods are observed and, moreover, to ensure that the consumer is not exposed to unacceptable residue levels.

Bibliography

Anonymous (1987) *Anabolic, Anthelmintic and Antimicrobial Agents.* The 22nd report of the Steering Group on Food Surveillance. The Working Party on Veterinary Residues in Animal Products. London: Her Majesty's Stationery Office.

Booth NH and McDonald LE (eds) (1988) *Veterinary Pharmacology and Therapeutics* 6th edn. Iowa: Iowa State University Press.

Brander GC, Pugh DM, Bywater RJ and Jenkins WL (1991) *Veterinary Applied Pharmacology and Therapeutics* 5th edn. London: Ballière Tindall.

Commission of the European Communities (1989) *The Rules Governing Medicinal Products in the European Community*, vol. V. Luxembourg: Office for Official Publications of the European Communities.

European Federation of Animal Health (Seminar) (1989) Rationale view of antimicrobial residues. An assessment of human safety. *Advances in Veterinary Medicine, supplement to the Journal of Veterinary Medicine* No. 42.

International Programme on Chemical Safety (1987) *Principles for the Safety Assessment of Food Additives and Contaminants in Food.* Environmental Health Criteria 70. Geneva: World Health Organization.

Rico AG (ed.) (1986) *Drug Residues in Animals.* London: Academic Press.

Woodward KN (1991) The licensing of veterinary medicinal products in the United Kingdom – the work of the Veterinary Medicines Directorate. *Biologist* 38: 105–108.

Kevin N. Woodward
Veterinary Medicines Directorate, Weybridge, UK

Residue Determination

Veterinary drugs are widely used both to prevent and to treat disease in animals, poultry, fish and bees. They can also be employed to increase weight gain and improve the efficiency of conversion of feed into animal tissue. In most countries of the world the use of drugs for these purposes is regulated to protect human and animal health, and maximum residue limits (MRLs) in foods of animal origin have been established for this purpose, typically in the range 1–1000 μg kg^{-1}. In addition, certain drugs may be banned. Thus, there is a need for methods of analysis to be used in monitoring residue levels, for application to surveillance of national food supplies and enforcement of regulations and quality control in food manufacture. This includes ensuring compliance with MRLs and also testing for the absence of antibiotics from raw materials intended for fermentation. This article will describe the principles and practice of veterinary drug residue analysis, which is a particularly exacting area of trace analysis due to the complexities imposed by drug metabolism and tissue matrices. *See* Legislation, Contaminants and Adulterants

Method Characteristics

Methods may be categorized as intended for screening, confirmation or reference. Screening tests should be rapid, of low unit cost and give rise to a minimum of false negative results; some level of false positives may be tolerated. Confirmatory methods provide unambiguous proof of identity of a residue in samples giving rise to a positive result in a screening assay, while reference methods must in addition be fully validated by collaborative exercise. They are employed in case of dispute and may be based upon instrumentation of skills which are not widely available.

Each of the various analytical objectives places differing requirements on method performance. Farm and abattoir screening methods must be fast, simple to carry out and robust. A manufacturer may wish to screen a large number of samples either for a specific drug or for the presence of a range of drugs. In both cases, important criteria will be sample throughput, cost per test and the incidence of false positive and negative results. The result could be a simple pass or fail at a level based upon the MRL and the performance characteristics of the testing method. Significant screening applications include testing liquid milk for antibiotic residues and monitoring compliance with sulphonamide MRLs in pig meat.

For regulatory purposes, it is necessary to establish conclusively the presence of violative residue concentrations, and sample throughput and assay cost become less significant. Most available confirmation and reference methods focus on individual drugs or at best on single families of drugs. Some multiresidue methods are available, but none of these are fully satisfactory in all aspects of the range of drugs detected, sensitivity, incidence of false positives or negatives, sample throughput and unit cost.

Most current methods are based on chromatographic, immunoassay or microbiological principles. These are compared in Table 1 and described individually below. Selection of a particular technique will depend upon the reasons for the analysis, the apparatus and skills available, and an appreciation of the constraints inherent in the individual methodologies. For example, immunoassay methods can in certain circumstances achieve a sensitivity that cannot be matched chromatographically, but antibodies may not be readily available. Microbiological methods may detect antibiotics for which no chromatographic method exists, while the latter are the only viable choice for confirmation, particularly in combination with mass spectrometry.

Table 1. A comparison of microbiological, chromatographic and immunoassay approaches for veterinary drug residue analysis in animal tissue

Method	Sensitivity	Specificity	Confirmation	Sample throughput		Clean-up	Availability
				Single	Batch		
Microbiological	1–4	1–2	1	1–2	4	3–4	3
Chromatographic	2–4	3	4	2	2	1	3–4
Immunoassay	3–4	3	2	2–3	2–4	1–3	1–2

Scale: 1, poor; 2, moderate; 3, good; 4, excellent.

Drug Standards and Reference Materials

Some drugs are readily available from laboratory chemical suppliers. Unfortunately, a considerable number can be obtained only by direct approach to the manufacturers, whose names and addresses can be found in compilations of product information. Quality assurance programmes benefit considerably from the use of standard reference materials and, in particular, tissue samples containing known levels of naturally incurred residues. None are currently available but the Reference Materials Bureau of the EEC has a programme to develop them.

Metabolism, Analyte Selection and Stability of Residues

Drugs are frequently extensively metabolized in the live animal. Pathways of importance to the residue analyst include oxidation and esterification (conjugation) to sulphates or glucuronides. Oxidation of benzimidazole anthelmintics containing a sulphide linkage gives rise to a residue containing a mixture of the parent compound, its sulphoxide and sulphone. Each of these compounds may be determined separately, or alternatively it is possible to oxidize the whole residue to the sulphone. The MRL is stated as the total of all three products. The formation of ester conjugates is of particular importance in hormone analysis. Anticipated hormone residue levels lie in the 0–10 $\mu g \, kg^{-1}$ range for the target tissue, liver, but this is distributed between a number of different conjugates. In order to facilitate the analysis all conjugates are hydrolysed, usually prior to extraction, and the total parent hormone determined. Conjugation is not extensive in muscle but hormone concentrations in this matrix are only 20% or less of those found in liver.

Drug metabolism may proceed to give protein-bound residues which are not extractable using normal approaches. These products are often considered to be of no significance toxicologically, but further work is required to establish this conclusively. It has been shown for example that part of the nitrofuran compound furazolidone becomes protein bound in a form which could possibly be cleaved during the digestive process.

Metabolic pathways and rates of elimination of residues from live animals vary considerably between drugs. For some compounds, such as carbadox, complete biotransformation of the drug occurs and it is necessary to test for the presence of a metabolite, quinoxaline carboxylic acid. The stability of residues in tissue samples is similarly variable. Some, such as tetracyclines and aminoglycosides, remain unchanged for periods of many months when held at $-20°C$. Others, including the nitrofurans, continue rapid metabolic transformation in frozen meat and all trace of the parent drug may be lost after only a few days. It may be possible to stabilize residues if the tissue is homogenized and enzyme activity inhibited by adjustment of pH or other treatment. Some metabolites revert to the parent drug on cooking or other processing.

Sampling

Residue concentrations in a carcass vary from tissue to tissue, and if possible the target tissue should be taken for analysis. This is frequently liver or kidney, where drug levels may be 3–10-fold greater than in muscle from the same animal. Individual animals of the same species and breed vary substantially in their metabolic rates, because of differences in enzyme expression. Based on limited evidence, the distribution of residue concentrations within a single organ from one animal is relatively uniform. However, in some circumstances 2–3-fold variations may be expected. For example, certain drugs are retained differently in the medulla and cortex of the kidney, while fat marbling may influence the uniformity of lipophilic drug residues.

Sample Preparation

Some microbiological and immunoassay methods may be applied directly to a core of tissue or to tissue exudate, but sample preparation is usually required. The approach depends upon the analytical method selected.

Initial extraction from the matrix is carried out with an appropriate organic solvent or buffer. This is a critical step and conditions must be selected with care to ensure a high and reproducible extraction of residues. Some drugs, including clenbuterol, are associated with matrix proteins in an undefined but probably noncovalent manner. In these cases it is necessary to break the protein binding, usually by digesting the sample with a proteolytic enzyme such as subtilisin, before extraction.

Subsequently, a sequence of chromatographic steps, often including liquid–liquid partition and solid phase extraction (SPE) may be used to isolate drug residues from coextractives and concentrate them. This phase of the analysis is generally carried out manually, and places heavy demands upon staff resources. There has therefore been considerable interest in automation, either by roboticization of existing manual methods or employing alternative approaches which typically integrate sample preparation in a continuous-flow system with the analytical step. A number of systems have been developed but none as yet has found widespread application. Automated dialysis of simple buffer extracts has been used successfully to eliminate proteinaceous interferences before valve-switching transfer of the dialysate to high-performance liquid chromatography (HPLC) for final separation and measurement. This is particularly successful for analytes capable of selective detection, such as fluorimetric determination of oxolinic acid in fish muscle. Supercritical fluid extraction is of interest but has not yet been adequately developed. A technique termed 'matrix solid phase dispersion' (MSPD), which involves grinding the tissue with reversed-phase silica materials and using the product analogously to an SPE cartridge has been found effective for spiked samples containing a range of drugs at levels of 50 μg kg^{-1} or higher but has not yet been fully validated.

Immunoaffinity chromatography has been employed very effectively for determination of hormone and β-agonist residues, principally in biological fluids but also in tissue. Antibody raised against the drug is bound to a gel and used as an SPE-type cartridge. Complete selectivity is not obtained because of nonspecific interactions with the gel matrix but a high degree of purification may be achieved. Gels may be used in-line with automated HPLC systems. Some capacity is lost during repeated use, but columns typically last for 10–100 cycles. The major drawback to wider application is a lack of sufficient quantities of the necessary antibodies. Some columns are available commercially.

Analytical Methods

Microbiological

Antibiotics may be detected by tests based upon their inhibition of bacterial growth. Such tests are widely used to monitor for the presence of benzylpenicillin in liquid milk and a number of systems are commercially available. Microbial inhibition methods are less easy to carry out on tissue samples and even under optimum conditions a 1–2% incidence of false positives may be expected. In addition, there is wide variation in the sensitivity for different antibiotic families and little indication of the individual antibiotic responsible for a positive result while potentially but microbiologically inactive metabolites will not be detected. The four-plate test (FPT) employs four agar plates seeded with different bacteria. Each plate represents a different combination of organism and incubation conditions selected to be sensitive to as wide a range of antimicrobials as possible. Cores of tissue are placed on or inserted into the agar and the plate is incubated, usually overnight. If the tissue contained antibiotic residues, these will diffuse out into the agar and produce a ring of inhibition of bacterial growth around the core. The test is positive if the zone of inhibition exceeds a certain diameter. Problems arise as the FPT cannot be made sufficiently sensitive to some compounds, including chloramphenicol and the sulphonamides, and because lysozyme and other tissue components can give rise to false positives. A piece of dialysis membrane may be placed between the tissue and the agar to avoid interference from lysozyme.

Chromatography

Chromatography is widely employed. The equipment is readily available and method development is relatively quick. The other outstanding advantage is the range of confirmation procedures available, including mass spectrometry. However, a combination of chromatographic processes is required to achieve adequate selectivity and overall sample throughput is low. Many drugs are polar molecules and HPLC is the preferred separation mode. Detection is typically by ultraviolet absorption, but to enhance selectivity fluorescence and electrochemical approaches should be selected where possible. Hormones and β agonists are amenable to gas chromatography (GC) and are often determined by selected ion monitoring gas chromatography/mass spectroscopy (GCMS) of silyl or perfluoroacyl derivatives. *See* Chromatography, High-performance Liquid Chromatography; Chromatography, Gas Chromatography; Mass Spectrometry, Principles and Instrumentation

Electrophoresis

Many drugs are charged at physiological pH and are therefore candidates for electrophoresis. Gel electrophoresis has been used to help identify individual antibiotics occurring in samples found positive by the microbiological FPT but is not always effective. Capillary electrophoresis is a very high-efficiency technique and would be of considerable interest if the loadability problem (most sample extracts contain substantial amounts of material in addition to the drug residue) could be resolved. *See* Electrophoresis

Immunoassay

Immunoassays have been used for residues of many drugs, but frequently the antibodies are not readily acceptable, while the very specificity of antigen–antibody interactions hinders application to multiresidue analysis. Cross-reactivity of antibodies with metabolites may be desirable or not. It is possible for a metabolite to give a signal much greater than that arising from the parent compound, potentially creating false positives. In addition, MRLs for many compounds are set in terms of the parent drug, excluding metabolites. For compounds with MRLs of perhaps 10 μg kg^{-1} or more, there is considerable potential for rapid enzyme immunoassay methods in a number of formats, and some of these are commercially available. There is no real alternative to immunoassay for determination of polypeptide residues such as bovine somatotrophin.

The perceived advantages of immunoassay include rapid analysis of ultra-low concentrations of analytes, such as hormone residues, but problems are often experienced with interference from coextractives. It has therefore often been necessary to employ extensive clean-up and the benefits of high sample throughput have largely been lost. HPLC is often employed to isolate individual hormones from sample extracts prior to immunoassay determination. *See* Immunoassays, Principles; Immunoassays, Radioimmunoassay and Enzyme Immunoassay

Other Assay Types

Receptor Assays

Preparations of bacterial cells containing receptors for different groups of antibiotics may be used in a competitive binding assay similar in principle to radioimmunoassay. One kit is available commercially for screening seven drug classes in liquid milk. A similar approach has been described for hormone analysis, utilising uterine hormone receptors.

Enzyme-based Assays

Another commercial screening method for β-lactams in liquid milk is based on an enzyme/substrate reaction which is inhibited in the presence of drug residues. There seems little scope for extending this to tissue matrices because of the high probability of interferences in the absence of extensive clean-up.

Method Validation and Quality Assurance

Any proposed method should be subject to validation before use to establish overall analyte recovery and its associated standard deviation, the limit of determination, sample throughput and method robustness. Quality assurance of analytical results implies careful continual monitoring of method performance by processing spiked blanks or reference materials in parallel with samples. It is important to allow spiked tissue to equilibrate with the added drug for an adequate period (at least 1 h) before extraction, although conditions must be chosen to avoid continued metabolism.

Bibliography

Bogaerts R and Wolf F (1980) A standardised method for the detection of residues of anti-bacterial substances in fresh meat. *Fleischwirtschaft* 60: 672–674.

Budavari S (ed.) (1989) *The Merck Index*, 11th edn. Rahway: Merck.

Crosby NT (1991) *Determination of Veterinary Residues in Food*. Chichester: Ellis Horwood.

Debuf YM (ed.) (1991) *The Veterinary Formulary*, 1st edn. London: The Pharmaceutical Press.

Morris BA, Clifford MN and Jackman R (eds) (1988) *Immunoassays for Veterinary and Food Analysis*. London: Elsevier.

Senyk GF, Davidson JH, Brown JM, Hallstead ER and Sherbon JW (1990) Comparison of rapid tests used to detect antibiotic residues in milk. *Journal of Food Protection* 53: 158–164.

Shepherd MJ (1991) Analysis of veterinary drug residues in edible animal products. In: Creaser CS and Purchase R (eds) *Food Contaminants: Sources and Surveillance*, pp 109–176. Cambridge: Royal Society of Chemistry.

Martin J. Shepherd,
MAFF Food Science Laboratory, Norwich, UK

ANTIOXIDANTS

Contents

Natural Antioxidants

The spontaneous reaction of atmospheric oxygen with lipids leads to complex chemical changes that eventually manifest themselves in the development of off-flavours in food. This process is known as autoxidation, and one of the characteristics is the occurrence of an induction period (Fig. 1), during which there is no detectable off-flavour development. Autoxidation is a free-radical process, and – in common with all free-radical reactions – the length of the induction period is sensitive to the presence of minor components which either extend the induction period and are known as antioxidants or shorten the induction period and are known as pro-oxidants. Although synthetic antioxidants are commonly added to foods, recent research has concentrated on the use of natural sources of antioxidants. *See* Fatty Acids, Properties; Oxidation of Food Components

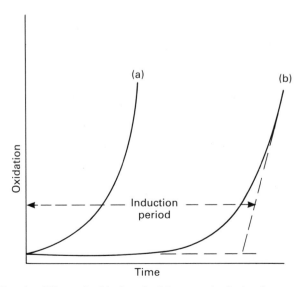

Fig. 1 Effect of added antioxidant on the induction period of fat: (a) no antioxidant; (b) with added antioxidant.

Oxidation (y-axis)
Induction period
Time (x-axis)

Classification of Antioxidants

In 1968 Ingold classified all antioxidants into two groups, namely primary or chain-breaking antioxidants, which react with lipid radicals to convert them into more stable products, and secondary or preventive antioxidants, which retard autoxidation by other mechanisms.

Primary antioxidants are usually compounds that donate a hydrogen atom to lipid free radicals to produce a relatively stable radical which is poor at propagating the chain reaction and hence interrupts the autoxidation process. Antioxidants of this type are mainly phenolic in structure and include tocopherols, gallic acid and derivatives, flavonoids – including quercetin, rhamnetin, kampferol, rutin and quercitrin, caffeic acid, carnosine, rosmaric acid and carnosic acid – and many other natural components. Primary antioxidants are consumed during the induction period, during which there is little change in the oxidative state of the fat. However, after the end of the induction period, the fat begins to deteriorate rapidly, liberating volatiles and generating hydroperoxides. Polymers may also be formed if the radical concentration becomes high, especially at elevated temperatures such as those that occur during deep-fat frying. *See* Colours, Properties and Determination of Natural Pigments

Secondary antioxidants are components that have no antioxidant action in pure fats but are effective in the presence of other minor components, either by improving the effectiveness of primary antioxidants or by inhibiting the effect of pro-oxidants. Natural antioxidants of this type include phospholipids which have a synergistic action with primary antioxidants such as tocopherols, and citric acid which chelates pro-oxidant metal ions and thereby has a dramatic effect on oil stability. *See* Phospholipids, Properties and Occurrence

Sources of Natural Antioxidants

A wide range of natural sources have been shown to contain antioxidants. These include plant extracts, herbs and spices and fermentation products (Table 1). In addition, naturally occurring chemical classes with antioxidant activity have been identified and some antioxidants have been found to be formed during the heat-processing of foods. These include Maillard reaction products formed by reaction of amino acids, peptides and proteins with carbohydrates.

Addition of Natural Antioxidants to Foods

The addition of antioxidants to foods in the UK is controlled by the Antioxidant in Food Regulations 1978, and similar regulations are in force in other countries. Tocopherols and L-ascorbic acid or its salts are listed as allowed additives. However, other natural antioxidants may be added as processing aids or as flavourings (e.g. rosemary extracts or citric acid). *See* Flavour Compounds, Structures and Characteristics

Most processed foods which require antioxidants have synthetic antioxidants added. Tocopherols may be added to animal fats and are naturally present in foods containing vegetable oils. Ascorbic acid or its sodium or calcium salts have been used to retard oxidation in a range of foods, including wines, beer, fruit, vegetables, butter, cured meat and fish products. Since ascorbic acid is very insoluble in oil, it is only used in aqueous systems or in emulsions. Ascorbyl palmitate is commonly used to stabilize edible oils because of its higher solubility (0·03% in oils at room temperature). It has been shown to be effective in stabilizing oils during deep-fat frying. *See* Vegetable Oils, Applications

Tocopherols

Mixtures of tocopherols occur with phospholipids in all plant and animal membranes. They are natural components of all isolated vegetable oils but do not occur at significant levels in animal fats. Addition of tocopherols to animal fats is a very effective method of increasing the stability of the fat. Addition of tocopherols to vegetable oils is often ineffective at increasing the oxidative stability of the oil, as the natural level of tocopherols in vegetable oils generally appears to be close to the optimum level required for oil stability. Addition of tocopherols above this optimum level often causes a reduction in oxidative stability. Thus addition of 1000 ppm DL-α-tocopherol to grape seed oil can reduce the Rancimat induction period at 100°C from 5 to 2 h. *See* Tocopherols, Properties and Determination

Natural tocopherols in vegetable oils are mixtures of α-, β-, γ- and δ-tocopherols, and the corresponding tocotrienols, although synthetic D-α-tocopherol is commonly used to stabilize animal fats. The antioxidant activity and stability of the tocopherols varies with their

Table 1. Plant extracts with antioxidant properties

Class	Material	Some active constituents
Herbs and spices	Rosemary	Carnosic acid, rosmarinic acid, carnosol, diterpenes, rosmaridiphenol, rosmariquinone
	Sage	
	Coriander	
	Clove	Gallic acid, eugenol
	Black pepper	
	Turmeric	Curcumin (and derivatives)
	Paprika	
	Betel	
	Oregano	
	Mace	
	Thyme	
	Basil	
	Nutmeg	
Fermented foods	Tempeh	Isoflavones
	Miso	
Oil seed	Soya meal	Saponins
	Cocoa bean husk	Catechin, chlorogenic acid
	Sesame seed	Sesamol, sesamolinol, sesaminol, etc.
	Defatted cottonseed flour	Flavonoids
	Sunflower seed protein isolate	
	Defatted cocoa solids	Epicatechin
	Peanuts	Flavonoids
Vegetables	Onion	
	Carrots	Lignin, β-carotene
	Tomato seed	
	Garlic	
Cereals	Oats	
	Rice	Orizanol
	Wheat gliadin	
Other plant materials	Green tea	Flavonoids
	Grape seed	
	Wood	
	Chia seed	
	Olive leaf	
	Horse radish	
	Mustard powder	
	Apple cuticle	
	Korum rind	
	Licorice	Flavonoids
	Birch bark	
	Carob pod	

structure. *In vivo*, the vitamin E activity of the tocopherols decreases in the order $\alpha > \beta > \gamma > \delta$, but in oil stabilization studies, δ-tocopherol has often been quoted as the most effective antioxidant.

One such study showed that α-tocopherol was consumed first, with β- and γ-tocopherols being consumed next and δ-tocopherol last during the induction period of soyabean oil tested under accelerated oxidation conditions. It therefore appears that the difference between α- and δ-tocopherol lies in the fact that the δ-tocopherol is consumed more slowly and is therefore active for a longer period of time, whereas α-tocopherol may be more active initially but is consumed more rapidly.

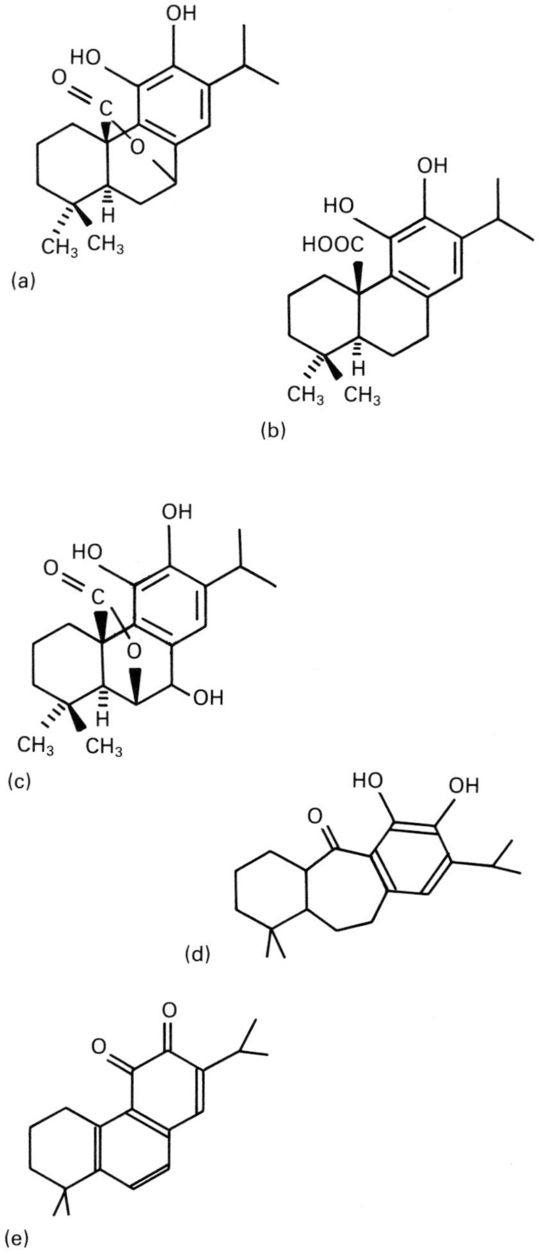

Ascorbic Acid

Ascorbic acid occurs in all tissues of living organisms and plays an essential role in normal metabolic processes. It is synthesized on a large scale for use as a food additive. Ascorbic acid acts as an antioxidant in several ways. First, in systems where oxygen is present in limited amounts, it acts as an antioxidant by removing oxygen as it is oxidized to dehydroascorbic acid. Ascorbic acid quenches various activated oxygen species (singlet oxygen, hydroxyl radicals, superoxide), and it also reduces free radicals and thereby inhibits the propagation of the autoxidation chain reaction. Ascorbic acid also reduces primary antioxidant radicals, and therefore shows synergistic effects with primary antioxidants, such as α-tocopherol. Ascorbic acid is commonly lost by oxidation by molecular oxygen in the presence of metal ions, and its antioxidant properties are therefore enhanced by chelating agents such as citric acid. *See* Ascorbic Acid, Properties and Determination

Herbs and Spices

The antioxidant activity of herbs and spices has been demonstrated in many studies over the last 50 years. Mace, black pepper, thyme, oregano, red pepper, basil, paprika and nutmeg are amongst the many plants in this group with antioxidant components, but sage and rosemary extracts have been found to be the most effective. The light petroleum extracts of rosemary and sage have been shown to be as effective as butylated hydroxyanisole. The antioxidant components can be extracted from rosemary by steam distillation to remove the essential oil, followed by ethanol extraction of the stripped leaves. The crude extract can then be purified by molecular distillation. Carnosol has been shown to be the most effective antioxidant in the rosemary extract, but other effective antioxidant components include carnosic acid, rosmanol, rosmaridiphenol and

Fig. 2 Some antioxidants occurring in rosemary: (a) carnosol; (b) carnosic acid; (c) rosmanol; (d) rosmaridiphenol; (e) rosmariquinone.

rosmariquinone (Fig. 2). *See* Herbs, Herbs and their Uses

Antioxidants with Other Functions

Tocopherols are the most common example of an antioxidant with vitamin activity. Indeed the antioxidant activity of tocopherols is believed to be the main source of their vitamin activity. The US National Academy of Sciences has recommended a daily allow-

Table 2. Effects of processing on the tocopherol content of soya bean oil

Processing step	Total tocopherols	Percentage loss
Crude	1132	—
Degummed	1116	1·4
Refined	997	11·9
Bleached	863	23·8
Deodorized	726	35·9

Data from Gutfinger T and Letan A (1974) Qualitative changes in some unsaponifiable components of soybean oil due to refining. *Journal of the Science of Food and Agriculture* 25: 1143–1147.

ance of 10 mg of RRR-α-tocopherol per day, although the vitamin E requirement is also dependent on other factors, such as the polyunsaturated fatty acid content of the diet. Clear deficiency of vitamin E is rare, although it may occur in the rare genetic disorder, abetalipoproteinaemia, or in other fat-malabsorptive conditions. *See* Tocopherols, Physiology

Vitamin C is also an essential nutrient. It has many specific physiological functions which are not dependent on its antioxidant properties. However, it has been suggested that vitamin C increases the effectiveness of α-tocopherol as an antioxidant in membranes by regenerating the α-tocopherol as it becomes oxidized. *See* Ascorbic Acid, Physiology

β-Carotene is a major pigment in fruits and vegetables. It contributes an orange colour to fruit, including apricots, palm fruit and peaches, or vegetables, including carrots. It is also present in green leaves, where its colour is masked by that of chlorophyll. β-Carotene is mainly active as a quencher of singlet oxygen which adds much more readily to unsaturated fatty acids than triplet oxygen which is the normal ground state of the molecule. However, it has also been shown that β-carotene acts as an antioxidant at low partial pressures of oxygen by adding to a lipid radical to form a more stable radical. *See* Carotenoids, Properties and Determination; Retinol, Properties and Determination

Effects of Processing on Natural Antioxidants

Losses of tocopherols from vegetable oils are normally quite small during the standard processing operations of degumming, neutralization, bleaching and deodorization (Table 2). Losses may increase dramatically during the deodorization stage if a good vacuum is not maintained, or if very high temperatures are used, as in physical refining of oils.

A rosemary extract has also been found to be adequately stable towards deodorization at 220°C, retaining its activity after this process.

Common antioxidants such as tocopherols are consumed relatively rapidly by oxidation and polymerization in frying oils at elevated temperatures. Citric acid is also thermally degraded, and it is necessary to add citric acid after the deodorization step when refining an edible oil in order for it to be active in the refined product.

Determination of Antioxidant Activity

In order to determine the activity of an antioxidant, it is necessary to determine the induction period of a fat with and without the antioxidant. Antioxidants are only effective if present in the fat before the end of the induction period, and the induction period ends when the antioxidant is consumed. The induction period may be determined by storing the sample in an oven and determining the oxidative state periodically by an accepted method such as peroxide value, sensory evaluation or the thiobarbituric acid (TBA) test. The Schaal oven test is a test in which this principle is employed.

The active oxygen method (AOM), or Swift test, and the Rancimat test are tests in which the oxidative deterioration of a fat is accelerated not only by the use of an elevated temperature (usually 100°C), but also by bubbling air through the sample. These tests are very useful in determining antioxidant activity because the stability of oil-containing antioxidants can be very high even at 100°C, and the practice of bubbling air through the sample shortens the induction period by a large amount. However, the activity of volatile antioxidants such as BHA (butylated hydroxyanisole) is underestimated by these tests because the antioxidant is lost from the sample by evaporation under these conditions. The AOM method has been standardized in the Official and Tentative Methods of the American Oil Chemists' Society, Method Cd 12–57. The AOM method requires determination of the peroxide value periodically but the Rancimat method is an automated method which relies on continuous monitoring of the electrical conductivity of the aqueous effluent to determine the induction period.

Analysis and Characterization of Natural Antioxidants

Tocopherol analysis has been simplified considerably by the use of high-performance liquid chromatography (HPLC). Normal-phase HPLC using a 25-cm column packed with 5-μm silica gel is commonly employed. A mobile phase comprising 1·5% 2-propanol in hexane is suitable, and fluorescence detection with excitation at 290 nm and emission at 330 nm provides a sensitive method of detection. *See* Chromatography, High-performance Liquid Chromatography

The method commonly used before HPLC for the analysis of tocopherols involved saponification of the oil prior to separation of tocopherols by TLC and a colorimetric determination using bathophenanthroline. However, considerable losses of tocopherols may occur during the saponification step if normal saponification procedures are used. *See* Chromatography, Thin-layer Chromatography; Spectroscopy, Visible Spectroscopy and Colorimetry

Numerous methods have been used to analyse the ascorbic acid content of foods. A common method involves a titration with 2,6-dichlorophenol-indophenol, but ultraviolet (UV) spectrophotometric, fluorometric, polarographic and colorimetric methods have also been used. In recent years, HPLC methods have been developed. Anion exchange or reversed-phase methods have been widely used. Ascorbyl palmitate has also been analysed by a variety of procedures, including gel permeation, thin-layer chromatography and HPLC.

In addition, HPLC is normally the preferred technique for analysing other natural antioxidants. Thus the polyphenols in olive oil have been analysed by HPLC mainly in order to identify components contributing to the oil flavour, but it is clear from the structures that many of these components also act as antioxidants in the oil.

Similarly, HPLC has been employed in the analysis of flavonoids in liquorice extracts which have been shown to have antioxidant activity.

Bibliography

Aruoma OI and Halliwell B (ed.) (1991) *Free Radicals and Food Additives*. London: Taylor and Francis.
Ball GFM (1988) Fat-soluble vitamin assays in food analysis. Essex: Elsevier Science Publishers.
Diplock AT (ed.) (1985) *Fat-Soluble Vitamins*. London: Heinemann.
Hamilton RJ and Rossell JB (1986) *Analysis of Oils and Fats*. Essex: Elsevier Science Publishers.
Hudson BJF (ed.) (1990) *Food Antioxidants*. Essex: Elsevier Science Publishers.
Ingold KV (1968) Inhibition of autoxidation. *Advances in Chemistry Series* 75: 296–305.
Kochhar SP and Rossell JB (1990) Detection, estimation and evaluation of antioxidants in food systems. In: Hudson BJF (ed.) *Food Antioxidants*, p 46. Essex: Elsevier Science Publishers.
Loliger J (1989) Natural antioxidants. In: Allen JC and Hamilton RJ (eds) *Rancidity in Foods*, 2nd edn. Essex: Elsevier Science Publishers.

M. H. Gordon
University of Reading, Reading, UK

Synthetic Antioxidants

When exposed to the air, fats, oils and fatty foods undergo auto-oxidation, which results in changes in flavour, degradation in quality and, under some conditions, formation of toxic compounds. The auto-oxidation reaction of a fat is thought to proceed as indicated in eqns [1]–[8], due to free radical chain reactions. When in contact with oxygen, an unsaturated fatty acid gives rise to free radicals (eqn [1]). Also, hydroperoxide, which exists in trace quantities prior to the oxidation reaction, breaks down to yield radicals (eqns [2] and [3]). An oxygen molecule binding to a radical (eqn [4]) becomes a peroxy radical, which, by abstracting a hydrogen atom from another molecule, becomes a hydroperoxide, producing a further radical (eqn [5]). This reaction, when repeated many times, produces an accumulation of hydroperoxide. When there is a reduction in the amount of intact unsaturated fatty acids present, radicals bond to one another forming a stable nonradical compound. This brings the chain reaction to a halt (eqns [6]–[8]). *See* Oxidation of Food Components

(1) Initiation
$$RH \rightarrow R\cdot + H\cdot \qquad (1)$$
$$RH \rightarrow R\cdot O_2 \rightarrow ROO\cdot \qquad (2)$$
$$2ROOH \rightarrow ROO\cdot + RO\cdot + H_2O \qquad (3)$$

(2) Propagation
$$R\cdot + O_2 \rightarrow ROO\cdot \qquad (4)$$
$$ROO\cdot + RH \rightarrow ROOH + R\cdot \qquad (5)$$

(3) Termination
$$R\cdot + R\cdot \rightarrow R-R \qquad (6)$$
$$R\cdot + ROO\cdot \rightarrow ROOR \qquad (7)$$
$$ROO\cdot + ROO\cdot \rightarrow ROOR + O_2 \qquad (8)$$

Foods contain factors that promote the oxidation of fatty acids. These factors include haematin compounds such as haemoglobin and myoglobin, colouring matter such as carotenoids, enzymes that contain metals such as iron, copper, cobalt, manganese and magnesium, and coenzymes.

Various synthetic antioxidants have been studied with the aim of preventing the oxidation of fats, and some of these have been used as food additives (Tables 1 and 2). Antioxidants that are used in foods must be extensively tested, e.g. for the absence of carcinogenicity and other toxic effects in the antioxidant itself, in its oxidized forms and in its reaction products with food components, for effectiveness at low concentrations, and for the absence of any propensity to impart unpleasant flavours or odours to the food in which it is used. Phenolic compounds are known to satisfy these conditions well, and are the most common food antioxidants.

Phenolic Compounds

Phenolic compounds perform the functions of capturing free radicals and halting chain reactions. Many of these compounds, including BHA, BHT, TBHQ and NDGA, contain large substituents that exhibit steric hindrance, resulting in more stable radicals. *See* Phenolic Compounds

BHA

Commercially available butylated hydroxyanisole (BHA) is a mixture of the 2-isomer and 3-isomer (2-BHA and 3-BHA). An excellent antioxidant, BHA has been used widely in fatty foods. However, the use of BHA has declined significantly since the publication of a report indicating that BHA exhibits carcinogenicity in the forestomach of rats.

BHA 3-isomer   BHA 2-isomer

Table 1. Permitted antioxidants in various countries

Countries	Tocopherol	Guaiagum	PG	BG	OG	DG	NDGA	BHA	BHT	THBP	HMBP	TBHQ
Australia			+		+	+		+				
Austria	+	+	+	+	+	+	+	+	+			
Belgium	+		+		+	+		+	+			
Brazil			+		+	+		+	+			+
Canada	+	+	+									
Czechoslovakia			+									
Denmark	+	+	+		+	+	+	+	+			
Finland	+		+		+	+	+	+	+			
France			+		+	+		+	+			
Greece			+		+	+						
Haiti			+				+	+	+			
Hong Kong			+		+	+		+	+			
India	+	+	+		+	+	+	+	+			
Italy	+		+		+	+		+				
Jamaica			+		+	+		+	+			+
Japan	+		+				+	+	+			
Korea			+					+	+			
Malaysia			+		+	+		+	+			
Mexico	+	+	+				+	+				
Morocco			+		+	+			+			
Holland	+		+		+	+		+	+			
New Zealand			+		+	+		+	+			
Nicaragua	+	+	+				+	+				
Norway	+		+		+	+	+	+	+			
Pakistan	+	+	+		+	+	+	+				
Peru			+		+	+		+	+			+
Poland	+		+									
Rumania		+			+							
South Africa	+	+	+		+	+		+				
Sri Lanka			+		+	+		+	+			
Spain			+		+	+		+	+			
Sweden	+	+	+		+	+		+	+			
Switzerland	+		+		+	+		+				
Turkey	+		+		+	+		+	+			
Taiwan			+		+	+		+	+			+
UK			+		+	+		+	+			
USA	+	+	+					+	+	+	+	+
USSR						+		+	+			
Yugoslavia			+		+	+	+	+				

Guaiagum, guaiacol gum; PG, propyl gallate; BG, butyl gallate; OG, octyl gallate; DG, dodecyl gallate; NDGA, nordihydroguaiaretic acid; BHA, butylated hydroxyanisole; BHT, butylated hydroxytoluene; PHBP, trihydroxybutylphenone; TBHQ, t-butyl hydroquinone; HMBP, hydroxymethylbutylphenol.
Data from Ohta S and Kusaka H (1979) The antioxidants for edible fats and oils. *Journal of the Japan Oil Chemists' Society* 28: 747–759.

Table 2. Japanese restrictions for the use of antioxidants

Antioxidants	Limitation or restrictions	Maximum permited level (mg kg^{-1})
Butylated hydroxyanisole (BHA)[a]	Butter	200
	Fats and oils	200
	Frozen fish, shellfish and whale meat (for dipping solution)	1000
	Mashed potato (dried)	200
	Salted fish and shellfish	200
	Dried fish and shellfish	200
Butylated hydroxytoluene (BHT)[b]	Butter	200
	Chewing gum	750
	Fats and oils	200
	Frozen fish, shellfish and whale meat (for dipping solution)	1000
	Mashed potato (dried)	200
	Salted fish and shellfish	200
	Dried fish and shellfish	200
Isopropyl citrate (as monopropyl citrate)	Fats and oils	100
EDTA CaNa$_2$, EDTA Na$_2$ (as EDTA CaNa$_2$)[c]	Canned or bottled soft drinks	35
	Canned or bottled food (except for soft drinks)	250
Erythorbic acid	Only for antioxidant use	
Sodium erythorbate		
Nordihydroguaiaretic acid	Butter	100
	Fats and oils	100
Propyl gallate	Butter	100
	Fats and oils	100
Resin guaiac	Butter	1000
	Fats and oils	1000
(±)-α-Tocopherol	Only for antioxidant use	

[a] If used in combination with BHT, total amount of both antioxidants.
[b] If used in combination with BHA, total amount of both antioxidants, except for chewing gum.
[c] To be chelated with calcium ions before completion of the final food.

BHT

Along with BHA, butylated hydroxytoluene (BHT) is the most widely used antioxidant among the phenolic antioxidants. Like BHA, BHT has been developed as a synthetic antioxidant to be used in petroleum and rubber products. BHT is known as a 'hindered phenol' because of its sterically hindered structure.

TBHQ

t-Butyl hydroquinone (TBHQ) was developed by the Eastman Kodak Corporation. Although hydroquinone itself has an antioxidant capacity, TBHQ, which contains a butyl group in a benzene ring, is an especially potent antioxidant.

Ethyl Protocatechuate

Ethyl protocatechuate has been used as an antioxidant in fats and oils. However, in Japan this compound was removed from the list of approved food additives in May 1970.

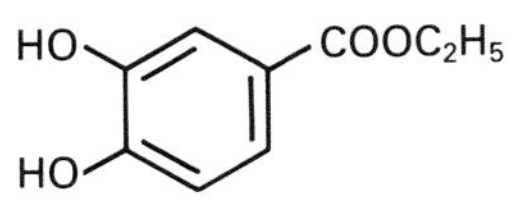

Propyl Gallate (PG)

Pyrogallol, which is also called gallic acid, occurs in nature as a constituent of tannin. The compound has been permitted as a food additive in the USA and Japan. Esters of gallic acid also exist, such as ethyl, butyl, amyl, octyl and dodecyl esters. *See* Tannins and Polyphenols

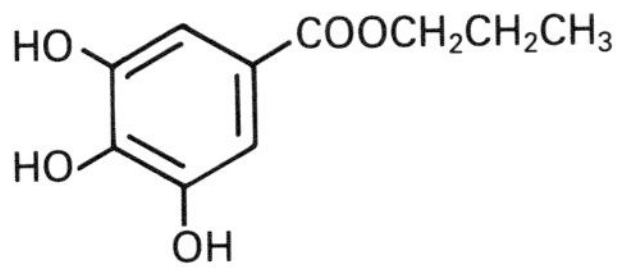

NDGA

Nordihydroguaiaretic acid (NDGA), was developed in the USA during World War 2. The compound is well known for having served as an antioxidant in military rations. The compound, which is obtained through extraction from the creosote bush, is expensive. Because of its high cost, the substance has been replaced by synthetic antioxidants in the postwar years. As its structural formula indicates, NDGA contains a branched alkyl group, which makes its synthesis difficult.

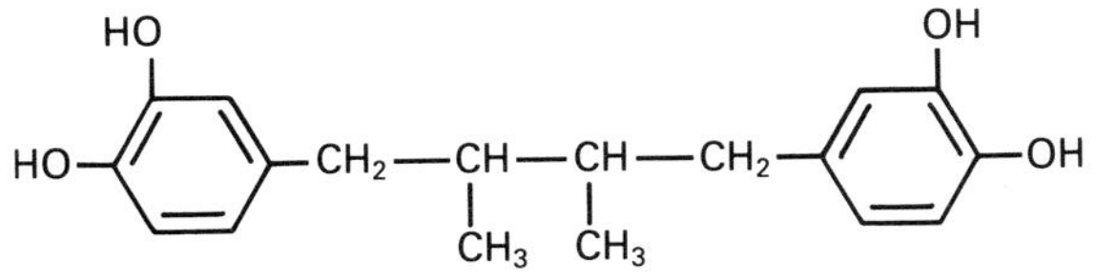

Among the bisphenol derivatives, 1,16-bis(2,5-dioxyphenyl)hexadecane (BDPH) is known to have a strong antioxidant property. When used together with other antioxidants (e.g. BHA), BDPH is known to exert a strong synergistic effect. However, the synergistic effect is especially pronounced when BDPH is used in combination with BHT and α-tocopherol.

Tocopherol and Trolox-C

Tocopherol (a member of the vitamin E group) occurs widely in plants and animals. Significant concentrations occur in plant oils. There are several tocopherols, including α-, β-, γ, and δ-tocopherols, and related tocotrienols. Although tocopherol is an excellent antioxidant, because of its relatively high cost the Hoffman-La Roche Corporation has developed Trolox-C, a substance which emulates tocopherol. *See* Tocopherols, Properties and Determination

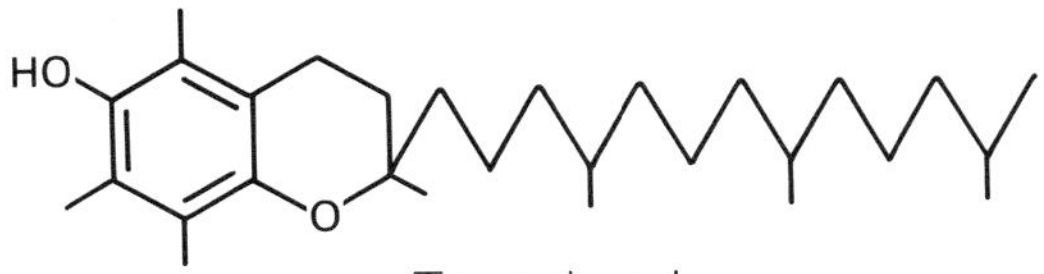

α-Tocopherol

Trolox-C has excellent antioxidant properties with plant and animal oils, showing considerable synergism when used in combination with ascorbic acid. When emulsified, the compounds formed from Trolox-C and amino acids show a stronger antioxidant effect than Trolox-C alone. Trolox-tryptophan methyl ester and Trolox-methionine methyl ester are especially effective antioxidants.

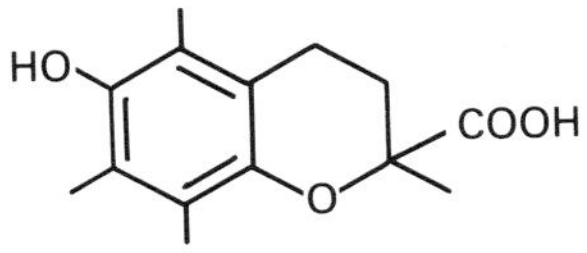

Trolox-C

Nitrogen Compounds

Among nitrogen compounds, amines are representative antioxidants, e.g. ethoxyquin, capsaicin and vanillylamide. As phenolic compounds, they act as inhibitors of free radical chain reactions. *See* Amines

'Ethoxyquin' is an abbreviation of 6-ethoxy-1,2-dihydro-2,2,4-trimethylquinoline, or EMQ for short. Although not permitted as a food additive in Japan, the compound is permitted in the USA and in EEC countries. When used in combination with lecithin (a phospholipid), EMQ shows a pronounced synergistic effect. When ingested in the body, it shows a biological antioxidant effect. *See* Phospholipids, Properties and Occurrence

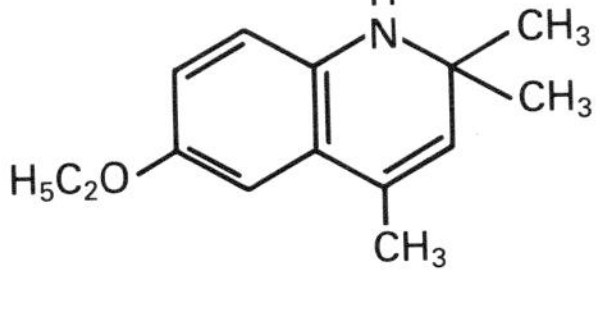

Sulphur Compounds

Some of the sulphur compounds, such as phenothiazine, exhibit strong antioxidant properties. However, because these compounds are unstable in food oil, and produce an offensive odour when heated, few have found practical utilization. Thiodipropionate and similar compounds have been approved for use as food additives in certain countries.

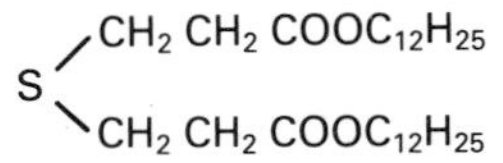

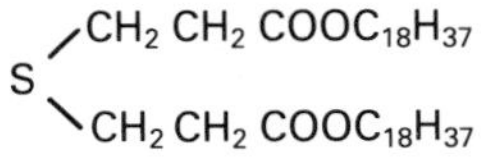

Polymer Antioxidants

These antioxidants are synthesized by polymerization, with an aluminum catalyst, of divinyl benzene, p-t-butyl phenol, p-hydroxyanisol and mono-t-butyl hydroquinone. A white powder with a molecular weight of about 50 000, with the 'Anoxomer', has been filed with the US Food and Drug Administration for approval as a food additive. Superior to BHA and BHT in antioxidant properties, the material is highly stable, even when heated to 300°C in air.

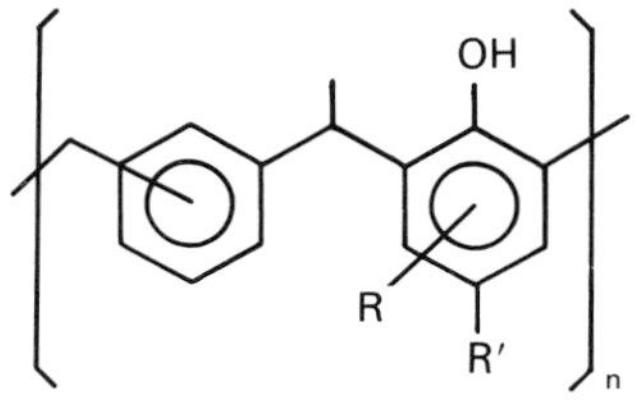

$R=$ —OH, — OCH$_3$
or — Alkyl
$R'=$—H or — Alkyl

Synergists

A substance which in itself has no or little activity but which enhances the activity of another compound when used in combination is called a synergist. Typical among the antioxidant synergists are citric acid, phosphoric acid and ascorbic acid.

Citric Acid and its Derivatives

Citric acid works as an antagonist of metals in fatty foods (i.e. it is a metal scavenger). In addition to citric acid, other hydroxy acids, such as tartaric acid and malic acid, are reported to work effectively. *See* Acids, Natural Acids and Acidulants

Phosphoric Acid and its Derivatives

Pyrophosphoric acid, hexametaphosphoric acid and other polyphosphoric acids are more effective than orthophosphoric acids as synergists for tocopherol

when used in oily or aqueous media. Phytic acid, which is the hexaphosphate acid ester of inositol, possesses a metal deactivation property. Lecithin, cephalin and other phospholipids also exhibit a synergistic effect with antioxidant substances.

Ascorbic Acid and Erythorbic Acid

Ascorbic acid exhibits synergistic effects when used in combination with a phenolic antioxidant. Ascorbic acid (AAH$_2$) and a phenolic antioxidant (QH) react as shown in eqns [9] and [10].

$$ROO \cdot + QH \rightarrow ROOH + Q \cdot \qquad (9)$$
$$Q \cdot + AAH_2 \rightarrow QH + AAH \cdot \qquad (10)$$

Erythorbic acid, a structural isomer of ascorbic acid, is claimed to be more effective than ascorbic acid itself in retarding the oxidation of products that are susceptible to oxidative degradation during processing or storage. *See* Ascorbic Acid, Physiology

In addition, sorbitols and other polyhydric alcohols are effective as metal deactivation agents. It has been reported that nitrogen compounds such as amines, amine oxides and amino acids also show synergistic effects when used in combination with an antioxidant.

Uses in Processed Foods

A common method for using an antioxidant is direct addition to oil and fats. However, in the case of fried foods, indirect addition has also been investigated because of the possibility of transfer of the antioxidant from the frying oil to the food product.

Direct Addition to Oils and Fats

Since BHA, BHT and related antioxidants are highly soluble in oil, they can be added directly to the oil. Similarly, an antioxidant can be prepared in the form of a highly concentrated solution, to be added in small quantities to the fat or the food product as necessary. *See* Vegetable Oils, Applications

Polyphenolic antioxidants, such as propyl gallate and NDGA, are not readily soluble in oil. Similarly, citric acid, ascorbic acid, phosphoric acid and other synergists are insoluble in oil. A common technique employed in dispersing these antioxidants in oil or food involves the use of solvents, such as propylene glycol, monoglycerides and lecithin.

Indirect Addition to Oils and Fats

Although antioxidants are extremely effective in preventing the oxidation of oils at high temperatures (as in

Table 3. Permitted levels for antioxidants in lard

		Maximum permitted level (mg kg^{-1})
Antioxidant	Propyl, octyl, dodecyl gallate	100
	Butylated hydroxyanisole (BHA)	200
	Butylated hydroxytoluene (BHT)	200
	Combination of BHA, BHT and gallates (gallates < 100 mg kg^{-1})	200
	Ascorbyl palmitate, stearate	200
	Dilauryl thiodipropionate	200
	Tocopherols	none
Synergist	Citric acid	none
	Sodium citrate	none
	Isopropyl, monoglyceryl citrate	< 100
	Phosphoric acid	< 100
	Combination of isopropyl, monoglyceryl citrate and phosphoric acid	< 100

Table 4. Permitted levels for antioxidants in margarine

		Maximum permitted level (mg kg^{-1})
Antioxidant	Propyl-, octyl-, dodecyl gallate	< 100
	Butylated hydroxyanisole (BHA)	< 200
	Butylated hydroxytoluene (BHT)	< 200
	Combination of BHA, BHT and gallates	< 200
	Ascorbyl palmitate, stearate	< 200
	Combination of ascorbyls	< 200
	Tocopherols	None
Synergist	Isopropyl citrate	< 100
Others	Citric acid	None
	Lactic acid, Na and K salts	None
	Tartaric acid, Na and K salts	None

the case of a frying oil) the antioxidant undergoes rapid losses. To counter this problem, the methods indicated below have been devised.

The techniques of spraying antioxidants on to fatty food by dissolving BHA and BHT in alcohol, of soaking the ingredients to be fried in a solution of antioxidants, and absorbing antioxidants in wrapping paper have been studied. Spraying is laborious, and the use of a flammable solvent presents obvious difficulties. Soaking is only applicable to foods that require a soaking operation. Using impregnated wrapping paper is technically difficult and expensive.

Addition to Food Oils

Antioxidants or synergists may be added to a food oil at the final stage of the deodorizing process.

Phenolic antioxidants have a more pronounced effect on animal fats than on plant oils. This may be due to the fact that plant oils already contain a significant amount of tocopherol.

Addition to Lards

An effective method involves addition of the antioxidant during the purification process. In this case, citric acid is often added as a synergist. Table 3 shows permitted levels for antioxidants in lard.

Addition to Margarines

BHA, BHT and a natural tocopherol mixture are added to the crude oil for the production of margarine. Direct addition of natural tocopherol mixtures to margarine is also permitted. The maximum amount of BHA or BHT that can be added, either singly or in total, is set at 200 mg per kilogram of oil. As a synergist, citric acid may also be added at a maximum level of 100 mg kg^{-1}. Since most margarine intended for domestic use is kept in refrigerators, some margarine products do not contain antioxidants. Table 4 shows permitted levels of antioxidants in margarine. *See* Margarine, Composition and Analysis

Synthetic Antioxidants

Addition to Shortenings and Lards

Shortenings are used as margarine substitutes in the production of biscuits and bread. To a considerable extent, quality is maintained by the addition of antioxidants.

For preservation of lard, the addition of antioxidants is an important consideration. Lard, which in the past was considered inferior, is now considered comparable to shortenings primarily because of the use of antioxidants.

Addition to Fish Products

BHA and BHT are used in dried small sardines to prevent 'oil burns'. In this type of application, antioxidants are mixed in the boiling water used in production. The concentraiton of antioxidant is 0·01% of the boiled water. *See* Fish, Spoilage

In salted fish products, the antioxidant is added at a rate of 0·01% of saline water, in the case of dip-salted products. In the case of sprinkled salting, the antioxidant is blended in the salt to 0·01–0·05%. In some cases the required amount of antioxidant is dissolved in propylene glycol which is then sprayed on to the table salt.

In the production of frozen fish or shellfish, the product is soaked in a solution of the antioxidant prior to freezing. Alternatively, the antioxidant is added to the water used for glazing. A commonly employed technique involves dissolution of the required amount of antioxidant in a small amount of alcohol or propylene glycol, which is poured, with stirring, into water, so as to make a suspension.

Addition to Meats and Their Processed Products

Although only ascorbic acid or tocopherol may be used on fresh meats, BHA and BHT can be used in oil and fats. Wherever possible, any natural tocopherol should be used at levels three to five times that of of BHA.

Various spices are used in the processing of meats, many of which have strong antioxidant properties. Further, many processed meats are smoked, and the smoke contains many constituents that are antioxidants. Thus, smoking affords an effective means of preventing the oxidation of food. Ascorbic acid and polyphosphoric acid are used to improve the colour, water content, and texture of meat products, and are helpful in preventing flavour changes in processed meats. *See* Meat, Preservation

Addition to Milk and Dairy Products

Compared with other animal fats or vegetable oils, milk fat has a complex fatty acid composition, which varies with the type of cow from which it is produced, its age, the season, and the animal feed ingested. Although BHT and octyl tartarate are effective in retarding the putrefaction of milk, few countries permit the use of phenolic antioxidants. Because milk fats produced in winter contain relatively low concentrations of tocopherol, some countries permit addition of ascorbic acid for arresting the production of an oxidation odour during storage.

Phenolic antioxidants are effective in preventing the putrefaction of butter. Some countries permit the use of BHA, BHT, guaiac resin, isopropyl citrate, NDGA and propyl tartarate in butter, although at present none of these antioxidants are used.

Addition to Starch-rich Foods

Phenolic antioxidants, such as BHA and dodecyl gallate, are used in the preservation of fats in biscuits intended for long-term storage. Heat-stable antioxidants, including Anoxomer, are capable of prolonging the shelf life of biscuits.

Addition to Potato Products

Instant mashed potato is made by peeling the potatoes, slicing them, gelatinizing them by dipping them into water at 65–73°C, and steaming. The resulting steamed product is mashed by adding pure monoglyceride at 0·2–0·3% of the final product, and BHT at 0·2%, followed by drying in a drum drier. The product made in this manner is highly flaky, and stable to quality degradation.

For prolonging the shelf life of potato flakes other methods for adding antioxidants have been studied. For example, antioxidants last longer when added as an emulsion rather than by spraying. The addition of a sodium hydrogenpyrophosphate to potato flakes can prevent colour degradation. This discovery has substantially improved the efficiency of potato flake production. *See* Potatoes and Related Crops, Processing Potato Tubers

Addition to Animal Feeds

The composition of animal feeds has a strong relationship to the quality of meat obtained from the animals so fed. Antioxidants are added to animal feeds to prevent the oxidation of fats, vitamin A and vitamin D among the feed constituents by oxygen in the air. Among the antioxidants used in mixed animal feeds in Japan are ethoxyquin, BHA and BHT. In the USA, antioxidants that are approved for use in human foods are also permitted as animal feed additives (Table 5).

Synthetic Antioxidants

Table 5. Antioxidants permitted for use in animal feeds in USA

Antioxidants	Maximum permitted level (%)
Butylated hydroxyanisole (BHA)	<0·02
Butylated hydroxytoluene (BHT)	<0·02
Citric acid	None
Ascorbic acid	0·02
Calcium ascorbate	0·02
Ascorbyl palmitate	0·02
Ethoxyquin	<0·015
Dilauryl thiodipropionate	<0·02 of fat content
Distearyl thiopropionate	<0·02 of fat content
Propylgallate	<0·02 of fat content
Resin guaiac	<0·1 of fat content
Thiodipropionic acid	<0·02 of fat content
Tocopherol	None
Potassium bisulphite	Not used in meat
Sodium sulphate	Not used in meat
Sodium bisulphite	Not used in meat
Sodium metabisulphite	Not used in meat

Addition to Essential Oils, Carotenoids and Vitamins

α-Tocopherol, NDGA and propyl gallate added to orange oil have produced favourable results. In lemon essence, NDGA and propyl gallate work effectively. Anoxomer has also been reported as an effective agent.

The stability of vitamin A and related carotenoids is significantly improved by the addition of an antioxidant, e.g. NDGA improves the stability of vitamin A in fish liver oil. The stability of vitamin A added to dried skim milk is also improved by the addition of an antioxidant.

Stability to Food Processing

The extent to which the antioxidants are lost during the purification of oil or during food processing is important for the preservation of product quality.

Behaviour of Antioxidants During Purification of Oil

Generally, purification of oil involves degumming, alkali refining, bleaching and deodorizing. Hydrogenation for hardening may be performed prior to the deodorizing process.

The degradation of antioxidants has been studied by adding 200 mg kg^{-1} of ($\pm$)-α-tocopherol and 100 mg kg^{-1} each of BHA and BHT to different crude oil samples and their fate followed during processing (Tables 6 and 7).

The higher the temperature of the deodorizing process employed, the more pronounced is the rate of disappearance. In the alkali refining process, some of the tocopherol breaks down when heated in the presence of alkali. During the bleaching process, some of the tocopherol is reportedly adsorbed by acid clay and activated charcoal. Reduction in the amount of tocopherol present during the deodorizing process appears to be attributable to losses by vaporization under reduced-steam distillation. However, even when treated at 250°C, approximately 50% of the original amount remains intact.

Both BHA and BHT showed a similar rate of survival, with little variation between them and from one raw material to another. During the alkali refining and bleaching processes, both BHA and BHT showed a smaller rate of decline compared with α-tocopherol. However, during the deodorizing process, both BHA and BHT disappeared completely, irrespective of the temperature employed, apparently due to complete volatilization during reduced-pressure steam distillation.

Citric acid should be added to oils after deodorizing, since the additive decomposes at deodorization.

During hydrogenation, changes in the concentration of tocopherol vary with the types of catalyst employed. The rate of decline increases in the following order: nickel < copper-nickel < palladium on charcoal < copper–chromium, with final concentrations varying from 69 to 33% of the initial values. There is little difference between BHA and BHT, both showing a concentration change from 91 to 86%.

Behaviour of Antioxidants During Storage

Changes due to temperature

The rate of survival of BHA, dissolved in methyl linoleate (4% BHA) and stored in a dark place at 50°C, has been studied with and without the addition of trimethylamine oxide (TMAO) (2%). According to the data, BHA and TMAO show a synergistic effect: in the presence of TMAO, BHA shows a higher rate of survival.

Similarly it has been reported that the rate of survival of TBHQ in methyl oleate under the accelerated oxidation method conditions is 10% after 1 h, and 5% after 2 h.

The amount of tocopherol present in hydrogenated soya bean oil under the AOM conditions has also been studied. According to these data, addition of citric acid can help prevent the breakdown of tocopherol.

Antioxidants in Freeze-dried Food

The amount of residual antioxidants, including BHA, BHT and TBHQ, after freeze drying of fatty model

Table 6. Survival of α-tocopherol during purification

Sample	Survival of α-tocopherol (%)			
	Beef fat	Fish oil	Soya bean oil	Palm oil
Crude oil	100·0	100·0	100·0	100·0
Alkali refining oil 1	100·0	98·7	95·7	96·7
Alkali refining oil 2	86·0	88·3	89·1	88·7
Bleaching oil 1	82·9	82·5	85·1	82·2
Bleaching oil 2	74·6	76·2	80·1	74·9
Hydrolysed oil	—	82·1	—	—
Deodorized oil 1	78·1	80·7	80·1	77·1
Deodorized oil 2	61·4	71·3	67·9	67·1
Deodorized oil 3	50·9	60·5	51·3	54·4
Deodorized oil 4	44·7	50·7	98·3	47·8

100 mg kg^{-1} of α-tocopherol were added to each sample.
Data from Kanematsu H, Maruyama T, Niiya I, Imamura I, Suzuki K, Kutsuwa Y, Murase Y, Mizutani H, Morita and Matsumo T (1976) *Journal of the Japan Oil Chemists' Society* 25: 234.

Table 7. Survival of BHA and BHT during purification

Sample	Beef fat (%)		Fish oil (%)		Soya bean oil		Palm oil (%)	
	BHA	BHT	BHA	BHT	BHA	BHT	BHA	BHT
Crude oil	100·0	100·0	100·0	100·0	100·0	100·0	100·0	100·0
Alkali refining oil 1	98·1	96·8	98·0	98·9	96·9	98·0	97·1	98·9
Alkali refining oil 2	95·2	944·6	96·0	93·6	94·8	94·1	93·3	93·5
Bleaching oil 2	90·5	93·5	91·2	91·5	89·1	92·2	90·6	90·3
Bleaching oil 2	83·8	86·0	83·3	90·4	80·4	82·3	83·8	83·9
Hydrolysed oil	—	—	91·1	91·7	—	—	—	—
Deodorized oil 1	0	0	0	0	0	0	0	0
Deodorized oil 2	0	0	0	0	0	0	0	0
Deodorized oil 3	0	0	0	0	0	0	0	0
Deodorized oil 4	0	0	0	0	0	0	0	0

100 mg kg^{-1} of BHA and BHT were added to each sample.
Data from Kanematsu H, Maruyama T, Niiya I, Imamura I, Suzuki K, Kutsuwa Y, Murase Y, Mizutani H, Morita and Matsumoto T (1976) *Journal of the Japan Oil Chemists' Society* 25: 234.

foods has been studied. Under slow freeze drying, the amounts of TBHQ, BHA and BHT remaining in the sample after the drying process were 32, 27 and 16%, respectively. Under rapid freeze drying, the amounts were somewhat lower, being 26, 14 and 22%, respectively.

Decomposition by Light

When benzene solutions of 2-BHA and 3-BHA are exposed to sunlight, 3-BHA breaks down more rapidly due to oxidation than 2-BHA.

The results of ultraviolet light irradiation of soya bean oil to which BHT is added in a 0·02% concentration, shows that the antioxidant prolongs the oxidation induction period of the oil. During the induction period,

BHT declines almost linearly. When BHT is exhausted, the rate of oxidation of oil increases suddenly.

Behaviour of Antioxidants During Frying

Table 8 shows results of adding 0·1% each of BHA, BHT, hydroquinone, PG and isoamyl gallate (IAG) to soya bean oil, heating the mixture at 170°C, and determining the amounts of antioxidants that remained. Heating at 170°C eliminated BHA in 30 min and IAG in 30 min.

Figure 1 shows the effect of heating BHA and BHT in liquid paraffin on the amounts of residual antioxidants. In a separate study, the heat tolerance of lard, to which BHA and natural tocopherol were added, was investi-

Table 8. The disappearance of added antioxidants in oil by heating

Heating time (min)	BHA	BHT	HQ	PG	IAG
10	+	+	+	+	+
30	+	+	+	−	−
45	+	+	±	−	−
60	−	+	−		
90	−	±	−		
120	−	−			

Antioxidants: BHA, butylated hydroxyanisole; BHT, butylated hydroxytoluene; HQ, hydroquinone; PG, propyl gallate; IAG, isoamyl gallate.
+, detected; ±trace; −, not detected.
Data from Kajimoto G, Inoue A and Yumoto H (1967) Studies on the preservation of oily foodstuffs by indirect method of antioxidant. *Nippon Shokuhin Kogyo Gakkaishi* 14: 72–75.

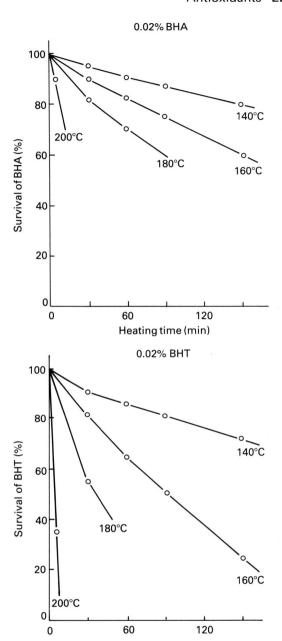

Fig. 1 Decrease of antioxidants in liquid paraffin with heating. Data from Ishitani T, Hirata T, Takai J and Kimura S (1976) Volatilization and decomposition of antioxidants by heating. *Nippon Shokuhin Kogyo Gakkaishi* 23: 244–249.

gated and the survival of BHA was shown to be less than that of tocopherol.

Experiments involving heating peanut oil and soya bean oil at 180°C have been carried out to study tocopherol stability. The peanut oil, which initially contained 70 ppm of α-tocopherol and 100 ppm of γ-tocopherol, showed complete loss of α-tocopherol after 1 h of heating and γ-tocopherol after 1·5 h. The soya bean oil, which initially contained 100 ppm of α-tocopherol, 550 ppm of γ-tocopherol and 22 ppm of δ-tocopherol, showed complete loss of α-tocopherol after 5 h of heating, and complete loss of γ-tocopherol and δ-tocopherol after 8–10 h.

Polymer antioxidants, such as Anoxomer, are stable even when heated. When such antioxidants are added to a mixture of cottonseed oil and soya bean oil and are heated at 190°C for 2 h, there is no appreciable loss.

The Fate of Antioxidants During Potato Crisp Production

Among various fried products, potato crisps are fried at a relatively low temperature. Since the process involves the vaporization of large quantities of water, the antioxidants added to the frying oil are lost by steam distillation. Any BHA added to oil undergoes a significant loss when potato crisps are fried in that oil. The extent of loss of tocopherol and TBHQ when potato crisps are fried in peanut oil and cottonseed oil at 160°C has also been studied. In the case of peanut oil, 55% of tocopherol and 54% of TBHQ were lost after 103 h total frying time. In the case of cottonseed oil, most of the antioxidants remained intact. The oil adhering to potato crisps, after the potato crisps were preserved for 6, 12 and 27 weeks at room temperature, retained more tocopherol if the potato crisps were fried in cottonseed oil rather than in peanut oil.

Factors Affecting the Loss of Antioxidants

When oil containing antioxidants is used for frying, the antioxidants are subject to loss due to thermal oxidation, evaporation and adsorption on to the ingredients which are fried. Such losses reduce the stability of the frying oil. Tocopherol mixed in a solid fat is especially prone to breakdown by thermal oxidation. BHA, which is volatile, is rapidly lost due to vaporization, and is therefore unsuitable for use as an antioxidant in frying oil. To minimize the loss of antioxidants, it is necessary to use antioxidants that are not very volatile. At the same time, it is important to prevent thermal oxidation. Although relatively immune to losses due to vaporization, tocopherol can undergo rapid losses due to thermal oxidation when used in a medium offering a large surface area in contact with air. Solid fats that contain high proportions of saturated fatty acids are extremely stable relative to auto-oxidation at low temperatures. Addition of trace quantities of antioxidants confers an even greater stability on these fats.

Bibliography

Finley JW and Given Jr P (1986) Technological necessity of antioxidants in the food industry. *Fd. Chem. Toxic.* 24: 999–1006.

Kahl R and Hilderbrandt AG (1986) Methodology for studying antioxidant activity for mechanisms of action of antioxidants. *Fd. Chem. Toxic.* 24: 1007–1014.

Katsura E (1979) Recent processing techniques of edible oils and fats. *Journal of the Japan Oil Chemists' Society* 28: 709–716.

Matsubara S (1979) Present status and future trends of refinings and deodorization technologies of fat and oils. *Journal of the Japan Oil Chemists' Society* 28: 670–688.

Murase Y (1979) Recent problems of hydrogenating oils and fats. *Journal of the Japan Oil Chemists' Society* 28: 689–699.

Namiki M and Matsushita S (eds) (1980) *Interaction Between Food Components.* Tokyo: Koudansha Press.

Ohta S (ed.) (1987) *Food and Antioxidants.* Tokyo: Shokuhin Shizai Kenkykai.

Totani Y (1980) Interaction between lipid peroxide and nitrogen compounds. *Journal of the Japan Oil Chemists' Society* 29: 323–329.

Tadokoro T (1982) Oilseed processing. *Journal of the Japan Oil Chemists' Society* 31: 820–825.

Yachigo S (1984) Suitable application of antioxidants. *Journal of the Japan Oil Chemists' Society* 33: 420–425.

You-Cheng Liu, Zheng-Li Liu and Zheng-Xu Han (1988) Radical intermediates and antioxidant activity of ascorbic acid. *Reviews of Chemical Intermediates* 10: 269–289.

H. Narita
Shizuoka Prefectural Institute of Public Health and Environmental Science, Shizuoka, Japan

Synthetic Antioxidants, Characterization and Analysis

Determination of Activity

The activity of an antioxidant is determined by adding the antioxidant to an oil, performing preservation tests on the mixture, and by measuring the extent of the resulting oxidation of the oil.

Methods for Measuring the Extent of Oxidation of Oils and Fats

Many methods, including chemical methods and sensory methods, have been proposed and used for the measurement of the extent of oxidation of oils and fats.

Chemical Methods

The extent of oxidation of a fat or oil can be determined by means of acid values, peroxide values and carbonyl values. The principles of these methods are shown in Table 1.

Sensory Methods

In many cases, the human senses are more sensitive than chemical analyses. Therefore, sensory tests are essential to the evaluation of the flavour of an oil. **See** Sensory Evaluation, Taste

The odour of an antioxidant itself can be detected by a sensory test. Thus, even if the antioxidant helps prevent oxidation, if its odour is detectable by a sensory test it may not be suitable for use in food. **See** Sensory Evaluation, Aroma

Methods for Testing the Stability of Oils or Fats

The first test that was proposed is the oxygen absorption test. Bakeries have developed an oven test, known as the 'Schaal oven test'. Subsequently, a method based on peroxide values was established, and advances occurred in procedures (the accelerated oxidation method (AOM)) for testing the stability of oils and fats.

AOM

The AOM equipment is described in detail in Section Cd-12-57 of the publication *Official and Tentative Methods.* This method is also referred to as the 'Swift stability test'.

The method involves placing 20 ml of a sample fat or oil in a 25×200 mm test tube, and injecting clean air, at a flow rate of 2.33 ml s^{-1}, into a thermostat tank maintained at $97.8°C$. A commonly used apparatus consists of a circular thermostat tank in which test tubes are arranged in a circular pattern. At specified time intervals, the odour of the exhaust gas from the test tubes is checked. Then, fat or oil samples are withdrawn, and their peroxide values are determined. As a general rule, the stability of a fat or oil is indicated by the time that it takes for the peroxide value to reach 100 mEq kg^{-1} in the case of vegetable oil, or 20 mEq kg^{-1} in the case of lard. An automated instrument, termed the Rancimat, has been developed which measures induction periods under similar conditions to the AOM.

Modified AOM

Instead of the 97·8°C heating level used in the AOM, a further method has been proposed wherein the water temperature is raised to 110°C, so as to reduce the time that it takes for a sample to reach the rancidity point.

Alternatively, the temperature may be increased to 125°C, and peroxide values measured by using the ferric thiocyanate method. Although increasing the tempera-

ture can shorten the incubation time, a possible drawback of the method is a reduced reproducibility due to breakdown of peroxides.

Oven Test

Originally, the oven test was used for shortenings used in biscuit and cracker manufacture. The method involves the use of a 63°C thermostat tank equipped with a ventilation device. A 50 g sample is placed in a 250 ml beaker. The beaker is placed in a glass container that can be covered with a watch glass or lid. Readings are expressed in terms of the number of days that it takes for the sample to undergo a deterioration detectable by a sensory test. Alternatively, readings can be expressed in terms of the number of days that it takes for the peroxide

Table 1. Analytical methods to determine the degree of oxidation of fats and oils

Property measured	Method	Principle of reaction
Acid value	Titration by alkali	R—CH$_2$—COOH + KOH $\longrightarrow$ R—CH$_2$—COOK + H$_2$O
Peroxide value	Iodometry	R—CH$_2$—CH(OOH)—CH=CH- + 2KI $\longrightarrow$ R—CH$_2$—CH(OH)—CH=CH— + I$_2$ + K$_2$O I$_2$ + 2Na$_2$S$_2$O$_3$ $\longrightarrow$ Na$_2$S$_4$O$_6$ + 2NaI
Carbonyl value	2,4-DNPH method	R—CHO + NO$_2$—C$_6$H$_3$(NO$_2$)—NH—NH$_2$ $\longrightarrow$ R—CH=N—NH—C$_6$H$_3$(NO$_2$)—NO$_2$ + H$_2$O R—CH=N—NH—C$_6$H$_3$(NO$_2$)—NO$_2$ $\longrightarrow$ R—CH=N—N=quinonoid ring (NO$_2$) N$^+$(O$^-$)=O
	Hydroxylamine method	R—CHO + H$_2$N—OH $\longrightarrow$ R—CH=N—OH
TBA number	Thiobarbituric acid method	2 (HS—pyrimidine(N)(OH)(OH)) + CH$_2$(CHO)(CHO) $\longrightarrow$ S=pyrimidine(N)(OH)—CH=CH—CH=—pyrimidine(HO)(SH)(OH) + 2H$_2$O
Amount of oxygen absorbed	Waerburg's manometer Oxygen analyser Measurement of weight	

2,4-DNPH, 2,4-dinitrophenylhydrazine; TBA, thiobarbituric acid

Table 2. Comparison of the AOM and oven test in lard

| Antioxidant | Amount added (%) | Stability | |
		AOM (h)	Oven test, 120°C (days)
Control	—	6	7
Resin guaiac	0·01	10	9
Resin guaiac	0·05	20	22
Resin guaiac	0·10	24	23
Control	—	6	7
PG	0·01	33	30
PG	0·03	50	60
PG	0·05	135	124
PG	0·10	145	135
Control	—	4	4
Tocopherol	0·02	16	15
Tocopherol	0·10	23	18
Control	—	5	6
NDGA	0·01	18	25
NDGA	0·02	35	32
NDGA	0·05	45	35

PG, propyl gallate; NDGA, nordihydroguaiaretic acid.
Data from Horne LW, Stevens HH and Thompson JB (1948) The effect of shortening stability on commercially produced army-ration biscuits. *Journal of the American Oil Chemists' Society* 25: 314–318.

value to reach a given limit. This test is conducted at a temperature somewhat more severe than the temperature under which the subject oil or fats are preserved. Compared with the conditions employed with the AOM, this temperature is closer to the temperatures prevailing under natural storage conditions.

Table 2 shows the stability of lard to which various antioxidants have been added, and a comparison with that of crackers made using such lard samples.

Light Beam Irradiation Method

The light beam irradiation method takes advantage of the fact that the oxidation of oils or fats is promoted by light. Samples of biscuits, fried confections, fried noodles, fried beans or other fatty processed foods, 80–100 g each, are placed in a polyethylene bag (low-pressure polyethylene film, 0·04 mm thick, 300 × 170 mm in dimensions) and hermetically sealed. On the sample table of the degradation test apparatus, the sample is irradiated under the following conditions: luminosity at the centre of one side, 15 000 lux; temperature, 50 ± 1°C. Panel members are used to perform sensory tests on a time series basis. The first time that a putrefaction odour is observed is designated as the odour onset time. If the food itself emits a strong odour, as in the case of a seafood, peroxide values of a fat or oil sample extracted

Table 3. Odour onset time and standard shelf life

Odour onset time, 15 000 lux, 50°C (h)	Standard shelf life
3–5	1 month
10–12	3–4 months
24	6 months
48	1·5 years

Data from Moser HA, Evans CD, Mustakas G and Cowan JC (1965) Flavor and oxidative stability of some linolenate containing oils. *Journal of the American Oil Chemists' Society* , 42: 811–813.

from the irradiated sample can be used as a reference point. These samples are packaged in a similar manner. The odour onset time that would result if the samples were stored under standard conditions (approximately 200 lux, room temperature, in-door storage and lights turned off at night) is determined. By taking subjective judgments into consideration, the odour onset time and standard shelf lives are determined as indicated in Table 3. *See* Storage Stability, Shelf-life Testing

The light irradiation method and the oven test method produce results that are in fair agreement with the results of sensory tests, but they are not always in good agreement with the result based on peroxide values.

Gravimetric Method

In this method, oil samples, 0·2–1·0 g each, are placed in beakers and covered with watch glasses. The beakers are placed in a thermostat tank maintained at 50–60°C. Weight changes are then determined gravimetrically.

Methods of Measuring the Amount of Oxygen Consumed

American Society for Testing and Materials (ASTM) bomb method

Here, 15 g of a solid fat sample, or 30 g of a liquid oil sample, is placed in a glass container of specified dimensions. The glass container, in turn, is placed in a stainless steel bomb, and sealed. Oxygen is pumped in at 690 kPa. The bomb is immersed in water, to check for the absence of any leaks, and is then placed in a boiling water bath. The pressure of oxygen is automatically recorded and the induction period is expressed in terms of the time that it takes for the sample to register a pressure drop of 13·8 kPa per hour. This method is superior to the AOM and the oven test method in the speed and accuracy of analysis. It is said to be 1·4 times faster than the AOM, and is 40–50 times faster than the oven test method.

Oxygen Absorption Method

In this method, using a Warburg's manometer, a specified amount of sample fat or oil is placed in a reaction flask, put in a water bath at a specified temperature, and then shaken. The amount of oxygen absorbed by the sample is measured with a manometer. The stability of the sample fat or oil can be determined from the rate of oxygen absorption.

Measurement of Dissolved Oxygen

In this method, an antioxidant is added to an emulsion composed of oil, water and the surfactant Tween 40. The electrodes on the analyser are set up and stirring is continued while setting the dissolved oxygen level at 100%. When a small amount of ferrous sulphate as a source of Fe^{2+} ions is added, the fat rapidly consumes the dissolved oxygen due to the catalytic action of Fe^{2+}. In the absence of an antioxidant, the level of dissolved oxygen falls to 5% in a matter of a few minutes at room temperature. Using the above method, the effectiveness of the antioxidants butylated hydroxyanisole (BHA), butylated hydroxytoluene (BHT), propyl gallate (PG) and citric acid has been compared. This method gives results that are in close agreement with antioxidant efficacy results obtained under the AOM conditions. This method, however, is not without drawbacks. Since Fe^{2+} tends to promote the reaction, if a chelating agent (eg EDTA) is used to inactivate Fe^{2+}, the chelating agent can be mistaken for the antioxidant. This problem, however, does not affect BHA and similar antioxidants that act as chelating agents.

Methods of Measuring Changes in Fat Quality by Chemiluminescence

Oxygen-containing compounds produced by oxidation, such as aldehydes, ketones and alcohols, have a low-level chemiluminescence capacity. Recent advances in optoelectronics have made the fabrication of 'weak light detection devices' possible, enabling researchers to measure the extent of oxidation of fats or oils.

To a hexane solution of an antioxidant is added 5 g of the methyl ester of a fatty acid, to give a final concentration of 0·02%. While allowing the passage of air through the sample, the resulting chemiluminescence is measured at 100°C for 60 min, which is reduced by an antioxidant. When compared with results obtained from the AOM and the oven test method, the results showed a high degree of correlation, except in the case of α-tocopherol. This affords a useful screening method for the development of antioxidants.

β-Carotene Test Method

This method involves spectrophotometric analyses of the extent of discoloration of β-carotene due to oxida-

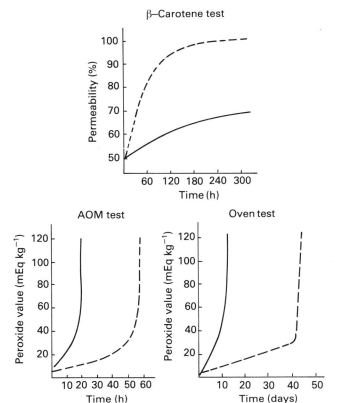

Fig. 1 Comparison of three tests (– – – – – –, sesamol; ————, tocopherol). Data from Isobe T, Kiyono H and Watanabe S (1980) *19th Annual Meeting of the Japan Oil Chemists' Society*.

tive degradation. *See* Carotenoids, Properties and Determination

Here, 2 g of β-carotene is dissolved in 10 ml of chloroform. To a round-bottomed flask containing 20 mg of linoleic acid and 200 mg of Tween 40 is added 1 ml of of the solution. After the chloroform is removed by evaporation, oxygen is introduced. Then, 50 ml of distilled water is added to the flask with stirring. A sample is withdrawn from this liquid, and an ethanol solution of the antioxidant is added to the sample. The absorbance is then measured on a spectrophotometer. After that, the cell is dipped in a water bath maintained at 50°C, and the absorbance measured at regular time intervals until the β-carotene becomes discoloured.

Fig. 1 shows a comparison of the β-carotene test method, the AOM and the oven test method. As shown in the figure, in some cases different results may be produced. For this reason, the β-carotene test method should be used in combination with other methods.

Measurement of the Consumption of Linoleic Acid

Lipoxidase is added to samples of linoleic acid with and without an antioxidant. The samples are enzymatically oxidized, and unreacted linoleic acid is quantitatively

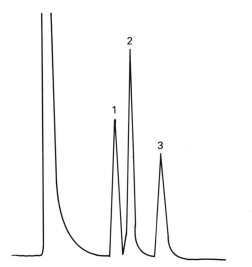

Fig. 2 Gas chromatogram of antioxidants extracted from salad oil. Column, 10% DC-200 on chromosorb W (3 mm internal diameter×2 m length); carrier gas, nitrogen, 60 ml min⁻¹; oven temperature, 160°C. Peaks: 1, BHA; 2, BHT; 3, fluorene (internal standard).

determined by means of gas–liquid chromatography (GLC). Reportedly, this method is simple to use and has a high degree of reproducibility. However, since antioxidants may inhibit lipoxidase activity to an extent which differs from that by which they stabilize an oil, results from the procedure should be treated with care.

Analysis and Characterization

Analysis of an antioxidant added to a food involves a pretreatment step, in which the antioxidant is extracted from the food, and an analytical step, in which the extracted and purified sample is identified and quantified.

Pretreatment

Solvent Extraction

Solvent extraction is a widely used pretreatment method. Various solvents are used according to the characteristics of a given sample and the antioxidant in question. A typical extraction process involves extracting the target antioxidant from an n-pentane or n-hexane extract of fatty food with acetonitrile.

Similarly, dimethyl sulphoxide has been used to extract BHA and BHT, the former from an n-heptane solution of a vegetable oil, the latter from a chewing gum homogenate. In fact, a wide range of extraction methods have been used, including direct extraction from oils or fatty foods with methanol.

Distillation

The solvent extraction method, which uses a large amount of solvent, necessarily involves a migration of the target fat from one medium to another, thus decreasing the accuracy of subsequent analyses. In such cases, steam distillation based on the use of an essential oil distillation apparatus can be useful.

This method, while requiring a certain length of time for the distillation process, needs a relatively small amount of solvent. With this method, the extent of migration of fat can be held to 0·2% even after 7 h of distillation. Thus, the method affords a viable technique for pretreatment, regardless of the form in which the target food item presents itself.

Column Chromatography

According to the Pharmaceutical Society of Japan's publication *Standard Methods of Analysis for Hygiene Chemists*, a polyamide column and a silica gel column should be used in combinaton for the purification of BHA and BHT. Also, a polyamide column is used for the purification of PG, isoamyl gallate (IAG), ethyl protocatechuate and nordihydroguairetic acid (NDGA). A Florisil column can also be used for the separation of BHT from a hexane solution of a vegetable oil. The same technique has also been used for the pretreatment of BHA and BHT present in fish samples, where high recoveries have been obtained. The technique eliminates the need for using acetonitrile distribution.

Sublimation

Sublimation has been used for the isolation of BHA and BHT from lard, but recoveries were not very high and the sublimate is always contaminated with fat.

Analytical Methods

Colorimetric Methods

There are several reports on quantitative colorimetric methods for the determination of BHA and BHT extracted from fat, butter or margarine with n-pentane, and purified by acetonitrile distribution. BHA forms a coloured derivative with 2,6-dichloroquinone chloromide, and BHT with o-anisidine, which may be quantified by colorimetry. Another quantitative colorimetric method, this one for PG, involves partitioning a fat sample between petroleum ether and an ammonium acetate solution containing 5% ethanol. After purification, a coloured derivative is formed using ferrous tartarate, and the absorbance measured at 560 nm. **See** Spectroscopy, Visible Spectroscopy and Colorimetry

Table 4. Recoveries (%) of added antioxidants from the foods by gas chromatography

Antioxidant	Oil	Butter	Margarine	Mayonnaise	Dried fish
BHA	89·0	85·7	84·5	85·7	84·6
BHT	99·8	97·8	97·9	99·6	87·4

Antioxidants were added at 100 mg kg^{-1}, $n=5$.
Data from Narita H, Kougo K and Kimura S (1976) Studies on the determination of antioxides. *Bulletin of the Shizuoka Prefectural Institute of Public Health and Environmental Science* 19: 55–57.

Thin-layer Chromatography (TLC)

TLC is primarily used for qualitative determinations. BHA, BHT t-butyl hydroquinone (TBHQ), tocopherol and eight other antioxidants from a 95% methanol extract of animal/vegetable oil have been separated using silica gel and polyamide plates. As a developing solvent for the silica gel plate, either benzene–petroleum ether–acetic acid or hexane–acetone–acetic acid was used. 2,6-Dibromoquinone-6-chloroquinone imide or ferric chloride-2,2-dipyridine was used for the colour development. As a developing solvent for the polyamide plate, methanol–acetone–water was used. In further studies the qualitative determination of BHA, BHT and TBHQ occurring in animal fats, vegetable oil, butter and margarine was investigated by means of silica gel plates. Hexane–acetic acid (30:5) was used as a developing solvent and 2,6-dichloroquinone 4-chlorimide, phosphomolybdic acid and dimethylamine for visualization. In particular, dimethylamine is useful for the detection of TBHQ, as it works specifically on this antioxidant, turning it red. *See* Chromatography, Thin-layer Chromatography

Gas Chromatography (GC)

Since BHA and BHT are volatile, and since other antioxidants can easily be made into volatile derivatives, analytical techniques based on GC have received much interest. *See* Chromatography, Gas Chromatography

Using 2% OV-17 and 5% SE-30 as columns, BHA, BHT and TBHQ occurring in cooking fats have been determined. Similarly, BHA and BHT, occurring in the scavenger fluid in the quantitative essential oil analyser for the analysis of cooking oil, butter and margarine, have been determined with the use of a 20% DC-200 column (Fig. 2, Table 4).

BHA, BHT, PG, IAG, ethyl gallate (EG) and NDGA occurring in cooking fats can be analysed on a 10% SE-30 column after trimethyl silylation of these substances. Alternatively, BHA, TBHQ and PG in a diethyl ether–benzene solution of cooking oil may be converted to their heptafluorobutyl derivatives in the presence of trimethylamine and analysed by using a 3% OV-3

column. Whereas previous reports used a flame ionization detector, highly sensitive analyses may be achieved, with fluoroderivatives, using an electron capture detector.

A problem which frequently hampers GC analysis is the presence of interfering peaks. To avoid this problem, columns of different characteristics should be used on a routine basis, and confirmation should be performed through the use of gas chromatography–mass spectroscopy (GCMS).

High-performance Liquid Chromatography (HPLC)

Recent rapid advances in HPLC techniques have produced numerous reports in this field, second only to the abundance of reports in the GC field. Although in some cases HPLC requires a solvent extraction or a purification by column chromatography, unlike GC it does not require preparation of derivatives. In the normal phase mode, HPLC has the advantage of direct analysis of antioxidants occurring in a given fat sample. For these reasons, HPLC is likely to become the most widely used technique for analysing antioxidants. *See* Chromatography, High-performance Liquid Chromatography

From hexane solutions of vegetable cooking oil, lard and shortenings, BHA, BHT, TBHQ, Ionox-100, THBP, PG, octyl gallate (OG), dodecyl gallate (DG) and NDGA can be extracted with acetonitrile. Then, using a Lichrosorb RP-18 column, which is a reversed-phase partitioning system, and either a 5% solution of acetic acid–acetonitrile or a 5% solution of acetic acid–methanol as the mobile phase, differing levels of separation may be achieved. The former mobile phase did not separate Ionox-100 from OG; however, it achieved an adequate separation of the remaining seven antioxidants. In contrast, the latter mobile phase did not achieve an adequate separation of THBP from TBHQ, Ionox-100 from OG, or DG from BHT. In a similar study, a μ-Bondapak C$_{18}$ column was used to analyse PG, OG, DG, BHA, BHT and TBHQ occurring in cooking oil, margarine and lard. For the mobile phase, a

Table 5. Recoveries (%) of antioxidants added to foods determined by HPLC

Antioxidant	Oil	Butter	Dried sardines	Frozen shrimps
PG	95·1	92·1	72·1	86·1
THBP	100·4	93·4	75·4	80·4
TBHQ	101·6	95·7	67·9	64·8
NDGA	93·7	93·7	70·5	84·7
BHA	93·8	94·9	84·6	88·0
HMBP	97·9	94·6	80·4	83·8
OG	92·7	94·4	78·6	88·2
BHT	88·1	91·0	72·6	80·7
DG	89·8	93·0	82·5	85·0

THBP, Trihydroxybutylphenone.
Antioxidants were added at 100 mg kg^{-1}, $n=3$.
Data from the Pharmaceutical Society of Japan (1991), pp 9–12.

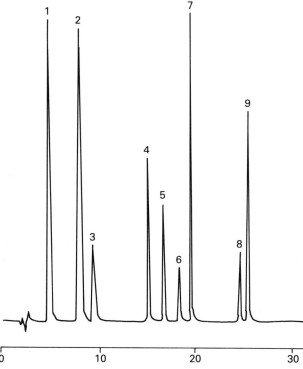

Fig. 3 HPLC chromatogram of antioxidants. Column, inertsil ODS-2 (4·6 mm internal diameter × 150 mm length); mobile phase, (A) acetonitril, methanol (1:1), (B) 5% acetic acid, liner gradient (A: 40–90%); flow rate, 1 ml min^{-1}; detector, ultraviolet 280 nm. Peaks: 1, PG; 2, THBP; 3, TBHQ; 4, NDGA; 5, BHA, 6, HMBP; 7, OG; 8, BHT; 9, DG. Data from the Pharmaceutical Society of Japan (1991), pp 9–12.

gradient method based on solutions of 1% acetic acid and 1% acetic acid–methanol were used. 2,4-Trimethyl phenol was used as an internal standard. The target substances were eluted in the following order: PG, TBHQ, internal standard substance, BHA, OG, BHT

Role of Antioxidant Nutrients in Defence Systems

and DG. The lowest rate of recovery of an additive from the sample was 90%, for BHT. In related studies, 15 antioxidants were extracted from food samples, using a solution of acetonitrile, 2-propanol, ethanol and oxalic acid, and then the substances separated on a Spherisorb ODS column. In a subsequent work, nine antioxidants were analysed as shown in Table 5 and Fig. 3. Whereas most reports used an ultraviolet detector (UVD), a method for TBHQ has been devised using a fluorescent light detector (FLD) to take advantage of the fact that TBHQ is fluorescent. There are reports of using an electrochemical detector (ECD) in addition to UVD and FLD. The ECD showed a higher sensitivity than UVD or FLD.

Bibliography

AOAC (1984) *Official Methods of Analysis*, 14 edn. St Paul: Association of Official Analytical Chemists.

Kitada Y, Nakazawa H and Fujita M (1985) The latest trend and analytical method concerning antioxidants as food additive (reviews). *Eisei Kagaku* 31: 145–155.

Kaneda T (1980) Recent topics on lipid peroxides. *Journal of the Japan Oil Chemists' Society* 29: 295–300.

Ministry of Health and Welfare (ed.) (1982) *Analytical Methods of Food Additives in Foods*. Tokyo: Kondansha.

Ohta S (ed.) (1987) *Food and Antioxidants*. Tokyo: Shokuhin Shizai Kenkukai.

Pharmaceutical Society of Japan (ed.) (1990) *Standard Methods of Analysis for Hygiene Chemists*. Tokyo: Kinbara Shuppan.

Shimazaki H (1980) Formation and determination of lipid peroxides. *J. Jpn. Oil Chem. Soc.* 29: 301–307.

Hiroko Narita
Shizuoka Prefectural Institute of Public Health and Environmental Science, Shizuoka, Japan

Role of Antioxidant Nutrients in Defence Systems

The control of free-radical-driven chemical reactions among biological macromolecules in living mammalian cells by a range of interacting nutrients and nutrient-derived factors is a new area of biochemistry that lies at the heart of the explanation of the aetiology of a number of human diseases and also probably the ageing process. This article will consider the nature of the free radical processes concerned, their control by antioxidant nutrients, and the role of these events in the aetiology of certain forms of cancer, cardiovascular disease and cataractogenesis, as well as in ageing. The evidence, largely epidemiological in nature, that links a high incidence of disease with low levels of intake of the nutrients concerned will also be considered. *See* Ageing – Nutritional Aspects

Free Radical Theory of Disease

It is customary to think of molecular oxygen as a benign, life-giving substance upon which animals depend to oxidize their food and release the energy contained within it in a packaged form that can be utilized at will for primary physiological events such as muscle contraction and nerve conduction.

This view of oxygen metabolism ignores its other face which, like that of Janus, is a malevolent one. The protection of mammalian organisms against damage caused by activated oxygen is a highly complex process that involves a subtly interrelated array of protective agents. Certain micronutrients, which are now often referred to as the 'antioxidant nutrients', occupy a central position in this protective mechanism. They include the trace minerals selenium, copper, zinc and manganese, vitamins E and C (and possibly vitamin A), as well as the carotenoids. The latter are now viewed as having an antioxidant role in their own right, independent of their provitamin A role. It is now possible to give a reasonably coherent account of the biochemistry of these protective mechanisms, understanding of which depends on a detailed knowledge of the way in which oxygen is metabolized. *See* Copper, Physiology; Retinol, Physiology; Selenium, Physiology; Zinc, Physiology

$$O_2 + 4H^+ \xrightarrow[\text{ADP} \quad \text{ATP}]{4e} 2H_2O \qquad (1)$$

The simple scheme for the reduction of oxygen to water given above does not disclose the possibility that the addition of electrons to the dioxygen molecule may occur in a stepwise fashion, with the intermediate production of activated oxygen species, some of which are very highly reactive. Oxygen permeates all intracellular sites and is even capable of penetrating the hydrophobic regions of biological membranes. The addition of two electrons to oxygen in a sequential fashion takes place readily, because dioxygen itself has two unpaired electrons, and this can occur as a random event whenever stray electrons are available. Thus, for example, electrons may be diverted from the mitochondrial and microsomal electron transfer chains at a number of points so that they do not reach their destination in the terminal cytochrome oxidase or cytochrome P-450 haemoproteins.

The first activated oxygen species formed by reduction of dioxygen is the superoxide anion radical $O_2^{\cdot-}$:

$$O_2 + e \rightarrow O_2^{\cdot-} \qquad (2)$$

A free radical is defined as an atom or molecule that has one or more unpaired electron(s), and it is this electron imbalance which gives rise to the very high reactivity, in many cases, of free radicals. As the reduction of oxygen proceeds, the electron deficiency of the superoxide anion radical is made up by the addition of a further electron

to form a peroxyl anion, which can then associate with protons from solution to form hydrogen peroxide.

$$O_2^{\cdot-} + e \rightarrow O_2^{2-} \xrightarrow{2H^+} H_2O \qquad (3)$$

The further reduction of hydrogen peroxide to water involves the addition of two more electrons. These electrons can be shown *in vitro* to be derived by the so-called Fenton reaction, from divalent cations such as iron and copper.

$$O_2^{\cdot-} + Fe^{3+} \rightarrow O_2 + Fe^{2+} \qquad (4)$$
$$H_2O_2 + Fe^{2+} \rightarrow OH^- + OH^{\cdot} + Fe^{3+} \qquad (5)$$
$$OH^{\cdot} + Fe^{2+} \rightarrow OH^- + Fe^{3+} \qquad (6)$$

It is attractive to suppose that such reactions are responsible *in vivo* for these reductions. However, this possibility is controversial at present because the Fenton reaction requires free, or low-molecular-weight-chelated, iron (or copper) and the intracellular iron is largely, if not exclusively bound to protein. As the debate about this continues one can envisage that, since the metal is acting as a catalyst, the amounts of free iron required are likely to be very small indeed, so that this small requirement for free iron may be provided even though most iron is protein bound.

The hydroxyl radical that occurs as an intermediate in this process is very highly reactive and potentially extremely damaging to living systems because it can pluck an electron from virtually any organic macromolecule situated in its vicinity. Because of its reactivity it cannot migrate and hydroxyl-radical-generated intracellular damage must occur close to the site of formation of the radical. However, it is the very high reactivity of the hydroxyl radical that is believed to be at the heart of the aetiogenesis of the biochemical changes that lead to pathology and disease. It is therefore necessary to enquire as to the likely targets for attack by the hydroxyl radical, which may give rise to degenerative disease, and as to the likely sources of hydroxyl radical *in vivo*. Before doing so it is necessary to mention briefly another reactive oxygen metabolite which, though not a radical, may be formed in living eukaryotic cells, namely singlet oxygen, $^1O_2$. This is formed as an excited state of dioxygen by energy capture from, for example, light radiation hυ

$$O_2 \xrightarrow{h\upsilon} {}^1O_2 \qquad (7)$$

A peripheral electron in the oxygen structure is excited to an orbital above that which it normally occupies. The resultant singlet state is highly reactive and may be of significance in certain normal biochemical processes such as the microbicidal activity of polymorphs, as well as contributing to the detrimental effects of oxygen metabolites in the aetiogenesis of disease. The energy captured in the singlet oxygen may be released to an organic macromolecule to cause a chemical change, and the oxygen returns to the ground state.

Role of Antioxidant Nutrients in Defence Systems

Targets for attack by hydroxyl radicals may be any organic macromolecule. Thus intracellular or extracellular proteins may be functionally damaged as the nature of specific constituent amino acids is changed and their normal role in the tertiary and quaternary structure of the protein modified or destroyed. However, there is little likelihood of secondary damage caused by such altered proteins and enzymes because they can be presumed to be efficiently removed from the system. There is ample evidence that, *in vitro*, the presence of a free-radical-generating system such as phagocytosing lymphocytes or xanthine oxidase in close proximity to DNA will result in extensive damage to the DNA structure. The potential for such damage in the multiplicity of events in the cancer process must therefore be self evident but direct evidence for a vital role in these events for free radicals is at present lacking. However, much circumstantial evidence suggests that free radical biochemistry must be considered to have major significance in carcinogenesis. *See* Carcinogens, Carcinogenic Substances in Food

The most detailed knowledge of a role for free radical-initiated pathology is in the field of the oxidation of membrane polyunsaturated fatty acids. The hydroxyl radical acts as an initiator of the process, abstracting a hydrogen atom from a methylene group, situated between two double bonds and forming a lipid carbon-centred radical.

$$LH + OH \cdot \rightarrow L \cdot + H_2O \qquad (8)$$

The lipid radical can then interact with molecular dioxygen to produce a lipid peroxyl radical which may be quenched by a lipid antioxidant such as vitamin E or, in the absence of antioxidants, may attack a further adjacent unsaturated fatty acyl group to give rise to further free radical species and the establishment of chain reactions.

$$L \cdot + O_2 \quad \rightarrow LOO \cdot \qquad (9)$$

$$either \quad LOO \cdot + E\text{—}H \rightarrow LOOH + E \cdot \qquad (10)$$

$$or \quad LOO \cdot + LH \quad \rightarrow LOOH + L \cdot \qquad (11)$$

If the lipid hydroperoxide is not removed by mechanisms described in the next section, it may undergo further iron-catalysed reactions, generating radical species that may be highly detrimental.

$$LOOH + Fe^{3+}\text{—}X \rightarrow LOO \cdot + H^+ + Fe^{2+}\text{—}X \quad (12)$$

$$LOOH + Fe^{2+}\text{—}X \rightarrow LO \cdot + OH^- + Fe^{3+}\text{—}X \quad (13)$$

(X denotes a haemoprotein.) The series of free-radical-initiated reactions among membrane polyunsaturated fatty acids described above are likely to have severe pathological consequences for living cells. Alterations in the structure of the phospholipids, in particular by the covalent attachment of oxygen in the hydrophobic region of the membrane will cause severe disruption to the normal membrane architecture which is likely to be of major significance in the development of disease. *See* Fatty Acids, Metabolism

Antioxidant Defences in the Body

The potential significance of the iron-catalysed generation of hydroxyl radicals (eqns [4] and [5]) cannot be overemphasized. It must follow that a major method by which such radical generation may be controlled, or even eliminated, is the efficient removal of the reactants O_2^- and H_2O_2. This process is carried out universally by enzyme systems; the removal of O_2^- is catalysed by a group of enzymes called superoxide dismutases (SODs). In the mitochondrial compartment of mammalian cells the SOD is a manganese-containing enzyme, whereas in the cytoplasm the SOD is an enzyme of different amino acid structure that depends for its activity on copper and zinc. Both enzymes catalyse the following reaction:

$$2O_2^- + 2H^+ \rightarrow H_2O_2 + O_2 \qquad (14)$$

Hydrogen peroxide is reduced to water in both intracellular compartments by glutathione peroxidase, an enzyme that depends for its activity on selenium:

$$H_2O_2 + 2GSH \xrightarrow{\text{glutathione peroxidase}} 2H_2O + GSSG \qquad (15)$$

(GSH is reduced glutathione and GSSG is oxidized glutathione.) Catalase, which is largely sequestered in peroxisomes, may have some significance in the general intracellular scavenging of hydrogen peroxide by disproportionation:

$$2H_2O_2 \rightarrow 2H_2O + O_2 \qquad (16)$$

The activities of SOD and glutathione peroxidase, since they depend on manganese and copper/zinc or selenium respectively, depend in turn on a ready availability of these 'antioxidant' minerals. A deficiency in the nutritional supply of these nutrients may then have consequences in terms of a failure of this first line of defence against oxygen-radical-induced damage.

It will be clear from consideration of eqns [10] and [11] that vitamin E is of major significance in the protection of biological membranes from attack by active oxygen species. In the process, vitamin E itself becomes a radical, following loss of its phenolic hydrogen to the lipid hydroperoxide. Regeneration of vitamin E from its radical undoubtedly takes place and the most likely mechanism for this, which remains to be proven, is a direct interaction with ascorbic acid. The dehydroascorbic acid (DHAsc) thus formed is probably regenerated by glutathione, the oxidized form of which is in turn reduced by NADPH.

$$E \cdot + Asc \rightarrow E + DHAsc \qquad (17)$$

$$DHAsc + 2GSH \rightarrow Asc + GSSG \qquad (18)$$

Role of Antioxidant Nutrients in Defence Systems

$$GSSG + NADPH + H^+ \rightarrow 2GSH + NADP^+ \quad (19)$$

Thus vitamin E and ascorbic acid act as a second line of defence against oxygen damage.

It is demonstrated clearly in eqns [12] and [13] that the lipid hydroperoxide is not a 'safe' end product. A third line of defence against the iron-catalysed formation of peroxyl or alkoxyl radicals from lipid hydroperoxides is provided by glutathione peroxidase. The formation of a lipid hydroperoxide in the hydrophobic region of biological membranes will result in disruption of the membrane architecture as the polar function of the hydroperoxide seeks to move towards a more hydrophylic environment. It is likely that this will cause an apparent activation of phospholipase A_2 so that the peroxidized fatty acid is removed from the covalent attachment to the membrane phospholipid. The peroxidized free fatty acid will then be reduced to a hydroxy acid by the catalytic activity of glutathione peroxidase, a process that also involves selenium:

$$LOOH + 2GSH \rightarrow LOH + H_2O + GSSG \quad (20)$$

Thus a nutritional supply of selenium is necessary also for this third line of defence against oxygen radical toxicity.

The potential for damage by singlet oxygen is at present difficult to assess. There is little reliable evidence to suggest how singlet oxygen may be generated in mammalian cells but the growing interest in the carotenoids as agents that ameliorate disease processes suggests that singlet oxygen may be involved in some of these processes. Carotenoids are excellent quenchers of singlet oxygen since they are able to capture the energy of the excited oxygen without chemical change because the carotenoids possess a conjugated double bond system. Vitamin A may also play a role in this connection.

Antioxidant Nutrients, Cancer and Cardiovascular Disease

Antioxidant Minerals

Little evidence exists to link a high incidence of cancer or cardiovascular disease to a low dietary intake of manganese, copper or zinc. Selenium is, however, highly likely to prove to be a major risk factor in the aetiology of certain forms of cancer; with respect to cardiovascular disease, none of the epidemiological evidence provides any convincing support for a role for selenium in the prevention of atherogenesis. There is much evidence derived from animal studies that, at high levels of intake, selenium can prevent or delay the onset of cancer. The protective amount of selenium, generally around 5 ppm in the diet, is much higher than the physiological requirement for the element, which is in the range 0·01–0·1 ppm. Indeed 5 ppm of selenium approaches the level

of intake at which selenium becomes toxic. Thus, although there is no doubt as to the veracity of the protective effect of selenium at these high levels against experimentally induced cancers in animals, there is no clear explanation of a mechanism and a sceptic would argue that these results are irrelevant to the prevention of human cancer. However, epidemiological evidence is now available that begins to argue for a role for selenium as a risk factor in certain specific cancers. Thus there is ecological evidence which frequently, but inconsistently, shows a correlation between high cancer incidence (or cancer-related death rate) and a low intake of selenium in the population concerned. *See* Cancer, Diet in Cancer Prevention

Case control evidence that shows a correlation between low blood selenium level and cancer risk in cancer patients is unreliable because it is never possible in such studies to distinguish cause from effect. Prospective studies, which provide the most reliable evidence of a link between low blood selenium level and subsequent high incidence of cancer, have now begun consistently to show such correlations. In several such studies there is, for a number of cancer sites, a good correlation between low blood selenium at the time when cancer may have been developing, and subsequent incidence of disease. These studies, however, are ongoing and the data preliminary; much more work is required before a firm conclusion can be reached.

Vitamin E

There are major inconsistencies in the literature concerning a possible relationship between low vitamin E nutritional status and high incidence of cardiovascular disease and cancer. Early epidemiological literature failed to find any such correlation, whereas more recent publications point to a highly significant preventive interaction of vitamin E in the cancer process. The explanation of this lack of consistency lies without doubt in flaws in the design and execution of earlier studies. In particular, two factors must be taken into account: (1) since cholesterol level may also be a variable in blood samples of diseased patients or those in a pre-disease state, as compared to normal controls, the blood vitamin E levels must be expressed as 'cholesterol standardized' values; (2) vitamin E is not very stable during prolonged storage of blood samples and in earlier prospective studies vitamin E measurements were made on samples that had been stored at either $-20°C$ or $-70°C$ for many years, because analysis was not undertaken until the subject concerned had been identified as having developed cardiovascular disease or cancer. Thus, in several recent prospective studies that have allowed for these potential defects, vitamin E has emerged as a risk factor in both cancer and cardiovascular disease. In one of these studies, coordinated from Basel, a further complication in interpretation has arisen. It has become apparent that a low level of intake of more than one antioxidant nutrient must also be considered since such multiple effects acting in concert may cloud the data derived from consideration of a single nutrient. Thus a particular level of vitamin E may appear to be adequate when the levels of all other antioxidant nutrients are also adequate: a fall in the level of another nutrient may result in an increased requirement for vitamin E. *See* Tocopherols, Physiology

Ascorbic Acid

The early evidence which identified ascorbic acid as a risk factor in the aetiology of some forms of cancer and cardiovascular disease was inferential rather than direct. There is a substantial body of evidence suggesting that the incidence of these diseases is lower in populations eating a diet containing large amounts of fresh fruit and green leafy vegetables. Furthermore, there is evidence that ascorbic acid is a powerful suppressant of carcinogen formation in model systems. More recently, however, evidence from prospective epidemiological trials has confirmed the early inferential evidence that ascorbic acid may be a risk factor in the aetiology of cancer and cardiovascular disease. *See* Ascorbic Acid, Physiology

Carotenoids

There is great interest in whether carotenoids have a disease-preventing role that is independent of their provitamin A function. A significant proportion of the total carotenoids in the human diet are absorbed unchanged, i.e. not converted by intestinal carotenoid oxygenases to vitamin A. Strong prospective epidemiological evidence now emerging implies a close correlation between high plasma carotenoid levels and a lowered incidence of cancer. Particularly significant correlations have been reported in two independent studies of carotenoids as risk factors in lung cancer and this relationship persisted strongly after adjusting for the number of cigarettes smoked, alcohol intake and other parameters. In these studies, serum retinol and vitamin E levels showed no correlations, and the possibility that carotenoids may have a significant protective effect against lung cancer in smokers is one that is currently exciting great interest. Early results from the Harvard Physicians' Health Study have recently indicated that intervention with 50 mg of beta carotene on alternate days in male physicians with a history of angina pectoris and/or coronary revascularization resulted in 44–49% lowering of all major sub-

sequent coronary events defined as myocardial infarction, revascularization or cardiovascular death. Evaluation of this important observation must await detailed publication of the study results but it suggests not only that beta carotene is likely to have a prophylactic role in cardiovascular disease but also that it may have some therapeutic significance. *See* Carotenoids, Physiology

Free Radicals and Cataracts

Cataract is one of the major causes of age-dependent visual impairment and blindness. Animal experiments have indicated that the ocular lens is physiologically damaged by exposure to activated oxygen species and the intraocular generation of oxygen radicals may constitute a significant or major factor in the pathogenesis of cataracts. This cataractogenic effect has been shown in animal models to be greatly reduced by treatment with vitamin E and ascorbic acid and it has therefore been suggested that these vitamins may offer a useful prophylaxis against senile cataracts in human subjects.

Recent epidemiological studies in elderly human subjects indicated that cataract patients tend to have lower plasma levels of vitamins E and C, and carotenoids, compared to carefully matched control subjects. Furthermore, in a comparison of supplementary vitamin taking, which was self reported in a group of cataract subjects and a corresponding matched group without cataracts, the control subjects who were free of cataracts took significantly larger amounts of vitamins C and E. These results have highlighted the need for a randomized controlled trial of vitamin supplementation in elderly subjects to evaluate the preventive effect of the vitamins against cataractogenesis.

Free Radicals and Ageing

Ageing in mammals appears to be the result of normal developmental and metabolic processes. The nature of the ageing process has been the subject of considerable speculation and one explanation of the process is the so-called 'free radical' theory of ageing, which suggests that progressive defects in the protective mechanism against free-radical-initiated damage to macromolecules eventually allow tissue damage to occur. It is suggested that the protective mechanism can cope with about 99·9% of 'normal' radical generation so that there is a progressive accumulation of damage which gradually builds up as the organism ages. A large body of experimental data have indicated a causative role for oxygen radicals in the ageing process and a positive correlation has been found between the tissue concentration of specific antioxidants and lifespan. These antioxidants include carotenoids, vitamin E and urate (a powerful endogenous antioxidant) and enzymes such as superoxide dismutase. The resistance of tissues to spontaneous autoxidation and the amount of oxidative damage to DNA that occurs are also shown to be inversely correlated to lifespan. These results have been interpreted as implying a role for oxygen radicals in the ageing process; extrapolating from the antioxidant status of an individual could be important in determining the frequency of age-dependent disease and the duration of general health maintenance. However, it must be stressed that this view is highly speculative and much further work is needed either to confirm or refute it.

Bibliography

Block G. Vitamin C and cancer prevention: the epidemiologic evidence. *American Journal of Clinical Nutrition* 53 (Supplement): 270S.

Comstock GW, Helzlsoner KT and Busch TL (1991) Prediagnostic serum levels of carotenoids and vitamin E as related to subsequent cancer in Washington County, Maryland. *American Journal of Clinical Nutrition* 53 (Supplement): 260S.

Cutler RG (1991) Antioxidants and aging. *American Journal of Clinical Nutrition* 53 (Supplement): 373S.

Diplock AT (1991) Antioxidant nutrients and disease prevention: an overview. *American Journal of Clinical Nutrition* 53 (Supplement): 189S.

Gey KF, Puska P, Jordan P and Moser UK (1991) Inverse correlation between plasma vitamin E and mortality from ischaemic heart disease in cross-cultural epidemiology. *American Journal of Clinical Nutrition* 53 (Supplement): 326S.

Jacques PJ and Chylack LT (1991) Epidemiologic evidence of a role for the antioxidant vitamins and carotenoids in cataract prevention. *American Journal of Clinical Nutrition* 53 (Supplement): 352S.

Knetk P *et al.* (1991) Vitamin E and cancer prevention. *American Journal of Clinical Nutrition* 53 (Supplement): 283S.

Luc G and Fruchart JC (1991) Oxidation of lipoproteins and atherosclerosis. *American Journal of Clinical Nutriton* 53 (Supplement): 206S.

Robertson JMcD, Donner AP and Trevithick JR (1991) A possible role for vitamins C and E in cataract prevention. *American Journal of Clinical Nutrition* 53 (Supplement): 346S.

Slater TF and Block G (eds) (1991) *American Journal of Clinical Nutrition* 53(supplement).

Stahelin HB, Gey KF, Eichholzer M and Ludin E (1991) Beta carotene and cancer prevention: the Basel Study. *American Journal of Clinical Nutrition* 53 (Supplement): 265S.

Anthony T. Diplock
Guy's Hospital, UMDS, London, UK

ANTISEPTIC PRODUCTS FOR PERSONAL HYGIENE

The role of environmental sites and skin surfaces (mainly the hands) in the transfer of infection has long been recognized. Under normal circumstances, the healthy adult in the community is relatively resistant to infection, but in situations where the environment provides an 'enrichment process', such as during the processing of foods, the survival and transfer of potentially pathogenic microorganisms is of considerable concern.

The healthy human skin possesses formidable powers of defence against microbial colonization and infection. Paradoxically, many of the traditional practices of skin care have tended to neutralize the natural defences. Recent investigations of the microbiology of human skin have provided a detailed understanding of the ecological processes which operate on the body surface, and have at least given a rational basis for the development of appropriate hygienic and antimicrobial procedures.

In this article, the hygienic significance of hand washing is reviewed, special attention being paid to the action of soap. The markedly diverse antimicrobial agents which have been introduced as topical antiseptics are then surveyed. The potential use of gloves is also examined.

Essentials of Personal Hygiene

The microflora on hands and outer garments of food handlers generally reflects the environment and habits of the individuals. Various workers suggest that humans shed from 10^3 to 10^4 viable microorganisms per minute. This flora would normally consist of microorganisms found on any object handled by the individual as well as some of those picked up from dust, water, soil and the like. In addition, there are several genera of bacteria that are specifically associated with the hands, arms, nasal cavities and mouth. Amongst these are the genera *Micrococcus* and *Staphylococcus*. While the genera *Campylobacter*, *Esherichia*, *Salmonella* and *Shigella* are basically intestinal bacteria, they may be deposited onto foods and utensils by food handlers if sanitary practices are not followed by the individual. Any number of yeasts and moulds may be found on the hands and garments of food handlers depending on the immediate history of each individual. One must also bear in mind the potential for virus transmission by hands. *See* Campylobacter, Properties and Occurrence; Food Poisoning, Tracing Origins and Testing; *Shigella*; *Staphylococcus*, Properties and Occurrence

The infected food handler is low on the list of factors which have contributed to outbreaks of food poisoning. Only in relation to *Staphylococcus aureus* food poisoning does the food handler play an important role, particularly with foods that are much handled during preparation and not reheated before final consumption. Food handlers who continue to work with active symptoms of gastroenteritis are a hazard in the food preparation area because of the increased risk of intestinal organisms reaching food. Many people who constantly handle raw foods, particularly those of animal origin, often become asymptomatic excretors and may carry organisms on their hands. Provided that they have good hand hygiene and pass formed stools, such individuals are not a major risk in food preparation. It should be noted that individuals suffering from infection by food poisoning bacteria and individuals who are carriers of food poisoning bacteria must not be allowed in the food area according to Food Hygiene Regulations (1970).

However, most people carry some type of food poisoning organism at one time or another, and food handlers have a moral and legal obligation to observe high standards of personal cleanliness to ensure that they do not contaminate food.

In commercial food processing environments critical contact surfaces not only include food and food preparation surfaces but also hand contact surfaces, such as waste bins, dishcloths and, in particular, handles in the toilet and bathroom. Incidences in which hand contact and transfer surfaces are implicated as the source or route of transfer of contamination are regularly reported. Thus appropriate disinfection procedures of inanimate objects or surfaces should be rigorously enforced as well as good personal hygiene.

Current evidence suggests that one of the most important routes of transfer of contamination is via the skin surface – mainly the hands. The subject of skin disinfection and its role in the prevention of cross-contamination has been recently reviewed (Reybrouk, 1986).

Food handlers can unwittingly pass on harmful food poisoning bacteria from their nose, throat, hair, skin, bowels and urinary tract or clothing, and this possibility of contamination underlines the importance of personal cleanliness and the adoption of hygienic practices by every member of staff. Open cuts or sores on the skin usually harbour harmful bacteria and must be covered by suitable waterproof dressing, preferably coloured blue or green to aid detection if they become detached. Cuts on fingers may need the extra protection of waterproof fingerstalls. Some people may be carriers of food poisoning bacteria even though they apparently seem fit and well. Food handlers must therefore take every precaution to ensure that harmful bacteria are not passed on to food or food contact surfaces. An obvious precaution is not to sneeze or cough over food, nor shake a handkerchief near it (disposable paper handkerchiefs should be used). A less obvious precaution is to avoid touching the lips or nose. Nose picking and finger licking are objectionable at any time, and wiping the hands on the apron should be avoided. Personnel must wear clean and washable overclothing, including head covering which completely encloses the hair. The use of any tobacco material is not allowed in any food room and food handlers should not eat sweets nor chew gum.

The principal danger, of course, comes from the hands. All food processing workers must realize that in their hands lies the health of their customers. It is desirable that they acquire a feeling of acute discomfort whenever their hands are unwashed. It is, therefore, imperative that fingers, hands and forearms should be meticulously clean. Nails should be kept short, well trimmed and clean and free from nail varnish. Jewellery and watches should not be worn at the site of work. Strong-smelling perfume should not be worn by food handlers, as it may taint foods, especially those of high fat content. Hands and wrists (and, for some food tasks, the forearms also) should be washed each time they enter the food preparation area, and frequently during the course of their work, particularly if they touch something unconnected with the task in hand.

The most important single rule of good food hygiene is as follows: always wash your hands after visiting the toilet or bathroom. This should be regarded by everyone as a necessary and well-mannered social habit. If this simple rule was universally followed, there would be a remarkable decrease in the spread of intestinal infections. Management should encourage their staff to obey it by providing fully equipped, clean washbasins – with hot and cold water supplies or hot water at a suitably controlled temperature, soap or other suitable detergent and nailbrush – close to the conveniences, and placing prominent 'Wash your Hands' notices as required by law. Hand-washing basins must not be used for washing food or food processing equipment, and food sinks must not be used for washing hands. Toilet paper is porous, and bacteria tend to lurk under finger nails, so that hand washing may not be fully effective without the aid of hot water and a nailbrush. Efficient drying of hands, which is also important, may be achieved by using disposable paper towels or continuous roller towels or hot air dryers. However, the latter can distribute microbes by aerosols and, of course, it is essential that the hand-drying surfaces of cloth towels are clean.

Frequent inspection should ensure that appropriate washing facilities are available and that notices are in position. Some managers carry out inspections at regular intervals in order to make sure that hands are being kept clean. There is, however, a tendency to resent such supervision and those who need it are probably unsatisfactory in other ways. The answer is appropriate food hygiene education. All food handlers must by law receive appropriate food hygiene education to ensure that they are aware of the dangers of poor food hygiene and that they have intimate knowledge of how to break the chain of events which may result in outbreaks of food poisoning. Posters on this and other aspects of food hygiene could, with advantage, be put in suitable places in the working environment. However, they should be pasted so firmly to the walls that they will not provide hiding places for dirt and insects.

To sum up, rules for personal hygiene in food handlers are necessary. If the rules are to be followed, they have to be explained and understood. This involves a training programme. The rules will be more meaningful and are more likely to be followed if they are linked with a cultural pattern of cleanliness in food preparation in particular.

Antiseptic Products

Removal or destruction of microbial flora from the skin, as opposed to hard surfaces, represents a particular problem. Experimental investigations indicate that, although reduction in skin flora can reduce the probability of contamination transfer, total elimination of bacteria from skin surfaces is not achievable.

The flora of healthy skin can be divided into two groups: the 'resident' and the 'transient' microorganisms. The residents are the true skin flora, whilst the transients include any microorganism which could survive after being deposited on the skin. Seen in relation to skin cleansing and disinfection, the important difference between resident and transient microorganisms is their ease of removal and killing. The numbers of transients may be quite effectively reduced by cleansing, and virtually eliminated by disinfection. However, cleansing alone is ineffective at reducing the numbers of residents, and disinfection is required to achieve this. The dividing line between these two groups of skin flora is not sharp, and the ease of removal or killing of transient microorganisms is likely to vary with the circumstances under which they become attached to the skin.

Soap

Washing with simple soap and water can be shown to have little effect on the resident microflora of the skin, unless vigorously performed for several minutes using a scrubbing brush, as in the ritual of the 'surgical scrub'. This procedure, however, damages the skin and encourages subsequent colonization by pathogenic microorganisms.

In contrast to the effect on resident microorganisms, washing with soap and water can be shown to reduce considerably the numbers of transient bacteria which have been applied to the skin and allowed to dry. The effect, however, if far less complete if the bacterial inoculum is first rubbed into the skin before being allowed to dry.

Apart from its generally poor antimicrobial effect, soap has other undesirable features. It is highly alkaline and, therefore, is not only relatively harsh but also tends to reduce the valuable acidity of the skin. Soap also decreases the concentration of another major component of the skin, the surface lipids, which have important physical and antimicrobial functions.

Synthetic detergents were introduced over 50 years ago as alternatives. They avoid the alkalinity of soap and do not precipitate calcium or magnesium salts in hard water. They do, however, have a tendency to degrease the skin excessively. This can be minimized by the addition of suitable emollients to the formulation, e.g. glycerol and lanolin. *See* Cleaning Procedures in the Factory, Types of Detergent

Recent reports of the isolation of microorganisms from used soap bars and bar soap dish fluids have raised concern that bacteria may be transferred from contaminated soap bars during hand washing. This concern can be eliminated by the use of liquid soaps or detergents from appropriate dispensers, and their use is recommended.

Microporous barrier creams are now available that prevent any material becoming ingrained in the skin. They are formulated to be effective shortly after application and last for periods up to 4 h, i.e. covering the normal break periods. They protect against contact allergies, dry chapped hands and maintain the ecobalance of the skin. During the 4-h period, protection is maintained through regular immersion in water. Soilage and bacteria are readily removed with soap and water. Silicone is used to seal in moisture and seal out problems. As with any product which comes into contact with food, they must be odourless, nontainting, nontoxic and nongreasy. The packaging of these creams should be given due consideration in that it is preferable to have dedicated tubes of cream than communal dispensers in order to minimize cross-contamination. The use of these creams in combination with a good cleansing regimen provides effective hand hygiene.

If hands are washed with soap and water and rinsed, a reduction of 10^3 in numbers of applied microorganisms may be obtained, whereas an application of 70% ethanol may give a reduction of 10^5. The question then is whether or not washing with soap and water is sufficient.

Hand disinfection is only necessary in critical situations, e.g. when the handling of high-risk food is unavoidable, or to protect food handlers such as fish filleters from developing septic cuts. In the majority of food handling situations, washing the hands properly in hot water using liquid soap is quite satisfactory. If hand disinfection is considered necessary it should be carried out after normal hand washing. Hand disinfectants should be fast-acting, rapid-drying, nontoxic and non-tainting to food and contain ingredients to protect the skin.

Choosing an Antiseptic

The choice of antiseptic depends on many factors, including the following:

1. Amount of soiling.
2. Contact-time available.
3. Type of microorganism that needs to be destroyed.
4. Way it is to be used.
5. Effect on the environment.
6. Cost.

The majority of formulations currently used for disinfection purposes are based on one or a combination of a limited range of chemical agents. They can be formulated with a detergent in a single cleansing and disinfection product but a two-step process is preferable. *See* Cleaning Procedures in the Factory, Types of Disinfectant

Alcohols

Alcohols commonly used for their disinfectant properties include ethanol and isopropanol. They have rapid action and their volatility is especially useful as a rapidly-drying skin disinfectant. Alcohols can be used as a base for other agents, such as chlorhexidine and Triclosan. Alcohol-impregnated wipes are available for convenience.

Ethanol is widely used for skin disinfection and a 70% solution is generally considered to be the most effective against a broad range of microorganisms. Higher concentrations are thought to precipitate surface proteins and thereby inhibit or retard penetration.

Isopropanol is more lipophilic and a little more active than ethanol. Many formulations contain 60–70% isopropanol.

Alcohols do not penetrate well into organic matter and should be used only on clean surfaces. They are, of course, inflammable and care should be taken to ensure they are stored and used correctly.

Amphoteric Surfactants

Amphoterics exhibit bactericidal activity in acid solutions. They are good detergents but are relatively expensive and exhibit limited antibacterial activity. Furthermore, they are inactivated by many materials. Despite these disadvantages they are used in skin disinfectants.

Bi(Di)guanides

Biguanides are cationic bactericides, similar in function to quaternary ammonium compounds (QACs) but with better all-round performance. They have no wetting properties and are therefore formulated with nonionic surfactants.

Chlorhexidine is gaining widespread international acceptance as an effective antiseptic. It is usually used as the dihydrochloride or digluconate; the digluconate being one of its most water-soluble forms. Although it shows higher activity against Gram-positives than Gram-negatives. The effect is thought to be less pronounced than that seen with QACs. It has good activity against fungi but is poor against spores and viruses. The high substantivity and rapid activity are important properties. It is inactivated by organic matter, soap and anionic detergents.

Chlorine-releasing Compounds

A large number of antimicrobial chlorine compounds are commercially available, but those used as a skin antiseptic and surface disinfectant fall into two main groups: hypochlorites and organic chlorine compounds. Both act by producing hypochlorous acid.

Properly used, these agents are amongst the most suitable for the food industry. The commonest are hypochlorites and the most useful is sodium hypochlorite which disinfects by oxidation of protein. Hypochlorous acid can also be generated in solution from organic solid compounds such as sodium dichloroisocyanurate. Their use can overcome storage instability problems associated with sodium hypochlorite solutions.

Sodium hypochlorite is normally supplied in solution containing 1–10% available chlorine (av.Cl) and should be diluted to between 100 and 1000 ppm av. Cl for disinfection of inanimate objects. For skin disinfection purposes they are used as short-time contact dips into isotonic solutions of 500 to 1000 ppm av.Cl.

Hypochlorites are relatively cheap and have a wide range of bactericidal, fungicidal and viricidal activity. They are anionic and unaffected by hard water. However, they have a pungent odour, exhibit staining or bleaching characteristics, are corrosive to metal and readily inactivated by organic matter. For this reason they are not used extensively for skin disinfection purposes. However, they may be used if hypochlorous acid is generally used in the food preparation area.

Quaternary Ammonium Compounds

Quaternary ammonium compounds now account for a significant proportion of antiseptic products in use. Well-known members of this group are benzalkonium chloride, cetalkonium chloride and cetrimide (often combined with chlorhexidine).

Cationic in nature, QACs are safe, odour-free, non-corrosive, stable and taint-free bactericides with inherent detergency properties. They have a narrow range of activity and are not very effective against Gram-negative bacteria. Activity against *Pseudomonas aeruginosa* is a major weakness of QACs, although most of the other antiseptics in common use also suffer from this. Activity can be enhanced by the addition of ethylenediaminetetraacetic acid (EDTA) to the formulation. They are more effective in alkaline solutions but are seriously affected by soaps, anionic detergents and organic matter.

Triclosan

Triclosan, which is frequently referred to by its trade name, Irgasan DP 300, is commonly included in soap and detergent formulations. It is more active against Gram-positives than Gram-negatives, and has little 'cidal' activity. It is slow-acting and, therefore, not suitable where single applications are intended. Triclosan's use lies mainly in formulations when repeat applications, leading to cumulative activity, are likely owing to its high substantivity. Single hand washing with triclosan-containing soap, for example, produces no greater reduction in skin flora than soap alone, whereas repeat applications do.

Other Agents

Modified phenolics are little used, except for chloroxylenols such as *p*-chloro-*m*-xylenol (PCMX). Halogenation of the phenol group increases its antimicrobial properties. Chloroxylenols have adequate activity against Gram-positive bacteria, but poor activity against some Gram-negative bacteria, which can be improved by the

addition of chelating agents such as EDTA. The spectrum of activity of PCMX is improved by the addition of Nonoxynol-9, an antimicrobial spermicide. These type of agents are easily inactivated by a wide range of materials.

At present there is no official UK standard for antiseptics in the food industry, and users should satisfy themselves that a product is suitable for the intended use. This situation is presently being addressed at the EEC level (Comité Européen de Normalisation-CEN/TC 216/Working Group 1) and will allow products for the skin to be evaluated and developed on a more rational basis, at the same time ensuring that products satisfy most user requirements at the outset.

Although 'in-use' disinfection failures associated with the occurrence of resistant organisms may be difficult to identify, the importance of 'limited activity' of most of the above agents is well illustrated by reports in which typically resistant Gram-negatives, such as the pseudomonads, are found as contaminants of the antiseptics themselves. The majority of such reports relate to phenolic-, QAC- or chlorhexidine-containing formulations. Perhaps one of the worrying aspects is the fact that despite considerable improvements in good manufacturing practice (GMP) involving handling, dilution, packaging, shelf-life control, etc., there is little evidence of any reduction in the frequency of occurrence of contaminated antiseptics in recent years.

Use of Rubber Gloves

Glove wearing by handlers of sensitive products may be rational, but work by the Heinz Company has shown that in one particular case, the stripping of chicken meat off bones, after the same period of time there was a higher bacterial count on the gloves than on bare hands washed regularly, so that in this process glove wearing is less satisfactory than regular hand washing. However, it should be noted that regular washing of gloved hands may well be effective, as found in health care studies. Other disadvantages associated with the use of gloves are hole formation, possibility of contact allergies, skin flora growth under occlusion, and loss of dexterity. It seems that the disadvantages outweigh the possible advantages, and hence wearing of gloves is not the solution.

Conclusion

Every person involved in the preparation of food must be aware that very few foods that enter the food processing area are sterile. Most foods will be contaminated to a greater or lesser extent according to the amount of heat processing and other manipulations. The majority of factors which contribute towards a relatively harmless food being made harmful can be grouped as either attributable to poor temperature control or to cross-contamination. Thus, although improvement in agricultural practices can lead to the reduction in the presence of some organisms in our foods (e.g. *Salmonella* and *Campylobacter*), good hygienic food preparation and education of food handlers are the final lines of defence in the prevention of most types of foodborne illness.

Bibliography

Block SS (1991) *Disinfection, Sterilization and Preservation.* Philadelphia: Lea and Febiger. London: Williams and Wilkins.

Doyle MP (ed.) (1989) *Foodborne Bacterial Pathogens.* New York: Marcel Dekker.
Nobel WC (1981) *Microbiology of Human Skin.* London: Lloyd-Luke.
Reybrouk G (1986) Handwashing and Hand Disinfection. *Journal of Hospital Hygiene Infection* 8: 5–23.
Russell AD, Hugo WB and Ayliffe GAJ (1982) *Principles and Practice of Disinfection, Preservation and Sterilisation.* Oxford: Blackwell Scientific Publications.
Springer RA (1991) *Hygiene for Management. A Text for Food Hygiene Courses.* Doncaster: Highfield Publications.

B. F. Perry
Procter & Gamble Ltd, Egham, UK

APPETITE

See Satiety and Appetite

APPLES

The apple is probably the most widely distributed of tree fruits cultivated in the world. The varieties of apple grown commercially today derive mainly from *Malus pumila* Mill., and are thought to have originated from natural mutations and hybridizations between *Malus* species growing in the Caucasus and the area around Turkestan. With subsequent cultivation, selection and hybridization by man, apple culture spread, in the period 2000–0 BC, via the 'Fertile Crescent' of the Middle East eastwards and also westwards to Europe, whence apples were later introduced into North America and the Southern Hemisphere.

Apples provide an important component of the fresh fruit industry, not only because there is a long span (*c.* 100 days) of maturation dates on the tree for fruits of different varieties but also because some varieties can be stored for long periods in refrigerated and controlled atmosphere (CA) conditions. Some varieties of apple, often with higher acid and tannin contents than dessert apples, are grown specially for hard cider production. Nutritionally, the apple provides sugars and useful amounts of dietary fibre, potassium and vitamin C. *See* Acids, Natural Acids and Acidulants; Ascorbic Acid,

Properties and Determination; Controlled Atmosphere Storage, Effect on Fruit and Vegetables; Dietary Fibre, Properties and Sources; Tannins and Polyphenols

Global Distribution

The principal areas of apple production are located approximately between the latitudes 30° and 60°, although apples are also grown in lower latitudes at higher altitudes, e.g. in Mexico and Central Africa.

Cropping varies annually according to climatic variations. However, about 35% of the annual world production of apples, which averaged around 40×10^6 t over the past 5 years, was accounted for by European orchards, mainly in France, Germany and Italy. A further 30% was attributable to Asian production, mainly in China, Korea and Japan. The annual production of apples in the USSR is slightly higher than that of North and Central America, which is dominated by the 4×10^6 t produced annually by the fruit industry in the USA, and double that of South America. *See* Fruits of Temperate Climates, Commercial and Dietary Importance

Exports of apples from Argentina, Chile, New Zealand, South Africa and Western Australia to the Northern Hemisphere fill gaps (April–August) and sell at a premium in markets where the regionally grown fruit has been stored for 6 months or more. Production of apples has expanded rapidly in some countries during the past few years, notably in Brazil, China, Korea and Turkey, as recently planted orchards have come into production.

Apple Varieties

Although there are now 2000–3000 named apple varieties, only a few are grown commercially. Apart from the obvious requirements of fruit growers for trees that are (1) resistant to adverse climatic conditions and to the various pests and diseases rife in orchards, (2) come into cropping rapidly and (3) consistently bear large numbers of good-quality fruit, the demands of the market have also to be met. The marketing chains of the developed countries, where much of the fresh fruit is handled, require constant supplies of firm, well-shaped, unblemished apples, of specified size and colour, which are free from pathological and physiological disorders. These requirements are apparently met by the 30 or so varieties that account for most of the world production of dessert and culinary apples, although these are not necessarily the most highly flavoured. At the head of the list are Golden Delicious and the various strains of Red Delicious, Granny Smith, Jonathan, McIntosh and Antonovka. The market dominance of these few varieties is likely to persist for some time because it takes many (12 or more) years for fruit breeders to demonstrate the commercial possibilities of a new variety, more for it to gain acceptance and even more for it to be grown widely. Varieties currently becoming more widespread are Jonagold, Elstar, Gala and Fuji.

Fruit breeders are now working to improve flavour, resistance to storage disorders (e.g. Spartan is resistant to low temperature breakdown; see Table 2), and long storage characteristics in apples (e.g. as in Malling Fiesta). Attention is also being given to improving rootstocks on which the scion varieties of apple are usually budded or grafted. Modern orchard systems favour dwarfing rootstocks, not only for precocity in production but also for ease of orchard management and harvesting. The future productivity of orchards may be increased by high-density plantings of the newly introduced columnar varieties (i.e. single-stemmed trees bearing heavy crops of apples on short spurs).

Apples are broadly categorized according to their use, i.e. dessert, culinary and cider varieties, although there are overlaps of usage in all categories. In some regions culinary apples are more acid (e.g. Bramley's Seedling in Table 1). Cider apples, often very old varieties, may be

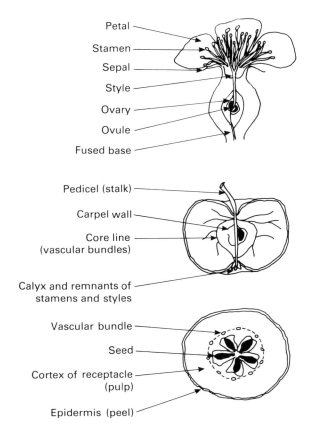

Fig. 1 Flower and fruit of the apple (diagrammatic representation). After Hulme AC and Rhodes MJC (1971) Pome Fruits. In: Hulme AC (ed.) *The Biochemistry of Fruits and their Products*, vol. 2, p 336.

sweet, bittersweet or sharp, and are usually blended prior to pressing to produce the finest hard ciders.

The Structure of the Fruit

The apple is a pome fruit consisting of five ovaries with carpellary tissues embedded in fleshy, edible tissue which is usually regarded as the swollen fused base of the calyx (sepals), corolla (petals) and stamens. With the exception of the petals, developed forms or remnants of all the original parts of the flower are to be found in the mature fruit (see Fig. 1). Alternatively, a pome fruit is sometimes regarded as a swollen receptacle.

Fruits might be described as roughly spherical, but they vary with species and variety from the extremely oblate to conical, and from about 0·5 to 30 cm diameter. In most cases surface colour is green, changing to yellow with ripening, suffused with varying amounts of red or brown. Their skins may be smooth or russeted.

The growth of the fruit from the flower is characterized by a short period of cell division of up to 6 weeks after full bloom, followed by cell enlargement and the development of intercellular spaces. The ovary and the

Table 1. The approximate chemical composition (per kg of fresh weight) of five varieties of apple measured soon after harvest

Variety	Dry matter (g)	Sugars Total (g)	Sugars Reducing (g)	Titratable acids (as malic) (g)	Starch (g)	Pectin (g)	N (mg)	K (mg)	P (mg)	Mg (mg)	Ca[a] (mg)
Golden Delicious	140	127	107	3·7	5	11	360	1060	100	40	50
Red Delicious	145	121	105	2·4	10	12	420	1150	80	50	47
McIntosh	137	116	86	5·6	5	9	400	1330	100	40	50
Cox's Orange Pippin	150	120	70	7·0	5	7	650	1300	130	50	50
Bramley's Seedling	125	90	60	12·5	4	8	550	1100	100	40	40

[a] Inversely related to mean fruit weight within a variety.
N, nitrogen, K, potassium; P, phosphorus; Mg, magnesium; Ca, calcium.

tissues within the core line develop more rapidly than the major portion of the outer cortex, which swells faster after the time when the seeds (numbering 0–25, depending on variety and orchard treatments) are fully grown. The layer of epidermal cells and the underlying layers of closely packed, thick-walled hypodermal cells become radially flattened and tangentially elongated, the cuticular layer of waxes over the epidermis thickens and extends between the epidermal cells, and openings in the peel (known as lenticels) develop. Water and nutrients pass into the fruit through the stalk, which divides into the vascular system, the main bundles of which delineate the core of the mature fruit.

Intercellular spaces, which account for about 25% of the volume of the parenchyma in mature apples, allow gases, including water vapour, to diffuse rapidly within the fruit and lower the specific gravity (compared with water at 4°C) of apples to below unity (e.g. 0·85 in Cox's Orange Pippin fruit). The numbers of lenticels varies within and between fruit varieties from hundreds to thousands per fruit. Lenticels may be open, or closed by suberin or cutin. The calyx 'eye' of the apple may also be open or closed according to variety. Apples with open calyces can be subject to fungal infections of the core. The layer of cutin may thicken and become more oily during the storage of apples.

The Chemical Composition of Apples

The greater part of the fresh weight of an apple is water. The remainder is referred to as dry matter or dry weight. Expression of analytical results on fresh matter (as in Table 1) is preferable to using a dry-matter basis, not only because of the difficulty of accurately measuring the concentration of apple dry matter (which is extremely hygroscopic) but also because the dry matter : water ratio in the whole fruit changes continuously on the tree and during storage, varies within the apple, and is altered by orchard treatments and climatic effects. The

mass of an apple when sampled provides a reasonable primary standard.

The dry matter is composed mainly of sugars, with lesser amounts of acids, sorbitol and the structural materials (cellulose, hemicelluloses and pectic substances), the reserve carbohydrate, starch, and protein. Here again, the ratios of these compounds vary continuously in the fruit, on the tree and during storage. Acid and starch concentrations decline progressively prior to and during harvest, as well as during storage. The metabolism of starch results in an increase in the concentration of sugars, mainly sucrose. *See* Starch, Structure, Properties and Determination; Sucrose, Properties and Determination

At harvest, the main sugars present are sucrose and fructose, in approximately equal amounts, with less glucose. About 90% of the acid is malic, the remainder being mainly citric. Additional to the constituents shown in Table 1 are cellulose and hemicelluloses (about 1·5% of the fresh weight) and fats (including oils and waxes) and protein, which (including soluble amino acids with the protein) each account for another 0·3% of the fresh weight of an apple. Phenolic compounds, some of which impart astringency to the fruit, contribute another 0·2%. The concentration of ascorbic acid (vitamin C) can range from 50 to 300 mg per kg, but it declines in store. Traces of chlorophyll, carotenoids and anthocyanins impart colour to the fruit, and aroma results from subtle blends of traces of the 250 or so volatile esters, alcohols, aldehydes, essential oils, etc., detected in apples. Potassium is the main mineral constituent (Table 1). *See* Cellulose; Colours, Properties and Determination of Natural Pigments; Essential Oils, Properties and Uses; Fructose; Hemicelluloses; Phenolic Compounds *see also* individual minerals

In addition to changes associated with ripening, the chemical composition of the fruit is altered by climatic conditions, cropping levels, orchard treatments and, in particular, by variety (Table 1). Concentrations of constituents also vary between fruits from the same tree and, to a greater extent, within individual apples. No gradients of concentration within an apple are the same for any two constituents, so that it is impossible to generalize. Concentration gradients occur transversely and longitudinally across apples and also around the calyx–stalk axes. The chemical composition of stalks and seeds differs greatly from that of the remainder of the fruit; hence they are usually removed prior to fruit analyses. The stalks approximate in composition to the wood of the tree. The seeds are high in dry matter (c. 50% of the fresh weight), mainly fats, protein and fibre, also some minerals, e.g. phosphorus, magnesium, iron and manganese. *See* Ripening of Fruit

One kilogram of fresh apples provides approximately 2100 kJ (500 kcal) of energy. Excluding the peel and cores of apples from the diet almost halves the amounts of vitamin C and dietary fibre available in the whole fruit (e.g. to about 30 mg per kg and 16 g per kg fresh weight of stored apples respectively) but makes little difference to the sugar content. *See* Dietary Fibre, Properties and Sources

Handling, Storage and Marketing

Apples bruise easily, so care must be exercised throughout harvesting and post-harvest handling. Thus careful hand-picking is the preferred method of harvesting apples for the fresh fruit market. Mechanical harvesters are available: tree or limb shakers combined with catching frames are used for larger trees when the apples are destined mainly for processing. Machines that comb or air-blast fruits onto padded conveyor belts can be used on specially formed rows of dwarf trees. Cider apples can be allowed to drop and be swept from the orchard floor using machines with spiked collectors or suction systems.

The first stage after harvesting is the removal of field heat from the crop as rapidly as possible. Apples are often transported from the orchard in bulk bins made of wood or plastic holding 300–700 kg of fruit, depending on varietal susceptibility to pressure damage. Apples can be stored in three ways. The simplest and most short-term procedure is barn or common storage: the fruit is kept in compartments (buildings or caves), ventilated with cool air. Refrigeration provides longer storage: the fruit is stacked in well-insulated chambers, cooled and maintained at the requisite temperature by circulating refrigerated air. The longest storage is provided by CA conditions: the fruit is sealed in gas-proof, refrigerated chambers maintained at the desired temperature with in-store concentrations of gases (oxygen, carbon dioxide, and nitrogen) kept at specified levels. For this method, provision must be made for monitoring and controlling gas concentrations in each chamber

and for continuous equilibration of internal and atmospheric pressures to prevent structural damage to the store. Gas samples can be withdrawn, analysed and recorded manually, and adjustments to gas concentrations made accordingly. However, modern instruments allow precise, continuous measurements and adjustments of carbon dioxide and oxygen concentrations automatically under computerized control. The latter procedure permits apples to be stored for the maximum period possible. Thus the oxygen concentration may be maintained slightly above the level (1–3% according to variety) at which anaerobic respiration, alcohol accumulation and rapid deterioration occur; checks may also be made on the level of alcohol vapour in the store. *See* Controlled Atmosphere Storage, Effect on Fruit and Vegetables; Storage Stability, Mechanisms of Degradation

The desired concentrations of gases may be achieved by allowing the apples, which are respiring rapidly before they are fully cooled, to reduce the oxygen concentration of the store to the required level over a few days. The resultant carbon dioxide is removed by scrubbing, i.e. pumping store gases through externally located, absorbent materials such as lime or activated carbon. Alternatively, the oxygen concentration in the store may be reduced rapidly, either by flushing with nitrogen or by burning off the oxygen, or by circulating the gas mixture via hollow-fibre membranes through which oxygen and nitrogen diffuse at different rates.

Recent research has shown that the maintenance of very low concentrations of ethylene (<0.1 ppm) in CA stores has the advantage of delaying fruit softening and the onset of physiological disorders.

Stores may be small or large (capacities of tens or hundreds of tonnes), their size being dependent on the rate at which the apples can be marketed after the store is opened. They may be owned and controlled by individual growers, or centralized, in which case the control of harvesting, storage and marketing is often vested in growers' cooperatives.

Apples put into stores should be preclimacteric (i.e. at the stage before their characteristic surge in respiration rate occurs) but not too immature. The object of storage is to reduce fruit respiration, delay ripening and minimize losses due to various disorders and shrivelling. The choice of storage conditions is governed by the susceptibility of any particular apple variety to injuries caused by low temperatures (e.g. freezing injury and low temperature breakdown) or gas concentrations (e.g. core flush and brown heart) and by interactions between storage temperature and gas concentrations. Recommended conditions, such as the examples shown in Table 2, differ for every apple variety and result from many years of experimental tests and commercial experience. In general, early apples (e.g. Discovery in Table 2) store less well than late maturing varieties such

Table 2. Recommended storage conditions for the main varieties of apple grown in England[a]

| | Air storage | | Controlled atmosphere (CA) | | | | | | |
| | | | | No scrubber | | Using a scrubber | | | |
Variety	Temperature (°C)	Terminate (month)	Temperature (°C)	Carbon dioxide (%)	Terminate (month)	Carbon dioxide (%)	Oxygen (%)	Terminate (month)
Bramley's Seedling	3·0–4·0	January	4·0–4·5	8–10	June	6	2	June
Cox's Orange Pippin	3·0–3·5	Mid-December	3·5–4·0	5	Early January	5	3	Mid-February
			3·5–4·0			<1	2	Late March
			3·5–4·0			<1	1·25	Late April
			3·5–4·0			<1	1·0	Early May
Mutsu	1·5–2·0	January	3·5–4·0	8	May	—	—	—
Discovery	3·0–3·5	End August	3·0–3·5	8	Mid-September	<1	2	Mid-September
Spartan	0–0·5	January	1·5–2·0	—	—	<1	2	March
			1·5–2·0	—	—	6	2	June

[a] Unless otherwise stated, the terminal date for each set of conditions allows for a further 2 weeks at ambient temperatures to cover grading and distribution.
Abridged from Table 1 of Sharples RO and Stow JR (1986) *Report of the East Malling Research Station for 1985*, pp 165–170. Courtesy of Horticultural Research International.

as Granny Smith. For any given variety of apple, length of storage and susceptibility to disorders is modified by climactic conditions and orchard treatments, and by the maturity of the fruit when harvested.

In addition to the injuries noted above, physiological disorders such as senescent breakdown, bitter pit and superficial scald can occur. Pathological disorders may also develop. Hence preventative measures are taken in the orchard (using sprays of calcium and fungicides) or, in certain countries, after harvest (using dips or drenches containing fungicides, calcium or antioxidants). Maturity tests (e.g. ethylene, starch and firmness) and analyses for nitrogen, phosphorus, potassium, calcium and magnesium on samples of apples taken in the weeks prior to harvest, and on samples of the harvested apples, facilitate the final choice of storage periods and conditions for particular batches of fruit. Good sampling and analytical techniques are required for mineral analyses of apples because small differences in mineral concentrations can lead to large differences in storage potential. Ten or so disorders, occurring in the orchard or in storage, are associated with deficiencies of calcium in the fruit. *See* Antioxidants, Synthetic Antioxidants; Fungicides

Apples may be stored in bins or graded and packed into smaller containers prior to storage. Size or weight grading is mechanized; grading for shape, blemishes and colour is normally done manually, although instrumental techniques are being introduced. At the grading stage, the natural wax is sometimes removed and replaced by artificial mixtures.

Apples are ideally marketed via a refrigerated chain. Modified atmosphere (MA) packaging further ensures that apples reach the consumer in perfect condition: MA packs are made of permeable plastic films chosen to provide ideal gas concentrations around the fruits sealed within. *See* Chilled Storage, Effect of Modified Atmosphere Packaging on Food Quality

Industrial Utilization

Juice from pressed apples may be marketed (sometimes blended with other fruit juices) or used to produce hard cider. This, in turn, may be distilled to make apple brandy (e.g. Applejack in the USA, Calvados in northwest France) or acetified to cider vinegar. The pressed residue, i.e. the pomace, is used as fodder for sheep and cattle, either in fresh, preserved or dried form, or as silage. Fresh or specially preserved pomace is used for the manufacture of pectin. Peel and cores discarded during apple processing also provide a rich source of pectin, which is at higher concentrations in these than in other zones of the fruit. Apple pulp is sliced, chopped, flaked or puréed and then canned, frozen or dried for direct sales or for further processing into sauces, baby foods, pies, etc. Pomace can also provide cellulose in the hydrogel form used in the food industry, as well as an extremely porous, low-ash carbon.

Bibliography

Alston FH (in press) Flavour improvement in apples and pears through plant breeding. Williams AA (ed.) Proceedings of the Conference on Bioformation of Flavours. Royal Society of Chemistry, Cambridge.
Bramlage WJ (ed.) (1987) Factors that influence commodity response to controlled atmosphere storage. *Hort Science* 22(5): 761–794.
Downing DL (ed.) (1989) *Processed Apple Products*. New York: AVI, Van Nostrand Reinhold.
Fidler JC, Wilkinson BG, Edney KL and Sharples RO (1973) *The Biology of Apple and Pear Storage*. Slough: Commonwealth Agricultural Bureaux.
Hulme AC (ed.) (1971) *The Biochemistry of Fruits and their Products*, vols 1 and 2. London: Academic Press.

Knee M (1985) Evaluating the practical significance of ethylene in fruit storage. In: Roberts JA and Tucker GA (eds) *Ethylene and Plant Development*, pp 297–315. Oxford: Butterworth.

Ministry of Agriculture, Fisheries and Food (1979) *Refrigerated Storage of Fruit and Vegetables*. Reference Book 324. London: Her Majesty's Stationery Office.

Perring MA (1989) Apple fruit quality in relation to fruit chemical composition. *Acta Horticulturae* 258: 365–372.

Smock RM and Neubert AM (1950) *Apples and Apple Products*. New York: Interscience Publishers.

Snowdon AL (1990) *A Colour Atlas of Post-Harvest Diseases and Disorders of Fruit and Vegetables*, vol. 1. London: Wolfe Scientific.

M. A. Perring
Bearsted, Maidstone, UK

APRICOTS*

Apricots are one of the most ancient crops produced by man and the fruit is grown on every continent of the globe. Most apricot production in the world is centred in Europe and Asia with lesser production in the Americas, Africa and Oceania. In the USSR, after years of collection and evaluation, there are as many as 1800 cultivars and forms of *Prunus armeniaca* and in China there are more than 2000 cultivars, many of which are purported to be widely adapted, large-fruited and of excellent quality. The apricot is generally adapted to narrow climatic areas. As a result of narrow adaptation, favourable local varieties are not always produced economically in other regions. Apricots are soft fruits with a hard stone (stone fruits) and are generally sensitive to disease and to high or low temperatures. Apricots have outstanding organoleptic qualities and the fruit is high in fibre and vitamins, making it ideal in the human diet. Consequently, this versatile fruit is consumed in fresh, canned, dried and other processed forms. The varied germplasm which exists in the world is being utilized to improve existing apricot cultivars, helping to ensure a continued supply of high-quality, healthy apricots for the world population.

Global Distribution and Relative Commercial Importance

Apricot production in the USSR is located primarily in Armenia, the Central Asian Republics (Uzbekistan, Tajikistan, Turkmenistan), the Northern Caucasus (Krasnodar region, Daghestan and Kabardino-Balkarsk ASSR). Smaller growing regions exist in Azerbaijan, Georgia, Kirghizia and Kazakhstan.

Apricots are grown in the Mediterranean region,

Spain, Tunisia, France, Italy, Yugoslavia, Turkey, Morocco, Greece, Israel, Portugal and Algeria. The central and western Mediterranean countries produce more than one third of the world's production of apricots. Apricot cultivars of the Near East include cultivars found in Iran, Iraq, Afghanistan, Pakistan and Turkey. Existing local varieties and ecotypes were developed by growers and horticulturists, and many small orchards today consist of wild seedlings mixed with cultivated forms. Turkey produces many of the world's apricots and there are an estimated 10×10^6 trees, of which about 50% are budded. Most of the fruit is consumed fresh; the remainder is dried and some of that is exported. In Iran there are an estimated 8996 ha (22 230 acres) of apricots. Most of the apricots are consumed fresh or dried both in Iran and in the previously mentioned countries. The apricots grown in Iraq and Pakistan are mostly generated by seed and consequently there is a wide variation in productivity from year to year.

In Australia and New Zealand, apricots are planted to a limited extent. In 1990, it was reported that approximately 27 300 and 7800 t of apricots were produced in Australia and New Zealand, respectively. Approximately 90% of Australia's apricots are produced in the River Murray irrigation areas in South Australia and Victoria and along the tributaries of the Murray in New South Wales and Victoria. Most of the apricots are dried. In New Zealand the main area of production (85%) is located in the South Island in the Central Otago region. Hawke's Bay is another apricot-producing area in New Zealand. In contrast to Australia, 60% of New Zealand's apricot production is sold fresh and 35% processed. South Africa produced approximately 46 000 t of apricots in 1990 (see Table 1).

China appears to possess the most extensive repository of apricot and related germplasm in the world. There are eight species in the *Armeniaca* genus located in China, four of which include the common apricot

---

* The colour plate section for this article appears between p. 556 and p. 557.

Table 1. Apricot production and utilization 1989–1990 in major producing/trading countries

Country and year	Total production (t)	Commercial production (t)	Domestic fresh consumption (t)	Processed (t)
France				
1989	130 000	114 000	101 200	15 000
1990	107 500	94 300	77 400	15 000
Greece				
1989	83 875	83 875	15 603	39 621
1990	113 360	113 360	10 273	41 880
Italy				
1989	189 000	181 000	166 725	30 000
1990	181 500	175 000	161 490	30 000
Spain				
1989	155 600	149 900	90 000	45 000
1990	115 200	110 600	63 800	40 000
Turkey				
1989	445 000	445 000	152 785	289 250
1990	400 000	400 000	137 000	260 000
Yugoslavia				
1989	46 000	37 000	20 879	23 000
1990	40 000	32 000	18 000	20 000
USA				
1989	120 000	113 000	18 000	95 000
1990	112 000	105 000	18 000	87 000
Argentina				
1989	16 550	16 550	7499	9000
1990	15 500	15 500	6950	8500
Australia				
1989	27 000	27 000	3300	23 700
1990	27 300	27 300	3500	23 800
Chile				
1989	14 000	13 500	6200	6300
1990	14 650	14 150	6500	6550
New Zealand				
1989	9000	6800	6500	2282
1990	7800	6000	4700	2500
South Africa				
1989	43 040	43 040	4652	37 709
1990	46 383	46 383	4650	40 650

Source: USDA (1990).

(*Armeniaca vulgaris* Lam. or *Prunus armeniaca* L.), the Siberian apricot (*P. sibirica* L.), the Manchurian apricot (*P. mandshurica* Koehne.), and the Tibet apricot (*P. armeniaca* var. *holoserice* Batal.). *P. mume* (mume), a related species, also originated in China. Much of the fruit which has been described in China is large-fruited with favourable dessert quality. The diversity of apricot germplasm in China, if utilized effectively in genetic improvement research, could substantially broaden the existing commerce of apricots in North America and the world. Japan is a producer of apricots and mume. Historically, the apricot and mume were utilized for medicinal purposes, but now the fruit is consumed in processed forms such as syrups, jams, pickles, and liquor. In 1986, mume production approximated 89 100 t and apricot about 1460 t.

Argentina and Chile are the two leading producers of apricots in the Southern Hemisphere, with production of 15 500 and 14 650 t, respectively, in 1990.

In North America, the USA is the leading producer of apricots, but they are produced to a limited extent in Canada and Mexico. Canadian apricot production is located primarily in the western part with some small production near the great lakes. In Mexico, apricots are grown in the high desert east of the Sierra Madre mountain range. In the USA, California is the leading apricot-producing state, followed by Washington and Utah with a smattering of production in Michigan,

Table 2. California acreage of selected apricot varieties

Variety	Acres (ha)	Harvest time
Blenheim/Royal	7303 (2955)	17 June
Castlebrite	986 (399)	7 May
Derby Royal	221 (89)	25 May
Flaming Gold	157 (64)	21 May
Improved Flaming Gold	118 (48)	21 May
Katy	319 (129)	15 May
Modesto	578 (234)	1 June
Patterson	3404 (1378)	12 June
Tilton	5922 (2397)	18 June
Westley	174 (70)	25 June
Other	584 (236)	

Colorado, Texas, New Jersey, Idaho, New York and the Carolinas.

In California, there are approximately 17 000–20 000 acres (6880–8094 ha) planted. Nonbearing acreage accounts for approximately 2700 (1093 ha) of that total. Stanislaus county is the leading apricot-producing county in California, with 7242 (2931 ha) bearing and 1620 (656 ha) nonbearing acres. Other important apricot-producing counties in California, in descending order of planted acreage, include San Joaquin, San Benito, Yolo-Solano, Merced, Contra Costa, Kern, Tulare, Fresno and Santa Clara.

Varieties

The most popular apricot varieties in California are described below, and their bearing acreages are listed in Table 2. The 'Patterson' apricot is being planted more widely and is a multi-use apricot, utilized primarily for canning (processing), but also frozen, dried and eaten fresh.

Castlebrite

Released as a very-early-ripening, fresh-shipping variety, the fruit is yellow-orange and attractive, with a red blush. It is firm, medium in size, but does not possess finest eating quality.

Derby

Derby or Derby Royal is principally grown in Yolo County, California. It originated from a chance seedling and was first planted in 1895. Derby is suitable for fresh shipping, but not for drying because the stone can cling to the flesh. The fruit may ripen unevenly. At least two distinct strains of the Derby have been recognized around Winters with differing fruit characteristics.

Flaming Gold

Originated in Modesto, California, by Floyd Zaiger, Flaming Gold was introduced in 1967 and was a seedling of Perfection. The fruit ripens early and has been used primarily for fresh shipping.

Katy

Large-to-medium-sized fruit developed by Floyd Zaiger, the Katy is yellow, firm, and an early ripening fruit used for fresh shipping.

Modesto

Originated in Le Grand, California, by FW Anderson, the variety was introduced in 1964 and was an F_2, open-pollinated seedling of Perfection. The fruit is firm fleshed, medium-to-large-sized, often with a red blush, and orange fleshed. The tree bears regularly, and the fruit ripens about the time of Royal and several days ahead of Patterson. Modesto is resistant to pit burning.

Patterson

Originated in Le Grand, California, by FW Anderson, the Patterson was introduced in 1968 and was an F_2, seedling of Perfection × unknown. The variety is firm, has orange flesh and skin, and is sometimes found with a red blush. The fruit is medium to large, and produces consistently good crops. It appears to be less affected by mild winters than the Tilton variety, and the fruit ripens evenly. Patterson is resistant to pit burning. It is a good variety for processing, makes a good dried product and is fair for fresh eating fruit.

Royal and Blenheim

The Royal and Blenheim varieties are considered together because they have lost their separate identities. The variety is utilized for fresh and canning but mostly for drying. It tends to bear alternately and unless properly thinned may have small fruit. It has excellent flavour when fully matured. It is rather soft and difficult to ship. The flesh is orange, and the skin is yellow orange; it often has a red blush. The fruit tends to pit burn and is not well adapted for the interior valleys of California. It can develop a condition known as fog spot in the coastal regions of California.

Tilton

The variety originated as a seedling in Kings County, California by JE Tilton in 1885. Tilton is one of the leading apricots for processing in California but is currently being replaced by Patterson. Tilton is adapted for canning, drying, and shipping, but the fresh flavour is only fair. The tree tends to bear alternately and is affected by mild winter temperatures. When properly thinned it may bear medium-to-large-sized fruit. The fruit is orange to yellowish and often has a red blush.

Westley

Originated in Le Grand, California, by FW Anderson, the variety was introduced in 1973 and was an F_2, of Perfection × Tilton. The fruit is medium firm, with good flavour, and is used for some fresh and drying. The tree tends to bear alternately.

Rootstocks

Apricots are grown commercially on apricot seedling, peach (*P. persica*), and plum (*P. cerasifera*, myrobalan seedling and 29C; *P. cerasifera* × *P. munsoniana. marianna 2624*) roots. The main plum rootstocks include myrobalan seedling, myrobalan 29C and marianna 2624. Plum rootstocks are characteristically resistant to wet and poorly drained soil conditions. The union between apricot and plum root reportedly is not as sound as apricot on peach or apricot root and occasionally some apricot varieties break off at the union during heavy wind storms. Apricots growing on plum roots may not be as productive as those grown on apricot or peach roots. Peach root for apricot is quite popular. The stocks include those propagated from Lovell and Nemaguard seedlings. Apricots grown on peach are productive, but peach cannot tolerate wet and poorly drained soil conditions as well as plum. Peach roots are very susceptible to *Phytophthora* root and crown rots. Apricots grown on apricot seedling roots are not as common as those on peach roots. Apricot roots are not as resistant to wet soil or *Phytophthora* as plum and also do not have the resistance to nematodes as does Nemaguard peach root. However, apricot roots are thought to occasionally impart better fruit quality and productivity to apricots. *See* Peaches and Nectarines

A new rootstock, developed by Floyd Zaiger and named 'Citation', is a peach × plum hybrid and has shown promising results in early testing. The rootstock may impart some tree size control to selected apricot varieties.

Morphology and Anatomy

Botany and Biology

The apricot belongs to the *Rosaceae* family and most cultivated apricots belong to the species *Prunus arme-niaca* L. Closely related species include *P. mume* Sidb. and Zucc., the Japanese apricot, *P. dasycarpa* Ehrh., the black apricot, *P. brigantiaca* Vill., the Briancon apricot from the French Alps, *P. ansu* Komar, *P. sibirica* L., and *P. mandshurica* (Maxim.). The apricot is diploid ($2n = 16$, $x = 8$). Flowers are borne singly or doubly at a node on very short stems (peduncles). Flowers have about 30 stamens with one pistil. The solitary flowers are white or pinkish. Most commercial cultivars in the USA are self-fertile, but Perfection and Riland are examples of self-incompatible cultivars. Trees generally produce vigorous upright growth, but not as upright as plum. Floral initiation occurs in summer (late May or June) and most of the flowers which set into fruit are produced on spurs. Spurs are productive for several (3–5) years. The highest quality fruit is borne on younger spurs. Apricots are the first deciduous fruit trees to produce flowers in the spring after almond, and because of that are subject to frost damage. Trees bloom over a period of approximately 1 to 2 weeks, depending upon weather conditions. Flowers are followed by the appearance of leaves, which are simple, alternate, and serrated, round-ovate to ovate and sharp-pointed. Apricot cultivars currently available require approximately 300–1200 h of chilling (temperatures below 7·2°C). Vegetative buds require less chilling than reproductive (flower) buds. In those years with insufficient winter (December and January) chilling, bud drop can occur. Apricots produce more flowers than are needed to ensure the production of an adequate crop and often require the removal of small fruit (thinning) to assure adequate fruit size. The apricot is a stone fruit (drupe). Other stone fruits in the genus *Prunus* include almond, cherry, nectarine, peach and plum. Other drupe fruit include olive, coconut, mango, etc. Botanically a drupe fruit is a fleshy, one-seeded fruit that does not split open of itself, with the seed enclosed in a stony endocarp, which is called a pit. The fruit of apricot consists of a stony endocarp, a fleshy mesocarp, and an outer exocarp (skin). *See* individual fruits.

Approximately 80% of all California apricots are processed (see Table 3). California represents nearly 100% of commercially processed fruit in the USA. Basic grower production is sold for processing to five different sources: canners, nectar processors, driers, freezers, and baby food processors. For the purpose of describing these processing methods, only canning, drying and freezing will be included since nectar and baby food processing are basically similar to the process for producing apricot concentrate or purée by canners.

Canned Apricots

The majority of apricots for canning are grown in Stanislaus and San Joaquin county. One major canner is

Table 3. Volume shares of apricots produced in the USA in 1990

Product type	Metric tonnage (t)	Percentage of total
Canned[a]	59 944	53
Dried	24 384	21
Fresh	18 288	16
Frozen	8128	7
Baby food	3048	3
Total	113 792	

[a] Includes canned apricots, nectar, purée.
Source: California Apricot Advisory Board, Walnut Creek, California.

located in this area and three others operate in the Santa Clara Valley. Most canning apricots consist of the Tilton and Patterson varieties, and the Patterson has now become the primary fruit for canning.

Canners' prices to the growers are negotiated between the canners and the growers' bargaining association. Current prices are based upon a price per (UK) ton for 'US No. 1s' with a downward sliding scale of five grades below this level. Grading is carried out by a third-party inspection programme approved by both parties.

Fruit is picked either by hand or, to a lesser extent, mechanically, and dumped into 272-kg bins. These bins are delivered to a weighing station where they are inspected for grade and weighed. The apricots are then delivered to the canning plant, where they are mechanically dumped into a water bath containing chlorinated water. They travel down an inspection belt for removal of any materials other than apricots (leaves, sticks, stones) or immature, green, overripe or rotted fruit. The apricots are then graded for size; the small fruits, unsuitable for canning, are collected and directed towards eventual use in concentrate and/or nectar-type product items.

The fruit is delivered to mechanical apricot cutters; these machines align the fruit in such a way that the cutting will take place on the apricot suture. Cut fruit is then opened and the loose pits drop through a stainless steel plate. Cut, pitted fruit is delivered to the sizer/grader to be mechanically sorted, resulting in uniformly sized fruit. Once the cans have been filled, a topping medium such as sugar water or fruit juice is added, then immediately sealed. The product is then ready to be cooked, rendering it commercially sterile. Later, when the product reaches the warehouse it will be labelled and cased as per the customer's request. Canned apricots are packed in heavy syrup, light syrup, juice pack (apricot or pear) and water pack.

Back in the processing plant, fruit that is unsuitable for cutting is delivered to a thermal screw, where it is heated to 98.9°C and delivered to a pulping unit, which will remove the pit. The heated pulp is pumped through a series of finishers that will remove some of the fibrous material, such as the skin of the apricot. Finished juice is then ready for the evaporation process or delivered to the nectar room where it is mixed with sugar, water and citric acid. The nectar is filled and sealed, similar to the cut-fruit canning process, and delivered to the warehouse. Fruit juice destined for the evaporator will be condensed resulting in 32° Brix (32%) fruit concentrate. The product is canned in 3.25-litre cans or aseptically filled in 250-litre drums. The concentrated product is ideally suited for nectar reconstitution or as an ingredient in various sauces.

There are a very few marketers of apricot nectar that purchase off-grade apricots directly from the grower and process their own concentrate or purée according to their own particular specifications. The concentrates are then diluted to an acceptable level as a drinkable apricot juice called nectar.

Dried Apricots

Dried apricots are produced from the plump, ripe, fresh fruit. The fruit is picked and sun-dried in June or early July. The Blenheim and Patterson apricots are the principal varieties used for drying. Other varieties are dried but most do not have the unique combination of high flavour density and solids-to-acid ratio that create the luscious, sweet-tart flavour of the California dried apricot.

Sun Drying of Fruits

The drying of apricots parallels methods used for processing other dried fruits (figs, peaches, pears, etc.). Stage of maturity of the fruit is important in selecting fruits for drying. If the fruit is picked too early, colour and flavour are lacking in the final product. When overripe, the final product loses shape and becomes slab-like in appearance. Much of the fine flavour of California dried apricots results from the fact that the dried fruit can be produced from fully tree-ripened fruit.

Preparation of the fresh fruit for sun drying is simple. The common predrying treatments applied to apricots are as follows: (1) selection and sorting of fresh fruit; (2) washing; (3) cutting into halves and removal of pits; (4) spreading of fruit on drying trays with the cut surface upward; (5) sulphuring with burning sulphur or gaseous sulphur dioxide; (6) placing of trays in full sun in the dry yard. *See* Drying, Drying Using Natural Radiation

Sulphuring

For many years sulphur dioxide (SO_2) has been used to preserve the colour of dried fruits. It is the only chemical added to dried apricots. Sulphur dioxide is recognized as safe for use in dried fruits by the US Food and Drug Administration (FDA). Apricots prepared for drying are usually exposed to gaseous SO_2 before being put in the sun for drying, but treatment with fumes of burning elemental sulphur is also practised.

In addition to preventing enzymatic browning, SO_2 treatment reduces destruction of carotene and ascorbic acid which are valuable natural nutrients in apricots; thus nutritional qualities are preserved.

Sulphured, dried apricots will contain a SO_2 level of about 2500 ppm. The amount of SO_2 must also be controlled because regulations on levels of SO_2 permitted vary from one country to the next. Sulphur dioxide in the fruit begins to dissipate as soon as applied and continues to diminish throughout storage, distribution and retail shelf-life of the product.

Sun Drying

After sulphuring, the trays are placed in the drying yard for sun drying. Sun drying is complete when the apricots have a moisture content of 15–20%. Drying time can vary depending on the condition of the fruit, air moisture and constancy of sun exposure. During drying the cut and sulphured fruit is left in full sun for 5 to 10 days, followed by further drying away from direct sunlight for a sufficient time to bring moisture to the desired level.

After drying, the apricots are transferred to boxes for curing and for bringing about equilibrium of moisture content. This requires from 2 to 3 weeks or even longer. The dried apricots are then ready for grading and final preparation for packing.

Screening, Inspection, and Washing

Size grading is required to obtain the desired piece size in the end product. Size grading is accomplished by passing the dried product over a shaking perforated metal screen and collecting the fractions separately. Each size fraction passes onto the final inspection operation.

Prior to packing, chopping, or grinding, the apricots are rigorously washed to remove dust, leaf particles, etc. Washing consists of a presoak in water, followed by mechanical scrubbing and rinsing. After washing, the fruit is spread on trays for a second treatment with SO_2 to assure optimum colour and keeping qualities. This postwashing treatment is accomplished with gaseous SO_2 or fumes from burning sulphur. At this point, control is critical to attain the proper final level of SO_2 in the finished product to meet shelf-life requirements, or requirements specified by the customer of bulk packs.

Storage

Dried apricots are protected from product decomposition caused by microbial or enzymatic deterioration. The relatively low moisture level, high natural sugar level, high acid content, SO_2 level, and low pH preclude these types of spoilage. *See* Storage Stability, Mechanisms of Degradation; Storage Stability, Parameters Affecting Storage Stability

The loss of SO_2 cannot be eliminated entirely, but it can be controlled so that it is of little consequence in normal commercial storage. The single most important factor in determining the storage life in dried fruit is temperature of the storage space. Temperature is so critical that the storage life is cut approximately in half for every 11°C increase above 4·4°C.

The following conditions and tips will help to obtain maximum storage life for dried fruits:

1. Store dried fruit at 4·4°C and 75% relative humidity for excellent keeping for at least 6 to 9 months (for washed and resulphured apricots).
2. Keep temperatures and humidity constant.
3. Be sure that the product is well wrapped and not exposed to air.
4. Protect dried fruit from strong direct light.

Frozen Apricots

Apricots for freezing include the Patterson and Blenheim varieties, with Patterson predominating.

Frozen apricots are processed for three different product types: sliced halves, slices, and a multiple scored apricot that is not completely sliced. The former two types are sold primarily to bakers, ice-cream makers and frozen-dessert makers. The latter type are processed for use in jams and jellies and are called 'machine pitted'.

Receiving

Apricots are received in approximately 363-kg bins. There are normally 48 bins per truckload. Each truckload is weighed and assigned a lot number. Bins from each lot are visually sampled for quality. The apricots are checked for ripeness, insect penetration, rot, flesh damage, and excess foreign materials such as leaves. Fruits are placed in high-temperature cold storage or left in receiving for ripening. As needed, bins of fruit are brought to the processing plant by truck.

Leaf Roller

The apricots are dumped onto a conveyor and pass over a series of parallel rollers. The rollers are separated by

Table 4. Nutritional composition (per 100 g of fruit) of apricots

	Fresh	Canned Heavy syrup	Canned Light syrup	Canned Juice pack	Nectar	Dried
Energy (J)	200	350	265	200	235	1000
Protein (g)	1	1	1	1	0	4
Carbohydrate (g)	11	21	16	12	14	62
Fat (g)	0	0	0	0	0	0
Sodium (mg)	1	4	4	4	4	10
Potassium (mg)	295	140	138	165	114	1378
Fibre (g)	2	0	0	1	1	8

Source: *Nutritionist III* (1990) (USDA Handbook No. 8-9, revised 1982).

small gaps through which leaves and twigs may fall. A worker is stationed there to remove leaves, foreign material, rot, and green fruit. The green fruit are held for rerunning when properly ripened.

From the leaf roller the apricots fall into the shaker-washer which agitates the apricots in water and propels them under freshwater sprays.

The shaker-washer discharges the apricots onto the first inspection belt. The fruit is examined for rot, leaves and green colour. From the first inspection belt, the fruit drops onto a cleated elevator which carries the fruit to a cross-belt. The cross-belt delivers the apricots to one of two apricot halvers. A shaker-feeder receives the apricots. Rotating scrubbers clean the apricots and single-file them into five lanes. The apricots from the five lanes are fed into pick-up pockets. The pick-up pockets feed the apricots to V trough belts in time with orienting fingers. The orienting fingers cause the apricots to rotate so that the suture is aligned with blades which cut the apricot in half in line with the suture.

A pit remover at the end of the blade is used to separate the pit from the two halves as they pass through. Approximately 85% of the pits are removed at this point.

A cross-belt carries the apricot halves to a conveyor, which transports them to a cup-up pit shaker. As the apricot halves move across the shaker pan they pass over holes which permit the remaining pits to fall through as they are shaken loose. As the apricot halves are discharged from the cup-up pit shaker they are aligned with the pit cavity facing up.

The cup-up pit shaker distributes the apricot halves onto the pit inspection belt. On the belt the apricots are inspected for pits and soft fruits. Soft fruits are placed into sort-out buckets and used to make purée. From the pit inspection belt the apricots are transported to a gang blade slicer. The slicer has parallel circular blocks separated by a 1·27-cm gap. The slicer cuts the halves into strips.

The sliced apricots fall onto a final inspection belt.

The apricots are inspected for pits, blemishes, and harmless extraneous material. Fruit from the final inspection belt is carried to a fill-weigh station. The fruit is placed in prelabelled tins and weighed. A depressor is placed on top of the fruit and 60° Brix syrup with ascorbic acid is added. The container is weighed again. A lid is placed on the can and it is passed through a can washer. The cans are coded, loaded on pallets, and tagged. The completed pallets are promptly moved to cold storage for freezing.

Apricot Usage

At the height of California apricot production in the 1930s and 1940s, the major usage was dried apricots. This was primarily because of the dried product's ability to remain shelf-stable for a relatively long period of time, its versatility as an out-of-hand snack, cooking and baking ingredient, and its sweet-sour flavour.

After World War II, the canning industry began its dynamic growth. Dried apricots gave way to the canned version because of a growing acceptance of canned fruits and vegetables as convenient and economical products, as well as the apricots' greater similarity to the fresh fruit. The dried apricot continued to be the largest usage type through the late 1940s but lost its position to canned apricot products (which included baby food, purée, and nectar) in 1950 and never regained its plurality.

Frozen apricots were introduced to the American public in 1943, diverting about 4064 t out of a total processed crop of 79 248 t, the smallest crop recorded up to that time. Apricots going into frozen production peaked in 1945 at 26 822 t out of a total of 161 544 t and have never regained that level. Today frozen apricots account for less than 10% of the pack.

Apricots sold fresh in retail and food-service outlets have been slow in developing into major usage. Their high point in sales was reached in the disastrous 1943 crop year with 21% of total production. Most years since 1909 have held at around 10% of the total crop. Since 1984, however, with substantially more marketing effort behind them, fresh apricots have been maintaining a 14–17% share of saleable tonnage.

In 1990, the last year reporting actual tonnage by use-type, the 113 792 t of apricots reported to the California Apricot Advisory Board were distributed as shown in Table 3.

Nutrition

Weight for weight, apricots provide more than three times the carotene of peaches, and three times the vitamin C of pears (based on a 1 cup serving of canned fruit, in juice pack with skin). They are also higher in potassium, calcium, phosphorus and iron than most other fruits (see Table 4). Apricots, especially dried apricots, are an excellent source of dietary fibre. They are low in sodium, calories and fat, and have no cholesterol. *See* individual nutrients

Bibliography

Bailey CH and Fredric Hough L (1975) Apricots. In: Janick J and Moore JN (eds) *Advances in Fruit Breeding*, pp 367–383 West Lafayette, Indiana: Purdue University Press.

CASS (1990) *California Fruit and Nut Acreage 1989*. Sacramento, California: California Agricultural Statistics Service.

Chandler WH, Kimball MH, Philp GL, Tufts WP and Weldon GP (1937) Chilling requirements for opening of buds on deciduous orchard trees and some other plants in California. *University of California Agricultural Experiment Station Bulletin* 611.

Chittenden FJ (ed.) (1956) Apricot *The Royal Horticultural Society Dictionary of Gardening*, vol. 1, pp 15–156. Oxford: Clarendon Press.

Coe FM (1934) Apricot varieties. *Utah Agricultural Experiment Station Bulletin* 251

Crosse-Raynaud P and Audergon JM (1987) Apricot rootstocks. In: Rom RC and Carlson RF (eds) *Rootstocks for Fruit Crops*, pp 295–320. New York: John Wiley.

Day LH (1953) Rootstocks for stone fruits. *California Agricultural Experiment Station Extension Service Bulletin* 736.

Glucina P, Hosking G and Mills R (1990) Evaluation of apricot cultivars for Hawke's Bay. *The Orchadist of New Zealand* 63: 21–25.

Hedrick UP (1922) *Cyclopedia of Hardy Fruits*. New York: Macmillan.

Hesse CO (1952) Apricot culture in California. *California Agricultural Experiment Station Extension Service Circular 412*.

Paunovic SA (ed.) (1988) Second International Workshop on Apricot Culture and Decline. *Acta Horticulturae* 209.

USDA (1990) *Horticultural Products Review*, Circular Series, November 1990, Washington, DC: US Department of Agriculture Foreign Agricultural Service.

Westwood MN (1978) *Temperate-Zone Pomology*. New York: WH Freeman.

Stephen M. Southwick
Pomology Department, University of California, Davis, California, USA
Eugene H. Stokes
General Manager, California Apricot Advisory Board, Walnut Creek, California, USA

AQUACULTURE

See Fish

AROIDS

See Vegetables of Tropical Climates

AROMA

See Sensory Evaluation

Apricots

AROMA COMPOUNDS

See Flavour Compounds

ARSENIC

Contents

Properties and Determination
Requirements and Toxicology

Properties and Determination

Chemical Properties

Properties of arsenic relevant to environmental chemistry, medicine and toxicology may be found in the reference works cited in the *Bibliography*.

Structures of some of the more important arsenic compounds are shown in Fig. 1.

Inorganic arsenic (As) occurs in three oxidation states, As(v) as in arsenate (AsO_4^{3-}), As(III) as in arsenite (AsO_3^{3-}) and As(−III) as in arsine (AsH_3). Assignment of the oxidation number −III to arsenic in arsine is arbitrary because arsenic and hydrogen have about the same electronegativities. International Union of Pure and Applied Chemistry (IUPAC) nomenclature, arsenate and arsenite are expressed as arsenate(v) and arsenate(III), respectively. In aerated water, arsenate is the stable form. Since arsenic(III) is considerably more toxic than As(v), the form in which arsenic exists, whether as arsenate or arsenite, is important. Doses of 70–180 mg of arsenic trioxide (As_2O_3) are fatal. Arsenic acid is a fairly strong acid, with pK_a values, 2·25, 7·25, and 12·30. Arsenous acid behaves in water practically as a weak, monobasic acid, with a pK_a of 9·23.

Arsenic forms a variety of organoarsenic compounds. Arsenic compounds of the types, R_3As, $RAs(OH)_2$, R_2AsOH, $RAsO(OH)_2$, $R_2AsO(OH)$ and $R_4As^+X^-$ are called arsines, arsonous acids, arsinous acids, arsonic acids, arsinic acids, and arsonium salts, respectively. It is believed that organoarsenic compounds are much less toxic than the inorganic arsenic. Biochemical conversion of inorganic arsenic compounds to organoarsenic compounds has been known for almost 100 years.

Arsenite is reduced in acid solution by zinc or sodium borohydride to form arsine (AsH_3), which is volatile and is stripped by the hydrogen generated during the reduction; it can be collected by a trap cooled in liquid nitrogen or by a dilute iodine or bromine solution. These properties are exploited in the determination of arsenic.

With zinc as the reductant, prior reduction of arsenate to arsenite is necessary for the conversion of arsenate into arsine. A mixture of potassium iodide and tin(II) chloride is used for the reduction of arsenate to arsenite. Tin(II) chloride also helps the reaction of zinc. In strongly acid solution, both arsenate and arsenite are converted by sodium borohydride to arsine.

Occurrence

Natural abundance of arsenic in the earth's crust is 1·5–2 ppm. Hot-spring and well waters sometimes contain appreciable quantities of arsenic, mostly in the form of arsenate. Arsenic is associated with sulphide ores. Waste water discharged from sulphide mines and ore-dressing plants often contains arsenic in appreciable quantities. Arsenic contamination caused by flue gases from lead and copper smelters has been frequently reported. In Taiwan, patients with blackfoot disease are found in areas where drinking water contains aresenic. Most authorities adopt a value of 0·05 mg l^{-1}, measured as arsenic, as the maximum permissible concentration in drinking water.

The arsenic levels in ocean water are around 2·6 µg l^{-1}. Although arsenate is the stable form in aerated waters, ocean water sometimes contains appreciable proportions of arsenite. It is believed that some bacteria are able to reduce arsenate to arsenite.

Because arsenic compounds were used as insecticides, herbicides and animal feed additives, there are possibilities that soils, vegetation, swine and poultry are con-

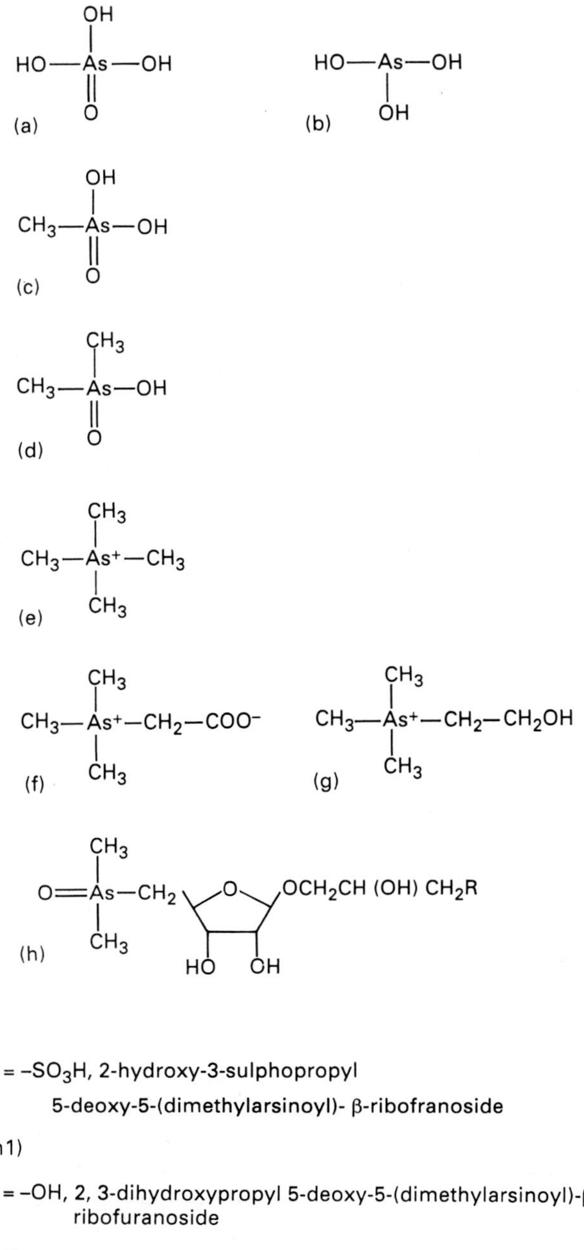

OH
|
HO—As—OH
‖
O
(a)

HO—As—OH
|
OH
(b)

OH
|
CH$_3$—As—OH
‖
O
(c)

CH$_3$
|
CH$_3$—As—OH
‖
O
(d)

CH$_3$
|
CH$_3$—As$^+$—CH$_3$
|
CH$_3$
(e)

CH$_3$
|
CH$_3$—As$^+$—CH$_2$—COO$^-$
|
CH$_3$
(f)

CH$_3$
|
CH$_3$—As$^+$—CH$_2$—CH$_2$OH
|
CH$_3$
(g)

CH$_3$
|
O=As—CH$_2$—〈 O 〉—OCH$_2$CH (OH) CH$_2$R
|
CH$_3$ HO   OH
(h)

R = –SO$_3$H, 2-hydroxy-3-sulphopropyl
5-deoxy-5-(dimethylarsinoyl)- β-ribofranoside

(h1)

R = –OH, 2, 3-dihydroxypropyl 5-deoxy-5-(dimethylarsinoyl)-β-ribofuranoside

(h2)

          O
          ‖
R = –O—P—O — CH$_2$CH (OH) CH$_2$OH,
          |
          O$^-$
                    3-'glycerophosphoryl'-2-hydroxy-1
                    -[5-deoxy-5-(dimethylarsinoyl)-β-
(h3)   ribofuranosyloxy] propane

R = –OSO$_3$H, (2S)-3-[5-deoxy-5-(dimethylarsinoyl)-β-
                    D-ribofuranosyloxy]-2-
(h4)   hydroxypropyl hydrogen sulphate

Fig. 1 Structures of some important arsenic compounds: (a) arsenic acid; (b) arsenous acid; (c) monomethylarsonic acid (methanearsonic acid); (d) dimethylarsinic acid (cacodylic acid); (e) tetramethylarsonium ion; (f) arsenobetaine; (g) arsenocholine; (h) arsenosugars.

taminated with arsenic. The value of 1 ppm, measured as As$_2$O$_3$, has been set in Japan as the maximum allowable limit for most fruits and vegetables. In Japan, soils containing more than 15 ppm arsenic are considered unsuitable for agriculture.

Edible marine organisms, such as lobsters, shrimps and brown kelps, contain appreciable concentrations of arsenic, frequently in the ppm range, occasionally at concentrations as high as several tens of ppm on a wet basis. Fortunately, however, the arsenic is mostly in the form of organoarsenic compounds, which are rapidly excreted and are relatively nontoxic to humans. On average, about 80% of the arsenic in marine living matter is found in the water-soluble fraction. Concentrations in freshwater plants and animals are usually lower than in marine species. *See* Shellfish, Contamination and Spoilage of Molluscs and Crustacea

In 1900, there was an outbreak of arsenic poisoning among beer-drinkers in England. The cause of poisoning was traced to the use of invert sugar produced by using arsenic-contaminated sulphuric acid. In 1955, there was an outbreak of an unusual disease and fatalities occurred in Okayama and Hiroshima Prefectures, Japan, among infants receiving a formulation made from powdered milk. The formulation contained As in concentrations of 20–30 ppm. The source of arsenic was traced to arsenic-contaminated sodium phosphate added as a stabilizer. The sodium phosphate had been produced from waste bauxite processing liquor and contained about 3% of arsenic.

Speciation of Arsenic in Food and Water

Arsenic in seafoods is mostly in the form of organoarsenic compounds, including arsenobetaines and arsenosugars. Many papers have been published on the speciation of arsenic in seafoods.

For the speciation of organoarsenic compounds in seafoods, the samples are usually extracted with methanol. The extract is evaporated, redissolved in water and subjected to gel permeation chromatography, ion exchange chromatography and preparative thin-layer chromatography. Buffered ion exchange chromatography, close to neutrality, is necessary as decomposition of the compounds to dimethylarsinic acid occurs at extremes of pH. *See* Chromatography, Principles; Chromatography, Thin-layer Chromatography

Arsenic compounds extracted with methanol from sea animals have been separated by liquid chromatography with inductively coupled plasma atomic emission spectrometric detection at wavelength of 193·7 nm. No single column was found to be satisfactory for separating all organoarsenic compounds present in the seafoods. Four compounds (Fig 1e,f,h2,h3) were found. Arsenobetaine (Fig 1f) was found in all sea animals tested. There is considerable evidence that arsenocholine and arsenobetaine are rapidly excreted and almost nontoxic to humans.

Arsenic(v) As(III), monomethylarsonic acid and dimethylarsinic acid have been determined in waters taken at various locations in Tone River, Japan. The mean concentrations expressed in ppb of As were as follows: As(v), 1·57; As(III), 0·61; dimethylarsinic acid, 0·04; monomethylarsonic acid, 0·021. It was noted that relatively high concentrations of organoarsenics were found in reservoirs located upstream where no special pollution sources were found. It was suggested that eutrophication is responsible for the formation of organoarsenics in reservoirs.

Sample Preparation and Isolation

For the determination of arsenic, the element must be brought into solution. Care must be taken during the destruction of sample to ensure that no arsenic is lost by vaporization of trivalent arsenic halides. Loss can usually be avoided by oxidizing the arsenic at an earlier stage by boiling with nitric acid under reflux.

Wet ashing of food samples with nitric acid plus sulphuric acid is incomplete. Yasui and Tsutsumi (1977) recommend the use of a mixture of nitric, sulphuric and perchloric acids. Monomethylarsonate, dimethylarsinate, arsenobetaine and phenylarsonate are decomposed. The following is the procedure recommended by Yasui and Tsutsumi.

Between 0·25 and 2·5 g (dry-weight basis) of the food sample is placed in a 100-ml beaker, 10 ml of nitric acid is added and mixed well. The beaker is covered with a watch glass, and gently heated on a hotplate (170–220°C). When violent reaction has ceased, the beaker is removed from the hot plate and cooled. After addition of 3 ml of nitric acid, 2·5 ml of sulphuric acid and 5 ml of perchloric acid (60%), the beaker is heated again on a hotplate (300–380°C). If the mixture darkens or blackens, the beaker is immediately removed from the hotplate, a small volume of nitric acid is added, and digestion continued. When the solution is transparent or faint yellow, the watch glass is removed and the solution evaporated until the volume is less than 1 ml. Oxides of nitrogen, which interfere with the determination of arsenic by the hydride generation method, are removed during the evaporation step, so that treatment with ammonium oxalate is unnecessary. After cooling, the contents are transferred to a 25-ml volumetric flask using 3 N hydrochloric acid and made up to volume with 3 N hydrochloric acid. An aliquot of this solution is used for the determination of arsenic by hydride generation atomic absorption spectrometry.

The procedure described by the Association of Official Analytical Chemists (AOAC; Article 973.33) adopts dry ashing at 600°C with magnesium nitrate for the destruction of meat and poultry. The ash is dissolved in dilute hydrochloric acid and then treated with potassium iodide and tin(II) chloride. The arsenite formed is then converted into arsine, which is collected in a dilute iodine solution and determined by the molybdenum blue method.

For the examination of arsenic contamination of soils in Japan, arsenic is extracted by shaking the soil with 1 N hydrochloric acid (50 ml per 10 g of sample) for 30 min at 30°C. The mixture is filtered through dry paper, and subjected to hydride generation atomic absorption spectrometry.

Low levels of arsenic in water can be enriched by coprecipitation with ferric hydroxide after being oxidized to the pentavalent state with potassium permanganate. Triton X-100 has been used to aid formation of large precipitates. It is claimed that both arsenate and arsenite are coprecipitated with iron hydroxide.

The hydride generation cold trap method is also useful for the isolation and enrichment of arsenic compounds.

Specific Methods of Analysis

There are several methods available for the determination of low levels of arsenic. Their approximate sensitivities are shown in Table 1.

Gutzeit Method

The Gutzeit method is becoming obsolete, although it is highly sensitive and has been used for many years for the detection and semiquantitative determination of traces of arsenic in foods, soils and fertilizers. The sample is brought into solution by wet ashing or by other means. Arsenic is reduced to arsenite with potassium iodide and tin(II) chloride and further to arsine with zinc in acid solution. The arsine is stripped by the hydrogen formed during the reduction with zinc, and passed through a tube containing a strip of paper impregnated with mercury(II) bromide. The paper darkens on reaction with arsine, and the length of the darkened area is proportional to the amount of arsenic.

Spectrophotometric Methods

There are two spectrophotometric methods frequently used for the determination of arsenic.

Molybdenum (Mo) Blue Method

Arsenate reacts with molybdic acid in the presence of a reducing agent to form heteropolymolybdenum blue.

Table 1. Approximate limits of determination of some analytical methods for arsenic

Method	Limits of determination[a] (mg l^{-1})
Spectrophotometry (molybdenum blue)	0·05
Spectrometry (silver diethyldithiocarbamate)	0·1
Flame atomic absorption spectrometry	0·2
Electrothermal atomic absorption spectrometry	0·004
Atomic fluorescence spectrometry	0·8
X ray fluorescence spectrometry	1
ICP emission spectrometry	0·2
Mass spectrometry	0·006
Neutron activation without chemical separation	0·002
Neutron activation with chemical separation	0·004
Direct current polarography	0·1
Linear sweep and cathode ray polarography	0·02
Pulse polarography	0·004
Inverse voltammetry	0·002

Source IUPAC (1982) *Pure and Applied Chemistry* 54: 1565.
[a] $(\bar{x}_b + 10\sigma_b)/$(slope of calibration graph), with $\bar{x}_b$ and σ_b mean of instrumental responses to blank and their standard deviation, respectively.

The colour develops slowly at room temperature but is stable. This method is interfered with by phosphate and silicate and is applied after isolation of arsenic by the hydride generation method. The following method is taken from AOAC 942.17. *See* Spectroscopy, Visible Spectroscopy and Colorimetry

Arsenic is converted into arsine. The arsine is passed through an arsine trap containing 3 ml of sodium hypobromite solution (50 ml of 0·5 N sodium hydroxide diluted to 200 ml with half-saturated bromine water). The collected material is transferred to a 25-ml volumetric flask and diluted to approximately 15 ml; 0·5 ml of ammonium molybdate–sulphuric acid solution (dissolve 5·00 g of $(NH_4)_6Mo_7O_{24}\cdot4H_2O$ in water, slowly add 42·8 ml of sulphuric acid and dilute to 100 ml) and 1·0 ml of 1·5% hydrazinium sulphate solution are added. The solution is made to volume, mixed and allowed to stand for 75 min. The absorbance at 845 nm is measured. If the mixture is heated to 50°C colour development is complete in 10 min.

Silver Diethyldithiocarbamate (AgDDC) Method

The AgDDC method involves arsine generation and bubbling the arsine formed through a trapping solution of 0·5% silver diethyldithiocarbamate solution in pyridine. An intense red colour is formed. To avoid nuisance from foul-smelling pyridine, a trapping solution prepared by dissolving 0·25 g of silver diethyldithiocarbamate and 0·1 g of brucine dihydrate in 100 ml of chloroform can be used. The wavelength for absorption maximum slightly changes with the composition of the trapping solution. The following procedure is similar to that recommended by AOAC Article 952.13.

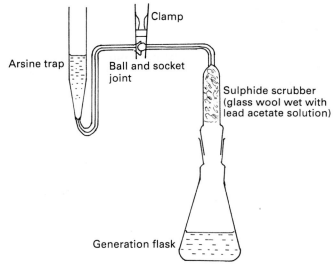

Fig. 2 Apparatus for AgDDC (silver diethyldithiocarbamate) method.

Figure 2 shows a typical apparatus used in this method. The glass wool in the sulphide scrubber is moistened with 10% lead acetate solution; 4 ml of AgDDC-pyridine solution is placed in the arsine trap.

An appropriate volume of sample solution is placed in an arsine generator flask and diluted to approximately 35 ml. Then 5 ml of hydrochloric acid, 2 ml of 15% potassium iodide and 8 drops of tin(II) chloride ($SnCl_2$: dissolve 40 g of $SnCl_2\cdot2H_2O$ in hydrochloric acid and dilute to 100 ml with hydrochloric acid) are added. The mixture is allowed to stand for more than 15 min at room temperature. Four grams of zinc metal (0·5 mm)

Properties and Determination

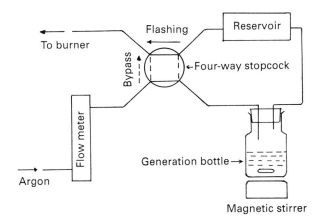

Fig. 3 Arsine generator for atomic absorption spectrometry (batch system).

are added. The generator bottle is immediately sealed and the tube connected as illustrated. The solution is allowed to react for 30 min. The trap is disconnected and the trapping solution mixed by gently drawing back and forth five times with an aspirator assembly. The solution is transferred directly to the spectrophotometer cell and the absorbance measured at 522 nm. If AgDDC-brucine-chloroform solution is used as a trapping solution, an appropriate volume of chloroform should be added to the trapping solution at the end of trapping operation to compensate for the loss of chloroform evaporation.

Atomic Absorption Spectrometry

Either a hollow cathode lamp or an electrodeless discharge lamp (EDL) is used as a light source. Absorption lines at 193·7 and 197·3 nm are used.

Direct nebulization air-acetylene flame atomic absorption spectrometry is impractical because of very poor sensitivity and because the flame strongly absorbs radiation at the wavelengths of sensitive absorption lines.

Fairly good sensitivity is obtained by the hydride generation technique, in which arsenic is introduced into a hydrogen-argon flame as arsine or into a heated tube atomizer for measurement of atomic absorption.

Hydride generators are sold by the manufacturers of atomic absorption spectrometers. The hydride generators are classified into batch and continuous-flow types. Directions by the manufacturer should be followed, but a brief description of these two types may be pertinent.

A batch hydride generator consists of a generator bottle, a gas reservoir and a four-way stopcock connected as illustrated in Fig. 3. An appropriate volume of sample solution (containing less than 1 μg As) is placed in a generation bottle with 4 ml of concentrated hydrochloric acid. Add 1 ml of 40% (m/v) potassium iodide

solution to eliminate interference from transition metals. Replace the air in the apparatus with argon. Remove the stopper and add a sodium borohydride tablet (0·25 to 0·3 g). Immediately place the stopper as illustrated and stir the contents with a magnetic stirrer. After a definite period of time (60 to 80 sec), turn the 4-way stopcock to the flashing position so that the arsine accumulated in the generation bottle and arsine reservoir is flashed into a burner by an argon stream and record the signal from the spectrometer.

In the continuous flow generator method, acidified sample solution is continuously mixed with sodium borohydride solution by means of a peristaltic pump. The mixture is led to a gas-liquid separator, and the gas phase is carried by a stream of argon into a burner or a heated tube atomizer. Because the response of arsenic(v) is lower in the continuous method, prior reduction to arsenic(III) is necessary.

Graphite furnace atomic absorption spectrometry can also be used. Successful results are obtained when nickel nitrate (10 mM) or magnesium nitrate (500 mg l^{-1}) is added as a matrix modifier to prevent loss of arsenic as the chloride during the ashing process and to reduce interference.

Inductively Coupled Plasma Atomic Emission Spectrometry (ICP/AES)

The sensitivity of direct nebulization ICP/AES for arsenic is high but not sufficient for the determination of traces of arsenic. A hydride-generation technique similar to that described for the atomic absorption spectrometry is used. A continuous hydride generator is convenient. Atomic emission at 193·7, 197·2, or 228·8 nm is measured. Atomic emission at 193·7 nm is less subject to interference. At 228·8 nm cadmium interferes.

A simple pre-concentration technique was proposed for direct nebulization ICP/AES, using a membrane filter soluble in sulphuric acid. To a 100 ml portion of sample is added 8 ml of molybdate solution (18 g Na$_2$MoO$_4$·2H$_2$O plus 100 ml sulphuric acid/400 ml) to convert arsenic(v) into a yellow arsenomolybdate. After 5 min, 2 ml of 0·02 M tetrapentylammonium bromide is added. The mixture is filtered through a nitrocellulose membrane filter, 25 mm in diameter, 0·45 μm nominal pore size. The arsenomolybdate is sorbed by the filter as the ion-associate with tetrapentylammonium ion. The filter and the arsenomolybdate sorbed are dissolved in 0·5 ml of concentrated sulphuric acid, diluted with water to 2 ml and nebulized into the plasma torch. Preconcentration up to 250-fold is possible by this technique. Tenfold preconcentration is sufficient to ensure drinking water safety. An emission line at 228·8 nm can be used. Interference from cadmium is eliminated because cadmium is not collected on the filter. Arsenic(III) does not form arsenomolybdate and is not determined.

Differentiation of Arsenic Species in Hydride Generation Method

Differentiation of various arsenic species is possible in the hydride generation technique with sodium borohydride as reductant. Conditions for the selective reduction and determination of various arsenic compounds, with a continuous-flow arsine generator and a heated tube atomizer, have been established.

Inorganic arsenic, monomethylarsonic acid and dimethylarsinic acid are reduced, in acid solution, to arsine, monomethylarsine and dimethylarsine, respectively, and collected in a cold trap. Differentiation of these arsenic compounds is possible by fractional volatilization of the arsines collected in the cold trap, because there are great differences in boiling point between arsine ($-55°C$), monomethylarsine ($2°C$) and dimethylarsine ($36°C$). Choice of a proper packing material in the cold trap is important for the mutual separation of these arsines. A silanized diatomaceous earth impregnated with phenylmethylsilicon (15%) or hydrofluoric-acid-etched glass beads (0·3 mm) have been used.

Bibliography

Anderson RK, Thompson M and Culbard E (1986) Selective reduction of arsenic species by continuous hydride generation. Part 1, Reaction media. *Analyst* 111: 1143.
Cullen WR and Reimer KJ (1989) Arsenic speciation in the environment. *Chemical Reviews* 89: 713.
Ferguson JF and Gavis J (1972) A review of the arsenic cycle in natural waters. *Water Research* 6: 1259.
Gerhartz W (ed.) (1985) *Ullmann's Encyclopedia of Industrial Chemistry* 5th edn, vol. A3, pp 113–141. Weinheim: VCH Verlagsgesellschaft mbH.
Helrich K (ed.) (1990) *Official Methods of Analysis of the Association of Official Analytical Chemists* 15th edn. Arlington: Association of Official Analytical Chemists.
Ishinishi N, Okabe S and Kikuchi T (eds) (1985) *Arsenic – Chemistry, Metabolism, Toxicology*. (In Japanese.) Tokyo: Koseishakoseikaku.
Morita M and Shibata Y (1987) Speciation of arsenic compounds in marine life by high performance liquid chromatography combined with inductively coupled argon plasma atomic emission spectrometry. *Analytical Science* 3: 575.
NRC (1977) *Arsenic*. US National Research Council, Committee on Medical and Biologic Effects of Environmental Pollutants. Washington, DC: National Academy of Sciences.
Tanaka S, Nakamura M, Kishi Y and Hashimoto Y (1986) Distribution of organic arsenic (methylarsonic acid, dimethylarsinic acid) and inorganic arsenic (As(III), As(V)) in river water. (In Japanese.) *Nippon Kagaku Kaishi* 727.
Yasui A and Tsutsumi C (1977) Adaptability of wet decomposition method to food samples for the determination of arsenic by arsine generation–atomic absorption spectrophotometry. (In Japanese.) *Bunseki Kagaku* 26: 809.

Noriko Hata, Issei Kasahara, Shigeru Taguchi and Katsumi Goto
Toyama University, Toyama, Japan

Requirements and Toxicology

Arsenic in the Environment

Arsenic is widely distributed in the natural environment. Virtually all soils and waters contain a variety of different arsenic compounds. As a by-product of melting copper, lead and several other metals, as well as by coal-fired power plants, high quantities of this metalloid are emitted into the atmosphere. Arsenic compounds are also used by the metallurgical and chemical industry. Phosphate fertilizer as well as many herbicides, fungicides, wood preservatives, insecticides and rodenticides contain arsenic. Thus agriculture contributes significantly to arsenic pollution. Legislation in countries with developed conservation systems attempts to minimize the quantity of these pesticides as well as other sources of arsenic pollution.

Owing to the ubiquity of arsenic in the environment, foodstuffs of plant and animal origin as well as drinking water also contain arsenic. The maximally permissible arsenic concentration in drinking water, vegetables, fruits and meat is regulated by law in most industrially developed countries. The US drinking water standard, for example, is fixed at $50\ \mu g\ l^{-1}$. However, several springs and spa waters contain 0·5–1·3 mg of arsenic per l.

The range of arsenic levels in foodstuffs in the absence of significant pollution is as follows: cereals, 0·05–0·4 mg kg^{-1}; fruits, 0·03–1·0 mg kg^{-1}; vegetables, 0·05–0·8 mg kg^{-1}; meat, 0·05–1·4 mg kg^{-1}; dairy products, 0·01–0·23 mg kg^{-1}. Higher concentrations – 1·5–15·3 mg kg^{-1} – are registered in seafoods because marine organisms accumulate arsenic in the form of nontoxic organic compounds. The average daily intake of arsenic is estimated in the range of 12–40 μg. When diets contain substantial amounts of seafood, as is usual in Japan, 70–170 μg could be the realistic daily intake. *See* Shellfish, Contamination and Spoilage of Molluscs and Crustacea

Arsenic Metabolism

Intestinal Absorption

Arsenic is generally well absorbed by the gastrointestinal tract, although the solubility of the compounds seems to correlate with the rate of absorption. Intestinal absorption of most inorganic and organic compounds of arsenic is a quick process. However, some unusual compounds, such as Na-P-N-glycolylarsenilate, given orally to humans, are poorly absorbed.

Arsenate is apparently absorbed by simple diffusion following a concentration gradient. Sharing a specific transport system with phosphate seems to be unlikely. Organic compounds of arsenic are also absorbed in a manner directly proportional to their concentration in the intestinal lumen over a wide range.

Arsenic in Human Tissues

Once absorbed, arsenic is quickly distributed to all organs and tissues, probably as a complex with α-globulins. Apart from inorganic arsenic, blood also contains methylated metabolites formed in the liver.

If the uptake of arsenic is low, no significant accumulation in the soft tissues occurs. However, in unexposed humans relatively high arsenic concentrations are usually found in skin, nails and hair. Because hair levels correlate with arsenic in the air as well as with renal arsenic excretion, hair concentration has often been used as an index of contamination with toxic amounts of arsenic. The median arsenic content of human hair was found to be $0.51 \mu g\, g^{-1}$. The hair of workers at plants with arsenic-containing emissions was found to be 10–31 μg of arsenic per g of hair. Values greater than 3 μg per g indicate toxic levels of uptake.

Arsenic Excretion

In general, the biological half-life of arsenic is short, the metalloid being excreted mainly in urine with a little in faeces. Some compounds, such as arsenobetaine, the form found in marine animals, pass through into the urine unchanged. For this reason, despite the high arsenic content, intoxication by seafood is unlikely. Different methylated compounds are the major urinary metabolites.

Excretion via the bile is low after dietary intake of arsenic, but can significantly increase when drugs containing arsenic are administered intravenously.

Biotransformation of Arsenic

Inorganic arsenic is methylated in the liver with *S*-adenosylmethionine as methyl (CH_3) donor. As the first step, arsenate is reduced to arsenite, which is methylated to di-methylarsenic acid with monomethyl-arsenic as a precursor. Investigations with germ-free animals have shown that methylation is mainly per-

formed by the liver cells, with little contribution from the intestinal microflora.

Some organic compounds, especially arsenobetaine, are excreted unchanged. Arsenocholine can be incorporated into phospholipids, replacing choline, but the major part of this compound is excreted by the kidney.

Some mould species are able to produce volatile neurotoxic compounds by biotransforming arsenical pigments contained especially in wallpapers. Some lethal poisoning cases have been described resulting from such toxic products of aerobic and nonaerobic fungi as well as other primitive organisms. Different species of the phytoplankton metabolize arsenate to nontoxic organic compounds that accumulate in marine animals consuming the plankton. The main compound produced is arsenobetaine. Some intermediates of this biotransformation, however, can be highly toxic.

Biochemical Function and Essentiality of Arsenic

Although a specific function for arsenic on a molecular level is unknown, some evidence has been accumulated indicating a distinct role for this element in several metabolic processes.

This could be the case in CH_3-group metabolism. Almost all organic forms of arsenic produced *in vivo* are methylated compounds. One of the trimethylated ones is arsenocholine, which can be incorporated into phospholipids, replacing choline. Choline is a methyl donor for different methylation reactions in intermediary metabolism. There is some evidence indicating that arsenocholine might have a similar function in labile methyl metabolism. As some experiments have shown that arsenic deprivation in the rat, chick and hamster affects labile methyl metabolism, it could be speculated that the role of arsenocholine cannot be fulfilled by choline.

Arsenic binds strongly to sulphydryl groups which are known to participate in hundreds of enzymatic reactions. In this context it behaves like heavy metals that impair enzymatic catalysis. It is likely that the biochemical basis is the inhibition of a wide range of SH-enzymes by arsenic. But it cannot be ruled out in advance that such an interaction is not only of toxicological but also of biological significance.

Some investigators have reported that arsenic can provide partial protection from chronic selenosis, with the vitamin E level influencing the incorporation of selenium into the tissues. It has been shown that selenium toxicity for cultured mice fibroblasts can also be counteracted by arsenic. Interactions between arsenic and cadmium have also been shown. Considering the common mode of action that these elements have at the cellular level, especially through interaction with SH-groups, these facts are not surprising. *See* Cadmium, Toxicology; Selenium, Physiology

Studies with chicks suggest that arsenic is closely related to the metabolism of zinc. Depressed growth caused by arsenic deprivation was alleviated when dietary zinc was given in excess. It seems, however, not only that interactions between arsenic and zinc exist but also that the arginine status of the chicks plays a distinct role in these complicated correlations between the two trace elements and the amino acid. There is support for the possibility that arsenic participates – in a way that has yet to be clarified – in utilizing amino acids for protein synthesis, or in protein degradation, as well as in uric acid metabolism. *See* Zinc, Physiology

Effects of arsenic on carbohydrate metabolism have been observed in experiments with guinea pigs. The most prominent finding after repeated arsenic (As_2O_3) administration was a marked decrease in total carbohydrate content of the liver, mainly owing to depletion of glycogen. *See* Carbohydrates, Digestion, Absorption and Metabolism

Some other biochemical facts in connection with arsenic – used in physiological as well as toxicological amounts – have been registered in the last few years. We are far from being able to classify the frequently conflicting facts and their significance for metabolism.

Since 1975, some conclusive evidence has been published supporting the suggestion of nutritional essentiality of arsenic. An element is considered essential if a dietary deficiency consistently results in a suboptimal biological function that is preventable or reversible by intake of a physiological amount of that element. Signs of arsenic deprivation were studied in four animal species – chick, goat, miniature pig and rat. Safe and adequate intakes of arsenic for these species are not precisely defined. However, a diet containing less than 50 μg of arsenic per kg is denoted as 'arsenic-deficient' ration in these animal experiments, whereas 350–500 μg kg^{-1} is considered a 'normal arsenic supply' and 3·5–5 mg kg^{-1} as a 'therapeutic dose'.

The essentiality of arsenic has been systematically investigated in growing, pregnant and lactating goats, as well as in miniature pigs and their offspring. Deficient rations contained less than 10 μg of arsenic per kg of semi-synthetic diet, and control rations 350 μg kg^{-1}. The following deficiency symptoms were described: feed consumption was reduced and this was correlated with diminished growth rates and milk production; a high abortion rate for goats and increased perinatal mortality for miniature pigs and rats were also registered; intra-uterine arsenic depletion in goats, miniature pigs and rats resulted in significantly reduced birthweight of the offspring.

The decreased milk-fat concentration could be a consequence of lowered triglyceride concentration in the blood serum of arsenic-deficient goats.

Histological changes, accompanied by ultrastructural alterations of the mitochondria, have been seen especially in skeletal muscles, the myocardium and liver tissue. Some modifications in the mineral composition of different organs with a remarkable retention of manganese were also connected to arsenic deficiency.

There is as yet no convincing evidence that arsenic is essential for humans, but the possibility cannot be ruled out. For definitive judgement of essentiality of arsenic further critical investigations are necessary.

Only data from animal studies are available for estimating the approximate amount of arsenic required by humans, if it is essential for humans at all. Cautious assessments support a daily requirement of about 12–15 μg for persons consuming 8·4 MJ per day. This amount is guaranteed by a mixed-food diet.

Beneficial effects of arsenic preparations have been known – or at least believed – for centuries. Arsanilic acid used to be incorporated into pig and poultry feed in pharmacological doses as a growth-promoting agent. Intake of relatively high amounts of inorganic arsenic salts by humans and horses was reported from several parts of Europe. 'Arsenic eaters' were convinced that these preparations had protective effects against diseases, and increased physical condition and virility. Regular daily intakes of 0·5 g of arsenic have been reported, a dose that can only be tolerated after being accustomed to arsenic for a long time. *See* Trace Elements

Toxicity of Arsenic

Arsenic has traditionally been associated with the poisoner and it was of interest to forensic medicine as a poison frequently used in suicide and homicide. Nowadays, intoxication mostly results from accidental intake of arsenic-contaminated food or beverages, or from environmental pollution. Depending on the dose, the nature of compounds and the health status of the individual incorporating the poison, arsenic can cause both acute and chronic poisoning.

Acute Toxicity

The smallest lethal dose reported is 130 mg of arsenic, but total recovery can occur even if the ingested dose is several times higher. Signs of intoxication can appear a few minutes after ingesting a solution containing arsenic, but when the arsenic is taken in solid form they can also be delayed for up to 10 h. After ingestion of a lethal dose, death occurs after 12–24 h.

Depending on the severity of exposure to arsine (AsH_3), haemolytic symptoms can occur in a few minutes or after about 24 h. After massive exposure nausea, vomiting and abdominal cramps begin within 2 h, followed by haematuria and the skin colour turning yellow within 24 h.

Chronic Toxicity

A maximum daily intake of arsenic that is well tolerated over a longer period of time without impairing health and wellbeing cannot be fixed precisely. The chemical form of arsenic strongly affects its toxicity and variations in individual susceptibility are large. It was reported that orchard workers ingested as much as 6·8 mg of arsenic per day, i.e. about 500 times the estimated daily requirement, for years without any signs of intoxication. The ratio of the toxic to nutritional dose for rats was found to be about 1250.

The toxicity of arsenic compounds has been classified in the following decreasing order:

1. Inorganic compounds (trivalent arsenicals, arsenite salts, pentavalent arsenate salts).
2. Organic arsenicals.
3. Arsine.

The mode of incorporation of arsenic can be by respiration, by oral intake with drinking water and food and by skin. For the latter route arsenic trichloride is the only compound of importance. Irritations of the respiratory tract are common in areas surrounding coal-burning power-stations, especially in eastern Europe where stations use coal that contains up to 200 times as much arsenic as average coal. Human exposure to arsenic in the air is likely to increase in the future.

In some areas of the world the concentration of arsenic in drinking water exceeds the fixed standards. However, the correlation of different disorders with drinking water containing arsenic in a range above the drinking water standards of 50 μg l^{-1} (0·6–6·0 mg l^{-1}) remains questionable. Most of the researchers (California, Oregon, Alaska) reported no adverse health effects, investigators from Minnesota, Taiwan and Chile presented data supporting circulatory and skin disorders from arsenic consumption through drinking water. Reasons for these regional differences may be the additional exposure to other chemicals and/or fungi that potentiated the observed effects. In addition, differences in the nutritional status of the populations investigated remains at issue.

Contamination of foodstuffs with arsenic can result from air pollution, soil pollution by agricultural measures or by accidental pollution. Use of arsenics as pesticides in vineyards resulted, in some cases, in poisoning by arsenic contaminated wine. Cirrhosis of the liver in vine-growers was assumed to have at least partially been caused by arsenic.

Until the first decades of the twentieth century a preparation of inorganic arsenic known as Fowler's solution was used for the treatment of dermatoses and even as a tonic against anaemia. The treatment often lasted several years and caused signs of chronic arsenic poisoning especially on the skin with a high incidence of skin cancer.

Clinical symptoms of long-lasting arsenic intoxication develop over weeks and months. The first signs occur in the skin, mucous membranes, gastrointestinal tract and neural system. The liver and circulatory system are affected later, if at all. The symptom complex resembles that of other progressive diseases, thus arsenic intoxication is difficult to diagnose. For this reason arsenic was one of the most common homicidal poisons for centuries.

Classical initial symptoms of chronic intoxication with arsenic are as follows: loss of appetite and, subsequently, weight; weakness; nausea; vomiting; dry throat; fatigue; gastrointestinal symptoms; icterus and skin erythema. As the disease progresses, further symptoms can be found: loss of hair, fragile and pigmented nails, eczema, hyperkeratosis, desquamation of the skin on hands and feet. Later, severe conjunctivitis, bronchitis, neurological symptoms, hearing disturbances and vascular disorders can occur. Some of the symptoms are reversible when exposure is interrupted, but individual variability is great, and neurological symptoms are particularly long-lasting.

Therapeutic Measures

The most common antidote to arsenic poisoning is 2,3-dimercaptopropanol (BAL). It is a dithiol which binds one arsenic molecule with its two SH- groups. Owing to the fact that this binding is more stable than binding of arsenic to the SH- groups of the amino acid residues, arsenic can be eliminated via renal excretion.

Successful treatments with BAL have been reported, especially in cases of dermatitis caused by arsenic intoxication. After injection of the drug a powerful stimulation of renal arsenic excretion is registered during the first 3–6 days, accompanied by an improvement of the skin lesions. A further chelating agent recommended in case of arsenic poisoning is D-penicillinamine. In severe cases of acute intoxication, exchange transfusion or haemodialysis might become necessary.

Teratogenic and Mutagenic Effects

Large doses of arsenic are reported to cause teratogenic alterations in different animal species. Embryotoxic effects of arsenite (1–40 μM) and arsenate (10–400 μM) on the development of mouse embryos during the early organogenesis have been registered in the form of growth retardation and malformations of the central nervous system and of the extremities. Although no direct evidence exists for embryotoxicity of arsenic in humans, it cannot be conclusively ruled out that this toxic element may be involved in 'unaccountable' early abortions and malformations claimed to be attributable to the toxicity of heavy metals.

Careful studies performed in the last decade point to the mutagenic potency of arsenic. Induction of chromosomal aberrations and sister chromatid exchanges have been described. A role of arsenic as a potential synergist to ionizing radiation, as well as inhibition of deoxyribonucleic acid (DNA) repair by this element have been supposed. The ability of arsenic to induce gene amplification may relate to its carcinogenic effects in humans since amplification of oncogenes is observed in many human tumours. *See* Mutagens

Arsenic and Carcinogenesis

A number of epidemiological studies have been performed to elucidate the correlation between chronic arsenic exposure and cancer. The results are controversial. *See* Cancer, Epidemiology

Inorganic arsenic causes a variety of benign skin lesions, including hyperpigmentation and hyperkeratosis. Some hyperkeratotic lesions and squamous cell carcinomas *in situ* may progress to invasive carcinoma and metastasize. Locally invasive but nonmetastasizing basal cell carcinomas may also occur. A dose–response relationship has been described between medicinally administered arsenic and the frequency of various skin lesions. Chronic intake of arsenical preparations for

psoriasis is reported to cause malignant lesions in skin, lung and liver.

A high incidence of carcinoma of the respiratory tract was registered in several epidemiological studies dealing with populations in areas highly polluted with arsenic. Factory workers exposed simultaneously to arsenic and sulphur dioxide ran a very high risk of developing multiple carcinoma.

In 1970 the Occupational Safety and Health Administration of the US government fixed the maximum concentration of inorganic arsenic in the air to $10~\mu g~m^{-3}$ for occupational exposure. On the basis of several studies performed in factories causing arsenic pollution the same institution predicted that the risk of lung carcinoma would rise exponentially with increasing pollution.

Bibliography

Anke M (1986) Arsenic. In: Mertz W (ed.) *Trace Elements in Human and Animal Nutrition* 5th edn, vol. 2, pp 347–372. Orlando: Academic Press.
Fowler BA (ed.) (1983) *Biological and Environmental Effect of Arsenic*. Amsterdam: Elsevier Science Publishers BV.
Lederer WH and Fensterheim RJ (eds) (1983) *Arsenic: Industrial, Biomedical, Environmental Perspectives*. New York: Van Nostrand Reinhold.
Nielsen FH (1990) Other trace elements. In: Brown ML (ed.) *Present Knowledge in Nutrition*, 6th edn, pp 294–296. Washington, DC: International Life Science Institute, Nutrition Foundation.

Gertrud I. Rehner
Institute of Nutrition, Giessen, FRG

ARTHRITIS

Although there are over 200 different sorts of arthritis, the two most common forms – osteoarthritis and rheumatoid arthritis (Fig. 1) – account for the vast majority of cases. Others include gout, ankylosing spondylitis, psoriatic arthritis and systemic lupus erythematosus. Cervical spondylosis and lumbar spondylosis are caused by osteoarthritis of the neck and lower spine.

Osteoarthritis

The term 'osteoarthritis' (OA) is one of a number of synonyms (e.g. degenerative joint disease) used to

describe a group of conditions characterized by focal loss of articular cartilage with overgrowth and remodelling of underlying and nearby bone. The resultant disruption in the joint can cause pain and stiffness, changes in the shape of the joint, loss of movement and loss of joint stability. Osteoarthritis affects many animal species and there is skeletal evidence that it has been present since the earliest history of man. It is extremely common: radiological (X ray) surveys suggest that about 10% of all adults have moderate or severe disease in one or more joints, although not all those with radiological changes have symptoms. About 75% of those people classified as disabled from arthritis suffer from OA, and the incidence increases with age. About 30% of arthritis problems in the working age group are due to OA. The natural history is of slowly progressive loss of articular cartilage with sclerosis (hardening) and reshaping of the subchondral bone (bone directly below the cartilage). At times there may be some inflammation of the synovial lining of the joint, and thickening and fibrosis of the joint capsule often develop. The articular cartilage in the early stages of experimental OA in animals shows an increase in water content with alteration in matrix proteoglycans and increase of metabolic activity of cartilage cells (chondrocytes). The long proteoglycan chains are split into small segments which are lost from the cartilage, and the collagen network in which they are embedded becomes disrupted. These changes reduce the ability of cartilage to withstand the stresses and strains normally transmitted through the joint. It cracks and becomes roughened and thin, and may be lost completely, exposing underlying bone. As the cartilage damage progresses, the subchondral bone becomes more vascular and sclerotic, and osteophytes – outgrowths of bone at the edge of the joint – develop. Cysts (holes) inside the bone ends may also develop, probably following death and necrosis of bone. The altered mechanics of the joint and episodes of synovial inflammation often result in production of excess, abnormal synovial (joint) fluid. *See* Bone

Factors Leading to OA

Osteoarthritis can be thought of as 'joint failure' which may be precipitated by several different mechanisms.

Genetic factors are important. There are gender and racial differences in expression of the disease: OA of the hand is common in Caucasian women, while OA of the hip occurs rarely in the Chinese. Heberden's nodes, associated with OA of the end joints of the fingers, has a particularly strong inherited component. Obesity, as well as being associated with more severe symptoms of OA in the legs, is associated with the development of OA in the knees and hands – but not the hips or ankles. This association is probably constitutional rather than mechanical.

Mechanical abnormalities in joint function may also predispose to OA. Menisectomy (removal of the extra cartilage 'cushion' found in the knee) results in the subsequent development of OA in about 40% of cases 15 years later. Severe trauma affecting the joint surfaces, or malalignment following limb fracture, can result in OA. Minor repetitive trauma over long periods in various occupations can lead to characteristic patterns of OA. Clearcut dysplasia (abnormal growth), leading to abnormalities in shape of joints such as the hip, is recognized as a further abnormal mechanical stimulus. The possibility that many cases of otherwise unexplained OA develop as a result of minor degrees of dysplasia has not yet been fully explored. Other permanent changes in joint mechanics, particularly following episodes of other forms of arthritis, will also result in the steady development of OA, often resulting in the progress of two types of arthritis at the same time.

Metabolic abnormalities that result in the formation of defective cartilage (ochranosis, iron deposition, acromegaly) or the deposition of calcium crystals (chondrocalcinosis) may result in OA.

While some patients have clear aetiological factors leading to the secondary development of OA, most appear to develop OA 'spontaneously' and probably have a combination of genetic, mechanical and inflammatory changes which determine pathogenesis.

Rheumatoid Arthritis

Rheumatoid arthritis (RA) is an inflammatory disease of the synovial membranes which line the joint (Fig. 1) and usually affects many joints from the outset. In addition, there are general features which show that many body systems may be involved. It is often accompanied by lethargy, tiredness, weight loss and anaemia, and sometimes by inflammatory lesions in blood vessels (vasculitis), nerves or pleura (lining of the lung), indicating that it may have far-reaching systemic manifestations. It is a common condition and has a worldwide distribution but is more prevalent in the temperate climates. It affects approximately one and half million people in the UK, the female to male ratio being about 3 : 1. The majority of patients have their first symptoms between the ages of 20 and 55 years of age, but the age range extends from early childhood to senility.

The joint lining (synovium), which is normally thin and delicate, becomes overgrown, developing folds and projections. It contains numerous inflammatory cells (such as polymorphs, lymphocytes and plasma cells), is highly vascular and has the histological characteristics of granulation tissue. It grows across and into the joint cartilage, forming a 'pannus' which releases proteolytic enzymes that digest cartilage and bone, thus allowing the pannus to burrow into and destroy these structures and giving rise to the classical X ray features of bony 'erosions' (Fig. 1). This process starts at the outer margins of the joint but gradually spreads across the articular surface and causes damage to the joint capsule and surrounding ligaments. In later stages of the disease the joints may become very deformed and the synovial membrane totally replaced by fibrous (scar) tissue which causes contracture of the joint capsule and adds to the general destructive process.

The synovial linings of tendon sheaths and bursae

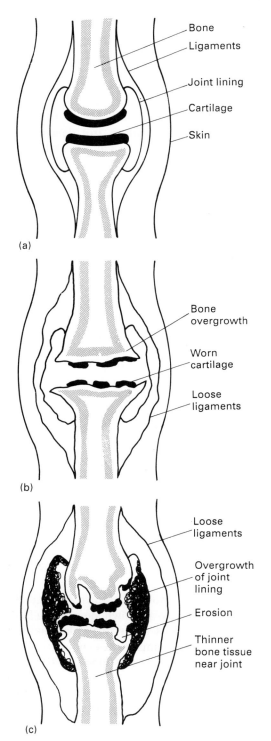

Fig. 1 Schematic representations of (a) a normal joint, (b) a joint with features of osteoarthritis, and (c) a joint with rheumatoid arthritis.

may also be affected, and this contributes to the characteristic hand deformities seen in this disease. The inflammatory process is driven on by a hyperactive immune system, which also produces antibodies that can be measured in the blood and are called 'rheumatoid

factors'. The stimulus that drives the immune system is unknown.

Factors Contributing to RA

Genetic factors appear to play a role, and the risk of developing RA is increased two- to threefold in first-degree relatives of patients with RA. The identical twin of a patient with 'seropositive' RA (i.e. with rheumatoid factor in the serum) has a 33-fold increased risk. Certain tissue typing (HLA) genes are associated with RA, of which the most striking are HLA-DR4 in Caucasians and HLA-DR1 in Asians. It is now known that the increased risk of disease resides in only a few amino acids crucial to the three-dimensional shape of the HLA gene proteins, but why this should be so remains conjectural.

Although various microbial infections may be followed by polyarthritis in both animals and humans, none have been shown to cause RA, and the polyarthritis usually resolves. It is possible that very small bacterial cell wall components remain in joints to act as potent immune stimulants that are capable of prolonged inflammatory reactions. Cytokines are small molecules which act as messengers between cells, particularly those involved in the immune system and inflammation. Recent intense interest in these cytokines has revealed the very complex interaction between these substances and has raised the possibility that RA may result from some abnormality induced in this system of cell control. The earliest event seen in the synovium is a mild proliferation of the lining layer. Subsequent increases in the vascularity are accompanied by obliteration of small blood vessels by inflammatory cells and organized thrombi (clots). The endothelial lining cells of the vessels are damaged and seem to play an important role in early inflammation. They also express HLA-DR antigens and various adhesion molecules that are recognized by inflammatory cells and assist their passage through the endothelial layer and into the inflamed tissues. The cytokines released from these inflammatory cells play a key role in the perpetuation of inflammation within the joint. This early phase is followed by a more chronic phase, associated with complex morphological changes and activation of T and then B lymphocytes. B lymphocytes secrete immunoglobulins (antibodies) which form complexes and may contribute to the perpetuation of the inflammatory reactions in RA. Erosions develop where cells such as fibroblasts and macrophages release prostaglandins, collagenases, and proteinases capable of tissue destruction. *See* Immunity and Nutrition

The pathogenesis of RA is complex and multifactorial (Fig. 2) but may be summarized as the initiation of an inflammatory cascade by unknown agents in genetically susceptible individuals, resulting in joint destruction and potential involvement of other nonarticular organs.

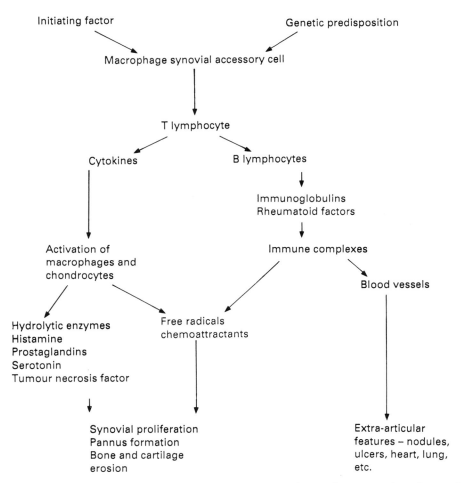

Fig. 2 The complex aetiopathogenic mechanisms involved in the initiation and perpetuation of synovial inflammation in rheumatoid arthritis.

Diet and RA

Several studies have shown a direct relationship between the severity of joint inflammation in RA and nutritional depletion. Three mechanisms probably contribute to poor nutritional status – reduced food intake, increased energy loss, and alterations in metabolism. Reduced food intake occurs as a direct consequence of loss of functional ability for activities of daily living. Destruction of the wrist joints, weakened fingers and hands, limited finger mobility, elbow and shoulder involvement, temporomandibular joint destruction, and lower limb arthritis can all limit the ability to self-feed, shop and prepare meals. These disabilities may lead to reduced food intake and an unbalanced diet. They also increase the energy requirement of normal activities, such as walking, and, as in other inflammatory conditions, there are metabolic changes during exacerbations of RA which result in protein loss and muscle wasting, perhaps mediated by tumour necrosis factor (TNFα).

Investigation of the dietary treatment of RA has not addressed the secondary nutritional deficiencies reported above, but has rather concentrated on finding a primary role for nutrients in the cause of the disease and hence in its control or cure.

Hopes that vitamins A, B_6 and C may play a role in the pathogenesis of RA have been dashed by experimental and clinical work which has shown no patient benefit after administration of supplements.

Osteoporosis is frequently seen in patients with RA, particularly those who require glucocorticosteroids to control their disease. The role of dietary calcium in preventing or reversing osteoporosis remains controversial but it seems prudent to ensure an adequate intake. For those who cannot consume milk and other dairy foods, calcium supplements may be necessary. *See* Calcium, Physiology; Osteoporosis

Interest in the role of copper in inflammatory disease was stimulated by raised serum and synovial fluid concentrations, but these almost certainly reflect a nonspecific response to inflammation and not a nutritional disturbance.

Inability to utilize iron in the normal way may result in anaemia in patients with RA, even when bone marrow iron stores are adequate. Some evidence suggests that iron deposition in the synovium may accentuate local inflammation.

Selenium deficiency is associated with a rare form of arthritis in China, but clinical studies in RA have not suggested therapeutic benefit, and the slightly low levels found in active RA return to normal when the disease is treated by other means. Plasma zinc levels are also reduced in active disease and return to normal when RA is treated.

Fasting can ameliorate joint symptoms in patients with rheumatoid arthritis at least in the short term. The effects of fasting on immune function in healthy volunteers include decreased neutrophil bacterial killing, depressed lymphocyte response to mitogens, decreased serum levels of several acute-phase reactants and complement factors, and increased serum cortisol levels. This depression in immune function may be the mechanism of action of fasting in rheumatoid arthritis, but at the present time fasting cannot be recommended. Not only would fasting be unacceptable to patients but it may lead to protein–energy malnutrition.

There have been a few well-documented patients in which food hypersensitivity triggers joint inflammation, but these are notable for their rarity. Almost all who claim 'allergy' to certain foods have no abnormal immunological response after ingestion and do not reproduce symptoms on blinded challenge with the implicated nutrient.

The Effects of Fatty Acids

The biological activity of prostaglandins, which play such an important role in inflammation, depends critically on the chemical series to which they belong, which in turn depends on the type of unsaturated fatty acid from which they derive. The fatty acids that are available as substrate via the diet determine this. *See* Essential Fatty Acids, Physiology; Fatty Acids, Dietary Importance; Prostaglandins and Leukotrienes

Linoleic acid (18:2 ω-6) is the predominant unsaturated fatty acid in a Western diet and is metabolized to produce leucotrienes and prostaglandins of the second series. Fatty acids from fish and fish oils are converted into leucotrienes and prostaglandins of the third series, which have much reduced inflammatory activity. Diets low in fat (reducing the total amount of inflammatory mediators available) or containing predominantly fish oil have been shown to reduce autoimmune disease severity in animal models of arthritis. Evening primrose oil (EPO) contains first-series precursors which also have less inflammatory activity. Clinical studies with large doses of EPO or fish oil have resulted in reduced requirements for anti-inflammatory drugs in patients with various types of arthritis. This effect may take several months to develop, and the general economic

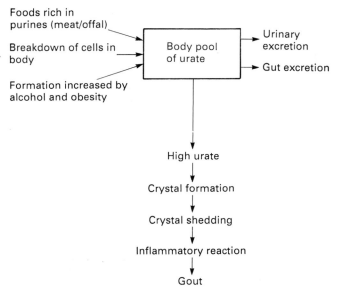

Fig. 3 Pathogenesis of gout.

and other health effects of such changes will need to be evaluated before such treatment can be recommended. *See* Fatty Acids, Gamma Linolenic Acid; Fish Oils, Dietary Importance

Gout

Gout usually causes recurrent attacks of very painful and inflamed arthritis in one joint – classically in the big toe. Each attack may last 10–14 days, unless treated. During an episode of gout there is an intense inflammatory reaction to crystals of monosodium urate which are present in the joint. These are related to the body pool of urate (Fig. 3) and occur more frequently in middle-aged, overweight men, and do not occur before puberty or before the menopause in women. Attacks can be precipitated by variations in serum urate concentrations caused by fluid balance changes, such as taking diuretics or dehydration.

Factors Contributing to Gout

Serum urate levels are not distributed normally in the population, so that about 10% of people have 'raised' levels. These are often above supersaturation, but crystals seldom form, implying some mechanism of prevention. Crystal formation becomes increasingly likely as serum urate levels increase. Crystal formation occurs preferentially in connective tissue, especially joints. Groups of crystals form intra-articular tophi. An acute attack is probably initiated by crystal shedding from cartilage or synovium, producing a shower of crystals, the charged surfaces of which interact with cells and proteins to activate acute inflammation. However, not everyone with high urate levels develops crystals, and not all with free crystals develop gout inflammation. The mechanisms by which crystal formation is inhibited, inflammation is prevented, or an acute attack brought under control, are currently unknown. It is possible that biological control of surface protein coating holds the key.

Bibliography

ARC (1991) *Diet and Arthritis*. London: Arthritis and Rheumatism Council.

Dieppe P (1988) *Arthritis* (Family Doctor Guides). London: British Medical Association.
Dieppe PA, Bacon PA, Bamji AN and Watt I (1986) *Atlas of Clinical Rheumatology*. Oxford: Oxford University Press.
Dieppe P, Cooper C, Kirwan J and McGill N (1991) *Arthritis and Rheumatism in Practice*. London: Gower Medical Publishing.
Kelley WN, Harris ED, Ruddy S, Sledge CB (eds) (1989) *Textbook of Rheumatology* 3rd edn. London: WB Saunders.

E. George and John R. Kirwan
Bristol Royal Infirmary, Bristol, UK

ASCORBIC ACID

Contents

Properties and Determination

Vitamin C, the antiscorbutic vitamin, is found in a large variety of foods but particularly in fruits and vegetables. Its two natural vitamers, L-ascorbic acid (AA) and dehydro-L-ascorbic acid (DHAA) form an oxidation–reduction system which is the basis not only of many of its physiological activities but also of its many technical applications.

This article concentrates on the physical and chemical properties of the vitamin, its occurrence in foods, its use as a food additive and the problems associated with its analytical determination in foods and physiological samples. It will be necessary to also discuss the diastereomer of ascorbic acid, D-isoascorbic acid (IAA) and the corresponding dehydro-D-isoascorbic acid (DHIAA) as these compounds are now being found in some processed foods since the isoascorbic–dehydroisoascorbic couple also forms an oxidation–reduction system and is being used in the food industry as a preservative.

The nutritional aspects and the biological role of vitamin C are discussed in a separate article.

Physical Properties

For our purposes, the structures of AA and DHAA can be drawn in the several ways shown in Fig. 1. Also shown is the ascorbate free radical known to be the intermediate in the transition from AA to DHAA.

Both AA and DHAA in the pure state are white crystalline solids, the former appearing as plates and the latter appearing as needles. The physical properties of both are listed in the *Merck Index* and those for AA are given in Table 1. DHAA exists as a dimer in the solid phase but in aqueous solution assumes a monomeric hemiacetal form (not shown). IAA and DHIAA have essentially the same structures as those of vitamin C except for the stereo configuration about carbon atom 5. IAA has at most 5% of the vitamin activity of AA.

Chemical Properties

AA is sensitive to heat and light, being rapidly converted to DHAA. The latter is further oxidized to diketogulonic acid (DKGA), shown in Fig. 1, which has no vitamin activity. DHAA can be prepared from ascorbic acid with activated charcoal, halogens, ferric chloride, hydrogen peroxide, 2,6-dichlorophenol–indophenol and other oxidizing agents, while it can be reduced to AA with reagents such as homocysteine, dithiothreitol, hydrogen sulphide and glutathione.

AA is most stable at a pH of 3·5–5. The decomposition is catalysed by the presence of such metals as iron and copper. Metal-chelating agents such as ethylenediaminetetraacetic acid (EDTA) and oxalic acid tend to reduce this catalysis. Enzymes found in foods, such as L-ascorbic-acid oxidase, catalyse the conversion of AA to DHAA.

There are several reactions of AA and DHAA which

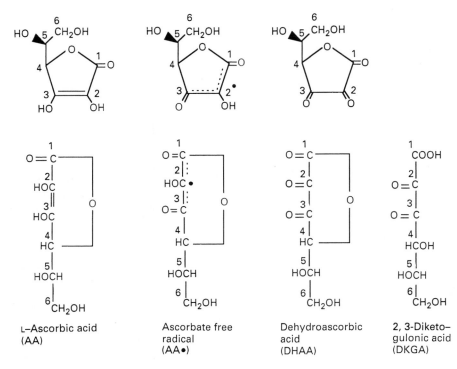

Fig. 1. Representative structures for ascorbic acid, the ascorbate radical, dehydroascorbic acid and diketogulonic acid.

Table 1. Physical properties of L-ascorbic acid

Property	Characteristics
Formula	$C_6H_8O_6$
Relative molecular mass	176·12
Appearance	White, odourless, crystalline solid
Crystal form	Monoclinic, usually plates, sometimes needles
Melting point	190–192°C
Density	1·65
Optical rotation	$[\alpha]_D^{25} = +20\cdot5–21\cdot5°$ ($c = 1$ in water) $[\alpha]_D^{23} = +48°$ ($c = 1$ in methanol)
pH	3 (5 mg ml^{-1}), 2 (50 mg ml^{-1})
pK_1	4·17
pK_2	11·57
Ultraviolet (λ_{max})	245 nm (acid solution) 265 nm (neutral solution)
Redox potential	First stage $E_0' = +0\cdot127$ (pH = 5)
Solubility	1 g in 3 ml water, 30 ml alcohol, 50 ml (ab. alcohol), 100 ml glycerol USP, 20 ml propylene glycol. Insoluble in ether, chloroform, benzene, petroleum ether, oils, fats, fat solvents

are of importance to food processors. AA can act as an O_2 scavenger, as shown in eqn [1].

$$AA + O_2 \rightarrow DHAA + H_2O \qquad (1)$$

In foods, free radicals, which are atoms or molecules containing unpaired electrons and are indicated in the text by ·, start chain reactions which can rapidly cause food spoilage. AA can intercept these radicals, thus stopping the chain reaction (eqn [2]).

$$\left. \begin{array}{l} R\cdot \\ ROO\cdot \end{array} \right\} + AA \rightarrow AA\cdot + \left\{ \begin{array}{l} RH \\ ROOH \end{array} \right. \qquad (2)$$

$$2AA\cdot \rightarrow AA + DHAA$$

Vitamin E is often used as a free-radical scavenger in fats and oils. AA (palmitate form) acts synergistically with vitamin E to maintain the latter's potency as illustrated in eqn [3]. *See* Tocopherols, Properties and Determination

$$E + ROO\cdot \rightarrow E\cdot + ROOH$$
$$E\cdot + AA \rightarrow E + A\cdot \qquad (3)$$
$$2A\cdot \rightarrow AA + DHAA$$

Nitrosamines, cancer-inducing agents, are generated in some food-producing processes as well as in tobacco smoke. These are formed by the action of nitrous acid with secondary and tertiary amines. AA can reduce the amounts of these generated nitrosamines by scavenging HNO_2 (eqn [4]). *See* Nitrosamines

$$2HNO_2 + AA \rightarrow DHAA + 2NO + 2H_2O \qquad (4)$$

The reaction of DHAA with glutathione (GSH) is thought to be important in the improvement found in gluten formation during breadmaking (eqn [5]).

$$DHAA + 2GSH \rightarrow AA + GSSH \qquad (5)$$

A reaction of importance in the low-temperature storage of fresh meat is that of AA with metmyoglobin (eqn [6]).

$$
\begin{array}{ccccc}
& AA & & O_2 & \\
MMB & \longrightarrow & Mb & \longrightarrow & MBO_2 \\
Fe^{3+} & & Fe^{2+} & & Fe^{2+} \qquad (6) \\
(Brown) & & (Purple/red) & & (Red) \\
Metmyoglobin & & Myoglobin & & Oxymyoglobin
\end{array}
$$

AA can also chelate with heavy metals, thus interfering with the ability to promote oxidation.

Occurrence in Foods

The vitamin C content of some of the more important food sources are shown in Table 2. Note that DHAA amounts to about 10–20% of the total vitamin C content in many vegetables. Although the values shown are typical of the observed levels found in these samples, they should not be taken as absolute. The vitamin C levels can vary tremendously in a given food product, as is shown in Table 3. Here, variations found in our laboratory are compared with those calculated from *USDA Handbook 8* (*Composition of Foods*) published by the US Department of Agriculture. To obtain the range from the handbook, the standard deviation is calculated from the reported standard error and the number of measurements, while the range has been taken to be four times the standard deviation. As can be seen, the calculated ranges are in agreement with those found in our laboratory.

This large variation in the nutrient from these sources has been known for some time. Genetic variety, maturity, climate, sunlight, method of harvesting and storage all can affect the levels of vitamin C. To make matters worse, there are variations within the fruit or plant depending on the amount of sunlight each part received during growth. While the variations are large for each individual source, the effects would be moderated for people eating a diversified diet where the nutrient would be assimilated from a variety of sources. The fluctuations from the individual sources would tend to balance out over a large number of typical meals. Such would not be the case, however, for human diet studies involving vitamin C where the nutrient sources are relatively few in number over a short period of time. There is evidence that such diet studies should include food analyses on a daily basis.

Cooking practices also influence the levels of vitamin C in any given source. The amount of water used, the temperature and the time of cooking have a direct influence on the retention of the vitamin, as does the acidity of the food. As a general rule, one can estimate that in microwave cooking of vegetables or boiling in sealed bags, the retention rate will be almost 80%. For boiling directly in water, the retention rates will be about 50%. Stir-fried vegetables are cooked at a high temperature so that the percentage retention is still only 50% even though the amount of water used is low. Frozen vegetables retain more vitamin (50–60%) than do canned vegetables (40–50%). Frozen juices retain their vitamin C content without significant loss for months. The above retention figures are only approximations as the percentages will vary from food to food. Acid vegetables, like tomatoes, for example, can have retention factors as high as 85%. Potatoes, no matter how they are cooked, appear to retain vitamin C at the 65% level. *See* Canning, Quality Changes During Canning; Cooking, Domestic Techniques

Role as an Additive in Food Processing

Often, AA is added to processed foods simply for restoration or fortification. For restoration, enough AA is added to replace the nutrient lost in processing. For fortification, the acid is added to enhance the nutrient intake of large portions of the population. The principal fortified foods are breakfast cereals, soft drinks, fruit juices and many processed fruits and vegetables. IAA cannot be used for this purpose because of its low vitamin activity. *See* Food Fortification

In fruit juices and beverages, AA is also added to stabilize the colour and flavour. It reacts as an antioxidant which scavenges oxygen from the head space in bottles and cans and it also scavenges oxygen which can permeate some of the plastic containers in use today.

It is added to processed fruits to inhibit the enzymatic oxidation of phenolic compounds which leads to browning. In this, it acts as an antioxidant. *See* Antioxidants, Natural Antioxidants

In fats, oils, margarine and butterfat, endogenous vitamin E serves as the primary free-radical scavenger which interrupts chain reactions leading to spoilage and rancidity. AA in its palmitate form (1), which is an ester of ascorbic acid and palmitic acid, is fat-soluble, and is added to act synergistically with vitamin E by eqn [3].

Table 2.   Vitamin C content of various food sources

	Concentration (mg per 100 g)[ab]		
	AA	DHAA	Total
Vegetables (fresh)			
Beans, snap	10·0± 0·0	2·0± 0·0	12± 0
Broccoli	89·0± 2·0	7·7± 0·6	97± 2
Cabbage	42·3± 3·4		42± 3
Carrots	4·7± 0·6	2·0± 0·0	7± 1
Cauliflower	54·0± 1·0	8·7± 0·6	63± 1
Coleslaw	23·1± 0·2	12·1± 0·6	35± 1
Collards	92·7± 2·6	—	93± 3
Cucumber	10·3± 1·2	4·0± 0·0	14± 1
Lettuce, iceberg	3·3± 0·6	3·0± 0·0	6± 1
Mustard greens	36·2± 2·4	—	36± 2
Peppers, green	129·0± 1·0	5·0± 0·0	134± 1
Peppers, red	151·0± 3·0	4·0± 1·0	155± 4
Potato, with skin			
Russet	9·0± 0·0	4·3± 0·6	13± 1
Idaho	6·7± 0·6	4·3± 0·6	11± 1
Maine	7·7± 1·2	5·3± 0·6	13± 1
Red-skinned	23·7± 0·6	3·3± 0·6	27± 1
Spinach	52·4± 2·5	—	52± 3
Tomato	10·6± 0·6	3·0± 0·0	14± 1
Juices			
Orange, frozen reconstituted	40·0± 0·0	2·0± 0·0	42± 0
Tomato	12·7± 1·5	2·7± 1·2	16± 2
Hi-C	28·5± 3·5	1·3± 0·6	30± 4
Tang	57·3± 0·6	2·0± 1·0	59± 1
Apple, unfortified	—	—	<1
Fruits			
Banana	15·3± 2·5	3·3± 0·6	19± 3
Cantaloupe	31·3± 0·6	3·0± 0·0	34± 1
Grapefruit	21·3± 0·6	2·3± 0·6	24± 1
Orange			
Florida	54·7± 2·5	8·3± 1·2	63± 3
California navel	75·0± 4·5	8·2± 1·6	83± 5
Watermelon	8·0± 0·0	1·7± 0·6	10± 1
Cereals			
Cornflakes	65·3± 2·1	—	65± 2
Product 19	247 ±22	33 ±10	290±24
Cheerios	66·0± 4·0	—	66± 4

[a] Values reported are mean±SD.
[b] Data taken from Vanderslice JT *et al.* (1990).

In the USA, it is permitted to use AA on pork which is prepackaged and stored under controlled conditions. This prevents browning due to metmyoglobin formation via eqn [6].

In the curing of meats, AA acts as a scavenger of oxygen, a scavenger of free radicals and an inhibitor of nitrosamine formation. With sausage, oxygen inhibits the development of colour. With canned luncheon meat, oxygen reacts with myoglobin to produce the brown metmyoglobin. The typical pink colour in cured ham or bacon is due to nitrosyl myochrome (NOMc), which is sensitive to the presence of oxygen. In all these cases, AA acts as an oxygen scavenger. Fat peroxides present in cured meat generate free radicals which dissociate the

Table 3. Range of vitamin C values (mg per 100 g) in some fruits and vegetables

Sample	Handbook[a]	Our data[b]
Apple juice	0– 2	<1
Bananas	7– 12	12– 19
Beans, snap, raw	11– 22	12– 18
Broccoli, raw	77–109	97–163
Cabbage, raw	31– 64	42– 83
Cucumber	0– 10	13– 14
Grapefruit, red	28– 48	21– 31
Lettuce	1– 7	5– 6
Oranges		
California navel	40– 74	52– 78
Florida	45	53– 63
Potatoes		
Idaho	0– 30	11– 13
Red-skinned		27
Spinach		
fresh	6– 50	25– 70
frozen	5– 44	25
Tomatoes	9– 26	14– 19

[a] Range obtained from mean value±twice the SD found from standard error and number of samples tabulated in *USDA Handbook 8*.
[b] Observed range of means from different samples.

pink pigment. AA in synergism with endogenous vitamin E inhibits the degradation. In the curing of meats, HNO_2 is added which reacts with metmyoglobin, eventually to produce NOMc. Not only does AA enhance the production of NO to form NOMc, it also scavenges excess HNO_2, thus partially inhibiting the production of nitrosamines. *See* Curing

AA has been used in breadmaking to improve the gluten structure. It is known that removal of free SH groups from a dough will strengthen a dough. Presumably, these SH groups can react with and break gluten S—S bonds which are partially responsible for its strength. DHAA, which is formed from AA during the processing of flour, reacts as an oxidizing agent to convert S—H bonds to S—S bonds. An example of such a reaction, that of glutathione which is present in flour, with DHAA has been given in eqn [5]. *See* Bread, Breadmaking Processes

IAA can replace AA in some of these applications but not in all. For example, it is used in some packaged luncheon meats as an antioxidant but it has not been found to be effective as a dough conditioner in breadmaking.

Analysis

Various methods have been used for the analysis of vitamin C in foods and biological materials. The

procedures to be discussed are equally applicable for foods, plasma or animal tissue. All methods, however, have the common problem of sampling, extraction and clean-up prior to analysis, commonly referred to as sample preparation. Each of these will be discussed in turn prior to discussions of the individual methods of analysis for the cleaned-up samples. Space does not permit a complete discussion of the many different procedures used for sample preparation, so those procedures which have been found to be satisfactory in the authors' laboratory will be emphasized.

Sample Preparation

Sample Selection and Initial Preparation

Ideally, an analyst would prefer to choose a sample representative of the particular food or biological sample that needs to be characterized. The levels of vitamin C found in a particular product are, in general, so variable (see Table 3) that, in most cases, it is impossible to choose a representative sample. The best that one can hope for in any given sample is to come close to the mean for that particular product.

Once the sample is in hand, the question arises as to how to get a representative value for that particular sample. Liquids, in general, do not cause problems. Vortexing under nitrogen, while withdrawing the necessary aliquot, is satisfactory. Solid samples do present problems as the distribution throughout the sample is normally not uniform. For small samples, the entire sample can be used. For large samples, such as cabbage, random sampling, discussed in statistics texts, can be used. However, the pieces should be as large as possible so as not to expose too much surface area to the atmosphere. In any case, homogenization of the solid sample should not occur unless it is immersed in the extracting agent. It has been our experience that homogenization prior to the addition of the extracting agent leads to very high values of DHAA, indicating that oxidation has occurred. The sample should be analysed as soon as possible after preparation. If this is not possible, the cleaned-up extract should be frozen at −40°C before analysis. For some samples, the loss of vitamin C will be about 5% during this time.

Extraction

The greatest loss in vitamins or the greatest conversion from one form to another normally occurs during the extraction and clean-up stages. These phases of the operation should be completed as quickly as possible. During these stages, oxygen will rapidly degrade the vitamin, particularly if metal ions are present. If the AA oxidase enzyme is present, this will also catalyse the conversion. While other workers have used a variety of extraction procedures, the authors have found that a solution of 5% metaphosphoric acid, 8% acetic acid and 0·005 M EDTA (10 ml per g sample) is satisfactory for blending of the sample. If fat is present in the sample, it is necessary subsequently to add an equal volume of hexane and vortex. If starch is present, it is necessary subsequently to add an equal volume of n-butanol and vortex.

Clean-up

We have not found it necessary to use any elaborate steps such as column clean-up to prepare a sample for final analysis. For samples without starch, centrifugation at 1200 **g** for 5 min with subsequent filtration through 45 μm filters was simple, fast and effective. For starchy samples, centrifugation at 48 400 **g** was necessary.

Plasma

Plasma presents special problems in that haemolysis of any erythrocytes during separation of plasma from whole blood will release oxyhaemoglobin which will very quickly oxidize AA to DHAA. The suggested procedures of haemolysing with water saturated with carbon monoxide or variants of this have not been found to be satisfactory in this laboratory. The most satisfactory procedure for the authors has been a simple centrifugation of blood at 4°C and 3500 **g** to separate the plasma which is then decanted and an aliquot used for extraction with the metaphosphoric acid solution. Care should be taken during sample collection and centrifugation that no haemolysis occurs.

Analytical Methodology

Many different procedures have been prepared by different investigators for the determination of vitamin C in biological materials. The literature on this subject is so vast that it is impossible to do justice to all who have contributed. It is suggested that the interested reader pursue the recommended readings at the end of this article for in-depth discussions of the available methods.

In general, the useful methods can be broken into two main categories—classical wet chemistry methods and high-performance liquid chromatography (HPLC). The classical methods have been with us for some time and innumerable refinements have been made on many of them. In the last few years, HPLC methods have been developed which have been applied successfully to a large variety of samples. *See* Chromatography, High-performance Liquid Chromatography

Most of the procedures either measure AA only or

total vitamin C (AA + DHAA). Most cannot cope with IAA if it is present in the sample along with AA. The methods normally measure only AA or only DHAA. To get the total vitamin content, either AA is converted to DHAA or DHAA is converted to AA, depending on the species being measured.

Classical Wet Chemistry Methods

Only the three most popular methods will be discussed.

2,6-Dichlorophenol–indophenol Reduction. 2,6-Dichlorophenol–indophenol (DCIP) is a blue dye which is reduced by AA to a colourless form. In the process AA is converted to DHAA. This is a simple titration method where the end-point is determined by a pink colour after all the AA has been oxidized. It is a simple, rapid and inexpensive method, which accounts for its popularity. In practically all applications, it measures only AA and can be used only when DHAA is at low levels. It cannot cope with the presence of IAA. As has been mentioned earlier, DHAA accounts for about 10–20% of the total vitamin activity in many samples. Some modifications of the method have been made to account for the presence of DHAA. Homocysteine is used to reduce DHAA to AA. Measurements of AA before and after reduction enable one to determine DHAA by difference. Unfortunately, the difference usually amounts to a small difference between two relatively large numbers. There are serious objections to this method. Most samples contain other reducing substances such as sulphur dioxide, tannins, cysteine and other sulphydryl compounds such as glutathione, ferrous and stannous ions, plant pigments, reductones and reductic acid, to name a few. Removal of these interferences requires a series of procedures and even then, it is not certain that all interferences have been eliminated. In addition, many materials contain natural or added colours which interfere with the end-point determination.

2,4-Dinitrophenylhydrazine Reaction. This is perhaps the most accurate classical method because of the many modifications made by Pelletier to account for interferences. 2,4-Dinitrophenylhydrazine (DNPH) reacts with the ketone groups of DHAA and DKGA to form osazones. The osazone colour is developed with nitric or sulphuric acid and its absorbance is measured at a wavelength of 520 nm. To obtain the total vitamin C content of a sample, it is necessary to make two measurements. In the first measurement, AA is oxidized to DHAA with DCIP; the osazone reaction is carried out and the absorbance is due to total vitamin C plus DKGA and interfering compounds. In the second measurement, no oxidation is performed, but a reduction of DHAA to AA is carried out with homocysteine; the osazone reaction is carried out and the absorbance is due only to DKAA plus interfering compounds. The difference in the two measurements corresponds to the total vitamin C content.

To determine the individual amounts of AA and DHAA present, a third measurement is required. No oxidation is performed; after osazone formation is complete, the absorbance is due to DHAA, DKGA and other interfering compounds. By difference the AA and DHAA contributions can be calculated.

The chief interfering substances are sugars, glucuronic acid, reductones, histidine and some other amino acids. In the latest procedures, most interferences are compensated for by parallel blank determinations. Pelletier has cleverly used the complexing properties of boric acid with AA and DHAA to substantially improve this method. The DNPH reaction is sensitive to temperature and time of reaction so special care must be taken in laboratory manipulations. It is claimed that IAA can be distinguished from AA by the different rates of osazone formation with DHAA and DHIAA. The concentration of each isomer can be calculated by the difference in osazone formation at 32 and 52°C.

o-Phenylenediamine Fluorescence. *o*-Phenylenediamine (OPD) forms a lactone with DHAA which fluoresces at 427 nm upon irradiation at 350 nm. Normally, AA is oxidized with activated charcoal (Norit) and the fluorescence after reaction with OPD is due to total vitamin C. Previous reports of interferences from DKGA are incorrect. It is usual to correct for interferences by running a blank. Boric acid is complexed with DHAA to prevent lactone formation so that the fluorescence observed after addition of OPD is due to interfering compounds. The method cannot be used with foods that contain high levels of dehydroreductones and dehydroreductic acids. The amount of DHAA in a sample can be determined by omitting the oxidation step and the boric acid. The measured fluorescence with the blank subtracted yields the DHAA concentration.

HPLC Methods

Gas-chromatographic methods have proven to be unreliable since the vitamins are unstable during the necessary derivatization step. HPLC procedures are the methods of choice. Ion exchange, normal and reversed-phase, and reversed phase with ion-pairing chromatography have all been used successfully in the analysis of vitamin C. Reversed-phase chromatography is the only approach so far that has been successful in the separation of IAA from AA.

Ultraviolet absorbance and electrochemical detection have been used to quantitate AA in samples. AA has a strong absorbance at 265 nm in ionic solutions and electrochemical detection is even more sensitive than ultraviolet measurements. DHAA has a poor or no response to these detectors. With these detectors, DHAA is normally reduced to AA for detection. The

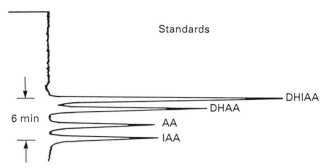

Fig. 2. Chromatographic trace showing separation of AA, IAA, DHAA and DHIAA.

amounts of AA and DHAA are quantified by measuring the response before and after reduction and DHAA measured by difference. This is usually a small difference between two relatively large numbers. AA and DHAA can, however, both be measured directly if one opts to use fluorescence. The authors have used this approach by first separating not only AA and DHAA but also IAA and DHIAA on a particular reversed-phase column with a phosphate buffer and subsequently oxidizing the elements to the dehydroxy compounds and reacting them with OPD to form the fluorescent derivatives. A typical chromatographic trace is shown in Fig. 2. This system, when combined with the extraction and clean-up procedures discussed earlier, has been used to quantify AA and DHAA in a large variety of foods, plasma and animal tissues. The traces from the samples are as clean as the traces for pure standards. In natural samples, where IAA is not present, IAA can be used as an internal standard for quantification purposes. Space does not allow for a discussion of other successful chromatographic procedures and the reader is referred to the bibliography. The method discussed, however, does illustrate the power of HPLC methods, when properly used, in quantifying the levels of vitamin C in biological samples.

Bibliography

Bui-Nguyen MH (1985) Ascorbic acid and related compounds. In: De Leenheer AP, Lambert WE and De Ruyter MGM (eds) *Modern Chromatographic Analysis of the Vitamins*, chap. 5. New York: Marcel Dekker.

Counsell JN and Hornig DH (1981) *Vitamin C, Ascorbic Acid*. London: Applied Sciences.

Friedrich W (1988) *Vitamins*. Berlin: Walter de Gruyter.

Jaffe GM (1984) Vitamin C. In: Machlin LJ (ed.) *Handbook of Vitamins. Nutritional Biochemical and Chemical Aspects*, chap. 5. New York: Marcel Dekker.

Pelletier O (1985) Vitamin C (L-ascorbic and dehydro-L-ascorbic acids). In: Augustin J, Klein BP, Becker D and Venugopal PB (eds) *Methods of Vitamin Assay*, 4th edn, chap. 12. New York: Wiley.

USDA (1982) *Composition of Foods. Fruits and Fruit Juices. Agricultural Handbook No. 8–9*. Washington, DC: Human

Nutrition Information Service, US States Department of Agriculture.

USDA (1984) *Composition of Foods. Vegetables. Agricultural Handbook No. 8–11.* Washington, DC: Human Nutrition Information Service, US Department of Agriculture.

Vanderslice JT and Higgs DJ (1990) Separation of ascorbic acid, isoascorbic acid, dehydroascorbic acid in food and animal tissue. *Journal of Micronutrient Analysis* 7: 67–70.

Vanderslice JT, Higgs DJ, Hayes JM and Block G (1990) Ascorbic acid and dehydroascorbic acid content of foods-as-eaten. *Journal of Food Composition and Analysis* 3: 105–118.

Windholz M, Budavari S, Blumetti RF and Otterbein ES (eds) (1983) *The Merck Index. An Encyclopedia of Chemicals, Drugs, and Biologicals*, 10th edn. Rahway, NJ: Merck.

J. T. Vanderslice and D. J. Higgs
Nutrient Composition Laboratory, US Department of Agriculture, Beltsville, USA

Physiology

Ascorbic acid is a vitamin (vitamin C) for only a limited number of species: man and the other primates, bats, the guinea pig, a number of birds and some fishes. Other species are capable of the synthesis of ascorbic acid, in considerably greater amounts than is required, as an intermediate in the pathway of glucuronic acid oxidation.

Ascorbic acid functions as a relatively non-specific, radical-trapping antioxidant, and it reduces the tocopheroxyl radical formed by oxidation of vitamin E; it also has a specific metabolic function as the redox coenzyme for dopamine β-hydroxylase and peptidyl glycine hydroxylase, and it is required to maintain the 2-oxoglutarate-dependent hydroxylases in the reduced state. *See* Antioxidants, Role of Antioxidant Nutrients in Defence Systems; Tocopherols, Properties and Determination

Biosynthesis of Ascorbic Acid

For those species for which ascorbic acid is not a vitamin, it is an intermediate in the gulonolactone pathway of glucuronic acid metabolism. This is a major pathway of glucuronic acid catabolism, and ascorbate is a metabolic intermediate whose rate of synthesis and turnover bears no relation to physiological requirements for ascorbate *per se*. It is impossible to extrapolate from the rate of synthesis of ascorbate in these species and derive a requirement for man.

Species for which ascorbate is a vitamin lack the enzyme gulonolactone oxidase, and have an alternative pathway of glucuronic acid metabolism.

Absorption

In rats and hamsters (for which ascorbate is not a vitamin) intestinal absorption is passive, while in guinea pigs and man there is sodium-dependent active transport of the vitamin at the brush border membrane, with a sodium-independent mechanism at the basolateral membrane. Dehydroascorbate is absorbed passively in the intestinal mucosa, and is reduced to ascorbate before transport across the basolateral membrane.

Iso-ascorbic acid (erythorbic acid) is not a substrate for active transport in the intestinal mucosa, but is absorbed passively; this presumably accounts for its relatively low biological activity.

In man some 80–95% of dietary ascorbate is absorbed at usual intakes (up to about 100 mg per day). The absorption of larger amounts of the vitamin is lower, falling from 50% of a 1·5 g dose to 25% of a 6 g and 16% of a 12 g dose. The unabsorbed ascorbate from high doses is a substrate for intestinal bacterial metabolism.

Transport and Tissue Uptake

Both ascorbate and dehydroascorbate circulate in the bloodstream in free solution and also bound to albumin. About 5% of plasma vitamin C is normally in the form of dehydroascorbate.

Tissue uptake mechanisms for the two vitamers differ. There is active uptake of ascorbate into cells, while dehydroascorbate only shows apparent concentrative uptake because it is reduced intracellularly to ascorbate. In addition, because it is lipophilic at physiological pH, dehydroascorbate may enter cells by diffusion.

About 70% of blood-borne ascorbate is in plasma and erythrocytes (which do not concentrate the vitamin from plasma). The remainder is in white cells, which have a marked ability to concentrate ascorbate; mononuclear leucocytes achieve 80-fold concentration, platelets 40-fold and granulocytes 25-fold compared with the plasma concentration.

There is no specific storage organ for ascorbate; apart from leucocytes (which account for 10% of total blood ascorbate), the only tissues showing a significant concentration of the vitamin are the adrenal and pituitary glands. Although the concentration of ascorbate in muscle is relatively low, skeletal muscle contains much of the body's pool of 900–1500 mg (5–8·5 mmol) of ascorbate.

Metabolism and Excretion of Ascorbic Acid

As shown in Fig. 1, oxidation of ascorbic acid proceeds by a one-electron process, leading to the monodehydroascorbate radical. The radical rapidly disproportionates to ascorbate and dehydroascorbate. Most tissues also have an NADPH-dependent monodehydroascorbate reductase, a flavoprotein which reduces the radical

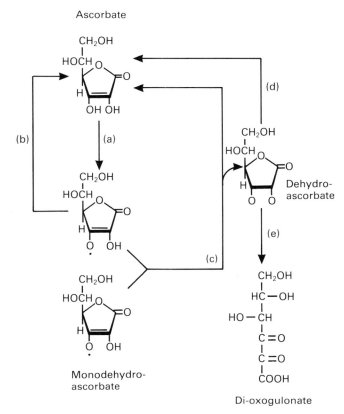

Ascorbate

Dehydro-
ascorbate

Monodehydro-
ascorbate

Di-oxogulonate

Fig. 1 The redox reactions of ascorbic acid: (a) reduction by substrate; (b) monodehydroascorbate reductase; (c) dismutation of monodehydroascorbate; (d) dehydroascorbate reductase; (e) non-enzymatic hydration.

back to ascorbate. Dehydroascorbate is largely reduced to ascorbate by either a glutathione-dependent or an NADPH-dependent reductase. (NADPH is the reduced form of nicotinamide-adenine dinucleotide phosphate.)

Dehydroascorbate can undergo non-enzymatic hydration to di-oxogulonic acid, followed by decarboxylation to xylose, thus providing a route for entry into central carbohydrate metabolic pathways. This is the major metabolic fate of ascorbate in those species for which it is not a vitamin, and also in the guinea pig. However, oxidation to carbon dioxide is only a minor pathway in man. The major fate is excretion in the urine, either unchanged or as dehydroascorbate and di-oxogulonate. *See* Carbohydrates, Digestion, Absorption and Metabolism

Both ascorbate and dehydroascorbate are filtered at the glomerulus, then resorbed, by sodium-independent, facilitated diffusion. It is when glomerular filtration exceeds the capacity of these transport systems, at a plasma concentration of ascorbate between 55 and 85 μmol l^{-1}, that the vitamin is excreted in the urine in amounts proportional to intake.

About 25% of the ascorbate intake is normally excreted as oxalate, and this accounts for some 40% of the total urinary excretion of oxalate. The pathway for oxalate formation from ascorbate is not known.

Metabolic Functions of Ascorbic Acid

Ascorbic acid has specific and well-defined roles in two classes of enzymes, copper-containing hydroxylases and the 2-oxoglutarate-linked, iron-containing hydroxylases. It also increases the activity of a number of other enzymes *in vitro*, although this is a non-specific reducing action rather than a reflection of any metabolic function of the vitamin. In addition, ascorbic acid has a number of less specific effects due to its action as a reducing agent and oxygen-radical quencher.

Dopamine β-Hydroxylase

Dopamine β-hydroxylase is a copper-containing enzyme involved in the synthesis of the catecholamines noradrenaline and adrenaline from tyrosine in the adrenal medulla and central nervous system. The active enzyme contains Cu^+, which is oxidized to Cu^{2+} during the hydroxylation of the substrate; reduction back to Cu^+ specifically requires ascorbate, which is oxidized to monodehydroascorbate.

Peptidyl Glycine Hydroxylase (Peptidyl α-Amidase)

A number of biologically active peptide hormones have a terminal amide, and amidation is essential for biological activity. The amide group is derived from a glycine residue in the precursor peptide, by proteolysis to leave a carboxy terminal glycine. This is hydroxylated on the α-carbon; the hydroxyglycine decomposes non-enzymatically to yield the amidated peptide and glyoxylate. Like dopamine β-hydroxylase, this is a copper-containing enzyme, and requires ascorbate as the electron donor.

2-Oxoglutarate-Linked, Iron-Containing Hydroxylases

A number of iron-containing hydroxylases share a common reaction mechanism, in which hydroxylation of the substrate is linked to decarboxylation of 2-oxoglutarate. Proline and lysine hydroxylases are required for the post-synthetic modification of collagen, and proline hydroxylase also for the post-synthetic modification of osteocalcin in bone and the $C1_q$ component of complement. Aspartate β-hydroxylase is required for the post-synthetic modification of protein C, the vitamin-K-dependent protease which hydrolyses activated Factor V in the blood-clotting cascade. Trimethyllysine and γ-butyrobetaine hydroxylases are required for the synthesis of carnitine.

Procollagen proline hydroxylase is the best studied of this class of enzymes; it is assumed that the others have essentially the same mechanism. The first step in the reaction is an attack on the substrate by oxygen, followed by condensation with 2-oxoglutarate, the release of the hydroxylated substrate and decarboxylation to release succinate.

There is oxidation of ascorbate during the reaction, but not stoichiometrically with the decarboxylation of 2-oxoglutarate and hydroxylation of the substrate. The purified enzyme is active in the absence of ascorbate, but after some 5–10 s (about 15 to 30 cycles of enzyme action) the rate of reaction begins to fall. At this stage the iron in the catalytic site has been oxidized to Fe^{3+}, which is catalytically inactive, and activity is only restored by ascorbate, which reduces it back to Fe^{2+}. This oxidation of Fe^{2+} is the consequence of a side-reaction rather than the main reaction of the enzyme. Nevertheless, ascorbate is essential for the activity of these enzymes *in vivo*.

Stimulation of Enzyme Activity by Ascorbate *in vitro*

A number of enzymes have been assumed to be ascorbate dependent because their activity is stimulated *in vitro* by the addition of ascorbate to the incubation medium. In general these reactions are not ascorbate dependent; ascorbate is just one of a number of reducing reagents which enhance the reaction. Ascorbate is also frequently added to the incubation medium to remove hydrogen peroxide formed during a variety of reactions. Again, a number of reducing agents have the same action, and *in vivo* this role would presumably be performed by catalase.

The Role of Ascorbate in Iron Absorption

Inorganic dietary iron is absorbed as Fe^{2+} and not as Fe^{3+}; ascorbic acid in the intestinal lumen will not only maintain iron in the reduced state but also chelate it, thus increasing absorption. A dose of 25 mg of vitamin C taken together with a semisynthetic meal increases the absorption of iron some 65%, while a 1 g dose gives a nine-fold increase. This is an effect of ascorbic acid present together with the test meal; neither intravenous administration of vitamin C nor supplements several hours before the test meal have any effect on iron absorption. The endogenous vitamin C in foods has the same effect on iron absorption.

This is not a specific effect of ascorbate; a variety of other reducing agents also enhance the absorption of inorganic iron. *See* Iron, Physiology

Inhibition of Nitrosamine Formation

Ascorbate reacts with nitrite and other nitrosating reagents *in vitro*, forming nitric oxide, nitrous oxide and nitrogen. This may be important in preventing the formation of carcinogenic nitrosamines by reaction between nitrites and amines present in foods in the acid conditions of the stomach. Again, this is an effect of ascorbate present in the stomach together with the dietary nitrites and amines, rather than an effect of vitamin C nutritional status. *See* Nitrosamines

However, while ascorbate can deplete nitrosating compounds under anaerobic conditions, the situation may be reversed in the presence of oxygen. Nitric oxide reacts with oxygen to form N_2O_3 and N_2O_4, both of which are nitrosating reagents, and can also react with ascorbate to form NO and monodehydroascorbate. It is thus possible for ascorbate to be depleted, with no significant effect on the total concentration of nitrosating species. It remains to be determined whether or not ascorbate has any significant effect in reducing the risk of nitrosamine formation and carcinogenesis.

Reduction of the Vitamin E Radical

One of the major roles of Vitamin E is as a radical-trapping antioxidant at membrane surfaces. α-Tocopherol reacts with lipid peroxides, forming the α-tocopheroxyl radical. This reacts with ascorbate in the aqueous phase, regenerating α-tocopherol, and forming the monodehydroascorbate radical, which reacts to yield ascorbate and dehydroascorbate. Vitamin C thus has a vitamin-E-sparing antioxidant action, coupling lipophilic and hydrophilic antioxidant reactions.

The antioxidant efficiency of ascorbate is variable. From the chemistry involved, it would be expected that overall 2 mol of tocopheroxyl radical would be trapped per mol of ascorbate, because of the reaction of 2 mol of monodehydroascorbate to regenerate ascorbate and yield dehydroascorbate. However, as the concentration of ascorbate increases, so the molar ratio decreases, and it is only at very low concentrations of ascorbate that it tends towards the theoretical 2:1. This is because, as well as its antioxidant role, ascorbate can be a source of hydroxyl and superoxide radicals.

At high concentrations, ascorbate can reduce molecular oxygen to superoxide, being oxidized to monodehydroascorbate. At lower concentrations of ascorbate both Fe^{3+} and Cu^{2+} ions are reduced by ascorbate, again yielding monodehydroascorbate. Fe^{2+} and Cu^+ are readily reoxidized by reaction with hydrogen peroxide to yield hydroxide ions and hydroxyl radicals. Thus, as well as its antioxidant role, ascorbate has pro-oxidant action; the net result will depend on the relative rates of formation of superoxide and hydroxyl radicals by auto-oxidation and metal-catalysed reactions of ascorbate, and the trapping of these radicals by ascorbate. Certainly in tissue culture ascorbate has a cytotoxic action as a result of radical-initiated DNA damage.

Table 1. Plasma and leucocyte concentrations of ascorbate as criteria of nutritional status

	Deficient	Marginal	Adequate
Whole blood ascorbate			
mg l^{-1}	< 3·0	3·0–4·9	> 5·0
μmol l^{-1}	< 17	17–28	> 28
Serum ascorbate			
mg l^{-1}	< 2·0	2·0–2·9	> 3·0
μmol l^{-1}	< 11	11–16·4	> 17
Leucocyte ascorbate			
mg l^{-1}	< 7·0	7–15	> 15
μmol l^{-1}	< 39	39–85	> 85
mg 10^{-6} cells	< 70	70–150	> 150
μmol 10^{-6} cells	< 390	390–850	> 850

Requirements and Recommendations

There have been two major studies of ascorbate requirements in depletion–repletion studies, one in Sheffield during the 1940s and the other in Iowa during the 1960s.

While the minimum requirement for vitamin C is firmly established, there are considerable discrepancies between the RDA (Recommended Dietary Allowance) published by different authorities, with figures ranging between 30 and 80 mg per day. This is the result of different criteria of adequacy, and reflects differences of opinion as to what represents an appropriate body pool of vitamin C.

Minimum Requirement

The minimum requirement for vitamin C was established in the Sheffield study, which showed that an intake of less than 10 mg per day was adequate to prevent the development of scurvy, or to cure the clinical signs. At this level of intake, wound healing is impaired. Optimum wound healing requires a mean intake of 20 mg per day. Allowing for individual variation, this gives an RDA of 30 mg per day, which is the WHO/FAO (World Health Organization/Food and Agriculture Organization) recommendation. *See* Scurvy

Plasma Concentration of Ascorbate

At intakes below 30 mg per day the plasma concentration of ascorbate is extremely low, and does not reflect increasing intake to any significant extent (see Table 1). As the intake rises, so the plasma concentration begins to increase sharply, reaching a plateau of 55–85 μmol l^{-1} at intakes between 70 and 100 mg per day, when the renal threshold is reached and the vitamin is excreted quantitatively with increasing intake.

The midpoint of the steep region of the curve, where the plasma concentration increases more or less linearly with increasing intake, represents a state where tissue reserves are adequate and plasma ascorbate is available for transfer between tissues. This corresponds to an intake of 40 mg per day – the basis of the British 1991 Reference Nutrient Intake.

Maintenance of the Body Pool of Ascorbate

Clinical signs of scurvy are seen when the total body pool of ascorbate is below 300 mg (1·7 mmol). It then increases with intake, reaching a maximum of about 1500 mg (8·5 mmol) in adults – 20 mg (0·11 mmol) per kg of bodyweight.

The basis of the 1989 US RDA of 60 mg is the observed mean fractional daily turnover rate of 3·2% of a body pool of 20 mg per kg of bodyweight, with allowances for incomplete absorption of dietary ascorbate and individual variation.

Because the mean fractional turnover rate of 3·2% per day was observed during a depletion study, and the rate of ascorbate catabolism varies with intake, it has been suggested that this implies a rate of 3·6% per day before depletion. On this basis, and allowing for incomplete absorption and individual variation, other authorities arrive at an RDA of 80 mg.

The need for a body pool as high as 1500 mg has been challenged. This figure was determined in subjects consuming a self-selected diet, with a relatively high intake of vitamin C, and cannot be considered to represent a requirement. There is good evidence that a body pool of 900 mg (5·1 mmol) is adequate; it is three-fold higher than the minimum pool required to prevent scurvy, and there is no evidence that there are any health benefits from a body pool greater than 600 mg. On the basis of maintaining a body pool of 900 mg, the RDA is 40 mg per day.

The rate of ascorbate catabolism is affected by intake, and the requirement to maintain the body pool cannot be estimated as an absolute value. A habitual low intake, with a consequent low rate of catabolism, will maintain the same body pool as a habitual higher intake with a higher rate of catabolism.

Groups at Risk of Vitamin C Deficiency (Scurvy)

The major determinant of vitamin C intake is the consumption of fruit and vegetables, and the range of intakes in healthy adults in Britain reflects this. The 2·5 percentile intake is 19 mg per day (men) and 14 mg per day (women), while the 97·5 percentile intake is 170 mg per day (men) and 160 mg per day (women).

Deficiency is likely in people whose habitual intake of fruit and vegetables is very low. Smokers may be more at risk of deficiency; there is some evidence that the rate of ascorbate catabolism is two-fold higher in smokers than in non-smokers. Clinical signs of deficiency are rarely seen in developed countries. *See* Smoking, Diet and Health

High Intakes of Ascorbic Acid

There is a school of thought which believes that human requirements for vitamin C are considerably higher than those discussed above. The evidence is largely based on observation of the vitamin C intake of gorillas in captivity, assuming that this is the same as their intake in the wild (where they eat considerably less fruit than under zoo conditions), and then assuming that because they have this intake, it is their requirement – an unjustified assumption. Scaling this to human beings suggests a requirement of 1–2 g per day.

Intakes in excess of about 80–100 mg per day lead to a quantitative increase in urinary excretion of unmetabolized ascorbate, suggesting saturation of tissue reserves. It is difficult to justify a requirement in excess of tissue storage capacity.

Pharmacological Uses of Ascorbic Acid

Ascorbate enhances the intestinal absorption of inorganic iron, and therefore it is frequently prescribed together with iron supplements.

A number of studies have reported low ascorbate status in patients with advanced cancer – perhaps an unsurprising finding in seriously ill patients. One study has suggested, on the basis of an uncontrolled open trial, that 10 g daily doses of vitamin C resulted in increased survival. Controlled studies have not demonstrated any beneficial effects of high dose ascorbic acid in the treatment of advanced cancer. *See* Cancer, Diet in Cancer Prevention

High doses of vitamin C have also been recommended for the prevention and treatment of the common cold. Again the evidence from controlled trials is unconvincing.

Scorbutic guinea pigs develop hypercholesterolaemia, which may lead to the development of cholesterol-rich gallstones. There is no evidence that increased intakes of vitamin C above requirements result in increased cholesterol catabolism. There is, however, evidence that monodehydroascorbate inhibits hydroxymethylglutaryl CoA reductase, resulting in reduced synthesis of cholesterol, and high intakes of ascorbate may have some hypocholesterolaemic action.

The Safety of High Intakes

Regardless of whether or not high intakes of ascorbate have any beneficial effects, large numbers of people habitually take between 1 and 5 g per day of vitamin C supplements. There is little evidence of any significant toxicity from these high intakes. Once the plasma concentration of ascorbate reaches the renal threshold, it is excreted more or less quantitatively with increasing intake.

Up to 5% of the population are at risk from the development of renal oxalate stones. The risk is from both ingested oxalate and that formed endogenously, mainly from the metabolism of ascorbate and glycine. Normally some 40% of urinary oxalate is derived from ascorbate. The capacity for catabolism of ascorbate is limited, and at high intakes a considerably lower proportion of the ingested ascorbate is metabolized to oxalate. It is thus unlikely that high ascorbate intakes are a significant source of additional oxalate in most subjects. However, some patients with recurrent oxalate stones do excrete significantly more oxalate after ascorbate loading, and for them high doses of ascorbate are a significant risk factor.

Since the rate of ascorbate catabolism increases with increasing intake, it has been suggested that abrupt cessation of high intakes of ascorbate may result in rebound scurvy, because of 'metabolic conditioning' and a greatly increased rate of catabolism. While there have been a number of anecdotal reports, there is no evidence that this occurs.

Bibliography

Basu TK and Scorah CJ (1981) *Vitamin C in Health and Disease*, London: Croom Helm.

Bender DA (1982) *Vitamin C*. In: Barker BM and Bender DA (eds) *Vitamins in Medicine*, Vol. 2 chapter 1, pp 1–68 London: William Heinemann Medical.

Bender DA (1992) *Nutritional Biochemistry of the Vitamins*, Cambridge: Cambridge University Press.

Chalmers TC (1975) Effects of ascorbic acid on the common cold: an evaluation of the evidence. *American Journal of Medicine* 58: 532–536.

Chatterjee IB (1978) Ascorbic acid metabolism. *World Review of Nutrition and Dietetics* 30: 69–87.

Prockop DJ, Kivirrikko KI, Turkman L and Guzman NA (1979) The biosynthesis of collagen and its disorders. *New England Journal of Medicine* 301: 13–23 and 77–85.

Rivers JM (1987) Safety of high-level vitamin C ingestion. *Annals of the New York Academy of Sciences* 498: 445–451.

Sato P and Udenfriend S (1978) Studies on vitamin C related to the genetic basis of scurvy. *Vitamins and Hormones* 36: 33–52.

David A. Bender
University College, London, UK

ASPARTAME

Aspartame, one of the most widely used intense sweeteners, was discovered accidentally in 1965 during the synthesis of a pharmaceutical product for ulcer therapy. It is an artificial sweetener composed of two amino acids, aspartic acid and phenylalanine, which combine to form a dipeptide that is subsequently methylated to a methyl ester (Fig. 1). Although it is not strictly a non-nutritive sweetener (it provides about the same amount of energy as sucrose on an equal weight basis, approximately 16.8 kJ g^{-1}), only very small amounts are needed in foods because of its intense sweetness, and thus its energy contribution to the diet is insignificant in most cases.

Sweetness

The intense sweetness of aspartame is unpredictable, considering the tastes of its constituent amino acids, because neither phenylalanine nor aspartic acid are sweet. Since it is very difficult to predict sweetness, most intense sweeteners such as aspartame have been discovered by accident. However, since the discovery of aspartame, extensive studies on many types of aspartame derivatives have suggested that the biochemical nucleus of aspartame sweetness lies with the L-aspartic acid group, although L-aspartic acid itself is not sweet. Table 1 lists a number of L-aspartic acid derivatives and their relative sweetness. The aminomalonic acid methyl fenchyl diester of L-aspartic acid is the most intensely sweet substance ever reported, either natural or synthetic. Of the series of L-aspartic acid derivatives described above, only aspartame has received approval for use in sweetening foods and drugs. *See* Sweeteners – Intense

The sweetness of aspartame has been studied in depth

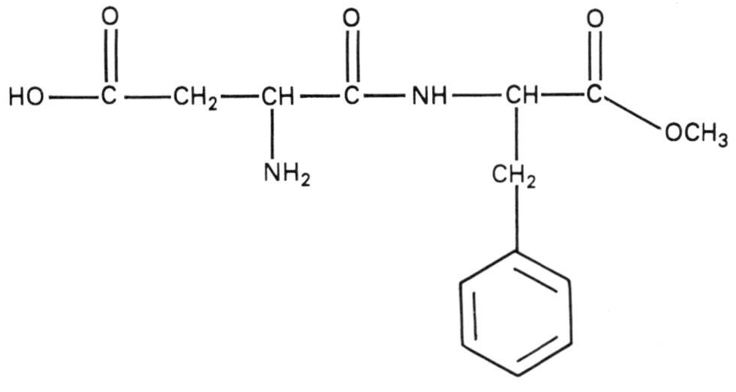

Fig. 1   Structure of aspartame.

Table 1.   Relative sweetness of L-aspartic acid derivatives

Compound	Relative sweetness[a]
Aspartyltyrosine methyl ester	50
Aspartyl-D-alanine *n*-propylester	170
Aspartylhexahydrophenylalanine methyl ester	225
Aspartyl-*S*-*t*-butylcysteine	900
Aspartylaminomalonic acid methyl, *trans*-2-methyl-cyclohexy diester	7300
Aspartylaminomalonic acid methyl fenchyl diester	33 000

[a] Relative to sucrose (1).

under many different conditions. The quality of taste is very similar to sucrose. The sweetener exhibits no bitter aftertaste like saccharin nor the liquorice aftertaste of several natural sweeteners such as glycyrrhizin, thaumatin or phyllodulcin. Aspartame does exhibit a lingering sweetness which may or may not be desirable depending upon the application. The prolonged sweetness can be minimized by blending aspartame with other sweeteners, or by adding naringin or salts such as aluminium or potassium sulphate. *See* Saccharin

The intensity of sweetness of aspartame depends upon the food system incorporating the sweetener. Its potency relative to sucrose increases in dilute solutions compared to more concentrated ones. For example, sweetness equal to a 0.34% sucrose solution is obtained using 400 times less aspartame. However, the equivalent sweetness of a 10% solution of sucrose is produced by 133 times less aspartame. *See* Carbohydrates, Sensory Properties

Since the perception of sweetness can be influenced by texture and the composition of a food, each application of aspartame must be tested on an individual basis to achieve the most palatable combination. For example, Table 2 lists sweetener equivalence data (equivalent to sucrose) for aspartame in a variety of food products. The aspartame concentration was adjusted to give the same intensity of sweetness, organoleptic properties and associated sensory characteristics as obtained with sucrose. The actual sweetening power of aspartame varies, depending upon the food and level of addition, from 130 to 250. Aspartame also exhibits some synergistic effects when mixed with other sweeteners, including both carbohydrate and artificial sweeteners. Combina-

Table 2. Aspartame sweetener equivalence data in typical food products

Food product	Sucrose content (g)[a]	Aspartame content (mg)[a]	Sweetening power
Beverages			
Carbonated cola	77	433	178
Carbonated lemon juice	103	433	239
Carbonated tonic	90	367	245
Concentrated fruit juice	84	417	201
Dairy			
Chocolate-flavoured milk	60	300	200
Yoghurt	105	500	210
Yoghurt drink	103	500	206
Vanilla ice cream	150	800	188
Chocolate ice cream	135	650	210
Frozen desserts			
Chocolate mousse	97	750	130
Confectionery			
Apricot jam	170	850	200
Powdered mixes			
Tomato soup	8	35	221
Chocolate pudding	53	289	183
Orange drink	100	761	153
Gelatin	100	500	200
Condiments			
Salad dressing	100	400	250

[a] Per litre or kilogram of product as consumed.

tions of aspartame and saccharin are commonly used in diet beverages in the USA.

In addition to sweetness, aspartame has some ability to enhance and extend flavours, particularly citrus flavours such as orange, lemon and grapefruit.

Physical and Chemical Properties

Aspartame is a white, odourless, crystalline powder which is only slightly hygroscopic under normal temperatures and humidity conditions. Its solubility in water is highly dependent on pH and temperature, ranging from about 0·5% at pH 5·2 (its isoelectric point) and 5°C to about 50% at pH 2·2 and 50°C. In the dry state aspartame is relatively stable under normal storage conditions. It can be stored at ambient temperatures (25°C) for 6 months or more with only a slight (0·1%) conversion to diketopiperazine (DKP), one of the major decomposition products of aspartame. However, at elevated temperatures aspartame undergoes a cyclization to form substantially increased amounts of DKP. Figure 2 illustrates the rate of conversion to DKP at

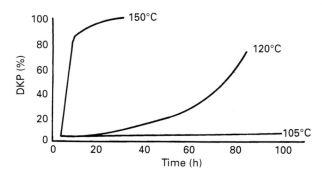

Fig. 2 Rate of conversion of aspartame to diketopiperazine (DKP) at 105°C, 120°C and 150°C.

105°C, 120°C and 150°C. This sensitivity to extremes of heat limits the use of aspartame to food uses where minimal heat treatment is employed. New formulations of the sweetener (particularly encapsulation) and careful timing of its addition to heated foods have in certain cases enabled it to be used in foods such as fruit jams, sauces, sweets and snack foods.

In aqueous solution the stability of aspartame is dependent upon time, temperature and pH and appears to follow first-order kinetics. It is most stable in the range of pH 3–5. Below pH 3 aspartame hydrolyses to the dipeptide, aspartylphenylalanine, and at pH values above pH 5 cyclization to DKP occurs. Both of these reactions result in a loss of sweetness. Figure 3 summarizes the conversion of aspartame to its decomposition products. The half-life of aspartame in solution at 25°C at pH 4·3 is about 300 days while at pH 2 and 6 the half-life is about 80 days. These half-lives decrease with increasing storage temperature. Figure 4 shows the effect of pH on the stability of aspartame in aqueous solution at 40°C: the rate of decomposition is substantial at pH 6 or greater.

The major decomposition products of aspartame are aspartylphenylalanine, DKP, aspartic acid, phenylalanine, methanol and, under certain conditions, the β-isomer of aspartame (in which phenylalanine is attached to the other carboxylic acid group of aspartic acid).

Food Uses

The most common use of aspartame in foods at present is in diet soft drinks where the pH is such that the products may be stored for up to 6 months without noticeable degradation of the sweeteners and loss of sweetness. In Canada, aspartame and sucralose are the only artificial sweeteners permitted for use in diet soft drinks, while in many other countries aspartame may be used in a blend with saccharin. Normal concentrations in diet soft drinks are about 0·03–0·09%.

Aspartame is used in a variety of dry products such as table-top sweeteners, cereals, chewing gum, pudding

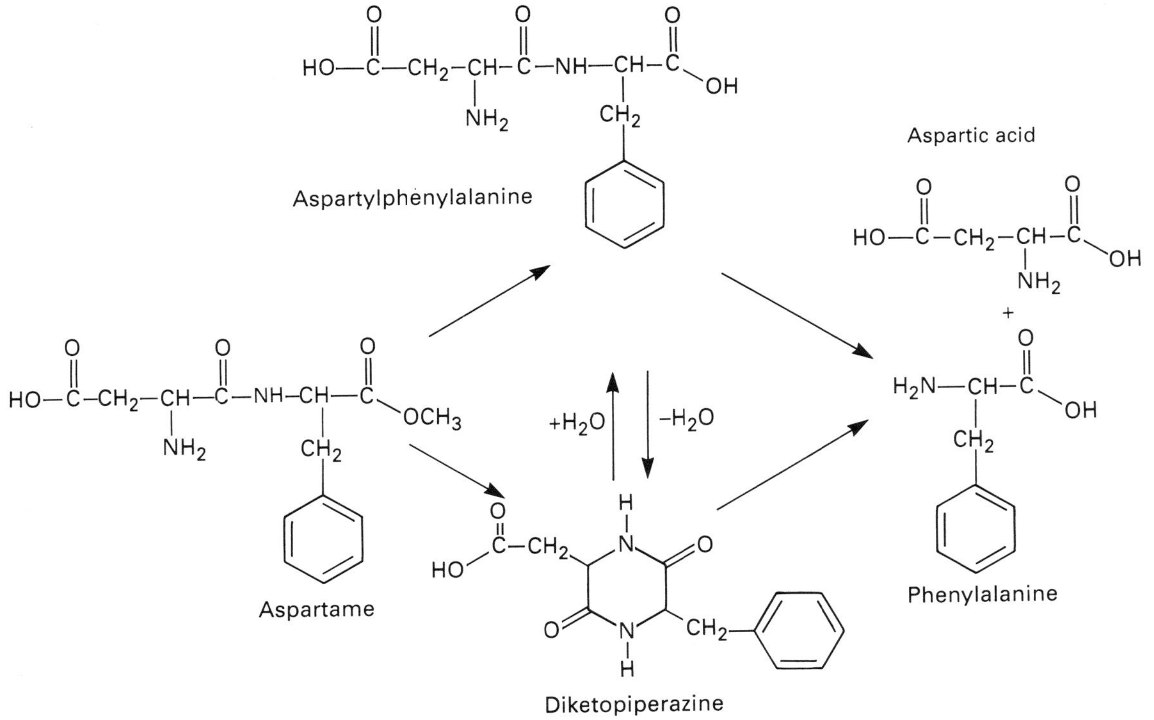

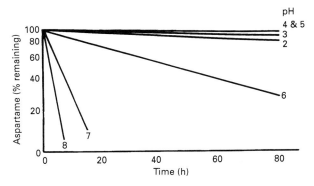

Fig. 3 Conversion pathways of aspartame to its decomposition products.

Fig. 4 Effect of pH on the stability of aspartame in aqueous solution at 40°C.

mixes, dry beverage powders, cocoa mixes, topping mixes, instant coffees and teas, natural fibre laxatives and milk and shake mixes. The application of aspartame to sweetening other food products continues to grow. It has already been successfully used for sweetening heat-treated products such as fruit purées and sauces, snack foods and confections, as well as salad dressings, pickles and relishes. Encapsulation of aspartame with a food-grade coating or carrier has been shown to protect the sweetener from decomposition during heat processing, but still allows the slow release of aspartame in the end product. This technology will enable aspartame to be used in many more baking applications than at present.

Metabolism

The metabolism of aspartame is similar to that of most proteins. It is converted to aspartic acid, phenylalanine and methanol, all of which are metabolized further. The energy content of aspartame is typical of protein, being about 16.8 kJ g^{-1}. The amount of aspartic acid and phenylalanine produced from a glass of aspartame-sweetened beverage is about 8–10 times less than that produced from a glass of milk. Both these amino acids are found in a variety of foods, including milk, meat, bread, fruits and vegetables. Phenylalanine is an essential amino acid which in healthy individuals is metabolized like other amino acids. However, in rare cases (one person in 10 000), owing to a metabolic disorder called phenylketonuria (PKU), phenylalanine cannot be metabolized; if untreated, this condition could lead to mental retardation. As a result, aspartame-containing foods must be labelled to indicate the presence of phenylalanine. *See* Amino Acids, Metabolism

Safety

The toxicology of aspartame has been extensively investigated. The results of the studies have been reviewed by many national and international organizations. Based on these, the FAO/WHO (Food and Agriculture Organization, World Health Organization)

Joint Expert Committee on Food Additives and other regulatory bodies and agencies in about 50 countries have assessed aspartame as being safe for consumption provided that the acceptable daily intake (ADI) by humans is less than 40 mg per kg bodyweight (ADI represents the maximum amount of aspartame that could be consumed daily for a lifetime without appreciable risk). In the USA the ADI is 50 mg kg^{-1}. *See* Legislation, Additives

Analysis

A number of methods for the determination of aspartame in foods have been reported. These include colorimetry, fluorescence, thin-layer chromatography, gas chromatography and, most commonly, high-performance liquid chromatography (HPLC). The last method is particularly suitable since most liquid foods such as soft drinks and juices can be analysed directly after filtration with little or no other sample treatment. Normally, reversed-phase chromatography with ultraviolet detection at about 210 nm is employed for the determination. The method is sensitive enough to detect very low concentrations of aspartame in most diet foods. Figure 5 shows typical results obtained from two diet beverages. High-performance liquid chromatography systems have been developed to enable the determination of aspartame and most of its degradation products in a single analysis. For nonliquid foods, aspartame is extracted with an aqueous buffer solution, after which it is removed from the solid matter and filtered before analysis by HPLC. Powders, such as beverage bases, pudding mixes and table-top sweeteners, are first dissolved in water before analysis. *See* Chromatography, Thin-layer Chromatography; Chromatography, High-performance Liquid Chromatography; Chromatography, Gas Chromatography; Spectroscopy, Visible Spectroscopy and Colorimetry; Spectroscopy, Fluorescence

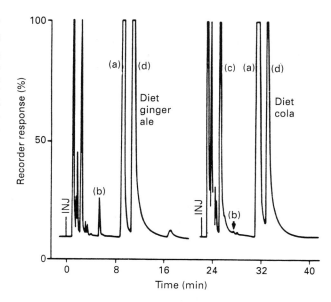

Fig. 5 High-performance liquid chromatography chromatograms of a diet ginger ale and a diet cola containing (a) aspartame, (b) β-aspartame, (c) caffeine and (d) sodium benzoate.

Bibliography

Franta R and Beck B (1986) Alternatives to cane and beet sugar. *Food Technology* 40: 116–128.

Homler BE (1984) Properties and stability of aspartame. *Food Technology* 38: 50–55.

Lawrence JF and Iyengar JR (1987) Liquid chromatographic determination of beta-aspartame in diet soft drinks, beverage powders and pudding mixes. *Journal of Chromatography* 404: 261–266.

Stegink LD and Filer Jr LJ (1984) *Aspartame, Physiology and Biochemistry*. New York: Marcel Dekker.

James F. Lawrence
Sir FG Banting Research Centre, Ottawa, Canada

ASSAYS

See Immunoassays and Specific Analytical Techniques

ATHEROSCLEROSIS

Definition

The lesions of atherosclerosis are known as atheroma. They consist of patches of thickening in the inner lining (intima) of the walls of arteries. This is due to deposition of lipids, proliferation of smooth muscle cells and the formation of fibrous tissue. Literally, the term atherosclerosis means 'hard porridge'.

Major Clinical Forms, Types of Lesion

Atheroma have similar characteristics wherever they are found in the arterial tree. It is assumed that the pathogenesis is identical even though certain risk factors appear to predispose to lesions in specific locations.

Subdivisions can be made on the basis of the size or state of the lesion (e.g. small, protruding, fissured, thrombosed), but this classification requires invasive investigation. Atheromatous lesions are therefore categorized according to their location in the vascular tree, the most important being coronary, cerebral and peripheral, affecting the lower limbs. It should be noted that atheromatous lesions are only clinically obvious when they cause a reduction in blood flow to such an extent that ischaemic symptoms develop. Acute cessation of blood supply produces the well-known clinical sequelae of heart attack, stroke and gangrene and significantly relates to the complications of the plaque.

Causation

Atherosclerosis is a multifactorial condition, the aetiology of which is poorly understood. There are various risk factors which predispose to atheroma formation and these are considered below.

Age and Sex

The presence of atheroma increases with age in both sexes. Atherosclerosis of the coronary and cerebral circulation tends to occur later in life in females, although this difference is less marked after the menopause. It is assumed that high levels of oestrogens and progestogens in some way account for the protective effect of female sex.

Hypertension

Hypertension (high blood pressure) accelerates the atherosclerotic process. A number of prospective studies have shown that a systolic blood pressure greater than 160 mm of mercury (mmHg) or a diastolic pressure above 95 mmHg carries a threefold increased risk of coronary heart disease (CHD) and an even greater risk of stroke, compared with levels below these figures (normotension). Even levels that are regarded as 'normal', however, impart some risk. *See* Hypertension, Physiology

The mechanism by which hypertension affects the atherosclerotic process is not understood. It is of interest that control of blood pressure has been shown to reduce the risk of stroke but has been disappointing with regards to CHD. The lack of treatment effect on heart attack has led to the proposition that atherosclerosis and hypertension are not causally related but are both a consequence of some common underlying abnormality (e.g. insulin resistance).

Hyperlipidaemia

The relationship between total plasma cholesterol concentration and CHD in men is strong and consistent over a large number of studies. It is the low-density lipoprotein (LDL) cholesterol fraction which imparts risk, whilst raised high-density lipoprotein (HDL) cholesterol levels protect against heart attack (Table 1). The relationship between high plasma levels of LDL cholesterol and cerebral or peripheral atherosclerosis is much weaker, perhaps because patients die from heart disease before developing significant lesions at these sites. Similarly, evidence supporting a link between levels of LDL cholesterol and CHD in women is not convincing and it appears that HDL cholesterol may be of greater importance than LDL cholesterol in females. An independent association between elevated fasting triglycerides and atherogenesis has yet to be demonstrated in either sex. *See* Cholesterol, Role of Cholesterol in Heart Disease; Hyperlipidaemia

Table 1.   Plasma lipids and their effects on cardiovascular risk

Plasma lipid	Risk of coronary heart disease
Total cholesterol	Increased
LDL cholesterol	Increased
HDL cholesterol	Decreased
Fasting triglycerides	? No effect

Cigarette Smoking

Large prospective studies have shown that men who smoke have an increased risk of stroke, myocardial infarction and intermittent claudication compared with nonsmokers. The risk is relatively greater in those under the age of 50 years and smoking acts synergistically with the other risk factors already discussed. Epidemiological studies and intervention trials have shown that substantial reductions in CHD death rates occur when smokers discontinue the habit. The benefits are most noticeable in those who have smoked less than 20 cigarettes per day, and 10 years after cessation their risk is similar to that of lifelong non-smokers. *See* Smoking, Diet and Health

Exercise

There is now good evidence that subjects who engage in regular exercise are less likely to suffer from heart attacks. Although exercise is difficult to quantify accurately, it appears that regular exertion has beneficial effects on blood pressure and HDL cholesterol levels, independent of any effect on body mass.

Personality and Stress

Some studies have shown that people with so-called type A behaviour (aggressive, ambitious, restless) have a greater risk of CHD and sudden death than more passive (type B) personalities. *See* Stress and Nutrition

Clotting Factors

Several studies have shown an association between high fibrinogen levels and CHD risk. Increasing age, smoking, obesity and the menopause are associated with increased levels of clotting factors.

Diabetes and Impaired Glucose Tolerance

Individuals with both type I (insulin–dependent) and type II (non-insulin-dependent) diabetes mellitus are at increased risk of atherosclerosis. The protective effect of female sex is eliminated by diabetes, making them seem more prone to this process. Atherosclerotic lesions account for a good deal of the morbidity (amputation, angina) and mortality from premature heart disease seen in diabetics. The mechanism by which diabetes accelerates the atherosclerotic process is unknown, although it is of interest that individuals with abnormal glucose handling, but without frank diabetes assessed by a glucose tolerance test, also have an increased risk of heart attack.

Obesity

Obesity confers an increased risk of death from atherosclerotic disease, as well as increasing morbidity from conditions such as hiatus hernia, osteoarthritis, etc. However, when the other risk factors are taken into account, body mass index is not an independent risk factor. The explanation for this finding is that obese individuals are more likely to have raised blood pressure, hyperlipidaemia and impaired glucose tolerance than individuals with a normal body mass.

Development

The earliest visible change in the walls of arteries which may be related to the development of atheroma is the 'fatty streak'. This is a collection of lipid, mainly cholesterol esters, in macrophages and smooth muscle cells ('foam cells') in the intima of an artery. Fatty streaks are present by the time of adolescence in all races that have been studied and are found in the aorta, cerebral and coronary arteries. It is of note that their location within these vessels shows little correlation with that of fibrous plaques and that they are found as frequently in groups with a high risk of future atheromatous disease as in those without. This has led to some debate as to whether the fatty streak is really a precursor of the atheromatous plaque.

Fibrous plaques are white lesions that usually protrude into the vessel lumen (Fig. 1). They consist of a core of cholesterol, cholesterol ester, phospholipid and necrotic cells covered by a fibrous cap of elastin and collagen. In individuals of advanced age, increasing amounts of calcium are also present.

Symptoms such as angina and intermittent claudication occur when the plaque has reached such a size that blood flow in the artery is reduced. During periods of increased oxygen requirement, such as exercise or excitement, blood supply cannot be adequately increased and ischaemia results. Gradual enlargement of a fibrous plaque will eventually produce symptoms at rest, but more often an acute event supersedes, producing a dramatic reduction in blood flow. this will produce the clinical sequelae of heart attack, stroke or peripheral gangrene.

The process that leads to an acute decompensation is thought to be rupture of the atherosclerotic plaque associated with partial or complete thrombosis and vessel occlusion. In the case of coronary artery plaques, it is often those lesions which produce only mild-to-moderate luminal narrowing that are liable to

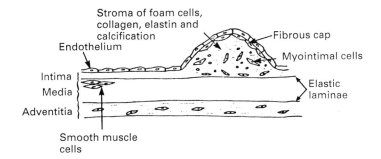

Fig. 1 Cross-section of an arterial wall demonstrating a fibrous plaque.

abrupt disruption. The other complications of plaque include rupture into an arterial wall (aneurysm) and calcification.

Pathogenesis of Atheroma

It is likely that an important event in the formation of atherosclerotic plaques is an alteration in the functional or structural barrier presented by the endothelial cell lining of arterial blood vessels. Lesions are commonly found at sites of turbulent blood flow such as bifurcations, especially those which are firmly supported and therefore prone to trauma. This has led to the suggestion that high-pressure turbulence injures the endothelium, resulting in increased permeability and platelet aggregation. Injured endothelial cells and platelets may then release growth factors, producing proliferation of smooth muscle cells. Conceptually, it is easy to imagine high levels of circulating cholesterol ester being deposited at such sites, leading to plaque formation.

It is now known, however, that fatty streaks can develop under an intact endothelial layer. Studies have shown that circulating white blood cells, known as monocytes, can penetrate intact endothelium, enter the intima and become loaded with lipoprotein-derived lipid. The process by which monocytes take up lipid and become 'foam cells' involves the uptake of modified LDL cholesterol via specific receptors which do not recognize native LDL cholesterol. The modification appears to involve peroxidation of polyunsaturated fatty acids in LDL lipids, a process which is usually inhibited by circulating antioxidants in the plasma. Oxidized LDL attracts circulating monocytes, inhibits the motility of tissue macrophages and is directly cytotoxic to endothelial cells.

Steinberg has proposed an alternative hypothesis, based on these studies, to explain the development of the fatty streak and its progression to a fibrous plaque. In the presence of high plasma levels of LDL, the concentration of LDL in the intima would be increased and, assuming that oxidation of LDL takes place at a constant rate, the intimal level of oxidized LDL would also be raised. The oxidized LDL would attract circulating monocytes to such areas, and then inhibit their subsequent migration. The newly formed macrophages would take up oxidized LDL via specific receptors and become foam cells. Subsequent release of oxidized LDL, perhaps as a result of cell death, could then promote loss of endothelial cells (through direct toxicity). At this point the sequence of platelet adhesion and aggregation with release of growth factors could promote the proliferation of smooth muscle cells and plaque development.

The effects of other known risk factors can easily be incorporated into these hypotheses. In the hypertensive individual, high pressures may increase vascular permeability, allowing increased deposition of lipid in the arterial wall. Some studies suggest that generation of free radicals, and hence lipid peroxidation, is increased in hypertensive individuals. Endothelial injury might be caused by a direct action of nicotine, or some other components of cigarette smoke, and cigarette smoking also results in increased platelet adhesiveness, fibrinogen levels and blood viscosity, which are associated with thrombosis. Furthermore, production of prostacyclin, an antiaggregatory prostaglandin, is reduced in smokers.

High-density lipoprotein cholesterol, high levels of which protect against heart attack, is thought to facilitate the removal of cholesterol ester from atheromatous sites, a process known as 'reverse cholesterol transport'. Although the mechanisms are poorly understood, exercise is known to increase levels of HDL cholesterol, whilst low levels are associated with smoking, hypertension and type II diabetes.

Significance for Health

In the Western world, clinical sequelae of atherosclerosis, CHD and stroke are the major causes of premature morbidity and mortality. It is clear from the list of risk factors that a change in lifestyle might effect a dramatic reduction in the development of atheromatous disease. ***See*** Coronary Heart Disease, Intervention Studies

Dietary Measures

The so-called prudent diet aims to reduce circulating cholesterol levels and hence slow the progression of atherosclerosis. The composition of the recommended diet is high in dietary fibre (40–45 g/24 h) with more than 50% of total energy in the form of unrefined carbohydrate. Dietary fat intake should be reduced to less than 25% of total energy, with less than 10% in the form of saturated fat. This diet will not only lower total cholesterol but has also been shown to produce a significant fall in blood pressure in hypertensive individuals. Glucose tolerance improves with such a regimen and may be normalized in some type II diabetics. *See* Dietary Fibre, Fibre and Disease Prevention

It should be emphasized that although this diet is now widely prescribed there is no evidence that it is of benefit to individuals with normal cholesterol levels. Furthermore, this regimen reduces total cholesterol by lowering both LDL cholesterol and HDL cholesterol; in women whose total cholesterol is not elevated, the deleterious effects of a fall in HDL cholesterol may outweigh the benefits of reducing LDL cholesterol levels. The prudent diet may not, therefore, be appropriate for all individuals.

An increased intake of oily fish has been shown to reduce the risk of further heart attack in men recovering from their first myocardial infarction. Omega-3 fatty acids are present in large quantities in oily fish (mackerel, salmon) and may be responsible for this beneficial effect. These compounds reduce the production of triglycerides and thrombotic prostaglandins whilst increasing production of vasodilator prostacyclins. The importance of these actions has yet to be fully assessed in clinical practice and it is possible that oily fish exert their beneficial effects simply by replacing meat in the diet. *See* Fish Oils, Dietary Importance

Vitamins C and E are natural antioxidants which circulate in the plasma. Since fatty acid peroxidation has been implicated in atherogenesis, some authors have suggested supplements of vitamin E and C as antiatherogenic agents. Once again, firm evidence is lacking and supplementation cannot be recommended at present. Weight reduction is recommended in obese subjects (Body mass index > 27 kg m^{-2}) since this will improve a constellation of cardiovascular risk factors. *See* Antioxidants, Role of Antioxidant Nutrients in Defence Systems

Exercise

Exercise will aid weight reduction and also have beneficial effects on HDL cholesterol levels. There may well be additional benefits in terms of CHD; thus regular exercise is recommended.

Smoking

All subjects should be advised to stop smoking.

Bibliography

Dodson PM and Horton RC (1987) The nature of atheroma. *Proceedings of the Nutrition Society* 46: 331–336.

Fuster V, Stein B, Ambrose JA, Badimon L, Badimon JJ and Chesebro JH (1990) Atherosclerotic plaque rupture and thrombosis. Evolving concepts. *Circulation* 82(II): 47–59

Grundy SM, Greenland P, Herd A *et al.* (1987) Cardiovascular and risk factor evaluation of healthy American adults. Position statement. *Circulation* 75: 1340A–1362A.

Halliwell B (1989) Current status review: free radicals, reactive oxygen species and human disease: a critical evaluation with special reference to atherosclerosis. *British Journal of Experimental Pathology* 70: 737–757.

McGill HC (1988) The cardiovascular pathology of smoking. *American Heart Journal* 115: 250–257.

Reaven GM (1988) Role of insulin resistance in human disease. Banting Lecture. *Diabetes* 37: 1595–1607.

Stehbens WE (1989) Diet and atherogenesis. *Nutrition Reviews* 47: 1–11.

Steinberg D (1989) The cholesterol controversy is over. Why did it take so long? *Circulation* 80: 1070–1078.

Steinberg D, Parthasarathy S, Carew TE, Khoo JC and Witztum JL (1989) Beyond cholesterol. Modifications of low-density lipoprotein that increase its atherogenicity. *New England Journal of Medicine* 320: 915–924.

Tall AR (1990) Plasma high density lipoproteins. *Journal of Clinical Investigation* 86: 379–384.

P. M. Dodson and S. C. Bain
East Birmingham Hospital, Birmingham, UK

AVOCADOS

The avocado (*Persea americana* Mill.) belongs to the family Lauraceae and is one of the major fruit crops in the world. They are indigenous to tropical America but are cultivated in nearly all tropical and subtropical countries. The fruit is a favoured article of diet and consumed mainly as a fresh fruit. It is very much relished for its dietary value, succulence and taste.

Morphology

The avocado (Fig. 1) is an evergreen tree; it grows to 20 m in height and can be equally wide. Leaves are variable in shape, from lanceolate to obovate, and spirally arranged. Flowers are small, 1–2 cm wide and equally deep, pea-green to yellow in colour with three whorls of three stamens and a one-celled ovary. The flowers are perfect in form, but exhibit a unique pollination mechanism referred to as 'dichogamy'. Each flower has two periods of opening: the first time it functions as a female, the second time as a male. The general tendency is for the pistil to be receptive before the pollen is shed. Varieties have been classified into two groups according to the time of flower opening: Group A are receptive in the morning but shed their pollen in the afternoon of the following day, giving a time lapse of more than 24 h; group B shed their pollen in the morning and are only receptive in the afternoon – the time lapse in this case is less than 24 h and the condition is not conducive to self-pollination.

Pollination occurs naturally by bees, but flies and

wasps also visit flowers and may contribute to this process. Fruits are mainly pear-shaped, but round to oval shapes are not uncommon. The colour ranges from green to purple. The pulp is firm at first, but on ripening it acquires a smooth, buttery texture. The large, round to egg-shaped central seed may be loose or closely appressed to the pulp.

Avocado Races and Varieties

There are three major recognized races of avocados: Mexican, Guatemalan and West Indian, usually adapted, respectively, to subtropical, semitropical and tropical climates. The Mexican race is native to the mountains of Mexico and Central America. Fruits are relatively small, weights ranging from 75 to 300 g with a thin, smooth skin and rich flavour. The Guatemalan race is native to the highlands of Central America and produces large fruits with average weights of 500–600 g with relatively thick, coarsely granular skin. The West Indian race is native to the lowlands of Central America. The cultivars of this race produce an intermediate size of fruits between the other two races with smooth, tough skin and flesh of good quality.

Mexican cultivars are the most cold-tolerant, West Indian stocks are very frost-sensitive, and the Guatemalan cultivars are intermediate in climate adaptation. Some Mexican selections have resistance to root rot, and some Guatemalan varieties are also apparently immune. In general, the cultivars of the Mexican race show low salt tolerance; the West Indian cultivars are the most resistant to salt.

Hybrids between the races are common and also commercially important. The frost-resistant Fuerte variety is a cross between Mexican and Guatemalan races. Varieties such as Lula, Booth7 and Booth8 (Table 1) are Guatemalan and West Indian hybrids, and are cold-sensitive.

Persea schiedeana, which is grown in southern Mexico and Guatemala, bears large, edible fruits.

Anatomy of the Fruit

The mature fruit of avocado is referred to as a berry and is comprised of soft pericarp and a single large seed. The pericarp consists of the exocarp, mesocarp and endocarp as the inner layer (Fig. 2). The exocarp is composed of a thin, wax-like cuticle as the outer layer, one layer of epidermis, two to three layers of hypodermal cells,

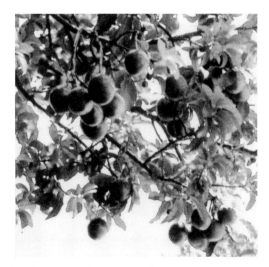

Fig. 1 Avocado (*Persea americana*).

Table 1.   Major avocado cultivars grown in various countries

Country/Regions	Cultivars
North America	
California	Hass, Zutano, Fuerte, Bacon, Anaheim
Florida	Waldin, Pollock, Booth7, Booth8, Lula, Taylor
Brazil	Pollock, Fuerte, Collinson, Waldin, Simmonds
Africa	
Lowlands	Booth7, Booth8, Collinson, Taylor, Lula
Highlands	Fuerte, Hass, Nabal, Puebla, Ettinger
Israel	Fuerte, Hass, Nabal, Ettinger, Reed
Australia	
Queensland, New South Wales	Fuerte, Hass, Edranol, Sharwil
Mildura	Fuerte, Helen, Rincon, Zutano, Edranol
Southeast Asia	Pollock, Waldin, Peterson

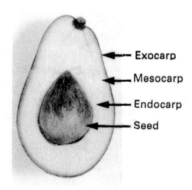

Fig. 2   Longitudinal section through the avocado fruit.

several layers of parenchyma cells, and a layer of sclerenchyma cells on the inner side of the skin. The mesocarp consists of a mass of nearly homogenous parenchyma cells which reach a diameter of about 60 μm in mature fruit and contain the major portion of the oil. In the mesocarp, some large cells with lignified walls are known as idioblasts, and these contain some of the oil. The endocarp consists of a few layers of parenchyma cells which are smaller than those of the mesocarp. The seed consists of two cotyledons, the plumule, hypocotyl and radicle, with two thin seed coats. The cotyledons consist of parenchyma tissue with oil and starch as the main storage compounds.

Compositional and Nutritional Value of Avocado Fruit

The avocado is an oleaginous fruit and the lipid level in the mesocarp varies from 10% to 30% in the mature

Table 2.   Average nutritional composition (on a fresh-weight basis) of the edible part of avocado fruit

Component	Fuerte[a]	Hass[a]	Anaheim[b]
Water (%)	71·2	74·4	79·3
Fat (%)	23·4	20·6	15·5
Protein (%)	2·0	1·8	1·8
Fibre (%)	1·9	1·4	1·7
Ash (%)	1·2	1·2	1·0
Sugars (%)			
Glucose	0·1	0·3	0·2
Fructose	0·1	0·1	0·2
Sucrose	0·0	0·1	0·1
Starch (%)	0·0	0·0	0·1
Organic acids (%)			
Malic	0·17	0·32	0·24
Citric	0·13	0·05	0·11
Oxalic	0·0	0·03	0·01
Energy (kJ per 100 g)	980	805	956
Vitamins (mg %)			
Ascorbic acid	9	11	14
Thiamin	0·07	0·07	0·08
Riboflavin	0·15	0·12	0·21
Pantothenic	0·9	1·2	1·11
Nicotinic acid	1·5	1·9	1·56
Vitamin B_6	0·61	0·62	0·39
Folic acid	0·03	0·04	0·018
Biotin	0·004	0·006	0·0034
Carotenoids (mg %)			
α-Carotene	0·36	0·29	0·24
β-Carotene	0·02	0·03	0·03
Cryptoxanthin	0·29	0·16	0·22
Minerals (mg %)			
Potassium	460	480	460
Phosphorus	29	27	29
Calcium	29	14	19
Magnesium	22	23	22
Sodium	2	2	2
Iron	0·6	0·7	0·6
Zinc	0·5	0·5	0·5

[a] Grown in Australia.
[b] Grown in California.

stage on a fresh-weight basis. Unlike other fruits, the avocado is high in fat, protein and minerals, but low in carbohydrates (Table 2). The fruit therefore serves as an important role in the diet as a source of energy, vitamins, minerals, and unsaturated lipids, especially monounsaturated fat.

Lipids

The oil content of avocados varies according to cultivar, growth conditions and period of storage. Mexican fruits have the highest oil content, West Indian the lowest, and

Table 3. Average fatty acid composition (as a percentage of total FAs) of Fuerte and Hass avocados

Fatty acids	Fuerte			Hass		
	Mature pulp	Ripe pulp	Seed	Mature pulp	Ripe pulp	Seed
Saturated						
Myristic ($C_{14:0}$)	0·05	0·04	0·9	0·07	0·06	0·7
Palmitic ($C_{16:0}$)	12·2	13·9	19·4	10·7	12·4	21·0
Stearic ($C_{18:0}$)	0·52	0·61	0·64	0·25	0·31	0·54
Arachidic ($C_{20:0}$)	0·16	0·19	0·21	0·19	0·20	0·21
Monounsaturated						
Palmitoleic ($C_{16:1}$)	4·6	3·9	3·7	6·4	5·2	3·6
Oleic ($C_{18:1}$)	72·8	69·9	26·2	70·5	68·5	29·2
Polyunsaturated						
Linoleic ($C_{18:2}$)	8·6	10·2	41·6	11·4	12·4	36·8
Linoleneic ($C_{18:3}$)	0·79	0·97	6·4	0·49	0·64	7·2
Arachidonic ($C_{20:4}$)	0·28	0·29	0·95	0·0	0·29	0·75
Total saturated fatty acids (SFA)	12·93	14·74	21·15	11·21	12·97	22·45
Total unsaturated fatty acids (UFA)	87·07	85·26	78·85	88·79	87·03	77·55
UFA/SFA	6·73	5·78	3·73	7·92	6·71	3·45

Guatemalan somewhat intermediate when grown in a given environment. The major fatty acid is oleic acid, followed by palmitic, linoleic and palmitoleic acids, while myristic, stearic, linoleneic, arachidic and arachidonic acids are present only in trace amounts (Table 3). Fatty acid compositions in seeds greatly differ from those of mesocarp. Seeds contain less oleic acid and more linoleic and linolenic acid. *See* Fatty Acids, Properties

Avocado lipid can be divided into four classes: glycerides, free fatty acids, phospholipids, and glycolipids. The glycerides represent the major fraction and about 85% of the lipids consist of triglycerides. Free fatty acid and phospholipid levels are found to be low. *See* Lipids, Classification; Phospholipids, Properties and Occurrence; Triglycerides, Structures and Properties

The contents of fatty substances increase during fruit development. The maximum accumulation of reserve lipids during maturation is mainly an increase in the triglyceride fraction. Oleic acid is the major acid synthesized during fruit growth. Palmitic, palmitoleic and linoleic acid contents increase slightly, while the content of linolenic acid remains constant. *See* Ripening of Fruit

Carbohydrate

The total carbohydrate content of avocado ranges from 1·5% to 9·5% (fresh-weight basis). The 7-carbon sugars, D-mannoheptulose, the 6-carbon sugars, glucose and fructose, and then disaccharide, sucrose, are present in mature and ripe fruit. The sugar alcohol, perseitol, is

also present in substantial amounts in fresh fruit. Several other 7-carbon and 8-carbon sugars have been identified in trace amounts. *See* Carbohydrates, Classification and Properties; Sugar Alcohols

During storage of avocado, there is a large drop in total sugar content from 2·7% to 0·6% in Fuerte avocados. The mannoheptulose and perseitol almost disappear, leaving glucose, fructose and sucrose as the major sugars after ripening.

Protein

The protein content in avocados ranges between 1·1% and 2·3%, which is higher than in the other fruits such as apple, peach, blackberry, olive and banana (average values of 0·1–1·1%). Asparagine, glutamine, glutamic acid and aspartic acid are the major amino acids found in avocado; serine, alanine, threonine, valine and cystine are also present in minor quantities. *See* Amino Acids, Properties and Occurrence; Apples; Bananas and Plantains; Peaches and Nectarines

Vitamins

In comparison with other fruits, avocado is an excellent source of vitamins B and E. It also contains vitamin C and carotene. The content of vitamin B_6 in avocados is the second highest following bananas. Vitamin B_6 occurs mainly as pyridoxine, pyridoxal and pyridoxamine forms, which comprise about 56%, 29% and 14% respectively. The pantothenic acid level is second highest among fruits, after passion fruit. *See* Ascorbic Acid, Properties and Determination; Pantothenic Acid, Properties and Determination; Vitamin B_6, Properties and Determination

Minerals

Avocado contains relatively high mineral content, ranging from 0·9% to 1·4% in Fuerte and Hass varieties. The fruit is a good source of iron and phosphorus, and this is considered to be valuable for people who have anaemic conditions. *See* Anaemia, Iron Deficiency Anaemia; Phosphorus, Properties and Determination

Volatile Compounds

In ripe Fuerte avocados, about 75% of the total volatile constituents are dominated by C_6 alcohols and aldehydes. Major components include *trans*-hex-3-en-1-ol (25·6%), *trans*-hex-2-en-1-ol (19·1%), hexan-1-ol (17·9%), *cis*-hex-2-enal (8·7%) and hexanal (4·5%). Most of the volatile compounds are derived from lipid oxidation or degradation.

Pests and Diseases

A number of insects attack the avocado, but they are not considered to be a serious problem in most countries.

The most serious problem in avocado production is root rot, caused by a fungus called *Phytophthora cinnamomi*. This fungus also causes seedling blight and stem canker. Cercospora spot, caused by *Cercospora purpurea*, is a serious problem in West Africa and Zaire. It causes sunken spots on leaves and stems, and brown spots on fruits. A virus disease called sunblotch is transmitted by vegetative propagation or by seed, and causes white patches on leaves, stems and fruit.

Post-harvest Diseases

Anthracnose is a latent fungal disease caused by *Glomerella cingulata* during storage. Symptoms are the development of light brown colour spots. In severe cases these spots enlarge rapidly changing the colour to dark brown with a sunken appearance. *Diplodia natalensis*, which causes stem-end rot, is a major problem in warm tropical countries. A dark brown to black rot develops at the stem end of ripening fruit and proceeds to the other end.

Fruit Maturity

Fruit will not mature while attached to tree; it must be harvested in order for it to soften and become edible. Correct determination of maturity is essential to ensure the keeping quality in storage and for processing. Avocados picked before the adequate attainment of maturity behave abnormally. They will not ripen properly and acquire a leathery consistency with shrivelled skin and undesirable flavour.

In many instances, the appearance of the fruit gives little indication of its maturity. Different factors, such as specific gravity, weight loss, days to softening, and seed coat colour, have been considered as criteria for determining maturity of fruits, but none of them has been found to be satisfactory.

Dry weight (21% minimum) or oil content (8% w/w minimum) are used as maturity standards.

Harvesting, Grading and Packing

Fruits can be harvested manually using telescopic poles fitted with a clipper blade and catch bag. In some California and Florida orchards a picking platform, operating independently or attached to a tractor, can be raised or lowered as necessary. Fruit can then be harvested by hand, which avoids bruising. Fruits should be harvested either by clipping or snapping, rather than plucking or pulling. Clipping and leaving a short stem reduces the chance of bruising the adjacent fruits. After picking, fruits are handled carefully to prevent bruising and damage, and are shaded to prevent damage by direct sunlight.

Harvested avocados are graded by hand and then sized by weight devices. Inspection grades are mainly based on similar variety characteristics, normal shape, colour, maturity, trimming of stems, defects and decay. Fruit is packed manually, usually into fibreboard containers. The majority of the crop is marketed as fresh fruits.

Transporting of avocados to distant markets is by refrigerated trucks within the country and by ships to foreign markets. Air freight is expensive and is used only in special cases. From Florida, transit time is usually 2–3 days to the markets along the East Coast of the USA and 3–5 days to the markets on the West Coast. Shipments from South Africa take as long as 2–3 weeks to UK and European markets.

Fruit Ripening

The avocado fruit is classified as a 'climacteric' fruit, which indicates a series of biochemical changes asso-

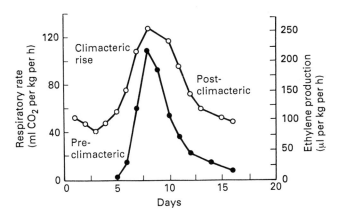

Fig. 3 Respiratory rate and ethylene production at 20°C in Fuerte avocados following harvest (O——O carbon dioxide; ●——● ethylene).

ciated with the respiratory rise. This is initiated by the autocatalytic production of ethylene making the changes from maturation to senescence and leading to ripening. In addition to a large increase in respiration, avocado shows increased ethylene production during ripening (Fig. 3).

Ethylene is a natural plant hormone which plays a major role in the ripening of avocados. Ripening occurs during the rise in respiration between preclimacteric minimum and climacteric peak; in general, fruit become soft and edible about 2–3 days after the peak respiratory activity. The best temperature for ripening of avocados is between 15°C and 20°C. Ripening at higher temperatures (> 30°C) leads to discoloration of the skin, uneven softening, and development of off-flavours.

Fruit Storage

Avocados are usually harvested and transported in the firm, preclimacteric condition and then ripened under ambient conditions. Successful storage of avocado is based on slowing down the respiratory rate or delaying the onset of ripening without causing physiological disorders and loss of quality. Such storage is achieved by altering the environment of the fruit immediately after harvest, mainly by lowering the temperature, by changing the composition of the atmosphere, by irradiation or by a combination of these treatments. *See* Storage Stability, Mechanisms of Degradation

Refrigerated Storage

The response of avocado to low-temperature storage mainly depends on storage temperature, duration and cultivar. Fruits of cold-tolerant cultivars can be stored for extended periods at 4.4°C, whereas fruits of cold

sensitive cultivars cannot be stored below 12.8°C without physiological stress. Avocados and many other tropical and subtropical fruits may develop chilling injury below a certain critical temperature level. Chilling injury in avocados is commonly characterized by grey-brown discoloration of the mesocarp, especially in the vascular tissue. In severe cases, abnormal ripening, surface pitting, darkening of the flesh and development of off-flavours and odours commonly occur.

Fuerte and Hass avocados stored at 4.4°C show no marked deterioration in quality when stored for 3 weeks, and subsequently ripen upon transfer to 20°C. Both varieties are affected by storage at 2°C, and the severity of chilling injury is proportional to the duration of cold storage. Storage at 12°C or slightly higher is the most suitable temperature for Pollock, Waldin and Fuchs avocados, but storage of these varieties at < 10°C results in chilling injury within 15 days.

Controlled-atmosphere Storage (CAS)

Controlled storage involves the addition or removal of gases in the storage atmosphere. These gas concentrations are regulated continuously during storage. By manipulating the amounts of oxygen, carbon dioxide and ethylene, ripening can be retarded. Controlled-atmosphere storage reduces the rate of senescence, ethylene sensitivity and incidence of decay through post-harvest pathogens.

Conditions of 2% oxygen with 10% carbon dioxide have been found to be more effective for avocados than any other combinations. Lula and Fuerte avocados can be stored at 7.2°C for 3 weeks in air, and for 6–8 weeks in 2% oxygen and 10% carbon dioxide. In this gas composition, chilling injury was substantially reduced in cold-sensitive varieties. Avocados stored in carbon dioxide concentrations above 15% and oxygen concentration below 1% developed skin discoloration and off-flavours during ripening. *See* Controlled Atmosphere Storage, Effect on Fruit and Vegetables

Modified Atmosphere Storage (MAS)

Modified atmosphere storage differs from CAS in the degree and method of control. Under MAS, the equilibrium gas concentrations are determined by the respiration of the product and the permeability of the packaging material or storage room.

Storage of Fuerte and Hass avocados in polythene bags at ambient temperature delayed the ripening by 4–5 days without affecting the quality. *See* Chilled Storage, Use of Modified Atmosphere Packaging; Chilled Storage, Effect of Modified Atmosphere Packaging on Food Quality

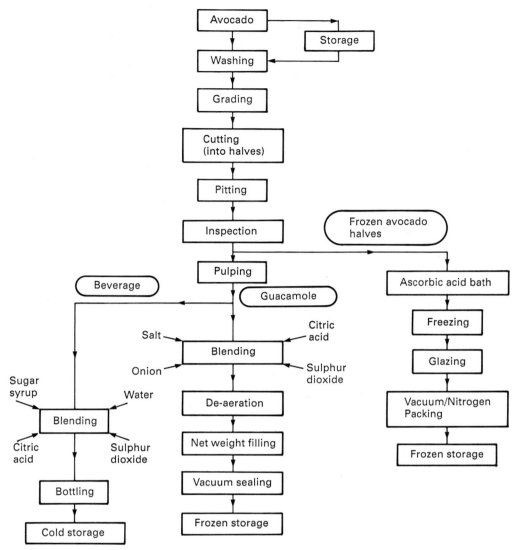

Fig. 4 Flow diagram showing processing of avocado products.

Irradiation

Post-harvest treatment of fruits with ionizing radiation has been found to delay the ripening and senescence. It also controls fungal infections. Avocado is one of the fruits that are sensitive to radiation, and doses in excess of 0·2 kGy (20 krad) cause brown discoloration in the mesocarp. *See* Irradiation of Foods, Applications

A radiation dose of 0·1 kGy resulted in an extension of storage life of Fuerte avocados by 4–5 days at 20°C. Fruits treated with 0·5 kGy did not ripen, the tissue remained hard and turned brown.

Industrial Uses

Avocado is generally consumed as a fresh fruit. It is mainly used as an ingredient in salads and on tortillas with lemon juice, pepper and salt. Avocado oil has considerable health value as it contains high amounts of unsaturated fatty acids, especially monounsaturated fatty acids (75–90%), and, in common with all fruits, no cholesterol. Pure avocado oil is a good product, light and delicate, and because of the mild flavour it mixes well with other foods. It is used in salads, sauces and stir-fry dishes. Compared to corn, almond, soya-bean and olive oils, avocado oil has the highest rate of skin penetration. It is therefore in great demand for the preparation of cosmetics and toiletries such as cleansing cream, bath oil, hair conditioner and make-up bases.

Avocados should not be cooked. Studies on the utilization of avocado in mayonnaise or salad cream have demonstrated that the flesh is very sensitive to enzymatic browning, which causes off-flavours. Enzymatic browning can be prevented by preserving avocados and their products by freezing.

Processing of Avocados (Fig. 4)

Frozen Avocado Halves

The avocado is cut in half along its longitudinal axis and the seed is removed. The open halves are inspected for any internal discoloration. The halves are then coated with an antioxidant, such as an aqueous solution of ascorbic acid (0·5%) or half-strength of lemon juice or a solution of citric acid, for 1 min to prevent browning of the fruit during freezing, storage and on thawing. After the treatment with the antioxidant, the halves are frozen quickly by immersion in liquid nitrogen or nitrous oxide. The time of immersion depends upon the maturity, variety, initial temperature and size of the avocado half and usually varies from 15 to 50 s. After removal from the liquefied gas, the avocado halves are placed in a cold environment, preferably as low as $-18°C$. *See* Antioxidants, Synthetic Antioxidants; Freezing, Freezing Operations

For maximum keeping qualities, frozen avocado halves are glazed with pure water to keep the fruit from having contact with oxygen in the package. After glazing, they are packed in nitrogen atmosphere or in vacuum and stored in a freezer.

Guacamole

Guacamole is a frozen savoury spread prepared from ripe avocados. Fruits are washed, surface-dried, halved and pulped. The pulp is then blended with dehydrated onion powder (10 g per kg), salt (14 g per kg), and sulphur dioxide (300 mg per kg). The pH of the mixture is adjusted to 4·9 by addition of citric acid (3%). Products are vacuum-packed in cans and blast frozen for 30 min at $-37°C$, then stored at $-18°C$.

Avocado Beverage

Avocado beverage is a delicious drink with excellent nutritive properties. It is commonly consumed at household level in developing countries, especially in the warm summer months. Fully ripe avocados are selected and washed. The fruit is sliced and the pulp is removed with a scoop. It is then blended with water, sugar, citric acid, and benzoic acid. The beverage is bottled in sterilized glass bottles and chilled. Avocado beverage contains 10% pulp, 0·3–0·5% acidity, and 200 ppm benzoic acid.

Bibliography

Ahmed EM and Barmore CR (1980) Avocado. In: Nagy S and Shaw PE (eds) *Tropical and Subtropical Fruits. Composition, Properties and Uses*, pp 121–156. Westport, Connecticut: AVI Publishing.

Biale JB (1941) The climacteric rise in respiration rate of the Fuerte avocado fruit. *Proceedings of the American Society for Horticultural Science* 39: 137–142.

Biale JB and Young RE (1971) The Avocado Pear. In: Hulme AC (ed.) *The Biochemistry of Fruits and their Products*, vol. 2, pp 1–28. New York: Academic Press.

Chambers' Encyclopaedia (1968) Oxford: Pergamon Press; 1968. Vol. 2, p 9.

Cummings K and Schroeder CA (1942) Anatomy of the avocado fruit. *California Avocado Society Year Book*, 26: 56–64.

Hall AP, Moore JG and Morgan AF (1955) B vitamin content of California-grown avocados. *Journal of Agricultural and Food Chemistry* 3: 250–252.

Hanson LP (ed.) (1976) Other fruits – avocados. *Commercial Processing of Fruits*, pp 276–282. New Jersey: Noyes Data Corporation.

Hatton TT and Reeder WF. Maintaining market quality of Florida avocados. Proceedings of the Conference on the Tropical and Subtropical Fruits; 1969 September 15–19. Tropical Product Institute, London; pp 277–280.

Lee SK (1981) A review and background of the avocado maturity standard. *California Avocado Society Year Book* 65: 101–109.

Samson JA (ed.) (1986) Avocado. *Tropical Fruits* 2nd edn, pp 235–255. New York: Longman.

Scudamore-Smith PD (1984) The utilisation of avocado as frozen savoury spread. *Food Technology in Australia* 36: 375–378.

Swisher HE (1988) Avocado Oil. *Journal of the American Oil Chemists' Society* 65: 1704–1706.

Wills RBH, Lim JSK and Greenfield H (1986) Composition of Australian foods. 31. Tropical and sub-tropical fruit. *Food Technology in Australia* 38: 118–123.

Acknowledgements

I wish to thank Dr AAP De Alwis (University of Reading) and Professor CA Schroeder (University of California) for their helpful advice and encouragement.

Thevaki Nagalingam
University of Reading, Reading, UK

BACILLUS

Contents

Occurrence

Occurrence in the Environment and Foods

Bacillus cereus spores and vegetative cells are frequently found in a wide range of environments, including soils, dust, water, vegetation and many foods. *B. cereus* can be found in cereals, dried foods, spices, starches, meat products, vegetables and vegetable sprouts. Ingredients such as spices, flour, starch and sugar have been incriminated as sources of spores (Table 1). These ingredients have caused *B. cereus* outbreaks in contaminated fermented sausages and canned food products. Investigators in the UK isolated *B. cereus* from 98 of 108 (91%) of rice samples. In Sweden, the reported *B. cereus* isolation rate from 3888 different samples of foods was reported to be 47·8%. Researchers in the USA found that *B. cereus* spores present in ready-to-serve moist foods could grow to large numbers if the products were temperature abused. *B. stearothermophilus* can cause spoilage in low-acid canned foods, and *B. coagulans* can cause spoilage in canned tomato products. *B. anthracis* causes anthrax in both animals and humans. *B. cereus* can be a problem in dairy products and is occasionally responsible for spoilage of raw and pasteurized milk. The spoilage of milk products is believed to be caused by the activity of *B. cereus* lecithinase. Researchers have demonstrated that *B. cereus* can often be present in infant formulae. If the formula is allowed to remain at room temperature for an extended period of time, *B. cereus* can grow to high numbers. *See* Milk, Processing of Liquid Milk

Although some *Bacillus* species can cause potential spoilage and health hazards, other species may be useful in foods or in food testing. Some *Bacillus* species can be used as a source of proteolytic enzymes that could be used to clot milk during cheese production. It might also be possible to use some bacilli in the production of single-celled protein. Several strains recognized by the American Type Culture Collection (ATCC) are used in sterility testing. *B. pumilus* (ATCC 27142) is recommended for determining the effectiveness of γ radiation sterilization. *B. stearothermophilus* (ATCC 7953) is used to test steam sterilization. *B. subtilis* (ATCC 6633) is recommended as the test organism for penicillin detec-

Table 1. Prevalence of *B. cereus* in some raw and processed products

Food products	No. of samples examined	% *B. cereus* positive	Range of *B. cereus* counts per g or ml
Raw rice	13	46	10^2–10^3
	108	91	Detected
	16	100	Detected
Boiled rice	32	38	10^3–10^7
	14	93	10^1–10^3
	252	10	10^2–10^5
Fried rice	14	86	10^1–10^3
	204	24	10^2–10^5
Raw milk	100	9	10^1–10^2
Pasteurized milk	100	35	10^1–10^3
Milk powder	120	27	10^1–10^2
	8	38	10^2–10^3
Infant formula	12	75	0·23–0·93
Nonfat milk	18	100	0·23–1·50
Spices	25	40	10^2–10^3
	51	10	10^2–10^3
	110	53	10^1–10^4

tion in milk and is also used for steam sterilization. Ethylene oxide sterilization testing is often done with *B. subtilis* var. *niger* (ATCC 9372). Another useful *Bacillus* species is *B. subtilis* var *globigii*, which is used to test the sterilization of hydrogen peroxide in aseptic processing equipment. *See* Cheeses, Chemistry of Curd Manufacture; Sterilization of Foods

Growth Factors/Conditions

The genus *Bacillus* belongs in the family Bacillaceae. The organisms are facultative aerobic, large Gram-positive rods that produce endospores Single endospores may be formed in central or paracentral position and do not swell the sporangium. The cells are typically $1 \cdot 0$–$1 \cdot 2 \, \mu m$ in diameter by $3 \cdot 0$–$5 \cdot 0 \, \mu m$ in length. The rods often occur in chains, and on agar medium the colonies have a dull or frosted appearance. The majority of the species are motile by peritrichous flagella, produce catalase, and produce acid but not gas from glucose.

The nutrient requirements for *Bacillus* species vary considerably from the simple to the very complex. *B. cereus* has an absolute growth requirement for amino acids but vitamins are not required. The pH range for bacilli is broad with pH $2 \cdot 0$ for *B. acidocaldarius* being the low tolerance level and pH $7 \cdot 5$–$8 \cdot 0$ for *B. alcalophilus* as the high tolerance level. *B. cereus* can grow over a pH range of $4 \cdot 9$–$9 \cdot 3$. Salt tolerance for the genus ranges from 2% or less for some species while others can grow at salt concentrations of 25%. There are psychrotrophs, mesophiles and thermophiles within the genus. Bacilli can grow from approximately 10 up to 75°C with the optimum for most species being 28–35°C. Generation time for most species in a rich culture medium ranges from 18 to 27 min at 35°C.

B. cereus is able to utilize glucose, fructose and trehalose, but not pentoses and many of the sugar alcohols. Some *Bacillus* strains can utilize sucrose, maltose, mannose, glycerol and lactose. The majority of the strains can hydrolyse starch, casein and gelatin. Different species in the genus are actively proteolytic, moderately proteolytic, or nonproteolytic, gas-forming or not, and lipolytic or not. This wide diversity within the genus can make identification difficult.

There has not been much research on the effect of water activity (a_w) on the growth of bacilli. The minimum a_w for growth has been reported to be $0 \cdot 95$; however, *B. cereus* is capable of growth in fried rice at an a_w of $0 \cdot 912$. In one study the limiting a_w for spore germination was $0 \cdot 95$ for glucose, sorbitol, and salt, but $0 \cdot 91$ when glycerol was used as the humectant. *See* Water Activity, Effect on Food Stability

The spores of the mesophile *B. subtilis* are less heat-resistant than spores of a thermophile such as *B. stearothermophilus*. Spores from strains of serotype 1, a serotype commonly involved in food poisoning outbreaks, were shown by researchers in the UK to have a D_{95} of approximately 24 min. Other serotypes have a broader range of heat resistance, with a D_{95} ranging from $1 \cdot 5$ to 36 min and an average z value of $9 \cdot 2$°C. Glycine or a neutral L-amino acid and purine ribosides are required for spore germination. L-Alanine is the most effective amino acid stimulating germination.

Mechanism of Introduction into Foods

Both vegetative cells and spores of *Bacillus* species can frequently be isolated from soils, dust, water and food. Low numbers of the organism are often present in foods, but do not cause a problem at a low level. Vegetative cells and spores of *Bacillus* species can enter the food chain via contamination on raw produce or in ingredients such as flour and sugar. It has been demonstrated that *Bacillus* species make up approximately 90% of the bacteria found in rice paddy soil. *B. cereus* is found in the soil, in rice plants and in finished polished rice. This close relationship of *B. cereus* to rice accounts for the frequent association of *B. cereus* food poisoning to fried rice.

Bacillus species can cause soft rot in vegetables by the action of pectinase enzymes. *B. thermosphacta* can grow on meat at pH $5 \cdot 4$ when incubated aerobically, but it cannot grow anaerobically at pH $< 5 \cdot 8$. This organism can predominate with lactobacilli in some types of vacuum-packaged meat products. The thermophilic *Bacillus* and *Clostridium* species are of the greatest importance in canned foods. The a_w, fat content, presence of salts and carbohydrates, and pH will all determine the heat resistance of *Bacillus* spores in canned foods. The incorporation of calcium chloride in the growth medium of *B. megaterium* spores will increase the heat resistance of the spores. *See* Canning, Principles; *Clostridium*, Occurrence of *Clostridium Perfringens*

The microbial flora of cereal products is low, but may be expected to be contaminated with bacteria found in soil and storage and processing environments. The a_w of most cereal products is low enough to restrict the growth of bacteria. If a_w conditions favour growth, *Bacillus* species and moulds will be the most common spoilage organisms. *Bacillus* species can produce amylase which allows them to utilize flour and related products as sources of energy. Bacilli are often present in low numbers on grain products, but will occur in high numbers only if the growth conditions become favourable.

Fate during Storage and Processing

Spores of *Bacillus* species are very stable under adverse conditions and can survive for extended periods in dried foods. The heat resistance of spores of *B. cereus* is greater than the heat resistance for other mesophilic spore-forming organisms; therefore, the food industry is concerned about the presence of this bacterium. Although spores of *B. cereus* have an increased heat resistance, low numbers of these spores in food do not pose a health hazard. Only if the product is not properly processed or if a prepared food is temperature abused will low numbers of *B. cereus* be able to grow to high enough numbers to pose a health threat. *See* Drying, Uses of Dried Foods

Bibliography

Banwart GJ (1989) *Basic Food Microbiology*, 2nd edn. Westport, Conn: AVI Publishing.

Frazier WC and Westhoff DC (1988) *Food Microbiology*, 4th edn. New York: McGraw-Hill.

Jay JM (1986) *Modern Food Microbiology*, 3rd edn. New York: Van Nostrand Reinhold.

Johnson EA (1990) *Bacillus cereus* food poisoning. In: Cliver DO (ed.) *Foodborne Diseases*, pp 128–135. New York: Academic Press.

Kramer JM and Gilbert RJ (1989) *Bacillus cereus* and other *Bacillus* species. In: Doyle MP (ed.) *Foodborne Bacterial Pathogens*, pp 21–70. New York: Marcel Dekker.

S. S. Sumner
University of Nebraska-Lincoln, Lincoln, USA

Detection

Detection in Foods

The isolation procedures of *Bacillus cereus* from raw and processed foods are identical. Isolation, detection and enumeration of *B. cereus* from foods involves direct agar-plating techniques. If the quantity of food to be examined is large, representative samples of 50 g each are taken from different parts of the suspected food because contamination may be unevenly distributed. In most food poisoning incidents, the sample of food will be limited in size.

Different plating media for *B. cereus* have been developed based on the ability of *B. cereus* to exhibit haemolysin production, lecithinase activity, and fermentation properties. The enumeration of *B. cereus* can be facilitated by the incorporation of selective agents into the medium to inhibit background flora. *B. cereus* is resistant to polymyxin; therefore, polymyxin is often added to isolation medium for *B. cereus*.

One medium that is commonly used for the isolation of *B. cereus* is mannitol–egg yolk–polymyxin (MYP).

MYP agar relies on the egg yolk reaction (lecithin hydrolysis) and negative mannitol fermentation for the isolation of *B. cereus*. After 24 h incubation at 30°C, *B. cereus* colonies are usually translucent to creamy white with a violet-red background surrounded by a visible zone of egg yolk precipitate. If reactions are not clear, the agar plates can be incubated for an additional 24 h. Only colonies exhibiting typical *B. cereus* reaction should be counted. This will give a presumptive plate count for *B. cereus*. Five presumptive colonies should be picked from MYP agar plates and transferred to nutrient agar slants for confirmation as *B. cereus*. MYP agar is the agar of choice in most laboratories in the USA and UK.

It is usually unnecessary to use enrichment procedures for the determination of *B. cereus*, since high numbers of the organism are often sought. A three-tube most probable number (MPN) technique using trypticase–soy–polymyxin (TSP) can be used for the detection of foods suspected to contain fewer than 10 *B. cereus* organisms per gram. The MPN procedure is also preferred for the examination of certain dehydrated starchy foods. Tubes showing growth are streaked onto MYP agar and examined for typical *B. cereus* appearance, as on MYP agar plates.

All suspect colonies of *B. cereus* must be confirmed. There are many different confirmation schemes that can be used. Typical colony types (lecithinase-positive and mannitol-negative) are picked from MYP agar plates and confirmed as large Gram-positive rods containing spores that do not swell the sporangium. Various confirmatory tests include anaerobic glucose fermentation (*B. cereus* is facultatively anaerobic), nitrate reduction (positive), Voges–Proskauer test (positive), citrate utilization (positive), tyrosine decomposition (positive), gelatin or casein hydrolysis (positive), and growth in the presence of 0·001% (w/v) lysoyme (positive). To differentiate *B. cereus* from *B. thuringensis* and *B. anthracis* the following tests can be done: motility test (positive); rhizoid growth (negative); haemolytic activity (positive).

Detection in Suspected Food Poisoning

Since spores of *B. cereus* are widely distributed in nature, it is not uncommon to find small numbers of the organism in foods. However, the isolation of high numbers ($> 10^5$ colony-forming units (CFU) per gram of food) of *B. cereus* from foods implicated in food poisoning suggest the involvement of this organism in the food poisoning outbreak. In order to implicate *B. cereus* in a food poisoning incident, large numbers of *B. cereus* ($> 10^5$ CFU per gram) should be isolated from the food, and isolation from the faeces or vomitus of the victims should be attempted. The isolates should be of the same phenotype to implicate the food.

Since the symptoms of diarrhoeal *B. cereus* food poisoning are similar to staphylococcal food poisoning and emetic *B. cereus* food poisoning is similar to *Clostridium perfringens* food poisoning, foods implicated in such outbreaks should also be examined for the presence of *B. cereus*. A brief history of the illness (symptoms, incubation and duration), details of the foods consumed, and information on preparation and handling of the food are all important data to collect. This information will assist the laboratory investigation of the food poisoning outbreak. *See Clostridium*, Food Poisoning by *Clostridium Perfringens*; *Staphylococcus*, Food Poisoning

Specimens, representative samples of at least 10 g of all food items and 10 g of faeces and vomitus from the victims, should be transported to the laboratory with the minimum amount of delay. Samples should be refrigerated. Refrigeration does not appear to decrease the numbers of *B. cereus*, but refrigeration will decrease the competitive background flora to make identification easier. Dehydrated foods may be stored at room temperature and shipped without refrigeration.

Case Histories and Statistics

B. cereus food poisoning accounted for 1% of the bacterial outbreaks in the USA from 1973 to 1987. *B. cereus* food poisoning is a rather mild illness and is less likely to be confirmed as the aetiologic agent in a food poisoning outbreak. There have been more outbreaks due to *B. cereus* in the UK than in the USA. This difference may be due to better reporting and a better surveillance system in the UK. The majority of *B. cereus* cases have been reported in northern and eastern European countries. The first large outbreak was described by Hauge and involved 600 cases. Patients and staff at a hospital in Norway complained of abdominal pain, profuse watery diarrhoea, and some nausea approximately 10 h after eating a meal. The dinner meal included chocolate pudding that contained a vanilla sauce. Both of these items had been prepared the day before and held at room temperature. Samples of the vanilla sauce contained high levels of *B. cereus* ($2 \cdot 5 \times 10^7$). *B. cereus* spores can be found in numerous environments; therefore, many foods have been implicated in outbreaks. Foods implicated include casseroles, sausages, other cooked meat and poultry dishes, råw and cooked vegetables, soups, milk and fried rice dishes. Spices can often contain large numbers of *Bacillus* spores, which may survive cooking and can germinate and cause problems in other foods, especially meat dishes. *See* Food Poisoning, Statistics

Bibliography

Banwart GJ (1989) *Basic Food Microbiology*, 2nd edn. Westport, Conn: AVI Publishing.

Frazier WC and Westhoff DC (1988) *Food Microbiology*, 4th edn. New York: McGraw-Hill.
Harmon SM (1984) *Bacillus cereus. FDA Bacteriological Analytical Manual*, 6th edn, pp 16.01–16.08. Washington, DC: US Food and Drug Administration.
Jay JM (1986) *Modern Food Microbiology*, 3rd edn. New York: Van Nostrand Reinhold.
Johnson EA (1990) *Bacillus cereus* food poisoning. In: Cliver DO (ed.) *Foodborne Diseases*, pp 128–135. New York: Academic Press.
Kramer JM and Gilbert RJ (1989) *Bacillus cereus* and other *Bacillus* species. In: Doyle MP (ed.) *Foodborne Bacterial Pathogens*, pp 21–70. New York: Marcel Dekker.

S. S. Sumner
University of Nebraska-Lincoln, Lincoln, USA

Food Poisoning

Of the 34 species in the genus *Bacillus*, only two, *B. anthracis* and *B. cereus*, are recognized as common pathogens. It was not until 1950 that Steinar Hauge in Norway proved the involvement of *B. cereus* in gastroenteritis. The first recognized outbreak occurred in the USA in 1969, while the first in the UK occurred in 1971. There have only been a few confirmed outbreaks and cases of *B. cereus* food poisoning in the USA (Table 1). Since the organism is so widely distributed in many environments and foods, it is commonly viewed as relatively harmless under most circumstances. In the 14 year period 1973–1987, the Centers for Disease Control (CDC) reported 58 *B. cereus* outbreaks in the USA or 1% of the diagnosed bacterial outbreaks (Table 2). There are two distinct types of illnesses attributed to the consumption of foods contaminated with *B. cereus*: a diarrhoeal illness and an emetic illness. The clinical features and characteristics of each illness are presented in Table 3. It is not routine procedure to analyse foods for *B. cereus*; therefore, the incidence of *B. cereus* food poisoning may be underestimated. *See* Campylobacter, Properties and Occurrence; *Clostridium*, Food Poisoning by *Clostridium Perfringens*; Food Poisoning, Statistics; Food Poisoning, Tracing Origins and Testing; *Staphylococcus*, Food Poisoning

Diarrhoeal Syndrome

This syndrome is rather mild with an incubation time of approximately 4–16 h, and lasting for 12–24 h. Symptoms consist of abdominal pain, nausea (with vomiting rare) and watery stools. The symptoms of this syndrome are similar to those caused by *Clostridium perfringens*. The foods involved in the diarrhoeal illness have been quite varied, ranging from vegetables and salads to meat dishes and casseroles.

Table 1. Confirmed *B. cereus* outbreaks reported in the USA from 1983 to 1987

Year	Outbreaks No.	Outbreaks %	Cases No.	Cases %	Deaths	Foods implicated (cases)
1983	—	—	—	—	—	—
1984	3	1·6	23	0·3	0	Beef Chinese food Multiple foods
1985	7	3·2	42	0·2	0	Shellfish Chinese food Fruits and vegetables Fried rice (2) Unknown (2)
1986	4	2·2	187	3·2	0	Fried rice Multiple foods (3)
1987	2	1·5	9	0·1	0	Unknown (2)

Table 2. Confirmed disease outbreaks by bacterial agent reported in the USA from 1973 to 1987

Aetiologic agent	Outbreaks	Cases	Deaths
Bacillus cereus	58	261[a]	0
Campylobacter spp.	61	6881	2
Clostridium botulinum	233	506	44
Clostridium perfringens	225	13 940	12
Salmonella spp.	789	54 635	89
Staphylococcus aureus	380	18 103	4

[a] Only number of cases from 1982–1987. From 1972–1982, 2·9% outbreaks (1·3% cases) were attributed to *B. cereus*. There were two large outbreaks in 1978: one outbreak in North Carolina involved 208 cases, and one outbreak in New York involved 118 cases.

The rapid onset time and the short duration of *B. cereus* food poisoning suggest that the illness is caused by toxins. Researchers at the University of Wisconsin-Madison demonstrated that the toxin responsible for the diarrhoeal syndrome is an enterotoxin. The enterotoxin probably consists of three proteins (M_r 43 000, 39 000 and 38 000, respectively). It causes fluid accumulation in rabbit ileal loops and is lethal in mice when injected at high concentrations. The enterotoxin is produced during the log phase of the growth cycle, and it is inactivated by trypsin and pronase. The toxin is relatively unstable to heat (destroyed at 55°C for 20 min).

Emetic Syndrome

This form of *B. cereus* food poisoning is more severe and acute than the diarrhoeal form. The incubation period is 1–5 h with resulting nausea and vomiting. The incubation period and symptoms mimic those of *Staphylococcus aureus* food poisoning. The emetic syndrome is most often associated with the consumption of contaminated boiled or fried rice dishes. Other foods that have been involved in outbreaks include pasteurized cream, spaghetti, mashed potatoes, and vegetable sprouts. Outbreaks of emetic *B. cereus* gastroenteritis have been reported in the USA, the UK, Canada, Finland, India, Japan, the Netherlands, Norway and Singapore.

The emetic syndrome is also caused by an enterotoxin, but its characterization has been hampered by the lack of an animal model to test its activity. The toxin causes emesis in monkeys, but this animal model is too expensive. The emetic toxin is a small protein (M_r < 10 000), and it is stable to heating at 126°C for 90 min.

Foodborne Illness Associated with *Bacillus* Species other than *B. cereus*

The requirements for identifying a microorganism as the causative agent in a food poisoning outbreak are extensive. Therefore, investigations of outbreaks involving *Bacillus* species other than *B. cereus* have been limited.

A large outbreak of food poisoning occurred in a Veterans Administration Hospital, Denver, Colorado, in which 161 staff members developed symptoms of gastroenteritis after eating turkey meat that had been held overnight at room temperature. Bacteriological examination of the turkey meat and patients stools revealed large numbers of aerobic spore-forming organisms, most likely *B. licheniformis*. The major symptoms, incubation period, and food vehicles involved in outbreaks associated with *B. licheniformis* are similar to *C. perfringens* food poisoning.

Table 3. Clinical features and characteristics

Agent	Aetiological agent	Incubation period; signs and symptoms	Foods involved
Bacillus cereus (gastroenteritis)	Diarrhoeal toxin	8–16 h; nausea, absominal cramps, watery diarrhoea	Custards, pudding, sauces, cereal products, meat products, soups
	Emetic toxin	1–6 h; nausea, vomiting, short duration 1 day	Fried rice, vegetables, vegetable sprouts, mashed potatoes
Staphylococcus aureus	Enterotoxin	30 min–8 h; nausea, vomiting, diarrhoea	Prepared salads, cooked meat and poultry
Clostridium perfringens	Enterotoxin	9–15 h; diarrhoea, gas pains	Cooked meat and poultry

There have also been reports of the isolation of large numbers of *B. subtilis* in foods implicated in food poisoning outbreaks. Most food poisoning outbreaks associated with the presence of *B. subtilis* are characterized by short incubation periods, nausea and vomiting. In all of the cases involving other *Bacillus* species, known pathogens have not been isolated from the food.

Control and Prevention

Since *B. cereus* is a spore-forming microorganism that is ubiquitous in nature and can survive extended storage in dried food products, it is not practical to eliminate it from our food supply. The presence of *B. cereus* in small numbers is usually not a problem. Control against *B. cereus* food poisoning should rely on the prevention of spore germination and prevention of multiplication of vegetative cells in prepared foods. Therefore, foods should be rapidly cooled to 4°C or maintained above 63°C, and they should be reheated thoroughly to a temperature above 74°C before reserving.

Since *B. cereus* is found in low numbers in many foods, it is questionable that application of *B. cereus* microbiological criteria is worthwhile. A microbiological criterion may be useful for foods such as cooked rice products that have clearly been identified as frequent vehicles in *B. cereus* food poisoning outbreaks. Low numbers of *B. cereus* in foods pose no direct health hazard, but if these products are mishandled, growth of this organism might result in a direct health hazard. Large numbers of *B. cereus* may produce enterotoxin in the food before it is consumed.

Bibliography

Banwart GJ (1989) *Basic Food Microbiology*, 2nd edn. Westport, Conn: AVI Publishing.

Frazier WC and Westhoff DC (1988) *Food Microbiology*, 4th edn. New York: McGraw-Hill.

Jay JM (1986) *Modern Food Microbiology*, 3rd edn. New York: Van Nostrand Reinhold.

Johnson EA (1990) *Bacillus cereus* food poisoning. In: Cliver DO (ed.) *Foodborne Diseases*, pp 128–135. New York: Academic Press.

Kramer JM and Gilbert RJ (1989) *Bacillus cereus* and other *Bacillus* species. In: Doyle MP (ed.) *Foodborne Bacterial Pathogens*, pp 21–70. New York: Marcel Dekker.

S. S. Sumner
University of Nebraska-Lincoln, Lincoln, USA

BACTERIA

See Microbiology and Specific Organisms

BAKING

See Biscuits, Cookies and Crackers, Bread and Cakes

BAKING POWDER

See Leavening Agents

BANANAS AND PLANTAINS

Bananas and plantains (*Musa* spp.) are grown extensively throughout the tropical and subtropical regions of the world. Together they represent the number one fruit crop in the world, in terms of both production and trade, exceeding grapes by 9×10^6 t per year (production) and oranges by 3×10^6 t per year (trade). Almost all of the exported fruit, which makes up only 12% of the total, are Cavendish-type dessert bananas. However, bananas and plantains which are cooked account for almost half of the world production. This article describes their global distribution and importance, the morphological and nutritional characteristics of the fruit, handling and storage and other uses of fresh and processed fruit. *See* Fruits of Tropical Climates, Commercial and Dietary Importance

The terms 'bananas' and 'plantains' require clarification at this point. The former refers to all the members of the genus *Musa*. In the narrow sense, plantains are a defined group within this genus which have the AAB genome and are characterized by the orange-yellow colour of both the compound tepal of the flower and the fruit pulp at ripeness. When ripe, a relatively high proportion of starch is present (10–25% of fresh weight) in the pulp. The fruits are slender, angular to pointed, and are generally, palatable only after cooking. Plantains, in the broad sense, include the other members of the genus *Musa* that are starchy at ripeness but which lack the other characteristics. In this article, plantains are referred to in the narrow sense, except when global world production figures are discussed, as these refer to plantains in the broad sense.

Global Distribution

Before international trade began a little over 100 years ago, bananas in temperate regions were merely a curiosity. Bananas are grown in commercial plantations, but more often in household gardens because of their almost universal appeal as a food, ease of growing, quick production and attractive plant appearance.

Bananas and plantains are suited to the warm, high-rainfall regions of the lowland tropics. They originated in Southeast Asia (including Papua New Guinea) and have been spread to other regions of the world in the past 2000 years. They are now grown from the equator to about 35°N and 30°S, and within these regions they may be grown in semiarid locations with the aid of irrigation or in large plastic greenhouses.

Bananas for export are produced mainly in Central and South America as well as the Philippines (Tables 1–4). Most exported fruit goes to North America, Europe and Japan, and in 1989 was valued at $3\cdot685 \times 10^9$. Exports of plantains are not significant. Other major areas of production are Southeast Asia and East Africa (according to FAO statistics*) but little of this is exported. Plantain production is most important in East and West Africa as well as South America.

Average world consumption of bananas and plantains in 1989 was about 13 kg per person per year. However, in much of Africa and Latin America it is 5–10 times this amount, and as much as 400 kg per person per year in some parts of East Africa.

The major export production areas are located close to the equator, where an even supply of fruit throughout the year is possible, and where they are less damaged by cyclones or typhoons.

The optimum temperature range for bananas is about 22–31°C. Chilling injury of fruit occurs when the latex coagulates at temperatures below 13°C. Bananas are susceptible to frost in subtropical regions and are often planted on hillsides to avoid it. The growth cycle is greatly prolonged outside of the tropics and productivity is reduced. The industries that have developed in the subtropics have largely done so because of proximity to markets.

---

* FAO (Food and Agriculture Organization) production statistics need careful interpretation because the meaning of the words 'bananas' and 'plantains' differs among countries, particularly in East Africa and South America. For instance, information from Burundi, Tanzania and Venezuela on bananas refers to plantains used for cooking purposes.

Table 1. World production of bananas

Region	Country	Percentage of total world production (44×10^6 t)
Asia	India	10·9
	Philippines	7·3
	China	5·6
	Indonesia	5·4
	Thailand	3·7
	Vietnam	3·4
	Other	4·0
South America	Brazil	12·8
	Ecuador	5·4
	Colombia	3·1
	Other	5·1
Central America	Mexico	3·7
	Costa Rica	2·9
	Honduras	2·4
	Panama	2·3
	Other	4·6
Africa	Burundi	3·4
	Tanzania	3·1
	Other	7·2
Other		2·8

Source: FAO (1989). *FAO Production Yearbook 1989*, Vol. 1.43. Rome: Food and Agriculture Organization.

Table 2. World plantain production

Region	Country	Percentage of total world production (25×10^6 t)
Asia		3·3
South America	Colombia	9·9
	Ecuador	3·8
	Other	4·2
Central America	Dominican Republic	3·2
	Other	4·2
Africa	Uganda	26·8
	Rwanda	8·6
	Nigeria	7·2
	Zaire	6·1
	Tanzania	5·4
	Cameroon	4·6
	Côte d'Ivoire	4·1
	Ghana	4·1
	Other	4·5

Source: FAO (1989). *FAO Production Yearbook 1989*, Vol. 43. Rome: Food and Agriculture Organization.

Table 3. World exports of bananas

Region	Country	Percentage of total world exports (8×10^6 t)
Asia	Philippines	10·4
	Other	1·7
South America	Ecuador	20·0
	Colombia	12·0
	Other	1·9
Central America	Costa Rica	15·6
	Honduras	10·5
	Panama	8·3
	Guatemala	4·7
	Other	9·5
Africa		2·7
Other		2·7

Source: FAO (1989). *FAO Trade Yearbook 1989*, Vol. 43. Rome: Food and Agriculture Organization.

Table 4. World imports of bananas

Region	Country	Percentage of total world imports (8×10^6 t)
Asia	Japan	9·4
	Other	4·2
North America	USA	37·3
	Canada	3·9
Europe	West Germany	10·6
	France	5·5
	UK	5·3
	Italy	5·2
	Other	13·8
Other		4·8

Source: FAO (1989). *FAO Trade Yearbook 1989*, Vol. 43. Rome: Food and Agriculture Organization.

Varieties

All the edible bananas belong the Eumusa section of the genus *Musa*, except for the Fe'i bananas of the Pacific region which belong to the Australimusa section (Fig. 1). The Fe'i bananas are characterized by erect bunches and pink-red sap, and an orange, slimy fruit pulp which requires cooking. The eating of Fe'i bananas changes the colour of the urine to pink. There are numerous wild, seeded species in each of the *Musa* sections.

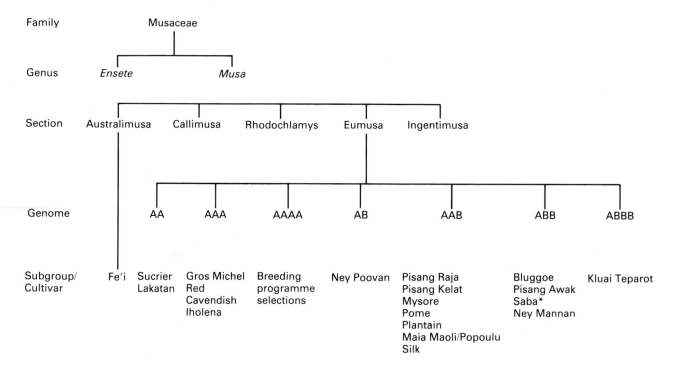

Family		Musaceae				
Genus	Ensete		Musa			
Section	Australimusa	Callimusa	Rhodochlamys	Eumusa	Ingentimusa	
Genome	AA	AAA	AAAA	AB	AAB	ABB	ABBB
Subgroup/ Cultivar	Fe'i	Sucrier Lakatan	Gros Michel Red Cavendish Iholena	Breeding programme selections	Ney Poovan	Pisang Raja Pisang Kelat Mysore Pome Plantain Maia Maoli/Popoulu Silk	Bluggoe Pisang Awak Saba* Ney Mannan	Kluai Teparot

*Considered as BBB in the Philippines.

Fig. 1 Systematic position of banana varieties. (Modified from Stover and Simmonds, 1987.)

Edible bananas and plantains belonging to the Eumusa section are believed to contain genomes from two wild species, *M. acuminata* (A) and *M. balbisiana* (B). Most cultivated bananas are triploid and are classified according to characteristics estimating the contribution of the two parent species. Because the binomial Latin nomenclature for edible varieties, e.g. *M. cavendishii* cultivar (cv.) Williams, proved unsatisfactory, they are referred to as, for example, *Musa* spp. (AAA Group, Cavendish Subgroup) cv. Williams. There are 200–500 varieties of bananas and plantains in existence, but about 150 are primary clones and the remainder are somatic mutants.

Bananas for export now come entirely from varieties of the Cavendish subgroup. From the 1940s to 1960s, these replaced cv. Gros Michel, which was devastated by a soil-borne fungus called Panama disease (fusarial wilt) in one of the largest disease epiphytotics that has ever occurred in crop plants. The greatest diversity of varieties occurs in Southeast Asia where particular varieties are especially favoured for various culinary uses (Fig. 2).

The leaf disease, black Sigatoka, and new races of Panama disease currently pose major threats to world banana and plantain production. As varieties with resistance to these diseases are developed by the conventional breeding programmes and by somacloning, further changes in the varieties cultivated can be expected.

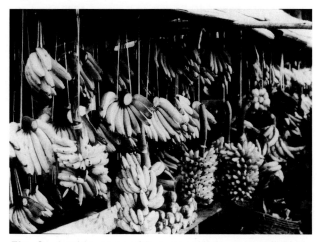

Fig. 2 A wide range of banana varieties are available in Southeast Asian markets.

Fruit Morphology and Anatomy

The banana plant is a large, tree-like, determinate perennial herb with a basal rhizome, a pseudostem composed of leaf sheaths, and a terminal crown of large leaves (Fig. 3). The terminal inflorescence is initiated near ground level and is then thrust up the centre of the pseudostem by elongation of the true stem. The basal flower clusters (hands) are female and form the fruit bunch. Distal flower clusters are male, do not produce fruit and are commonly deciduous. The banana has the ratio increases, in part as a result of water movement from the peel to the pulp associated with an increase in osmotic pressure in the pulp caused by the hydrolysis of starch.

Nutritional Composition

Ripe dessert bananas are considered by many to be a complete food if taken in association with a protein source such as milk. They are favoured as food for young babies and elderly folk because they are easily digested and very nutritious. They are excellent for people with stomach complaints, particularly ulcers, and are ideal for diets with low levels of cholesterol, fats and sodium salts. The potassium concentration is about 350 mg per 100 g of pulp with trace amounts of sodium (Table 5). Bananas are also recommended in the treatment of infant diarrhoea, coeliac disease and colitis. They are also a good source of vitamins C and B$_6$ (Tables 5 and 6). A major feature is the high sugar to acid ratio (100:180) compared with 7:10 for citrus. This is confirmed by the carbohydrate levels shown in Tables 5 and 7. If we assume 20·2% of the fresh banana pulp is sugar and 75·7% water, then 83% of the dried solids are sugar (Tables 5 and 7). This is why bananas have recently received much attention from sportsmen and women because of the high carbohydrate content capable of rapidly releasing energy necessary for vigorous sporting events. The sugars present are almost entirely glucose, fructose and sucrose, in a ratio of 20:15:65. The high sugar content of bananas is only exceeded in fresh fruit by that of dates, jujube, tamarind and carob. *See* Coeliac Disease; Colon, Diseases and Disorders; Exercise, Metabolic Requirements; Infants, Nutritional Requirements *see also* individual nutrients.

The characteristic aroma of bananas has received considerable attention with more than 350 volatile compounds having been identified. The major constituents appear to be amyl and isoamyl esters of acetic, propionic and butyric acids.

The major differences between bananas and plantains are as follows: (1) the lower moisture percentage of the pulp in green plantains compared to ripe bananas (Tables 5 and 7); (2) the lower sugar concentration of the solids in ripe plantains compared to ripe bananas; and (3) plantains are a much richer source of vitamin A than bananas (Tables 5 and 6). These differences are valid for the edible product, but are less important if fruits are compared at the same stage of ripeness. For example, the moisture percentage can increase from about 60% in preclimacteric banana fruit to 70% after ripening and 75–80% at the stage of senescence. In addition, there are major inconsistencies in the literature regarding the conversion of starch to sugar in plantains, with some references indicating only traces of starch in the ripe

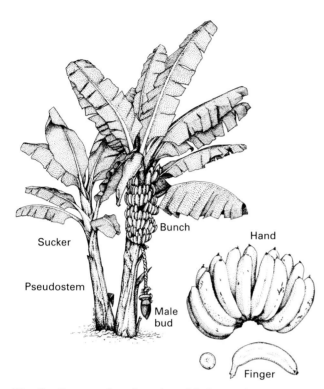

Fig. 3 Banana plant, bunch and fruit morphology.

largest inflorescence of any plant grown as a crop. The world record for a mature fruit bunch is 121 kg, obtained in northern Australia.

Banana bunches have from one to twenty hands and take 2–6 months to reach maturity. Bunches are pendant or subhorizontal and usually weigh between 10 and 60 kg. Individual fruits (fingers) can number up to 300 on a bunch. Fingers of different varieties can be anywhere from 6 to 60 cm in length and from 50 to 1000 g in weight, but are more usually 15–30 cm long and weigh 50–200 g. The curve often seen in the fruit is caused by a negative geotropic growth response. Immature bananas are usually green, and when mature they ripen to a yellow colour. Young fruits are somewhat angular, but this disappears with maturity in the AAA varieties. AAB and ABB varieties may still be angular at maturity.

The fruit develops from the inferior ovary of the female flower. It is a parthenocarpic berry, i.e. it develops without the stimulus of pollination. The ovules shrivel early but can still be recognized as brown specks in the central part of mature fruit. Most varieties are sterile or have very low fertility. If a pollen source, such as a wild species, is nearby, some varieties will set an occasional dark hard seed about 3–5 mm in diameter. These are a hazard to the teeth of consumers so it is fortunate that seeds are an extremely rare event.

In the growing fruit, the pulp:peel ratio varies from about 1:1 to 4:1, depending upon variety and maturity at harvest. When the mature fruit ripens, the pulp:peel

Table 5.   Compositional data per 100 g edible portion of plantains (unripe) and bananas (ripe)

Components	Proximate analysis (g)		Minerals	Mineral content (mg)		Vitamins	Vitamin content	
	Plantain	Banana		Plantain	Banana		Plantain	Banana
Water	67·5	70·7	Sodium	4	1	Retinol (μg)	0	0
Sugars	5·7	16·2	Potassium	500	350	Carotene (μg)	360	200
Starch	23·7	3·0	Calcium	9	7	Vitamin D (μg)	0	0
Dietary fibre	2·3	3·4	Magnesium	37	42	Thiamin (mg)	0·10	0·04
Total nitrogen	0·18	0·18	Phosphorus	36	28	Riboflavin (mg)	0·05	0·07
Protein	1·1	1·1	Iron	0·5	0·4	Nicotinic acid (mg)	0·7	0·6
Fat	0·3	0·3	Copper	0·08	0·16	Ascorbic acid (mg)	15·0	10
			Zinc	0·1	0·2	Vitamin E (mg)	0·20	0·2
			Sulphur	15	13	Vitamin B_6 (mg)	0·30	0·51
			Chlorine	80	79	Vitamin B_{12} (mg)	0	0
						Folate (μg)	22	22
						Pantothenate (mg)	0·26	0·26

Sources: Paul AA and Southgate DAT (1978) *McCance and Widdowson's The Composition of Foods* 4th edn. London: Her Majesty's Stationery Office.
Holland B, Unwin ID and Buss DH (1991) *Vegetables, Herbs and Spices.* Fifth supplement to *McCance and Widdowson's The Composition of Foods* 4th edn. London: Ministry of Agriculture, Fisheries and Food.

Table 6.   Nutrient content of the fruit pulp of banana varieties

Nutrient	Percentage of US RDA[a] per 100 g		
	Gros Michel[b]	Cavendish[c]	Horn plantain[c]
Vitamin A	3·8	5·1	61·6
Ascorbic acid	13·3	20·0	26·7
Vitamin B_6	25·0[c]	NA	NA
Thiamin	3·3	2·6	2·9
Riboflavin	3·8	5·3	5·9
Nicotinic acid	4·7	4·8	4·0

[a] US Recommended Dietary Allowance.
[b] Source: USDA (1963) *Composition of Foods.* Agriculture Handbook 8. Washington, DC: US Government Printing Office.
[c] Source: Anonymous (1959) *Bananas: Versatile in Health or Illness.* Boston: United Fruit Co.

Table 7.   Proximate analysis (g per 100 g) of banana and plantain

	Banana		Plantain	
	Edible portion	Oven-dried solids	Edible portion	Oven-dried solids
Water	75·7	—	66·4	—
Carbohydrate	22·2	91·4	31·2	92·8
Protein	1·1	4·5	1·1	3·3
Fat	0·2	0·8	0·4	1·2
Ash	0·8	3·3	0·9	2·7

Source: USDA (1963) *Composition of Foods.* Agriculture Handbook 8. Washington, DC: US Government Printing Office.

fruit. Some of the differences are probably due to different ripening conditions and the stage of ripeness selected for measurement. *See* Ripening of Fruit

Fresh Fruit Handling and Storage

Handling procedures vary substantially in the different banana-producing countries and depend upon whether fruit is to be exported. What follows largely applies to commercial plantings producing fruit for export and gives an understanding of the considerations involved.

Bananas travel best and receive a minimum of mechanical damage while they are in the hard, green condition. It is necessary to transport the fruits to the marketplace in this hard, green state so that they can be uniformly ripened with ethylene gas (1000 mg l⁻¹) in humidified rooms at 15–18°C. This greatly facilitates marketing. Fruits can take from a few days to 3 weeks to reach the marketplace, and so must have sufficient greenlife (the period after harvest for which the fruit stays in a hard green condition). No post-harvest treatment can improve upon this greenlife, but it can reduce its rate of decline. In general, the earlier the harvest in the life of the fruit the greater is the fruit greenlife, but any gain in greenlife must be weighed against the loss in bunch weight (5–10% per week). A bunch which would ripen in the field 5 months after it emerged may be harvested and ripened satisfactorily as early as about 10 weeks (pulp:peel ratio of 1:1), when

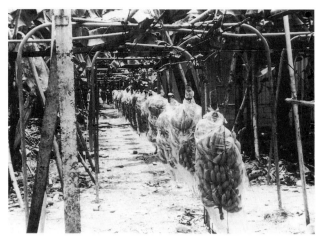

Fig. 4 Bananas for export are usually transported to the packing shed by cableways to minimize skin blemishes due to mechanical damage.

the fingers are still quite thin. A key to profitable banana growing is to maximize yield without premature ripening occurring. Other considerations are that greater fruit maturity leads to a higher proportion of edible pulp and possibly an increase in fruit flavour. In practice, maturity standards are varied, so that more mature bunches are harvested for nearer markets and less mature ones for more distant markets.

Maximum greenlife for a particular finger diameter (grade) at harvest is achieved by manipulating the plant and environment to obtain the maximum possible rate of fruit filling. Finger diameter, bunch age and degree of fruit fullness (loss of angularity) are used as criteria for harvest. The combination of age–grade control for determining time of harvest ensures the production of high-quality fruit with sufficient greenlife at harvest. To minimize the risk of premature ripening after harvest, it is important to keep the fruit as cool as possible (but above 13°C to prevent chilling injury) and not to expose it unnecessarily to light.

Banana bunches are harvested by hand and usually carried on the shoulder to nearby cableways (Fig. 4) or to tractor-drawn, padded trailers. The plastic sleeve, known as a bunch cover, which is applied to the young bunch to improve fruit quality, is retained to minimize mechanical damage during handling. In the packing shed, the bunches are dehanded, usually into tanks of water, sorted and graded, divided into clusters of 4–10 fingers, weighed, labelled and packed into fibreboard cartons containing plastic liners. The water in the washing tank may contain a systemic fungicide to reduce fungal rots, or the fungicide may be applied in a separate operation before the fruit is packed. Cartons hold from 12 to 18 kg of fruit. The packed fruit is sent by refrigerated transport to the marketplace and usually involves transport by rail, road and sea. The transport system is highly integrated and regular (at least weekly)

so that fruit of uniform maturity is marketed. This has the effect of avoiding the need for storage beyond the shipment period. *See* Fungicides

Bananas are usually consumed within 3 to 4 weeks from the day of harvest, with no long-term commercial storage possible, as for citrus and pome fruits. It is possible to delay the onset of the ripening by a few weeks by the use of modified atmosphere storage with high carbon dioxide (5%) and low oxygen (2%) and with ethylene scrubbers, such as potassium permanganate, but because banana fruit is available year round there is usually no advantage in doing this. However, in places where the expensive technology of refrigeration is not available, this technique may be valuable for marketing fruit in distant markets.

Once the fruit ripens, the period over which it may be eaten, its shelf life, is relatively short. It is usually of the order of 2–10 days depending upon variety and ambient temperature. The extremely perishable nature of banana is associated with its high rate of metabolism – the rate of respiration during the climacteric is 100–180 ml of oxygen per kg of fruit per hour and 40–60 whilst green. This is higher than apples and pears, which have a respiration rate of 6–40 ml of oxygen per kg per hour at similar temperatures. Lower temperatures will reduce the metabolic rate, but chilling injury occurs when the fruit is kept for a long period below 13°C.

Fruit Utilization

Almost half of the bananas and plantains produced are eaten raw as a dessert fruit; the other half is cooked, usually by frying, boiling, roasting or baking. Virtually all varieties of bananas and plantains may be either eaten raw when ripe, or cooked when either green or ripe. Cultural preferences govern the choices made.

Bananas can also be processed in various ways so that they may be stored for longer periods and utilized for other purposes. Fruits which are unmarketable because of small size or peel blemishes are suitable for processing.

Banana purée is by far the most important processed product made from the pulp of ripe fruit. The purée is canned and used as an ingredient in dairy desserts, bakery items, drinks, processed foods and sauces, and as a part of special diets in hospitals and nursing homes. Ripe bananas are also sliced and canned in an acidified syrup and are used in desserts, fruit salads, cocktail drinks and bakery items.

Chips are made by deep-frying thin slices of unripe fruit, with the optional addition of various flavourings, and sold as a snackfood like potato crisps. Ripe bananas may be dried (known as banana figs in some regions) and are said to store satisfactorily for over 10 years without the addition of preservatives. This would presumably be due to their high sugar content which is in excess of 50%. The ripe fruit is ideal for ice-blocks (water ices, ice lollies), when peeled and frozen, with the optional addition of toppings such as chocolate and chopped nuts. It is also an excellent base for ice creams because of its creamy consistency.

The other major processed products are flour made from dried unripe fruit, and essence which is extracted from the pulp of ripe fruit. When ripe fruit is fermented it makes a low-alcohol beer. Beer manufacture is confined to East Africa, with consumption being as much as 1·2 l per person per day in Rwanda. Less important processed products include a clarified juice, powder, jams, flakes, freeze-dried slices, ketchup 'filler', vinegar and wine. Unripe bananas have been used to make starch, but none is currently produced.

Green banana fruit, pseudostems and foliage are suitable as animal feed. They mainly provide a source of energy and require supplementation with a protein source. Bananas are only economical as a source of animal feed when the livestock are nearby, because of the high cost of transport. The corms, shoots and male buds find widespread use as an animal food in Asia and Africa.

Conclusion

Bananas have become the major fresh fruit consumed around the world, even in the temperate zone where they are not grown, despite the fact that they cannot be stored for more than a few weeks. This has been possible because they are available the year round, are competi-

tively priced, come packed in hygienic, easily opened peel, are extremely convenient to eat in virtually all situations and, as William Forsyth put it, 'The suave melting texture of a fully ripe banana combined with its distinctive mellow flavour makes a delicious combination'.

Bibliography

Champion J (1963) *Le Bananier*. Paris: Maisonneuve et Larose.

Forsyth WGC (1980) Banana and plantain. In: Nagy S and Shaw PE (eds) *Tropical and Subtropical Fruit*, pp 258–278. Westport, Connecticut: AVI Publications.

Hassan A and Pantastico EB (eds) (1990) *Banana – Fruit Development, Postharvest Physiology, Handling and Marketing in ASEAN*. Jakarta: ASEAN-COFAF.

Israeli Y and Blumenfeld A (1985) Musa. In: Halevy A (ed.) *CRC Handbook of Flowering*, pp 390–409. Boca Raton, Florida: CRC Press.

Marriott J (1980) Bananas – physiology and biochemistry of storage and ripening for optimum quality. *CRC Critical Reviews in Food Science and Nutrition* 13: 41–88.

Soto M (1985) *Bananos Cultivo y Comercialización*. Costa Rica: Litogratia e Imprenta LIL.

Stover RH and Simmonds NW (1987) *Bananas* 3rd edn. London: Longman.

Von Loesecke HW (1950) *Bananas*. New York: Interscience Publishers.

Jeff Daniells
Queensland Department of Primary Industries,
South Johnstone, Australia

BARLEY

The Crop and its Importance

Barley is one of the major cereal crops in the world. This article reviews its origin, botany, distribution, chemical composition and uses as food and feed. Utilization of barley in the malting and fermentation industries (brewing, distilling, alcohol production) is covered in other articles.

Botany

Barley is a member of the grass family Gramineae, the subfamily Festucoideae, the tribe Hordeae and the genus *Hordeum*. Cultivated barleys belong to the subspecies *vulgare*, whereas the wild forms of barley belong

to the subspecies *spontaneum*. The basic chromosome number of the genus *Hordeum* is 7 and all cultivated barleys are self-fertilizing, diploid annuals ($2n = 14$).

The spike or head of barley consists of a series of spikelets that are attached – in sets of three, at nodes – to alternating sides of the rachis. Each spikelet contains a floret. In six-rowed barley (Fig. 1a), each floret is fertile and develops into a kernel, leading to the formation of six rows of kernels. Only the central kernel in each triplet is symmetrical; the lateral kernels are twisted to varying degrees. Therefore two thirds of the kernels in a sample of six-rowed barley will be nonsymmetrical. In two-rowed barley, the lateral florets are not fertile, so that only the central floret in each triplet develops into a kernel (Fig. 1b), leading to the formation of two rows of symmetrical kernels in the mature spike. All cultivated barleys are either two- or six-rowed, but some six-rowed cultivars appear to have only four rows of kernels; thus reference is sometimes made to four-rowed barleys, although these are really six-rowed barleys.

The barley kernel consists of many different tissues; some of these are shown in Fig. 2. Outer layers of the kernel and the area between the embryo and the starchy endosperm are shown in detail in insets (a) and (b). In botanical terms, the barley seed is that part of the kernel enclosed by the testa. Hence the testa is often referred to as the seed coat. Surrounding the testa and fused tightly to it is the pericarp, the outer tissue of the grain or caryopsis. Since a caryopsis is a fruit, barley is a fruit containing a seed. The hull or husk completely surrounds the grain and adheres tightly to the pericarp in most barley cultivars. In some cultivars, however, the so-called naked or hull-less types, the hull is loosely attached to the grain and is removed during threshing. *See* Wheat, Grain Structure of Wheat and Wheat-based Products

Origin, Adaptation and Production

Neither the place of origin nor the progenitor of cultivated barley are known with certainty. There is archaeological evidence that from about 7000 BC barley was cultivated in the fertile crescent of the Middle East. This area includes present-day Israel, Jordan, Syria and Iran. There is evidence also that barley may have been cultivated even earlier than that in the Nile valley of Egypt, but considerably later in India and China. It is probable, but by no means certain, that two-rowed *Hordeum spontaneum* is the ancestor of cultivated barley, but this subspecies may be an intermediate between the actual barley progenitor and cultivated barley. Six-rowed forms of barley are thought to have developed from early two-rowed forms through mutation and hybridization.

Barley is a widely adapted crop and grows under a wider range of environmental conditions than any other cereal. It appears to require fewer heat units than other cereals to reach physiological maturity and can therefore be grown successfully at higher latitudes and altitudes than other cereal crops. Barley is relatively tolerant to drought and to alkaline and salt conditions, but grows best in temperate regions of the world where growing seasons are long, cool and moderately dry.

Winter barley is less cold-tolerant than either winter wheat or winter rye. Nevertheless, in some countries with temperate climates, such as the UK, most of the barley is grown during winter. In countries such as Australia and Spain, which experience hot summers, a significant proportion of the barley is grown during the winter. Conversely, the harsh winters of North America

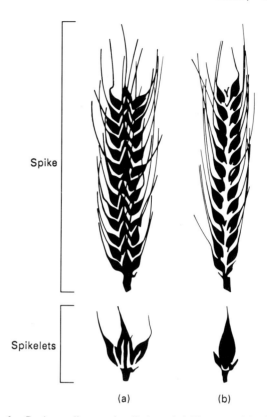

Fig. 1 Barley spikes and spikelets. (a) Six-rowed barley; (b) two-rowed barley.

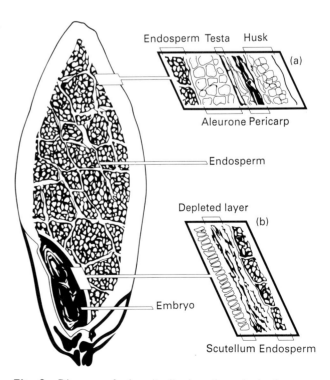

Fig. 2 Diagram of a longitudinal section of a barley kernel. (a) Outer layers of kernel; (b) junction between the embryo and endosperm.

preclude the growing of winter barley, except for some areas in the southern USA.

Over the past 10 years, worldwide production of barley has averaged 171.5×10^6 t (Table 1). This places barley fourth after wheat, maize and rice in terms of total annual production. In 1989, barley accounted for 9·4% of the world's total cereal production. The USSR is the largest producer of barley, but it is all consumed internally. Canada, the USA and Australia each produces much smaller quantities but they, as well as members of the EEC, are major barley exporters. *See* Cereals, Contribution to the Diet

Composition

The major constituent of barley kernels is starch, which is present in the endosperm in the form of discrete granules (Fig. 2) and represents, on average, 60–64% of the weight of the kernel (Table 2). Starch consists of two high-molecular-weight polymers of glucose: amylose and amylopectin. Amylose is composed of long chains of glucose residues linked by α-(1,→4) bonds with a few side-chains joined to the main chains through α-(1,→6) bonds. Amylopectin contains much shorter unit chains of α-(1,→4)-linked glucose residues which are inter-linked through α-(1,→6) bonds. In other words, amylose is lightly branched and amylopectin is heavily branched. In general, barley starch contains about 75% amylopectin and 25% amylose. However, starch from 'waxy' barley cultivars contains 95–100% amylopectin, and starch from high amylose barley cultivars may contain more than 40% amylose. These starches have different functional properties, but they have not yet been utilized widely in the food industry.

Arabinoxylans are polymers of xylose and arabinose and are present mainly in the cell walls of endosperm and aleurone in soluble and insoluble forms. They absorb many times their own weight of water and form viscous solutions in water. The major component of endosperm cell walls is the polysaccharide, (1,→3), (1,→4)-β-D-glucan; this forms viscous solutions which may cause filtration problems during brewing and digestive problems when untreated barley is fed to chickens. Small amounts of cellulose are present in the outer tissues of the kernel.

Only small amounts of the simple sugars, glucose and fructose, are present in the kernel; the major sugars are sucrose and raffinose, which are present mainly in the embryo. Varying amounts of fructosans, which are fructosyl polymers of sucrose, are also present in the mature kernel.

Barley contains a large number of proteins which can be separated into four major groups on the basis of solubility. Albumins and globulins (15–30% of barley protein) are soluble in water and salt solutions, respect-

Table 1. World production of barley

Country	Average production, 1981–1990 ($\times 10^3$ t)
USSR	47 867
Canada	12 404
USA	10 695
France	10 231
UK	9578
FRG	9337
Spain	8556
China	6365
Turkey	6093
Denmark	5232
GDR	4131
Australia	3879
Poland	3836
Other	33 314
Total	171 518

From *Canadian Grains Industry Statistical Handbook* (1990) Winnipeg: Canada Grains Council.

Table 2. Barley composition

Component	Content (%, dry weight)
Starch	60–64
Arabinoxylans	4·4–7·8
β-Glucans	3·6–6·1
Cellulose	1·4–5·0
Simple carbohydrates (glucose, fructose, sucrose, maltose)	0·41–2·9
Oligosaccharides (raffinose, fructosans)	0·16–1·8
Proteins	8–15
Lipids	2–3
Minerals	2–3

Barley also contains small quantities of the B-complex vitamins, including thiamin (B_1), riboflavin (B_2), nicotinic acid, pyridoxine (B_6) and pantothenic acid, biotin, folic acid and vitamin E.

ively; hordeins (35–50% of barley protein), the major storage proteins in barley, are soluble in aqueous alcohol solutions; glutelins (15–20% of barley protein), a mixture of storage and structural proteins, are soluble in alkali. Although aleurone cells are rich in protein, most of the barley protein is in the endosperm, especially in the subaleurone region.

About 70% of barley lipid is present in the endosperm, 20% is in the embryo and the remainder is in the outer layers of the kernel.

Minerals such as magnesium, sulphur, sodium, potassium, zinc and calcium are concentrated in the outer layers of the kernel. Phosphorus is present, mainly, as phytic acid in the aleurone. *See* individual nutrients *See* Cereals, Dietary Importance

Uses

Animal Feed

The largest use of barley, worldwide, is as animal feed, especially for cattle and pigs. Barley provides a good balance of high energy, because of its starch content, and reasonable protein quality and content. Hulled barley is less desirable than other cereal grains, such as maize, for chicken feed formulations because of its relatively high fibre content.

Malting, Brewing and Distilling

The proportion of the total barley production used for malting varies widely among countries, but worldwide utilization is about 15% of total production. This aspect of barley utilization is discussed more fully in another entry. *See* Beers, Ales and Stouts, Preparation of Wort; Malt, Malt Types and Products; Malt, Chemistry of Malting

Human Food

Less than 5% of total barley production is used for human food in most developed countries, but in some countries in the Far East, Middle East and North Africa, barley products form an important part of the diet. The most common products are blocked, pot and pearl barley, barley flakes and barley flour. Blocked barley is prepared by lightly scarifying the grain between abrasive discs to remove the husk. More severe treatment (pearling) results in removal of the outer kernel layers and rounding of the grain to produce pot barley, which amounts to about 65% of the starting material. Extensive pearling leads to removal of the outer endosperm layers and the embryo to leave pearled barley, which is only about 35% of the original barley. These products are used in soups, breakfast cereals and stews, as tea or coffee substitutes after roasting, and as rice extenders. They can also be milled into flour and used in baby foods, porridge and some baked goods when blended with wheat flour. Barley may be puffed by heating it under pressure to gelatinize the starch, and then releasing the pressure suddenly. The loss in pressure allows rapid expansion of the water vapour and significant puffing of the grain. Barley flakes are made by cooking the barley, rolling the hot, moist product between heavy rollers and drying the flakes to about 10·5% moisture content. *See* Cereals, Breakfast Cereals

Nutrients are not distributed uniformly throughout the barley kernel. Vitamins, minerals and lipids are concentrated in the outer layers and embryo of the grain, and peripheral regions of the endosperm have significantly more protein than central regions. During pearling, therefore, the nutritive value of the product decreases as the outer layers of the kernel are removed. Pearl barley, for example, is nutritionally inferior to pot barley because it does not contain the embryo or any of the nutritionally rich outer layers of the kernel.

Sound, bright, uniformly plump kernels with high test weight (> 60 kg hl^{-1}) are preferred for all barley uses. In general, barley cultivars possessing yellow aleurones are also preferred, but there is a small demand for malts prepared from blue-aleurone barley.

Storage

The end-use quality of grain stored under high moisture conditions deteriorates through loss of viability and attack by insects and microorganisms. The temperature recommended for safe storage depends on the moisture content of the grain. Dry grain (12–13% moisture) can be stored safely at 17°C, but grain at higher moisture contents deteriorates and should be dried with cool, dry air before storage. Barley intended for malting should not be dried at temperatures over 45°C because the germination potential of the grain may be damaged. For food and feed uses, however, temperatures up to 60°C may be used without impairing quality of the grain. Ideally, barley should be stored at about 12% moisture and at 15°C or less. Grain may be treated with insecticides and pesticides, but some of these may leave unacceptable residues on the grain. It is possible to store grain under anaerobic or low oxygen conditions (e.g. under carbon dioxide or nitrogen), thus slowing down or inhibiting the development of microorganisms and insects. Such treatment does not impair the germination potential of the grain, nor does it leave residues on the grain. *See* Cereals, Handling of Grain for Storage; Cereals, Bulk Storage of Grain

Bibliography

Briggs DE (1978) *Barley*. London: Chapman and Hall.
Henry RJ (1988) The carbohydrates of barley grains – a review. *Journal of the Institute of Brewing* 94: 71–78.
Hockett EA (1991) Barley. In: Lorenz KJ and Kulp K (eds) *Handbook of Cereal Science and Technology*, pp 133–198. New York: Marcel Dekker.

Kent NL (1983) *Technology of Cereals* 3rd edn. Oxford: Pergamon Press.

Rasmusson DC (ed.) (1985) *Barley*. Madison: American Society of Agronomy, Crop Science Society of America, Soil Science Society of America.

USDA (1968) *Barley: Origins, Botany, Culture, Winterhardiness, Genetics, Utilization, Pests*. USDA Agriculture Handbook 338. Washington, DC: US Department of Agriculture.

A. W. MacGregor
Grain Research Laboratory, Canadian Grain Commission, Winnipeg, Canada

BARRELS*

Oak wood is used in cooperage for its mechanical properties (strength, hardness and flexibility) which makes it possible to shape staves, for its impermeability to liquids (extensive tyloses), for its extractable compounds and also for its porosity to air which enhances oxidation processes. There are many varieties of oak in the world, but only a few such as the pedunculate oak and sessile oak in Europe and the American white oak are used for making casks for ageing spirits and wines.

This article principally covers the chemical composition of oak wood, the construction of barrels and their use for wines and spirits.

Oak Wood

Varieties of Oak

Oaks belong to the genus *Quercus*, which is divided into two subgenera, *Cyclobalanopsis* and *Euquercus*. The subgenus *Euquercus* is divided into six sections. The section *Lepidobalanus* is widely distributed, being found in Europe, Asia, North Africa and North America, and includes the important species used in cooperage.

Quercus robur (= *Q. pedunculata*), the pedunculate oak, and *Q. petraea* (= *Q. sessiliflora*), the sessile oak, are found in Europe. *Quercus alba*, the white oak, is native to North America.

The pedunculate oak requires light and moisture; it grows throughout Europe from the northern half of the Iberian peninsula to the Urals and the Caucasus.

The sessile oak will grow in poorer soils (acid or calcareous) than the pedunculate oak; it is fairly tolerant to waterlogging, has better resistance to drought, requires less light and often grows as high forest. Its geographical area is smaller than that of the pedunculate oak. The population ecologies of the two oak varieties are compared in Table 1.

Separate groups of sessile and pedunculate oaks are found but, in the areas covered by both species, they are often found in the same forest. Users of oak wood must therefore be aware that they will often have a mixture of logs from the two species.

White oak comes from the central and eastern USA – mainly from Indiana, Tennessee and Missouri.

Anatomical Structure

Oak wood has a marked porous structure in which the earlywood vessels are of much larger diameter than the latewood vessels. Raw sap moves in the vessels, whose walls are dotted with pits for the translocation of substances to and from other parts of the wood. The area with large vessels is called earlywood, in contrast to latewood in which the vessels are narrower and surrounded by dense fibrous tissue. The fibres constitute reinforcement and make the wood strong and rigid. There are also parenchyma cells, which form vertical wood parenchyma near or in contact with the vessels, and ray parenchyma (horizontal ligneous parenchyma), which may be in uniseriate or multiseriate rays.

When the sapwood has become heartwood, the large vessels are blocked by tyloses – membranous growths originating in the parenchyma cells near the vessels – which make the wood impermeable during the storage of wines and spirits. Not all species of oak produce tyloses and such oaks are therefore too porous for the storage of wines and spirits and cannot be used for cooperage. An alteration in colour, tending towards dark brown, appears during the change to heartwood; the cell walls are also impregnated with substances produced by the vertical and ray parenchyma cells.

Oak Wood Chemistry

Wood has two main components: lignin (22–32%) and polysaccharides (64–72%). These two materials are polymerized and complex. From 5 to 12% is extractable

---

* The colour plate section for this article appears between p. 556 and p. 557.

Table 1. Population ecology of pedunculate and sessile oaks

	Pedunculate oak	Sessile oak
Mineral nutrition	Fairly demanding	Hardier; it will grow in poorer, acid or calcareous soils
Drought	Poor resistance, especially after waterlogging	Much better resistance both in permeable soils and soils with temporary groundwater
Light	Extremely demanding	Less demanding
Competition	Poor resistance	Better resistance
Soil water	Withstands surpluses well	Fair tolerance to waterlogging
Production objectives	Girth 70 cm at 100–110 years old	Girth 70–80 cm at 140 to 200–220 years old according to the fertility of the site

Data from Becker M, Levy G and Lafouge R (1990) Chêne sessile, chêne pédonculé et chêne rouge d'Amérique en forêt française. *Revue Forestière Française*, numéro spécial, 2: 148–154, 269–275.

Table 2. The distribution of wood components

Wall components (macromolecular substances)	Extractables (low-molecular-weight substances)
Polysaccharides (holocellulose)	Phenolic compounds (phenols, tannins, phenolic acids, lignans, coumarins)
Cellulose	Aliphatic compounds (acids, alcohols, hydrocarbons)
Hemicelluloses (polyoses)	Terpenes
Lignin	Lactones
	Furans
	Steroids
	Norisoprenoids
	Inorganic substances
	Miscellaneous

by alcohol–water mixtures; this fraction consists mainly of ellagic tannins (castalagin, vescalagin, roburin, etc.) and has a 0·3% mineral content.

The distribution of wood components is shown schematically in Table 2.

Table 3 shows the chemical composition of the different varieties of oak wood.

Method of Manufacture

Preparation of Stave Wood

Oak is used in a number of industrial areas, including veneering, cabinet making and joinery. 'Stave wood' is used in cooperage and is from trees with a girth of at least 35 cm; the trees are 100 years old or more according to the species and growth rate. The timber is selected for its mechanical properties, its suitability for shaping and its porosity.

Perfect straight-grained logs are used. These are split into quarters and only the heartwood is used. Cooperage must withstand pressure at right angles, and so the greatest strength is sought with the least thickness. Fibres are kep undamaged so that the staves are as strong as possible. This is achieved by cutting the wood radially, that is to say, the jointing edges are parallel with the growth rings and the inner and outer faces of

Table 3. Total phenolic compounds and lignin contents expressed as methoxyl groups of different varieties of oaks (mg g^{-1} of wood)

Country/type	Methoxyl content	Total phenolic compounds
French		
Tronçais	53·8	135
	58·6	96
	57·1	84
Limousin	60·1	73
	53·6	154
	62·3	89
Gascony	55·9	111
	55·7	153
	59·9	120
	54·3	105
	53·3	150
	54·8	80
	55·7	82
	61·1	81
Bulgarian	55·9	79
Russian	58·6	105
White American	62·6	39

Data from Puech J-L (1984) Characteristics of oak wood and biochemical aspects of Armagnac aging. *American Journal of Enology and Viticulture* 35: 77–81.

the staves are radial. Five cubic metres of logs are required for 1 m^3 of stave wood. The staves are about 3 cm thick.

Drying

The outdoor drying time of oak depends in particular on the density, the origin of the wood and the stacking technique used. In France, stave wood is traditionally stacked for 3 years, as it is considered that drying takes place at the rate of 1 cm of stave thickness per year. During this period, weather conditions (rain and sun) causes changes in the physical (density and shrinkage), mechanical (compression and bending) and biochemical (monomers and polymers) properties of the constituents and also in the colour. Oven drying is sometimes used to complement a shorter period of air drying because of financial constraints.

Different drying techniques are also used for American oak. In air drying, the staves are placed in a drying oven and the temperature increased according to a typical kiln drying schedule. For example, the drying temperature is increased from an initial 35°C to 77°C at the end of the drying period. Staves are sometimes air dried for an average of 12 months and the moisture content subsequently reduced to about 15% in drying kilns.

Barrel Manufacture

Making barrels for wines and spirits is semimechanical since a perfect seal is required and frequent monitoring is necessary. Barrels are made in several stages: preparation of the wood, making the staves, 'raising' the barrel, bending under heat, bevelling, grooving and placing heads, hooping and checking (Fig. 1).

Assembly and Shaping

Barrels are made up of different wooden parts. The number depends on the irregular width of each one. An average of 28–32 staves and 12–16 head pieces are used. A normal barrel is 27 mm thick at the top and 24 mm thick in the middle (the bilge).

In the first phase of manufacture, the staves are cut to the same length. They are then planed, hollowed, shaped and jointed. Planning renders the outer surface of each stave convex. The inside of the stave is hollowed to give the barrel a regular, concave shape. The staves are shaped to make them narrower at the ends than in the middle.

'Raising' the barrel is the operation in which the staves are assembled in a 'truss hoop' before tightening.

Bending

Bending is a very important part of the barrel-making process since it governs to a great extent the quality and longevity of the barrel; poor heating can lead to defective products.

In Europe, bending is generally performed using a wood fire, whereas steam is used in the USA. In the wood fire technique, the cooper burns oak chips and off-cuts in a brazier to make a fierce fire inside the barrel. As the barrel begins to grow hot, the cooper windlasses the base of the barrel while continuing to feed the fire. He takes special care to heat the central part of the staves so that they bend without breaking. The cooper may also use a lid to cover the barrel shell, to concentrate the heat inside. Bending gives perfect jointing to reduce leakage to a minimum.

The wood is heated to temperatures of up to 200°C during the bending operation. Such temperatures modify the thermoplasticity of certain polymeric constituents of wood (polyoses and lignin), allowing it to bend without splitting or breaking. The inside and outside of the barrel are dampened during bending to prevent warping and difficulties when the heads are inserted.

The barrel is then turned and new hoops fitted. They are hammered on quickly while the barrel is still hot to tighten the staves and make the joints perfectly liquid tight. Some coopers soak the barrels in boiling water to ensure good penetration of moisture into the wood. Once the shell has been formed, European coopers heat the barrels.

Heating

Light, medium or strong heating gives the substances in the wood particular organoleptic qualities. Light and medium heating differ mainly in the exposure of the surface of staves to heat (5–10 minutes); temperatures generally vary from 150 to 200°C. Strong heating is stopped when exothermic reactions begin, that is to say at about 280°C, because the barrel may catch fire at higher temperatures. Traditionally, only the shells of barrels are heated. The heads, forming nearly 25% of the barrel surface in contact with the liquid contents, do not generally receive heat treatment.

Charring

In the USA, the barrels are steamed before shaping. They are then put over firing pots to dry the staves and remove the surface moisture acquired in the steam box. Next, they are sent to the charring fires. The inside of each barrel is treated for 15–45 s to achieve light, normal or heavy char. Barrel heads are also charred on a heading char machine.

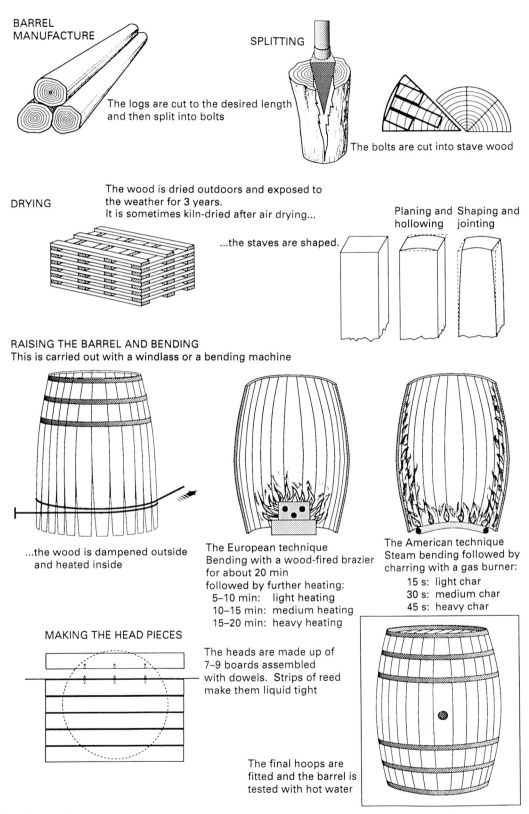

BARREL
MANUFACTURE

The logs are cut to the desired length
and then split into bolts

SPLITTING

The bolts are cut into stave wood

DRYING

The wood is dried outdoors and exposed to
the weather for 3 years.
It is sometimes kiln-dried after air drying...

...the staves are shaped.

Planing and   Shaping and
hollowing   jointing

RAISING THE BARREL AND BENDING
This is carried out with a windlass or a bending machine

...the wood is dampened outside
and heated inside

The European technique
Bending with a wood-fired brazier
for about 20 min
followed by further heating:
  5–10 min: light heating
  10–15 min: medium heating
  15–20 min: heavy heating

The American technique
Steam bending followed by
charring with a gas burner:
  15 s: light char
  30 s: medium char
  45 s: heavy char

MAKING THE HEAD PIECES

The heads are made up of
7–9 boards assembled
with dowels. Strips of reed
make them liquid tight

The final hoops are
fitted and the barrel is
tested with hot water

Fig. 1   Barrel manufacture.

Final Assembly

The heads are assembled with wooden dowels; a length of reed is fitted in each joint to give a good seal. They are then cut to the required size and fitted to each end of the barrel. The barrels are now crozed – a groove is cut in the ends of the staves to hold the head.

The truss hoops used during assembly are removed and replaced by the final hoops. The bung hole is drilled and boiling water or steam is injected to check for any leakage.

Large Barrels and Vats

Large barrels and vats are made in the same way as barrels. Shaping is performed over a wood fire and requires several hours of heating. After assembly in the cooper's workshop, each part is marked before dismantling for transport. They are filled with water to check liquid tightness after final assembly in the warehouse.

The Influence of Heat Treatments

The various heating and charring operations modify the macromolecular structure of the constituents to varying degrees. Changes thus occur in the chemical composition of the stave face in contact with liquids. These changes depend on the intensity and duration of treatment. As a result, the porosity, accessibility to solvents and the proportion of substances extractable by water–alcohol mixtures are deeply modified. These differences affect beverage quality and must be taken into consideration in the light of the type of wine or spirit to be stored in the cask.

Hydrothermolysis and pyrolysis cause the degradation of polysaccharides (cellulose and hemicellulose) and polyphenols (lignin, hydrolysable tannins); this can lead to the appearance of new classes of odoriferous volatile substances which are not present in uncharred wood (furans, pyrazine, phenols, etc.) or additional amounts of pre-existing substances.

During heating, the most thermosensitive polymer hemicelluloses in oak wood are partially degraded, causing the appearance of furfural. In the case of cellulose, a decrease in the degree of polymerization and the production of oligomers (cellobiose, glucose, etc.) are observed; this can lead to the formation of characteristic furan-type substances. The thermal degradation of lignins results in the appearance of oligomers and monomers with phenolic structures (cinnamic aldehydes or benzoic acids). The thermolysis of tannins involved in parietal structures may lead to permeability and increased accessibility of solvents to extractable compounds.

Traditional Uses

At one time, the cooperage industry manufactured barrels in chestnut or other woods, such as acacia, for transporting beverages or dry goods. Today, the industry only produces casks for ageing wines and spirits. Traditionally, great red wines – and sometimes whites – are kept in wooden casks from end of vinification until bottling. Ageing in the wood depends on the wine desired and its structure; the cask must contribute subtle fineness and aromatic complexity, and 'respect' the wine. Heating appears to be a determinant factor in this ideal aromatic contribution made by the wood. Choice of the type of heating will depend on the type of wine, its structure and character. In general, the barrels used for wines are less burned than those for spirits. In addition to the aromatic substances in the wood, storage in barrels involves special oxidation–reduction conditions. Wooden barrels enable weak, but continuous, contact between the wine and the outside atmosphere, so allowing a constant dissolution of oxygen. Some wines, and especially sherry, are aged in oak butts using the solera system. After use, these barrels are much sought-after for ageing Scotch whisky. *See* Brandy and Cognac, Brandy and its Manufacture; Sherry, The Product and its Manufacture; Wines, Production of Table Wines; Whisky, Whiskey and Bourbon, Products and Manufacture

American or European oak barrels are used according to spirit type: grain, wine or sugar cane. American whiskies are aged for 3 years in charred oak (*Q. alba*) barrels. These barrels are then reused for ageing Scotch whisky and also rum. The spirits may remain in barrels for 3 to over 10 years. Some coopers reburn the insides of barrels for fresh use. Spirits from wines are stored in European oak with a coarse grain, i.e. with mainly spring vessels, and thus more porous than fine-grain oak woods. The spirits are first lodged in new barrels for a few months and then in increasingly older barrels. Ageing periods may range from 3 years to several decades. While it is in the wood, the spirit acquires colour and its bouquet becomes rich with complex perfumes. *See* Rum

The mechanism of the maturation of spirits consists of the following features:

- partial integration of the macromolecules contributing to the structure of the wood – lignin, cellulose and hemicellulose – and the dissolution in the spirit of the resultant compounds; *See* Cellulose; Hemicelluloses; Lignin
- degradation of the solubilized compounds in the spirit and oxidation of the tannins; *See* Tannins and Polyphenols
- direct extraction of oligomer or monomer compounds in oak wood.

The internal charring of the barrel may serve as an adsorbent for the volatile substances formed during distallation.

During storage in wood, spirits preferentially extract certain wood constituents and only a very small fraction of the lignin becomes dissolved in the spirit; this is 4% of the total amount in the woods. In contrast, the percentage of total phenolic compounds is 55% of the level in the wood. Other wood extractables which affect the characteristics of wines and spirits include lactones (*cis*- and *trans*-β-methyl-γ-octalactone), volatile phenols, furans and pyrazines. *See* Phenolic Compounds

Future Developments

Variability in wood of genetic origin or resulting from forestry treatment and interactions with the environment appears through the structural, physical, chemical and mechanical aspects. In future, foresters must therefore accurately define the properties required to produce stave wood whose quality is optimal for use in the maturation of wines and spirits.

Research on kiln drying should define the optimal physical parameters to be applied to the wood. In addition, studies on the biochemical mechanisms which occur during air or kiln drying will lead to a rational combination of the two methods. Barrel making has always been empirical but should now be monitored and optimized. Stave heating and charring – which change the chemical composition of the wood – must also be supervized and controlled. As a result, the origin of the timber, the cutting of the stave wood, drying, barrel manufacture, heating and charring of barrels must be appropriate for each wine (origin, type and structure) or spirit (grain- or sugar cane-based beverages) and the final product features required.

Bibliography

Keller R (1987) Différentes variétés de chêne et leur répartition dans le monde. *Connaissance de la Vigne et du Vin*: 1–38.
Maga J (1989) The contribution of wood to the flavor of alcoholic beverages. *Foods Reviews International* 5: 39–99.
Puech J-L and Moutounet M (1990) Oak wood chemistry and extractable substances. In: Campbell I (ed.) *Proceedings of the Third Aviemore Conference on Malting, Brewing and Distilling*, pp 209–225.

J.-L. Puech and M. Moutounet
Institut National de la Recherche Agronomique, Montpellier, France

BEANS

Throughout human history, more than 3000 species of plants have been used as foods. On a global basis, plants provide 65% of food protein and over 80% of food energy, and account for 85% of gross tonnage. Excluding the large number of fruit and vegetable species, only about 50 crop species make a significant contribution to human diet. Of these, cereals are the largest group, followed by legumes, in terms of global production. However, because legumes contain almost two to three times more protein than cereals, their dietary importance as a protein source is well appreciated. Of more than 1300 species of legumes, only about 20 are most commonly consumed by humans. Among these, the common dry bean, *Phaseolus vulgaris*, is consumed in the largest quantity on a worldwide basis. Dry beans are low in fat (excluding oilseeds) and sodium, and contain no cholesterol. They are a rich source of proteins, complex carbohydrates, fibre, vitamins, and certain minerals. On a caloric basis, dry beans are more nutrient-dense than cereals. In addition, dry beans are less expensive than animal food products, and have considerably longer shelf life than several animal, fruit and vegetable products when stored properly. Since legumes have the ability to fix atmospheric nitrogen and therefore add nitrogen to the crop-soil ecosystem, they are important in soil conservation as well as in maintaining soil quantity. *See* Cereals, Contribution to the Diet; Cereals, Dietary Importance; Legumes, Legumes in the Diet

Global Distribution, Varieties, and Commercial Importance

The word 'legume' is derived from the Latin word, *legumen*, which means seeds harvested in pods. The term 'pulse' (from Latin word, *puls*, meaning pottage) is used for legume seeds, which contain small amounts of fat, while for those containing large amounts of fat (such as soya beans and peanuts) the term 'leguminous oilseed' is used. According to the Food and Agriculture Organization (FAO), the word 'legume' is used for all leguminous plants. Those legumes most commonly used as human food are listed in Table 1. *See* Peanuts; Pulses; Soya Beans, The Crop

Although legumes have been cultivated for several thousand years, the chronology and origins of domestication of food legumes is almost impossible to reconstruct. Some legumes (e.g. lentils) have been dated back to 7000–6000 BC. Leguminosae (or Fabaceae) is the third largest family of flowering plants (after Compositae and Orchidaceae) in size and economic importance, and is second only to the grasses (Gramineae). Current estimates indicate that Leguminosae has about 16 000–19 000 species in about 750 genera. The subclassification is somewhat controversial. The generally accepted subclassification is shown in Fig. 1. Almost all of the domesticated legumes used as food are members of Papillionoideae. All of the common beans belong to the tribe Phaseolaeae. *See* Peas and Lentils

In terms of global production, legumes (including oilseeds) rank fifth in annual world grain production. Dry beans account for approximately 27% of the total world legume production (Table 2). On a worldwide basis, the common beans (*Phaseolus* spp.) are the number one crop among dry beans (excluding oilseeds) in both production and consumption, and are therefore economically an important crop. Asia produces the largest quantity (43·16% of total world production) of dry beans, followed by South America (19·25%), northern Central America (17·81%), and Africa (12·96%). The major importers of legumes are the Europeans and Asians, accounting for 49·59% and 29·80% respectively, of the total dollar value; Europe and Asia account for 32·18% and 33·35% (dollar value) of the total exports on a global basis. North and Central America are the net exporters of legumes and legume products (Table 2).

Morphology of the Pods and Seeds

Regardless of the fat content, most legume seeds have similar structure. Mature legume seeds have three major components: the seed coat, the cotyledons, and the embryo axis. In most dry seeds, they respectively account for 8–20%, 80–90%, and 1–2% of the seed weight. The majority of the nutrients are present in cotyledons. Typical seed structure and various anatomical parts of legume seeds are shown in Fig. 2. The outermost layer of the seed is the seed coat or testa. The external seed structure includes the hilum, micropyle and raphe. The hilum is a scarlike structure (usually oval-shaped) near the middle edge where the seed breaks away from the stalk. The micropyle is the small opening in the seed coat where the pollen tube enters the valve. The raphe is the ridge at the side of hilum opposite to the

micropyle and represents the base of the stalk that fuses with the seed coat upon seed maturation. In most legumes, the endosperm is short-lived and shrinks to a thin layer surrounding the cotyledons (or embryo). On soaking the seeds, the endosperm is easily removed along with the seed coat. The remainder (embryo) of the seed consists of shoot (which contains two cotyledons) and a short axis above and below the cotyledons, and terminates in the shoot tip. The plumule or embryonic stem is well developed in the resting seed and lies between two cotyledons.

The outermost layer of seed coat is the cuticle, which has papillae or papillae-like growth in some legumes (e.g. green gram) but in most legumes it is a smooth structure. The thickness of the seed coat is quite variable, depending upon the type of bean. Generally, seeds containing thick seed coats tend to have high fat content. Both hilum and micropyle are important in water imbibition by testa. Palisade cells, which are derived from the outer epidermis of the outer integument and lie next to the cuticle, are either loosely packed or densely packed, depending upon the seed maturity, and may affect seed hydration. Next to palisade cells are the hourglass cells. Hourglass cells vary in shape from bottle (guar), to dumbbell (broad beans) to hourglass (soybeans). Only a few legume species (such as *Dolichos*, *Cajanus* and *Vigna*) have more than one layer of hourglass cells. The remainder of the testa contains primarily mesophyll cells.

Legume cotyledons are primarily composed of parenchyma cells which have variable size (70–100 μm) and act as storage sites for most nutrients. Each cell of the cotyledon is bound by the cell wall and the middle lamella. Vascular bundles in cotyledons are generally devoid of any filling material. Vascular bundles are often used as key structures in the identification of different plant types.

Chemical and Nutritional Composition

The majority of nutrients in dry beans are primarily located in the cotyledons and account for up to 90% of the total nutrititive value. Typically, dry beans provide 300–350 kcal per 100 g of dry seeds. The majority of constituents of cotyledons are proteins and carbohydrates, which respectively account for 15–25% and 50–75% of the total seed weight. The remainder consists of fat, minerals, fibre and vitamins. With the exception of oilseeds, dry beans generally contain low amounts (1–3% of seed weight) of fat. Although most minerals are present in cotyledons, some (such as calcium and iron) may be present in seed coat in significant proportion. Typical nutrient composition of several *Phaseolus* beans is shown in Table 3. Dry beans contain not only significant amounts of nutrients, but also several

Table 1. Grain legume species commonly used for food purposes[a]

Name	Common name
Aracahis hypogaea	Groundnut, peanut, monkey nut, goober pea, nguba
Cajunus cajan	Pigeon pea, arhar, red gram, tur, *toovar*, Angola pea, gandal, ambre vade, alverja
C. indicus	Pigeon pea, congo pea, yellow dhal
Canavalia ensiformis	Jack bean, horsebean, gotani bean, haba de burro, chickasaw, lima
C. gladiata	Sword bean, maxima
Cicer arietinum	Chickpea, bengal gram, chana, deshi chana, kabuli, chiche
C. minotinum	Chana, garbanzo
Cyamopsis tetragonoloba	Cluster bean, guar, aconite, cyamopse
Dolichos biflorus	Horse gram
D. lablab	Hyacinth bean, bonavist, field bean, caballeros, Indian butter bean, Egyptian kidney bean
Ervum vulgaris	Lentils, masur dhal
Faba vulgaris	Windsor bean
Glycine max	Soya bean, soja
G. hispida	
G. soja	
Lablab niger	Lablab bean
L. purpureus	Kidney bean, hyacinth bean, Indian bean, lubia bean
Lathyrus sativus	Grasspea, kasari dhal, vetch, chickling vetch, chicaro
Lens esculenta	Lentils, masur dhal, red dhal, lentille, split pea, lentija
L. culinaris	
Lupinus spp.	Lupins, tarwi, tarin, pearl lupin, wolf bean, tremoco
Macrotyloma uniflorum	Horse gram, Madras gram, Kallu, Kulthi bean
Mucuna pruriens	Velvet bean, cowage, Mauritius bean, stizolobia
Phaseolus aconitifolius	Moth bean
P. acutifolius	Tepary bean, pavi, Yorimuni, dinawa
P. angularis	Adzuki bean, *feijao*
P. aureus	Mung bean, green gram, golden gram, chiroko, chicka sano pea
P. calcaratus	Rice bean, frijol arroz
P. lunatus	Lima bean, sieva bean, Madagascar bean, sugar bean, Burmabean, towe bean, pole bean, caraota, panguita
P. mungo	Mung bean, mungo bean, urd dhal, black gram, *urad*, woolly pyrol, kambulu
P. radiatus	Mung bean, golden gram, green gram
P. vulgaris	Dry bean, haricot, common bean, kidney bean, navy bean, pinto or snap bean, feijao, opoca, *rajma*, French bean, chumbinho
Pisum sativum	Dry pea, green pea, garden pea, field pea
P. angularis	
P. arvense	
Psophocarpus tetragonolobus	Winged bean (humid tropics), Goa bean, asparagus bean, Colombo, four angled bean, princess bean
Sphenostylis stenocarpa	Yam bean
Stizolobium spp.	Velvet bean
Tetragonolobus purpureus	Winged bean (Europe)
Trigonella foenumgraecum	Methi, fenugreek
Tylosema esculentum	Marama bean
Vicia faba	Broad bean, horsebean, faba bean, field bean, Windsor bean
V. sativa	Vetch
Vigna aconitifolia	Moth bean, matki, mouth bean, mat, math
V. aureus	Mung bean
V. radiata	
V. mungo	Black gram, *urd, urad*, kambulu, pyrol
V. sinensis	Dry cowpea
V. umbellata	Rice bean, red bean, mambi bean
V. unguiculata	Black-eyed cowpea, black-eye pea, cowpea, kaffir bean, Hindu pea, asparagus pea
Voandzeia subterranea	Bambara groundnut, Madagascar groundnut, earthpea, Congo goober, kaffir pea, jugo bean, haricot pistache

[a] Compiled from Deshpande and Srinivasan (1990) and Doughty and Walker (1982).

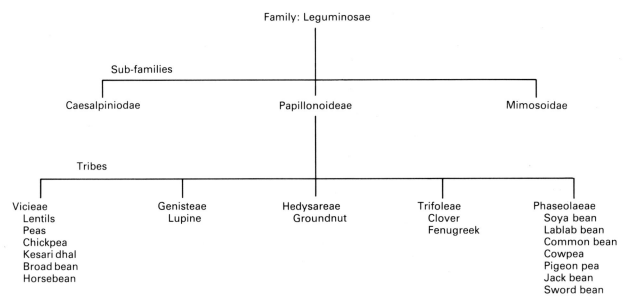

Fig. 1   Botanical classification of food legumes.

Table 2.   Acreage, production, yield, and import/export data for legumes[a]

	Total legumes							Dry beans		
	Area harvested ($\times 10^6$ ha)	Yield (kg per ha)	Production ($\times 10^3$ t)	Import[b] ($\times 10^3$ t)	($\times 10^3$ $)	Export[b] ($\times 10^3$ t)	($\times 10^3$ $)	Area harvested ($\times 10^6$ ha)	Yield (kg per ha)	Production ($\times 10^3$ t)
World	68·403	807	55 200	5 773 827	2 245 257	6 044 651	2 071 857	26·207	563	14 750
Africa	10·872	646	7026	385 505	203 396	433 546	6669	2·592	737	1911
North and Central America	3·944	937	3694	329 225	147 735	1 066 920	421 064	3·138	837	2627
South America	6·690	471	3153	208 674	94 315	254 346	102 098	6·218	457	2839
Asia	35·709	688	24 551	1 826 774	669 045	2 171 964	690 890	12·894	494	6366
Europe	3·243	1632	5294	2 980 817	1 113 505	1 815 955	66 676	1·293	642	830
Oceania	0·936	1145	1072	18 539	10 241	532 836	106 564	0·006	1078	7
USSR	7·008[c]	1485	10 410[c]	24 293	7020	60 084	17 896	0·065	2615	170

[a] Data from FAO (1986).
[b] Data from FAO (1988).
[c] FAO estimate.

undesirable components and attributes: inhibitors of enzymes such as trypsin, chymotrypsin, subtilisin, amylases and elastase; lectins; phenolic compounds including tannins; phytates; toxic amino acids, mimosine and djenkolic acid; cyanogenic glycosides which produce hydrogen cyanide; flatulence factors such as oligosaccharides raffinose, stachyose and verbascose; lipoxygenases, which catalyse the development of rancidity; and beanlike, grasslike or paintlike odours.

Proteins

Phaseolus beans are valued for their protein content because they are a major protein contributor to the human diet on a global basis. In certain parts of the world they are the sole source of dietary protein. Dry bean proteins can be classified as storage and metabolic proteins. The original protein classification proposed by Osborne was based on solubility of proteins in a series of solvents. In this scheme the water- and dilute-salt-soluble proteins were termed as albumins and globulins, respectively. Dry beans contain 40–60% globulins and 20–40% albumins, based on Osborne's protein classification. Globulins are exclusively storage proteins, while the albumin fraction contains both storage and metabolic proteins. The protein content of dry beans is usually calculated by multiplying Kjeldahl nitrogen content by a factor of 6·25. Because dry beans contain 10–15% of total nitrogen as nonprotein nitrogen, most

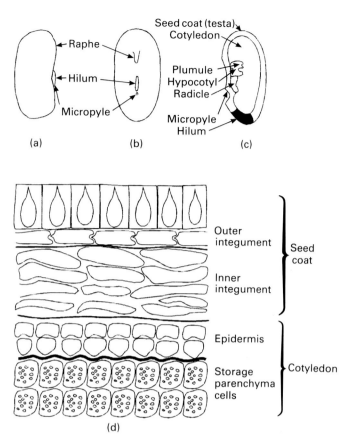

Fig. 2 Dry bean (*Phaseolus vulgaris*) seed. (a) External side view; (b) external face or edge view (viewing at hilum side); (c) cross-section (one cotyledon removed); (d) detailed cross-section across seed coat and cotyledon.

dry bean protein values are typically overestimated by 1–2%. *See* Protein, Chemistry; Protein, Food Sources; Protein, Digestion and Absorption of Protein and Nitrogen Balance

The major storage proteins in dry beans have been identified by several names and therefore their nomenclature is somewhat confusing. Based on the nomenclature using ultracentrifugation sedimentation coefficient (s), dry beans contain both $7s$ (vicilin-like) and $11s$ (legumin-like) storage proteins. Depending on the bean variety, the relative proportion of these two types of proteins varies considerably. The $11s$ type proteins typically are nonglycosylated proteins with estimated molecular weight (mol. wt) in the range 300 000–400 000. They are usually composed of six subunits (mol wt 60 000) each consisting one acidic (mol. wt 40 000) and one basic (mol. wt 20 000) polypeptide linked by disulphide bond(s). Usually, $11s$ proteins are present in minor amounts in *Phaseolus* beans. The $7s$ globulin in *Phaseolus* beans has also been referred to as glycoprotein II, globulin 1, euphaseolin, globulin, and phaseolin. Depending on the type of bean, the $7s$ globulin type and quantity varies considerably. In *Phaseolus* beans the $7s$ globulins are, however, the major storage proteins and account for 40–60% of the total proteins. The three major types of $7s$ proteins that have been identified, biochemically purified, and characterized are (1) phaseolin, (2) lectin (also called glycoprotein II, phytoagglutinins or phytohaemagglutinins, and protein II), and (3) Arcelin in wild bean accessions from Mexico (named after the town Arcelia in Mexico, where some of the accessions were collected). All the $7s$ globulins are glycosylated and contain D-mannose and D-glucosamine as the major sugar constituents.

Phaseolin

Phaseolin is the major globulin in domesticated *Phaseolus* beans. It is soluble in 0·5 M NaCl at all pH values. It undergoes reversible, pH-dependent dissociation-association with sedimentation coefficients of $3·0s$ (pH 12·0), $7·1s$ (pH 7·0), and $18·2s$ (pH 3·6) known as peptides (mol. wt 44 000), protomers (mol. wt 163 000), and tetramers of protomers (mol. wt 653 000). Phaseolin consists of a group of subunit polypeptides with mol. wts 43 000–54 000 and isoelectric points from pH 5·6 to 5·8, depending on phaseolin type. Among *Phaseolus* beans, three distinct types of phaseolins – named after cultivars tendergreen (T), Sanilac (S), and Contender

Table 3. Proximate composition of *Phaseolus* beans[a]

Bean	Moisture (%)	Protein (%)	Carbohydrates (%)	Fat (%)	Ash (%)	Crude fibre (%)
Adzuki	11·0	20·2	49·8	1·9	4·39	4·9
Black beauty	10·41	22·87	70·79	4·48	1·86	—
Black gram	10·2–10·9	19·7–24·0	56·6–63·4	1·3–1·6	3·2–3·4	4·4–6·4
California small white	9·65	25·90	58·00	0·25	—	—
Cranberry	12·71	23·43	71·26	1·09	4·22	—
Great Northern	8·5–13·3	21·0–24·37	61·2–71·07	1·0–3·48	3·5–4·86	6·7
Lima						
Baby	13·30	20·40	62·10	0·80	3·40	6·0
Large	8·90	22·30	63·80	0·80	4·20	7·4
Mung						
Green	17·92	27·12	62·85	1·53	4·01	4·5
Black	13·64	25·68	64·20	0·45	4·32	5·3
Navy	9·41–18·2	23·13–24·65	61·2–66·19	1·5–4·3	2·90–4·27	3·4–6·6
Pinto	9·05–14·70	18·8–24·97	61·8–69·47	1·2–3·6	3·07–4·10	3·9–6·3
Red kidney						
Light	10·52	20·89	73·20	1·52	4·39	—
Dark	13·22	20·32	73·68	1·58	4·42	—
Rice bean	—	18·0–25·0	60·0–77·0	1·0–1·6	3·8–4·3	3·3–4·8
Roshina G₂	9·89–11·11	25·77–26·30	63·33–64·02	1·85–2·00	3·19–3·79	4·6–5·1
Roshina pink	4·90	19·40	68·80	3·50	3·40	4·6
Sanilac	11·61	18·98	75·09	1·65	4·28	—
Tepary	—	21·0–25·0	70·0–73·0	0·8–0·9	4·1–4·8	—
Small red	13·12	22·45	71·97	1·43	4·15	—
Small white	13·03	19·73	74·34	1·99	3·94	—
Viva pink	12·69	21·30	73·23	1·06	4·41	—

[a] Data compiled from Sathe *et al.* (1984) and Salunkhe and Kadam (1989). Data expressed on a dry-weight basis.

(C) – have been identified. Screening of 107 cultivars has revealed that S, T, and C type phaseolins accounted for 69%, 25%, and 6% respectively of the total cultivars. These types can be easily distinguished by one-dimensional or two-dimensional gel electrophoresis using sodium dodecyl sulphate (SDS) polyacrylamide gel electrophoresis (PAGE) for one-dimensional or isoelectric focusing in first dimension, followed by SDS-PAGE in the second dimension for two-dimensional gel electrophoresis. The C-type phaseolin is believed to have originated from T and S types. Regardless of type of phaseolin, phaseolin contains 3–5% carbohydrates and its amino acid composition is dominated by acidic amino acids (30–40% of total). Sulphur-containing amino acids (notably methionine) are the limiting amino acids in phaseolin as well as other major storage proteins in *Phaseolus* beans. The secondary structure of phaseolin in 0·5 M-NaCl typically has a low α-helix (10%) and β-turn (9·0%) contents, and high β-sheet (48·0%) and random coil (33·0%) contents. Native phaseolin is quite resistant to digestive proteases such as pepsin, trypsin and chymotrypsin, and is degraded to polypeptides with mol. wts 24000–28000. Heat-denatured phaseolin, however, is easily digested by these proteases. *See*

Amino Acids, Metabolism; Protein, Determination and Characterization

Lectin

Bean lectins agglutinate erythrocytes due to their ability to bind with cell surface glycoproteins and glycolipids. Although the precise function of lectins in beans is unknown, they are thought to offer protection to the plant. Since lectins are toxic, they are of nutritional concern. Lectins occur in both albumin and globulin fractions. Certain bean cultivars lack lectins. When present, lectins represent 6–12% of total protein. In addition to agglutinating activity, many bean lectins have mitogenic activity. Most lectins of *Phaseolus* beans have subunits of mol. wts 29000–36500 with isoelectric pH in the range 4·9–7·9 (most are in the pH range 5–6). A majority of the native lectins have tetrameric nature (mol. wts of 100000–150000), although some (e.g. lima beans) have dimeric nature. A majority of *Phaseolus* lectins have 4–6% carbohydrate, low sulphur-containing amino acids, and sugar specificity towards D-acetyl-galactosamine. Lectins are very resistant to common digestive proteases and are slowly hydrolysed *in vitro* even after extensive heat denaturation. Proper moist heat denaturation can completely inactivate the biological activity of lectins and can therefore render them nontoxic. *See* Plant Toxins, Haemagglutinins

Arcelin

Arcelin was first discovered in wild accessions of Mexican *Phaseolus* beans. It also occurs in lines which contain phaseolin as well as lectin. Because it is present in equal or greater levels than phaseolin in certain lines, it is one of the major storage proteins in *Phaseolus* beans. The mol. wts of arcelin subunit polypeptides range from 35 000 to 42 000, depending on the variant, and are more basic than both lectin and phaseolin. The native arcelin has a mol. wt of 89 000 and is therefore a dimeric protein. Arcelin has many similarities with lectin (including agglutinating activity) with respect to chemical composition.

Other Proteins

Phaseolus beans contain trypsin inhibitors (many of them also inhibit chymotrypsin), amylase inhibitors, lipoxygenases, and several other minor protein components. Most of these proteins are a part of albumins. Trypsin and chymotrypsin inhibitors in *Phaseolus* beans typically account for up to 10% of the total proteins and are generally rich in sulphur-containing amino acids. The mol. wts of these inhibitors range from 2000 to 23 000. Most *Phaseolus* beans lack Kunitz type (inhibitors with 170–200 amino acids with mol. wt of approximately 20 000) trypsin inhibitors. Amylase inhibitors in dry beans have been characterized from only a few cultivars and therefore have not yet been extensively studied. The mol. wt of kidney bean amylase inhibitor (a glycoprotein) has been shown to be 50 000. Appropriate moist heat treatment (such as cooking or autoclaving) can inactivate both the protease and amylase inhibitors.

Carbohydrates

Total carbohydrates in *Phaseolus* beans contribute 50–70% of the seed weight and include mono-, di- and oligosaccharides, starch, and other polysaccharides. Starch is the most abundant nutrient in *Phaseolus* beans, accounting for up to 70–80% of total carbohydrates. Among the simple sugars, oligosaccharides (raffinose, stachyose, verbascose, and ajugose) are the major constituents (up to 10% of seed weight) and are at least partially responsible for flatulence production. Crude fibre is primarily composed of cellulose, hemicellulose, lignins (not a carbohydrate), and other nonstarchy polysaccharides such as arabinogalactans, arabinoxylans, glucomannans, galactomannans, and pectins. The

hypocholesterolaemic effect of dry beans is partially attributed to the presence of nonstarchy polysaccharides. *See* Carbohydrates, Classification and Properties; Dietary Fibre, Properties and Sources

Phaseolus bean starch granules are quite variable in shape (round, oval, oblong, elliptical, spherical, kidney-shaped, and irregular, and size (5–60 μm) and typically contain 10–45% (of total starch) amylose. The average degree of polymerization for amyloses, and the chain lengths for amylopectins of *Phaseolus* bean starches are 1600–1900 glucose units and 22–26 glucose units respectively. Based on X-ray diffraction spectra *Phaseolus* dry bean starches are mostly C type – a mixture of A (typical of cereal starches) and B (typical of root and tuber, and high amylose cereal starches) type. These starches have restricted swelling, a gelatinization temperature range of 60–89°C, high solution viscosities, and good thermal stabilities. Upon gelatinization they produce opaque gels. Dry bean starches (especially if cooked) are well digested (digestibility is comparable to those of many cereal and tuber starches) by humans. Because dry bean starches are digested slowly, however, they are hypoglycaemic and therefore useful in the diets of diabetics. *See* Starch, Structure, Properties and Determination

Vitamins and Minerals

Phaseolus beans are a good source of B vitamins, especially thiamin, riboflavin, nicotinic acid and folacin. Typically, thiamin, riboflavin, nicotinic acid and folacin contents (on a dry-weight basis) of *Phaseolus* beans are, respectively, 0·5–1·14, 0·1–0·25, 0·4–3·14, and 0·037–0·676 mg per 100 g. Vitamin E content ranges from 0·72 to 1·97 g per 100 g and B_6 content ranges from 0·2 to 0·659 mg per 100 g. *Phaseolus* beans are not good sources of carotenes and vitamin C.

Phaseolus beans are excellent sources of several minerals, including calcium, iron, copper, zinc, phosphorus, potassium and magnesium (Ca, Fe, Cu, Zn, P, K and Mg). Typically raw beans contain 70–260, 0·5–1·40, 3·34–13·5, 160–320, 1·0–2·1, 380–570, 1320–1780, 4·0–21·0 and 1·9–6·5 (all expressed as mg per 100 g, dry-weight basis) of Ca, Cu, Fe, Mg, Mn, P, K, Na and Zn, respectively. The low-sodium and high-potassium contents of raw beans make them a desirable constituent of human food (especially for people with hypertension). *See* individual minerals and vitamins

Antinutritional Factors

In addition to protease inhibitors and amylase inhibitors, *Phaseolus* beans contain several other antinutritional and antiphysiological factors, such as phytic acids, tannins, cyanogenic glycosides, saponins and allergens. Because these components are usually present in small quantities (less than 5% of the total seed weight), they do not pose a serious health hazard under normal conditions (i.e. when beans are a part of total diet and are properly processed prior to consumption). Of these antinutritional factors, phytates and tannins are of particular concern because both of them are heat-stable and cannot be easily removed from beans during normal home processing. Phytate is a general term used for mono-to-dodeca anions of phytate, along with esters lower than hexaphosphate. Calcium–magnesium salts of phytic acid – myoinositol 1,2,3,4,5,6-hexakis (dihydrogen phosphate) – are referred to as phytin. In most dry beans, phytate phosphorus accounts for up to 80% of the total phosphorus. The amount of phytate in *Phaseolus* beans ranges from 0·6 to 2·1% (by weight) of the total seed weight. Because phytates are chelating agents, they may interfere in mineral utilization. Germination, fermentation and soaking, followed by cooking (if both soak- and cook-water are discarded), are effective methods of removing phytates (50–80% reduction). *See* Allergens; Phytic Acid, Properties and Determination; Phytic Acid, Nutritional Impact

Tannins (especially condensed tannins) are heat-stable compounds that are present in *Phaseolus* seeds (especially in coloured varieties) up to 2% of total seed weight. Because of their ionic character, they may interact with other constituents (notably proteins) and adversely affect the nutritional bioavailability of that constituent. Tannins are thought to offer protection to the plant from insects and pests. *See* Tannins and Polyphenols

Lipids

Phaseolus beans contain 1–3% lipids (by weight), depending upon the species. Neutral lipids (30–50% of total) and phospholipids (25–35% of total) are the major constituents, and glycolipids may account for up to 10% of the total lipids. Regardless of the variety, *Phaseolus* bean lipids primarily contain palmitic, oleic, linoleic and linolenic acids. Polyunsaturated fatty acids and saturated fatty acids typically account for 55–87% and 12–28% of total lipids. *See* Fatty Acids, Properties; Lipids, Classification

Grading, Handling, and Storage

Dry beans are usually harvested at maturity. The seeds are removed either manually or mechanically from the pods, cleaned to remove dirt, stalks, leaves, blemished and wrinkled seeds, and packaged prior to storage. The grading of seeds is usually based on external characteristics, such as colour, gloss, seed size, seed soundness, seed firmness, and presence of contaminating substances. The seeds are stored at farmer, trader or government levels. Typically, farmers hold up to 8% of harvested seeds until next season so that they can be used as planting seeds if crop failures occur. In developed and developing nations, a majority of the seeds are stored by traders and/or governments to protect against subsequent crop failures (or low yields), price fluctuations, and fluctuations in supply (change in demand, shortages, and famines).

Losses in seeds occur both pre- and post-harvest. The normal preharvest losses are mainly due to birds and mammals feeding on bean plant seeds. Drought or floods, insects, and rodents can also contribute to pre-harvest losses. In developed nations pre-harvest losses are usually small (as low as 1% of the crop). A majority of the losses occur during post-harvest handling and storage, and can range from 8% to as high as 50% of total crop. It is estimated that as much as 48% of food produced in the world is lost as a result of pre- and post-harvest losses. Factors which influence post-harvest losses of legumes include moisture, temperature, respiration rate, insect damage, microbial spoilage, and damage caused by mites and rodents.

Properly packaged dry beans should be stored at low relative humidity and temperature conditions. High relative humidity and temperature favour the 'hard-to-cook' beans. These conditions also favour the growth of moulds and insects. Three major insect genera that cause much of the damage to stored legumes are *Bruchus*, *Acanthoscelides* and *Callosobruchus*. Dehusked, split stored pulses are also damaged by *Rhizopertha*, *Trogoderma* and *Tribolium* species. Pests usually seem to have preference for the type of bean they infest, although the basis for such preference (or the lack of it) has not been elucidated yet. The major microbial problem during bean storage is contamination by aflatoxin-producing moulds (*Aspergillus flavus* and *A. parasiticus*). Mites can consume food up to their own weight (6–8 μg) and because of their large numbers can cause serious losses. Rodents cause twofold damage to stored legumes by not only consuming but also contaminating (up to 20 times the amount they would eat). Because rodents are carriers of many communicable diseases, they pose serious damage to stored beans. The species that most commonly cause damage include *Rattus rattus*, *R. norvegicus*, *Bandicota indica*, *B. bengalensis* and *Mus muscalatus*. *See* Insect Pests, Insects and Related Pests; Insect Pests, Problems Caused by Insects and Mites; Spoilage, Moulds in Food Spoilage; Storage Stability, Parameters Affecting Storage Stability

Processing and Food Uses

Phaseolus beans are processed and used in a variety of ways. The processing of beans is mostly at the household level in developing and underdeveloped countries, while in most developed countries the majority of the processing is done at the industrial level. Home-processing methods include milling, soaking, cooking, frying, germination, fermentation (either alone or in combination with cereals), roasting, puffing, parching, extrusion and frying, and toasting. The method(s) used for home processing depend on regional preference for bean variety and the desired end product. For example, mung beans in sprouted form are popular on global scale and germination is therefore one of the preferred home-processing methods used. Black gram, on the other hand, is extensively used for preparation of *idli*, a breakfast food popular in India and Sri Lanka, after fermenting it with rice. Industrial processing includes freezing (e.g. green French beans, snap beans), milling (production of flours and high-protein flours), baking (baked beans), cooking and frying (refried beans), and canning (alone in salt water or tomato juice, or in combination with meats such as beef and pork). In developing countries dehusking and splitting to produce *dhal* is also done on an industrial scale. *See* Freezing, Freezing Operations

In developing and underdeveloped countries, *Phaseolus* beans are used in numerous ways, depending on the type of bean and regional preference: they may be eaten as raw, immature seeds; cooked as green vegetables (e.g. French beans); consumed as parts of salads; used in making curry; used as a soup ingredient; cooked, mashed, mixed with condiments and spices and used as gruels and porridges; prepared as pastes to be extruded to prepare fried snack products; sprouted; puffed or roasted and eaten as snack foods; and fermented to prepare numerous fermented products.

In developed countries, *Phaseolus* beans are consumed as salad and soup ingredients, as sprouts, or canned, frozen, or refried. They are also extensively used in the preparation of Mexican style preparations, such as burrito, chimichanga, taco, bean dips, and tamale, and often canned with meats such as beef and pork. In many South American countries, cooked black beans are a preferred part of breakfast.

Although there is a good potential for the preparation of protein concentrates and isolates, and for the development of food starches, *Phaseolus* beans have not been used on a large scale for such purposes. In many countries, especially the developed ones, *Phaseolus* beans have been extensively used as animal feed. In developing and underdeveloped countries, the green foliage, deseeded pods, and roots and shoots of bean plants are used as natural fertilizers, especially after composting. Because the legume roots fix nitrogen, they help to conserve soil quality. For this reason, in many developing countries they are extensively used for soil quality conservation.

Bibliography

Derbyshire E, Wright DJ and Boulter D (1976) Legumin and vicilin, storage proteins of legume seeds. *Phytochemistry* 15: 3–24.

Deshpande SS and Srinivasan D (1990) Food legumes: chemistry and technology. *Advances in Cereal Science and Technology* 10: 147–241.

Doughty J and Walker A (1982) Legumes in human nutrition, Food and Nutrition Paper 20. Rome: Food and Agriculture Organization.

FAO (1986) *Production Yearbook*, vol. 40, pp 67–69, 99–103. Rome: Food and Agriculture Organization.

FAO (1988) *Trade Yearbook*, vol. 42, pp 149–151. Rome: Food and Agriculture Organization.

Osborn TC (1988) Genetic control of bean seed proteins. *CRC Critical Reviews in Plant Sciences* 7: 93–116.

Patwardhan VN (1962) Pulses and beans in human nutrition. *American Journal of Clinical Nutrition* 11: 12–30.

Reddy NR, Pierson MD and Salunkhe DK (1986) *Legume-Based Fermented Foods*. Boca Raton, Florida: CRC Press.

Salunke DK and Kadam SS (1989) *Handbook of World Food Food Legumes: Nutritional Chemistry, Processing Technology, and Utilization*, vols I, II and III. Boca Raton, Florida: CRC Press.

Sathe SK, Deshpande SS and Salunkhe DK (1984) Dry beans of *Phaseolus*. A review. Part 1. Chemical composition: Proteins. *CRC Critical Reviews in Food Science and Nutrition* 20: 1–46.

S. K. Sathe
Florida State University, Tallahasee, USA
S. S. Deshpande
Research Station, Mordern, Manitoba, Canada

BEEF

Beef is 'the flesh of ox, bull or cow' (*Oxford English Dictionary*). *Boef* (Anglo-French) is derived from the Latin *bos*, *bovis* (ox), and until the 18th century beef meant both animal and meat. The etymology suggests that the meat was for the Norman ruling class, and was not commonly eaten by Anglo-Saxon folk even in the late 13th century as Middle English was forming.

Beef has enjoyed a special status since *Bos* spp. were domesticated in Neolithic times in Southwest Asia. The bull was a totem for warrior nomads; eating his flesh transferred his power. The docility and strength of draft oxen, the versatile milk, the valuable hides and attractive meat, have made the *Bos* genus economically vital to humans.

Today beef cattle are raised all over the world (Table 1). The natural environment of *Bos taurus* is temperate grasslands. *B. indicus* prefers savannah. Crossbreeds such as 'Santa Gertrudis' grow well in hot dry areas, such as the southwest USA.

Different breeds have been developed over the centuries to maximize returns under local conditions. The compact, early-fattening Aberdeen Angus and Hereford

Table 1. World production of beef and veal[a]

Region	Live ($\times 10^3$)	Slaughtered ($\times 10^3$)	Carcass weight (kg, mean)	Production (kilotonnes)
1979–1981				
World	1 218 277	223 143	198	44 090
Africa	172 203	20 683	142	2932
North/Central America	173 510	48 911	254	12 402
USA	112 152	37 292	271	10 092
South America	239 246	34 023	201	6853
Asia	350 404	21 382	114	2435
China	52 567	2350	75	177
India	186 500	1710	80	137
Europe	133 377	48 037	220	10 551
France	23 825	7841	234	1832
Germany[b]	20 672	7353	259	1890
UK	13 321	4097	260	1063
Oceania	34 790	12 715	173	2198
USSR	114 748	37 391	180	6720
1989				
World	1 281 472	236 577	209	49 436
Africa	185 794	23 277	148	3455
North/Central America	166 999	52 631	267	14 028
USA	99 180	36 376	293	10 655
South America	261 096	34 006	209	7100
Asia	391 556	29 599	119	3532
China	661 141	6658F	99	662F
India	195 500	2925	80	234F
Europe	125 569	43 388	242	10 500
France	21 780	6900F	249	1716F
Germany[b]	20 369	7814	258	2005
UK	11 902	3374	284	958
Oceania	30 858	10 375	195	2021
USSR	119 600	43 300F	203	8800F

'F' is Food and Agriculture Organization estimate.
All data from FAO (1989).
[a] Average per annum.
[b] Summed over FRG and GDR figures.

are productive in harsher nutritional and climatic environments. The great draft cattle of Europe, like Charolais and Chianina, put on muscle quickly in larger quantity and are heavier at slaughter. They are leaner, more productive and are gradually replacing the earlier-maturing breeds.

Many European countries, and New Zealand, produce beef from the dairy herd, whose cows are selected mainly for milk production. Beef bulls on surplus heifers produce beef calves. Pure dairy calves may be raised for beef, in the UK, Ireland and New Zealand, or veal, in France and the Netherlands, or pet food, in the USA.

Modern economic pressures intensify and concentrate animal production. Many once strong local 'rare breeds' are facing extinction; in the British Isles and USA alone about 30 are listed. Their rich gene pool must be maintained so a wide genetic base will be available to accommodate future natural or market constraints on production.

Comparison of systems converting feed into saleable meat is complex. Prices of land, stock and feed change yearly. Support schemes alter markets. Health and diet are important to consumers, so a demand for 'natural' feeding has reinforced economic pressures towards increased use of grass and less use of animal-derived feeds.

Typical Production Systems

2-Year-Old Spring Born Steer (Friesian/Friesian Cross). This tightly managed semi-intensive system is suitable for northwest Europe. In February, male calves are bought and finished cattle are sold. In early April yearlings start grazing 45% of the farm; 55% is closed for silage. By mid-May the calves are grazing ahead of the yearlings. In late May silage is cut, 45% of the farm is closed for a second cut, taken in mid-July, then slurry is spread. The calves are castrated in late September. Finishing cattle are housed in mid-October, weanlings in early November.

50 cattle may be produced off 22 ha. The main inputs per animal sold per year are the 0·45 ha of productive grassland, to provide grazing and 10 tonnes of silage; the fertilizers are 110 kg of nitrogen equivalent, 41 kg of potassium, and 11 kg of phosphorus. Each animal receives 25 kg of reconstituted milk powder, roughage and concentrates *ad lib*. In the first winter the weanlings are fed silage and concentrates (150 kg). Yearlings receive 600 kg of concentrates during a 150 day finishing period.

Liveweight gains are from 0·6–0·9 kg per day. Slaughter weight (Friesian) is about 600 kg, to give a carcass of 320 kg, with about 220 kg of saleable lean beef, some 55 kg of bone and 45 kg of fat trim. Charolais × Friesian reach 680 kg, dressed 380 kg; giv-

ing 270 kg of lean meat, 60 kg of bone and 50 kg of fat trim.

Suckler Beef. This is extensive and more common on marginal land. Calves suckle dams; a 'cow unit' consists of cow, calf and yearling. Cows are cross-bred Hereford or Limousin on Friesian to give adequate milk with low maintenance requirements. Mating is to a third breed. Hereford, Aberdeen Angus or Limousin for the first calving and large breeds, Charolais or Simmental for later pregnancies.

Calving takes place in February to April. Calves grow rapidly on the milk, reaching about 300 kg at weaning in November. Each cow unit grazes 0·32 ha in April–June, with 0·45 ha reserved for silage. Then, until August, 0·48 ha is grazed; 0·29 ha is for silage. Thereafter 0·77 ha is grazed until housing in November. Silage is cut, in late May and late July, totalling 37 tonnes ha^{-1}. About 175–225 kg ha^{-1} of nitrogenous fertilizer is applied yearly.

Housed yearlings have silage *ad lib* with 1 kg per head per day of concentrates. After the second summer on grass, the heifers are slaughtered, at 20 months, in November–December, finishing on silage and 3 kg per day of concentrates. Slaughter at 500–600 kg gives carcasses of 260–330 kg. Steers are fed silage and 4 kg per day of concentrates to finish in early spring at 24 months, at a live weight of 620–680 kg and a carcass weight of 340–380 kg.

Bull Beef. In Europe, except the British Isles, most male beef cattle are bulls. From about 4 months they grow up to 8% faster than steers, giving perhaps 40 kg more carcass. Bulls kill out at about 57% (dressed weight as percentage of carcass), 2% more than comparable steers, with carcasses up to 15% heavier. About 74% of a bull's carcass is lean meat, compared to 66% for steers. Bulls have a heavier forequarter, but a higher yield of high-price cuts.

Most bull beef is from the dairy herd, being Holstein/Friesian dual-purpose and dairy beef crosses. Calves bought at 1–3 weeks of age reared to 100–150 kg on 25–50 kg of milk replacer, concentrates and roughage. Slaughter at 12 months requires a high-cereal or -fodder beet diet, giving a daily gain of 1·1–1·4 kg and a carcass weight of 180–220 kg. The meat is very pale. Slaughter at 18–21 months requires maize silage with 15–20% concentrates or beet pulp. Friesians reach 550 kg, dual-purpose and crosses may attain 600 kg.

In France, Spain and Italy the suckler herd is an important source of bull beef. 'Veau de Lyons' is Limousin, and at 12 months the slaughter weight is 450 kg; the meat is pale and not marbled. Slaughter at 18–21 months requires a diet like the dairy bull, but with more concentrates (25–30%). Carcass weights are 300–430 kg, depending on the region and breed.

Nearly all bulls are housed, usually loose in pens of 2–5 m^2 per bull with up to 25 per pen. Farmers raising bulls must ensure safety, with secure housing and fencing, warning notices, and careful work practice.

Bovine spongiform encephalopathy (BSE) is a progressive, fatal neurological disease. Since 1986 some 26 000 cases have been recorded in Britain, with sporadic cases in other countries. BSE presents, in adult dairy cows, as abnormalities of behaviour and gait. The causal agent was in meat and bone meal in concentrates fed to calves. In 1988, feeding ruminant protein to ruminants was banned, and notification and compulsory slaughter were introduced. These measures are expected to eliminate the disease by the late 1990s. There is no evidence for the transmission of BSE, or the analogous sheep 'scrapie', to human beings. *See* Bovine Spongiform Encephalopathy (BSE)

Meat Trade – Transport and Slaughter

The trade is closely controlled both nationally and internationally, e.g. by the EEC. Feeds and therapeutics must not endanger consumers' health. Cattle handling must be humane, so animals must be led, not driven, and moved in production groups with minimal goading and noise. Journeys should be short and packing must allow fallen cattle to rise. A 12 m lorry will take 22 650-kg cattle.

Humane treatment improves meat quality and reduces cross-contamination; nervous over-frequent defecation increases *Salmonella* and other infections. Lairage at the meat plant must have drinking water and shelter. Groups should not be mixed as this causes fighting. Stock must not be fed for 24 h before slaughter.

'Western' slaughter is preceded by stunning with a blow or captive bolt. The unconscious animal is hoisted by a hind-leg, over a 'bleeding trough' and 'stuck' in the arteries of the throat. Delayed sticking allows blood pressure to rise, arteries in muscles burst so meat is 'blood splashed' and unsightly at sale. *See* Meat, Slaughter

Jewish or Muslim ritual slaughter, 'kosher' or 'halal', despatches the conscious animal with one cut across the throat; slaughtermen must be licensed by the religious authorities. Bleeding-out takes about 10 min. Blood supports microbial growth and its removal is important for increasing meat shelf life.

The carcass, suspended by both hind legs, is dressed 'on the line'. A moving chain carries it past successive work stations. Hooves and head are removed. The oesophagus and rectum are tied and freed before the ventral abdominal wall is opened. The 'green offal', the alimentary tract, and the 'red offal', the heart, lungs and liver, are removed onto conveyors. All parts are inspected by veterinarians. The carcass is flayed and split with a power saw into two 'sides'. Trimming is to specifications agreed with the farmers' associations.

Sides are weighed 'hot' and graded for fatness and 'conformation' (shape) by public inspectors. Payment is generally on 'hot weight minus 2%' to accommodate evaporative weight loss in the chills. Sometimes grade will affect price.

Sides are washed and pass into the chill room about 1 h post-mortem. Chilling is mandatory. Chilling rates are determined by carcass weight and fatness and by air speed and temperature. Faster cooling facilitates throughput and reduces bacterial growth and evaporative weight loss, but is more expensive in equipment and energy. 'Cold toughening' may result if muscle cools below 10°C sooner than 10 h post-mortem.

Cutting

EEC regulations stipulate that, before cutting, sides must be chilled to below 7°C. A 140 kg side of average fatness will achieve 7°C in the centre hip, in about 32 h under air of 0°C at 1 m s^{-1}, but this rate could cause cold toughening in the 'striploin', (longissimus dorsi, LD), so a slower chilling may be required.

Chilled beef sides are 'quartered' according to local usage, often near the end of the rib cage, and go for shipping, to the boning hall or retail shops. The 'primal cuts' of the side differ slightly by country, but are based on convenient anatomical divisions, eating quality and costing.

Figure 1 shows 'London and Home Counties' cuts. Vacuum-packed, usually boneless, primals now predominate over quarters for distribution.

Beef differs in eating quality depending on the cut, the age of the animal and pre- and post-mortem handling. The relative price of sides and cuts depends chiefly on expected tenderness. Prime 2-year-old steer is more expensive than 7-year-old culled cow. Fillet (psoas major) is always tender, and is the most expensive, striploin and rump (gluteus medius) are slightly tougher, more unpredictable, and are cheaper in cost. Shin beef is cheapest of all. *B. indicus* meat is tougher than that from *B. taurus*, but breed differences are not large; reports of tougher bull meat are now attributed to faster cooling in the leaner sides.

Butchers, and customers, may identify different cuts, but once the beef is off the bone and trimmed of fat it is difficult to distinguish lean beef from, for example, adults of different ages or from fast- and slow-cooled sides. This has made beef marketing less transparent than that of other meats.

The trade has developed empirical techniques for improving quality. 'Prime beef' is from 18–36-months-old cattle. 'Ageing', holding in chill for some days, effects some improvement in tenderness, but will not make cold-toughened beef as tender as slow-cooled beef.

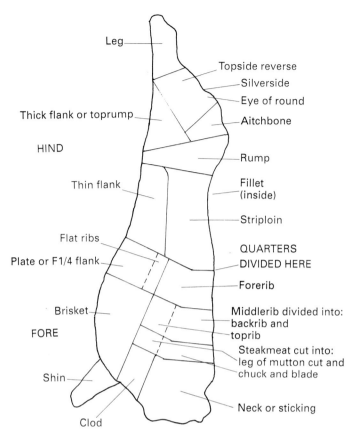

Fig. 1   'London and Home Counties' primal cuts. Adapted from Gerrard F *et al.* (1977).

Muscle biochemistry now provides explanations for much meat quality variation. In cattle, prolonged stress pre-mortem depletes muscle glycogen reserves and post-mortem production of lactic acid from glycogen is inadequate to bring the physiological pH of muscle from 7 to 5·4–5·6, the normal level 48 h after slaughter. Stressed cattle give meat of above pH 6·0 that is described as 'dark, firm and dry' (DFD). Consumers react against the darker appearance compared to the customary bright cherry-red due to oxymyoglobin at pH 5·4–5·6; the higher pH facilitates microbial spoilage. *See* Meat, Structure

Young bulls, and most cattle in the autumn, are more prone to stress and thus to produce DFD meat. Biopsies have shown that depleted muscle glycogen is not replaced in life for several days after the stress insult. Stressed cattle must be rested before slaughter. Humane handling will prevent most DFD meat.

Tenderness variation among muscles is partly due to differences in connective tissue collagen content. More collagen implies lower tenderness (Table 2(a)). Decreasing tenderness with age is due to increasing collagen molecular cross-linking. Solubility is an inverse measure of cross-linking and is less in older cattle. Table 2(b) shows that extraction, that is, solubility, of collagen falls significantly with increasing animal age.

Cold toughening seems to invoke two mechanisms.

Early exposure to a temperature of about 10°C causes the release of Ca^{2+} ions, which stimulate contraction in slack muscles like LD. As the muscle contracts into rigor, extra bonds are formed between the thick and thin filaments of the contractile myofibrils, and the strength and toughness of the meat is increased. This is 'cold shortening', and is confirmed by micrometry of the 'sarcomeres', units of the myofibrils.

Although ultra-fast cooling may enhance tenderness, normal cold inhibition of protein-splitting enzymes during the very early period, 2–4 h post-mortem, probably causes more tough beef in commerce than cold shortening. A near-physiological temperature should be maintained up to 4 h post-mortem to maximize tenderness. Lower temperatures reduce tenderness *pro rata*. Subsequent ageing at low temperature, and low pH, may not facilitate the splitting of particular protein links in the myofibrils which would be critical in providing re-entrant cracks for the breaking of connective tissue during chewing. *See* Meat, Preservation

Fillet is always consistently tender because it is low in collagen, it is stretched giving minimal thick–thin filament overlap and, being inside the rib cage under kidney fat, cools slowly.

A coherent explanation of beef tenderness is awaited; the synergy of temperature, pH and Ca^{2+} concentration in controlling enzyme activity and shortening is com-

Table 2.   Collagen and tenderness

(a) Differences between muscles

Muscle	Cut	Collagen (%)	Tenderness
Psoas major	Fillet	2·24	6·7
Longissimus dorsi	Striploin	2·76	5·2
Gluteus medius	Rump	3·64	4·5
Semimembranosus	Topside	4·09	3·3
Semitendinosus	Eye of round	4·75	3·6
Biceps femoris	Silverside	5·07	2·8

Collagen is expressed as per cent fat-free dry matter (Dransfield E, 1977). Tenderness is on a linear scale: 0, extremely tough; 8, extremely tender (Joseph RL and Connolly J, 1977).

(b) Collagen cross-linking and age

Extraction temperature of medium (°C)	Animal age groups			
	I (40–49 days)	II (403–495 days)	III (5 years)	IV (10 years)
60	544 ± 29	168 ± 10	82 ± 1	38 ± 1
70	863 ± 34	409 ± 26	171 ± 4	82 ± 1

Figures are average ± SE μg collagen extracted from samples into medium (Goll DE *et al.*, 1964).

Table 3.   Contribution of 100 g of beef to recommended daily allowances (RDAs)

Nutrient	US RDA	From Beef	% RDA
Energy	11·3 MJ	2·4 MJ	21·0
Protein	56 g	31·1 g	55·5
Calcium	800 mg	22·6 mg	2·8
Phosphorus	800 mg	312·8 mg	39·1
Iron	10 mg	4·7 mg	47·0
Magnesium	350 mg	31·7 mg	9·0
Vitamin A[a]	1000 μgRE	455 μg RE	45·5
Vitamin C	60 mg	1·16 mg	1·9
Thiamin	1·4 mg	0·50 mg	35·7
Riboflavin	1·6 mg	0·43 mg	26·9
Niacin	18 mg	7·95 mg	44·2
Vitamin B_6	2·2 mg	0·59 mg	26·8
Vitamin B_{12}	3·0 μg	5·23 μg	174·3
Folacin	400 μg	17·5 μg	4·4
Zinc	15 mg	7·1 mg	47·3
Copper	2·0–3·0 mg	0·21 mg	10·5

[a] 1 retinol equivalent (RE) = 3·3 international unit (IU) of vitamin A activity.

plex, as is the interaction of connective tissue, myofibrils and cooking.

Electrical stimulation (ES) of pre-rigor carcasses, was patented 40 years ago to improve tenderness. ES causes muscular contractions, depleting the glycogen and other energy reserves in muscles, so preventing the cold shortening of slack muscles like LD. It may toughen muscles if the concomitant fast pH fall inactivates certain proteolytic enzymes. Its effect may be compounded by the tearing of opposing simultaneously contracting muscles. The New Zealand lamb industry and the North American beef industry use ES, but it is not widely used elsewhere.

Nutritional Value

Beef is central in most societies for celebrations and family meals, but has lost a little ground to white meats recently. Beef is an excellent food, supplying most nutritional requirements save fibre (Table 3); its vitamin B_{12} content promotes vitamin absorption from other sources. The three essential unsaturated fatty acids account for 3–6% of total fatty acid in lean beef. Trace elements (iodine, manganese, zinc, cobalt, selenium, nickel, chromium, molybdenum, fluorine, vanadium, silicon, arsenic) occur in beef so a normal diet will ensure an adequate supply. *See* Meat, Dietary Importance; *see also* individual nutrients

The culinary uses of beef are numberless and it does not pall. Stock from beef and bones is the 'fond de cuisine'. The beefburger has been universally accepted by the world's youth. Charqui ('biltong'), sun-dried salted beef, provides protein and salt throughout the tropics. Salamis were developed to preserve beef, and other meats with salt and spices; now thousands of varieties are available. The 'roast beef of old England' still forms the centrepiece of state banquets. Beef is indeed the universal meat.

Bibliography

de Boer H and Martin J (eds) (1978) *Patterns of Growth and Development in Cattle.* The Hague: Martinus Nijhoff.

Dransfield E (1977) Intramuscular composition and texture of beef muscles. *Journal of the Science of Food & Agriculture* 28: 833–842.

FAO (1989) *FAO Yearbook of Production*, vol. 43. Rome: Food and Agriculture Organization.

Gerrard F, Mallion FJ and Quin (eds) (1977) *The Complete Book of Meat.* London: Virtue.

Goll DE, Hoekstra WG and Bray W (1964) Age associated changes in bovine muscle connective tissue. II. Exposure to increasing temperature. *Journal of Food Science* 29: 615–628.

James SJ and Bailey C (1990) Chilling of beef carcasses. In: Gormley TR and Zeuthen P (eds) *Chilled Foods – the Ongoing Debate.* Amsterdam: Elsevier.

Joseph RL and Connolly J (1977) The effects of suspension method, chilling rates and post mortem ageing period on beef quality. *Journal of Food Technology* 12: 231–247.

Lawrie RA (1985) *Meat Science*, 4th edn. Oxford: Pergamon.

Pearson AM (1981) Meat and health. In: Lawrie RA (ed) *Developments in Meat Science*, vol. 2, ch. 8. London: Applied Science Publishers.

Tarrant PV (1989) Animal behaviour and environment in the dark-cutting condition in beef – a review. *Irish Journal of Food Science and Technology* 13: 1–21.

Wallis D (1986) *The Rare Breeds Handbook*. Poole: Blandford.

R. L. Joseph
The National Food Centre (Teagasc), Dublin, Ireland

BEEKEEPING

See Honey

BEERS, ALES AND STOUTS

Contents

Types

Characteristics of Ales and Stouts

The main feature that differentiates ales and stouts from lagers is the fact that they use top-fermenting yeasts as opposed to bottom-fermenting yeasts. Traditionally, top fermentations take place at 15–24°C compared to 8–12°C for a typical modern lager fermentation. During the fermentation the yeast is collected and removed from the top of the fermented beer, compared to lager fermentation where the yeast collects at the bottom of the fermented beer.

Other differences between ales/stouts and lagers will be described below but, essentially the differences are due to the types of water, cereals, hops, yeast and temperature regimes encountered during production.

The following section outlines the main characteristics of a range of top-fermented beers. A summary is shown in Table 1.

Ale

The term 'ale' causes some considerable confusion. The term was used to describe all beer styles in England up until the 15th century. Flemish immigrants then started

Table 1.   Summary of typical characteristics of top-fermented beers

	Country of origin	Town of origin	Alcohol content (% ABV)	Colour (EBC)	Bitterness (EBU)	Flavour characteristics
Bitter ale	England	Various	3–5	25	30–40	Bitter, malty
Pale ale	England	Burton	5	22	25–30	Bitter, sulphury, malty
Mild ale	England	Birmingham	3–4	100	20–25	Sweet, toffee, dry
Porter	England	London	6	40–50	25–30	Rich, fruity
Scotch ale	Scotland	Edinburgh	3–7	20	20	Creamy, full
Bitter stout	Ireland	Dublin	4–5	150–200	40	Bitter, roasted, smooth
Milk stout	England	Various	2·5–3	325	20–25	Sweet
Russian stout	England	London	11	300	40	Burnt, bitter, alcoholic
Brown beers	Belgium	Various	4–6	70		Dry, sweet
Trappist/abbey beers	Belgian	Various	6–10			
Kolsch	FRG	Cologne	4	7	25–30	
Alt	FRG	Dusseldorf	4	35	32	Malty, estery
Barley wine	UK	Various	7–10	20–30	40	Alcoholic, sweet
Weisse	FRG	Berlin	4–5	10–12	25	
Weisen	FRG	Munich	2·5–3	6	20	Estery, yeasty

ABV, alcohol by volume; EBC, European Brewing Convention Units; EBU, European Brewing Convention Units.

to introduce beer produced with hops. The term 'ale' continued to describe beer produced without hops. In present times, all beers produced in the UK are made using hops and the word 'ale' is used to describe a range of products. The main categories of ale found today in the UK are as follows:

Bitter Ale

This is the commonest of the ale family in the UK. Nearly every brewery in the UK produces its own bitter ale, usually simply referred to as 'bitter'. It is the most traditional of all the beer styles produced in the UK and is the main product of most of the smaller independent breweries left in the UK. A typical bitter is produced from malted barley and sometimes cereal/sugar syrups may be used along with other cereal adjuncts. English hops are used and the overall bitterness level is relatively high compared to other beer types. The process of 'dry hopping' is also common with bitter ales. The yeast used is often a traditional strain or mixture of strains found only in that brewery. In particular, the strain of yeast used has a marked effect on the overall product, and bitters produced in the UK show a wide range of characteristics. The presentation of bitter ale in the glass also varies throughout the UK, with bitters from the north being served with 2–3 cm of head foam whilst some bitters from the south are served with little or no head foam. *See* Malt, Malt Types and Products; Malt, Chemistry of Malting

The majority of bitter served in the UK is on draught. Draught bitter is either termed 'bright' or 'cask conditioned'. Bright beer is conditioned in the brewery and is sterilized by a mixture of filtration and pasteurization before packaging the beer into kegs. Cask-conditioned beer is racked into casks whilst still retaining a proportion of live yeast. This yeast conditions the beer in the cask before serving. Connoisseurs of bitter normally prefer the cask-conditioned version and there has been a significant swing from bright bitter to cask bitter in the UK since the 1970s. However, cask beer needs careful management and handling at all stages and has a much shorter shelf life than bright bitter. This is discussed further in the section on future trends. *See* Barrels

Pale Ale

There is a certain degree of overlap between the terms 'bitter ale' and 'pale ale'. In present times, the term 'pale ale' is usually used to describe a premium bitter ale product with a typical ABV (alcohol by volume) content of about 5%. In addition, most pale ales are bottled rather than draught products. They also tend to be slightly paler in colour than bitter ales.

Because pale ales are often bottled, they tend to be 'bright beers'. There are exceptions to this, however, and Bass Worthington White Shield is a classic example of a beer conditioned in the bottle.

A small but significant proportion of pale ale produced in the UK is for export to northern Europe, in particular Belgium. In the last century a lot of pale ale was exported to India and the term 'India Pale Ale', or 'IPA', is still used today to describe some pale ales in the UK. Like bitter ale, the major ingredient in pale ale is malted barley.

Types

Mild Ale

'Mild ale' is the term used to describe a beer type that is darker, less bitter and less alcoholic than bitter ale. The level of sweetness varies and some milds can be as bitter as bitter ale. Mild tends to be a minor brand in most UK breweries, accounting for less than 5% of the total beer produced. There are, however, notable exceptions to this and some breweries in the Black Country (the Midlands) and, to a lesser extent in the northwest of England, sell as much mild ale as they do bitter ale.

Mild ale has always been considered the 'poor relation' to bitter ale and sells for a lower price.

Mild that is bottled tends to be termed 'brown ale'. Mild ale is mainly produced from malted barley. Its colour is usually derived from caramel, although dark-coloured malts may also be added.

Porter

Porter was first brewed in London in the 18th century. It was brewed to create a beer encompassing several different styles of beer popular at that time.

At the present time very little porter is brewed or drunk in Europe. A number of smaller breweries produce porter as a speciality beer. In the UK, a porter beer is now usually more alcoholic, darker and less bitter than a bitter ale and has a rich and fruity taste. Porter is produced in Sweden in bottle at 3·5% ABV.

Scotch Ale

The main markets for Scotch ale tend to be in its home market of Scotland and Belgium. In Scotland, 'Scotch ale' is a term used to cover a wide range of strengths of beer, typically from 3–5% ABV. Scotch ales brewed for sale in Belgium tend to be somewhat stronger at 5–7% ABV. Scotch ale normally has a relatively low bitterness level and lacks any marked hop character. The beer tends to be creamy and smooth. Many Scotch ales include the term 'shilling' (derived from the UK currency system pre-1971) in their names, the shilling value being related to the traditional duty system of the tax per barrel of beer brewed.

Bitter Stout

Bitter stouts are very dark (black) in colour and have a characteristic creamy head, due to dissolved nitrogen. They are brewed using roasted or black malt and have relatively high bitterness levels. Bitter stout originates from Ireland where several well-known brands, including Guinness, are brewed to an alcohol content of 4–5% ABV. Bitter stout is also popular in the Caribbean and various parts of Africa where the alcohol contents are typically 7–8% ABV. Bitter stouts tend to be very full bodied, bitter with a dry, sometimes burnt, palate and very smooth.

Sweet Stout

Sweet stout is still produced in the UK in small quantities. The alcohol content tends to be lower than for bitter stout at 3–5% ABV. The fermentation of sweet stout is stopped early and the beer is also often sweetened by sugar addition before leaving the brewery. Both these factors result in a sweet palate in the final product.

Russian Stout

Russian stout is rarely brewed at present and tends only to be found as a bottled speciality beer. The beer was first brewed in the 18th century and exported to the Baltic region. Russian stout has an alcohol content of about 10% ABV and is rich, fruity and bitter in taste.

Barley Wine

Barley wine is a term given to a family of strong beers of 7–10% ABV brewed in the UK. Most barley wines are bottled but some may be served in small measures on draught. Barley wines vary in colour and character but tend to be relatively dark and sweet. Some barley wines are only brewed around Christmas time and are termed 'winter warmers'.

Trappist/Abbey Beers

Trappist beers are brewed at six breweries in Europe, five of which are in Belgium. Trappist beers are relatively strong (6–10% ABV) and can vary in colour from copper to dark brown. Trappist beers tend to be full flavoured and well hopped. Abbey beers are based on existing or monastic recipes, but are brewed under licence in conventional breweries. Because of this, the quality perception by Belgian consumers of abbey beers is lower than that of Trappist beers, which outsell the abbey beers by over two to one.

Lambic/Fruit Beers

Lambic/fruit beers are derived from wheat beer. The beer is matured for varying lengths of time and contains a rich flora of naturally occurring microorganisms. Cherries are added to produce a derivative known as kriek beer. These beers are an acquired taste and tend to be sharp, acidic, fruity and sometimes fizzy due to the bacterial fermentation occurring within the beer. The beer is typically 5–8% ABV.

Brown Beers

Brown beer (ambree) is a popular speciality beer in Belgium. These beers can be similar in character to UK brown ale (see above) but can be stronger at up to 7%

Table 2.   UK beer sales from 1987 to 1990 and forecast from 1991 to 1995

Year	Total beer market (million barrels)	Total change (%)	Ale/stout volume (million barrels)	Ale/stout market share (%)	Ale/stout change in market share (%)
1987–1988	39·11	+2·1	20·72	53	−2
1988–1989	38·89	−0·6	19·90	51·1	−4
1989–1990	38·73	−0·4	19·05	49·2	−4·3
1990–1991	37·27	−3·8	17·60	47·2	−7·5
1991–1992	37·07	−0·6	16·97	45·8	−3·6
1992–1993	36·59	−1·3	16·32	44·6	−3·8
1993–1994	36·55	−0·1	15·90	43·5	−2·6
1994–1995	36·49	−0·2	15·48	42·4	−2·6

ABV. Levels of sweetness tend to vary between different brands.

Alt Beer

Alt beer typically has a bitter taste and a malty aroma. It is usually a red/bronze colour similar to a bitter ale although some varieties have colours more associated with a lager beer. The alcohol content tends to lie between 3·8 and 4·2% ABV. Most Alt beer (90%) is brewed and consumed in the Dusseldorf area of the FRG.

Kolsch Beer

Kolsch beer is mainly produced in the Cologne area of the FRG. It has a similar colour to Pils and an alcohol content of about 3·7% ABV.

Wheat Beers

Wheat beers are produced by top fermentation and hence are included in this section. There are various types of wheat beer available, ranging in alcohol content from 2·5 to 5% ABV. Wheat beers tend to be lightly hopped and fruity with a relatively delicate but very characteristic palate. Examples are weizen beers originating from Bavaria in the FRG with a typical alcohol content of 3·4–4·4% ABV, weisse beer from Berlin in the FRG with an alcohol content of 2·5–3% ABV and 'white' beer now produced in Belgium with an alcohol content of about 5% ABV. Wheat beers are often served with a dash of fruit juice. Wheat beers are produced both with and without yeast present in the final product.

Low-Alcohol/Nonalcoholic Beers

Low-alcohol and nonalcoholic beers are brewed using various techniques by which alcohol formation is restricted or alcohol is removed from the beer. Legislation throughout the world and even within Europe varies on the definition of what constitutes a low-alcohol and nonalcoholic beer.

Types

In the UK a nonalcoholic beer has an alcoholic content of less than 0·05% ABV and a low-alcohol beer has an ABV% of less than 1·2% ABV.

Production Statistics and Future Trends

Throughout Europe, the total volumes of top-fermented beers are decreasing as overall beer consumption slowly declines and consumers continue to switch from top-fermented beers to bottom-fermented lagers.

This trend is clearly shown in the UK (see Table 2) and is expected to continue into the mid-1990s.

Each type of beer will be considered in turn below.

Bitter Ale

Sales of bitter ale are declining in the UK. Table 3 shows the decline since 1982. Table 4 shows that the premium end of the market is holding up better than the standard end. A significant recent trend has been a swing from keg bitter to cask-conditioned bitter. This trend started in the 1970s and, currently, about 60% of draught bitter in the UK in cask conditioned. Sales of canned bitter, particularly at the premium end of the market are showing a slow growth in market share while bottled bitter shows a steady decline.

Pale Ale

As mentioned previously, there is some overlap between pale ale and premium bitter ale described above. Generally, sales of bottled pale ale are declining as bottled ale sales in general reduce. The export market for pale ale, particularly Belgium, is also declining. Exports of pale ale from the UK to Belgium in 1989 were only 47% of the level exported in 1981. This is due in large part to local brewing of pale ale in Belgium. The only real growth in this market is for premium canned pale ales, which form a relatively small portion of the overall pale ale market.

Table 3. Percentage market share of ales/stouts from 1982 to 1989

	1982	1983	1984	1985	1986	1987	1988	1989
Draught bitter, pale ale, stout	47·1	45·2	43·4	41·8	39·8	37·7	36·3	34·8
Draught mild	8	7·3	6·9	6·4	5·9	5·3	4·9	4·4
Bottled bitter/pale ale	3·6	3·5	3·5	3·3	3·3	3·3	3·1	2·95
Canned bitter/pale ale	3·8	4·2	4	4·1	4·2	4·3	4·4	4·6
Bottled/canned brown ale	1	0·9	0·7	0·7	0·6	0·6	0·5	0·4
Bottled/canned stout	2·6	2·3	2·1	2·1	2	1·8	1·7	1·8
Barley wine	0·4	0·4	0·4	0·4	0·4	0·3	0·3	0·24
Low-alcohol and nonalcoholic beer	—	—	—	0·2	0·3	0·6	1·1	1·1
Total market share (%)	66·5	63·8	61	59	56·5	53·9	52·3	50·4

Source: Brewer's Society.

Table 4. UK draught beer sales in 1990 (market share expressed as percentage of on-trade sales)

Product	ABV	Current market share (%)	Volume (million barrels)	Change in market share 1990–1991
Standard bitter	3·8	33·0	12·5	−4
Premium bitter	5·8	7·6	2·9	−1
Stout	4·5	4·6	1·7	+8
Mild	3·5	7·7	2·9	−5
Total		52·9	20·0	

Mild Ale

Table 3 shows how draught mild in the UK has declined from 8% of the total UK market in 1982 to half that in 1989. Table 4 shows that the mild market share fell by 5% in 1990. Brown ales show a similar trend (see Table 3). The only area of the UK where mild sales remain relatively stable is in the Midlands.

Porter

Volumes of porter brewed in Europe are currently minimal. A number of small independent breweries in the UK product porter as a speciality brew. A bottled 3·5% ABV alcohol version of porter is produced in Sweden. No market forecasts on porter sales are currently available.

Scotch Ale

Sales of Scotch ale are currently in decline. In its home market in Scotland there is a strong trend towards lager drinking. Exports of Scotch ale to Belgium have fallen by 50% over the last 10 years.

Bitter Stout

Sales of bitter stout are currently enjoying a revival in the UK market. Table 4 shows the draught stout market share up by 8% in 1990. These sales are shared between three leading brands, all of Irish origin, although two are now brewed in the UK. Guinness has about 86% of the draught bitter stout market in the UK.

Table 3 shows that bottled stout sales have declined since 1982. A recent recovery of the packaged stout is currently being driven by 'draught in can' versions of bitter stout which recreate a draught character product in the can by using nitrogen injection.

In other parts of the world, draught stout, particularly Guinness, holds a significant market share, especially in Africa and the Caribbean. The potential for selling bitter stout into the European 'speciality' market is also starting to be realized.

Sweet Stout

Most sweet stout in the UK is sold in packaged form. Table 3 shows the decline in sales from 1982. This rate of decline is expected to continue.

Russian Stout

Russian stout is now only brewed in very small quantities for the speciality beer market and packaged in bottles. There is no evidence for a sales recovery of this beer as the consumer switches to products of a lighter colour and lower alcohol content.

Barley Wine

Most barley wine is sold in bottled form. Table 3 shows how sales have declined since 1982. This rate of decline is expected to continue.

Trappist/Abbey Beers

The speciality beer market in Belgium is the one growing sector in an otherwise stagnant market and, as such, Trappist and abbey beers are showing small but significant growth.

Total production volumes of Trappist and abbey beers are about 600,000 hl per annum with both types of beer produced in equal amounts. Whereas most of the Trappist beer is consumed in Belgium, about 50% of abbey beer is exported. Together, Trappist and abbey beers make up nearly 4% of the Belgian market.

Lambic/Fruit Beers

These beers are included in the Belgian speciality market. Gueuze beer currently has about 2·9% of the Belgian market whilst acides beer (fruit beer) has 1·4%. Total production volume for beer in this category is just over 500 000 hl per annum, most of which is consumed in Belgium.

Brown Beers (Ambree)

Ambree beers are the largest contributor to the Belgian speciality market. About 854 000 hl are produced annually. Sales are showing modest growth in line with the rest of the speciality market.

Alt Beer

About 6 million hl of Alt beer are produced annually. Alt beer showed tremendous growth during the 1970s, increasing volume of sales by 50% between 1970 and 1983. Sales have currently levelled out. The majority of alt beer is consumed in the Dusseldorf area. Efforts are now being made to market the product in other areas of the FRG, which could provide further growth in the future.

Kolsch Beer

Over the last 20 years, sales of Kolsch beer have increased 10-fold to a current level of 3·5 million hl per annum. Sales are split equally between draught and bottle which is unusual for FRG beers. Sales volumes of Kolsch were 12% up in 1990 compared to 1989.

Wheat Beers

Sales of weizen beer have doubled in the last 5 years to about 7 million hl per annum, giving it a national market share of 8% in the FRG. About 90% of weizen beer is sold in bottles. Sales are still increasing, with Bavaria being the strongest market.

Sales of weisse beer from Berlin have shown a gradual decline over the last 5 years and are currently around 100 000 hl per annum.

A potential market for wheat beers outside the FRG is apparent and sales of 'white' beer in Belgium are showing strong growth from a small base.

Low-Alcohol/Nonalcoholic Beers

These beers have showed tremendous growth from a zero base since 1985. The sales growth now appears to have levelled off, some way short of original expectations. As brewing technology advances to produce a closer match to its full strength counterpart, sales are expected to increase gradually.

The majority of these beers in Europe are based on bottom-fermented lagers, although some low-alcohol bitter ale products are available in the UK, mainly in bottles.

Bibliography

Baille F (1974) *Bristol Brewers and Beer Types, The Drinkers Companion*. David and Charles (Holding).

De Clerck J (1957) *A Textbook of Brewing*, vols 1 and 2. London: Chapman and Hall.

Hough JS, Briggs DE and Stevens R (1982) *Malting and Brewing Science*, vols 1 and 2. London: Chapman and Hall.

Jackson M (1982) *The World Guide to Beer*. Burlington Books.

Lloyd Hind H (1950) *Brewing Science and Practice*, vols 1 and 2. London: Chapman and Hall.

Pollock JRA (ed.) (1980) *Brewing Science*, vols 1–3. London: Academic Press.

S. Oakland
Courage Ltd – Brewing, Reading, UK

Preparation of Wort

Wort Production

During the wort production, raw materials are taken into the brewery and converted into a sterile nutrient solution capable of supporting yeast fermentation. The basic raw materials and principles of extract production are similar for ales, stouts and lagers, but traditionally there were differences in plant and procedures, largely to accommodate the differences in quality of the raw materials for lager and ale production, particularly the

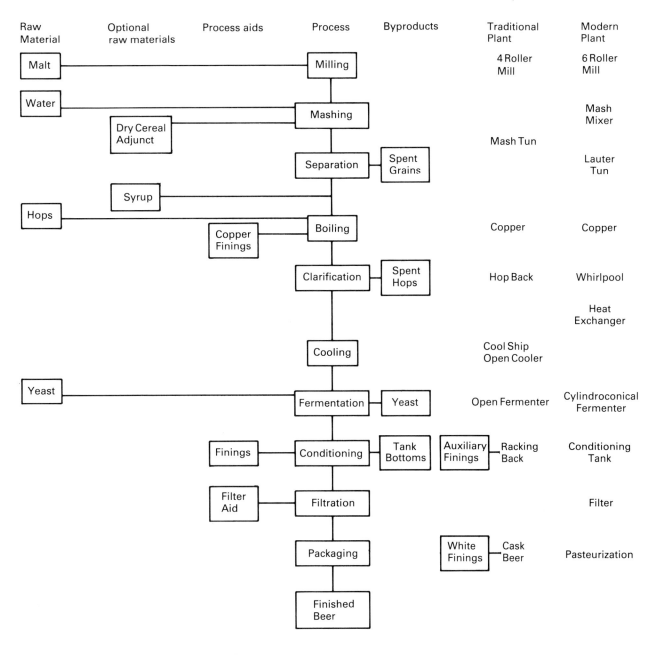

Fig. 1   Schematic of ale brewing process.

malt used. These are summarized in the schematic of the brewing process (Fig. 1). Traditional ale and stout production methods are largely restricted to the UK and Ireland, with a few other countries producing specialist beers. The UK now produces substantial amounts of lager and many plants are adapted to produce both types of beer side by side.

Raw Materials

Water is the principal raw material, accounting for 95% of beer volume. The mineral content of brewing water

has long been recognized as making an important contribution to the flavour of the beer. Historically this has played a key role in determining the location of breweries specializing in producing different types of beer (see Table 1). Burton-on-Trent became famous for pale ales, while Dublin is famous for stouts, whereas places with water with a low ionic concentration, such as Pilsen, specialized in lager production. Now the composition of brewing water can be determined scientifically and can be adjusted to brew any style of beer anywhere.

Malt, the next major ingredient, is made from barley varieties especially selected for their brewing properties.

Preparation of Wort

Table 1.   The ionic composition of various brewing waters (ppm)

Town	Type of beer	Na^+	Mg^{2+}	Ca^{2+}	Cl^-	SO_4^{2-}	HCO_3^-
Burton	Pale ale	54	24	352	16	820	320
Dublin	Dry stout	12	4	119	19	54	319
London	Porters and stouts	24	14	90	18	58	123
Pilsen	Light lager	32	8	7	5	6	37

The barley is malted, a process designed to release the enzymes necessary for converting the starch granules in the barley into sugar. The degree to which the barley corn structure is degraded is called modification, and traditional ale and stout brewers require well-modified malt. Malt provides many of the flavour components in the beer and also provides the brewer with a starch source capable of being broken down into fermentable and nonfermentable sugars. It is also a source of protein products for yeast nutrition and foam production. Much of the colour of beer is derived from the malt, which is determined during the kilning process. In addition to standard ale malt, there is a variety of speciality malts, which are made by applying additional heat during the normal kilning process, by roasting after normal kilning or by 'stewing' the malt during the early part of kilning. The effect of these treatments is to produce a darker malt which not only adds colour, but also contributes to the flavour, smoothness, fermentation, foam and stability of the product. Typical examples of these malts are given below:

- Crystal malt (colour 140 EBC). A sweet, caramel-flavoured malt where the starch is crystallized into sugar during kilning.
- Black/roasted malt (colour 1300 EBC). Produced by roasting normal specification malt; for use in dark beers and stouts to give colour and roasted flavour.
- Roasted barley (colour 1400 EBC). Not a malt, but made directly by roasting barley; it gives a unique colour and flavour to stouts, with a flavour similar to dark roasted coffee beans, giving a smooth taste.
- Amber malt (colour 55 EBC). Produced from light roasting of pale ale malt; gives a warm biscuit flavour and a golden colour to the beer. *See* Malt, Malt Types and Products; Malt, Chemistry of Malting

Other cereals, referred to as 'adjuncts', can also be used as a source of extract, replacing part of the extract which would normally have come from the malt. In order to be used in the mash tun the adjuncts must be pregelatinized or added as brewing syrup directly to the copper (the boiling vessel).

Hops (*Humulus lupulus*)

Hops are the dried flowers (specifically the cones derived from the inflorescence) of the female hop plants, which are grown on a climbing stem in a similar manner to grapes or runner beans. Hops are cultivated in a variety of temperate parts of the world solely for the use of the brewing industry.

The cone contains the lupulin gland which holds the hop character, while the rest of the leaf material is used in a traditional brewery as a natural filter bed to retain the hot trub in a hop back. The addition of hops has the following effects:

(1) provides the beer with a bitter taste;
(2) gives hop aroma to the beer;
(3) promotes head formation and retention;
(4) promotes shelf life through its antiseptic action (particularly for cask beers);
(5) modifies yeast performance during fermentation;
(6) aids protein coagulation during the boil;
(7) acts as a filter medium in the hop back.

The bitterness from the hops gives beer its characteristic flavour which sets it apart from other malt drinks. The bitterness potential of hops is derived from the α-acids, which are usually present at between 4 and 14% of the total weight of the cone.

The α-acids require to be chemically changed or 'isomerized' before they can be extracted and give their bitter tastes. This occurs normally during wort boiling. The utilization rate is relatively poor in that between 20 and 40% of the total α-acids available ends up in the beer, (this largely depends on the wort boiling procedure used). In general it takes up to 60 min to achieve the optimum hop utilization during the wort boil; therefore when adding kettle hops (hops added just minutes before the end of boil) only a proportion of the available bitterness will be recovered.

The essential oils or aroma compounds of certain hops can provide a delicate fragrance to beer to create an interesting and very fresh aroma; however, during the course of boiling many of the volatile compounds are lost. Hence special procedures such as adding hops at the end of boil, called kettle hopping, have to be adopted in order to retain the volatile hop character. *See* Essential Oils, Properties and Uses

Grist Preparation

Since only a few breweries still have maltings on the brewery site, most malt is delivered to the brewery in sacks or in bulk vehicles for storage in silos. Between malt intake and milling, the malt has to be screened to remove unwanted materials such as dust, stones and metal objects which would interfere with milling performance and could cause damage to the rollers, including the risk of explosion.

The principal objectives of malt milling are:

(1) To split the malk husk longitudinally to expose the starchy endosperm, while at the same time maintaining husk integrity to aid wort separation.
(2) To crush the endosperm, making its contents accessible to enzyme action.
(3) To keep the amount of fine particles (flour) to a minimum to avoid clogging the bed during wort separation.

Different types of mills have been developed to meet the requirements of different types of wort separation systems and to accommodate malts with different degrees of modification. Most mills used in breweries are roller mills, which rely on a mixture of direct pressure and shear forces to crack the malt. The composition and grind of the malt will influence the particle size distribution and hence its suitability as a filter bed: if it is too fine it can result in a poor wort separation rate; if it is too coarse then the full extract potential of the malt will not be recovered.

Four-roller Mill

These are the traditional mills favoured for well-modified malts, usually used in conjunction with a mash tun. They consist of two pairs of smooth or slightly fluted rollers with gaps of approximately 1·2 mm for the top pair of rollers and 0·8 mm for the bottom pair.

Six-roller Mill

This mill was developed for the less well-modified lager malts, where a finer grind is required to release the full extract contained in the malt. These mills involve effective separation and differential size reduction; the output from each roller is sieved and separated with only the appropriate section of grist going onto the next pair of rollers. In this way it is possible to maintain the integrity of the husk, while producing a finely ground

endosperm. A typical roller setting would be: top pair, 1·2 mm; middle pair, 0·95 mm; and bottom rollers, 0·6 mm.

Malt Conditioning

The effectiveness of both the four- and six-roller mills may be enhanced by warm water or steam (steep) conditioning of the malt, where about 1·2% additional moisture is added almost entirely to the husk on the way to the mill a few minutes before crushing, making the husk more pliable and hence less likely to shatter.

Wet Milling

The idea of malt conditioning is carried a stage further in wet milling, which involves presteeping the malt for about 20 min before milling, so that both the husk and the endosperm become saturated with 25–30% moisture. The wet malt is then passed through a single pair of rollers with a gap setting of 0·4 mm, and the endosperm is squeezed out of the husk, leaving the husk almost entirely intact. Although wet milling is used by a number of ale brewers, steep conditioning has found little application in ale brewing.

Starch Hydrolysis

During mashing, the ground malt is mixed with water at a precise temperature and allowed to stand, thus permitting the natural enzymes in the grain to continue breaking down the starch, a process which was initiated during the germination stage of malting and which was suspended during kilning.

In well-modified malts (malts where the enzymatic conversion is allowed to proceed throughout the entire grain) there is a much higher breakdown of structure, with as much as 60% of the protein breakdown occurring during malting. With poorly modified malts there is very little structural modification in malting, and this has to be completed by a proteolytic stand in the mashing vessel before saccharification can occur.

The malt can be considered as a package of enzymes awaiting the optimum mashing conditions to carry out its work. The extent of the enzyme breakdown can be controlled by varying factors such as time, temperature, pH and calcium salt concentration, to determine the extent of the starch degradation and hence the fermentability of the worts produced. Each enzyme has an optimum working temperature (see Table 2).

The principle saccharification enzymes are α-amylase and β-amylase, which break the α-1,4 links present in amylose and the unbranched parts of amylopectin, the

Table 2.   Upper limits of thermal activity of malt enzymes

Malt enzyme	Upper thermal limit (°C)
Proteases (hydrolyses proteins to amino acids)	58
β-Glucanase (breaks down gummy β-glucans into short chains)	62
β-Amylase (attacks the end of starch chains to yield maltose)	64
α-Amylase (random hydrolysis of starches to dextrins)	68

two polymeric sugars present in starch. α-Amylase hydrolyses the starch chain at random, while β-amylase breaks off maltose units starting from the reducing end of the starch molecule. Neither enzyme can break down the α-1,6 links, leaving unfermentable branched higher sugars in the wort which are called dextrins.

Although the structure of the corn is altered by malting, very little of the starch itself is broken down, with the starch being stored in granules in the endosperm. Before the enzymes can attack the starch it has to be gelled, which occurs in malt at a temperature of 62–64°C; this temperature must be exceeded prior to the enzymatic degradation of the starch granules.

Isothermal Mashing

Traditionally in the UK, brewers have been fortunate in having well-modified malts, and are able to select a single mashing temperature of 65°C, which is called 'isothermal (or same-temperature) mashing', and mash directly into a single vessel which is also used for wort separation, called a mash tun. The single temperature selected is above malt starch gelatinization temperatures, being in the optimum range for α- and β-amylase activity. This temperature is too high for very much proteolytic activity, and maltsters are relied upon to provide most of the proteolysis – producing up to 60% of the nitrogen compounds present in the worts.

It is also traditional to mash with a low ratio of water to malt of around 2–2·5 litres of water to 1 kg of crushed malt; this is usually referred to as the liquor-to-grist ratio. The thicker the mash, the greater the stability of the more heat-labile enzymes, and hence, at the usual temperature of 65°C, there may be a marginal improvement in proteolytic activity, but a marked improvement in β-amylase activity and that of other enzymes which are operating outside their optimum temperature range.

To achieve a temperature of 65°C in the mash tun requires a strike, or water, temperature of around 68°C, depending on ambient conditions. After the initial mashing, the mash is allowed to rest for between 1 and 2 h, depending on malt quality and the requirements of the brewer, or at least until all the starch has been converted. At the end of the mash stand no starch should remain, as this will present major problems in clarifying the beer.

In other parts of Europe and North America where the malts are not so well modified, the mashing procedures have to be optimized to encourage protein breakdown before the gelatinization of the starch. This is accomplished through a series of temperature rises and stands conducted in a separate mash mixing vessel. The initial mashing temperature will provide a protein hydrolysis stand before the temperature is raised gradually to between 76 and 78°C, after which the contents of the mash mixer are transferred to the lauter tun for wort run-off. This temperature rise effectively halts most enzyme activity, in particular that of β-amylase, which would otherwise continue to produce more fermentable sugars. In contrast, the mash in a mash tun is not heated after the mash conversion stand, and hence conversion continues during the run-off. Therefore, for a similar malt, a more fermentable wort will be produced using a mash tun as opposed to a mash mixer and lauter tun, because conversion is allowed to occur over a longer period.

A large volume of ales produced in the UK use Continental-style brewhouses, where the malt is mashed into the mash mixing vessel at 65°C and going through a final temperature raise to 78°C before being transferred to the lauter tun for run-off.

Wort Separation

Compared with the complex biochemical changes which occur during mash preparation, wort separation is a relatively simple procedure, involving the filtration of the converted sugar through a filter bed made up of the insoluble malt husks, to produce a clear wort. Once most of the dense sugar solution has been extracted, then further hot water, at a temperature of between 76 and 78°C, called 'sparge', is sprayed onto the top of the mash bed to aid the extraction of the rest of the sugars. The amount of sugar present in the wort is measured as specific gravity multiplied by 1000, commonly referred to as the original gravity. The wort run-off and sparging usually continues until the required original gravity is achieved in the copper, or until the gravity of the solution leaving the mash tun has fallen below 1004, whichever comes first.

Filtration of the wort is usually the slowest procedure

in the brewhouse, and involves straining the wort through a bed made up of husk material, which retains the solids. The flow rate has to be controlled to maintain the flow of wort through the grain bed without clogging or setting the bed. In the traditional ale brewhouse, this process is carried out in the same mash tun as is used for mashing. Mashing-in is usually via a coarse screw called a 'Steele's masher', which introduces air into the coarse grist along with the mashing water. Mashing-in, coupled with the high original gravity of the wort resulting from the low water to grist ratio, causes the bulk of mash in a mash tun to float; hence, most of the sugar extraction is by diffusion along a liquid density gradient. In contrast, ales which are mashed into a mash mixing vessel are transferred to the lauter tun for wort separation where the mash sits on the lauter tun plates, due to lower levels of entrained air and lower mash gravities, and where sugar extraction is by leaching. Mechanical arms called 'rakes' are used to maintain the porosity of the grain bed.

Whichever system is used, there is a need to produce clear wort to ensure both the flavour and stability of the beer and adequate fining performance for cask-conditioned beers.

Wort Boiling

The stability of ales is largely determined during the course of the wort boiling process. For cask-conditioned beers this is the major area for protein removal and beer stabilization, since fermentation is not followed by cold conditioning and filtration. Any problems which arise through inadequate boiling persist into the finished beer and cannot be easily rectified at a later processing stage.

Other reasons for wort boiling include:

(1) evaporating water (i.e. increasing original gravity);
(2) terminating enzyme action;
(3) sterilizing the wort;
(4) removing unwanted, harmful, volatile flavours;
(5) encouraging wort colour production;
(6) isomerizing (making soluble) the bitter (alpha) hop acids;
(7) reducing wort pH;
(8) coagulating large protein/polypeptide molecules to form insoluble particles called 'hot break' which would otherwise promote haze in finished beer.

It is essential to promote a vigorous boil of at least one hour's duration to ensure the right conditions for protein coagulation before a gentle transfer of the worts to the hopback or whirlpool.

The vigour of the boil is traditionally related to the heat input to the wort, which is reflected by the amount of evaporation, for traditional ales 10% evaporation is considered necessary. Heat transfer falls off as the heating surfaces become fouled with each successive brew, and to achieve consistently good breaks it is necessary to ensure good heat transfer which, for most conventional coppers, will require a full caustic clean at least every third to fourth brew.

Wort Clarification and Wort Cooling

After the wort has been boiled, but before the yeast can be added at the beginning of the fermentation, three steps have to be completed:

(1) The excess protein/tannin compounds in the wort will precipitate out and should be removed.
(2) The wort has to be cooled from boiling point to the temperature required at the start of fermentation, usually between 14°C to 20°C depending on the type of beer being produced.
(3) The wort has to be aerated to encourage healthy yeast growth.

Wort produced from the brewhouse is an ideal growth medium for yeast and other micro-organisms. After the boil the wort is sterile, but as soon as it is cooled to 30°C or below, it can be readily infected by beer and wort spoilage organisms. It is therefore essential that the processes described above are carried out under the most hygienic conditions.

When leaf hops are used these have to be removed in either a 'hop back', which is a similar vessel to a mash tun, where the hops form a bed through which the wort is strained and which also filters out the coagulated solids, or through a screw conveyor, which presses the hops and squeezes out the wort. When pelletized hops are used, or after going through the screw conveyor the wort is introduced tangentially to a whirlpool vessel where centrifugal force causes the hop debris and coagulated proteins called 'trub' to spin to the centre and settle after about 30 min, thus enabling clear wort to be drawn from above the trub level. On cooling there is a second precipitation of insoluble protein called the 'cold break', which is largely proteinaceous. The volume of cold break can be reduced with improved trub separation.

It is better to avoid trub carryover where possible since excess carryover causes fouling on the cooling surfaces and dirty yeast heads where more than 15% of the vessel surface is covered with a greenish-brown crust. It also tends to impart a sulphury aroma to the beer.

Following clarification the wort passes into wort cooling. The most common cooler is a counter-current plate heat-exchanger using water as the cooling medium. The hot water thus generated is then used in the brewhouse for mashing.

Some traditional breweries still use large open coolers

called 'coolships' or open coolers. As well as cooling the beer 'cold break' settles to the bottom of the cooling vessel where it is left behind on transfer thus reducing the quantity of cold break being carried forward into the fermenter.

At this stage air or oxygen is added to achieve a dissolved wort oxygen level of between 6 and 12 ppm before the wort proceeds to the fermentation stage.

Bibliography

De Clerck J (1957) *A Textbook of Brewing*, vols 1 and 2. London: Chapman and Hall.
Hough JS, Briggs DE and Stevens R (1982) *Malting and Brewing Science*, vols 1 and 2. London: Chapman and Hall.
Lloyd Hind H (1950) *Brewing Science and Practice*, vols 1 and 2. London: Chapman and Hall.
Pollock JRA (ed.) (1980) *Brewing Science*, vols 1–3. London: Academic Press.

T. O'Rourke
Courage Ltd – Brewing, Reading, UK

Fermentation Systems

Fermentation is perhaps the most critical stage in the whole of the brewing process and has a major influence on the flavour characteristics of the final product. During fermentation, wort is turned into beer by live yeast, which carries out a series of complex biochemical reactions which not only produce alcohol from sugar, but a variety of other flavour compounds in smaller quantities which determine the overall character and flavour of the product. It is the subtle balance and quantities of these flavour compounds which help to distinguish the many and varied types of beer. Each brewery will use its own strain of yeast which will be slightly different to any other brewing yeast. Each yeast has its own characteristics which help to create a unique blend of flavours for each brewery's beer.

In simplified terms the main biochemical reaction which converts sugars in the wort to alcohol to produce beer is given in eqn [1].

$$C_6H_{12}O_6 \longrightarrow 2\,CO_2 \quad + 2\,C_2H_5OH$$

| Glucose | Carbon dioxide | Ethanol | (1) |

Every molecule of glucose or an equivalent produces two molecules of ethanol (alcohol) and two molecules of carbon dioxide. Some of the carbon dioxide gas dissolves in the beer, and the remainder being lost to the atmosphere or collected for use in the later stages of the brewing process.

Having stressed the critical nature of fermentation

whereby yeast is used to turn wort into beer, the factors affecting yeast behaviour can now be discussed in order to demonstrate how yeast is controlled in order to produce a beer of both consistant quality and character.

Fermentation Conditions and Yeast Characteristics

Oxygen is required by yeast to synthesize certain sterol compounds which are an integral part of the yeast cell membrane. During a normal top fermentation, three to five times as much yeast as originally added will be produced. This magnitude of yeast replication is necessary to ferment the wort to the desired level in a standard time. Failure to add sufficient oxygen results in poor yeast growth and both slower fermentation times and a failure to achieve the correct alcohol level.

Oxygen is added to the wort on the cold side of the heat exchangers, typically in the range 5–15 mg l^{-1}. Oxygen levels are obtained using pure oxygen or compressed air, which is injected into the wort stream. Different strains of yeast have different oxygen requirements to achieve the same degree of replication. It is vital that the oxygen requirements of the yeast are known, either by laboratory analysis or by practical experience, such that the oxygen level in the wort matches the yeast's oxygen requirement. Yeast in a good physiological state will rapidly take up the oxygen, such that up to 15 mg l^{-1} will be completely removed after 2–3 h in the fermentation vessel.

Temperature Control

Generally, the temperature of the wort prior to yeast addition is in the range 15–17°C, which is achieved by control of the heat exchangers. After the yeast is added, heat generated during fermentation causes the temperature to rise, typically to 20°C and, in some instances, to 22°C in ales and up to 26°C in stouts. Higher temperatures tend to have deleterious effects on the physiological state of the yeast, and hence give rise to poor flavour. In modern, temperature-controlled, fermentation vessels, the maximum temperature to be achieved is preset, and a system of probes monitor temperatures constantly and open and close cooling jackets to keep the beer at the desired temperature. In open vessels, temperature control is affected by passing cool water through attemperating coils in the fermentation vessel. This is less sophisticated, and the fermentation temperature tends to be controlled by normal ambient temperatures such that fermentations are warmer in summer and colder in winter, and therefore less control is exerted. When fermentation is complete the beer is cooled to 10°C, and often to 3°C in a modern system, to help yeast settlement and help prevent damage to the yeast.

Yeast Addition

The amount of yeast added should be controlled as this has a major influence on fermentation performance. Generally, the yeast addition rate or pitching rate is 0·15–0·3 kg of pressed yeast per hectolitre, which equates to 5–10×10^6 yeast cell per millilitre. The higher the rate, the faster the fermentation will proceed. It is vital that the yeast is properly dispersed throughout the wort in order for fermentation to proceed correctly.

During fermentation the yeast grows and multiplies, forming new yeast cells. During the first 8–10 h, the yeast does not increase in number and is in the lag phase. Here the yeast firstly takes up oxygen in the wort and adapts to its new surroundings. After 10 h the yeast starts to form buds, which eventually grow into new cells. This phase is called the exponential or growth phase, during which cell numbers increase from 10×10^6 to 50×10^6 cells per millilitre. As the yeast metabolizes the sugars the growth rate slows and eventually ceases, and the yeast enters the stationary phase. One key characteristic of brewing yeast behaviour is the ability to flocculate. At the onset of the stationary phase, the yeast cells clump together – i.e. flocculate. The aggregation of cells into clumps causes them to rise to the top of the fermentation vessel. The size of the clumps formed varies between yeast strains, some being more flocculant than others. In fact, brewing yeasts can be classified into four distinct groups depending on the degree of flocculation exhibited. Flocculation is genetically determined, but it is also influenced by environmental conditions. The production process in one particular brewery will have been developed to fit in with the flocculation behaviour of the yeast or yeasts used in that particular brewery. In traditional plants, the yeast will, in fact, be a mixture of up to six strains of yeast; which makes control of the process more difficult. Modern plants use a single strain of yeast, which will invariably have been isolated from the original mixture of strains. *See* Flocculation

Fermentation Monitoring

The most common way of monitoring a fermentation is by measuring the specific gravity. During the course of a fermentation, the specific gravity decreases as carbon dioxide is lost from the beer and alcohol is formed. The specific gravity is measured by withdrawing samples every 4 or 8 h to verify that the process is proceeding as expected. Any slight deviations can be corrected early in the fermentation to give production consistency. The fermentation profile of a typical ale with an original gravity of 1040 and a final gravity of 1010 is illustrated in Fig. 1. Generally, an ale fermentation takes 48 h to reach one-third of its original gravity and then a further

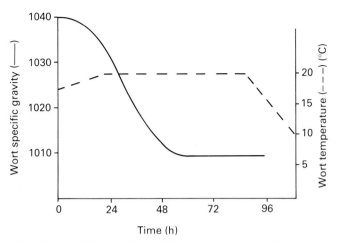

Fig. 1   Specific gravity profile of a top fermentation.

24 h to reach its final gravity. The beer may then spend another 48 h in the vessel, during which time it is cooled to allow further yeast cropping before moving to the maturation stage.

Traditional Top-fermentation Systems

Traditionally, ales and stouts are produced by a top-fermentation system. The yeast used is a species called *Saccharomyces cerevisiae*, and its main characteristic is that it rises to the top during fermentation, forming a thick creamy head which is supported by carbon dioxide gas evolving from the fermenting beer below. This makes the system distinctly different from lager fermentations, which use a bottom-fermenting or sedimentary yeast which sinks to the bottom of the vessel during fermentation. This key difference in yeast behaviour accounts for some of the operational and plant differences encountered in top fermentations which have evolved to suit the behaviour of the yeast involved. Bottom fermentation or lager fermentation has spread from the FRG to all over the world, with the result that traditional top-fermentation techniques have virtually disappeared from all countries except the UK, where it still accounts for 50% of the beer produced. Top-fermentation systems can also still be found in the FRG, USA, Belgium, Canada and Australia, but their proportion of the market is small and confined to specialist rather than mainstream beers.

Fermentation Vessel Design

The most widespread system of top fermentation uses a single vessel open to the atmosphere. These vessels were constructed originally of stone, wood, slate or copper, and are either rectangular, square or spherical in shape. Any recent vessels will invariably have been made of stainless steel, and have been enclosed to facilitate cleaning and general hygiene control. With open vessels, the yeast rises to the surface of the beer during the course of the fermentation and is removed by a suction pump or is skimmed off the surface, in what is termed a skimming system. A variation on this system is a dropping system whereby the beer is fed by gravity from one vessel to another. The movement of beer can take place after 12–24 h of fermentation, which leaves mainly trub in the initial vessel, or after 48 h, which leaves the yeast in the initial vessel for harvesting or cropping.

Traditional vessels made of stone, slate, wood or copper are usually around 2·4 m deep and of small capacity (25–150 barrels). More modern stainless steel vessels often have a capacity of 250–500 barrels. The gradual change to larger, enclosed stainless steel vessels has become necessary to increase brewery throughput, and also to improve general hygiene levels and minimize the problems of beer infection. Traditional, wood, stone or slate fermenting vessels either have a porous or uneven surface which makes cleaning and sterilization of vessels virtually impossible. In this way, any infecting microorganisms are perpetuated by passing from one fermentation to the next. In addition, the open nature of the vessels also facilitates airborne transmission of infecting microorganisms. Changing to open stainless steel vessels improved hygiene, but the actual cleaning of vessels still had to be carried out manually by entering the vessels and literally scrubbing them clean. A further change to an enclosed system with a fixed sprayball cleaning system as an integral part of the design enabled 'in place' cleaning, which is both safer and more effective.

Fermentation Conditions

The wort is pumped into the fermentation vessel and oxygen introduced (as described earlier), and fermentation started when the yeast is added or pitched into the vessel. Traditionally, yeast was pressed into a cake form and weighed out in a tub as pressed yeast to add at a rate of 0·15–0·30 kg hl^{-1} (0·5–1 lb barrel^{-1}). The yeast was then slurried with some of the wort to give a thick slurry and added by tipping into the fermentation vessel during filling. More modern systems do not press the yeast but simply dose in an equivalent volume of yeast in line from a yeast slurry storage tank. Usually, wort is pitched at 15–16°C and allowed to rise to 18–21°C as the heat generated by the fermentation raises the overall temperature.

In an open vessel, an experienced brewer can monitor the fermentation visually merely by observing the appearance of the foam head. The first stage of fermentation is noted by the slow production of carbon dioxide bubbles, which start to form a froth. This is followed by so-called 'rocky heads', whereby the carbon dioxide foams the wort into characteristic sharp points of foam. Initial heads are dark, containing trub, and these heads can be skimmed to improve beer quality later in the process. As fermentation proceeds, 'rocky heads' give way to 'cauliflower heads' and, finally, to a 'yeast head' as the yeast rises to the surface. At this stage the yeast must be skimmed off, otherwise, if left after fermentation and carbon dioxide evolution has ceased, the head may collapse and sink, making it difficult to harvest the yeast. Yeast is removed by suction into a mobile yeast cart which can be moved from one vessel to another, or by a conical collector or parachute which is attached to each vessel. The parachute is lowered to just below the yeast head and paddles used manually to push the yeast into the conical collector. Pipework leads from the parachute through the base of the vessel to a yeast cart situated below. The initial crop will contain trub and is usually discarded, and it is only yeast from the second crop which is kept for repitching. A third crop to improve beer clarity may also be taken but this yeast is also sent to waste.

Yeast removed is collected in a storage tank which is refrigerated to keep the yeast at < 5°C. The yeast can then be pumped to a sheet filter press and the intrained beer recovered, leaving a solid yeast cake which is stored in a refrigerator at < 5°C prior to reuse. Alternatively, the yeast slurry can be pitched directly to the next fermentation vessel. After yeast removal, the beer can be moved to undergo its maturation process. At this stage the beer will have been cooled to 3–10°C and have a yeast count of less than 5×10^6 cells per millilitre. The yeast concentration will vary according to the flocculation characteristics of the yeast.

Special Fermentation Systems

The fermentation systems described are widespread throughout the UK; however, there are some specialized systems.

Burton Union System

As the name suggests, this system originated in Burton-on-Trent. Fermenting wort is dropped into a series of oak union vessels of 7 hl capacity. The vessels are arranged in adjacent rows of 12, each one equipped with a swan neck pipe which, during fermentation, feeds yeast and beer into a trough above the casks. Yeast sediments in the trough but the beer is returned to the union. At the end of fermentation, most of the yeast will be in the trough and the beer will be in the union, and it can then be moved to the 'racking back' for the next stage in the process.

To suction pump to remove yeast

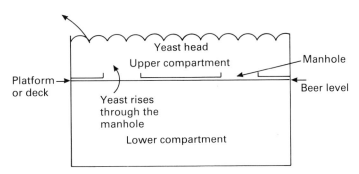

Fig. 2 A Yorkshire square fermentation vessel.

Yorkshire Stone Squares

Originally, these vessels were made of stone then slate, and are of small capacity (30 barrels) (Fig. 2). More recent vessels are constructed of stainless steel and have a larger capacity (120–240 barrels). The key feature is that the vessel has an upper and lower compartment separated by a deck. The deck has one or two main manholes connecting the two compartments. The vessel is filled with wort to a level of 2·5 cm above the deck. During fermentation, yeast rises through the manholes and remains supported on the deck, leaving beer to drain back to the lower compartment. Strongly flocculant yeasts are used with this system, such that a rousing system for pumping yeast back into the beer has to be used to achieve the correct final gravity. The rousing is then stopped, allowing yeast to be skimmed. Finally, relatively clear beer with a yeast count of $1–2 \times 10^6$ cells per millilitre is left in the lower compartment.

Recent Developments

All the systems described are still in use in traditional cask beer breweries. However, modern production techniques are also applied to beer production.

Cylindro-conical Vessels

These vessels are in use throughout the world for both bottom and top fermentations. Each vessel consists of a tall, thin, cylindrical vessel with a steeply angled cone at the base. They are fitted with cooling jackets for temperature control and have their own cleaning system. Top-fermenting yeasts can be used in such vessels. In these instances, the yeast head collapses under its own weight and the yeast sinks to the bottom of the vessel. Cropping can only take place from the base of the vessel. If the yeast is strongly flocculant, antifoam is added to prevent the formation of a strong yeast head and to aid yeast settlement.

Bibliography

Baille F (1974) *Bristol Brewers and Beer Types. The Drinkers Companion*. Newton Abbott: David and Charles (Holding).

De Clerck J (1957) *A Textbook of Brewing*, vols 1 and 2. London: Chapman and Hall.

Hough JS Briggs DE and Stevens R (1982) *Malting and Brewing Science*, vols 1 and 2. London: Chapman and Hall.

Jackson M (1982) *The World Guide to Beer*. London: Burlington Books.

Lloyd Hind H (1950) *Brewing Science and Practice*, vols 1 and 2. London: Chapman and Hall.

Pollock JRA (ed.) (1980) *Brewing Science*, vol 1–3. London: Academic Press.

S. Loseby
Courage Ltd – Brewing, Reading, UK

Maturation and Distribution

'Green' beer at the end of fermentation has a yeast count of up to 5×10^6 cells per millilitre, giving it a cloudy appearance, a low carbon dioxide content and an undeveloped taste.

Cask-conditioned Ales

A cask-conditioned ale is one where the maturation and conditioning stage takes place in the container (known as a cask) from which the beer is dispensed for sale. This is the traditional method of ale production dating back to the early 19th century when it became common for beer to be transported from brewery to alehouse rather than brewed on site. Casks are still traditionally made from wood, manufactured by skilled coopers, but today most brewers choose to use steel or aluminium casks which are lighter and easier to clean. There are several cask sizes commonly used, these are pins at 4·5 gallons, firkins at 9 gallons, kilderkins at 18 gallons, barrels at 36 gallons and hog heads at 54 gallons. Kegs are also available in most of these sizes as well as metric sizes of 50 and 100 litres. *See* Barrels

Postfermentation Treatment

Beer is transferred to a vessel known as a racking back at the end of fermentation. These vessels are usually held under slight carbon dioxide top pressure to maintain this gas in solution and minimize the risk of microbiological infection. Priming sugars are often added to the racking back to promote secondary fermentation in the cask which will increase the carbonation level. Typical addition rates are $0.5–1.5\,l\,hl^{-1}$ of a sugar with specific gravity approximately 1150, such as sucrose, invert sugar or hydrolysed starch. Stouts and milds tend to have higher addition rates because the primings also add to the sweetness of the beer. Hops may also be added at this stage to improve the aroma and flavour of the beer; these will be in the form of whole dry hops, either loose or compressed pellets or hop oil extract. Beer will usually be held in the racking back for a maximum of 24 h before racking.

Cask Racking

'Cask racking' is the brewing industry term for cask filling. Empty casks are returned from the trade and the old vent plug and tap plug, known as the 'shive' and 'keystone', are removed manually. They are then washed thoroughly in a multistage washer that forms an integral part of the racking line. Typical stages of the wash are cold rinse, hot detergent wash with caustic or acid at 80°C, hot water rinse also at 80°C and direct steaming, to leave a clean sterile cask. New keystones are added manually before the casks pass to the racking heads. Most plants have 4–10 racking heads fed by a single line from the washer, depending on the relative speeds of the washers and cask fillers. At the racking head, the cask is laid on its side and the racking head lowered through the shive hole. The beer is then metered into the cask and a new shive hammered in manually.

Fining

In order to produce a beer of acceptable clarity, yeast and large protein and tannin molecules suspended in the beer must be removed. This is done by adding isinglass finings, which are traditionally produced from the swim bladders of certain fish species native to oriental waters. These fish are caught by local fishermen, dried out and sold to merchants who ship them to Western countries, where they are processed by reacting with weak acid.

The resultant material is viscous, translucent and rich in collagen. Collagen has a positively charged helical structure which sediments slowly in the beer, taking negatively charged yeast cells and tannins with it. The rates of addition vary from 0.3 to $1\,l\,hl^{-1}$, working best when the yeast count of the beer is $0.5–2 \times 10^6$ cells per millilitre prior to fining. The yeast count after fining should be 1×10^2 to 1×10^3 cells per millilitre. Once the beer has been fined it is important to move it as little as possible, since each time the beer is shaken the action of the finings is less efficient. If the beer is fined in the brewery, the finings will have to act at least five times as the beer is moved from the brewery to the warehouse, from the warehouse to the distribution depot, from the depot to the distribution vehicle, from the vehicle to the public house and from the public house cellar to the stillage. Adding an excess of finings will help to ensure that the beer is bright, but can lead to a large volume of unsaleable bottoms in the cask, so is not favoured by publicans. Instead, some brewers choose to delay fining as long as possible, often fining at the secondary distribution depot from where the beer will be delivered directly to the public house. Auxiliary finings consisting of silicates or alginates may also be added at rates of around $0.3\,l\,hl^{-1}$. These have a net negative charge and help to increase the electrostatic action between proteins and isinglass finings. They are most often used for beers with a low yeast count. Alginate finings must be added at least 4 h prior to isinglass finings, but silicate finings can be added immediately before or after isinglass finings as they act much more rapidly.

Dispense

However good the quality of a cask beer when it leaves the brewery, the way in which it is handled once it has been delivered to the public house will have a great effect on the quality of the product in the glass. Casks should be stored at 12–14°C to maximize shelf life. Casks are laid on their sides, kept steady using chocks or a gantry and left for 24–48 h to allow the sediment to settle. During this phase, secondary fermentation will continue and carbon dioxide will be produced which will carbonate the beer. To avoid overcarbonation, a soft wooden peg called a spile is inserted into the core of the shive to allow some of the carbon dioxide and hydrogen sulphide gases to escape. When fermentation is complete, a hard spile is inserted to maintain the carbon dioxide level. Beer is occasionally served directly from the cask by hammering a tap into the keystone hole, but more usually pumps are used to raise the beer up from the cellar to bar level. Manual and electric pumps are used for this purpose. The manual type uses a suction pump at bar level; in England, one pull of the handle usually delivers half a pint of beer in the south or a quarter of a pint in the north. Electric pumps are located at cellar level and activated by pressing a button or operating a tap at bar level. Some dispense a metered amount of beer, others operate continually whilst the tap is pulled. The spouts are usually fitted with nozzles called sparklers which can be opened or closed to vary the consistency of the head according to local preference. Beers served in the north of England have a tight frothy head produced with a partly closed sparkler, whereas the majority of southern beers have a loose-foaming head often produced with a fully open sparkler. This is to accommodate customer preference. Once casks have been tapped they should be used within 3 days, and stock levels in the cellar should not exceed 10 days. Casks should be used in strict order for racking dates. To maintain quality, throughput should be no less than two casks per week. This factor will be taken into account by the publican when deciding which cask size to order.

To minimize the risk of microbiological infection, the beer left in the lines should be pulled through the taps and replaced with water at the end of each session. The lines should be cleaned with detergent at least weekly.

Brewery-conditioned Ales and Stouts

Maturation

With the growth in licensed clubs which have cellars that were not purpose designed, or no cellars at all, where beer was often served by untrained volunteers, market pressure developed for ales with a longer shelf life, which did not need such strictly attemperated cellar conditions and were simpler to serve at premium quality. This, together with competition from Continental-style lagers, led to the development of brewery-conditioned ales and stouts. Draught brewery-conditioned beers have a shelf life of approximately 6 weeks or more compared to a 3 week life for cask beers. Bottled beers can be kept up to 9 months and some canned beers up to 12 months. Brewery-conditioned beers are matured in a similar way to lagers. The fermented beer is transferred to a conditioning vessel where it undergoes a maturation phase similar to that which would occur in a cask. The precise conditions for maturation vary from brewery to brewery, depending on the type of beer being produced. Those which require secondary fermentation are initially held at 12–16°C for around 3 days in a stage known as 'warm conditioning'. Secondary fermentation may rely on residual carbohydrates, or priming sugars may be added. Flavour modification occurs as some volatile components are purged by the carbon dioxide produced. The beer is clarified by chilling to −1 to 3°C, at which temperature the yeast settles and protein–tannin colloids are precipitated. This cold conditioning

phase must take place at a temperature lower than the serving temperature to ensure that the chill haze precipitates in the tank and not in the glass. Finings and auxiliary finings can be added to promote clarification and reduce conditioning times. Conditioning times for ales are usually shorter than those for lagers, typically 5–14 days in the UK and as low as 2–4 days in the USA. Stouts tend to have a long conditioning time at around 10°C, with one of the main aims being the reduction by the yeast of undesirable flavour components, such as vicinal diketones, e.g. 2,3-butanedione (diacetyl), which has a butterscotch flavour. *See* Colloids and Emulsions

Further Processing

Most draught stouts are packaged at the end of the maturation phase without any further processing, but the majority of draught, canned and bottled ales are treated in a similar manner to lagers. The beer is filtered, usually using a diataomaceous earth filter, to remove yeast and other suspended solids. This can be done using a conventional plate and frame filter, or a more modern filter such as a pressure leaf or candle filter. Care must be taken to filter at a low temperature to ensure that chill haze is removed. *See* Filtration of Liquids

Packaging

Brewery-conditioned ales and stouts can be packaged into kegs (known in the industry as containers), cans and bottles using the same packaging lines as for lagers, including a pasteurization stage. One notable difference is that stouts are packaged using nitrogen to produce the top pressure, and sometimes with nitrogen injection to form a creamier head when the beer is served. *See* Pasteurization, Principles

Bottle-conditioned Ales and Stouts

Many popular bottled stouts and some ales are brewed in the same manner as cask ales, fined and then bottled so that secondary fermentation takes place in the bottle. The bottles are stored in the brewery at 15–20°C for around 1 week while the yeast ferments residual carbohydrates and/or priming sugars. In some cases, fresh yeast is added for the secondary fermentation, whereas in other cases there is enough yeast remaining from the primary fermentation.

If bottle-conditioned beers are carefully packaged and correctly stored they can enjoy a very long shelf life, with some of the very high-gravity beers being sound after 100 years, having matured and mellowed like a strong wine.

Bibliography

Baille F (1974) *Bristol Brewers and Beer Types. The Drinkers Companion*. Newton Abbott: David and Charles (Holding).

De Clerck J (1957) *A Textbook of Brewing*, vols 1 and 2. London: Chapman and Hall.

Hough JS, Briggs DE and Stevens R (1982) *Malting and Brewing Science*, vols 1 and 2. London: Chapman and Hall.

Jackson M (1982) *The World Guide to Beer*. London: Burlington Books.

Lloyd Hind H (1950) *Brewing Science and Practice*, vols 1 and 2. London: Chapman and Hall.

Pollock JRA (ed.) (1980) *Brewing Science*, vol 1–3. London: Academic Press.

S. Potter
Courage Ltd – Brewing, Reading, UK

Biochemistry of Fermentation

Yeast metabolism during beer fermentations is principally directed towards the anaerobic conversion of wort carbohydrates to ethanol and carbon dioxide. The remaining nutrient pools are channelled towards cell growth and a repertoire of secondary metabolites which determine key flavour attributes. Growth and fermentation are interdependent, and the biochemistry of fermentation represents the expression of a complex network of essential pathways.

The Fermentation Process

Beer is produced from the alcoholic fermentation of malted grain extracts by yeasts of the genus *Saccharomyces*. The traditional beer fermentation is a two-stage batch process. The primary fermentation cycle is conducted under conditions which support wort attenuation, intermediary metabolism and cell growth, as illustrated in Fig. 1. A secondary fermentation then matures the young beer under conditions of limited metabolic activity.

Cell division during the primary fermentation ceases

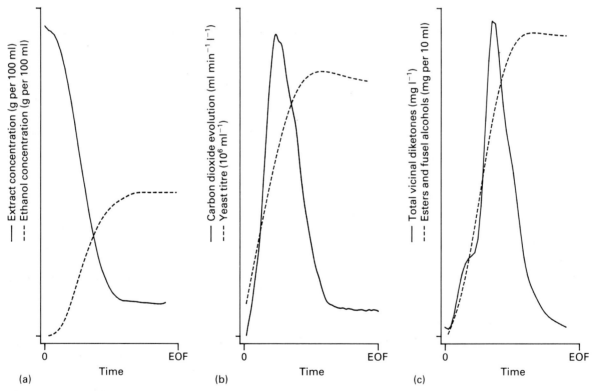

Fig. 1. Time course of fermentation. The patterns of gross changes in the medium from pitching until end of fermentation (EOF) are illustrated for a generic lager fermentation. (a) Wort attenuation and alcohol synthesis. Sugars and amino acids (fermentable extract) assimilated by the yeast are converted to ethanol, which is subsequently expressed into the beer. Approximately 1·6 mol of ethanol are produced per mole of glucose consumed (80% of theoretical yield). (b) Cell growth and fermentation rate. The rate of fermentation (measured by carbon dioxide evolution) increases rapidly with increasing cell number and process temperature early in the fermentation cycle, then declines as substrates are consumed. Cell division proceeds throughout the aerobic phase, but ceases as oxygen is depleted. (c) Secondary metabolite expression. Most volatile flavour components are coupled to cell growth. Alcohols, esters and organic acids accumulate during the course of fermentation, and maintain a nearly constant level after the end of cell division. Vicinal diketones are reassimilated by the yeast late in the process.

Table 1. Principal yeast metabolites in beer[a]

Primary fermentation products		Secondary yeast metabolites							
		Fusel alcohols		Organic/fatty acids		Volatile esters		Other volatiles	
Compound	Level (%,w/v)	Compound	Level (mg l^{-1})	Compound	Level (mg l^{-1})	Compound	Level (mg l^{-1})	Compound	Level (mg l^{-1})
Ethanol	~4–9	Isoamyl	⩽100	Acetic	⩽150	Butyl acetate	⩽50	2,3-Butanedione	⩽5
Glycerol	⩽1·5	2-Phenylethyl	⩽50	Butyric	⩽150	Ethyl acetate	⩽50	2,3-Pentanedione	⩽5
Carbon dioxide		Amyl	⩽25	Isobutyric	⩽150	Isobutyl acetate	⩽25		
Yeast biomass		Isobutyl	⩽25	Citric	⩽150	Isoamyl acetate	⩽10	Acetaldehyde	⩽50
		Propyl	⩽25	Pyruvic	⩽75	Amyl acetate	⩽5		
		Tyrosol	⩽25	Malic	⩽50	2-Phenylethyl acetate	⩽5	Dimethyl sulphide	Trace
		Butyl	⩽10	Succinic	⩽25	Ethyl caprylate	⩽5	Ethyl mercaptan	Trace
		Tryptophol	⩽10	Caprylic	⩽10	Ethyl butyrate	⩽5	Hydrogen sulphide	Trace
		s-Butyl	⩽5	Valeric	⩽10	Ethyl caprate	⩽5	Methyl mercaptan	Trace
		Isopropyl	⩽5	Isovaleric	⩽10	Ethyl caproate	⩽5	Sulphur dioxide	Trace
				Capric	⩽5	Ethyl propionate	⩽5		
				Caproic	⩽5				

[a] A small number of the yeast metabolic by-products expressed in beer are listed according to their chemical class. The concentration estimates represent approximate maximum levels or concentration ranges for 'typical' beers, and indicate the relative magnitudes of these compounds (e.g. trace vs 5 mg l^{-1} vs 100 mg l^{-1}) rather than the precise concentration for any particular product. Ales in general contain higher levels of esters and fusel alcohols than lagers.

as oxygen is exhausted, but the conversion of wort nutrients to ethanol continues until the wort extract is nearly depleted. Flavour development also proceeds beyond the growth phase, as a multitude of secondary metabolites are released into the beer. The principal yeast derivatives present in the beer are summarized in Table 1. As the initial fermentation subsides, a secondary fermentation is induced to attenuate the residual wort sugars*. Nutrient limitations depress most further intermediary metabolism, but the yeast does assimilate specific compounds which contribute undesirable flavours and passively adsorb wort polymers which contribute to haze formation. In contemporary brewing practice, these functions are more often accomplished by extending the primary fermentation cycle and ageing the beer after removal of the yeast in lieu of a second fermentation.

Carbohydrate Metabolism: The Pathway of Fermentation

The principal function of brewing fermentations is the synthesis of ethanol from wort sugars. Glucose and α-1,4-linked dimers (maltose) and trimers (maltotriose) of

glucose are the principal fermentable carbohydrates in wort. The yeast imports glucose through facilitated diffusion, mediated by hexose carrier proteins. Maltose and maltotriose are actively transported by separate permease systems and then hydrolysed to glucose by a cytoplasmic maltase activity. The culture does not utilize significant quantities of maltose or maltotriose until glucose assimilation is nearly complete: the glucose carrier systems are constitutively expressed, but the maltose and maltotriose permeases must be induced. Because of this lag in the onset of transport and the abundance of maltose and maltotriose relative to glucose, oligoglucoside assimilation is typically the rate-limiting step of fermentation.

Glucopyranoside transport is coupled to glucose phosphorylation by hexokinase, and subsequent catabolism by the routes summarized in Fig. 2. Most of the carbon derived from glucose is transformed to pyruvate through glycolysis. Until the wort is depleted of oxygen, the pyruvate pool is partitioned between acetyl-CoA, the entry point of the tricarboxylic acid cycle, and acetaldehyde, which is reduced to ethanol at the terminal step of the Embden–Meyerhoff–Parnas pathway. Yeast generally expresses both fermentative and respiratory pathways in aerated media when substrate sugar concentrations are high, a property known as the Crabtree effect. This phenomenon is especially pronounced in brewer's yeasts, and the ethanol pathway is

* **Attenuation** The reduction in the extract content and density of the wort which results from the assimilation of soluble nutrients and the release of ethanol by the yeast.

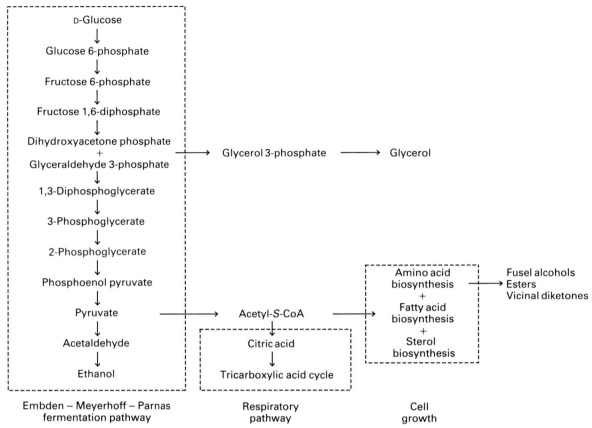

Fig. 2. Pathways of carbon catabolism. The Embden–Meyerhoff–Parnas alcoholic fermentation pathway is the primary route for the metabolism of wort sugars, and is highly expressed even during the early aerobic phase of the fermentation cycle. Glycerol synthesis provides an alternate end-point as intermediates accumulate in later stages of fermentation. Respiration via the tricarboxylic cycle is oxygen-dependent and principally functions in support of cell growth.

highly expressed even under the aerobic conditions found early in fermentation. When the wort oxygen is consumed, the ethanol pathway is the sole mechanism for the production of adenosine triphosphate (ATP) from glucose. As a result, typical brewing yeasts convert 80% or more of the carbon available in fermentable wort sugars to ethanol.

Pyruvate decarboxylase (PDC) and alcohol dehydrogenase (ADH) are the key enzymes of alcoholic fermentation. These activities catalyse the cleavage of pyruvate to acetaldehyde and carbon dioxide, and the subsequent reduction of acetaldehyde to ethanol, respectively. Yeast encode multiple forms of ADH; the principal isozyme active in fermentation (ADHI) is constitutively expressed and refractory to carbon catabolite repression.

A branch point in the glycolytic pathway produces significant quantities of glycerol during the anaerobic phase of fermentation (Fig. 2). This may consume up to 10% of the assimilated sugar, depending upon the relative efficiency of α-glycerophosphate dehydrogenase and ADH in competing for nicotinamide-adenine-dinucleotide dehydrogenase (NADH). The glycerol

produced is essential for proper texture and mouth feel in the finished beer.

Oxygen Utilization and Yeast Growth

Although respiration diverts carbon from ethanol synthesis, brewing fermentations require limited aerobic metabolism to support cell growth. Yeast possesses alternative anaerobic mechanisms for many biosynthetic reactions that normally occur aerobically. However, oxygen is absolutely required to produce the sterol (ergosterol) and fatty acid ($C_{16:0}$, $C_{16:1}$, $C_{18:0}$ and $C_{18:1}$) precursors for cell membrane synthesis.

Yeast assembles fatty acids and sterols from acetate in the form of acetyl-CoA. Respiratory cleavage of pyruvate is a primary source of acetyl-CoA, although anaerobic mechanisms exist for early steps in condensation of the carbon skeletons. The ergosterol pathway can progress to squalene in the absence of oxygen, but the subsequent epoxidation reaction is oxygen-dependent. Saturated fatty acids may also be synthesized anaerobically, but the desaturase activities which con-

Biochemistry of Fermentation

vert them to functional, unsaturated forms require oxygen as a terminal electron acceptor. Key reactions of sterol and fatty acid synthesis are localized in the mitochondrion, which degenerates as oxygen is depleted and the yeast adapts to wholly fermentative metabolism.

Flavour Development and Cell Growth

Wort provides a limited supply of free amino nitrogen, and yeast growth during fermentation depletes the pools of several essential amino acids. Cellular amino acid synthesis is induced as extracellular substrate declines, and by-products of the synthetic pathways are excreted into the beer. These secondary metabolites include key determinants and potentiators of beer flavour: fusel alcohols, organic acids, esters, diketones and volatile sulphur compounds (Table 1).

Fusel Alcohols

Although ethanol and glycerol are the primary alcoholic components of beer, a variety of higher-order alcohols are excreted at low levels during fermentation (Table 1). These fusel alcohols are formed by two mechanisms related to amino acid metabolism. The amino acids taken up by the yeast cell are not directly incorporated into protein. Instead, the α-amino group is donated to an α-keto acid as the terminal step of amino acid synthesis, and the carbon backbone is recycled. One mechanism for processing the carbon skeleton proceeds by decarboxylase cleavage of the α-carboxyl group, followed by reduction of the resulting aldehyde to alcohol by ADH. The fusel alcohol produced is one carbon atom shorter than the precursor amino acid, but the branch structure of the backbone is preserved. This sequence of deamination, decarboxylation and reduction (the Ehrlich pathway) accounts for 50–80% of fusel alcohol synthesis in fermentation.

The existence of an alternate alcohol synthesis mechanism was deduced from the presence of alcohols whose amino acid precursors are not found in wort. The decarboxylation and reduction steps of the Ehrlich pathway may be separated from the initial deamination, and α-keto acids derived from glucose catabolism may be converted directly to fusel alcohols. This alternate path is also coupled to the nitrogen cycle: the α-keto acid substrates normally serve as amino acceptors for the terminal transamination step of amino acid synthesis.

The isoleucine–leucine–valine (ILV) pathway for branched-chain amino acid synthesis is particularly significant for the higher-order alcohol content of beer. Intermediates of the ILV pathway are precursors of the more abundant fusel alcohols: propanol, amyl alcohol, isoamyl alcohol and isobutanol (Table 1). Amyl alcohol, isoamyl alcohol and their ester derivatives are also particularly significant flavour elements in beer.

Organic Acids and Acetaldehyde

The acidic character of beer is determined by a variety of organic acids (Table 1), which are produced as intermediates of respiratory glucose metabolism and as precursors of amino acid synthesis. Yeast also accumulates pyruvic acid and acetaldehyde as intermediates of the alcoholic pathway. Organic acids are released into the wort until the end of cell growth, when the pH reaches its minimum value. The final levels of the acid components are sufficient to acidify the wort by 1·5 pH units or more, depending upon the wort buffering capacity.

Yeast also liberates a number of fatty acids during fermentation (Table 1). Caproic, caprylic and capric (C_6, C_8 and C_{10}, respectively) acids constitute approximately 80% of this material. These shorter-chain fatty acids are toxic to *Saccharomyces*, and their excretion is of considerable physiological importance to the cell.

Esters

A portion of the fusel alcohols and organic acids formed during fermentation combine to produce volatile esters, which exhibit low sensory thresholds and contribute a characteristic fruity note to the beer. Since ethanol is the most abundant beer alcohol, and acetate is the principal organic acid, ethyl acetate is the ester expressed at the highest concentration. The acetate esters of butyl, amyl and isoamyl alcohols are also present at relatively high levels. Ethyl esters of various fatty acids form at lower concentrations, but are significant flavour elements (Table 1).

Ester formation during fermentation is mediated by the yeast. Intracellular acids are enzymatically activated by the formation of the corresponding acyl-*S*-CoA intermediates. These in turn serve as acyl donors to alcohols in condensation reactions mediated by alcohol-acetyl transferase (AAT). The number and specificity of yeast AAT activities is not known. Ester synthesis begins after the initial burst of cell growth at the start of fermentation, and increases after oxygen depletion halts fatty acid and sterol synthesis. The kinetics of ester excretion into the medium follow the expression of fusel alcohols and organic acids (Fig. 1).

Volatile Sulphur Compounds

Most of the sulphur compounds found in beer originate in the malting and brewing processes, and persist through fermentation. However, yeast metabolism is a significant source of hydrogen sulphide, sulphur dioxide, dimethyl sulphide and mercaptans (Table 1). Elevated levels of the volatile sulphur compounds are generally associated with sensory defects, but sulphur dioxide is important in stabilizing normal beer flavours. The routes of sulphur metabolism are less well understood than the carbon and nitrogen pathways, and the reactions by which yeast produces excreted sulphur compounds are not clearly defined.

Hydrogen sulphide, sulphite and mercaptans are associated with amino acid synthesis in the growth phase of fermentation. The sulphur requirement for methionine and cysteine synthesis is supplied by the wort methionine and inorganic sulphate pools. Sulphur is normally bound to carrier intermediates throughout the sulphate reduction and amino acid synthesis pathways. However, a portion of the pool may be captured as hydrogen sulphide or as sulphite and released into the medium. The sulphite is recovered as sulphur dioxide at normal beer pH. Thioredoxin may donate sulphur to alternate acceptors in side reactions of the amino acid synthetic pathways, and volatile metabolites may also be produced by minor routes for intracellular cleavage of sulphur-containing amino acids.

The formation of dimethyl sulphide during fermentation is not coupled directly to amino acid biosynthesis. Wort normally contains small amounts of dimethyl sulphoxide, produced by the thermal degradation of S-methylmethionine during brewing. The sulphoxide is assimilable under fermentation conditions, and is transformed directly to dimethyl sulphide by the yeast.

Diketones

2,3-Butanedione (diacetyl) and 2,3-pentanedione are perhaps the most closely studied of the yeast metabolites found in beer. These vicinal diketones (VDKs) are of particular interest because diacetyl contributes a strong buttery flavour, and can be a detrimental sensory note at high concentrations. Diacetyl and 2,3-pentanedione derive from the branched-chain amino acid pathway intermediates α-acetolactate (valine) and α-aceto-α-hydroxybutyrate (isoleucine), respectively. A common acetohydroxy-acid synthase generates both precursors in excess, and significant amounts of each are excreted. The beer pH at later stages of yeast growth is sufficiently low to convert chemically the free α-aceto acids to the corresponding diketones. Cells rapidly assimilate diacetyl and 2,3-pentanedione, and VDK levels are controlled through extended contact with the yeast after active fermentation and cell growth are completed. Levels of VDK synthesis and final VDK concentrations vary widely among yeast strains and product formulations (Table 1).

Secondary Fermentation

The rate of fermentation declines as yeast growth ceases and the wort approaches its attenuation limit (Fig. 1). In traditional brewing processes, a secondary fermentation is induced at this point by kræusening the end-fermenting wort.* Secondary fermentation serves four purposes: to complete the assimilation of residual fermentable sugars; to stabilize the physical quality of the beer by removing haze-forming components; to carbonate the brew; to develop the proper balance of flavour compounds. Lagers are cooled after kræusening and matured for prolonged times at temperatures which limit yeast metabolism and growth. Ales are aged at temperatures near that of the primary fermentation.

The biochemistry of beer maturation is principally concerned with the control of product flavour. Carbohydrate assimilation is of limited importance during maturation, as most wort fermentable sugars are consumed during the primary fermentation. Sugar metabolism during the secondary fermentation is restricted to the anaerobic pathways leading to ethanol and glycerol. The physical removal of haze precursors from the wort is a commercially important function of the maturation process. However, the adsorption of haze-forming polyphenols to the yeast cell is a passive process requiring no metabolic activity; comparable results may be obtained by downstream processing after removal of the yeast from the brew.

The maturation of beer flavour involves both the reassimilation of metabolites expressed during the primary fermentation, and the excretion of additional by-products into the beer. Yeast continue to assimilate VDKs at low temperatures, and accomplish a net reduction in the extracellular VDK content during lagering. The same is true of ale maturation, although the rate of assimilation is higher at the elevated temperature. The levels of volatile sulphur compounds also decline during ageing, but the role of yeast assimilation in this process is not established. Amino acids which are not normally assimilated during active fermentation may be extensively absorbed in the maturation cycle.

Low temperature inhibits *de novo* biosynthesis of flavour compounds during lagering.† The ale maturation process permits a higher level of intermediary metabolism, and the pathways active in primary fermentation may continue during ageing. However, the extent of further metabolism is subject to nutrient limitation, as carbon and nitrogen sources are depleted soon after kræusening. Most of the flavour-active materials excreted into the beer during maturation are accumulated during the primary fermentation, and slowly leach

* Kræusening   The induction of secondary fermentation by addition of a small amount of fermentable sugar or a small volume of fermenting wort to an exhausted or slowly fermenting culture.
† Lagering   Traditional term for ageing beer by a secondary fermentation at reduced temperatures which limit intermediary metabolism.

from the yeast under prolonged storage conditions. The materials released into ageing beer typically include short-chain fatty acids and free amino acids. Fusel alcohols, esters and organic acids normally reach a stable concentration in primary fermentation and do not accumulate thereafter.

Process Parameters

The chemistry of flavour development during fermentation is coupled to cell growth, and moderated by the regulatory systems which control various biosynthetic enzymes. Growth is primarily limited by oxygen, and is readily stimulated by increasing wort aeration. More abundant yeast growth typically depletes the wort of nitrogen, induces *de novo* amino acid synthesis, and consequently enhances the levels of fusel alcohols, esters, vicinal diketones and volatile sulphur compounds. The fermentation temperature profile also strongly influences the rate and extent of cell growth, and the timing of the expression of growth-related pathways. Worts are typically pitched at low temperatures of about 10–12.8°C, which rise due to the heat of fermentation until normal process temperatures of about 15.6°C (lagers) to 20°C (ales) are reached. Cell growth and the net levels of volatile by-products generally increase at higher final temperatures, and the proportions of specific components may also vary with the rate and extent of the temperature rise. The fusel alcohol and ester content of the beer is particularly sensitive to temperature effects. It should be noted that the impact of aeration and temperature upon specific metabolites varies significantly among yeast strains and wort formulations.

Many pathways of yeast metabolism are physiologically regulated by substrate composition, and the wort formulation is critical to the character of the final product. The ratio of carbon to nitrogen, the distribution of nitrogen among the various amino acid pools, and the proportion of fermentable sugar as glucose each influence the distribution of specific alcohols, acids, esters, and sulphur compounds excreted in fermentation. Low molar fractions of branched-chain amino acids produce elevated levels of vicinal diketones, butanol and amyl alcohols; methionine pools determine the concentration of sulphur metabolites; and high glucose to maltose ratios favour high levels of acetate esters. As with aeration and temperature, the effect of wort composition upon specific metabolites is highly dependent upon the yeast strain.

The chemistry of fermentation comprises two major components: the conversion of wort carbohydrates to ethanol and carbon dioxide; and the metabolism and synthesis of amino acids during cell growth. The most important flavour elements expressed by the yeast derive from the carbon and nitrogen cycles, and the modulation of these pathways in response to process conditions determines the character and quality of the beer.

Bibliography

Hardwick WA (1989) Beer. In: Reed G (ed.) *Biotechnology—A Comprehensive Treatise in 8 Volumes. Food and Feed Production with Microorganisms,* vol. 5. Verlag Chemie, Weinheim.

Reed G and Nagodawithana TW (eds) (1991) *Yeast Technology.* Van Nostrand Reinhold, New York.

Strathern JN, Jones EW and Broach JA (eds) (1982) *The Molecular Biology of the Yeast* Saccharomyces—*Metabolism and Gene Expression.* Cold Spring Harbor Laboratory, New York.

Stewart GG and Russell I (1986) One hundred years of yeast research and development in the brewing industry. *Journal of the Institute of Brewing* 92: 537–558.

C. B. Ball and Etzer Chicoye
Miller Brewing Company, Milwaukee, USA

Chemistry of Brewing

Brewing Ingredients

The list of ingredients that are required to make beer is quite short. Water, malted barley, an additional carbohydrate source such as corn or rice (optional), hops and yeast are all that are required. Malted barley or malt serves two major purposes: a source of starch and the only source of the enzymes needed to break down the starch into simple sugars. Most beers employ additional carbohydrate sources often called adjuncts. These adjuncts are usually dry milled degermed corn grits or dehulled polished white rice. Hops give beer its characteristic bitter taste and distinctive aroma. Yeast converts the simple sugars supplied by malt and the other grains to alcohol, carbon dioxide and some of the trace flavour components important to beer.

From Barley to Malt

Although rarely regarded as a part of brewing, the first step in the brewing process is the production of malt from barley. For the most part, malting involves the germination of barley in a manner so as to produce the enzymes required for the brewing process. First, the barley is 'steeped' in large tanks of water until root formation begins. The steeped grain, separated from excess water, is then covered to the germination equipment where it rests on a slotted floor through which humid air passes. The biochemical reactions taking place in the growing grain produce heat so the temperature of the air must be controlled to maintain optimum conditions. When 'modification' is complete, the grain is transferred to the kiln, which slowly removes moisture in a stepwise controlled manner. After the malted barley has been dried, it is stored prior to shipment to the brewery. *See* Malt, Malt Types and Products; Malt, Chemistry of Malting

In addition to production of the enzymes which are required during later brewing steps, there are substantial differences in the chemical compositions of barley and malt. In Table 1 the relative amounts of the major components of barley and malt are given. By far the most abundant constituent of barley is starch (65%). Other complex carbohydrates make up another 14% of the total. Proteins comprise about 10%. The differences between malt and barley are largely due to conversion of some of the complex carbohydrates to simple sugars. For example, the data in Table 1 shows a 5% decrease in starch and a 3% increase in reducing sugars. The breakdown of complex sugars to simple sugars in the malt kernel will resume on a much larger scale during mashing. *See* Barley

Malted barley, as well as unmalted barley and other

Table 1. The chemical composition of European two-rowed barley and malt

Fraction	Proportions (% dry weight)	
	Barley	Malt
Starch	63–65	58–60
Sucrose	1–2	3–5
Reducing sugars	0·1–0·2	3–4
Other sugars	1	2
Soluble gums	1–1·5	2–4
Hemicelluloses	8–10	6–8
Cellulose	4–5	5
Lipids	2–3	2–3
Crude 'protein' (nitrogen × 6·25)	8–11	8–11
Albumin ⎫ salt-soluble protein	0·5	2
Globulin ⎭	3	—
Hordein – 'protein'	3–4	2
Glutelin – 'protein'	3–4	3–4
Amino acids and peptides	0·5	1–2
Nucleic acids	0·2–0·3	0·2–0·3
Minerals	2	2·2
Other substances	5–6	6–7

Compiled from various sources by Harris (1962) In: *Barley and Malt* (Cook AH, ed), p. 431. London: Academic Press.

Chemistry of Brewing

grains, contains starch, which is a mixture of two classes of polysaccharides called amylose and amylopectin. Amylose is a straight chain polymer of glucose units attached by α-1,4 bonds (Fig. 1). Amylopectin is similar to amylose in that it contains glucose connected by α-1,4 linkages, but it also contains some α-1,6 bonds which give amylopectin a branched structure (Fig. 2). Starch is the major energy-storing component of plants; the energy stored within starch (actually the glucose units in starch) will fuel the process of fermentation. Malted barley contains a supply of various enzymes; only a few of the enzymes active in brewing will be mentioned. Some enzymes are employed in the brewing process for the degradation of starch to simple fermentable sugars and are often referred to as diastatic enzymes or simply diastase. Other enzymes include the proteolytic enzymes involved in generating free amino acids and various polypeptides, and also certain β-glucanases which are enzymes that are important to filtration. *See* Enzymes, Uses in Food Processing; Starch, Structure, Properties and Determination

Malt Enzymes and their Action

α-Amylase catalyses the hydrolysis of α-1,4 linkages of both amylose and amylopectin. It randomly attaches itself to a region of the polysaccharide that is spatially removed from either branch points or chain ends and catalyses the breaking of the chain at that point. α-Amylase activity slows as long chains are broken into smaller pieces. β-Amylase attacks nonreducing starch chain ends and catalyses the sequential removal of maltose, which is a fermentable oligosaccharide containing two glucose units attached by an α-1,4-glucosidic bond. Degradation usually continues until a glucose unit containing a branch point is encountered. More accurately, as hydrolysis approaches to within about six glucose units of the branch point, the action stops. The two enzymes operate in a synergistic fashion because the action of α-amylase produces more nonreducing chain ends which β-amylase can attack. On the other hand, α-amylase can catalyse the hydrolysis of α-1,4 bonds of amylopectin that are within α-1,6 branch points; this polysaccharide can, by the action of both enzymes in consort, be degraded to relatively small oligosaccharides held together by α-1,6 linkages, 'limit dextrin'.

It should be noted that the relative levels of β-amylase in the barley and malt kernel are about the same, i.e. there is little or no net synthesis of this enzyme during malting. However, β-amylase is more difficult to extract from barley than from malt and it becomes easier to extract after the 'modification' which occurs during the malting process. In contrast, there is little α-amylase in the barley kernel. Virtually all of the enzyme is synthesized during malting. The same is true for the various components of the β-glucanase system.

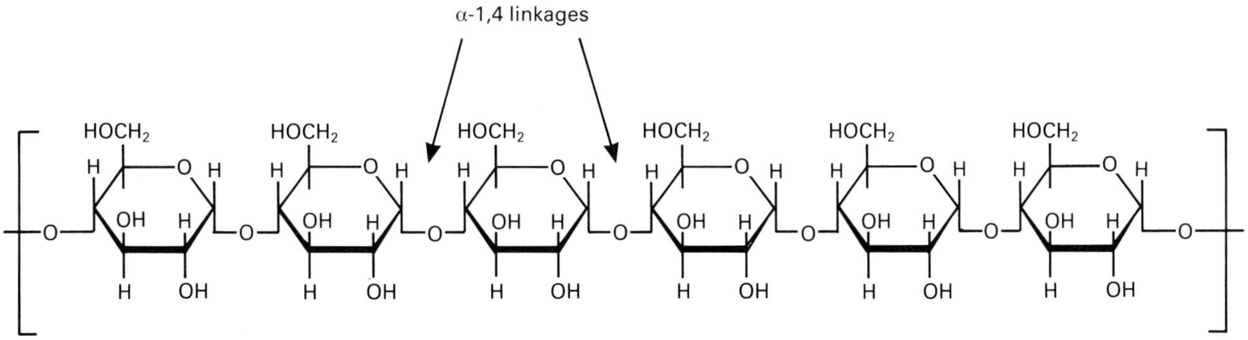

Fig. 1   α-1,4 bonds in amylose.

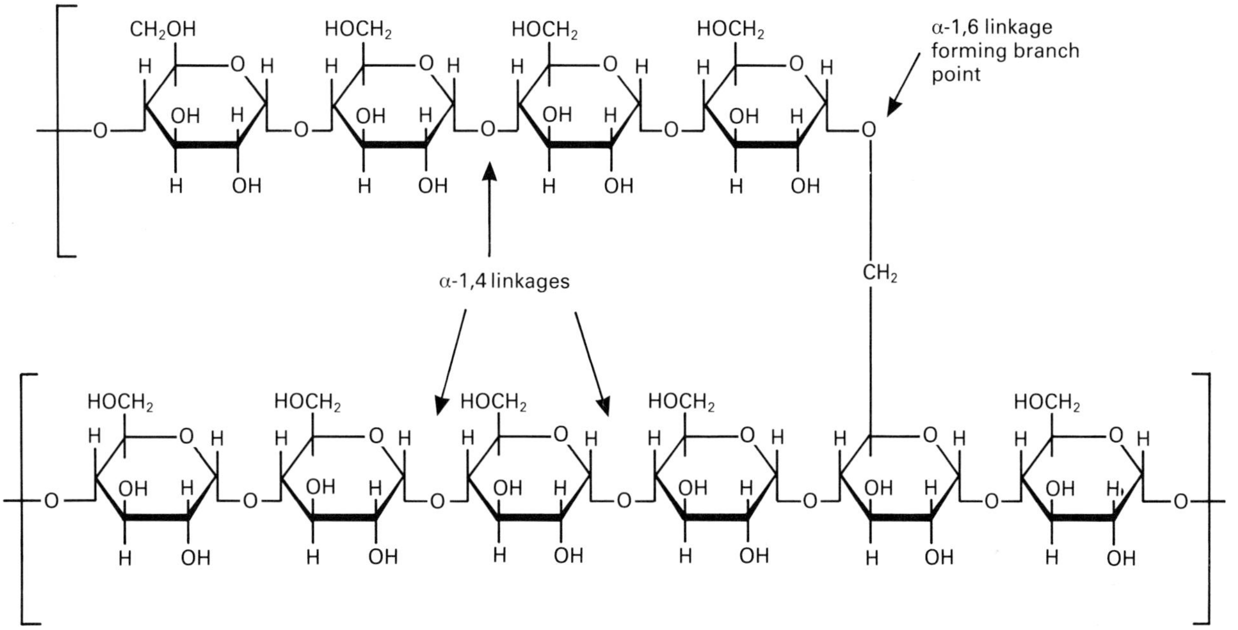

Fig. 2   α-1,4 and α-1,6 bonds in amylopectin.

A whole arsenal of other enzymes, including additional carbohydrases, proteases and phosphorylases, exist in malt. Although not completely obvious from Table 1, proteolysis of grain proteins such as hordein and glutelin provides less complex nitrogen compounds such as smaller peptides and amino acids. This breakdown of proteins during the malting process is made more difficult to follow due to the recombination of amino acids, often in sites removed from the original breakdown, to new proteins. Malt also provides other noncatalytic proteins which not only supply nitrogen for fermentation but play the central role in the formation and stability of beer foam. During the early part of the mash cycle (see later), conditions can be manipulated to favour the development of a protein profile favourable to good foam properties.

Mashing

The first operation performed in the brewing process is mashing. In a modern brewery, which employs a cereal grain adjunct, mashing usually involves two vessels and is called 'double mash upward infusion'. In the cereal cooker, water, the adjunct grain and a small amount of malt are combined. After a short rest period, during which α- and β-amylases are extracted from the malt, the temperature in the cereal cooker is increased to the boiling point. The high temperature causes gelatinization of the starch while α-amylase catalyses starch liquefaction. At the same time, a second vessel, the mash tun, is charged with water and the remainder of the malt. The contents of the mash tun are held at moderate temperature (40–50°C) for a period of time. This process is referred to as the protein rest. During protein rest, both α- and β-amylases are extracted from the malt. This extraction can be carried out under conditions that favour the generation of protein fractions of different molecular weight ranges. In general, a prolonged protein rest at low temperature favours the 'peptidases', which produce short-chain peptides. A shorter protein rest at higher temperature produces larger proteins generally favourable to good foam stability.

After protein rest the contents of the cereal cooker are transferred to the mash tun. Transfer of the boiling cooker contents to the main mash causes a temperature increase of the latter to what brewers term the conversion temperature. Typical conversion temperatures range from 60 to 70°C, depending on (1) the protein rest temperature in the main mash, and (2) the relative volumes and mash densities of the two vessels. Generally, the contents of the mash tun are rested at the conversion temperature for a period of time prior to 'mashing off'. During the rise to and hold at the conversion temperature, the bulk of the saccharification of the malt and adjunct starches and dextrinization of the malt starch occur.

After conversion rest, the contents of the mash tun are raised to about 75°C, i.e. to the 'mash off temperature'. Mashing off completes dextrinization of the starches and makes the mash more fluid, which facilitates wort separation as described below.

In the course of mashing of both adjunct and malt, we have seen that α- and β-amylases require the action of each other. From the earlier discussion, it is apparent that, optimally, the action of α-amylase should begin to take place prior to the action of β-amylase. For β-amylase to function, it must find nonreducing chain ends. Due to the fact that both starch polysaccharides have relatively few chain ends, as compared to internal glucose units, β-amylase cannot function to any large degree until the polysaccharide is first broken apart due to the catalytic action of α-amylase.

Unfortunately for the brewer, the temperature optimum for α-amylase is higher than that for β-amylase. As the brewer reaches the optimum temperature for β-amylase (50–60°C) there is little opportunity for it to function optimally due to the very small number of nonreducing end glucose units. When the temperature has risen to the optimum for α-amylase (65–67°C), and internal cleavages occur, the temperature optimum for β-amylase has been passed. Luckily, both enzymes display some activity, albeit not optimal activity, at a wider temperature range; the brewer must carefully control heating rates in the cereal cooker and mash tun in order to achieve the desired balance of saccharification (fermentable sugar production) and dextrinization (nonfermentable sugar production), which in turn determines the ratio of alcohol to residual dextrin in the fermented product.

Lautering

The converted mash must be subjected to a physical process by which the liquid wort is separated from the mash solids. This is usually accomplished in the lauter tun, which is a filtering device. Other equipment, such as a mash filter, has been used for the same purpose. The ease of this operation depends in large measure on the availability of β-glucanase activity, which is required to break down gums which may interfere with good filtration. The product of lautering is the wort. *See* Filtration of Liquids

The Wort

Wort solids consist mostly of carbohydrates (about 90%). Proteins and other nitrogen-containing organic and inorganic compounds make up about 5% of the wort. Lipids, inorganic salts, organic acids, phenolic materials and trace organic compounds such as vitamins make up the remainder. Carbohydrates are often designated as fermentable and nonfermentable; the former are the most abundant. The fermentable sugar in largest excess, by far, is the disaccharide maltose, which was formed during mashing by the action of β-amylase. The other major fermentable sugars in wort are the monosaccharide glucose and the trisaccharide maltotriose, while trace quantities of sucrose are also present. The unfermentable sugars, of higher degree of polymerization (DP) than maltotriose, consist of dextrins, which are the undegraded remnants of starch, and the β-glucans, which are derived from the grain cell walls. The dextrins' contribution to beer flavour is subtle, at most. Some of these sugars can be metabolized by humans. In the production of many low-calorie beers the dextrins are enzymatically degraded to fermentable sugars prior to or during fermentation.

Physical and Chemical Reactions During Kettle Boil

Wort boiling is the next major step in the brewing process. While mashing may be thought to be the province of biochemistry, wort boiling involves little or no enzyme-catalysed chemistry. The reason for this is that the temperatures within the brew kettle prevent almost all biological and biochemical activity. Not only are all the enzymes deactivated by heat, any microorganisms that might be present from the brewing ingredients are killed. This is very important because wort is an excellent medium for microbial growth. In addition to the cooker adjuncts described above, many brewers also use a variety of liquefied adjuncts such as corn syrups, commonly referred to as liquid adjuncts.

Chemistry of Brewing

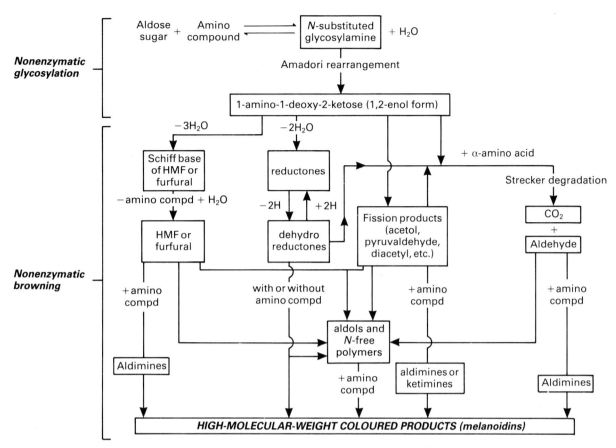

Fig. 3 Browning reaction. HMF, hydroxy methyl furfural. From Meyer LH (1960).

These syrups are usually obtained by an acid/enzyme or enzyme/enzyme process designed to achieve a suitable carbohydrate profile, which is usually two-thirds fermentable. Syrups are added to the wort during kettle boil.

Wort boiling produces a number of physical changes. The most obvious is that a number of volatile compounds are removed by evaporation, the most prevalent being water. During kettle boil, 5–10% of the water is removed. Wort boiling also coagulates certain proteins to produce an insoluble mass often called the 'hot break', which is removed from the wort later on. The coagulation and subsequent removal of those proteins, along with all the triglycerides from the wort, affect the clarity and physical stability of the finished beer. This coagulation is enhanced by complexation reactions between the proteins and naturally occurring tannins in the wort. A number of reducing agents are generated during kettle boil as a result of the browning reaction, which will be discussed later. These reducing agents play a major role in protein coagulation. Their presence is often supplemented by the addition of certain 'kettle aids', which contain bisulphites. *See* Tannins and Polyphenols

The high temperatures of the brew kettle also cause chemical changes which are essential to the proper flavour development of the beer. For example, certain sulphur-containing amino acids are converted to products which will form volatile sulphur compounds such as dimethylsulphide or sulphur dioxide. When formed in excess, volatile sulphur compounds may be detrimental to beer flavour.

Other important reactions during kettle boil involve polymerization, complexation with proteins, and precipitation of certain polyphenols such as the derivatives of hydroxybenzoic and hydroxycinnamic acids, some flavonols, anthocyanogens and catechins. Both the proteins and the polyphenols tend to become oxidized and precipitate out.

Another kettle boil reaction involves the simple sugars and secondary amines, to form maltol, an important flavouring substance. *See* Amines

Several hexose sugars also react with secondary amines, yielding desirable 'reductones'. The reductones, which are very strong reducing agents containing the $-C(OH)=C(OH)C=O$ group, enhance beer flavour stability.

A very important reaction series known as the 'browning reaction' takes place during the kettle boil. Low-molecular-weight carbohydrates react with some free amino acids in a very complex scheme as illustrated in Fig. 3. Free amino nitrogens from amino acids and short peptides react with aldose sugars to yield aldosamines. The aldosamines undergo chemical rearrangement. Some condense with other aldose sugars to form brown pigments which affect wort colour; others can react with α-amino acids to undergo the so-called 'Strecker degradation', which results in the loss of a carbon atom and the amino group from the amino acids. Many strong flavouring aldehydes, such as the isobutyl aldehydes, are the end results. *See* Browning, Nonenzymatic

Still other transformations occur during kettle boiling. The pH of the wort becomes more acidic. This is due to the reaction of calcium ions and the phosphates in the wort. In low-calcium worts or with high-bicarbonate brewing water, the drop in pH may be minimal due to competing reactions. During boiling, any bicarbonates will be converted to carbon dioxide and carbonate ions. Carbon dioxide is driven off, resulting in an increase in pH.

Hops – Chemistry and Contributions to Beer Flavour

Hops (*Humulus lupulus*), which are grown in temperate zones throughout the world, are an important ingredient in the production of beers; they are added during kettle boil, often in two or three portions. While the chemistry of the hops' bittering components is fairly well known, the fate of the aromatic constituents and their contribution to beer aroma is only now being elucidated. Special varieties such as the Hallertauer Mittelfreu are used for their aroma. The aromatic fraction of hops has been shown to be extremely complex and is made up of hydrocarbons and oxygenated compounds. The hydrocarbon portion is the largest by volume but is considerably less aromatic than the oxygenated compounds. The hydrocarbon portion is made up of two groups of compounds; the first are terpenes (consisting of two condensed five-carbon isoprene units, forming a branch dimer or a cyclic compound) and the second is the sesquiterpenes (consisting of three condensed isoprene units). The most common terpenes are myrcene, humulene, farnesene and the pinenes. The oxygenated part of the hop oils is comprised mostly of alcohols of carbonyls and various esters. Aroma compounds found in the oxygenated part are linalool, humulene epoxide, humulenol and many esters. These minor compounds are extracted into the wort and oxidized during kettle boiling. Many are lost by evaporation, polymerization or steam distillation. The remaining compounds play an important role in the development of the 'kettle hop aroma'. Thus, this aroma is not so much the result of the formation of new compounds, but is due to minor aroma constituents being 'unmasked' by the loss of more volatile ones. This

is not the case for traditional ales in which part of the hopping occurs after fermentation (dry hopping). *See* Flavour Compounds, Structures and Characteristics

Hop soft resins (nonvolatile) consist of the α-acids and β-acids, often called humulones and lupulones, respectively, and are precursors to the major bittering components in the finished beer.

When hops are added to boiling wort, the α-acids undergo isomerization, the products of which are called iso-α-acids or isohumulones; these compounds are partially responsible for beer bitterness. The β-acids undergo less well-characterized oxidation reactions which produce hulupones and other products which are also bitter and are minor bittering components of beer (Fig. 4). Hulupones have also been identified in stored hops. In addition to their flavour contributions, the isohumulones play an important role in the formation of beer foam and its stability. As an additional minor function, isohumulones are thought to be useful for promoting microbiological stability in beer; it is for this final consideration that hops were probably originally added to beer.

Modern brewing practices include the use of hops in many different forms. Hops are pelletized and enriched in the useful hop resins. In other cases hop extracts are made, preferably using liquid or super-critical carbon dioxide. These are used in the kettle like conventional hops. In other technological developments α-acids are pre-isomerized and compounded in a soluble form suitable for addition after fermentation. The iso-α-acids can be structurally modified by reduction processes, resulting in products with increased light stability in beer. ρ-Isohumulone or tetrahydroisohumulones are in that category.

Flavour Constituents Formed During Fermentation

After kettle boil, fermentation is the next major step in the brewing process. A large number of beer constituents associated with flavour are formed during fermentation. They are believed to be associated with amino acid metabolism and include a wide variety of higher alcohols, ethyl esters and short-chain carboxylic acids. The predominant higher alcohols are n-propyl (9–18 ppm) isobutyl (8–14 ppm), s-butyl (3·5 ppm), isopentenyl (35–52 ppm) and active amyl (11–17 ppm) alcohols. The fatty acids go from formic (C_1) to decanoic (C_{10}) acids, with the dominant compounds being formic (20–35 ppm), acetic (80–130 ppm), propionic (3·1–4·1 ppm), hexanoic (3·1–5·6 ppm), octanoic (5·6–8 ppm) and decanoic (0·4–1·7 ppm) acids. Beer flavour is also affected by a number of esters, primarily ethyl esters of the various fatty acids mentioned above and acetates of the various higher alcohols.

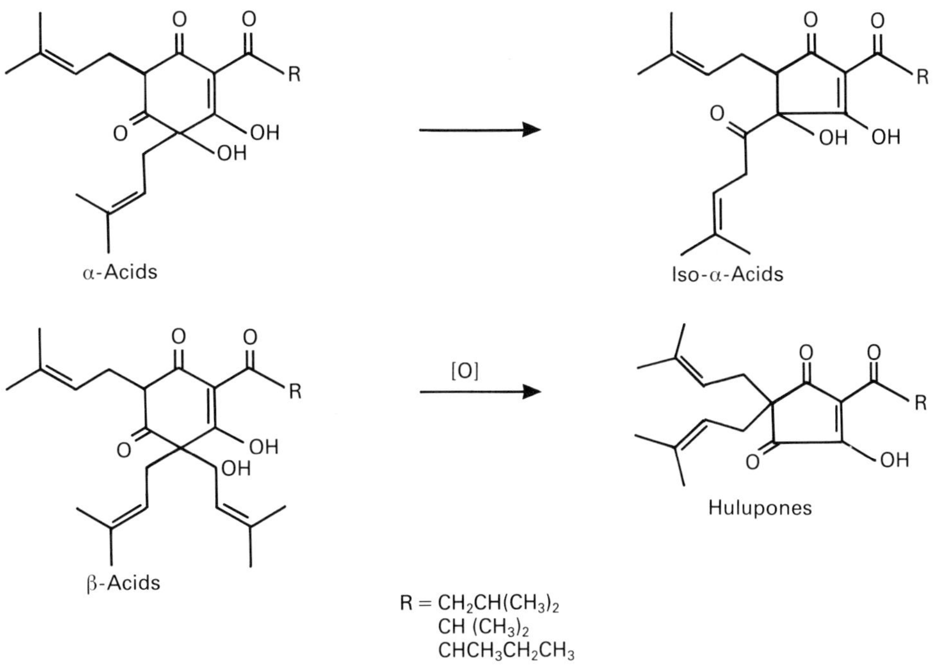

Fig. 4 Reactions of soft resins.

Beer Flavour – Development, Characterization and Deterioration

The flavour impact of a given constituent is a function of its concentration and its flavour threshold value. For example, certain natural sulphur-containing compounds in beer may be present in parts per trillion levels and still greatly influence beer flavour, whereas acetaldehyde content in beer has little influence on flavour unless present in tens of parts per million. Modern analytical methodologies such as headspace gas chromatography, gas chromatography–mass spectroscopy (GC–MS) and high-performance liquid chromatography (HPLC) can identify hundreds of compounds in beer; however, sensorial relevance for many of these compounds generally remains a mystery. To complicate things even more, a single compound may be present in beer at a level well below its flavour threshold but, as a member of a group of compounds, acting in synergy, it may play an important role in beer flavour. *See* Chromatography, High-performance Liquid Chromatography; Chromatography, Gas Chromatography

Some compounds or groups of compounds in beer are detrimental to beer flavour; two classes may be cited. One class of defect compounds is beneficial to beer flavour at certain levels, but at higher levels has the opposite effect. The second class of compounds, much rarer than the first, plays no beneficial role and is a problem at concentrations above the threshold levels. Esters, fusel oils, vicinal diketones, oxidized terpenoids and sulphur-containing organic compounds are examples of the former. If, for instance, certain esters are present in beer at too high a level, the product is described as being 'fruity'. This may be caused by improper temperature control during fermentation. When vicinal diketones such as diacetyl are present above 0·5 ppm, for example, the resulting beer has a buttery flavour. This may be caused by too short a fermentation. Beers stored for too long a time, at temperatures which are abnormally high or are packaged with high oxygen content, may exhibit a cardboard-like aroma and taste, which is called 'oxidized'. Although the compounds responsible for this have not been well characterized, it is generally thought that various carbonyl compounds including *trans*-2-nonenal play a role. The average beer drinker will probably never experience any of these defects because the art and science of modern brewing has developed in such a manner as to preclude their formation.

Brewing Aids and Additives

Although most large breweries try to avoid the use of additives, some are still used. Water treatment is very common. A certain hardness is believed desirable and is achieved by appropriate addition of calcium salt. Hydrogen ion concentration is often adjusted with sulphuric acid.

Kettle aids to promote formation of kettle break contain bisulphites. In the mash tun, β-glucanases may be used to facilitate lautering. Zinc salts are used as a major ingredient in yeast foods to enhance fermentation and yeast viability. Glucoamylases of fungal origin are sometimes used in fermentation or prior to fermentation to break down residual dextrin and achieve beers lower in residual carbohydrates and calories.

Haze is produced when polyphenols, formed via oxidative polymerization, achieve a certain molecular size; these complex with certain proteins to produce particles which become visible when the beer is chilled. Papain, a natural proteolytic enzyme, has been used to insure that the chilled product does not display a proteinaceous haze. Avoidance of chill haze can also be accomplished by the use of phenolics such as gallo-tannins. In this case the haze-forming proteins are precipitated by the tannins and filtered out. A similar result can be achieved by using appropriate adsorbants such as silica hydrogels or bentonite to remove the proteins. Yet another approach is to remove the poly-phenols with a treatment of polyvinylpyrolidone.

Oxidation has been prevented by employing antioxidants such as potassium metabisulphite. Kelcoloids, which are alginates derived from seaweed, have been employed to enhance beer foam. Caramel and roasted malt are commonly used to enhance colour and achieve certain flavour characteristics. This is particularly true in the production of certain dark beers such as stout. *See* Antioxidants, Natural Antioxidants; Antioxidants, Synthetic Antioxidants; Caramel, Properties and Analysis

Although the number of ingredients that go into the making of beer are few, the chemistry of brewing is complex. From a cursory and rather simplistic point of view, the production of beer involves the (malt) enzyme-catalysed saccharification of starch (malt and adjunct) to fermentable sugars followed by the conversion of these sugars to alcohol and carbon dioxide by yeast. Hops provide bitterness through the isomerization of humulones to isohumulones. From this basic chemical framework, the brewing scientist continues to develop a much deeper understanding of the chemistry of brewing. It is through this understanding that the brewer will produce better beers which will meet higher and more demanding quality standards.

Bibliography

Broderick HM (ed.) (1977) *The Practical Brewer*, Madison: Master Brewers Association of America.
Hough JS, Briggs DE, Steven R (1971) *Malting and Brewing Science*. London: Chapman and Hall.
Meyer LH (1960) *Food Chemistry*. New York: Reinhold.
Pollock JRA (ed.) (1979) *Brewing Science*. London: Academic Press.

Etzer Chicoye and Henry Goldstein
Miller Brewing Company, Milwaukee, USA

Analysis and Sensory Evaluation

Analysis and Sensory Evaluation

Beer is an extremely complex solution with important compounds present at concentrations varying from tens of grams per litre to fractions of a nanogram per litre. Routine analytical schemes never attempt to embrace this complexity fully, but are guided by a mixture of legal requirements and the need to define the product. The legal aspect is stronger with beers than for many food and drink products as, in general, beer is a source of taxation in the countries where it is sold. Analysis then becomes not just a matter of ensuring compliance with food regulations such as use of specified ingredients or absence of a contaminant, but an important day-to-day financial issue for both the producer and the government. In addition to protocols for this type of analysis which are laid down by the government, three bodies publish recommended methods for beer analysis which are based on best practice and the results of interlaboratory collaborative trials. These are The Institute of Brewing, The European Brewery Convention and the American Society of Brewing Chemists.

Determination of Beer Strength

The exact definition of what constitutes beer strength varies, but there are two main possibilities from a legal viewpoint: original gravity (specific gravity of wort prior to fermentation) or ethanol concentration. In most countries beer strength is defined as ethanol concentration and this is the most significant characteristic as far as the drinker's physiology is concerned. Currently in the UK, taxation is collected on the basis of original gravity but the beer containers have to carry the concentration of ethanol as percentage by volume (% ABV) to conform to EEC labelling legislation. January 1993 has been set for the UK to come into line with EEC legislation and use %ABV for taxation purposes as well. *See* European Economic Community, The Common Agricultural Policy

Ethanol Content

The method in use in the UK is specified by the Laboratory of the Government Chemist. Carbon dioxide is first removed from the beer at 20°C by filtration through a medium-fast qualitative filter paper with the funnel covered with a clock glass to reduce evaporation of ethanol. One hundred millilitres of the degassed beer is distilled in a specified glass apparatus to collect approximately 85 ml of distillate. The distillate is then made up to 100 ml and the specific gravity measured at 20°C using a 50 ml pycnometer. The density is calculated from the following equation:

$$\text{density in air (kg m}^{-3}\text{) at }20°C = \\ \text{specific gravity at }20°C \times 997·17. \quad (1)$$

Ethanol content by volume or by weight can be found from the density using the Laboratory Alcohol Table issued by HM Customs and Excise in 1979 (ref. RDC80/267/04).

For control purposes the density can be determined using an Anton–Paar densitometer operating at 20°C.

The above methods are unsuitable for low-alcohol or alcohol-free products, and in these cases it is recommended that the analysis should be carried out using the Boehringer test combination for the determination of ethanol in foodstuffs. This method measures the increase in the absorbance at 340 nm (NADH synthesis) catalysed by the enzyme alcohol dehydrogenase.

Original Gravity (OG), Residue Gravity (RG) and Present Gravity (PG)

PG simply refers to the specific gravity of the beer at 20°C without any treatment other than degassing, and can be determined either by a pycnometer or densitometer.

The method for OG and RG determinations proceeds exactly as for the determination of alcohol described in the previous section except that both the distillate and the residue in the distillation flask are made up to 100 ml and the specific gravity of both determined. The specific gravity of the residue (RG) represents the material originally present in the wort but unfermented. In order to calculate the OG the specific gravity of the distillate is used to calculate the 'spirit indication' $(1000 \times (1·00000 - \text{specific gravity of the distillate}))$. The corresponding degrees of gravity lost during the fermentation can be obtained from the statutory Degrees of Gravity Lost Table. The sum of the RG and the degrees of gravity lost gives the OG.

The above method is capable of giving the true OG, as determined on the wort before addition of yeast, to within 1% but gives erroneously high results if beers have had postfermentation treatments, such as addition of priming sugars, which increase the RG value. If the beer was made by a high-gravity procedure then the method will give the theoretical OG equivalent to the diluted beer strength rather than the actual OG as it was in the fermenter.

The legal procedure as described is time-consuming and requires technical skill, so in practice more rapid methods are used for control purposes. A common and economical method is to use refractometric measurements of the beer in conjunction with the PG. The refractometric reading for degassed beer is found at 20°C on the Zeiss–Pulfrich scale and the PG is converted into excess degrees $(1000 \times (\text{specific gravity of the beer} - 1·0000))$. The OG in excess degrees can then be calculated from the following equation:

$$OG = 3·24 - 1·644PG + 2·597 \times \text{refractometric reading.} \quad (2)$$

The equation is an average for a range of commercial beers and more accurate results can be obtained if the equation is derived for the particular beer in question.

A number of automatic and semiautomatic instruments are available for the measurement of OG. All seem to rely on the same basic principles. Beer is injected into the instrument, which determines the PG and the ethanol content either by refractometry or by thermal conductivity. The OG is then calculated from eqn [2], which rests on the average relationship between OG, alcohol content, degrees of gravity lost and PG.

In many countries the specific gravity is not used directly as in the UK, but is converted to a system of named degrees based on the density of sucrose solutions according to an official sugar table. For example, °Plato represent the percentage of sucrose (w/w) in a solution at 20°C; a specific gravity of 1·032 is approximately equivalent to 8·1°Plato whilst 1·040 is equivalent to 10·0°.

Degree of Attenuation

The degree of attenuation can be a useful process control and beer quality indicator as it describes the proportion of the original extract which has been fermented:

$$\text{degree of attenuation} = \frac{OG - RG}{OG} \times 100, \quad (3)$$

where OG and RG are in excess degrees.

Calorific Value

Though not a required measurement at the moment, the calorific value of beer is of interest in diet control and may become necessary if labelling regulations change in the future:

$$\text{calorific value per 100 ml} = \\ (\text{grams of ethanol} \times 7) + (\text{grams of carbohydrate} \times 4) + \quad (4) \\ (\text{grams protein} \times 4).$$

Carbohydrate is determined by the anthrone/sulphuric acid method and protein is calculated from the Kjeldahl nitrogen figure. Beers are typically in the 30–40 kcal per 100 ml range and the calorific value correlates roughly with the OG regardless of the degree of attenuation.

Determination of Physical Properties

Several physical properties of beer are of the very highest importance to quality and product definition.

Clarity

The majority of beers are required to be clear to the eye and in the case of lighter-coloured beers they should appear bright without the slightest suggestion of a haze or opalescence. Clarity is normally measured in EBC formazin haze units, referring to a standard hazy solution made by mixing hexamethylene tetramine with hydrazine sulphate. A measure of 1·0 EBC unit represents a just detectable haze and is equivalent to 69 ASBC formazin units or 40 Helm units. The Radiometer haze meter, which has been widely used internationally since the early 1960s for the laboratory measurement of beer clarity, is now being replaced by several other instruments. The Radiometer depended on measuring the amount of green light scattered at 90° in relation to the amount of transmitted light and, although undoubtedly a very successful instrument, this made it more sensitive to small haze particles than is the human eye. The result was occasional recording of clear beers as hazy; the so-called invisible haze. The new generation of instruments use a forward scattering angle of 120°, which tends to reduce this problem. *See* Sensory Evaluation, Appearance

Colour

Colour is a major determinant of beer quality and type and arises either entirely from the raw materials and the processing or from the addition of food-grade caramel. There is no connection between beer colour and strength. The recommended method to determine colour is to measure the absorbance at 430 nm, which is multiplied by 25 and any dilution factor to give EBC colour units. Alternatively, the beer can be compared by eye against standard coloured discs in a simple comparator. *See* Caramel, Properties and Analysis; Colours, Properties and Determination of Natural Pigments

Beer Foam and Head

The appearance and longevity of the foam formed on the top of a glass of beer on pouring is considered a major indicator of product type and quality. Unfortunately, as yet, there is no recommended method for measurement of foam properties and most brewers use a technique which measures head retention, i.e. the longevity of the foam when produced under standard conditions. In the UK, the Rudin method is popular. Here the beer is placed in a glass column and foamed by passage of carbon dioxide through a sintered glass disc in the bottom of the column. The rate of increase in the volume of the liquid beer phase during collapse of the foam is measured and reported as a half-life in seconds. Techniques of this type are not very reproducible from one laboratory to another and seem to give only a good, bad or average type of classification. The value obtained may not relate to the performance of the beer at the point of sale. The problem is that the technique measures the rate at which beer drains from the foam. This is a composite of the bubble size, column diameter and beer viscosity, and the situation is significantly different from that seen by the customer. In this case more important aspects are the carbon dioxide and nitrogen contents of the beer, its temperature, the mode of pouring and degree to which gas break-out is encouraged and, vitally, the cleanliness of the glass.

A subsidiary aspect of beer foam considered important by many is the phenomenon of lacing. this refers to the net of foam which is retained on the surface of the glass as the beer is drunk. The important prerequisites for a good lacing pattern are, first of all, good foam formation on pouring, then the presence of hop bittering compounds at concentrations over about 20 ppm and a clean, uncharged and properly hydrophobic glass surface.

Measurement of Specific Compounds

In addition to the overall properties of beers, in many cases a close correlation has been found between individual compounds or groups of compounds and specific product properties.

Residual Carbohydrates

The amount of residual carbohydrates in a beer is considered by many to be important in the 'palate' or 'fullness' of the beer. It may certainly contribute to sweetness and in some cases can be an indicator that all is not well with the fermentation system. A higher than normal residual carbohydrate content indicates an incomplete fermentation and, possibly, altered beer flavour properties. It may also make the beer more open to microbiological infection during packaging and storage. *See* Carbohydrates, Sensory Properties; Flavour Compounds, Structures and Characteristics

Until recently the only methods available were based on RG, total carbohydrate content using the anthrone/sulphuric acid method or taste. None of these is very discerning but the situation has been changed completely by the advent of high-performance liquid chromatography (HPLC). Simple systems are available which will give a qualitative and quantitative analysis of the full range of residual carbohydrates. Thus, the desired profile of the beer carbohydrate fraction can be defined precisely. *See* Chromatography, High-performance Liquid Chromatography

Residual Amino Acids

Most worts have limiting amounts of amino acids so beers tend to be relatively free of amino acids other than proline. Although amino acids can be separated and estimated by automatic ion exchange chromatography, this is rarely done in the control context and determination of free amino nitrogen using the ninhydrin reagent is sufficient. Higher than expected levels of residual amino acids, as with the carbohydrates, indicates an incomplete fermentation which may have consequences for beer properties including flavour and certainly makes the beer more open to infection by *lactobacillae*. *See* Amino Acids, Determination

Compounds Derived from Hop Resins

Beers contain a considerable number of compounds derived from hop resins during wort boiling and the overall concentration of these compounds correlates well with the perceived bitterness of beer. Although HPLC techniques have now made a sophisticated analysis of hop compounds possible, for ordinary control purposes a simple extraction of acidified beer (10 ml beer + 3 ml of 3M hydrochloric acid) with optically clear iso-octane (20 ml) is normally sufficient. The absorbance of the iso-octane layer at 275 nm multiplied by 50 gives the bitterness units of the beer.

Carbon Dioxide

Carbon dioxide is important in giving beers much of their perceived qualities. Evolution of gas bubbles gives the poured beer its characteristic head of foam, gives the impression of liveliness in the glass, brings out the aroma of the beer and results in a sharpness in the mouth during drinking. In a tank or container where carbon dioxide is the only gas present, then the excess pressure in relation to the temperature accurately defines the amount of gas dissolved in the beer. In packaged beer it will be necessary to measure carbon dioxide in other ways to obtain accurate results. In this case the most difficult thing is to obtain a representative sample. The beer should be chilled to 0°C, opened very carefully and 40% w/v sodium hydroxide solution added immediately at the rate of 10 ml per 250 ml of beer followed by careful but thorough mixing. In the recommended method a sample of the alkaline beer is transferred to a sealed glass apparatus. Acid is then added to release the carbon dioxide and the amount of gas is estimated manometrically. In everyday practice it is more likely that a Corning carbon dioxide meter will be used. Again a sample of the alkaline beer is injected and acid is added to liberate the carbon dioxide, but in this case the

amount is estimated from the thermal conductivity of the gas phase. Both types of apparatus must be calibrated with standard sodium carbonate solutions. Commercial beers usually contain carbon dioxide in the range $3 \cdot 5$–$4 \cdot 5$ g l^{-1}. In the older UK system, 1 volume per volume is equivalent to $1 \cdot 96$ g l^{-1}.

Sulphur Dioxide

A certain amount of sulphur dioxide is produced during yeast fermentation, so it is a natural constituent of beer, but in some cases sodium metabisulphite is added directly or indirectly along with finings. The amount of sulphur dioxide allowed in foodstuffs is controlled by law and there is a general tendency at the moment to reduce the legally defined maximum concentration. It is therefore important to determine the sulphur dioxide levels in commercial beer before sale.

Several methods for the determination of sulphur dioxide have been recommended, but the one which appears to give the most reliable results is based on the Monier–Williams procedure. Fifty millilitres of beer are distilled under reflux with a flow of carbon dioxide or nitrogen in an air-free glass apparatus. The evolved sulphur dioxide is trapped in a receiver containing 10 ml of 10% neutralized hydrogen peroxide. In the receiver the gas is converted to sulphuric acid which can be estimated by titration with $0 \cdot 02$ M sodium hydroxide using bromophenol blue as the indicator.

Volatile Organic Compounds

A range of volatile organic compounds is produced by yeast during fermentation and each compound has potential significance in beer flavour. Production of these compounds is very susceptible to the exact conditions of fermentation so variation in the beer can indicate inadequate control in the brewery.

Higher Alcohols and Esters

n-Propanol, isobutanol, 2-methylbutanol, 3-methylbutanol and phenylethanol are the commonest of the higher alcohols produced and occur in the tens of milligrams per litre range. Their synthesis is very much involved with the metabolism of the equivalent amino acis with one more carbon atom. The relationship is exactly the same as that between alanine and ethanol. Esters arise from the alcohols through intracellular reaction with acyl-CoA derivatives. Ethyl acetate is synthesized in the same way from ethanol and acetyl-CoA. All these compounds can be estimated by gas chromatography (GC) under relatively simple conditions, e.g. a Carbowax column operating isothermally at about 100°C and flame ionization detector (FID) with either headspace or direct injection. A temperature profile may be needed if esters of longer-chain such as caproate or caprylate are under investigation. *See* Alcohol, Properties and Determination

Vicinal Diketones

Two vicinal diketones, butane-2,3-dione (diacetyl) and pentane-2,3-dione, arise in beer as the result of the spontaneous decomposition of α-acetohydroxy acids which leak from the cells. The diketones can be determined individually by using GC separation and an electron capture detector. For routine control the recommended colorimetric method is usually used. This technique does not distinguish between the two diketones or indeed their precursor α-acetohydroxy acids, but this is quite acceptable within the practical brewing context as it is this total value which is the relevant criterion. One hundred millilitres of undegassed beer is distilled in a glass apparatus to collect 15–20 ml of distillate in 5–10 min. This is made up to 25 ml with distilled water and a 5 ml aliquot mixed with 1·0 ml of 4% α-naphthol in isopropanol and 0·5 ml of a solution of 0·3 g of creatinine in 80 ml of 40% aqueous potassium hydroxide. After making up to 10 ml the mixture is shaken for 1 min and the absorbance at 530 nm measured within 5 min. The concentration of vicinal diketones and their precursors is then read from a standard curve constructed with purified diacetyl.

Dimethylsulphide

Dimethylsulphide is an important component of traditional lager flavour but can also arise from bacterial infection. As for the other higher alcohols and esters there is not a recommended method, but the compound is normally measured by a GC technique. *See* Chromatography, Gas Chromatography

Inorganic Ions

Recommended methods (either colorimetric or using atomic absorption spectroscopy) are available for iron, copper, zinc, arsenic, lead, nickel, sodium, calcium, chloride and sulphate. *See* Spectroscopy, Visible Spectroscopy and Colorimetry

Miscellaneous Contaminants

On occasion, unwanted compounds occurring as contaminants or arising from the process, e.g. pesticides or nitrosamines, are discovered in beer. Techniques for the measurement of such compounds are best found in the research literature such as the *Journal of the Institute of Brewing* or the *Journal of the American Society of Brewing Chemists*. When such a case arises, work concentrates on discovering the source of the unwanted compound and then procurement and processing procedures are adapted to eliminate the compound from further beer production. *See* Contamination, Detection

Assessment of Flavour

Because of the large size of modern breweries, multisite production of the same brand, sometimes under licence from another company, and the market-led approach to development of new brands, flavour assessment of beers has to be carried out in a formalized and reliable way. At each stage it is vital that all criteria are met or a considerable effort can be put into obtaining meaningless results. *See* Sensory Evaluation, Taste

The two main areas of assessment are, on the one hand, determination of consumer preferences and, on the other, analytical assessment for the purposes of control and development. The people used must suit the purposes: potential customers for the preference tests and trained brewery personnel for the analytical tests. In either case care must be taken to select the assessment technique most suited to the problem, which must, itself, be clearly identified. The procedure must be carried out with at least the defined minimum number of tasters and the results must be collected and correlated immediately. In analytical testing it is good practice to blend assessment sessions with continuing training and discussion sessions.

Selection of the Assessment Panel

In the case of consumer preference testing, the assessors will most likely be volunteers from a club or organization or invited in from the street. The important thing is to obtain a large number of people who are potential customers. *See* Sensory Evaluation, Practical Considerations

For analytical assessment it is normal to obtain volunteers from the brewery staff and then use simple taste tests to screen out individuals who have poor sensitivity to the basic characteristics of beer, e.g. sweetness, bitterness and acidity. The selected group can then be trained to the level necessary. This varies considerably, depending on the assessment techniques to be utilized.

Selection of the Assessment Technique

Possibly the commonest problem to occur in beer assessment is whether or not two beers can be distinguished on the basis of their flavour. The simplest approach is to apply the paired comparison or two-glass test. A glass of each beer is presented to the assessor under carefully controlled conditions. The question 'Is there a difference?' should be answered yes or no. Reference of the number of yes votes to a statistical table shows the level of certainty that the panel could detect a difference. Take note that it is impossible to say that two beers are the same. This type of test requires a minimum of seven assessors, but 10 is a more realistic minimum and a panel with at least 15 members would be preferred. The test can be made more sophisticated by changing the question to ask which of the two beers has a higher intensity of a named flavour characteristic. This gives the test a directional aspect but the analysis of the results is carried out in the same way. Tests of this kind are common in determining consumer preferences.

In the analytical situation, simple difference testing is more likely to use a version of the triangular or three-glass test, as fewer tasters are required to achieve any given level of statistical significance. In this case the assessor is presented with three glasses containing the beers in any order, e.g. ABB, ABA, AAB, etc. The question to be answered asks which of the beers is different from the other two. The number of positive replies for a given glass are referred to a statistical table to obtain the significance of the results. The minimum number of assessors is five, and 10 makes a satisfactory working group. This test is particularly prone to transfer bias, i.e. the effect of tasting one beer on the perception of another, and it is important that all the possible combinations of order of beers are tested.

As the questions asked become more sophisticated so does the assessment technique and the degree of training required of the panel. Ranking tests can be used to put up to four beers in order on the basis of a single defined characteristic. Descriptive tests allow a wide degree of information about a beer to be assessed and presented. Such tests vary from description of a few flavour notes in, say, returned beer based on the opinion of only one or two people to statistically validated fully quantitative descriptions of all the flavour notes present. Work of the latter type may require up to 100 highly trained assessors. The most commonly applied descriptive test in brewery situations is probably the flavour profile type which requires 6–8 people and provides a semiquantitative description. *See* Sensory Evaluation, Sensory Rating and Scoring Methods; Sensory Evaluation, Descriptive Analysis

Bibliography

Analysis Committee of the EBC (1987) *Analytica EBC*, 4th edn. Zurich: Brauerei- und Getranke-Rundschau.

Broderick HM (ed.) (1977) *The Practical Brewer*, 2nd edn. Madison: Master Brewers Association of the Americas.

Hough JS, Briggs DE, Steven R and Young TW (1982) *Malting and Brewing Science*, vol. 2. London: Chapman and Hall.

Institute of Brewing (1982) *Recommended Methods of Analysis: Worts and Beers*. London: Institute of Brewing.

J. C. Slaughter
Heriot-Watt University, Edinburgh, UK

BEHAVIOUR AND DIET

Nutritional Effects on Behaviour

Behaviour other than eating and drinking can be influenced by physiological effects of the constituents of foods and beverages. Indeed, consumers' attributions of effects on their subjective feelings or objective performance appear to be among the major determinants of the acceptance or refusal of certain items of the diet. This aspect of the many relationships among food, nutrition and behaviour is the topic of this article.

Scientific Study of Effects of Diet on Behaviour

The possible influences of diet on behaviour have attracted a considerable amount of public and professional attention in recent years, and yet reliable scientific information on such effects remains very limited.

This is partly because studies claiming positive findings are often open to serious criticism of their design and also of the theory behind them. Even arguably supportable findings have frequently failed to be substantiated after some years, at least on the scale initially claimed. A field that acquires a dubious reputation, or at best an air of scientific intractability, will naturally have difficulty attracting much good research. Nevertheless, definite scientific progress could be made by close collaboration among social cognitive psychologists, applied nutritionists and food technologists.

The measurement of behavioural performance or experiences is not the real difficulty in studying dietary effects on behaviour, despite a widespread misconception to the contrary. Even the answers to questions about personal viewpoints, which seem such 'soft' data to biologists and chemists, can be shown, by the well-established criteria of multivariate psychometrics, to reflect underlying determinants. Such adequately scaled instruments provide valid and reliable expressions of differences in emotional state and in judgements of one's own ability. Sound measurements of intellectual performance, such as ability to concentrate or remember, or indeed physical performance,such as athletic endurance, can be constructed at least as easily as self-ascription scales such as mood or ability by cognitive or exercise scientists.

The greatest difficulties arise in the design and interpretation of investigations of real-life psychological phenomena and, indeed, in measuring the composition of the everyday diet as well. as in any other area of science, effective research requires a good theoretical grasp of the mechanisms involved and hence of the methods for obtaining evidence of their operation. There are no standardized tests for effects of diet on behaviour and there never will be, any more than there can be standardized tests for dietary effects on children's growth or for consumer perception of food quality.

Hence what follows is an impressionistic sketch of the theoretical issues of how diet might affect behaviour, with brief comments on the current state of evidence for the mechanisms involved. Detailed reviews referring to original studies are included in the *Bibliography*.

Long-term Effects of Diet on Behaviour

There are broadly speaking two ways in which consti-tuents of the diet could have long-term psychological effects. They may affect the general physical growth or deterioration of the nervous system. Alternatively, diet might permanently affect the functioning of the brain, via short-term effects on changes within specific neural connections that have long-term psychological conse-quences.

Brain Development

The nerve cells in the human brain have virtually all been formed prior to birth. Considerable elaboration of interneuronal connections occurs postnatally, however. Maternal nutrition might therefore affect the fetus or the breast-fed infant. Nevertheless, the brain is very effec-tive at extracting essential nutrients from the blood supply and is not susceptible to overdevelopment. Hence there is reason to think that only metabolic disorder or extreme deficiency in the diet is liable to prejudice development of the brain.

In the rare inherited metabolic disorders, the accumu-lation of unusual catabolites damages the brain unless prevented by dietary or genetic engineering. As well as neurological disorders, more or less severe learning difficulties (mental handicaps) can result. *See* Inborn Errors of Metabolism

Possibilities under study include psychological seque-lae of neurological defects, prematurity or very low birthweight, to which maternal deficiency (such as in folic acid) might contribute. There is concern that some fatty acids in breast milk may be needed in infant milk formulae, at least in premature babies, in order for the brain to develop to full intellectual potential.

Energy–protein deficiency early in childhood is asso-ciated with slow intellectual development. It is difficult to disentangle effects of malnutrition and disease on brain growth from functional handicaps arising from effects of economic and social disadvantage. Nutritional supplementation and psychosocial stimulation exert separate effects. In addition, school failure in low-income areas is associated with missing breakfast. However, regular provision of supplements or break-fasts can be an important environmental change, aside from its physiological effects. *See* Breakfast – Role in the Diet; Protein, Deficiency

Brain Damage

Nutritional factors have repeatedly been proposed for schizophrenic and other psychiatrically diagnosed dis-orders. None has yet been substantiated, however, when subjected to controlled investigation. Thiamin defi-ciency produces neurological symptoms, and lack of this and other B vitamins is generally considered to contri-bute to some encephalopathies that involve several memory defects. Therapeutic effects of supplementation remain to be established. *See* Thiamin, Physiology

Toxic contaminants of the diet may damage the brain, with psychological sequelae. Nevertheless, no long-term psychological effect of the present dietary levels of residues, heavy metals, etc., has been established to date. Ingestion of flakes of paint or contaminated dust can contribute to an accumulation of lead in the brain but this generally results from hands or objects being brought to the mouth, not from dietary consumption. *See* Heavy Metal Toxicology

Short-term Mediation of Long-term Effects

Long-term psychological effects of dietary constituents on children, such as those on intelligence quotient (IQ), personality or behaviour disorders, are likely to be mediated by acute psychological effects of the daily diet. For example, if school performance were permanently improved by regular provision of breakfast, it could be because each meal facilitated learning that morning.

Additives and Hyperactivity

Feingold's initial hypothesis that intolerances to food additives such as colourings cause widespread behavioural problems in children was narrowed at an early stage to tartrazine and salicylates. Much subsequent investigation has established the very low incidences of food intolerances and the infrequency and transience of proven allergenic reactions to food proteins in young children. Moreover, recent work has shown no systematic behavioural effect when a toxicological sensitivity has been provoked. *See* Food Additives, Safety; Food Intolerance, Types; Food Intolerance, Food Allergies; Food Intolerance, Lactose Intolerances

Vitamins and IQ

Several recent reports have provided data interpreted as supporting the hypothesis that supplementation with one or more unspecified vitamins and/or minerals prevents a supposed slowing of the normal rise in nonverbal intelligence test scores (IQ) in schoolchildren whose diets are alleged to be deficient in those micronutrients.

As yet, however, there is no satisfactory evidence that those whose IQ scores appear to respond to supplements are deficient in micronutrients, because the only relevant dietary data are the children's dietary records and these are likely to be confounded by factors that influence scores in IQ tests. Furthermore, children who are estimated to be consuming less than recommended levels of a micronutrient generally appear also to have inadequate energy intakes. The accuracy of these records is therefore suspect. Alternatively, these children may be chronically hungry or reacting to other sorts of deprivation. This might account at least in part for the fidgetiness and apparent lack of attention that has been reported in children having the poorer dietary records, which in turn could make for poor learning and hence slowed development of performance in some IQ tests. *See* Energy, Measurement of Food Energy

Another (not incompatible) hypothesis is that the high sugar intake of some children might have acute sedative effects. This could result in difficulty in thinking clearly, so that the child becomes restless when faced with an intellectual challenge. *See* Sucrose, Dietary Importance

No biochemically sound mechanism has yet been proposed by which moderate vitamin or mineral deficiency could affect non-verbal learning. Theory is hardly feasible in any case because, although some speculations have been offered, the neural bases of individual differences in human 'intelligence' are as yet unknown.

Short-term Effects of Diet on Behaviour

The acute effects on behaviour of a constituent of a drink or even of the composition of a meal are both theoretically and methodologically much more accessible than chronic dietary effects. Even so, they pose formidable multidisciplinary challenges to investigators, in design and analysis of characteristics of the diets, the consumers and the situations to be observed.

Design of Investigations

The Foods

When the issue is physiological effects in the brain, the postingestional effects of the diet must be distinguished from its sensory effects. This is crucial in principle because a flavour or texture may suggest effects to the consumer (e.g. filling, nutritious, junk food, luxury) that could confuse the search for physiologically mediated effects. The distinction has become demonstrably necessary in some cases, such as reduction of distress – just the taste of sugar can quieten a baby and raise the pain threshold. Hence differences in dose of the hypothesized active constituent must not be detectable to the subject. If the agent cannot be swallowed in a capsule, demonstration of effective sensory matching or masking is necessary. *See* Sensory Evaluation, Sensory Characteristics of Human Foods

For major constituents of the diet, the technological requirements to design unambiguous research protocols may be so unusual and difficult as to be impossible at reasonable expense. Experimental cognitive psychology can provide a way round by measurements that pick out the effects of sensorily triggered expectations, but this demands sophisticated design and analysis (and a modicum of good luck).

The Eaters

Individuals may vary from one another physiologically in susceptibility to a dietary factor. They will certainly differ in prior experiences with foods and drinks containing the component(s) of interest.

Where the psychological effect being studied is known to the public, and especially if it is commonly sought or avoided, the effectiveness of a study is likely to depend on designing and analysing it around the participants' uses of items and the occasions when they are consumed. This will not only help to accommodate differences in both physiology and experience; it can also enable differences to be exploited. For example, disguised variations of a constituent, around the level at which an individual normally consumes it with the expectation of a relevant psychological effect, are likely to be a more sensitive design than the same levels imposed on everyone tested, without regard to their normal expectations.

The Test Tasks and Situations

A psychological effect may be wanted only in certain situations by a given consumer. Indeed, the effect may only occur in specific circumstances. That can be because the effect is part of conventional behaviour and experience in those circumstances or because the user personally discovered something, when the conditions were right, that the item could do for mood or performance. It may well be crucial, therefore, that the setting investigated and the state of mind of the research participant is suited to the mood or performance under study and that the behavioural tests measure those particular benefits that each participant obtains during normal use of the dietary item.

Alcohol

Alcoholic beverages have been an important part of the diet in many cultures from time immemorial. The alcohol content is widely regarded as a source of good cheer on social occasions and soothing or even emotionally anaesthetic at times of distress. However, incapacitating effects of alcohol are also well known, as is the risk of problems from its continuous heavy use. *See* Alcohol, Metabolism, Toxicology and Beneficial Effects

Neurophysiological evidence suggests that ethanol has psychoactive effects by acting on the GABA (γ-aminobutyric acid) receptor system at inhibitory synapses throughout the nervous system. Such neural inhibition is critical to the precision of information processing. Thus the postingestional psychological effects of ethanol are likely to be protean. It may be that all forms of fine control, including precise physical movements (walking down a straight line), vigilance against subtle dangers (crossing in front of approaching traffic), and self-critical social performance (ethical inhibitions and fears for self-esteem), are rendered less competent.

However, ethanol has been regarded in animal pharmacology as specifically anxiety-reducing at subsedative doses. The benzodiazepines (such as Valium), that also act on the GABA system, are used as antianxiety agents, as well as muscle relaxants and sedatives. Thus the neural actions of ethanol may be more effective at reducing tensions than at incapacitating generally.

Many of the effects of common levels of consumption of alcoholic beverages on mood and social behaviour appear to have at least as much to do with the drinking situation as with neural actions of ethanol. Merriment and perhaps sexual predation are what is expected at parties; personal aggressiveness and vandalism became a norm for soccer fans, and gloom is natural for the lone(ly) drinker. All these effects have been seen in experimental studies, but there tend to be large 'placebo' or expectancy effects too. It seems that ethanol contributes some disinhibition or incapacitation but a participative spirit achieves the rest.

The behavioural effects of ethanol in the diet are therefore complex to investigate. The sensory qualities of ethanol and the aftereffects of its ingestion on bodily sensations and mental and physical abilities are well known to experienced drinkers. This weakens the interpretations of sophisticated experiments on the behavioural effects of ethanol (as also for other familiar substances).

One example is the so-called 'balanced placebo' design. This has four conditions, two drinks with ethanol and two without, where one of each pair is stated by the investigator to contain alcohol and the other is said not to. The presence and absence of alcohol are supposed to be masked but, when the sensory disguise is checked, it is often found to have been ineffective. Furthermore, characteristic effects of ethanol are liable to be noticed some minutes after ingestion of the ethanol-spiked drink that was alleged to be an alcohol-free drink. This is likely to provoke an emotional reaction and to change the strategy in the task set by the experimenter. An experienced user not feeling the usual effects when the drink was falsely said to contain alcohol is also likely to react to that disparity but in a different way, perhaps more disappointed than angry. Thus the effects on behaviour of stated and actual alcohol contents cannot be separated out by analysis of this two-by-two design on an additive model: it is not balanced and placebo control is impracticable (as generally for familiar psychoactive substances). Detailed evidence is needed on the cognitive processes after drinking more or less alcohol with the normal approximate knowledge of amount.

Traditional dose–response studies of behavioural effects of alcohol are subject to similar problems, even when the variations in alcohol content are not detected during consumption and aftereffects are hard to distinguish, e.g. within the lower range of doses. Sensitive tests of psychomotor performance can show deficits at low doses that are proportionate to those at higher doses, thus justifying an argument for a zero blood alcohol limit on drivers. However, the consumer of a known amount of alcohol before driving or working may pay closer attention to the task and put extra effort into control and decision. In some circumstances, such an effort can overcompensate for the detrimental effect of ethanol, associating a low dose with objectively improved performance. Of course, such an effect should not be confused with the personal belief that a little alcohol has improved one's performance, since that is liable to be an illusion fostered by ethanol's disruption of self-critical abilities. Nevertheless, this phenomenon does illustrate how actively people use the effects of food and drink; they are not just affected passively or automatically.

Caffeine

Caffeine is thought to be able to act as a mild alerting agent by blocking synaptic receptors for endogenous adenosine, which is sedative. However, the experimental literature on human behaviour has been confused by the use of large doses relative to those obtained through normal coffee, tea and cola drinking, by differences between people in responsiveness to caffeine, and in the benefits to performance or mood habitually obtained from such drinks, and by unrealistic tests for such benefits. *See* Caffeine

Recently, by using normal doses, Lieberman and colleagues have shown quite strong and consistent effects of caffeine (at a dose as low as 32 mg) on tests of mental concentration (attentive and integrative thinking), effects which the participants themselves noticed in ratings of their state. Furthermore, in one study the participants rated themselves also to be more cheerful and less anxious, perhaps because they felt that they were doing better at the cognitive tests. Such conscious benefits may mediate some of the attractions of caffeinated drinks, over and above cultural norms and advertisers' implications.

A remaining weakness in even these studies is a lack of dose–response relationships. As recognized by physiologists, engineers and others, if an effect does not become stronger with increasing strength of an influence, that is a sign we are not looking at the actual mechanism. Grouped designs may sample a wide range of personal dose optima, depending on the benefits habitually gained from the use of caffeine in particular contexts by different individuals. Hence studies of behavioural effects of caffeine (and of other dietary constituents) should investigate individuals' habitual uses at doses ranging around that which is usual for each person in that situation.

Blood Glucose and Behaviour

Hypoglycaemia has been blamed for aggressiveness in members of societies subsisting on low energy intakes and for restlessness and poor attention in children consuming large amounts of sucrose. However, such claims are not well supported by measurements of blood glucose levels. Hypoglycaemia is in fact quite rare, in contrast to the prevalences claimed for such problematic behaviour. *See* Hypoglycaemia for Nutrition

The consumption of sucrose with relatively little complex carbohydrate and other nutrients might indeed lead to reactive hypoglycaemia, arising from overstimulation of insulin secretion. However, the behavioural aftereffect of consuming a large amount of sugar is if anything drowsiness, not agitation. Sucrose challenges specifically to children diagnosed as suffering from 'attention-deficit hyperactivity disorder' have mostly shown no effect on physical activity. However, the sedative effects could acutely impair attention and, in theory, a child's awareness of this might exacerbate problem behaviour in attention-demanding situations. It must be noted, on the other hand, that a parent's or institution staff's concern about the sugar intake of a problem child may be no more than a desperate hope for some remedy for the unmanageable behaviour. These relations between diet and behaviour also need careful sociopsychological analysis before biomedical investment.

Somewhat paradoxically in the light of the above, it has been recently suggested that administration of glucose might improve memory in the elderly, perhaps via noradrenaline systems in the brain. However, animal experiments have involved administering concentrated glucose solutions; these are stressful and may improve memory simply by alerting the rat.

Dietary Effects on Monoamine Neurotransmitters

A meal that is high in carbohydrate and low in protein content stimulates insulin secretion in the rat. The insulin facilitates uptake by muscle of circulating branched-chain amino acids (BCAAs; leucine, isoleucine and valine). These amino acids compete with other large neutral amino acids (LNAAs) for transport from the blood into the brain. The LNAAs include tryptophan, the precursor of the neurotransmitter 5-hydroxytryptamine (5-HT, or serotonin), and phenylalanine and tyrosine, precursors of the catecholamine transmitters dopamine and noradrenaline. The supply of precursor can limit the rate of synthesis of the transmitter, especially in the case of 5-HT. Thus reduced competition by BCAAs for brain tryptophan uptake is liable to increase the activity of serotonergic (5-HT-transmitted) synapses. *See* Amino Acids, Properties and Occurrence

Serotonergic neurons are important in the control of sleep. Oral administration of a substantial dose of tryptophan is sedative. This tryptophan supply effect on brain 5-HT probably explains why a high-carbohydrate meal promotes postprandial sleep in the rat. *See* Carbohydrates, Requirements and Dietary Importance

The LNAAs are abundant in protein mixtures of high biological quality. Thus, although a high-protein, low-carbohydrate meal also provokes insulin secretion in the rat, plasma levels of BCAAs are kept high by absorption and are not reduced enough to have a substantial effect on competition with tryptophan for transport into the brain. Hence the high-protein meal does not increase 5-HT activity and induce sedation by that mechanism. *See* Protein, Requirements

Relatively modest dietary levels of protein, e.g. 10–15% in the rat, keep the ratio of tryptophan to other LNAAs in blood plasma low enough to have no effect on brain 5-HT levels. However, as little as 4% protein keeps the plasma ratio low in human subjects. Few eating occasions provide that little protein. Even chocolate and sugar confectionery may contain a milk protein and/or grain protein. Hence it is unlikely that carbohydrate-rich foods induce sedation or other mood changes in people via the 5-HT mechanism.

This is a difficulty for the suggestion that drugs and psychiatric disorders affecting serotonergic activity induce a craving for carbohydrate via the action of carbohydrate-rich foods on tryptophan uptake, 5-HT and mood. Another difficulty is that many of these foods are sweet, an oral sensation that by itself apparently dampens distress via opioid mechanisms. In addition, the high-carbohydrate foods reportedly 'craved' are high-fat foods, and the creaminess or crispiness, with or without sweetness, makes them highly palatable. They can therefore be pleasurable and cheering to eat, independently of postingestional factors.

Finally, in a further illustration of the need for psychosocial analyses of diet and behaviour, these craved foods are generally convenience products that are recognized as nutritionally less desirable (so-called junk foods). Hence they may be avoided and as a result become tempting and craved for. Their consumption could then have the powerful impact on mood of any guiltridden sensual indulgence ('naughty but nice'), by purely cognitive processes with no particular neurotransmitter mediation.

Meals

A modest amount of food is widely regarded as mentally and physically energizing or refreshing. However, a heavy meal is expected to make one drowsy (while not necessarily promoting a good night's sleep). Recent behavioural research has provided some support for these conventional beliefs but the physiological mechanisms involved remain obscure.

There is a semicircadian rhythm of arousal, including a period of reduced performance in midafternoon as well as a more profound reduction in the small hours after midnight. A series of experiments by Smith and colleagues has shown that a substantial lunch tends to depress objective and subjective alertness further for a few hours. Going without lunch can therefore improve cognitive performance in midafternoon, although other consequences may not be desirable. Caffeine helps to counter the 'postlunch dip' and alcohol makes it worse. Different aspects of attention are affected by different protein:carbohydrate ratios in the meal. There is as yet no clear basis for this theory, in terms of either the cognitive processes or the physiological actions of food involved in these effects.

Breakfast is reputed to improve performance at work, although the evidence has been largely correlational with accident rates or school reports. Such effects are likely to depend on the size and composition of the breakfast, the physiology, personality and attributions of the consumer and the activities and tasks that follow the meal. *See* Breakfast – Role in the Diet

Bibliography

Bendich A and Butterworth CE (eds) (1991) *Micronutrients in Health and in Disease Prevention.* New York: Marcel Dekker.

Blane HT and Leonard KE (eds) (1987) *Psychological Theories of Drinking and Alcoholism.* New York: Guilford Press.

Dews PB (ed.) (1984) *Caffeine.* Berlin: Springer-Verlag.

Heuther G (ed.) (1988) *Amino Acid Availability and Brain Function in Health and Disease.* Berlin: Springer-Verlag.

Lieberman HR, Wurtman RJ, Garfield GS, Emde GG and Coviella ILG (1987) The effects of low doses of caffeine on human performance and mood. *Psychopharmacology* 92: 308–312.

Shepherd R (ed.) (1989) *Handbook of the Psychophysiology of Human Eating.* Chichester: John Wiley.

Smith AP, Leekam S, Ralph A and McNeill G (1988) The influence of meal composition on post-lunch changes in performance efficiency and mood. *Appetite* 10: 195–203.

Thayer RE (1989) *The Biopsychology of Mood and Arousal.* New York: Oxford University Press.

D. A. Booth
University of Birmingham, Birmingham, UK

BERIBERI

Aetiology

Beriberi is caused by a deficiency of the vitamin thiamin, one of the water-soluble B-group vitamins. There is very little free thiamin in the tissues and most of it is present in the phosphorylated active coenzyme forms bound to cell enzymes. Consequently, the experimental withdrawal of thiamin is very quickly followed by biochemical and clinical abnormalities and humans are dependent on a constant supply of this vitamin in the diet to meet their daily requirements. *See* Coenzymes; Thiamin, Physiology

The principal sources of thiamin in the diet are either cereals or starchy roots and tubers, which may contribute from 60% to 85% of dietary thiamin in the developing world. In developed countries, animal, dairy and other foods make a greater contribution. However, in the British diet, cereal products provide 45% of dietary thiamin, this somewhat artificial situation arising because white flour is fortified to the extent of 2·4 mg of thiamin per kg of flour. *See* Thiamin, Properties and Determination

Within the cereal grain, the germ and bran portions contain most of the thiamin; thus intake is closely related to milling practices. Rice which is parboiled before milling retains most of the thiamin that would otherwise be lost, whereas highly milled (polished) rice is particularly low in thiamin (80 μg of thiamin per 100 g) and was associated with widespread beriberi in Asia and the Far East at the end of the nineteenth and early part of the twentieth century. Endemic beriberi, however, has also occurred in communities subsisting on white wheat flour in China, India and Newfoundland, and should not therefore be linked specifically with rice but with impoverished or restricted diets in which the cereal is refined and is virtually the sole food item.

Food spoilage resulting from dampness and fungal attack undoubtedly contributes to thiamin losses both during storage and cooking. Cooking temperature above 100°C and alkaline conditions will cause loss of thiamin but leaching into cooking water is probably a more important cause of loss than chemical destruction.

Widespread beriberi dates from the introduction of the steam-powered rice mill in the nineteenth century but this was aggravated by socioeconomic conditions at the time – large sections of the community might live in closed or controlled communities where normal eating habits were prevented. In 1958, Platt revealingly described the feeding conditions of factory workers (aged 10 years and older) in Peking pre-1937: highly milled rice, sometimes stored for long periods, became infected with mould which matted the grains together in large lumps; in order to use this rice, the lumps had to be broken, remilled and washed thoroughly, resulting in the loss of most of the thiamin. *See* Rice

Polished rice is preferred by Chinese and Japanese communities to brown (undermilled) rice, while parboiled rice is preferred by Indians. The advantages of parboiled rice were clearly seen in Malaysia, where in the latter part of the nineteenth century there was a large-scale immigration of young able-bodied Chinese labourers to work in the tin mines, and of Indians for the rubber plantations. In both cases, the immigration workers very often lived in remote regions where there was little local production of food and where they were dependent on imported rice. In these conditions it was the Chinese who, because of their dietary preference for highly milled rice, contracted beriberi and died in enormous numbers.

While endemic beriberi has now largely disappeared, isolated outbreaks in developing countries still occur both within the community and, more often, in jails or boarding schools where normal eating practices are prevented and food choice is restricted.

Types of Beriberi

Beriberi is a state in which both cardiac and nervous functions are disturbed. However, the more serious the nervous lesion, the greater the muscular pain and weakness and the more likely the patient is to rest at an early stage in the attack and reduce the risk of severe cardiac beriberi. There are four main forms of beriberi: wet (cardiac, oedematous), dry (chronic polyneuropathy), infantile and the Wernicke–Korsakoff syndrome.

It is suggested that severe beriberi more often attacked the more active, stronger or supposedly better-nourished members of a poor community, and men appear to be more susceptible than women. Compare, for example, the recent outbreak of beriberi in The Gambia, where most of the people affected were aged between 20 and 40 years and attack rates were higher in men (9·3%) than women (3·4%).

Infantile beriberi received less attention than adult forms, although reports from Madras, Indonesia, Burma and Hong Kong indicated that it was a serious problem. It was also particularly characteristic of breast-fed infants in this region, and in the Philippines in

1910 it was pointed out that nowhere else had such a high mortality (448 per 1000) been recorded in breast-fed infants.

Wernicke's encephalopathy and Korsakoff's psychosis are common neurological disorders and the association with thiamin deficiency was established in the 1930s. They represent two facets of the same syndrome and appear to arise as a result of moderate to severe dietary restriction, usually of long duration and usually associated with alcohol abuse. The syndrome is primarily a neurological disorder and overt signs of beriberi heart disease are rarely observed.

Clinical Features

The name 'beriberi' is said to mean 'sheep' because the partial paralysis of the disease caused patients to walk like sheep. Endemic beriberi in adults is usually described as either 'wet' or 'dry' according to the presence or absence of oedema. Early symptoms include an ill-defined malaise and weakness of the legs which may be accompanied by a variety of symptoms associated with a developing polyneuritis (inflammation of many nerves; multiple and peripheral neuritis) or impaired cardiac function and many mothers whose infants had beriberi showed these signs. Acute forms of beriberi in which the cardiovascular symptoms predominate tend to occur in the younger, more active or stronger members of the community, whereas dry forms in which muscular atrophy and polyneuritis occur tend to be more frequent in the older adult.

Subacute Wet Beriberi

The course of disease is extremely variable. The predominant form, which is typically seasonal in endemic areas, is subacute wet beriberi. Anorexia is common but not characteristic. Constipation is more common than diarrhoea. The first cause of complaint in male labourers is an aching pain, stiffness or cramps in the calf or associated muscles. Pain is commonly experienced on squeezing the calf; there is increasing muscular tenderness and pain may occur especially at night before sleep. There may be diminished, bilateral reflexes of ankles and knees. In women, hypoaesthesia or paraesthesia in the fingers is frequently a first cause of complaint. Oedema (the presence of excessive amounts of fluid in the intercellular tissue spaces of the body) of the feet and legs is frequently an early symptom in both sexes and may also appear on the back of the hands and as a puffiness of the face. The heart is usually enlarged with tachycardia (rapid action of the heart, in excess of the normal limits which range from 40 to 100 beats per min) and a bounding pulse. There may be raised venous pressure and percussion may reveal dilatation of the right auricle and ventricle and a downward and outward displacement of the apex beat. Systolic heart murmurs may be present. There is commonly dyspnoea (discomfort or distress occurring when the increased need for pulmonary ventilation obtrudes unpleasantly into consciousness) on exertion and there may be palpitations, dizziness and giddiness. The extremities may be cold with peripheral cyanosis (blue appearance of the skin and mucous membranes) or, if the circulation is maintained, they may be warm owing to vasodilation. Electrocardiograms are often undisturbed but inversion of T waves may indicate disturbed conduction. In ambulatory prisoners of war, nocturia was noted following oedema during the day. Albuminuria is uncommon.

Fulminating Wet Beriberi

The clinical features of acute fulminating wet beriberi, which include sudden, intense pain, are dominated by insufficiency of heart and blood vessels. However, all other features of the subacute form tend to be present and accentuated. In addition, vomiting is common and usually indicates the onset of acute symptoms. There is often intense thirst but drinking initiates vomiting. The pupils are dilated with an anxious expression on the face. The patients are severely dyspnoeic, have violent palpitations of the heart, are extremely restless and experience intense precordial agony (relating to the precordium which is the anterior aspect of the thorax overlying the heart. Aphonia is frequently present and the patient's moans take on a special character believed to be because of the paralysis of the laryngeal muscles. There are widespread and powerful undulating pulsations visible in the region of the heart, epigastrium and neck owing to tumultuous heart action. Facial cyanosis is more marked during inspiration. The pulse is moderately full and even, with a frequency of 120–150 beats per min. The liver is enlarged and tender and the epigastric region is spontaneously painful. On percussion the heart is usually enlarged to both the left and right, and the apex beat may reach the axilla. Raised systolic and low diastolic pressure gives a 'pistol shot' sound on auscultation (listening to and interpreting the meaning of sounds within the body, usually by means of the stethoscope) over the large arteries. Oedema may cover legs, trunk and face with associated pericardial, pleural and other serous effusions. There is oliguria or anuria but no albuminuria or glycosuria. Death is accompanied by a fall in systolic blood pressure to 80 or 70 mmHg, the pulse becomes thinner and the veins dilate. The rough, whistling respiration deteriorates and rales (abnormalities sounds accompanying the breathing sounds heard during auscultation) appear. The patient dies intensely dyspnoeic but usually fully conscious.

Dry Beriberi

Dry beriberi is essentially a chronic condition showing muscular atrophy and polyneuritis and generally occurring in the older adult. Walking may be difficult because of weak, wasted and painful musculature and in the later stages feeding and dressing may also become impossible. In the later stages the patients also become very susceptible to infections when bedridden and cachetic (extreme state of general ill health, with malnutrition, wasting, circulatory and muscular weakness). Sensory nerve disturbances are evident from hypoaesthesia in the extremities and these progressively extend over the outer aspects of legs, thighs and forearms. Anaesthesia may become almost complete. Motor nerve disturbances likewise begin in the extremities and ascend progressively. Flaccid paralysis of the extensor muscles precedes that affecting the flexors and results in 'wrist drop' and 'foot drop'. Hypoactivity of the Achilles tendon reflex usually precedes an impaired patellar reflex. Cerebral manifestations are uncommon but were reported among Caucasian prisoners of war in Japanese camps.

Infantile Beriberi

Infantile beriberi occurs mainly between the first to the fourth month of life. The onset is sudden and the cardiovascular symptoms predominate as the most important features. The whole condition can deteriorate rapidly in a matter of a day or two. The infants are generally pale, oedematous and ill-tempered on admission. There is abdominal distension, colicky pain, vomiting and paroxysmal screaming. Constipation and water retention occur, leading to oedema. There follow tachycardia (200 beats per min), tachypnoea (undue rapid breathing which is quick and shallow), dyspnoea and aphonia (inability to produce sound via the laryngeal mechanism). The aphonia is recorded as being particularly striking on the observer. The soundless cry of infantile beriberi is attributed to either laryngeal nerve paralysis or oedema of the vocal cords. Cyanosis, signs of right-sided cardiac enlargement and failure, congestion of lungs and engorgement of the liver occur later. Finally, signs of increasing intracranial pressure are evident, with meningism, rigidity, twitching, drowsiness, coma and then death.

There are very few reports on juvenile beriberi, and the symptoms resemble those of the chronic condition with motor disturbances of the lower extremities rendering gait difficult. In addition, there are cerebral disturbances, nasal voice, hoarseness, difficulty in hearing and occular signs, blepharoptosis (drooping of the upper eyelid because of paralysis of the muscles or nerve), strabism (squint), and nystagmus (a condition in which the eyes are seen to move in a more or less rhythmical manner, from side to side, up and down, or in a rotatory manner from the original point of fixation). There is some cardiovascular involvement but cardiac dilatation and oedema are relatively rare.

Wernicke–Korsakoff Syndrome

Wernicke's encephalopathy may be defined as a neurological disorder of acute onset characterized by the following features in various combinations: nystagmus; abducens and conjugate gaze palsies; ataxia of gait; global confusional state. In addition, resting tachycardia and liver disease are present in 50% or more of patients. Overt signs of beriberi are rare but dypsnoea on exertion is commonplace, and sudden cardiovascular collapse may occasionally follow mild exertion. Polyneuropathies are present in most patients, mainly affecting the legs. Common symptoms include weakness, paraesthesia pain, loss of tendon reflexes and loss of sensation and motor power. Korsakoff psychosis refers to an abnormal mental state in which memory and learning are affected more severely than other cognitive functions in an otherwise alert and responsive patient.

Metabolic Effects

Some of the earliest studies on the biochemical defects produced by a lack of thiamin were performed by Sir Rudolph Peters in pigeons. Lactate levels were elevated in the brain and other tissues and it was shown that oxygen uptake by the avitaminous brain tissue was reduced *in vitro*. The metabolic acidosis results from an impairment of carbohydrate metabolism in thiamin deficiency. Thiamin in its active form, thiamin pyrophosphate (TPP), is of critical importance for the decarboxylation of pyruvic acid to acetyl coenzyme A and linking the Embden–Meyerhof glycolytic pathway with the tricarboxylic acid cycle for the efficient utilization of carbohydrate in energy production. *See* Carbohydrates, Digestion, Absorption and Metabolism

Approximately 10% of the body's thiamin is in the form of thiamin triphosphate (TTP) in nervous tissues. Thiamin triphosphate may be the neurophysiologically active form of thiamin which is pathogenically important in chronic beriberi and Wernicke's disease. It has been suggested that TTP may be involved in the binding of TPP to apoenzyme moieties or in ion movements in nervous tissue, but the true function still requires clarification.

Treatment and Prognosis

There is a dramatic improvement within a few hours following intramuscular or intravenous administration of 50–100 mg of thiamin hydrochloride to a patient with beriberi. Treatment should be followed by 5–10 mg orally for several days. In the case of infantile beriberi, the thiamin status of the mother should also be checked and similar treatment given to correct any deficiency. Once recognized and treated, the outlook as far as a full recovery is concerned is excellent.

The symptoms of Wernicke's disease all usually respond to treatment with thiamin regardless of the presence of alcohol, but the Korsakoff component responds only slowly or not at all.

The specific test for thiamin status is the transketolase stimulation test on a red cell haemolysate and can be made on samples of finger-tip blood. The ratio of stimulated to unstimulated activity is called the activation coefficient and is indicative of thiamin deficiency if greater than 1·25. Apo-transketolase (containing no TPP) is unstable both *in vitro* and *in vivo* and both the degree of unsaturation and basic enzyme activity should be used in interpreting results.

Prevention

Endemic beriberi in Asia and the Far East has declined greatly in recent years, reflecting changes in diet, food distribution, socioeconomic factors and the knowledge that the disease is caused by a vitamin deficiency and not by toxins or bacteria, although there is still some debate about the extent to which other factors may be of aetiological importance.

Outbreaks of beriberi among African communities, where traditional millet or corn diets are being replaced by rice, are disturbing. The ease of preparation of rice makes it a popular food as it reduces the workload of women, on whom much of the responsibility for maintaining both family and farm depend. Government agencies and medical authorities must be aware of this trend and be able to recognize and treat the symptoms if seasonal shortages develop and outbreaks of beriberi occur in unusual circumstances.

Alcohol reduces the efficiency of thiamin absorption as well as having many general effects on the metabolism of the liver, brain and other tissues. Alcohol abuse may occur for a variety of social, economic and other reasons, such as response to bereavement, but, whatever the reason, it may impair dietary intake and precipitate a downward sequence of events leading to nutritional deficiencies and mental impairment, possibly culminating in the Wernicke–Korsakoff syndrome. Preventing this condition therefore requires action at many levels in society as it is not simply a dietary deficiency.

Bibliography

Bray GW (1928) Vitamin-B deficiency in infants: its possibility, prevalence and prophylaxis. *Transactions of the Royal Society of Tropical Medicine and Hygiene* 22: 9–42.

Fehily L (1940) Infantile beriberi in Hong Kong. *Caduceus* 19: 78–93.

Inouye K and Katsura E (1965) Clinical signs and metabolism of beriberi patients. In Shimazono N and Katsura E (eds) *Beriberi and Thiamin*, pp 29–63. Kyoto University, Kyoto: Vitamin B Research Committee of Japan.

Platt BS (1958) Epidemiology and clinical features of endemic beriberi. Proceedings of a conference on beriberi, endemic goitre and hypervitaminosis A. *Proceedings of the Federation of the American Societies of Experimental Biology* 17(supplement 2): 3–20.

Tang CM, Wells JC, Rolfe M and Cham K (1989) Outbreak of beriberi in the Gambia. *Lancet* ii: 206–207.

Thurnham DI (1978) Effect of specific nutrient deficiencies in man: thiamin. *CRC Handbook: Nutrition and Food*, section E, vol. 3, pp 3–14. West Balm Beach, Florida: CRC Press. Florida.

Williams RR (1961) *Towards the Conquest of Beriberi.* Cambridge, Massachusetts: Harvard University Press.

David I. Thurnham
Dunn Nutrition Centre, Cambridge, UK

BIFIDOBACTERIA IN FOODS

The potentially beneficial roles of bifidobacteria in the human intestine have been mentioned in many publications. As a result, a variety of fermented milk products containing bifidobacteria have been developed. The consumption of these products shows a trend of steady increase in many countries throughout the world, especially in Europe. *See* Fermented Milks, Types of Fermented Milks; Fermented Milks, Products from Northern Europe; Fermented Milks, Kefir; Microflora of the Intestine, Probiotics

Biology of Bifidobacteria

Bifidobacteria are found in the human intestine, mouth and vagina, and in the alimentary tract of various animals and honey bees; they also occur in sewage. They have characteristic morphology, physiology, biochemical characters and other properties:

1. Morphology: non-motile and non-spore-forming rods; variable in appearance; Gram-positive; methylene blue may stain internal granules, but not the entire cell.
2. Physiology: anaerobic.
3. Biochemical characters: major products of glucose fermentation are acetic and L(+)-lactic acids in a molar ratio of 3:2; not fast-acid producers; gas (carbon dioxide) not produced from glucose; negative tests for catalase, nitrate reduction, formation of indole and liquefaction of gelatin; acid not produced from rhamnose, sorbose, adonitol, dulcitol, erythritol and glycerol; positive for fructose 6-phosphate phosphoketolase in cellular extracts.
4. Cell wall composition: the cell wall peptidoglycan is not uniform; the basic amino acid in the tetrapeptide can be either ornithine or lysine; there are various types of cross-linkage.
5. Phospholipid composition: polyglycerolphospholipid and its lyso derivatives; alanyl phosphatidylglycerol; lyso derivatives of diphosphatidylglycerol.
6. DNA-base composition: guanine plus cytosine $(G+C)$ content, 55–67 mol%.
7. Growth temperature: optimum, 37–41°C; maximum, 43–45°C; minimum, 25–38°C.
8. pH Relations: optimum pH for initial growth, 6·5–7·0; no growth occurs at 4·5–5·0 or 8·0–8·5.

Bifidobacteria have been classified into 24 species, 9 occurring in humans, 12 in animals and 3 in honey bees. Those in the human species include the following: *Bifidobacterium bifidum* biovars a and b; *Bif. longum* biovars a and b; *Bif. breve; Bif. infantis; Bif. adolescentis* biovars a, b, c and d; *Bif. angulatum*; *Bif. catenulatum*; *Bif. pseudocatenulatum* and *Bif. dentium*. All these are able to utilize glucose, galactose, lactose and, generally, fructose as carbon sources, and ammonia as the sole source of nitrogen. Many strains require riboflavin and pantothenate or pantethine for growth, whereas requirements for other vitamins vary among the different species.

In the manufacture of fermented milk products, *Bif. bifidum* is the species most often used, then *Bif. longum* and *Bif. breve*. Some pharmaceutial preparations also contain *Bif. infantis*. Bifidobacteria are usually used in combination with other lactic acid bacteria because of their slow acid production. Acid production is increased following the addition to the culture media of growth-promoting substances such as yeast extract or autolysate, whey protein, pepsin-digested milk, cysteine, maize extract, etc. Some strains of bifidobacteria show a weak proteolytic activity in milk, but there are considerable differences in the activity of most strains. *See* Lactic Acid Bacteria

Types of Bifidobacteria-Containing Fermented Milk Products – their Technology and Manufacture

Bifidobacteria-containing products can be divided, according to their utilization, into two categories: baby foods and other fermented milk products.

Baby Foods

Bifidobacteria are the predominant intestinal organisms of breast-fed babies. The potentially beneficial roles of these bacteria in the intestine include the following: competitive antagonism against pathogens; production of acetic and L(+)-lactic acids; inhibition of nitrate reduction to nitrite; improvement of nitrogen retention and weight gain in infants; protection against enteric infection or side-effects of antibiotic therapy; and aid in the therapy of intestinal disorders and enteric infections.

Bif. bifidum is the species most often used, either alone or together with its *in vivo* growth-promoting substances. The best known products are Lactana B, Femilact, and Bifiline. The dried formula called Lactana-B (developed in Germany) contains lactulose and viable *Bif. bifidum*, and is produced from partially adapted milk. The dried formula product called Femilact (developed in Czechoslovakia) is made by fermenting heat-treated cream (12% fat) with a mixed culture (2–5%) consisting of *Bif. bifidum*, *Lactobacillus acidophilus* and *Pediococcus acidilactici* (1:0·1:1 ratio) at 30°C to the desired acidity, followed by cooling; heat-treated vegetable oil, lactose, whey protein and vitamins are added, and the mixture is homogenized and spray-dried. The final product, when reconstituted, contains 0·25% lactic acid and 10^8–10^9 viable culture bacteria per ml; the number of viable cells declines by a factor of 10 during storage for 2 months. The liquid formula product called Bifiline (developed in the USSR) is made from a milk formula called Malutka and selected strains of bifidobacteria. The product is prepared by fermenting the heat-treated, homogenized formula with a starter culture (5%) containing 0·5% maize extract at 37°C for 8–10 h until coagulation has taken place. After cooling, the final product is reported to contain about 0·60% lactic acid and 10^7–10^8 viable bifidobacteria per g. *See* Infant Foods, Milk Formulas; Starter Cultures

Fermented Milk Products Containing Bifidobacteria

Fermented milk products are prepared with bifidobacteria alone, or in combination with lactic acid bacteria.

Table 1. Fermented milk products containing bifidobacteria

Product name	Culture organisms
Bifidus milk	*Bifidobacterium bifidum* or *Bif. longum*
Bifighurt	*Bif. longum, Streptococcus thermophilus*
Biogarde	*Bif. bifidum, Lactobacillus acidophilus, St. thermophilus*
Biokys	*Bif. bifidum, L. acidophilus, Pediococcus acidilactici*
Yoghurt with bifidus bacteria	*Bif. bifidum (Bif. longum), St. thermophilus, L. bulgaricus*
Special yoghurt with bifidus and acidophilus bacteria	*Bif. bifidum (Bif. longum), L. acidophilus, St. thermophilus, L. bulgaricus*
Cultura	*Bif. bifidum, L. acidophilus*
Cultura drink	*Bif. bifidum, L. acidophilus*
Mil-Mil	*Bif. bifidum, Bif. breve, L. acidophilus*
Progurt	*Lactococcus lactis* biovar. *diacetilactis, Lac. lactis* biovar. *cremoris, L. acidophilus* and/or *Bif. bifidum*

Thermophilic or mesophilic lactic-acid-producing bacteria are added in order to help acidification (Table 1). Fermented milk products containing bifidobacteria can be divided into several groups.

Type 1: Bifidus Milk

The product is named according to the bacteria (former name *Lactobacillus bifidus*) used in the fermentation. Bifidus milk is produced in small quantities in some European countries, but its consumption is linked to alleged dietetic and therapeutic values rather than to its organoleptic properties.

The manufacture of bifidus milk involves standardization of milk to the desired fat content, increasing the protein content, homogenization, and heat treatment at 85–120°C for 5–30 min. The milk is then inoculated with about 10% of a starter culture, and incubated at 37–41°C until coagulation occurs; this is followed by cooling.

Bifidus milk can be produced as a set or stirred product. The final product has a pH of 4·3–4·7 and contains 10^8–10^9 viable bifidobacteria per ml; these numbers decline by two log cycles during refrigerated storage for 1–2 weeks. Bifidus milk has a mild acid taste and distinct flavour, slightly spicy, and different from the flavour of other fermented milks.

A bifidus milk with yoghurt flavour is obtained by fermenting whey-protein-enriched skim milk with a culture of *Bif. bidifum*, or *Bif. longum*, or *Bif. infantis*. The processing technology of this product was developed in the UK. The product is made by mixing equal volumes of the retentate of ultrafiltered sweet whey (concentrated by a factor of 8) and ultrafiltered skim milk (concentrated by a factor of 2), then pasteurizing the mixture at 80°C for 30 min and cooling to 37°C, followed by the addition of threonine (0·1%) and starter (2%). The incubation is at 37°C for 24 h, followed by cooling to 4°C, and cold storage. The final product has about 15% total solids, including 7·3% protein and 1·3% fat, a pH of about 4·7 and an acetaldehyde concentration between 29 and 39 ppm. It contains 10^9 viable bifidobacteria per ml; these numbers decline during storage for 21 days at 4°C to 10^6–10^7 viable cells per ml.

Type 2: Bifidus-Acidophilus Milk

Fermented milks with intestinal strains of bifidobacteria and acidophilus bacteria have been developed in recent years. A product called Cultura (developed in Denmark) is made by fermenting homogenized, heat-treated, protein-enriched whole milk with *Bif. bifidum* and *L. acidophilus* at 37°C for about 16 h until the desired acidity is obtained, followed by cooling. It is made by the set method, and the final product contains more than 10^8 *L. acidophilus* per ml and more than 10^8 *Bif. bifidum* per ml. It has a characteristic flavour, mild acid taste and firm consistency. Cultura has a shelf life of at least 20 days after production, and is sold in plastic containers of 150 ml. By fermenting partially skimmed milk, a beverage is obtained.

A similar drink, called 'Mil-Mil' (developed in Japan), is made by fermenting the heat-treated milk with a starter consisting of *Bif. bifidum, Bif. breve* and *L. acidophilus*.

Type 3: Bifidus-Thermophilus Milk

Bifighurt (developed in Germany) is made by fermenting heat-treated milk with 6% of a starter consisting of *Bif. longum* (no indication about the ecological origin of the strain) and *Streptococcus thermophilus* at 42°C for about 4 h. The product has a pH of about 4·7, mild acid taste and may contain 10^7 *Bif. longum* per ml as well as a large number of *St. thermophilus*.

Type 4: Bifidus-Acidophilus-Thermophilus Milk

Biogarde (Sanofi Company) is obtained by fermenting milk with a starter consisting of *Bif. bifidum, L. acidophilus* and *St. thermophilus*. The process for creating the bulk starter is as follows: the special nutrient medium for Biogarde culture (1·5%) is dissolved in water; this solution is added to the bulk starter milk, heated to 90°C for 10 min, and cooled to 42°C; it is inoculated with liquid, freeze-dried or deep-frozen culture, then incubated for 4·5–6·5 h at 41–42°C, depending on the quantity of starter inoculum; finally, it is cooled to, and stored at, approximately 8°C.

The manufacture of Biogarde involves standardization of the milk, homogenization, heat treatment (90°C for 10 min or 95°C for 5 min), tempering and inoculation with a bulk starter (6%), mixing well, packaging and incubating at 42°C for about 3–5 h until coagulation, then cooling.

Biogarde is also used in the preparation of various other products, including buttermilk, sauces, muesli (breakfast cereal), beverages, fresh cheeses, and ice cream. The final product contains 0·85–0·90% L(+)-lactic acid.

Type 5: Bifidus-Acidophilus-Pediococcus Milk

Biokys (developed in Czechoslovakia) is obtained by fermenting milk with a mixed culture of bifidobacteria, acidophilus bacteria and *Pedicoccus acidilactici*. The first two cultures are human intestinal strains, while *P. acidilactici* is incorporated to help the acidification.

The manufacture of Biokys is as follows: standardized milk (15% total solids including 3·5% fat) is homogenized and heat-treated, then fermented to the desired acidity with 2–5% of a starter consisting of *Bif. bifidum*, *L. acidophilus* and *P. acidilactici* (1:0·1:1 ratio) at 30–31°C; this is followed by stirring and cooling. The product has a sour-cream-like viscosity, and a clean, mild acid taste.

Type 6: Bidifus-Yoghurt or Bifidus-Acidophilus Yoghurt

The combination of yoghurt culture bacteria with bifidobacteria, and the addition of *L. acidophilus*, has led to the development of products which have a characteristic flavour. There are two types of such yoghurts: the first sub-group contains only bifidobacteria and yoghurt organisms. These products are produced in Germany, the USA, Japan, France and several other countries. *See* Yoghurt, The Product and its Manufacture; Yoghurt, Yoghurt-based Products

The first type of yoghurt is made either by a simultaneous fermentation of the standardized, heat-treated, homogenized milk with a starter (5–10%) consisting of a yoghurt culture and bifidobacteria (*Bif. bifidum*, or *Bif. longum*, or *Bif. infantis*) at 40–42°C until coagulation, followed by cooling, or by mixing into cultured yoghurt, at the desired ratio, a separately cultured bifidus milk followed by stirring and cooling. The former method may ensure better viability of the bifidobacteria. A more recent example of this type of product is 'B*A' (bifidus-active), which is prepared with

a human strain of *Bif. longum* and a yoghurt culture; it is made in France, the UK and several other countries.

The second subgroup of products is usually made by a simultaneous fermentation of the heat-treated milk with cultures of *Bif. bifidum* and/or *Bif. longum* and/or *Bif. infantis*, *L. acidophilus* and the yoghurt microorganisms. The products have a characteristic mild acid flavour, which may be masked or modified in fruit-flavoured varieties. A more recent example of this type of product is Ofilus, which is prepared with human intestinal strains of bifidobacteria and acidophilus bacteria; it is produced in France and numerous countries.

Type 7: Bifidus-Acidophilus-Mesophilic Streptococci Milk

A protein-enriched product called Progurt is prepared by fermenting pasteurized skim milk with 1–3% of a mixed culture of *Lactococcus lactis* biovar. *diacetilactis* and *Lac. lactis* biovar. *cremoris* (ratio 1:1) until 0·7–0·8% lactic acid is produced. The product is then subjected to a partial whey separation, the addition of cream and 0·5–1·0% of *L. acidophilus* and/or *Bif. bifidum* cultures (no indication about the ecological origin), homogenization and cooling. The product contains 5% fat, 6% protein and 3% lactose, and has a pH of 4·4–4·5.

A product made in France, called Ofilus Double Douceur, contains *Bif. bifidum*, *L. acidophilus*, *Lac. lactis* and *Lac. lactis* biovar. *cremoris*.

Pharmaceutical Preparations

Freeze-dried pharmaceutical preparations containing bifidobacteria, alone or in combination with other organisms, are prepared by the pharmaceutical and food industries. They contain human intestinal microorganisms. In general, these preparations are utilized for the treatment of gastrointestinal disorders (e.g. diarrhoea, and side-effects of antibiotic and radiation therapy), as special preparations for certain liver diseases, and as a protective means against imbalance in the intestinal microflora.

Some examples of pharmaceutical preparations are: Bifidogene (France); Bifider (*Bif. bifidum*; Japan); Inflora Berna (*L. acidophilus* and *Bif. infantis*; Switzerland); Eugalan Toepfer forte and Lactopriv (with bifidobacteria; Germany); Liobif (*Bif. bifidum*; Yugoslavia); Lyobifidus (*Bif. bifidum*; France), and Life Start II (*Bif. bifidum*; the USA).

Bifidobacteria in Other Foods

The utilization of bifidobacteria in other foods is in the early stages of research and development.

Fresh Cheese (Quarg)

Separate inoculation of pasteurized milk with cultures of mesophilic lactic acid bacteria and bifidobacteria (e.g in a ratio of 1:1) is used in the production of quarg.

Unripened White Cheese

The procedure is the same as that used with fresh cheese, showing good survival of bifidobacteria.

Fermentation of Fish Hydrolysates

It may be possible to ferment fish hydrolysates using cultures of bifidobacteria.

Fruit Juices

Some fruit juices may be fermented using bifidobacteria cultures, but there is a problem with the survival of bifidobacteria.

Sausages

Bifidobacteria cultures are used in the ripening of sausages.

Bibliography

IDF (1988) *Fermented Milks. Science and Technology*. IDF Bulletin 227. Brussels: International Dairy Federation.

Kurmann JA, Rašić JLj and Kroger M (1991) *Encyclopedia of Fermented Fresh Milk and Related Products*. New York: Van Nostrand Reinhold.

Rašić JLj and Kurmann JA (1983) *Bifidobacteria and their role*. Basel and Boston: Birkhauser Verlag.

Robinson RK (ed.) (1991) *Therapeutic Properties of Fermented Milks*. Essex: Elsevier Science Publishers.

J. A. Kurmann
Agricultural Institute, Grangeneuve-Posieux, Switzerland
J. Lj. Rašić
Food Research Institute, Novi Sad, Yugoslavia

BILE

Bile is a complex aqueous solution of organic and inorganic compounds secreted by the liver. It contains bile acids, a class of detergent-like molecules that exert their biological functions as lipid solubilizers within the biliary tree and the gut lumen. The bile acids are restricted to the enterohepatic circulation, so as to reutilize many times these biologically valuable molecules. This article reviews the composition and the physicochemical properties of bile, and the function of bile acids as solubilizers of biliary and dietary lipids.

Composition of Bile

Human bile flow varies from 1·5 to 15·4 μl min^{-1} kg^{-1}, depending on bile acid secretion rate. The driving force for movement of water into the bile canaliculus is provided by an osmotic gradient, mainly generated by active bile acid transport into the canaliculus. This mechanism accounts for the so-called bile-acid-dependent bile flow, representing about 60% of total canalicular bile flow. Extrapolation of the linear regression function relating bile acid secretion rate and bile flow to

a value of zero bile acid secretion rate yields a positive intercept. According to the two-components theory of canalicular bile flow generation (Fig. 1), this linear extrapolation identifies the so-called bile-acid-independent bile flow (about 40% of total canalicular bile flow). Bile-acid-independent bile flow is generated by active transport of Na$^+$ and HCO$_3^-$ into the canalicular lumen. The finding of a curvilinear relationship at very low bile acid secretion rates in animal models has challenged the concept of bile-acid-independent bile flow, and supports the one-component theory (Fig. 1). According to this theory, the whole canalicular bile flow is generated in the presence of bile acid secretion.

Inorganic compounds in human hepatic bile comprise electrolytes in concentrations similar to those in plasma, with the noticeable exception of HCO$_3^-$ concentration which is higher in bile. The osmolarity of human hepatic bile is also similar to plasma osmolarity, at about 300 mosmol l^{-1}.

Organic compounds in bile comprise protein and bile pigments in addition to the three biliary lipids – bile acid, cholesterol, and phospholipid. Proteins account for 4·5% of organic compounds in bile, and their

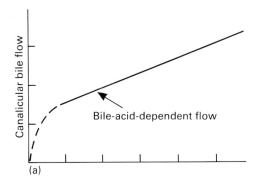

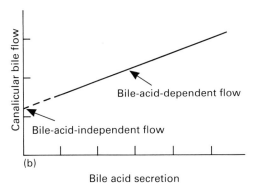

Fig. 1 (a) One-component and (b) two-component theory for canalicular bile flow. According to the former theory, bile acids account for all canalicular bile flow; according to the latter, a fraction of bile flow is generated in the absence of bile acids. (From Erlinger S, 1988.)

concentration ranges between 0.3 and $3.0 \, \mathrm{g \, ml}^{-1}$ in typical human bile. The most abundant biliary protein is albumin derived from the plasma pool. In general, the biliary concentration of other plasma proteins is inversely related to their molecular weight. Bile also contains immunoglobulin A, lysosomal enzymes, and plasma membrane enzymes. The secretion of these latter proteins is influenced by bile acid secretion rate.

Bile pigments constitute less than 0.3% of organic compounds in bile, and their concentrations range between 0.8 and $3.2 \, \mathrm{mmol \, l}^{-1}$ in human hepatic and gall bladder bile respectively. Conjugation with glucuronic acid is essential for biliary bilirubin excretion, and bilirubin diglucuronide is the major pigment in human bile. Maximal bilirubin excretion capacity depends on bile flow, and is increased during enhanced bile acid secretion rates. About 30% of bilirubin excretion is thought to be bile-acid-independent, suggesting that incorporation of bilirubin into mixed micelles is not essential for its biliary excretion.

Many other endogenous substances are present in human bile in addition to those listed above. These include vitamins (mainly D_2, B_{12}, folic acid) and steroid (oestrogens) and thyroid hormones. Exogenous compounds, such as contrast media, some antibiotics (ampi-

cillin, metronidazole), cardiac glycosides and opiates, may also be excreted in bile and undergo some degree of enterohepatic circulation. *See* Cholecalciferol, Physiology; Cobalamins, Physiology; Folic Acid, Physiology; Hormones, Thyroid Hormones; Hormones, Steroid Hormones

Biliary Lipid Chemistry and Physicochemical Properties

Bile Acids

Bile acids comprise a class of molecules derived from the hepatic catabolism of cholesterol. More than 200 bile acids have been isolated in human bile, and 92–99% of total bile acids is constituted by mono-, di- and trihydroxy derivatives of a 24-carbon steroid, cholanoic acid (Fig. 2). The brief and systematic names, and the relative proportions of individual bile acids in human bile are shown in Table 1.

Virtually all biliary bile acids are amidated in humans, almost exclusively with glycine or taurine at a ratio of about $2:1$. Sulphation on the steroid nucleus of bile acids occurs to a significant extent in humans only for lithocholic acid, and glucuronidation is a trace metabolic pathway.

From a physicochemical point of view, bile acids are planar amphiphiles in that they exhibit both hydrophilicity with one part of the molecule, and hydrophobicity with the remainder. In commonly occurring bile acid molecules, the hydrophobic face is constituted by the β side of the steroid nucleus, and the hydrophilic face by the α side of the nucleus and by the side-chain. The relative potency of the hydrophilic and hydrophobic functional groups in affecting the physicochemical properties of bile acids is referred to as the hydrophilic–hydrophobic balance. The order of decreasing hydrophilicity, as assessed by high-pressure liquid chromatography, follows the order taurine conjugates, glycine conjugates, unconjugated bile acid, and trihydroxylated, dihydroxylated, monohydroxylated bile acids.

Bile acid solubility is strongly dependent on amidation. Unconjugated bile acids ($pK_a \, 5.0$) are insoluble at a pH below 6–7, and glycine ($pK_a \, 3.8$) and taurine conjugates ($pK_a < 1.0$) are soluble at pH 4–5 and below 2, respectively. Fully ionized common bile acids are present in physiological solutions as their sodium salts. They are extremely water-soluble, with a monomeric solubility of $1–3 \, \mathrm{mmol \, l}^{-1}$ (Fig. 3). They are present in diluted water solutions as monomers in the bulk water phase, and as an unstable film on the water surface. Upon concentration, a critical monomeric concentration is reached called the critical micellar concentration (CMC), at which bile acid monomers self-associate to form multimolecular aggregates known as micelles.

Micelle formation involves back-to-back agglomeration of the hydrophobic side of the bile acid molecules, with the hydrophilic side facing water. At concentrations above the CMC, bile salts micelles have the capacity of incorporating and solubilizing otherwise insoluble compounds, thus acting as detergents. In general terms, hydrophobic bile acids form micelles at lower concentration than hydrophilic bile acids, and the CMC ranges between 0.5 and 11 mmol l^{-1} for common bile acid (Table 1).

Phospholipids

The most abundant biliary phospholipid species are phosphatidylcholines (lecithins), which account for 80–95% of phospholipids in human bile. Phosphatidylcholines are insoluble, swelling amphiphiles, with a mono-

meric solubility in water of about 1 pmol l^{-1} (Fig. 3). Upon hydration ($>45\%$ water), phospholipids swell to form liquid crystalline phases consisting of choline bilayers with interposed water layers. These liquid crystalline phases may fold and aggregate to form vesicular structures.

Cholesterol

From a physicochemical point of view, cholesterol is an insoluble, nonswelling amphiphile, with a monomeric solubility in water of about 1 nmol l^{-1} at 37°C (Fig. 3). Upon hydration, crystals of cholesterol monohydrate are in equilibrium with water-containing monomers of cholesterol monohydrate.

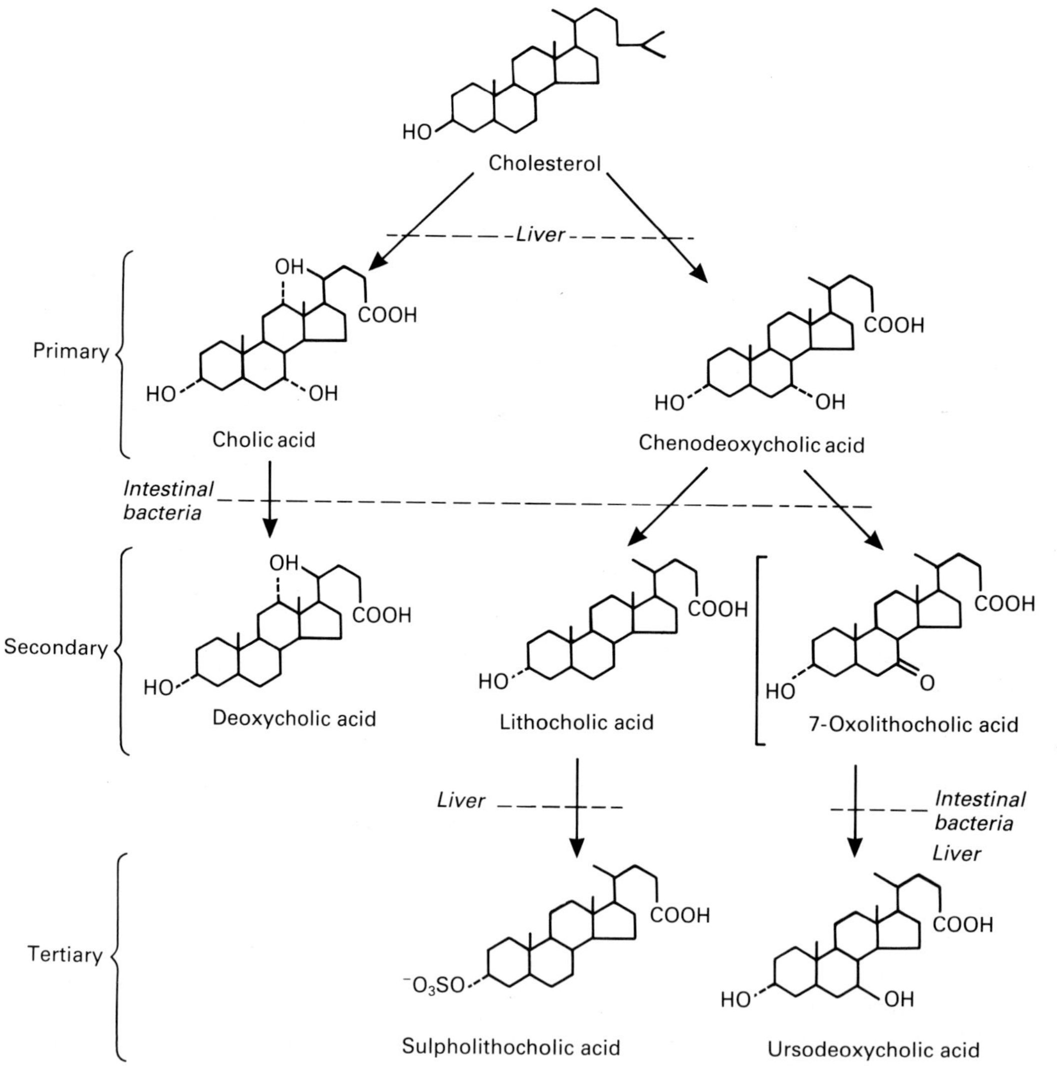

Fig. 2 Structural formulae, sites of synthesis and of metabolism of common bile acids in humans. (From Carey MC and Cahalane MJ, 1988.)

Table 1   Name and composition of biliary bile acids of typical human bile

Bile acids		CMC	
Brief name	Systematic name	(mmol l^{-1})	Percentage in bile[a]
Cholic	$3\alpha,7\alpha,12\alpha$-Trihydroxy-5-cholanoic acid	11	35
Chenodeoxycholic	$3\alpha,7\alpha$-Dihydroxy-5-cholanoic acid	4	35
Deoxycholic	$3\alpha,12\alpha$-Dihydroxy-5-cholanoic acid	3	24
Ursodeoxycholic	$3\alpha,7\beta$-Dihydroxy-5-cholanoic acid	7	tr–4
Lithocholic	3α-Monohydroxy-5-cholanoic acid	0·5	tr–3

CMC, critical micellar concentration; tr, trace.
[a] Refers to individual bile acids as a percentage of total bile acids.

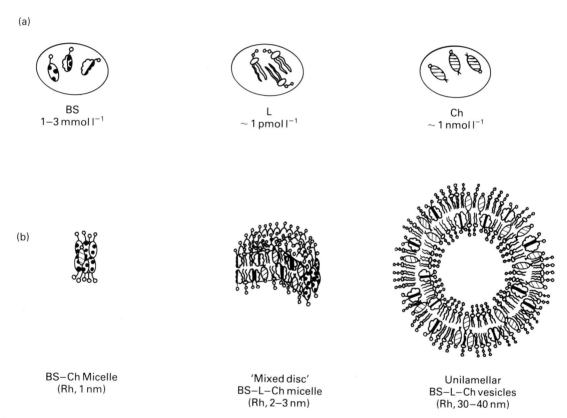

(a)

BS
1–3 mmol l^{-1}

L
~1 pmol l^{-1}

Ch
~1 nmol l^{-1}

(b)

BS–Ch Micelle
(Rh, 1 nm)

'Mixed disc'
BS–L–Ch micelle
(Rh, 2–3 nm)

Unilamellar
BS–L–Ch vesicles
(Rh, 30–40 nm)

Fig. 3   Molecular models of (a) monomeric and (b) aggregated biliary lipids. Monomeric solubility in water and mean hydrodynamic radius (Rh) of aggregated lipids are also shown. BS, bile acids; L, lecithin; Ch, cholesterol. (From Carey MC and Cahalane MJ, 1988.)

Bile Acid Synthesis and Enterohepatic Circulation

Bile Acid Synthesis

Biliary bile acids are derived from two sources, *de novo* hepatic synthesis and hepatic recycling via the enterohepatic circulation. The former mechanism compensates for daily fecal loss of about 200–600 mg. The liver is the unique site for bile acid synthesis, and cholesterol is the obligatory precursor. Bile acid synthesis involves both nuclear and side-chain transformation of cholesterol molecules, and about 25 intermediate compounds have been isolated along this pathway. 7α-Hydroxylation of cholesterol, a process catalysed by microsomal 7α-hydroxylase, is the rate-limiting step in bile acid synthesis. The end products of this synthetic pathway in man are two bile acids, cholic and chenodeoxycholic acid, conventionally called 'primary' bile acids (Fig. 2). Bile acis resulting from subsequent bacterial modification of the two primary bile acids in the enterohepatic circulation are termed 'secondary' bile acids (see below). Bile acids resulting from hepatic sulphation of lithocholic and hydrogenation of 7-oxolithocholic acid are termed 'tertiary' bile acids (Fig. 2).

It is generally agreed that bile acids returning to the liver via the enterohepatic circulation regulate their own synthesis by a negative feedback mechanism. Bile acid synthesis may increase as much as 20-fold during interruption of the enterohepatic circulation in a rat with bile fistula, and an opposite effect is achieved by increasing bile acid return to the liver. Inhibition of both cholic and chenodeoxycholic acid synthesis accompanies intraduodenal or intravenous infusion of either bile acid in a rat with bile fistula. Individual bile acids appear to exhibit a specific inhibitory capacity for synthesis, which is less marked for the more hydrophilic bile acid.

Enterohepatic Circulation and Gall Bladder Storage of Bile

The movement of bile acid molecules is mainly restricted to the biliary tree, intestinal lumen, portal blood and liver, topographically referred to as the enterohepatic circulation. The driving force for the enterohepatic circulation is provided by two chemical pumps and two mechanical pumps. The chemical pumps are provided by the active transport processes underlying ileal absorption and hepatic uptake, and the mechanical pumps are gall bladder emptying and small intestinal transit. *See* Liver, Enterohepatic Circulation

Gall bladder motor function is the major factor affecting delivery of bile into the intestine, thus influencing bile acid recycling frequency in the enterohepatic circulation. As a result of gall bladder storage and emptying functions, duodenal bile acid output typically varies from 5 μmol kg h^{-1} in the interdigestive period to 25 μmol kg^{-1} h^{-1} postprandially. Low duodenal bile acid output during the interdigestive period is accompanied by diversion of about 90% of hepatic bile into the gall bladder (absolute filling). Absolute gall bladder filling alternates with gall bladder emptying, occurring synchronously with the periodic aboral progression of the intestinal interdigestive migrating motor complexes. This alternation of filling and emptying also occurs postprandially, and this 'bellows' effect may play a role in mixing of gall bladder content during each 24-hour period. *See* Gall Bladder

The net effect of these alternating episodes of filling and emptying is that the gall bladder only stores about 50% of the hepatic bile that enters it during overnight fasting. As a result of net gall bladder storage of bile, about 50% of the bile acid pool size (1·3–4·0 g) is stored in the human gall bladder during fasting, thus providing a physiological interruption of the enterohepatic circulation.

Given a capacity of 20–40 ml, the gall bladder would very soon be filled during fasting beyond its storage capacity if it were not for its marked capacity for active reabsorption of sodium chloride and sodium bicarbonate, and passive water reabsorption.

Functions of Bile Acids

Bile

Despite the very low solubility of both phospholipid and cholesterol in water, bile is an optically clear solution which does not contain a macroscopically detectable solid phase in healthy individuals. At physiological bile-salt:lecithin:cholesterol molar ratios (approximately 75%:15%:5%), cholesterol monomers are solubilized in large, mixed micelles having a mixed disc structure (Fig. 3). This structure envisages bile acid covering the external surface of the micelles, but also dispersed inside the micellar core together with phospholipid.

The amount of cholesterol in a given bile sample may exceed the solubilization capacity of the micellar mechanism as determined from *in vitro* studies on model bile solutions (supersaturated bile). Hepatic bile is normally supersaturated with cholesterol at low bile acid secretion rates (< 10–15 μmol kg^{-1} h^{-1}) and gall bladder bile is often supersaturated in healthy subjects. Cholesterol monohydrate crystals are not found in these supersaturated biles when analysed immediately following collection. However, if these supersaturated biles are stored under appropriate laboratory conditions, phase separation and cholesterol crystal formation occur within days or weeks (nucleation time). These observations indicate that bile behaves as a metastable system, and that a nonmicellar mechanism of cholesterol transport must be involved to account for this prolonged metastability. This mechanism involves formation of spherical unilamellar vesicles composed mainly of cholesterol and lecithin (ratio ranging between 1:1 and 5:2; Fig. 3). The proportion of cholesterol carried in vesicles, relative to that carried in mixed micelles, is about 50% in hepatic bile, and 40% in gall bladder bile. This proportion is not constant, and the vesicular system prevails at low bile acid secretion rates. The degree of metastability of supersaturated human bile, as assessed by *ex vivo* nucleation time, is greater than that predictable from the nuclation time of model bile systems. A protein component of bile, probably a lipid-containing bile protein, may act as a 'stabilizer' of supersaturated normal biles.

Phase transition occurs during passage of bile down the biliary tree and during storage in the gall bladder. Cholesterol–phospholipid vesicles are probably excreted by the biliary canaliculus as such by a mechanism independent of that involved in bile acid monomer secretion. As soon as the excreted bile acid concentration reaches the CMC within the biliary canaliculus, vesicular lipids are dissolved in mixed micelles. Supersaturated mixed micelles in hepatic bile rapidly form stable cholesterol–lecithin vesicles, probably unsaturated with cholesterol. On entry into the gall bladder, this lipid fraction may be slowly redissolved into mixed micelles, unsaturated with cholesterol. This latter effect occurs as a result of the increased total lipid concentration in concentrated gall bladder bile, and this is known to enhance the micellar capacity for cholesterol. In supersaturated gall bladder bile, cholesterol-rich vesicles may remain stable as a result of protein–vesicle interaction.

Small Intestine

According to the classical theory of Hofman and Borgstrom, normal fat digestion can be divided into two closely related events: a chemical event – lipolysis; and a physical event – aqueous solubilization. Pancreatic lipolysis of dietary fat is a prerequisite for its micellar solubilization, and micellar solubilization is a prerequisite for its absorption. Bile acids play a key role in both these events.

From a physicochemical point of view, fat droplets consist of long-chain triglyceride stabilized mainly by phospholipids in natural food, and by other emulsifiers (arabic gum, mono- or diglycerides) in processed food. Dietary triglyceride is hydrolysed by pancreatic lipase (lipolysis) to monoglyceride and fatty acid. In the absence of bile acids, access of lipase to lipid droplets is prevented by the emulsifiers surrounding the oil droplets. Bile acids have the ability to wash these off the oil droplets, thus giving access to lipase. Bile acids would also wash off the lipase, a phenomenon prevented by colipase. This coenzyme binds to lipase and bile acid, thus fixing the lipase molecule in contact with the underlying triglyceride. *See* Triglycerides, Structures and Properties

Following digestion, the products of lipolysis are kept in solution by the natural detergents, bile acids, mainly in the form of mixed bile-acid–phospholipid–fatty-acid–monoglyceride micelles. Unilamellar vesicles, consisting of the products of lipolysis, have been observed under the microscope to 'bud off' the lipid emulsion surface following lipase digestion. These vesicles are rapidly dissolved by biliary micelles freshly delivered by bile, so that during intestinal fat digestion saturated mixed-disc micelles coexist with vesicles of the same lipid composition. Both micelles and vesicles contribute to transport of solubilized lipids across the intestinal unstirred water layer lining the gut lumen. It is not known whether lipid absorption involves monomeric absorption or vesicle fusion with the plasma membrane of the enterocyte.

Bile Acids and the Colon

Every day, 200–500 mg bile acids escape the enterohepatic circulation and enter the colon. In the human colon, bile acids are exposed to obligate anaerobes – bacteria that are capable of producing hundreds of metabolic products of bile acids. The vast majority of these products are poorly characterized, and account for only about 3% of faecal bile acid. The two main biotransformations of bile acids in the colon are bacterial deconjugation and 7α-dehydroxylation. As a consequence of the former biotransformation, conjugated bile acids are totally absent from the colon. As a result of 7α-dehydroxylation of the primary bile acids, cholic and chenodeoxycholic acid, the majority of faecal bile acids consist of deoxycholic acid (about 50%) and lithocholic acid (33%) (Fig. 2). Since these two bile acids are reabsorbed and resecreted in bile along with the two primary bile acids, they are termed 'secondary' bile acids. The two primary bile acids account for about 7–8% each of faecal bile acid, and the remaining 2–4% is mainly constituted by oxo-bile acid. *See* Colon, Structure and Function

Most of the bile acids precipitate in faeces, since the slightly acidic pH of faeces is lower than the pK_a value for unconjugated bile acids. Bile acid concentration in faecal water is about $0.5 \ \text{mmol} \ l^{-1}$ and a small proportion of these bile acids are reabsorbed from the colonic mucosa by passive nonionic diffusion and re-enter the enterohepatic circulation. If the value of $1.5 \ \text{mmol} \ l^{-1}$ for bile acid concentration in faecal water is exceeded, bile acids exert a cathartic effect by inhibiting water absorption and, at higher concentrations, by promoting colonic electrolytes and water secretion. The cathartic effect of bile acids depends on bile acid structure, and it is maximum for α-dihydroxylated bile acids.

In addition to the cathartic effect, dihydroxylated bile acids may also increase colonic permeability. Increased colonic absorption of dietary oxalate, and the consequent hyperoxaluria, accompanies increased exposure of the colon to bile acids in conditions causing bile acid malabsorption. This effect of bile acids on colonic absorption has raised the possibility that they may enhance colonic absorption of environmental and dietary carcinogens, thus contributing to development of colonic cancer. Furthermore, bile acids are known to enhance the carcinogenic effect of substances such as azoxymethane and dimethylhydrazine, thus acting as cocarcinogens in animal models. On the basis of this information, increased exposure of colonic mucosa to bile acids has been put forward as an explanation for the greater incidence of colonic cancer following cholecystectomy. However, the evidence relating cholecystectomy to increased risk of cancer is conflicting, and a causal relationship between bile acids and colonic cancer in humans is far from proven. *See* Colon, Cancer of the Colon

Bibliography

Borgstrom B, Barrowman JA and Lindstrom M (1985) Roles of bile acids in intestinal lipid digestion and absorption. In: Daniellsson H and Sjovall J (eds) *Sterols and Bile Acids*, pp 405–425. Amsterdam: Elsevier Science Publishers.

Carey MC and Cahalane MJ (1988) Enterohepatic circulation. In: Arias IM, Jakoby WB, Popper H, Schachter D and Shafriz DA (eds) *The Liver: Biology and Pathobiology* 2nd edn, pp 573–616. New York: Raven Press.

Erlinger S (1988) Bile flow. In: Arias IM, Jakoby WB, Popper H, Schachter D and Shafriz DA (eds) *The Liver: Biology and Pathobiology* 2nd edn, pp 643–661. New York: Raven Press.

Hofmann AF (1988) Bile acids. In: Arias IM, Jakoby WB, Popper H, Schachter D and Shafriz DA (eds) *The Liver: Biology, and Pathobiology* 2nd edn, pp 553–572. New York: Raven Press.

Lanzini A and Northfield TC (1988) Gallbladder motor function. In: Northfield T, Jazrawi R and Zentler-Munro P (eds) *Bile Acids in Health and Disease*, pp 83–96. Lancaster: Kluver Academic Press.

A. Lanzini
University of Brescia, Brescia, Italy
T. C. Northfield
St George's Hospital Medical School, London, UK

BIOAVAILABILITY OF NUTRIENTS

Concept and Definition of Bioavailability

Bioavailability (biological availability) is a term used to describe the proportion of a nutrient in food that is utilized for normal body functions. Although the overall concept is simple, it is very difficult to describe the bioavailability of most nutrients in quantitative terms. Therefore, to facilitate its measurement and interpretation of the data, the bioavailability of nutrients can be subdivided into its three constituent phases: (1) availability in the intestinal lumen for absorption, (2) absorption and/or retention in the body, and (3) utilization. The reasons for studying bioavailability are to evaluate the nutritional quality of foods and diets and to provide data for establishing dietary requirements for nutrients.

The amount of any nutrient that is available for absorption depends upon the form in which the nutrient is presented to the absorptive cells of the intestine. This is dependent on dietary composition and luminal events, namely the digestive processes to which the food has been subjected, and is relatively constant for any food or mixture of foods. On the other hand, the proportion of absorbable nutrient which is taken up and used by the body is very variable, being largely dependent upon regulatory mechanisms in the intestinal mucosa that reflect the individual's physiological need for the nutrient. This is particularly true for many of the micronutrients, notably certain minerals.

Low absorbability of some minerals and vitamins may be the underlying cause of certain nutritional inadequacies. If intakes are well in excess of physiological requirements but bioavailability is a limiting factor, nutritional deficiency disorders may occur, as for example with iron.

Determinants of Bioavailability

There are many factors, both dietary and physiological, that influence nutrient bioavailability. Examples include (1) the physicochemical form of the nutrient in a foodstuff and its solubility in the lumen, (2) the presence of proteolytic enzyme inhibitors (commonly associated with legumes such as soybeans) which reduce the body's ability to digest protein, and (3) the presence of enzymes such as thiaminase which partially hydrolyses thiamin and makes it less biologically active.

Diet-related factors include:
- Physicochemical form of the nutrient
- Oxidation state
- Enhancers, e.g. ascorbate (for iron), some organic acids, sugars, amino acids, fatty acids
- Inhibitors, e.g. phosphates (especially phytate), polyphenols (including tannins), oxalate, carbonate
- Competition for transport proteins or absorption sites, e.g. between metals.

Physiological factors are:
- Gastric acidity
- Intestinal secretions
- Gut motility
- Luminal redox state

- Body status (e.g. tissue levels, nutrient stores)
- Short-term homeostatic mechanisms mediated through the mucosal absorptive cells
- Anabolic demands (e.g. growth in infancy and childhood, pregnancy and lactation)
- Endocrine effects
- Infection and stress
- Genetic influences, inborn errors of metabolism
- Gut microflora.

Certain food constituents have the ability to bind nutrients, thereby rendering them more or less absorbable. For nutrients that are transported into the mucosal cell by means of a carrier-mediated pathway, the degree of binding is an important determinant of bioavailability. If the chelating compound has a higher affinity for the nutrient than the specific carrier molecule, then the net effect is a reduction in bioavailability. Conversely, a weak chelator may act as an absorption promoter by holding the nutrient in a suitably soluble form ready to be taken up into the intestinal mucosal cells. Chelating compounds that impair vitamin bioavailability include avidin in egg white, which binds biotin making it biologically unavailable.

Competitive inhibitors of nutrient metabolism make up another category of dietary factors affecting bioavailability. It has been suggested that minerals with similar chemical properties may compete for common binding sites or carriers. Transition metals such as iron, zinc and copper are typical examples of competitive inhibitors. This will only take place at high levels of intake when the sum of ionic species present at the site of absorption exceeds the critical threshold relating to the absorption kinetics of the minerals in question. *See* Copper, Physiology; Iron, Physiology; Zinc, Physiology

The absorbability of a nutrient also depends upon certain physiological factors, such as the composition and volume of gastric and intestinal secretions. The absorption and utilization clearly depend upon a number of host-related variables. Most of these are key participants in the body's homeostatic regulatory mechanisms such as nutritional status, developmental state, gastric and intestinal secretions, mucosal cell regulation and gut microflora.

Methods of Determining Bioavailability

Various techniques have been employed to assess the bioavailability of nutrients. The best estimate is probably obtained by combining the results from several different methods. By and large, the methods chosen depend on the resources available since detailed human studies on nutrient bioavailability use specialized techniques which can be very expensive.

In Vitro Techniques

These range from simple measures of chemical solubility and fractional dialysability following simulated digestion, to measures of uptake and transport by mucosal tissue from experimental animals. The substance of unknown bioavailability is incubated with a variety of intestinal preparations, including intestinal rings, everted loops (sacs), isolated mucosal cells from cell culture, and vesicles. Uptake of the nutrient into the tissue is determined and equated with absorbability. Perfused loops, with an intact blood supply, can be used to measure the transport of the nutrient into the body.

Generally speaking, *in vitro* techniques are reproducible and are useful for studying dietary factors that affect nutrient bioavailability. They are relatively simple and inexpensive, but their relevance to actual utilization in humans is questionable. Results obtained from *in vitro* studies are a measure of the amount of a nutrient that is available for absorption.

Balance Studies

This is the classical technique used to measure nutrient absorption and retention from the diet by the body over a period of time. Subjects are fed a diet containing a known amount of the nutrient and the difference between what is taken in and what is recovered from the faeces is calculated as apparent absorption. If urinary excretion is added to the faecal figure, retention can be calculated, and with an allowance for endogenous losses it is possible to calculate true absorption.

Balance studies have a number of limitations. They can only be used to assess absorption of a nutrient from the whole diet, and not to study individual foodstuffs. They are prone to errors on both the intake and excretion side, and with a nutrient that is poorly absorbed (e.g. iron) this may result in erroneous values for absorption. The measurement of endogenous losses of nutrients is a difficult task, but without this figure absorption may be significantly underestimated (e.g. zinc). Finally, balance techniques do not give information on the utilization of the nutrient in the body, merely its retention.

Bioassays

The response of experimental animals or man to graded levels of the nutrient in the diet can be used to assess bioavailability. The response criteria employed should specifically reflect the utilization of the nutrient of interest, either by direct measurement of the nutrient or its metabolites in tissues, blood or urine, or by employing functional measurements, such as enzyme levels.

For water-soluble vitamins it is possible to measure the 24-hour excretion following the ingestion of the food(s) containing vitamins of unknown bioavailability and comparing this with a reference dose. Certain assumptions have to be made when using this methodology regarding the kinetics of absorption, distribution, and excretion of the test and reference materials, and large quantities are needed to elicit a readily quantified response. Alternatively, a chronic administration regimen can be employed which parallels the dietary situation rather better.

Isotopes

Many of the problems of lack of measurement specificity can be overcome by using radio- or stable isotopes. Foods can be labelled with isotopes, and the fate of the labelled nutrient following ingestion monitored in the body. Isotopes can be used to measure the absorption, and sometimes the utilization, of nutrients in the body from different foods and under different dietary and physiological conditions. The method used to label the food is an important consideration. Extrinsic labelling, as used for haem and non-haem iron, is the preferred technique. The isotope is mixed into the food just before consumption and is assumed to fully exchange with the nutrient in the food. However, intrinsic labelling, in which the isotope is incorporated into the foodstuff whilst it is growing, may be necessary.

The use of radioisotopes for human studies is restricted by ethical considerations. The hazards associated with exposure to ionizing radiation preclude the use of radio-isotopes in infants, children and pregnant women. Since these groups are most vulnerable to nutritional deficiency, they are the subject groups for whom nutrient bioavailability is of particular interest. Thus alternative methods to study bioavailability have been sought using stable isotopes, which are safe and ethically acceptable. The main disadvantages of stable as compared to radio-isotopes stem from the larger quantities that have to be employed, usually far exceeding the tracer amounts required for radioisotope studies, and the difficulties associated with their measurement. *See* Immunoassays, Radioimmunoassay and Enzyme Immunoassay

Minerals

For many nutrients the bioavailable fraction is high (i.e. 90% or more), but for a number of micronutrients, primarily inorganic elements, it is low and variable. Examples of ionic species that have a low ($< 25\%$), medium (25–75%) and high ($> 75\%$) absorption are:

Low, Fe, Mn, Cr, Ni, V;
Medium, Ca, Mg, Zn, Cu, Se, Mo, Co, PO₄;
High, Na, K, Cl, I, F.

Iron

Iron deficiency is a worldwide problem, yet iron is one of the most abundant elements in the earth's crust. This paradox can be explained in terms of bioavailability. The main factors that influence the bioavailability of iron from the diet are the amounts of haem and non-haem iron, the presence and amounts of dietary factors influencing iron absorbability, and the iron status of the individual. *See* Iron, Physiology

Haem and non-haem iron are absorbed by two separate pathways: the haem complex is absorbed intact into the mucosal cell, whereas non-haem iron is bound to a transport protein. The absorption of non-haem iron is very variable and generally much less than haem iron. Absorption of haem iron is relatively constant (approximately 25%), the only dietary factor that significantly alters its bioavailability is meat, which has a promoting effect. Dietary factors that influence non-haem iron absorption include meat, ascorbic and certain other organic acids, all of which increase iron bioavailability; tannins, phytate and calcium decrease bioavailability. *See* Ascorbic Acid, Physiology; Phytic Acid, Nutritional Impact; Tannins and Polyphenols

Physiological variables have a profound influence on iron bioavailability, notably body iron status. Previous dietary iron intake will also affect the bioavailability of subsequent iron, probably mediated via mucosal cell regulation. Iron is one nutrient for which it is possible to estimate true bioavailability because absorbed iron is utilized for haemoglobin production. Therefore the incorporation of isotopically labelled food iron into red blood cell haemoglobin can be measured to assess dietary iron bioavailability. Another method involves measuring the rate of haemoglobin regeneration in deficient subjects in response to different dietary sources of iron compared with a control substance (e.g. ferrous sulphate).

Zinc

A number of dietary factors affect zinc bioavailability. Phytate is probably the most important zinc antagonist, especially in the presence of calcium, as it forms a chelate with zinc which is unavailable for absorption. Other cations with similar physicochemical properties (copper and cadmium) or mutual affinity for carrier protein (iron) also reduce zinc bioavailability. Some proteins have been shown to improve zinc bioavailability, but the mechanisms for the effect are not yet clear. *See* Cadmium, Toxicology; Copper, Physiology; Zinc, Physiology

Zinc homeostasis in the body is controlled by alterations in efficiency of absorption coupled with changes in the quantities of endogenous zinc secreted into the intestine. Thus, body zinc status plays an important role in determining dietary zinc bioavailability.

Calcium

Calcium absorption is vitamin D dependent; therefore bioavailability depends upon vitamin D intake and status. Dietary inhibitors of calcium absorption include substances that form complexes in the intestine, such as phytate and oxalate. Protein also modifies calcium bioavailability; high levels of protein increase urinary calcium excretion, and this is accompanied by an increase in intestinal absorption. The net result is a reduction in the proportion of dietary calcium utilized by the body, i.e. lower bioavailability. Lactose, on the other hand, promotes calcium absorption. *See* Calcium, Physiology; Cholecalciferol, Physiology; Protein, Interactions and Reactions Involved in Food Processing

Vitamins

A number of vitamins are not fully bioavailable to the human body. The more important ones are folate, vitamin B_6, niacin, vitamin A, carotenoids, and vitamin E.

Folate

Folate exists in nature primarily as reduced one-carbon substituted forms of pteroylpolyglutamates. The polyglutamyl form of folate makes up approximately 80% of dietary folate and must be cleaved to the monoglutamate form for absorption. Polyglutamate folate is utilized 70–80% as efficiently as the monoglutamate form.

Numerous dietary and physiological factors influence the deconjugation and absorption of folate, and its subsequent utilization in the body. Dietary factors that reduce folate bioavailability include conjugase inhibitors in foods, as found for example in pulses, folate-binding proteins in milk, and dietary fibre such as wheat bran. Physiological factors include intraluminal pH (maximal absorption occurs at pH 6·3), the fall in intestinal conjugase enzyme activity associated with aging, and certain nutrient deficiencies, including zinc, vitamin B_{12}, and folate deficiency. *See* Cobalamins, Physiology; Folic Acid, Physiology

Vitamin B_6

Vitamin B_6 (3-hydroxy-5-hydroxymethyl-2-methyl-pyridine) exists in foods as either the free or phosphorylated form of pyridoxine, pyridoxamine, and pyridoxal. Plant foods also contain pyridoxine glucoside, and it has been suggested that the observed lower bioavailability in plant than animal foods is associated with this form of vitamin B_6. Dietary substances that have been shown to reduce vitamin B_6 absorption include orange juice, the active component probably being a low molecular weight binder, and wheat bran. *See* Vitamin B_6, Properties and Determination

Niacin

Niacin deficiency is associated with diets containing high levels of maize because the niacin is chemically bound to carbohydrate by ester linkages and unavailable for absorption. However, alkali treatment, as used by certain cultural groups when processing foods in the traditional way, renders the niacin more bioavailable. Other grains, such as sorghum, wheat, barley and rice, contain niacin in chemically bound forms. *See* Niacin, Physiology

Vitamin A, Carotenoids, Vitamin E

The absorption of these vitamins depends upon the presence of fat. When diets are adequate in fat and not excessively high in dietary fibre, especially pectin, they are all well absorbed. Fat stimulates bile flow and facilitates their transport into mucosal cells; bile salts assist in the formation of micelles, which are more readily absorbed than emulsions. Dietary proteins are believed to improve vitamin A absorption because of their ability to act as surface-active agents. Thus protein or protein–calorie malnutrition is often associated with malabsorption of vitamin A. Zinc deficiency, alcohol and certain food additives, e.g. nitrites, are associated with reduced vitamin A utilization. *See* Retinol, Physiology

In addition to the level and type of fat, a number of other dietary and physiological factors influence the bioavailability of carotenoids in foods. These include the digestibility of the food, the presence of antioxidants and certain types of dietary fibre, protein or zinc deficiency, and vitamin A status. The actual absorption of carotenoids from uncooked foods can be as low as 1%. Mild cooking can enhance absorption by increasing the digestibility of the food and its constituent carotenoids. For example, some of the carotenoids in green leafy vegetables are complexed with protein. Mild heating is believed to dissociate the complexes, releasing the free carotenoids, which are then more available for absorption. However, it has been observed that overcooking can drastically reduce carotenoid bioavailability. *See* Carotenoids, Physiology

There are at least eight compounds of plant origin that have vitamin E activity, but α-tocopherol accounts for almost all of the vitamin E activity in foods of animal origin. This isomer has by far the highest biological activity of all the natural isomers. Under normal dietary conditions only about 20–40% of ingested vitamin E is absorbed, and the absorption efficiency decreases with its dietary level. Polyunsaturated fatty acids are known to decrease vitamin E absorption and utilization, probably because of their tendency to oxidize. It has been demonstrated in rats that high levels of pectin and wheat bran reduce vitamin E bioavailability. Dietary constituents such as vitamin A, iron, selenium and zinc may affect vitamin E utilization. *See* Tocopherols, Physiology

Nutritional Implications of Bioavailability

The ultimate goal in nutritional science is to understand the interactions between diet and health. This requires a detailed knowledge of nutrient bioavailability, without which it is impossible to relate dietary intakes to indices of physiological function used to assess health. Estimates of dietary requirements cannot be made without the appropriate 'bioavailability' factors. Where diets are marginal or inadequate in one or more micronutrient it is often possible to improve the quality of the diet by increasing the bioavailability of the nutrients in question, with consequent improvements in the nutritional status of people consuming it. Future research should utilize recently developed techniques to quantify the different phases of bioavailability, differentiating where possible between dietary and physiological factors. The ultimate goal is to combine all the information to form a coherent picture of bioavailability of nutrients for different foods and diets.

Bibliography

Allen LH (1982) Calcium bioavailability and absorption: a review. *American Journal of Clinical Nutrition* 35: 783–808.

Dintzis FR and Laszlo JA (eds) (1989) Mineral absorption from the monogastric GI tract. New York: Plenum Press.

Hazell T (1985) Minerals in foods: dietary sources, chemical forms, interactions, bioavailability. *World Review of Nutrition and Dietetics* 46: 1–123.

Kies C (ed) (1982) *Nutritional Bioavailability of Iron.* Washington DC: American Chemical Society.

Solomons NW (1982) Biological availability of zinc in humans. *American Journal of Clinical Nutrition* 35: 1048–1075.

Southgate DAT, Johnson I, Fenwick GR (eds) (1989) *Nutrient Availability: Chemical and Biological Aspects.* Cambridge: Royal Society of Chemistry.

Susan J. Fairweather-Tait
AFRC Institute of Food Research, Norwich, UK

BIOCHEMICAL PATHWAYS

See Tricarboxylic Acid Cycle and Oxidative Phosphorylation

BIOGENIC AMINES

See Amines

BIOMINERALIZATION

This article will discuss the possible beneficial effects of the biomineralized mass as an additional component in the diet. This review is also concerned with the significance of mineral elements in lactic acid bacteria, bifidobacteria and propionibacterial mass. *See* Bifidobacteria in Foods

Definition

The term 'biomineralization' is commonly used to describe the intracellular mineralization of crystals in microorganisms and in other organic cells or tissues. It involves a range of minerals and trace elements. Biomineralization has global consequences and has helped to mould the Earth.

As bacteria rely entirely on diffusion, they are designed for maximal diffusion. They also have the highest surface area to volume ratio of any life form. Soluble minerals and trace elements will inevitably reach and interact with their cell walls. The bacterial surface possesses metallic ions in some form. They are often an important component of the cell wall. Calcium and magnesium are the preferred minerals of gram-positive cell walls. Some bacteria bind more minerals from laboratory media than others. There is also some evidence that capsules protect bacterial cells from the toxic effect of heavy metals. The sorption of soluble minerals can be so efficient that visible precipitates inside bacterial cells can be seen by electron microscopy. It is evident that bacteria have a greater capacity to absorb and precipitate metal ions from solution than any other form of life.

In addition to this, mineral and trace elements in the cell mass of certain beneficial bacteria could also play a role in nutrition through their increased bioavailability from, for example, fermented milk products and similar foods. *See* Bioavailability of Nutrients

Metabolic disturbances in the availability of minerals and trace elements can lead to diseases, e.g. anaemia and rickets, which can be cured as the regulatory systems are known even on a cellular level. But further information is needed and there is still considerable interest in the nutritional significance of minerals and trace elements, partly because of their potential beneficial effect in the prevention of osteoporosis, hypertension, cancer and cardiovascular diseases. *See* Hypertension, Hypertension and Diet

Incorporation of Minerals into Biomass

Soil bacteria are an example of biogeochemical agents which convert complex organic compounds into simple inorganic compounds or their constituent elements. This is called mineralization. It ensures a continuous supply of nutrients for plants and animals including man. Bacteria play an essential role in the transformation of nitrogen, carbon and sulphur, through assimilation and dissimilation. The production of acids – a metabolic activity of microbes – solubilizes phosphate, for example, from insoluble iron and aluminium phosphates. Bacteria also change insoluble oxides of iron and manganese to soluble salts. Bacterial cells cannot grow in the absence of all mineral and trace elements, because many metabolic processes rely on metal ion activation, and metals are incorporated into the structure of several cell substances. The functions of mineral and trace elements in the bacterial cell are varied and not always known. Teichoic acids, for example, bind magnesium ions and there is some evidence that they help to protect bacteria from thermal injury. The following ions are known to act as cofactors for various enzymes: magnesium, iron, zinc, molybdenum, manganese and copper.

Only a few references concerning the mineral and trace element contents of lactic acid bacteria, bifidobacteria and propionibacteria can be found in the literature. The requirement for special ions in their metabolism is well known. Magnesium and manganese are special growth factors for lactic acid and bifidobacteria. In propionibacteria, iron stimulates the production of propionic acid. Magnesium and manganese also accelerate the decarboxylation of succinate. These mineral and trace elements along with cobalt act as cofactors in propionate fermentation and vitamin B_{12} synthesis. *See* Coenzymes

The mineral and trace elements needed by bacteria for their growth and metabolism are obtained from the growth substrate and are partly fixed in the bacterial cell mass. In Tables 1 and 2 the concentrations of some selected mineral and trace elements in different *Lactobacillus*, *Bifidobacterium* and *Propionibacterium* species are presented.

Looking at the figures it can be noted that in bacterial mass potassium and magnesium concentrations are of another order of magnitude than those for other mineral and trace elements. There are also considerable differences in concentration between strains, species and genera.

In *Lactobacillus acidophilus* mass the potassium con-

Table 1. Concentrations (mg kg^{-1}) of mineral elements in some lactic acid bacteria, bifidobacteria and propionibacteria

Bacteria	Ca	Mg	K	Fe	Mn	Cu	Zn
Lactobacillus acidophilus 74	10·2	3372·0	19 400	5·4	32·9	44·4	92·5
L. acidophilus 145	54·6	3290·0	14 600	0·3	40·0	85·7	90·0
L. delbrueckii ssp. *bulgaricus*	84·0	1890·0	760	12·5	114·0	50·0	14·0
Bifidobacterium bifidum	60·0	6190·0	4000	5·8	90·0	25·0	104·0
B. longum	460·0	985·0	370	6·6	200·0	90·0	85·0

Table 2. Total concentrations of trace elements in *Propionibacterium freudenreichii* mass

Trace element	Average weight of dry matter (mg kg^{-1})
Mg	2190
Fe	535
Ca	366
Mn	267
Zn	159
Cu	102
Co	44
Ni	9
Cr	1·4
Cd	0·1
Se	0·1

tent is particularly high. *L. delbrueckii* ssp. *bulgaricus* shows the highest concentration of iron and the second highest concentration of calcium and manganese. *Bifidobacterium bifidum* contains very high levels of magnesium and zinc, but low levels of copper. *B. longum* again shows high concentrations of calcium and manganese as well as copper. When comparing the amounts of mineral and trace elements above with those of *Propionibacterium freudenreichii* it is apparent that iron, manganese, copper and zinc occur in considerably higher concentrations. They seem to be quite strongly bound in the bacterial mass.

Although the same laboratory growth medium is used for lactic acid and bifidobacteria (MRS-broth), and that used for propionibacteria (LY-broth) is less rich in nutrients, there are significant differences in the mineral and trace element concentrations of the bacterial cell mass, which can be traced from differences in their metabolic capacity to use mineral and trace elements.

Probiotics and Nutritional Supplements

For many decades, lactic acid, bifido- and propionibacteria have been used as probiotics, in both humans and animals, to achieve therapeutic and growth-promoting effects. They are often used to correct a disturbed microbial balance in the large intestine after antibiotic therapy or diarrhoea. The effect of these bacteria is based on their acid production, antibacterial, antitumoral, anticarcinogenic and anticholesterolaemic agents. The mineral and trace element contents might also act as a contributory factor. In healthy adults a dietary supplement of intestinal *Lactobacillus* and *Bifidobacterium* strains does not replace other intestinal bacteria, but helps to maintain a proper balance of the resident flora. The organisms survive for some time in the gastrointestinal tract and sometimes even colonize and multiply before excretion in the faeces. Regularly consuming fermented milk products, which contain these bacteria, ensures a continual passage through the gut. But only biotypes specific to a particular animal species can be used. Biotypes of bifidobacteria differ between human infants and adults. *See* Microflora of the Intestine, Probiotics

The therapeutic preparations used are mostly freeze-dried, pure bifidobacteria or mixed preparations containing bifidobacteria and other intestinal bacteria. Some producers prefer fresh preparations.

The role of propionibacteria as probiotics in swine fodder is evident. Their growth-promoting effect is absolutely clear even in excellent swinery conditions and the effect is stronger in a less hygienic environment. The influence on the decrease of gastrointestinal disturbances follows the same trend. It could be tentatively assumed that the mineral and trace element – especially manganese, zinc, copper, iron and calcium – contents of propioni- and also bifidobacterial mass may contribute to this beneficial effect.

Effect of Fermentation on Absorption

It has been speculated that the intestinal absorption of calcium from cultured dairy products is superior to that from milk, because lactic acid would increase the utilization of calcium. However, no significant evidence has yet been shown to support this theory. An important matter in the intestinal absorption of essential mineral and trace elements from milk products is the effect of lactose. It stimulates the absorption of calcium and may also improve the intestinal absorption of phosphorus, magnesium, zinc and iron. It is presumed that the fermentation of lactose could alter the bioavailability of mineral and trace elements by changing the physicochemical nature of the milk. Lactose enhances the diffusion of calcium and magnesium across the ileum wall. The lower pH of milk fermented by lactic acid bacteria may help to lower gastric pH and hence increase mineral solubility and absorption. This is especially beneficial for elderly people with reduced gastric acid production. *See* Lactose

There are no data indicating that fermentation significantly improves the bioavailability of zinc and other trace elements. However, this does not exclude the significance of the mineral and trace elements of the bacterial mass.

Absorption of 'Organic Minerals' Compared to Inorganic Forms

The intrinsic properties of the dietary source of mineral or trace element may alter its absorbability. It seems obvious also that the form in which the mineral or trace element is present in various foodstuffs and probiotic preparations contributes to the differences.

Some minerals are equally well absorbed from organic and inorganic salts, e.g. magnesium. On the other hand some investigators have shown that zinc is more easily absorbed from foodstuffs of animal origin. Some chelates of zinc with animal proteins might protect the trace element from inhibitory influences in the food, while much of the zinc is associated with metalloenzyme proteins. This is not always the case in different experimental animals.

Selenium absorption is dependent on the chemical form found in food or probiotic preparations. It is clear that the more reduced forms have superior biological availability. Selenium is relatively well absorbed from the gastrointestinal tract by humans as discrete selenium compounds, Se-selenomethionine is somewhat more efficiently absorbed than Se-selenite (99% as opposed to 81%).

The site of manganese absorption in the gastrointestinal tract is not precisely known. It can probably be absorbed along the extent of the small bowel. The manganese content of bacterial mass forms a considerable source of this element, particularly in bifido- and propionibacteria. Manganese shows several mineral–mineral interactions at the level of intestinal absorption. Zinc and copper do not have any effect, but iron seems to be the major inhibitory factor in manganese absorption. Mercury also decreases manganese intake.

The bacterial mass represents such a source of 'organic minerals and trace elements' and they could be assumed to be better absorbed in the intestinal tract of man and animals. Besides, there are significant differences in the ability of lactic acid, bifido- and propionibacteria to incorporate minerals and trace elements from their growth substrates into their cells. According to this it would even be possible to choose a probiotic preparation that meets varying mineral or trace element needs. Therefore a combined effect of mineral and trace elements in the mass of those bacterial species as additional factors in the bioavailability of fermented milk products could be relevant. However, scientific evidence is still needed.

Bibliography

Beveridge TJ (1989) Role of cellular design in bacterial metal accumulation and mineralization. *Annual Review of Microbiology* 43: 147–171.

Mann S, Sparks NHC, Frankel RB, Bazylinski DA and Jannasch HW (1990) Biomineralization of ferrimagnetic greigite (Fe$_3$S$_4$) and iron pyrite (FeS$_2$) in a magnetotactic bacterium. *Nature* 343: 258–262.

Mantere-Alhonen S and Vuorinen A (1989) Mineral elements in the cell mass of lactic acid bacteria and bifidobacteria. *Milchwissenschaft* 44 (12): 758–760.

O'Dell BL (1984) Bioavailability of trace elements. *Nutrition Review* 42 (no. 9): 301–308.

Schaafsma G (1989) Bioavailability of minerals and micronutrients from fermented milks. Les laits fermentés. *Actualités de la Recherche* 147–152.

Solomons NW and Rosenberg IH (eds) (1984) *Absorption and Malabsorption of Mineral Nutrients*, vol. 12. New York: Alan R. Liss.

Vuorinen A and Mantere-Alhonen S (1982) On trace elements in *Propionibacterium freudenreichii*-mass. *Meijeritieteellinen Aikakauskirja* (Finnish Journal of Dairy Science) XL: 53–59.

Säde Mantere-Alhonen
University of Helsinki, Helsinki, Finland

BIOTECHNOLOGY IN FOOD PRODUCTION

Fundamental discoveries in molecular biology in the 1960s and 1970s sparked a scientific revolution which, in the 1980s, resulted in the first generation of biotechnology derived products based on recombinant DNA and cell fusion techniques.

Today, technical advances continue to drive production costs down, and earlier commercial successes in pharmaceuticals and chemicals will be repeated in areas of food and agriculture. Indeed, advances in modern biotechnology, together with the increased activity in areas of traditional biotechnology such as fermentation and screening, are poised to have a profound impact on key segments of the food production chain. Currently the main emphasis of new biotechnology is on raw materials and food ingredients whereas the traditional biotechnology prevails in the processing of other food products (Fig. 1).

The driving forces for the food industry's investment in biotechnology include:

- Consumer demand for convenient, superior quality food products at 'value-for-money' prices. The key elements of food quality include:
  taste and appearance,
  healthiness (natural, additive-free, nutritious),
  safety (microbiology, toxicology).
- The need to develop more efficient processes with reduced environmental impact.
- Competition between food companies for improved shares of both traditional and emerging markets.

Table 1 Required technologies in the food industry

Physical	Chemical	Biological
Separation	Hydrogenation	Breeding
Drying	Preservation	Fermentation
Blending	Modification	Screening
Extrusion		Enzyme/protein engineering
Precipitation		Cell fusion
Concentration		Cell/tissue culture
Extraction		Anti-sense RNA technology
Distillation		Antibody technology
Chromato-		Biosensors
graphy		Immobilization
		Hygienic processing
		Biocatalysis

Clearly, those companies which are able to manage all these factors successfully will be well positioned to compete in the market place of the future. Although conceptually straightforward, success will require, among other things, very sophisticated technological skills in all of the relevant (bio)technological disciplines (Table 1).

In this article, progress and opportunities in (modern) food biotechnology, for key segments of the food production chain, are evaluated.

Raw Materials

Raw materials used in food production generally originate from plants and animals. Traditional (bio)technologies such as classical breeding, and physical and chemical processing, have dominated this segment of the food chain for many years. Although such traditional technologies will continue to be important, modern biotechnology will have an increasingly important role, as hitherto unapproachable targets come within range.

The recombinant DNA tools of modern biotechnology are now being generally applied to plants, in order to create species in which plant metabolism is 'tailored' to provide superior raw materials with respect to quality, functionality and availability. However, the application of recombinant DNA technologies to provide tailored, transgenic animals is much further away.

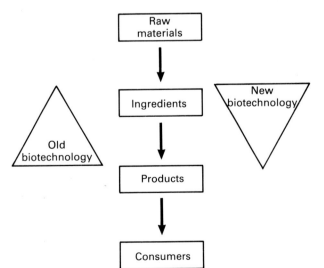

Fig. 1 Implications of biotechnology for the food chain.

Plants

Current and future opportunities in the engineering of plant-derived raw materials include:

- higher crop yield;
- altered product composition (e.g. fatty acids, polysaccharides, proteins, flavour, colour, etc.);
- improved nutritional composition;
- introduction of new genes (e.g. proteins, nitrogen-fixing system);
- improved 'keepability' (e.g. storage/shelf life);
- improved ease of processing (e.g. flour);
- improved resistance (e.g. diseases, herbicides, frost, drought, temperature);
- removal of undesired components (e.g. caffeine);
- reduction of process waste streams.

In some species these targets are already being achieved. A striking example is the 'anti-sense tomato' of Imperial Chemical Industries. The keepability of this tomato has been improved by suppressing, via anti-sense RNA technology, the expression of the enzyme endopolygalacturonase, which causes the pericarp to degrade during ripening. Furthermore, some insect-, virus- and herbicide-resistant plants have been created and are now being evaluated in field trials. These examples involve single gene transformations but, in the longer term, more complex characteristics will be introduced, such as improved drought and temperature tolerance.

Animals

Commercial realization of the potential applications of modern biotechnology to animal-based raw materials are far more difficult to predict. Research on transgenic animals is in its infancy and developments will be strongly influenced by ethical considerations.

Potential targets for animal food production include:

- higher yield (e.g. meat, milk);
- improved resistance (e.g. diseases);
- tailored milk or meat (e.g. lactose-free/low-fat milk and the protein composition of meat).

Not unexpectedly, progress in plant biotechnology has been much more rapid than progress in animal biotechnology. The first generation of commercial transgenic plants is expected within 5 years, whereas the time required for commercialization of transgenic animals for food production will be much longer.

Ingredients

A second group in the food chain, often referred to as food ingredients, includes:

- proteins;
- enzymes;
- cultures;
- stabilizers/thickeners;
- emulsifiers;
- colours;
- sweeteners;
- preservatives;
- flavours.

The application of biotechnology to this group is proving particularly successful. In a relatively short time-frame, a number of technical targets have been realized, and novel and/or improved products are being rapidly commercialized. Many of these ingredients are still produced by traditional fermentation technology, using strains obtained by routine screening or from classical mutagenesis. To date, only a handful are produced via recombinant DNA technology, and few have as yet completed the approval procedure for use in food (e.g. chymosin and improved baker's yeast). This situation will change, but the traditional (bio) technologies will continue to advance, and will therefore remain important to sustain progress. For example, important advances have been made in designing improved fermentation equipment, automated control techniques, and monitoring devices. Furthermore, new downstream processing technologies have been developed, which enable the isolation of bioproducts under mild conditions, in a controlled, cost-effective manner (e.g. (selective) membranes and chromatography materials). Whether or not a technology is traditional or modern is not important; the key to success is being able to apply the right combination of available technologies to produce food ingredients which are of benefit to the consumer.

Progress can be expected in the following areas:

- upgrading of waste streams to useful ingredients;
- overproduction of well-defined ingredients by microorganisms, plant/animal cell (tissue) culture, or by genetically modified systems;
- search for novel, superior food ingredients;
- development of milder, safe and cost-effective processing methods;
- high solid and solid-state fermentation processes.

Although many of the skills are already in place to address these opportunities, major breakthroughs are still needed in the areas of plant and animal biotechnology in order to achieve commercial success. The same applies to high solid concentrations or solid-state fermentations, where the current rather phenomenological approach could benefit from a sound scientific input.

Products

Ultimately, raw materials and ingredients are processed and packed to provide consumer products. In the same way that biotechnology has had an impact on raw materials and food ingredients, the implications of biotechnology on the end product (with respect to processing, quality control, microbial stability, packaging and healthiness) are becoming increasingly evident.

Hygienic processing is one of today's key technologies in food production. The main driving forces for the rapid developments in this area are the need to produce high-quality, microbiologically safe products under mild conditions, and the growing demand for fresh, chilled and shelf-stable food products. Particularly important is the design of automated process equipment, where the risk of microbial contamination is minimized. Also, hygiene kits are being developed which facilitate direct and rapid monitoring of critical control points in the production cycle (HCCP). *See* Hazard Analysis Critical Control Point

The rapid growth of automated on-/in-line quality control systems will continue. Instead of controlling the quality of the end product, the process will be controlled and where necessary corrected. In this way production problems will be minimized, and cost savings achieved. *See* Computers – Use in Food Processing

New advances in quality control also include the development of detection systems based on monoclonal antibodies and DNA probes. In comparison with existing detection systems (e.g. enzyme immunoassay (EIA) and radioimmunoassay (RIA)) they are easier to use, faster and are generally more sensitive. *See* Immunoassays, Radioimmunoassay and Enzyme Immunoassay; Quality Assurance and Quality Control

Packaging serves many purposes. It is necessary to safeguard the quality of the product during transport and storage, it is generally designed to attract the attention of the consumer, and is also used to provide information about the contents. In the future it might be possible, for example, to coat or to impregnate packaging materials with biomolecules to improve food preservation. A likely impact of biotechnology will be the development of biodegradable packaging materials. Promising results have been obtained using polyhydroxybutyric acid produced by fermentation, although as yet the production costs are a limitation.

The Consumer

Food consumption patterns throughout the world are changing rapidly as a result of economic, social and political factors. Changing lifestyles influence eating habits, including not only the individual's choice, but also where and how food is prepared and eaten. Consumers are increasingly aware that they are what they eat, and that diet and health are inextricably linked.

In the Western world there is a trend towards families eating fewer meals together, partly a consequence of more women going out to work, and people dedicating more time to leisure and sporting activities. Consequently, there is a growing demand for food products which offer convenience, quality and variety. *See* Convenience Foods, Definition and Classification

Convenience includes not only the planning and preparation of meals, but also food purchase and packaging. Increasingly, consumers are prepared to pay more for quality and variety. Also, ethnic foods, especially Oriental, Italian and Mexican, appeal to the changing and increasingly sophisticated taste of consumers, providing new opportunities for those who enjoy entertaining, and for those who regard cooking as a leisure activity rather than an essential function.

Not only is the profile of the food consumer changing, the food-processing industry itself is undergoing dramatic change, particularly as a result of company acquisitions. Acquisitions provide advantages such as increased market-share, or new products, but they can also provide the opportunity to 'leap-frog' into new technologies, such as biotechnology. Indeed, it has been suggested that, by the year 2000, at least four-fifths of food industry sales could be dominated by a few multibillion dollar conglomerates.

Concern for personal 'health and well-being' is reflected in a growing consumer demand for food items which project a healthy image. Products labelled as 'natural', 'low-fat', 'low-calorie', 'fresh' and 'nutritious' have become the hallmark of the health-conscious consumer. *See* Health Foods, Definition and Dietary Importance

Such trends are being exploited around the world, particularly in Europe and North America, and also in Japan, where in 2 years the market for healthy, functional foods grew from zero to US\$ 600 million.

'Healthy' includes food products which help:

- body defence mechanisms (e.g. hypoallergenic and immunoactivating foods);
- prevent diseases (e.g. hypertension and diabetes);
- recovery from diseases (e.g. by controlling the cholesterol level);
- slow down the ageing process by suppressing oxidation mechanisms.

Although at this time there is somewhat limited medical evidence that such foods do what they suggest, a clear trend is emerging.

The growing impact of biotechnology on the food industry is clearly shown by the rapid increase in patent applications. At present, biotechnology patents make up approximately 20–25% of the total number of food patents. Although most of these patents are still based on traditional biotechnologies and process developments, the importance of modern biotechnology is increasing.

Products of biotechnology intended for food use are

subject to the national requirements relating to safety. Within the EEC, food additives have to be assessed for both safety and 'case-of-need', and only when both are accepted can a material be used. In addition, regulations are under discussion concerning the production of novel foods and ingredients which will involve both notification and assessment. The handling and use of genetically modified organisms is already addressed by the requirements of the directives concerning both contained use and deliberate release. Outside the EEC, national regulations apply. Unfortunately they have, to some extent, developed independently, and hence are not identical to those of the EEC. In the USA, for instance, there is a move to consider products of biotechnology within the existing legislative framework rather than exact specific requirements. *See* European Economic Community, International Developments in Food Law; Legislation, International Standards

Perhaps more important than legislation is the public acceptance of products produced by or containing recombinant organisms. The few surveys that have been carried out indicate a mixed public perception. It is important that reliable information is available to the public in order to avoid misinformed reaction. Industry, through its biotechnology associations, is helping to provide such information, and is working openly with governmental bodies and consumer organizations to ensure that all the necessary information is available.

Bibliography

Bartle IDG (1991) ICI seeds – A marriage of bioscience and conventional plant breeding. *Biotechnology Forum Europe* 8: 1–2.
Cole M (1991) When food meets medicine. *Food Manufacture* January: 26–27.
Fowler MW, Warren GS and Moo-Young M (1990) *Plant Biotechnology*, 2nd suppl. to *Comprehensive Biotechnology*. Oxford: Pergamon Press.
Hamstra AM (1991) Biotechnology in foodstuffs, towards a model of consumer acceptance. *SWOKA Research Reports*, No. 105. The Hague: Internal SWOKA Report.
Harlander SK (1989) Biotechnology opportunities for the food industry. In: Rogers PL and Fleet GH (eds) *Biotechnology and the Food Industry*, pp 1–16. New York: Gordon and Breach.
Keuning R (1989) Biotechnology in the flavour and food industry in Europe. In: Lindsay RC and Willis BJ (eds) *Biotechnology Challenges for the Flavor and Food Industry*, pp 101–130. Amsterdam: Elsevier.
MAFF (1989) *Advisory Committee on Novel Foods and Processes, Annual Report*. Ministry of Agriculture, Fisheries and Food, UK.
Smith CJS, Watson CF, Ray J, Bird CR, Morris PC and Grierson D (1988) Antisense RNA inhibition of polygalacturonase gene expression in transgenic tomatoes. *Nature* 334: 724–726.
Webber DJ (1990) *Biotechnology: Assessing Social Impacts and Policy implications*. Greenwood Press.

C. Laane and B. J. Willis
Quest International, Bussum, The Netherlands

BIOTIN

Contents

Properties and Determination

In 1901, Wildiers observed that yeasts required a factor present in meat extract for growth. He named this factor 'bios'. In the following years 'bios' was fractionated and the different components identified. One component of this complex mixture was shown to be identical to biotin, a substance isolated from egg yolk by Kögl in 1936. However, it was observed that raw eggs in the diet are toxic to animals and caused skin lesions, which can be cured by treatment with a 'protective factor X' found in liver by György and named vitamin H. Later, it was found that vitamin H and other essential factors such as coenzyme R_1 and factor S were identical to biotin. The structure of this vitamin was established in 1942 by du Vigneaud and confirmed in 1945 by Harris who achieved its chemical synthesis. Biotin is a coenzyme for vital processes such as biosynthesis of fatty acids, glucose and amino acid metabolism. Therefore, biotin which is present in most plants and animal tissues is an important nutritional factor. Biotin is produced industrially by chemical synthesis. *See* Amino Acids, Metabolism; Coenzymes; Fatty Acids, Metabolism; Glucose, Function and Metabolism

Physical Properties

Biotin is soluble in dilute alkali and hot water, slightly soluble in dilute acid, cold water and alcohol and practically insoluble in most organic solvents. In contrast to the lability of most of the vitamins, crystalline biotin is stable in air, daylight and heat. Aqueous solutions are relatively stable if weakly acidic or alkaline and can be autoclaved without being affected. Biotin resists autoclaving in dilute sulphuric acid, conditions which are used to extract biotin from biological samples. However, biotin can be easily oxidized into biotin sulphoxides. This process, which is negligible in concentrated solutions, can become significant in very dilute solutions. Biotin sulphoxides are inactive in animals but active in certain microbial species.

Chemical Properties

The formula of biotin is $C_{10}H_{15}O_3N_2S$, its molecular weight is 244·31 Da and it has an optical rotation of $[\alpha]_D = +92°$. Biotin results from the fusion of an imidazolidone ring with a thiophane ring bearing a valeric acid side-chain (Fig. 1). The imidazolidone and thiophane rings are fused in the *cis* configuration. (The two hydrogens bound to the C3 and C4 carbons are on the same side of the rings.) The valeric chain attached to the thiophane ring (at C2) is *cis* with respect to the ureido ring. The molecule contains three asymmetric carbon atoms. Among the eight possible stereoisomers, only D-biotin is biologically active. The absolute configuration of D-biotin was established by X-ray crystallography studies.

The first total synthesis of biotin was achieved

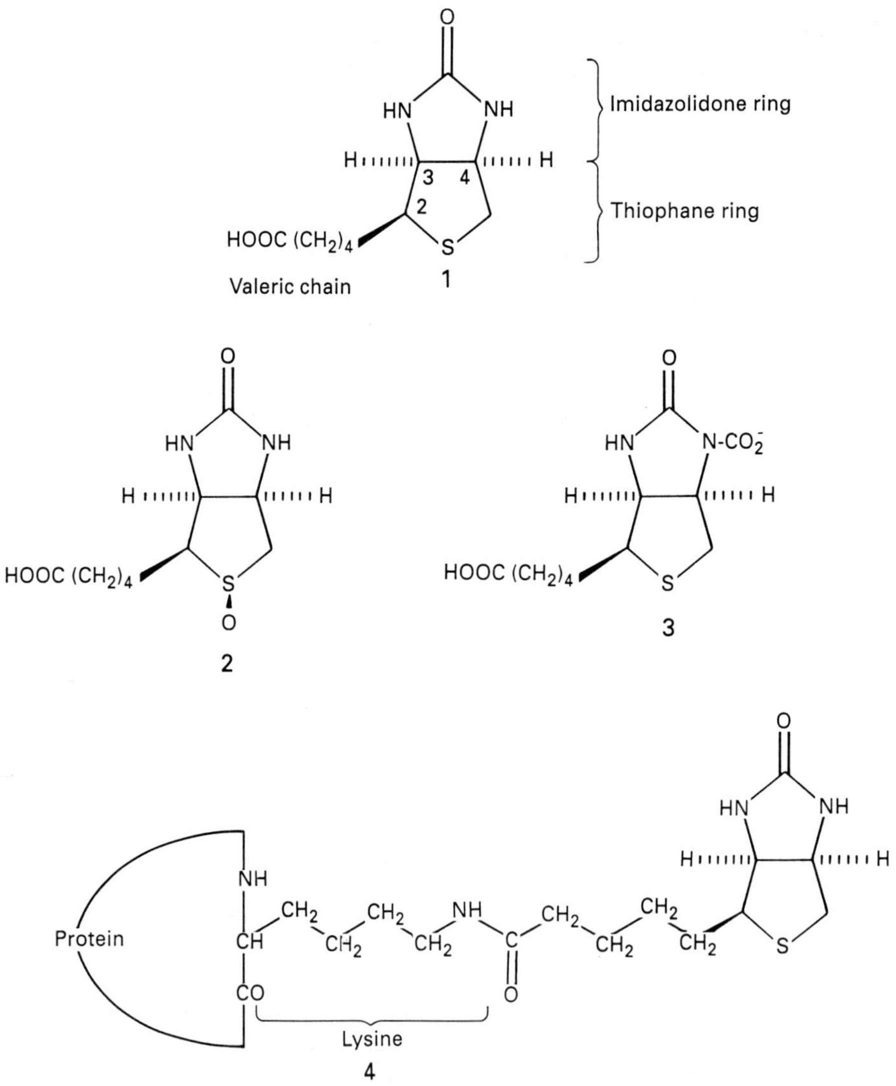

Fig. 1 Structures of D-biotin (1), l-biotin sulphoxide (2), N-carboxybiotin (3) and of biotin covalently linked through the amino group of lysine to protein (4). (The product resulting from the condensation of biotin and lysine is named biocytin.)

Properties and Determination

between 1943 and 1945. In 1949, the laboratories of Hoffman-La Roche developed a new synthesis by which biotin is prepared commercially. In the past 20 years, many other stereospecific syntheses for biotin have been described which use various starting materials.

Biotin exhibits normal reactivity at the functional groups of the molecule. The carboxyl group can be esterified normally, using classical reagents. Through this carboxylic function, biotin is bound to protein or peptides when it participates in metabolic reactions. In all the enzymes examined, the biotin has been shown to be linked through an amide bond to the ε-amino group of a lysine (Fig. 1). Biocytin which results from the condensation of biotin and lysine is biologically active. Reactions of the ureido ring occur preferentially at the N1 atom. N-Carboxybiotin (Fig. 1) is an important intermediate in enzymatic reactions catalysed by biotin. The biotin-dependent enzyme group includes three classes of enzymes: carboxylases, transcarboxylases and decarboxylases. In all these reactions, biotin acts as a CO_2 carrier, to activate CO_2 and transfer it to a substrate as in carboxylases, or to transfer a CO_2 moiety between two substrates as in transcarboxylases, or to abstract the CO_2 from a substrate as in decarboxylases. In the three cases, N-carboxybiotin is an intermediate. The sulphur atom can be oxidized with various reagents yielding sulphoxide. Biotin sulphoxide (Fig. 1) and some components bearing a structural relationship to biotin present some biological activity of biotin, but with a lower efficacy.

Proteins exist which can bind biotin to form a stable complex which is not degraded in the gastrointestinal tract. Among these proteins, streptavidin and avidin, which have been isolated respectively from *Streptomyces* and egg white, have been used extensively to induce biotin deficiencies and as a tool in molecular biology or in biotin determinations. It has been established that the toxicity of raw eggs is due to avidin. *See* Protein, Interactions and Reactions Involved in Food Processing

Nutritional Requirement

As mentioned above, biotin deficiency can be induced in animals by feeding them with raw egg whites, which contain avidin. However, cases of spontaneous biotin deficiency in humans were not detected until 1976, but since then several cases have been observed. The clinical symptoms (alopecia, skin rashes, presence of metabolites in urine, etc.) linked to low or even absent carboxylase biotin-dependent activities, can be eliminated by biotin absorption. The presentation of this deficiency has been classified into two groups: the neonatal form characterized by an unusually low carboxylase activity and the late-onset form which is characterized by a low level of plasma biotin.

The evaluation of the nutritional requirements of biotin is complicated. This is due in part to the fact that biotin-producing microorganisms exist in the intestinal microflora. Furthermore the intestinal flora is influenced by the composition of the food and the amount of biosynthesized biotin may vary. Therefore the significance of the contribution of the intestinal biotin to the biotin requirement is not fully established. *See* Microflora of the Intestine, Role and Effects

Biotin given orally is well absorbed. However, only free biotin can be absorbed; biotin bound to protein is released in the intestine.

In 1980, the Food and Nutrition Board of the US National Academy of Sciences estimated an adequate daily dietary intake of biotin to be 30–50 μg for infants up to 1 year old, 65–100 μg for children 1–10 years old and 100–200 μg for adults. As biotin deficiency in humans is unlikely and daily requirements are low, in many countries it is assumed that the diet and intestinal synthesis by microorganisms supply the biotin requirement, so dietary allowances have not been recommended.

Occurrence in Foods

Biotin is widely distributed in food products. In animal tissues, yeast and plant seeds, biotin is present partly bound to protein, whereas in milk, vegetables and fruit it is present in the free form. Microbiological tests have demonstrated a higher concentration in liver and a lower content in meat (beef, veal, pork). Brewer's yeast, soya beans, peanuts and eggs are good sources of biotin, whereas fruit and vegetables are relatively poor sources. Cereals (barley, rice wheat) are also poor sources. The biotin content of breakfast cereals varies with the type of cereal and the degree of milling. The largest amounts of biotin are found in oatmeal and wheat germ. Some protein sources declared suitable for infants, e.g. cow's milk or casein preparations provide small quantities of biotin. Similarly, the biotin content of human milk is sometimes insufficient to supply the infant's requirement for biotin. In this case it is recommended that the mother takes supplementary vitamins. Preservation and food processing reduce the biotin content of foods. For example, reduction of the biotin availability was observed in preserved baby foods. The biotin content of various types of food are listed in Table 1.

Isolation

Biotin may be isolated as its methyl ester from egg yolk, beef liver and milk. It is extracted from eggs with acetone, precipitated with ethanol and dissolved in water. Impurities are removed by several precipitations

Table 1. Biotin content of various types of food ($\mu g\ kg^{-1}$)

Fruit			Meat	
Apples	10		Beef	30
Apple juice	5		Pork	50
Oranges	10–19		Chicken	110
Orange juice	3–8		Liver (beef, pork)	1000
Peaches	20			
Peaches (canned)	2		*Fish*	
Grapefruits	30			
Grapefruit juice	7		Tuna (canned)	30
Bananas	40		Mackerel (canned)	180
Raisins	50		Sardines	240
Peanuts (roasted)	340			
Walnuts	370		*Miscellaneous*	
			Chocolate	320
Vegetables			Brewer's yeast	800
			Soya beans	600
Potatoes	1			
Lettuce, carrots	30		*Cereals (cooked, whole)*	
Onions, tomatoes	40			
Spinach	70		Rice (brown)	120
Peas (fresh)	95		Wheat	160
Peas (canned)	20		Oats	240
Mushrooms	160		Barley	310
Cauliflower	170			
Dairy products				
Cow's milk	20			
Cheese	30–50			
Eggs (whole)	200			

Data from Hardinge MG and Crooks H (1961) *Journal of the American Dietary Association* 38: 240 and Documenta Geigy (1975).

with lead acetate, mercuric chloride and phosphotungstic acid. The extract may be purified further by absorption on charcoal, and elution with a mixture of acetone–ammonia. After transformation as its methyl ester, biotin is obtained as a crystalline product: in one particular experiment 4 mg of biotin was isolated from 1000 egg yolks. In liver, biotin exists mainly as bound biotin. Therefore, liver has to be autoclaved with dilute acid or digested with papain prior to beginning the extraction procedure. Methods similar to those used in the case of egg yolks were used to isolate and purify biotin from liver.

Extraction

In biological materials, such as blood, bacteria or cells, biotin exists either free or bound and the isolation of total biotin implies, as above, acidic treatment of the biological sample. Biotin is then absorbed on active charcoal. Elution can be performed with an ethanol–

ammonia mixture. Following concentration, biotin is extracted with ethanol and purified on an ion exchange column. *See* Chromatography, Principles

Ion exchange chromatography is a technique which can be used for the purification and concentration of traces of weak acidic materials such as biotin. This method has been used to isolate and purify biotin from the culture filtrate of many microorganisms, including moulds, yeast and bacteria. The same chromatographic technique proved to be a good method to monitor and titrate biotin in biological media.

Specific Methods of Analysis

Animals as Test Organisms

Biotin can be evaluated using rats or chicks as test organisms.

Rat Method

Incorporation of raw egg white or avidin in a synthetic diet results in biotin deficiency in the animal. Biotin forms an unabsorbable complex with avidin and the biotin requirement is not provided by the synthesis of the vitamin by the intestinal microflora. After a 6–7 week depletion period, the rats show a cessation of growth and manifestations of biotin deficiency. They then receive the amount of biotin contained in the test sample by injection. Pure biotin serves as the reference standard. The bioassay is based on the growth response: the gain in weight during the test period is a function of the dose of biotin assigned.

Chick Method

The chick test is used to assay biotin in grains and feeds. The chicks are prepared by giving them biotin-free feed and the biotin is estimated, as in the case of the rat test, on the basis of weight gain. Furthermore, biotin can be calculated from the blood level of pyruvate carboxylase, a biotin-dependent enzyme. In this test, the sample and standard vitamins may be given orally.

Microbiological Tests

The most commonly used assay for biotin is the microbiological test, in which biotin-dependent microorganisms are employed. For these microorganisms biotin acts as a growth factor. The microbiological methods are technically simple. However, most of the microorganisms used for the assay of biotin will respond only to free biotin and not to its bound form. Thus, test samples must be prepared by enzymatic or acid hydroly-

Table 2.   Activity of biotin derivatives versus growth of microorganisms

	Lactobacillus plantarum	*Lactobacillus casei*	*Saccharomyces cerevisiae*
Biotin	+	+	+
Biotin methyl ester	0	0	+
Biotin sulphoxide	+	0	+
Biocytin	0	+	+

sis in order to obtain all the biotin in free form. Unsaturated fatty acids interfere with the assay and have to be removed by either filtration or ether extraction. Standards of known biotin concentration and unknown samples are added to tubes containing an appropriate medium. After inoculation and incubation the biotin content of the test materials is evaluated by measuring the growth response of microorganisms turbidimetrically by comparison with standards.

Several microorganisms which require biotin as a growth factor, have been used in microbiological assays. Of these microorganisms, *Lactobacillus plantarum* and *Saccharomyces cerevisiae* are the most widely used. The specificity of the test organisms to various derivatives is summarized in Table 2.

Yeast assay methods (*S. cerevisiae*) for biotin are simple and less time consuming than the use of *Lactobacillus*, but yeasts are generally less specific in their response to biotin. *S. cerevisiae* is widely used to estimate biotin and its metabolites.

In natural food products, biotin is present at only very low concentrations. Its estimation, until the development of chromatographic techniques, has been carried out using its biological effect in animals and microorganisms.

Other Methods

The high affinity of avidin for biotin has been used extensively in biotin determinations. Several methods are based on the fact that biotin changes either the affinity of avidin with dyes or the properties of a fluorescently labelled avidin. Several radioisotope dilution techniques have also been proposed.

Finally, biotin can be assayed by means of chromatographic techniques. Thin-layer chromatography can be used for the determination of biotin in the presence of other water-soluble vitamins. The best detection agent is *p*-dimethylaminocinnamaldehyde, which is quite a specific reagent for biotin. Liquid chromatography (LC) is a very specific technique for the analysis of thermostable and nonvolatile compounds such as biotin. However, the limitation of LC lies in the availability of a suitable detection system. Biotin does not absorb in the ultraviolet region and only refractometer detection can be

applied to direct analysis. Satisfactory results have been obtained despite the usual low sensitivity due to the detector. In order to facilitate the analysis of small quantities of biotin, convenient derivatizations for ultraviolet or fluorometric detection have been used. These LC methods are helpful in qualitative and quantitative analysis even if the detection limits of biotin are higher than those observed in the case of microbiological techniques. *See* Chromatography, Thin-layer Chromatography

Bibliography

Bonjour JP (1984) In: Machlin LJ (ed.) *Handbook of Vitamins, Nutritional, Biochemical and Clinical Aspects.* New York:- Marcel Dekker.
Frappier F and Gaudry M (1985) In: De Leenheer AP, Lambert NE and de Ruyter MGM (eds) *Modern Chromatographic Analysis of Vitamins.* New York: Marcel Dekker.
Friedrich W (1988) *Vitamins.* Berlin: Walter de Gruyter.
Sebrell Jr WM and Harris RS (eds) (1968) *The Vitamins Chemistry, Physiology, Pathology, Methods,* Vol. II, New York: Academic Press.

F. Frappier
Muséum National d'Histoire Naturelle, Paris, France

Physiology

Biochemical Function

Biotin is a required, covalently bound prosthetic group for four mammalian carboxylases (Fig. 1); each catalyses an essential step in intermediary metabolism. The four carboxylases are acetyl-CoA carboxylase (ACC), pyruvate carboxylase (PC), propionyl-CoA carboxylase (PCC), and methylcrotonyl-CoA carboxylase (MCC).

The cytosolic enzyme, ACC, catalyses the incorporation of bicarbonate into acetyl-CoA to form malonyl-CoA. This C_3 compound then serves as the rate-limiting substrate for the fatty acid synthetase complex; the net result is the elongation of the fatty acid substrate by two carbons and the loss of the third carbon as carbon dioxide. It has been proposed that deficient activity of ACC is an essential step in the pathogenesis of the cutaneous manifestations of biotin deficiency, which resemble the cutaneous manifestations of essential fatty acid deficiency. *See* Fatty Acids, Metabolism

The mitochondrial enzyme, PC, catalyses the incorporation of bicarbonate into pyruvate to form oxaloacetate, an intermediate in the tricarboxylic acid cycle. Thus PC catalyses an anapleurotic reaction. In gluconeogenic tissues (i.e., liver and kidney), oxaloacetate can be converted to glucose. Deficient activity of PC has been proposed as the cause of the lactic acidaemia, central nervous system (CNS) lactic acidosis, and abnormalities in glucose regulation observed in biotin deficiency and biotinidase deficiency.

Another mitochondrial enzyme, PCC, catalyses the incorporation of bicarbonate into propionyl-CoA to form methylmalonyl-CoA, which, in turn, is isomerized

to succinyl-CoA and enters the tricarboxcylic acid cycle. The third mitochondrial enzyme, MCC, catalyses an essential step in the degradation of the branch-chained amino acid, leucine. Deficient activity of PCC leads to increased urinary excretion of 3-hydroxypropionic acid and 2-methylcitric acid. Deficient activity of MCC shunts the substrate 3-methylcrotonyl-CoA to an alternative metabolic pathway, producing 3-hydroxy-isovaleric acid (3-HIA) and 3-methylcrotonyl glycine, which are then excreted in increased quantities in urine.

Deficiency

The fact that the normal human has a requirement for biotin has been clearly documented in two situations: (1) parenteral nutrition without biotin supplementation in

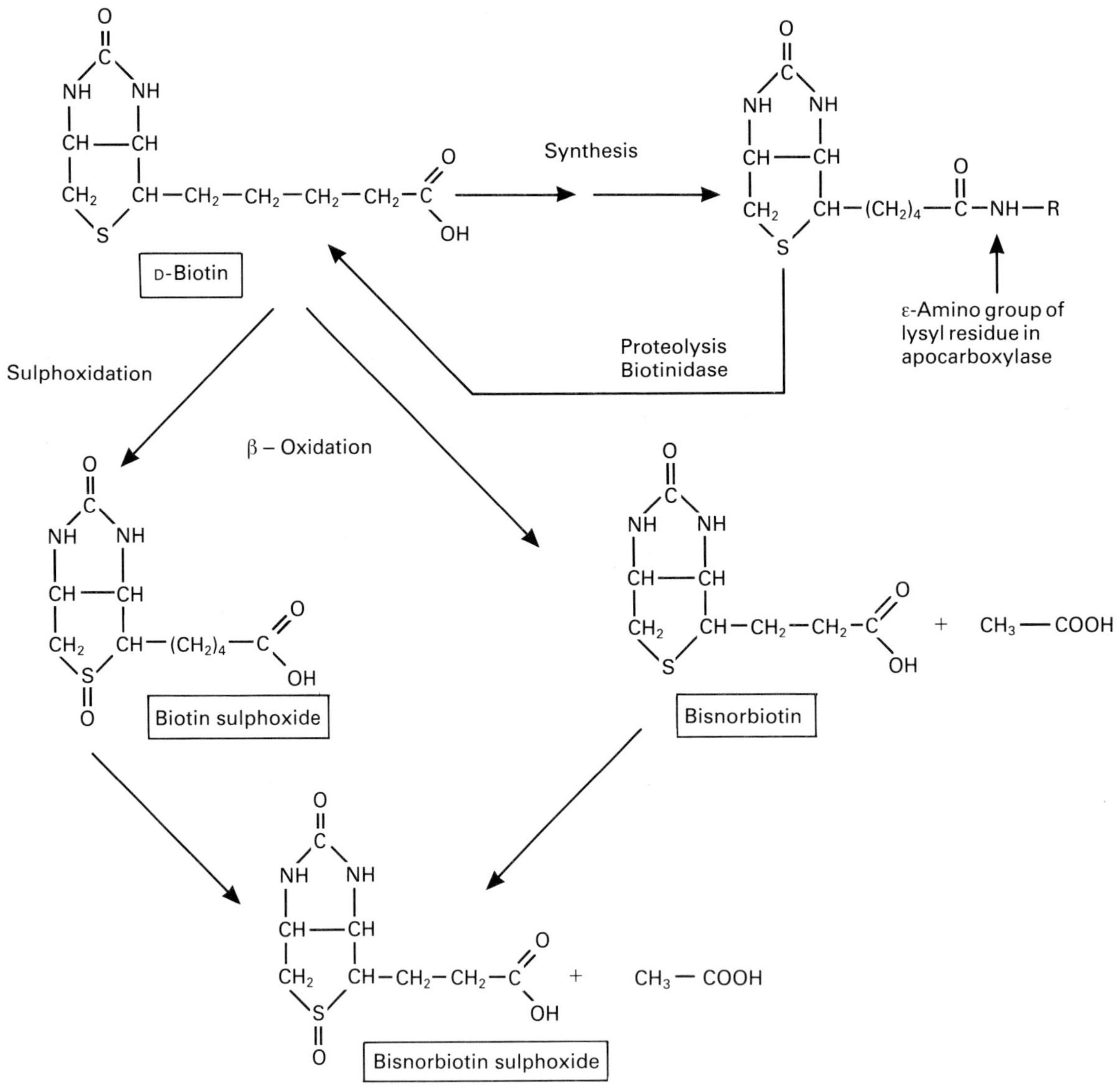

Fig. 1   Metabolism of biotin.

Physiology

patients with short-gut syndrome and other causes of malabsorption; (2) prolonged consumption of raw egg white. The critical event in this 'egg white injury' is a highly specific and very tight binding ($K_b = 10^{15}$ M^{-1}) of biotin by avidin, a glycoprotein found in egg white. Avidin is resistant to intestinal proteolysis in both the free and the biotin-bound form. Thus dietary avidin binds and prevents the absorption of biotin. Cooking denatures avidin, rendering it susceptible to digestion and hence unable to interfere with absorption of biotin. *See* Eggs, Dietary Importance

Biotin deficiency has been clearly demonstrated in biotinidase deficiency. A significant part of the biotin present in some foods and most tissues is covalently bound to protein. Biotinidase is probably required for efficient salvage of biotin at the cellular and renal level as well as efficient release of bound dietary biotin. Many of the clinical findings and biochemical abnormalities associated with biotinidase deficiency are probably the consequence of a secondary biotin deficiency. Common findings include periorificial dermatitis, conjunctivitis, alopecia, ataxia, and developmental delay. However, the reported signs and symptoms of biotin deficiency and biotinidase deficiency are not identical. Seizures, irreversible neurosensory hearing loss, and optic atrophy have been observed in biotinidase deficiency but have not yet been reported in human biotin deficiency. Cerebral atrophy and apparent stretching of the optic nerve were reported in one patient with biotin deficiency. Moreover, two groups have reported that biotin deficiency causes impaired auditory brain-stem function in young biotin-deficient rats.

Accumulating data provide evidence that long-term anticonvulsant therapy in adults and children can lead to biotin depletion severe enough to interfere with amino acid metabolism. This diagnosis of biotin deficiency was originally based on decreased plasma concentrations of biotin as determined by the *Lactobacillus plantarum* bioassay; the incidence of biotin concentrations below the normal range was approximately 75% in a cumulative study group of 274 adults undergoing long-term therapy with a variety of anticonvulsant drugs. The diagnosis of biotin deficiency was strengthened by the demonstration of increased urinary excretion of the characteristic organic acids (e.g. 3-HIA) in adults receiving long-term anticonvulsant therapy. *See* Drug–Nutrient Interactions

The mechanism of biotin depletion during anticonvulsant therapy is not known. The anticonvulsant drugs implicated include phenobarbital, phenytoin, carbamazepine and primidone. These drugs each have a carbamide (-NH-CO-) moiety in their structure, as does biotin; in some cases they incorporate a full ureido group (-NH-CO-NH-). Physiological concentrations of primidone and carbamazepine specifically and directly inhibit biotin uptake by brush border membrane vesi-

cles from human intestine. This finding suggests that impaired intestinal absorption of biotin may contribute to biotin deficiency. In addition, phenobarbital, phenytoin and carbamazepine displace biotin from biotinidase and thus conceivably could have an effect on plasma transport of biotin, renal handling of biotin, or cellular uptake of biotin. Recently increased urinary excretion rates of biotin sulphoxide and bisnorbiotin have been demonstrated in children receiving long-term anticonvulsant therapy, raising the possibility that accelerated catabolism of biotin contributes to the biotin deficiency associated with long-term anticonvulsant therapy.

Biotin deficiency has also been reported or inferred in several other circumstances, including Leiner's disease, sudden infant death syndrome, pregnancy, individuals undergoing dialysis, and individuals suffering from chronic gastrointestinal disease.

Whether caused by egg-white feeding or omission of biotin from parenteral nutrition, the clinical findings of frank biotin deficiency in adults and older children are similar to those reported in a study of adults fed raw egg-white. Typically, the findings began to appear gradually after an interval of 6 months to 3 years of parenteral nutrition and after an interval of 6 weeks to several years of egg-white feeding. Thinning of hair, often with loss of hair colour, was reported in most patients. A skin rash described as scaly (seborrhoeic) and red (eczematous) was present in the majority; in several, the rash was distributed around the eyes, nose and mouth. Depression, lethargy, hallucinations and paraesthesias of the extremities were prominent neurological symptoms in the majority of adults.

In infants who developed biotin deficiency, the signs of deficiency began to appear within 3–6 months after initiation of total parenteral nutrition. The rash initially appeared around the eyes, nose and mouth; ultimately, the ears and perineal orifices were involved. The appearance of the rash was similar to that of cutaneous candidiasis (i.e. an erythematous base and crusting exudates); typically, candida could be cultured from the lesions. The character and distribution of the biotin deficiency rash is quite similar to the rash of zinc deficiency. In some infants, hair loss can progress to total baldness, including eyebrows and lashes. The most striking neurological findings in biotin-deficient infants were hypotonia, lethargy, and developmental delay. Peculiar withdrawn behaviour was noted and may reflect the same CNS dysfunction diagnosed as depression in adult patients.

Bioavailability

As judged by percentage of total biotin that can be extracted into aqueous solutions, the proportion of free and protein-bound biotin in foods is quite variable. The majority of biotin in meats and cereals appears to be protein-bound, whereas approximately 95% of the biotin in human milk is free. The bioavailability of biotin in various dietary sources and the effect of protein binding on bioavailability of biotin have not been studied directly in human subjects. Studies of the bioavailability of biotin in cereals using animal growth tests have revealed that only part of the analytically determined biotin was available to weanling pigs, turkeys and chickens. Assessment of the bioavailability of biotin from various foods is complicated by the fact that the published estimates of biotin content in particular foodstuffs differ considerably. In order to be detected by either bioassays or avidin-binding assays for biotin, protein-bound biotin must be quantitatively released with minimal degradation using either acid or enzymatic hydrolysis. However, recent studies of human milk suggest that substantial degradation of biotin occurs with commonly used acid hydrolysis measures, and completeness of release has been difficult to assess quantitatively until the recent development of [^{3}H]-biotinylating agents. *See* Bioavailability of Nutrients

To date, the only reported covalent bond between biotin and protein is an amide bond between the carboxyl group of biotin and the ε-amino group of a specific lysyl residue of the various apocarboxylases, *trans*-carboxylases, and decarboxylases (Fig. 1). In the normal intracellular turnover of proteins, holocarboxylases are degraded to biotin linked to lysine (biocytin) or biotin linked to an oligopeptide containing at most a few amino acid residues. Because the amide bond between biotin and lysine is not hydrolysed by cellular proteases, biotinidase is required to cleave the amide bond to the lysine. *See* Protein, Synthesis and Turnover

Biotinidase may play a critical role in the release of biotin from covalent binding to dietary protein. The release of biotin might occur in or near the intestine mucosa via the action of mucosal biotinidase, or biotinidase in pancreatic juice might release biotin during the luminal phase of proteolysis. Theoretically, biotinyl oligopeptides might also be absorbed directly, either by a specific biotin transporter or by a nonspecific pathway for peptide absorption. The mechanism remains to be established. Biotinidase is present in pancreatic juice and in intestinal mucosa, but the activity is not enriched in intestinal brush border membranes. In patients with biotinidase deficiency, doses of free biotin – e.g. 150 μg (0·6 μmol) per day – that do not greatly exceed the dietary intake (approximately 70 μg per day) prevent the signs and symptoms of biotinidase deficiency by preventing biotin deficiency. These observations are consistent with the hypothesis that impaired intestinal digestion of protein-bound biotin contributes to biotin deficiency caused by biotinidase deficiency.

Intestinal Absorption

Insight into the mechanism of intestinal absorption of biotin has increased substantially in the last decade. The majority of the evidence suggests that, contrary to earlier conclusions, passive diffusion is neither the only nor the most important process for the intestinal absorption of biotin. Instead, a picture is emerging of a specific, regulated system. Based on studies in the rat there are indications that intestinal uptake of biotin occurs by two distinct systems. The first is a saturable, structurally specific transporter located in the brush border membrane. This carrier is dependent on sodium ions (Na^+), energy, and temperature, and is electroneutral. As judged by the V_{max} of the transport process, the transporter is appropriately up- and down-regulated by biotin deficiency and biotin excess, respectively. In the rat, biotin transport is most active in the upper small bowel; activity of biotin transport declines proceeding from the jejunum to the ileum to the colon. However, activity in the colon is still 3% of jejunal values, leaving open the possibility that biotin synthesized by enteric flora might contribute to absorbed biotin.

The second process is not saturable and appears to be mediated by passive diffusion; this is probably the system observed by early investigators who were unable to work at physiological biotin concentrations owing to the low specific activity of radiolabelled biotin available for early studies. In the rat, activity of the biotin transporter increases with age from suckling to weanling to young adult (aged 3 months) to old adults (aged 24 months). As with the other changes observed in the biotin transporter, the mechanism leading to increased transport appears to be an increase in the number or activity of the carriers, rather than changes in the affinity of the carrier.

A very similar biotin transporter in the human intestine has been identified and characterized. This transporter is saturable, electroneutral, Na^+-dependent and capable of accumulating biotin against a concentration gradient. The anatomical distribution along the gastrointestinal tract is similar to that observed in the rat. Changes in transport activity appear to be mediated primarily by an increase in the number or activity of transporters, rather than by changes in the affinity of the transporter. The exit of biotin from the enterocyte (i.e. transport across the basolateral membrane) is also carrier-mediated but is independent of Na^+, electrogenic, and cannot accumulate biotin against a concentration gradient.

Clinical studies have also provided evidence that biotin is absorbed from the human colon. When biotin is instilled directly into the lumen of the colon, the plasma concentration of biotin increases; however, when the same dose of biotin is given orally, the increase in plasma concentration is greater.

Transport of Biotin from the Intestine to Peripheral Tissues

The mechanism for transport of biotin from the intestine to the liver and peripheral tissues remains controversial. It was originally hypothesized that biotinidase might serve as a biotin-binding protein in plasma or perhaps even as a carrier protein for the transport of biotin into the cell. Using [³H]biotin, ammonium sulphate precipitation, and equilibrium dialysis, it was concluded that biotinidase is the only protein in human serum that specifically binds biotin. They identified two biotin-binding sites on biotinidase. One had an equilibrium dissociation constant (K_d) of 3 nmol l^{-1} and a maximum binding capacity (B_{max}) of 0·065 mol of biotin per mol of biotinidase; the other had a K_d of 59 nmol l^{-1} and a B_{max} of 0·79 mol mol^{-1}. For comparison, the substrate concentration for half maximal velocity (K_m) of the substrate biocytin is 6·2 μmol l^{-1}. Thus the product of the reaction (biotin) binds at least 100-fold more tightly than the substrate (biocytin); this surprising result led these investigators to speculate that the K_m for biocytin may be decreased *in vivo* by a modifier, or that in plasma biotinidase may function primarily as a biotin carrier rather than as a hydrolytic enzyme.

Using published binding parameters, theoretical calculations predict that 88% of the total pool of free and reversibly-bound biotin should be bound to biotinidase at the known plasma concentrations of biotinidase and free biotin. However, studies using tracer [³H]biotin and centrifugal ultrafiltration to examine reversible binding in human plasma, evidence found that less than 10% of the total pool of free plus reversibly-bound biotin is reversibly bound to plasma macromolecules (presumably protein) under physiological conditions during relevant time intervals (minutes to days). This reversible binding of biotin to plasma protein did not saturate at biotin concentrations three orders of magnitude greater than physiological concentrations; hence the system appeared to be low-affinity and high-capacity. A similar biotin-binding system was detected in experiments with physiological concentrations of human serum albumin.

The proportion of the total biotin in human plasma that is bound to protein either reversibly or covalently also remains uncertain. Some studies have detected a sixfold increase in biotin after acid hydrolysis, leading to the suggestion that most of the biotin in human plasma is bound to protein. However, some studies provide evidence that covalently-bound biotin accounts for only 20% of the total of covalently-bound, reversibly-bound and free biotin in plasma. Reversibly-bound biotin accounts for approximately 6% and free biotin for the rest (approximately 75%). These investigators have proposed that the increase in biotin after acid hydrolysis detected by an avidin-binding assay for biotin is an artefact attributable to unknown products produced during acid hydrolysis.

Transport of Biotin in Liver and Peripheral Tissues

The mechanism of biotin uptake by the liver remains uncertain. Based on studies using rat hepatocytes isolated by collagenase perfusion, biotin uptake is transported into the liver by saturable system which is dependent on Na$^+$, temperature and adenosine triphosphate (ATP). It has been proposed that this system is an acid-anion carrier (e.g. ligandin). Studies with mouse fibroblasts suggest that biotin is taken up both by a saturable carrier-mediated process and by diffusion, whereas the uptake of biotin by a human cell line has been reported to occur by fluid-phase pinocytosis.

Biotin is reabsorbed from the glomerular filtrate by a saturable, Na$^+$-dependent, structurally specific transport system which operates against a concentration gradient and is dependent on temperature. Based on animal studies, it has been reported that (1) biotin is transported across the blood–brain barrier by a saturable system which is structurally specific, and (2) that biotin is taken up into the neurons by a specific saturable transport system, after which it is slowly incoporated into brain protein.

Biotin concentration in human milk is approximately 20 pmol ml^{-1} (approximately 20-fold greater than plasma concentrations). Almost all the biotin is free in the aqueous phase; thus biotin must be transported against a concentration gradient into human milk. The mechanism for transport has not been elucidated.

Metabolism and Excretion

Contrary to the tacit assumption of many early biotin balance studies, it now appears that a significant proportion of biotin undergoes metabolism before excretion (Fig. 1). Using paper chromatography to separate biotin analogues and bioassays based on *Neurospora crassa* and *L. plantarum* for detection of biotin, biotin metabolites in human urine have been identified. This semiquantitative study detected significant amounts of the metabolites biocytin sulphoxide and biotin sulphoxide; however, the authors speculated that the biotin sulphoxide might have been produced artificially during the chromatographic procedure. In subsequent studies, rats were injected intraperitoneally with biotin labelled with ^{14}C in the carbonyl moiety. Radioactive metabolites in urine were fractionated using ion exchange chromatography and were identified as biotin l-sulphoxide, biotin D-sulphoxide, bisnorbiotin, and biotin. The absence of production of ^{14}CO$_2$ and

[^{14}C]urea provided evidence that biotin is not immediately degraded to these simple compounds; instead, it appears that, although the side-chain carbons and the sulphur ring undergo oxidation, the bicyclic ring is excreted largely intact. During incubation of [^{14}C]biotin with rat liver homogenates, the same four biotin metabolites were produced, although in different proportions. The bisnorbiotin was thought to result from the mitochondrial β-oxidation of the side-chain and the sulphoxides from oxidation of the thioether sulphur, perhaps by a microsomal monooxygenase. *See* Chromatography, Principles

Using a combination of high-pressure liquid chromatography (HPLC) and an avidin-binding assay to determine biotin and biotin analogues, it has been reported that approximately half of the total avidin-binding substances in urine and ultrafiltrates of human plasma are attributable to biotin analogues rather than to biotin *per se*. On the basis of HPLC retention times and chemical conversion studies, the principal biotin metabolites were identified as biotin, bisnorbiotin, and biotin sulphoxide. *See* Chromatography, High-performance Liquid Chromatography

The relationship of the metabolite profile to biotin nutritional status has not been defined. In the rat, it has been observed that a greater portion of [^{14}C]biotin is excreted as biotin metabolites rather than as the unchanged vitamin when a small amount (e.g. 0·5 vs. 1000 μg biotin per 100 g bodyweight) is injected intraperitoneally.

Requirements, Allowances and Intakes

Data providing an accurate estimate of the biotin requirement for infants, children and adults are lacking; as a result, Recommended Dietary Allowances (RDAs) or Dietary Reference Values (DRVs) have not been formulated. The recommendations that have been made are conflicting. The Food and Nutrition Board of the US National Academy of Sciences has proposed safe and adequate intakes ranging from 35 to 200 μg per day with increasing age (Table 1). In the UK a safe intake of 10–200 μg per day has been set. An important factor in the current uncertainty concerning the biotin requirement is lack of information concerning the nutritional significance of biotin synthesized by enteric bacteria. Some nutritional authorities have recommended against dietary supplementation on the grounds that it might diminish enteric synthesis.

Data providing an accurate estimate of the requirement for biotin administered parenterally are also lacking. In this instance, uncertainty about the dietary requirement for biotin is compounded by lack of information concerning the effect of infusing biotin systemically and continuously. Despite these limi-

Table 1.   US recommended intake of biotin

	Safe and adequate biotin intake (μg)	Daily parenteral supplement (μg kg^{-1})
Preterm infants	NA	8
Infants		
< 6 months	35	20
Up to 1 year	50	20
Children		
1–3 years	65	20
4–6 years	85	20
Older children, 7–10 years	120	20
Older children (> 11 years) and adults	100–200	60

NA, not available.

tations, recommendations for biotin supplementation were formulated in 1975. A study of parenterally supplemented infants reported normal plasma biotin concentrations in term infants supplemented with 20 μg per day and increased plasma concentrations of biotin in preterm infants supplemented at 12 μg per kg per day.

There are substantial discrepancies between recommended and actual intakes. Whether recommended intakes are too high or actual intakes are too low is not clear. Breast-fed infants provide an example. Using the *L. plantarum* bioassay, urinary excretion of biotin from birth to 7 days was measured, and urinary biotin decreased to undetectable amounts by 7 days, despite increasing biotin intake, as a result of increased intake of human milk of increasing biotin concentration. Decreasing plasma concentrations of biotin from 1 week to 3 weeks of age in breast-fed infants was also reported. Other studies have suggested that the biotin intake of infants beyond the neonatal period might also be inadequate. In a study of infants 1–2 months old, it was found that the average biotin intake of exclusively breast-fed infants (measured by *L. plantarum* bioassay) was only 4·4 μg per day, which is about 10% of the recommended safe and adequate intake (Table 1). These investigators also found that the large individual variation in biotin concentrations in human milk from individual donors would result in many infants receiving amounts that were undetectable. One interpretation of the results of these three studies is that the biotin available from human milk (plus intestinal flora, if any) was not adequate to maintain biotin nutritional status. However, overt findings of biotin deficiency have not been clearly documented in any breast-fed infant. If the intake of breast-fed infants is adequate, the recommended intake is too large by a factor greater than is usually allowed in calculating safe and adequate intakes.

Biotin is widely distributed in foodstuffs, but the content of even the richest sources is low when compared to the content of most other water-soluble vitamins. Foods relatively rich in biotin include egg yolk, liver, and some vegetables. The average dietary biotin intake has been estimated to be 70 μg per day for the Swiss population. These data are in reasonable agreement with the estimated dietary intake of biotin in a composite Canadian diet (62 μg per day) and the actual analysis of the diet (60 μg per day). Calculated intake of biotin for the British population was 35 μg per day. Daily doses up to 200 mg orally and up to 10 mg intravenously have been given to treat biotin-responsive inborn errors of metabolism and acquired biotin deficiency; toxicity has not been reported at any dose.

Bibliography

Acuta Murthy PN and Mistry SP (1977) Biotin. *Journal of Progress in Food Nutritional Science* 2: 405–455.

Bonjour JP (1977) Biotin in man's nutrition and therapy – a review. *International Journal of Nutrition Research* 47: 107–118.

Bonjour JP (1991) Biotin. In: Machlin LJ (ed.) *Handbook of Vitamins*, pp 393–427. New York: Marcel Dekker.

Dakshinamurti K and Bhagavan HN (1985) *Biotin*. New York: New York Academy of Science.

Mock DM (1986) Water-soluble vitamin supplementation and the importance of biotin. In: Lebenthal E (ed.) *Textbook on Total Parenteral Nutrition in Children: Indications, Complications, and Pathophysiological Considerations*, pp 89–108. New York: Raven Press.

Mock DM (1989) Biotin. In Brown M (ed.) *Present Knowledge in Nutrition*, pp 189–207. Blacksburg, Virginia: International Life Sciences Institute – Nutrition Foundation.

Sweetman L and Nyhan WL (1986) Inheritable biotin-treatable disorders and associated phenomena. *Annual Review of Nutrition* 6: 317–343.

Donald M. Mock
University of Iowa Hospitals, Iowa City, USA

BISCUITS, COOKIES AND CRACKERS

Contents

Nature of the Products

Biscuits and biscuit-like products have been consumed by humans for hundreds, perhaps thousands, of years. Although in existence for a very long time, the difference between a biscuit, cookie and a cracker is still often less than clear. This is due to a recognized overlap between the boundaries used to define each of the categories. The intent of this summary is to present a definition of the terminology, enumerate the types of product in each category, and describe the features common to the various products.

Definition of a Biscuit

The term 'biscuit' is derived from the Latin '*bis coctus*' or the Old French '*bescoit*', meaning twice cooked. This refers to the practice, generally abandoned in the 18th century, of first baking the product in a hot oven and then transferring to a cooler oven to complete the drying process. The word cookie is derived from the Dutch '*koekje*', meaning little cake. Crackers likely derived their name from the sound made while being eaten.

The name 'biscuit' is regarded differently based upon geographic location. In the USA the term 'biscuit' describes a chemically leavened product which has no true parallel elsewhere but bears some similarity to what in the UK is a scone. In contrast, those products recognized in the UK as 'biscuits' would be termed 'cookies' or 'crackers' in the USA. The products described in this work will be those recognized as biscuits in the UK, and cookies and crackers in the USA.

The characteristic that all biscuits have in common is their general composition. All are based on cereals, the most common cereal being soft wheat flour. However, these products differ from other cereal-based products (breadstuffs) in that they are baked to a moisture content of less than 5%. The low moisture content serves two purposes. It ensures that the products have a relatively long shelf life without risk of microbiological spoilage. Further, it confers a crisp texture deemed to be desirable in most biscuits and crackers. *See* Cereals, Dietary Importance

In addition to flour, the two principal ingredients that all biscuits have in common are shortening and sugar. While water is common to all formulae, it is not considered a principal ingredient because it is utilized to modify the raw product's rheology during processing and is then driven off during baking.

Types of Biscuits

Biscuits can be classified based upon their formulation, their method of manufacture, their dough rheology and/or finished product texture or their name. In the UK, biscuit doughs are characterized as either 'hard doughs' or 'short doughs'. Hard doughs are those possessing a continuous, three-dimensional gluten network formed during mixing and processing. Such doughs are usually elastic with some degree of extensibility. The doughs are sheeted and then cut to form the desired product shape. In the USA these doughs are usually referred to as 'cutting machine doughs', a name which reflects the equipment utilized in processing. Regardless of the name given to the doughs, finished products in this group are referred to as crackers and semisweet biscuits.

All cookies are classified as 'short doughs'. Short doughs are distinct from hard doughs in that the former are neither elastic nor extensible. Wheat flour along with shortening, sugar and a relatively low level of water create a plastic, cohesive dough with minimal gluten network formation when subjected to limited mixing. Short doughs are formed into finished biscuits in a number of ways: rotary molding, wire cutting, extrusion and sheeting/cutting. Cookies formed by the extrusion method are sometimes called soft doughs or deposited biscuits. In the UK these products may be referred to as sweet biscuits. The internal structure of the baked cookie is a mixture of a discontinuous protein phase, starch and the sugar in glass form. The fat is present in large globules or as interconnecting masses between the starch and protein. *See* Extrusion Cooking, Principles and Practice

Description of the Products

Soda Crackers

The term 'soda' or 'saltine' describes a very particular type of cracker. Popular in the USA and in areas with a strong US influence, this type of cracker has been produced in the USA for more than 150 years. The soda

cracker is an unsweetened, long-fermented and laminated dough product. A typical soda cracker is a square biscuit approximately 50×50 mm with a thickness of 4 mm. Individual saltines are not formed and baked. Instead, wide dough sheets are perforated by scrapless cutters prior to baking. After baking, these perforations form lines of weakness which enable the sheet to be broken into individual units. An additional feature of the product is the nine docker holes arranged in three rows of three which serve to tie the layers of dough together at those points. During baking, a good quality soda cracker puffs (springs) uniformly at every space between the docker holes as well as at the edge of the cracker. The top's blisters are uniformly brown while the bottom surface is nearly flat with many small blisters. The internal structure of the product consists of a series of layers between each docking hole generated by lamination during the manufacturing process. The cracker usually weighs 3–3·5 g and has a moisture content of 2·5%. The cracker is usually bland in flavour but with a unique crisp texture. The texture is the result of the laminar structure and low moisture content.

Soda crackers are made from a dough that is lean relative to the other products is this category. A typical formulation has 8–10% shortening in the dough, up to 0·5% yeast, plus salt, and, optionally, malt or malt syrup. The crackers are produced in a sponge and dough process with a lengthy sponge fermentation followed by neutralization with soda before sponge mixing and fermentation. The pH of the product does not drop appreciably during the dough fermentation, resulting in a slightly alkaline product; hence, the name 'soda' cracker.

Cream Crackers

Cream crackers originated in the 1880s from an Irish firm named Jacobs. They are popular in the UK and in most countries having a UK influence except the USA. Although the product name implies that there is cream in the product, there is none. It seems that the name is traditional with no reference to the ingredients utilized to make the product. The cracker is similar to a soda cracker in that it is created from an unsweetened but long-fermented, laminated dough. However, there are a significant number of differences between the two products. The cream cracker is usually relatively large (65×75 mm) and rectangular in shape. Its surface is pale with lightly browned blisters on both the top and bottom surfaces. The puffing and blistering give the product its uneven surfaces and a flaky layered structure that should be even throughout the interior. The finished moisture content is approximately 3–4%, slightly higher than for saltines.

All cream crackers have a simple formula containing

flour, shortening (12–18%), salt (0·9–1·5%), water and yeast (1·0–2·4%). The dough is mixed in a single stage and fermented for a length of time defined by the manufacturer which ranges from 4 to 16 h. As with saltines the product is laminated, but in this case a fine cracker dust is added between layers prior to cutting and baking. The cracker dust filling, which consists only of flour, shortening and salt, is thought to facilitate separation between the layers of rather wet dough (approximately 26% moisture) during the processing. During baking, the laminations lift apart, form the irregular layers and give rise to the characteristic blisters and flaky structure. As is true for the production of saltines, a very hot oven is preferred to provide rapid expansion from steam and to dry the product.

The texture of a cream cracker should be soft so that it melts in the mouth and does not shatter. The texture is a result of both the fat content and the degree of separation of the layers. Because there is no chemical leavening, the product's flavour is bland and slightly nutty.

Snack Crackers

This group of biscuits may also be termed savoury or fat-sprayed crackers. They are made in a wide variety of sizes and shapes, but the essential feature that defines the group is that they are oil sprayed while still hot from the baking process. The products may also be salted or dusted with a flavoured powder after the oil spraying. The flavourings may range from herb or savoury to cheese powders.

The products in this group may be generated by a range of manufacturing methods. As a rule, the doughs are usually not fermented although exceptions exist which employ a one- or even two-stage fermentation. Generally, those products that have been fermented are also laminated; products generated without fermentation may be laminated or simply sheeted and cut.

Depending on the process utilized to create the dough, the products are either yeast or chemically leavened with most being chemically leavened. The texture of the products in this group depends on the manufacturing process utilized and differs from that of either saltines or cream crackers. In general, they have a more dense structure than that of either saltines or cream crackers and a relatively soft bite. Snack crackers have a finished moisture content that should not exceed 2%. The flavour of the product comes primarily from the fat spray and the topping applied. Surface oil sprays improve the mouth feel and enhance the appearance. It is common for a small amount of sugar or syrup to be included in the formulation. The sweetener acts to reduce the dry mouth feel and also as a flavour enhancer. *See* Leavening Agents

Hard Sweet and Semisweet Biscuits

The biscuits comprising this group are colloquially called 'hard dough' biscuits. They originate from the UK. All doughs of these products are characterized by a well-developed gluten network which is the result of a relatively high water content, relatively low amount of fat and sugar, and vigorous mixing. The usual formula is quite simple, containing only flour, sugar, shortening, molasses or corn syrup, chemical leavening and water. The sugar content is usually 18–20% of the flour weight for the semisweet biscuits. In hard or semihard biscuits the shortening is present in about the same proportion as the sugar. Corn syrup or molasses is present at 8–9% while water varies at up to 20% of the flour weight.

These biscuits receive a very short rest period once out of the mixer, and may or may not be laminated. Following the cutting operation, the dough may be washed with milk or an egg/milk mixture to enhance the glossy appearance obtained during baking. The biscuits may also be garnished with sugar or other granular material.

The visual characteristics of this product are a smooth surface with a slight sheen and a pale colour. The products are always docked and usually include a product name and identifying pattern stamped into the top surface of the biscuit. The texture of the products is highly dependent on their formulation, ranging from a hard to a delicate bite. However, all products have an open texture. The higher the flour protein content and the lower the formula sugar level, the harder the resulting texture of the biscuit. As the sugar level increases, the texture becomes more delicate and the flavour is modified.

Most products have a mild vanilla or butter flavour which is derived from the ingredients, not developed by baking. This is particularly evident when butter is used in the formula. Artificial flavours are rarely added to the product.

Rotary Cookies

The origin of rotary or rotary moulded cookies can be traced to monastery kitchens where sweet baked products were hand formed and inscribed with a design on the top surface before baking. The desire for more consistency from piece to piece as well as for an increase in productivity led to the development of the rotary moulder, a metal die roll which has the desired design in reverse relief on the forming roll.

In general, rotary cookies are thin and smooth with no cracks or irregularities in the surface. The formulation must be controlled so that the product does not change shape during baking, causing the design to blur or distort. Thus, a formulation in which there is essentially no spread, no lift or flow of the dough is desired. Doughs that meet these requirements are generally high in shortening and sugar, and low in moisture. Ingredients that would contribute moisture and provide a means for either gluten development or encourage dimensional change such as water, milk, syrups and eggs are limited. The only other ingredients included are flavours, colours and chemical leaveners.

The nature of these products also affects the selection of the ingredients. Flour for rotary moulded cookies is tyically very weak, ranging in protein content from 7·1 to 9·2%. Sugar may be pulverized to aid quick dissolution in the limited amount of water. Shortening may be either in liquid or solid form.

Wire-cut Cookies

The origin of this type of cookie may be traced to the Dutch who first popularized machine-made cookies. The key to the success of this product is to control the rheology of the cookie dough to produce the form desired after the action of a wire cutter on the production line. It is imperative that the dough consistency be such that it is easily extruded, cut by the wire, and dropped cleanly onto the baking belt.

Surprisingly, the dough composition can be varied over a wider range for wire-cut cookies than for any other type. Dough formulae may contain up to 100% shortening and several hundred per cent sugar (both based on flour weight). The resulting doughs can range in consistency from being too stiff to mould by hand to a very thick batter. As a consequence, products having a range of textures can be generated using a single process. Wire-cut cookies are generally described as having a more open texture than rotary moulded cookies but lacking their dimensional uniformity and surface design. However, wire-cut cookies do have a more uniform shape than those created in the deposited, soft dough process (see below).

The critical ingredient for wire-cut cookies is a flour having a protein content less than 9·5%. Stronger flours will require the use of higher amounts of sugar and shortening. Other ingredients common to most formulae are eggs, syrups, milk, salt and chemical leaveners. Some products also contain flavourings, oatmeal, fruits or nuts.

Deposited or Soft Dough Cookies

The doughs utilized in this process must be just soft enough to be just pourable. The cookie pieces are formed by extrusion through a nozzle, which may be shaped to give the product a pattern. The dough must have a consistency such that it breaks away from the nozzle and adheres to the baking band.

Deposited dough is rich, generally high in fat or based on egg whites which have been whipped to a stable foam. Butter is commonly used, as are ground almonds, coconut flour and cocoa. The ingredients are more expensive than those used in other types of cookies and the production rates are usually low. Consequently, products in this group usually fall in the fancy or luxury category. Most products have a soft, delicate texture that melts in the mouth. This same texture makes the product quite fragile so cookies in this category are also subject to breakage.

Ingredient form and type are critical to generate the consistency necessary to provide an unobstructed flow from the nozzle. Thus, coarse particle sizes of any ingredient must be avoided. The sugar particle size must be fine to aid in dissolution in the limited water and to provide the desired eating texture.

Deposit cookies generally have 35–40% flour, 65–75% shortening and 15–25% liquid whole eggs. The flour is from soft wheat having a protein content of 8–8·5%. The flour should be capable of carrying the sugar and shortening without allowing too much spread during baking or distortion of the design generated by the nozzle.

Bibliography

Bohn RM (1957) Biscuit and Cracker Production – *A Manual on the Technology and Practice of Biscuit, Cracker and Cookie Manufacture, Including Formulas*, 1st edn. New York: American Trade Publishing Company.
Hoseney RC, Wade P and Finley J (1988) Soft wheat products. In: Pomeranz Y (ed.) *Wheat Chemistry and Technology*, 3rd edn, vol. II, pp 407–456. St Paul, MN: American Association of Cereal Chemists.
Manley D (1991) *Technology of Biscuits, Crackers and Cookies*, 2nd edn. Chichester: Ellis Horwood.
Matz SA (1984) *Snack Food Technology*. 2nd edn. Westport, CT: AVI.
Smith WH (1972) *Technology, Production and Management. Biscuits, Crackers, and Cookies*, vol. I New York: Magazines for Industry.
Wade P (1988) *The Principles of the Craft. Biscuits, Cookies and Crackers*, vol. I. London: Elsevier.

Linda Doescher Miller
The Pillsbury Company, Minneapolis, USA

Methods of Manufacture

The manufacturing process used to produce all biscuits, cookies, and crackers consists of a mixing step, a shaping or forming step and a baking step. The mixing and baking steps are common to the manufacture of all types of these products. What is distinct for the products are the shaping or forming steps. In this article the processes used to produce these products will be described.

Mixing

Mixing is commonly defined as a process designed to blend separate materials into a uniform, homogeneous mixture. In the context of cookie and cracker doughs the term takes on a broader meaning in that it also applies to the development of gluten from hydrated flour proteins, the aeration of a mass to give a lower density, and the dispersion of solids in liquids. One or more of the functions is required for the formation of cookie and cracker doughs. These processes are accomplished with three principal types of mixers: vertical spindle mixers, horizontal drum mixers, and continuous mixers. *See* Bread, Dough Mixing and Testing Operations

Vertical Spindle Mixers

Vertical mixers were used extensively before the development of the high-speed mixer. Although usage has decreased overall, this type of mixer is still used for crackers and semisweet doughs for which the vertical spindle design is particularly well suited. The feature that all vertical mixers have in common is the portable dough trough which serves as the mixing vessel. The trough is usually a wheel-mounted, heavy tub with vertical sides, round ends and a flat bottom. The trough is designed so that it may be wheeled into position below the mixer head and locked into place. Mounted on an overhead frame are the drive mechanism and spindles with horizontal paddles or arms. Most mixers of this type are equipped with two or three spindles. The spindles are lowered into the trough and move in either a planetary or a stationary, circular motion when activated. The shape of the arms forces the dough upwards and downwards in the trough, generating a mixing action. The mixer blades are designed to provide a cutting action rather than kneading or stretching the dough.

The advantage of vertical spindle mixers is that they can be used for almost any product. They are very well suited for products such as soda cracker doughs. These doughs require a two-stage mixing sequence separated by a fermentation period. The sponges and doughs do not have to be transferred in and out of the trough at each mixing stage. Instead they remain in the same trough for the entire mixing/fermentation sequence. Because there is almost no heat generated during the mixing process, this mixer is ideal for doughs that must remain cool. The mixing action is very gentle. Doughs containing ingredients or particulates that are easily damaged may be safely mixed with this mixer type.

The primary disadvantage of vertical mixers is their slow operating speed. The spindles rotate over a limited range at two or three speeds, up to a maximum of approximately 20 rpm. For doughs requiring the development of a gluten network, the mixing time required may be as long as 90 min. Because this is slow relative to the speed of the remainder of the processing line, several mixers may be needed to maintain an uninterrupted dough supply. Other disadvantages include lack of uniformity of the mix, and the labour-intensive nature of the system's design. The latter disadvantage relates to the fact that the dough troughs are very heavy, requiring special equipment to move, lift and tilt the tubs at each stage of the process.

Horizontal Mixers

The feature that all mixers of this type have in common is a horizontal bowl mounted on a rigid frame that encloses the drive motor. The bowl may be stationary with a vertical front wall that slides down so that the dough may be ejected. More commonly, the mixer bowl is designed to tilt and the dough is ejected from the tilted position. In both designs, the top cover is fixed so that mixing takes place in an enclosed space.

The blades of horizontal mixers are mounted on a horizontal shaft and may have any of several different shapes depending on whether a cutting, scraping or kneading action is needed. Mixing times for cookie and cracker doughs range from 5 min for soft cookie doughs to 30 min for the hard doughs which require gluten development. Most mixers of this type are fitted with a jacket surrounding the mixing chamber. This allows a coolant to be circulated so that dough temperatures can be controlled. Without such control, horizontal mixers can increase the dough temperatures to the point where dough handling and finished product properties are adversely affected.

The advantages of horizontal mixers are their high speed, ability to supply dough to a processing line continuously, uniformity of the mixes they produce, and their potential for complete automation. Horizontal mixers may be operated at speeds of 15–80 rpm. Commonly, their power train is equipped for two-speed rotation. Unlike most vertical spindle mixers, ingredients may be added with the blades in motion and the discharge of the dough from the mixer is simple. Accurate control of dough temperature is possible because there is a continuously circulating refrigerant.

Horizontal mixers require that all ingredient charging spouts be located overhead or that ingredients be added manually. Charging the mixer with ingredients is typically a significant portion of the total mixing cycle time. During mixing the blades may throw material to the top of the chamber so that it is never fully incorporated.

With the shaft and mixing blades located in the centre of the bowl, dough discharge is not always rapid and may occur in several large fragments. Only one operation (charging, mixing or discharging) may be performed at any one time so that fast cycling of the dough batches may not be possible.

Horizontal mixers usually have capacities of up to 550 kg. The weight and the vibrations generated by their relatively high operating speeds place special design demands on the production facility. In addition to a reinforced floor, special mounts are necessary to secure the mixer in place.

Continuous Mixers

Continuous mixers are best described as a rotor or screw operating within a barrel jacketed for temperature control. The ingredients are fed continuously, either from one end of the barrel or in successive ports at intervals along its length. The mixing action may be altered from gentle blending and dispersing to vigorous or high-intensity kneading by varying the arrangement of different mixing arms along the length of the barrel. The amount of work put into the dough during its transit may be controlled additionally by restricting the dimension of the outlet orifice, creating a back pressure inside the barrel.

Continuous mixers are favoured in some plants because they are capable of providing a constant supply of dough to production line, all of uniform age. Continuous mixers are small in size relative to horizontal mixers and are suitable for complete automation. In spite of this advantage, continuous mixers are not common in cookie or cracker plants where a single line may be required to produce a variety of products. They are usually used only on high-output lines having a single purpose or similar product types.

The primary disadvantages of this mixer type are its high cost and the additional cost of the associated automated, continuous ingredient feeding systems. Beyond this, continuous mix systems are not particularly flexible; different products usually require completely different types of machines. In addition, the initial process set-up can be difficult, requiring considerable experimentation to determine optimum mixing conditions and sequences. Finally, starting and stopping the process is difficult in the event of any problem along the rest of the production line.

The Forming Process

While the same mixing and baking process may be used for many types of cookies and crackers, the forming step is specific to each product type. There are three processes used to form cookie and cracker doughs: (1) cutting or stamping from a continuous sheet of dough, (2) rotary moulding by shaping dough in die cavities cut into the surface of a metal cylinder, and (3) extruding dough through a shaped die.

For each of these methods the rheology of the dough is different, and designed to be compatible with the process. In general, doughs that are to be sheeted possess a significant gluten network as a result of mixing, and are both elastic and extensible. Those destined for rotary moulding lack gluten development and are best described as cohesive. Doughs intended for extrusion are soft, frequently high in shortening, and spread while baking.

Sheeting and Cutting

The most common and versatile method to form cookie and cracker doughs is by sheeting and cutting. This method consists of the production of a thick sheet of dough, evenly reducing the thickness of the sheet, cutting out the desired shapes, and returning the scrap dough to be reincorporated either in the mixer or early in the sheeting process. This method is used for the production of cracker, semisweet biscuit, and selected soft doughs.

After mixing, the dough is fed into a hopper, below which lie the sheeting rollers. There typically are three rollers below the hopper arranged in a triangular fashion (Fig. 1). At least one of the top two rollers,

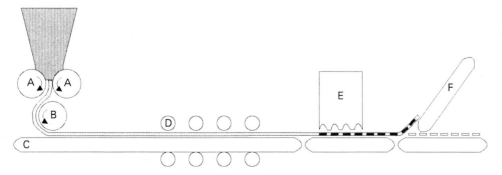

Fig. 1   Sheeting and cutting process. See text for explanation.

Methods of Manufacture

known as forcing rollers (labelled A in the figure), is grooved so that a positive feed is provided to the gauge or gauging roller. The gauging roller (B), which is always smooth, serves to deliver the dough to the conveyor belt (C). The purpose of the sheeting unit is to compact the mass from dough hopper uniformly and provide a sheet of even thickness having the width of the processing line.

The relatively thick dough slab from the sheeter then passes through a series of reduction or gauge rollers (D). These are smooth steel rollers used to reduce the dough sheet to the thickness which is desired before cutting of the finished dough piece. The gauge rollers occur in pairs mounted vertically. For products having sticky or adherent doughs it may be necessary to mount a scraper blade against one or both of the rollers to release the sheet of dough. On most process lines there are two to three pairs of rollers. This ensures that the thickness is reduced no more than 50% at any one rolling operation.

Some doughs, such as those of saltines and cream crackers, are laminated before cutting. The lamination occurs by lapping the dough back upon itself in the process direction. At the lapper, the take-away conveyor lies at a 90° angle relative to the line delivering the dough. The number of layers is controlled by the relative rate of the lapper and take-away conveyor. The lapped dough then passes through several more sets of gauging rollers to bring the dough sheet to the desired thickness prior to cutting.

The repeated working of the dough in one direction results in an accumulation of stress. If the dough was cut at this point the resulting pieces would shrink to relieve the stress and misshapen or distorted products would result. Therefore, it is normal to relax the dough after reduction and before cutting. The relaxation is accomplished by transferring the dough to a conveyor, still moving in the same direction, but at a slower speed.

Once the dough has been relaxed it passes onto the cutting operation. Two different types of cutting methods exist: reciprocating cutters and rotary cutters. The reciprocating cutters are heavy block cutters that stamp out one or more pieces at a time. The cutter head (E) may have a dual action whereby the cutter drops first, followed by a docking head or an embossing plate. The equipment operates via a swinging mechanism so that the dough sheet moves at a constant speed, the cutter drops and moves with the dough, then it rises and swings back to the original position. The second type of cutter, the rotary cutter, consists of a rotating metal cylinder. On the face of the roll are formed the desired shapes with a sharp metal edge. As the cutter rotates with the dough conveyor, the metal edges cut into the dough sheet to form the product. The product pieces are then conveyed into the oven.

As a result of either cutting process, from 20 to 60% of the dough sheet remains as scrap. The scrap dough (F) is lifted way from the cut dough pieces and returned either

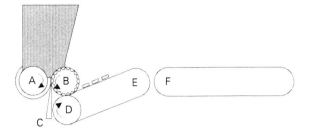

Fig. 2 Rotary moulding process. See text for explanation.

to the mixer or to the sheeter. Return to the mixer permits uniform incorporation of the scrap into the dough mass. However, most systems route the scrap back into the sheeter either along the full length of the hopper or at the back side of the hopper. If dough is incorporated behind the new dough, imperfections will be on the bottom side of the dough sheet and will not be visible on the finished product.

Rotary Moulding

The principle of rotary moulding is illustrated in Fig. 2. Three rollers are placed in a triangular arrangement below a dough hopper. A roller called the forcing or feed roller (A) has deep grooves designed to pull dough down from the hopper. The dough is forced into the cavities of the engraved roller (B) by the forcing roller. A scraper blade (C) is mounted against the engraved roller to remove any excess dough and return it to the hopper via the forcing roller. Beneath the engraved roller is a rubber-covered extraction roller (D) that serves to drive the take-away belt (E). The extraction roller applies pressure to the engraved roller via the belt, causing the dough to adhere preferentially to the conveyor belt. Dough pieces are dropped from the take-away belt into pans or directly onto the baking belt (F).

The rotary moulding process is suitable only for dry, crumbly doughs. This process offers advantages over sheeting and cutting in that there is no scrap to recycle, and there are very low labour requirements to run the process.

Extrusion

There are two types of devices used in the production of extruded cookies: wire-cut machines and bar/rout-presses. Both systems are very similar in design (Fig. 3). A hopper is placed over a system of two or three rollers (A) that force dough into a pressure chamber (B). The rollers may run continuously or intermittently to force dough out of the pressure chamber at the die. For wire-

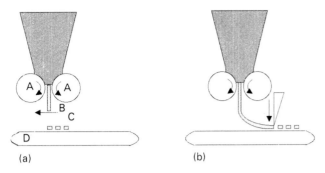

Fig. 3 Extrusion process: (a) wire-cut machine; (b) bar/rout-press. See text for explanation.

cut cookies, the dough is extruded through a row of dies and a wire or blade (C) mounted on a frame moves through the dough just below the die nozzle outlet. The cut dough pieces then drop into a conveyor band (D) for transport to the oven. The wire usually moves only in one direction through the dough, opposite that of the conveyor. The wire-cut machines operate at rates of up to 100 strokes per minute. Difficulties encountered with this type of production are distortion of the extruded dough piece during cutting, and inconsistent placement or drop of the cut piece onto the conveyor. *See* Extrusion Cooking, Principles and Practice

The design of the bar- or rout-press is very similar to the wire-cut machine. The hopper rollers and pressure chamber are essentially identical to their wire-cut counterparts. Unlike the wire-cut machine, the base of the pressure chamber has a die plate that is inclined in the direction of the extrusion. A continuous ribbon of dough is extruded from a nozzle which is shaped to impart the desired finished product design. The dough ribbon can be cut into individual pieces by a vertically operating guillotine before the oven or after baking. If the product can be baked as a continuous ribbon the dough is extruded directly onto the oven band, otherwise it is extruded and cut onto a conveyor belt.

Baking

The cookie and cracker industry relies almost exclusively on band or travelling ovens to bake its products. The band oven is essentially an insulated, heated tunnel equipped with a continuous conveyor. The ovens vary both in length (from 30 to 150 m) and in band width (from 1·0 to 1·5 m). More modern ovens frequently consist of a series of modular units or zones. Each of the zones is equipped with its own set of controls so that the temperature and air flow may be controlled within that zone. The oven band is typically continuous, passing onto a drive drum at the end of the oven and returning underneath the baking chamber to a tension drum at the feed or input end of the oven. The chamber through which the oven belt returns may or may not be enclosed. Frequently, the oven band serves as the baking surface for the product. Depending on the product type the oven band may be solid or any of a variety of open wire-mesh types. Choice of mesh is a critical factor in the process as it affects the heat transfer at the bottom of the product. This, in turn, can have a marked effect on quality of the finished product.

There are three basic types of ovens: direct fired, indirect fired and fully indirect fired. Ovens are usually heated by the combustion of gas, although there are a few manufacturers who use oil or electricity for economic reasons. The most common type is the direct-fired oven in which gas is burned inside the baking chamber itself. In these ovens, the burners are placed across the width of the oven at regular intervals, both above and below the oven band. In other oven types, termed 'indirect ovens', the gas or oil is burned outside the baking chamber and the heated combustion gases are circulated into and throughout the baking chamber. Indirect-fired ovens typically have a single burner for each section. The hot gases from the burner pass along pipes parallel to the length of the oven, both above and below the oven band. The products of combustion are circulated throughout the baking chamber by large fans. Fully indirect ovens are those in which the heat source is independent from the baking chamber and heat transfer occurs via a heat exchanger. None of the products of combustion circulate inside the baking chamber. This type of oven is not common except when oil is used as a combustible material. If circulated, the products of this type combustion would impart an unacceptable flavour to the products.

Cooling

Products hot from the oven must be cooled prior to packaging for several reasons: the products may not be firm enough to withstand the packaging process while warm, the packaging material may shrink around a warm product, or the quality of the products would deteriorate if palletized while warm because the cooling rate across the pallet would be quite slow.

The normal method of cooling products is to place them on an open conveyor and transfer them a distance 1·5–2 times the length of the oven. The products cool naturally in the ambient factory atmosphere. In a few cases, it is necessary to provide forced air to aid the cooling process.

Bibliography

Almond N (1989) *The Biscuit Making Process. Biscuits, Cookies and Crackers*, vol. 2. London: Elsevier.

Manley D (1991) *Technology of Biscuits, Crackers and Cookies*, 2nd edn. Chichester: Ellis Horwood.

Matz SA (1978) *Cookie and Cracker Technology*, 2nd edn. Westport, CI: AVI.

Matz SA (1988) *Equipment for Bakers*. McAllen, TX: Pan-Tech International.

Pyler EJ (1988) Baking Science and Technology, 3rd edn, vol. II. Merriam, KS: Sosland.

Smith WJ (1972) *Technology, Production and Management. Biscuits, Crackers and Cookies*, vol. I. New York: Magazines for Industry.

Wade P (1988) *The Principles of the Craft. Biscuits, Cookies and Crackers*, vol. I. London: Elsevier.

Linda Doescher Miller
The Pillsbury Company, Minneapolis, USA

Chemistry of Biscuit Making

What is a biscuit? Depending on the part of the world in which you live, the answer will vary. In the USA it would be described as a chemically leavened bread-type item similar to a scone in the UK. However, in the UK a biscuit is equivalent to a cookie or cracker in the USA. The term 'biscuit' will be used here to include biscuits, cookies and crackers.

Most biscuits differ from other baked cereal products by having a very low moisture content. Finished breads and cakes typically have moisture contents of 35–40% and 15–30%, respectively, whereas biscuits usually contain only 1–5% moisture. Wheat flour, sugar and fat are basic ingredients, but thereafter the variety is almost endless. Biscuits can be grouped in many ways, based on their texture and hardness, their change in outline during shaping and baking, the extensibility or other characteristics of the dough, or the ways that the doughs are handled prior to biscuit formation. The groups often overlap, so it is important to see how several types of biscuits are related, based on their proportions of fat, sugar and water, and then to compare their typical characteristics and processing means.

The greatest fundamental difference among the biscuit groups is the development or absence of gluten within a dough. These two types are called hard and soft doughs, respectively. Hard doughs possess a gluten matrix. They are stiff, tight doughs that require extensive mixing (work) with a resulting increase in dough temperature. These are similar to bread doughs, exhibiting viscoelastic properties. Hard doughs are usually laminated and sheeted before cutting. The formed pieces will generally shrink because of the extensible quality of the gluten. During baking, the biscuits may continue to shrink in outline, but become thicker. *See* Bread, Chemistry of Baking

Soft doughs do not have a formed gluten structure, because of their high levels of shortening and sugar, and are generally mealy or sandy in texture. They are usually formed by compressing into dies (rotary moulded) or by extruding and cutting, but some types can be sheeted then cut. Dough pieces formed from soft doughs tend to retain their shape until baking, but then they spread or flow, becoming thinner.

Deposit biscuits are the machine-made counterpart of the hand-bagged or 'drop' version. Such formulae have been successfully adapted to automated production. Deposit biscuits contain about 35–40% sugar, 65–75% shortening and 15–25% eggs and possess a spread factor of 79–80 (percentages based on 100 parts flour). Formulations should be such that excessive spread does not occur and the top design of the biscuit is preserved during baking. Adequate adhesive characteristics of the dough are also needed, so that it will adhere to the band and separate from the main tube of dough when deposited (Fig. 1).

Dough Composition

Wheat Flour

Wheat flour is unique among the cereal grain flours in that, when mixed with water, its protein components form an elastic network capable of holding gas and developing a firm spongy structure during baking. The protein substances contributing these properties (gliadin and glutenin), when combined with water and mixed, are known collectively as gluten. The suitability of a flour for biscuit making is generally determined by its gluten. Gluten characteristics are determined by

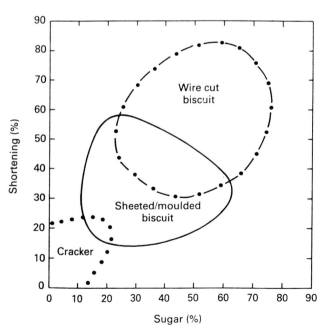

Fig. 1 Biscuit composition in relation to sugar and shortening, based on 100 parts flour. (Each dough is processed according to its consistency or water content.)

genetics, the wheat's growing conditions, and the milling process. *See* Flour, Dietary Importance

Wheats are described by millers as hard, medium or soft, based on the grain's physical characteristics. Hard types tend to have higher protein quantity and quality. They generally have a vitreous endosperm, with starch granules tightly packed in a protein matrix. During milling, some starch grains are damaged, resulting in an increased surface area that leads to higher water absorption. The softer wheats possess a less compact starch/protein complex that allows less starch damage and lower water absorption. The protein levels of soft wheats are usually lower, producing a less resistant, more extensible dough. These 'weaker' flours are traditionally deemed more suitable for biscuit making than the harder flours used for breads. *See* Flour, Roller Milling Operations; Flour, Analysis of Wheat Flours

Flour protein levels needed for biscuit making typically range from 7 to 10%, and are often affected by functionality for end use, price and availability. Flour should contain no more than about 14% moisture. Biscuit flours are typically left unbleached and unchlorinated.

Sweeteners

All biscuit formulae contain sweeteners, which constitute the bulk of dissolved materials in most doughs. Sugars impart sweetness, act as vehicles for other flavours, and create an attractive finish. They increase tenderness, crust colour, volume and moisture retention, while maintaining the proper balance between liquids and solids responsible for product contour. Machining properties and baking characteristic are also closely related to sugar. Sweeteners tenderize the finished product by interfering with gluten hydration and starch gelatinization. *See* Sweeteners – Intense

High-fructose corn (maize) syrups are becoming increasingly important, but sucrose from sugar cane or beet is still the major sweetener. Commercial sugars are categorized as granulated or powdered. Granulated sugars range from coating sugar (extremely fine grain) to coarse. Powdered sugars are made by grinding granulated sugars and screening through fine bolting cloths. Corn starch or other anticaking agents are often added. Generally, as the size of the crystal increases, the size and symmetry of the biscuit decrease, while the thickness and colour increase.

Sucrose may be hydrolysed (inverted) to glucose (dextrose) and fructose (laevulose) by heating it in the presence of a dilute weak acid or mixing it with invertase enzyme. Sucrose is the standard for sweetness, with a rating of 100. Fructose is rated at 170 and glucose at 74. Their combined sweetness in a completely inverted sugar is 127, sweeter than the starting sucrose. Inverted

sugars are used primarily for their hygroscopicity. *See* Carbohydrates, Sensory Properties

Shortenings and Emulsifiers

Fats are the third major component used in biscuit making, but are considerably more expensive than flour or sugar. Besides being used in the doughs, fats are used as surface sprays, in cream fillings and coatings (such as chocolate), and as release agents. In doughs, they tenderize (impart shortness to) the crumb by being dispersed in films and globules during mixing, which interferes with gluten development. Shortening also aids dough aeration. The overall effect improves palatability, extends shelf life, improves flavour and, of course, adds energy. *See* Fats, Uses in the Food Industry

Animal fats, primarily lard, were originally used by bakers. Compound (part animal and part vegetable source) shortenings and all-vegetable shortenings were then developed. Soya bean, cottonseed, palm, coconut and peanut oils are the primary vegetable sources used in shortening production. The new products were more consistent. Continued advancements in purification and hydrogenation developed vegetable oils that could replace animal fats with equal or better flavours, melting points and availability. Because of current health concerns, most bakeries have switched to fats of plant origin. *See* Vegetable Oils, Applications

Surfactants (surface-active agents) are given many names by bakers: crumb softeners, emulsifiers, antistaling agents or dough conditioners. Examples include lecithin, mono- and diglycerides, diacetyl tartaric acid esters of fatty acids, polysorbate 60 and sodium stearoyl 2-lactylate. Surfactants at low concentrations act to modify the surface behaviour of liquids. They are believed to complex with the protein–starch structure, thereby strengthening the film, and to delay dough setting during baking. The behaviour of surfactants is due to their amphoteric (possessing both hydrophilic and hydrophobic molecular regions) properties. Their behaviour varies according to the charges on the molecules, their solubility, the hydrophilic – lipophilic balance, and the type of functional groups involved. *See* Emulsifiers, Uses in Processed Foods

Surfactants modify dough consistency and reduce stickiness. The greasiness of biscuits with high fat content is also reduced by surfactants. They appear to react with gluten and increase its gas-retaining properties. Crumb softeners also complex with the starch molecules to delay retrogradation and texture staling. The grain pattern and volume of the finished product are often improved.

Antioxidants retard the development of certain off-flavours during storage of fat-containing foods. They are usually added to bulk shortenings and are important for preserving low-moisture products, which are expected to remain edible for several months. *See* Antioxidants, Natural Antioxidants; Antioxidants, Synthetic Antioxidants

Is Water an Ingredient?

Water is often thought of as a processing aid or catalyst, rather than as an ingredient. It is incorporated at the dough stage but driven off during baking. Water functions in several ways, including hydrating flour proteins and starch, dissolving sugars, salts and various leavening chemicals, and aiding in ingredient distribution. Water also helps control dough temperature.

A dough's consistency is directly related to its water content, or absorption. Many factors affect dough absorption. About 46% of the flour's total absorption is associated with the starch, 31% with protein and 23% with the pentosans. Acceptable dough consistency can be obtained only after sufficient water is present to hydrate the flour. This is regarded as bound water and controls the dough's consistency. As bound water layers are 'stacked up', some of the water is held less and less strongly, resulting in water that escapes and travels as free water.

Making Biscuits Lighter

Leavening agents aerate the dough or batter to make it light and porous. The leavening action is responsible for good volume, improved eating quality and a uniform cell structure. Leavening can be achieved by various methods, including yeast fermentation, the mechanical incorporation of air by mixing and creaming, formation of water vapour during baking, and the creation of carbon dioxide and/or ammonia by chemical leaveners. *See* Leavening Agents

Small products like biscuits that bake quickly need a fast-acting leavener that will release the gas before the structure sets. The most widely used source of carbon dioxide in chemically leavened systems is the reaction of sodium bicarbonate or baking soda ($NaHCO_3$) and an acid, usually the acidic salt of a weak mineral acid. The leavening acid promotes a controlled and nearly complete evolution of carbon dioxide from sodium bicarbonate in an aqueous solution. Some examples include monocalcium phosphate monohydrate (CaH_4 $(PO_4)_2 \cdot H_2O$), sodium acid pyrophosphate ($Na_2H_2P_2O_7$) and potassium acid tartrate ($KHC_4H_4O_6$). When these agents combine with water, they react to form controlled amounts of carbon dioxide. Sodium bicarbonate also raises dough pH.

Ammonium bicarbonate (NH_4HCO_3) generates carbon dioxide, ammonia and steam when heated. It increases spread and gives a larger, more desirable surface 'crack' in some types of hard, high-sugar biscuits. However, it can be used only with low-moisture biscuits that are baked sufficiently to drive off all residual ammonia.

Other Ingredients

Milk products, eggs and salt are added for variety. Milk and eggs are viewed as wholesome ingredients by consumers, but they are also some of the most expensive.

Milk and whey are usually added in the dried form. They add flavour and nutrients, improve texture, crust colour and keeping qualities, and control spread. *See* Whey and Whey Powders, Production and Uses

Eggs contribute colour, structure, nutritional value and some flavour. They affect texture as a result of their emulsifying, tenderizing, leavening and binding actions. The form of eggs used can be fortified or whole components (yolks and whites) in the liquid, frozen or dried state, or combined with sugar.

Salt performs two principal functions in biscuit doughs. The first is flavour. It accentuates the flavour of other ingredients (e.g. the sweetness of sugar is emphasized), and it removes the flatness or lack of flavour in other foods. Moreover, salt has a slight effect on the consistency of hard doughs, because it has a strengthening effect on gluten. Salt also controls fermentation and aids in suppressing undesirable bacteria.

Minor ingredients include malt, proteases, mould inhibitors, spices and flavourings. Though used in relatively small amounts, these ingredients have quite important effects on the sensory and physical qualities of biscuits.

Malt is prepared from barley by sprouting it, then drying it at elevated temperatures. Malt provides enzymes that break starch into simple sugars and add flavour and colour. *See* Malt, Chemistry of Malting

Proteases are important in crackers (low sugar). They are often added to modify the gluten framework. The effect of a protease is to make the dough less elastic, so that shrinkage does not occur during sheeting and cutting. Proteases may occasionally be used in cookie production. A dough containing gluten that is too strong will decrease biscuit spread, so proteases can improve the spread ratio. *See* Enzymes, Uses in Food Processing

Mould inhibitors are not generally used in low-moisture cookies and crackers, but some types higher in moisture may benefit from their inclusion. Other food products used in biscuits (i.e. fillings, toppings and creams) may require an inhibitor. Some examples include sodium diacetate ($Na_2C_2H_3O_2 \cdot HC_2H_3O_2 \cdot \frac{1}{2}H_2O$), calcium propionate ($Ca(CH_3CH_2COO)_2$) and sodium propionate (CH_3CH_2COONa).

Chemistry of Biscuit Making

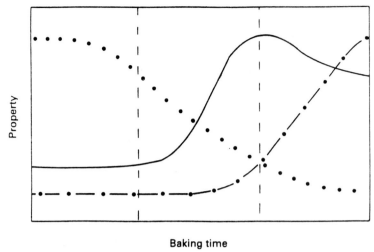

Fig. 2   Physical changes in biscuits during baking. Key: –·–, colour; ——, thickness; ·····, weight.

Added Flavours

Our choice of food is largely influenced by taste and flavour. Smell, taste, touch and sight are all influenced by the chemical and physical properties of the food. Sweet bakery foods are often selected for this reason. Therefore, selecting the correct flavour is extremely critical. Selection of the best flavour is most often achieved through experience and trial and error. *See* Flavour Compounds, Structures and Characteristics

Biscuits may be flavoured in one or more of three ways: adding the flavouring to the dough before baking; dusting or spraying the flavour on after baking; or by flavouring a nonbaked portion such as cream filling, icing or jam that is applied after baking.

Spices are aromatic vegetable products (tree bark, seeds, fruits and roots), and are usually finely ground. They improve quality through smells and tastes. The most commonly used spices are cinnamon, mace, nutmeg, caraway, anise, allspice, poppy seed, coriander, ginger, cloves and fennel.

Flavourings are alcohol extracts from fruits or beans. Vanilla is the most common because it blends with other flavours. Flavourings, such as vanilla or almond, can be either natural or synthetic. Because flavourings are volatile, much of them may be lost during baking.

Added Colours

Colour additives are used in biscuits and in fillings, icings and coatings to create a perception of quality and richness. *See* Colours, Properties and Determination of Natural Pigments; Colours, Properties and Determination of Synthetic Pigments

Chemical Changes during Baking

Biscuits are usually baked in a tunnel oven. They are placed on either a flexible metal or wire mesh band that travels continuously through the oven's length, which may reach 100 m. Baking is controlled by varying the temperatures in the 'zones' within the oven. Baking time is regulated by the band speed. Crackers and some biscuits are docked by pressing blunt pins into the dough sheet. Docking dough pieces before baking creates air passages through the crust and seals the top to the bottom, reducing big blisters.

Dough undergoes several changes during baking (Fig. 2). Changes in dimension and texture, loss of moisture, and colour and flavour development are the most important. Baking is divided into three phases. The first involves dough expansion and the start of moisture loss. Dough expansion and water loss reach maximum rates and colour development starts during the second phase. The third phase concludes baking with a lower rate of moisture loss, thinning of the biscuit, and increasing surface colour.

Dimension and Texture Changes

As dough pieces enter the oven, sugars and fats melt. The matrix becomes an aqueous sucrose solution. Water evaporation causes the solution to become more concentrated, and the dough temperature increases. Leaveners and steam increase the dough volume (expansion). Starch and proteins are heated sufficiently that swelling, pasting and denaturation occur and structures set.

Doughs rich in fat and sugar, but containing little water, often have unhydrated proteins and ungelatinized starch when baked. The rigid structure is replaced by a soft sugary matrix, which does not set properly, resulting in a large expansion in dough followed by a collapse that is responsible for the characteristic cracked surface.

Chemistry of Biscuit Making

Moisture Loss

Dough moistures average 11–30% before baking and 1–5% after. Moisture can be lost only from the biscuit surface. It migrates from the centre to the surface of the biscuit by capillary action and diffusion. The free water is evaporated very readily, but part of the bound water will also be liberated, in association with colour development. Moisture content is critical and directly influences storage life.

Colour Changes

One of the most important colour reactions is the Maillard reaction. It involves the interaction of reducing sugars with amino groups in the proteins, mainly from lysine, and produces an attractive reddish-brown hue. It is also associated with the dextrinization of starch and the caramelization of sugars. These reactions require very high temperatures, which are reached only at the biscuit surface. *See* Browning, Nonenzymatic

Storage and Staling

Most freshly baked biscuits are cooled before packaging or secondary processing, though snack crackers are sprayed with oil first. The cooling period is usually 1·5–2 times longer than the baking period. During cooling and storage, the biscuit continues to undergo texture changes. Hard dough biscuits are rigid and crisp immediately after baking. Soft dough products are still flexible at the end of baking, but become firm and crisp after cooling.

Changes in Moisture Distribution

The residual moisture is not uniformly distributed as a biscuit leaves the oven. Most of the moisture lies in a lamella near the centre, leaving the surface and the outer periphery almost dry.

'Checking' is a change associated with uneven moisture distribution. Dimensional changes within the biscuit after baking cause it to crack. The centre shrinks as it loses moisture, but the rim expands as it absorbs moisture. Checking can happen in almost any type of biscuit or cracker, but is most commonly found in semisweet products.

Bibliography

Blanshard JMV, Frazier PJ and Gailliard T (1986) *Chemistry and Physics of Baking. Special Publication*, No. 56. London: The Royal Society of Chemistry.

Bohn RM (1957) *Biscuit and Cracker Production*. Rahway: American Trade Publishing.

Fennema OR (1976) *Principles of Food Science*. New York: Marcel Dekker.

Manley DJR (1983) *Technology of Biscuits, Crackers and Cookies*. Chichester: Ellis Horwood.

Matz SA (1978) *Cookie and Cracker Technology*, 2nd edn. Westport: AVI.

Matz SA (1991) *The Chemistry and Technology of Cereals as Food and Feed*, 2nd edn. New York: Van Nostrand Reinhold/AVI.

Pomeranz Y (1978) *Wheat Chemistry and Technology*, 2nd edn. St Paul: American Association of Cereal Chemists.

Pyler EJ (1988) *Baking Science and Technology*, 3rd edn. Merriam: Sosland.

Smith WH (1972) *Biscuits, Crackers, and Cookies: Technology, Production, and Management*. Barking: Applied Science.

Stauffer CE (1990) *Functional Additives for Bakery Foods*. New York: Van Nostrand Reinhold/AVI.

Sultan WJ (1986) *Practical Baking*, 4th edn. Westport: AVI.

Wade P (1988) *Biscuits, Cookies, and Crackers*. New York: Elsevier.

J. L. Hazelton and C. E. Walker
Kansas State University, Manhattan, USA

Wafers*

Wafers are baked as sheets, cones and sticks or with different fancy shapes.

Characteristic features in respect to other bakery products are as follows:

1.   They are very thin biscuits; the overall thickness is usually between <1 and 4 mm. They often carry the typical 'wafer pattern' on one surface or on both.
2.   The texture is delicate and crisp. The product density is approximately $0·25 \text{ g cm}^{-3}$. In cross-section the matrix is highly aerated and primarily of gelatinized starch.
3.   The surfaces are smooth and precisely formed, with the dimensions and all the details – engravings, logos, etc. – of the baking moulds.

Basic Wafer Types

There are two basic types:

1.   No- or low-sugar wafers. The finished biscuits contain from zero to a low percentage of sucrose or other sugars. Typical products are flat and hollow wafer sheets, moulded cones, and fancy shapes.
2.   High-sugar wafers. More than 10% of sucrose or other sugars are responsible for the plasticity of the

---

* The colour plate section for this article appears between p. 556 and p. 557.

freshly baked sheets. They can be formed into different shapes before sugar recrystallization occurs. Typical products are moulded and rolled sugar cones, rolled wafer sticks, and deep-formed fancy shapes.

In both wafer types, the main ingredient is usually wheat flour. Wafers fit very well into current dietary recommendations to consume more cereals, as they are high-carbohydrate, low-fat products. *See* Cereals, Dietary Importance

The baking of 'wafers' between hot metal plates has been known since medieval times, but these first wafers were more like our waffles or pancakes in their high fat and egg contents and their texture.

Modern wafers are low-fat cereal products, very similar to the altar breads for Christian churches, and are basically made out of flour and water.

The first wafer ovens were built after World War I, but automatic manufacturing lines have been available since the middle of the 1950s.

Wafer Recipes

Before creating a wafer recipe, two main questions have to be answered:

1. What is the end use of the wafer? If it is part of a cream-filled, chocolate-covered biscuit, where the typical bite is far more important than the taste of the wafer itself, recipes with few components are recommended. If the wafers are to be consumed directly as wafer bread or wafer sticks, more sophisticated recipes are chosen.
2. What kind and quality of raw materials are available? Low-protein wheat flours with low water uptake work best, especially for no-sugar wafers. Problems with suboptimal flours must be balanced by variations in minor ingredients in the recipe. The use of wholemeal flour is possible, and in some regions other cereals, such as rice or corn, are used for wafer production.

Table 1 lists the common ingredients for both types of wafer.

Wafer Production

Wafers are often part of different products in the market, both with savoury or, mostly, with sweet tastes.

Typical production schemes for two of the currently most important products are shown in Table 2.

In-line Manufacturing of Wafer Biscuits

Ingredient Mixing (Fig. 1, process 1)

After mixing for a few minutes, the water-soluble components are dissolved and the farinaceous ingre-

Table 1. Wafer batter ingredient ranges (weight parts; flour=100)

	No (low)-sugar	High-sugar
Wheat flour	100	100
Water	130–160	100–140
Sucrose	0–4	25–70
Milk powder	0–2	0–2
Oil or fat	0·5–2	2–6
Soya lecithin	0·2–1	0·2–1·5
Sodium bicarbonate	0·1–0·5	0–0·3
Salt	0–0·6	0–0·6

Optional minor ingredients: other cereal flours, soya flour, starches, other sugars, eggs; ammonium bicarbonate, yeast, caramel, cocoa powder, spices, flavours, colours.

Table 2. Scheme of wafer production lines

Step	No-sugar wafer (e.g. sandwiched wafer biscuits) (See Fig. 1)	High-sugar wafer (e.g. rolled sugar cone)
1	Ingredient mixing	Ingredient mixing
2	Batter transport and depositing	Batter transport and depositing
3	Oven baking of a sheet	Oven baking of a sheet
4	Release and cooling	Release and forming
5	Conditioning[a]	Cooling
6	Creaming and book building	Stacking
7	Cooling and cutting	Packaging
8	Enrobing or moulding[a]	
9	Cooling[a]	
10	Packaging	

[a] Optional.

dients made up into a homogeneous suspension ('wafer batter'). *See* Bread, Dough Mixing and Testing Operations

Batter Transport and Depositing (Fig. 1, process 2)

From a storage tank, the batter is pumped to a depositor head and spread onto the baking mould.

Oven Baking (Fig. 1, process 3)

The baking of wafer sheets is performed in 'tongs', i.e. pairs of cast-iron metal plates with a hinge and latch on opposite (shorter) sides. The precisely machined baking plates carry reedings or other engravings ('flat' wafer

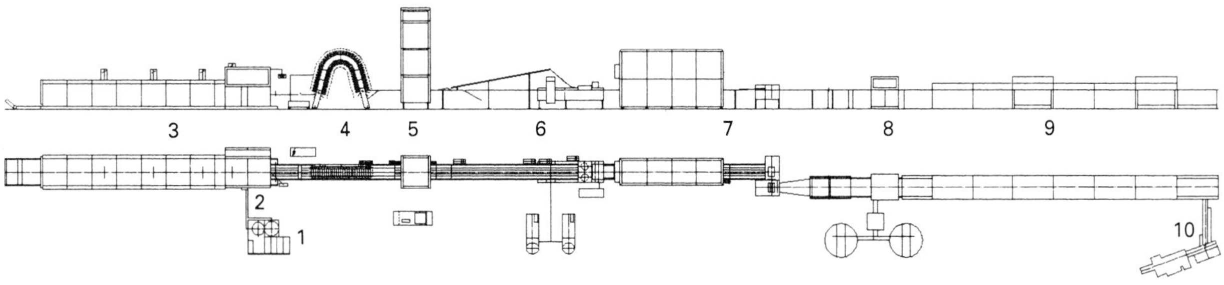

Fig. 1   Manufacturing line for creamed and enrobed wafer biscuits. Numbers refer to different processes: see text for explanation.

sheets). The plates can also carry special figures (nuts, sticks, hemispheres, fancy shapes) up to a depth of approximately 20 mm. This kind of sheets are called 'hollow wafers'. The plates can be surface-plated, e.g. with chromium. The plates are edged with metal strips to give a closed baking mould, except for small venting channels for steam release. Baking plate sizes up to 350×700 mm are available. Wafer baking ovens have 32 to 120 of these pairs of plates, continuously circulating on a chain. They can be gas or electrically heated and operate at temperatures between 160°C and 180°C.

The Baking Process

A few seconds after deposition of the batter, the baking moulds close and are locked. At first, the batter is distributed mechanically, but then it is spread completely by the steam which evolves. Small 'bobbles' of batter are extruded through the venting strips as the pressure rises. Aeration of the batter and gelatinization of starch start immediately. *See* Extrusion Cooking, Principles and Practice

When most of the water has been driven off by evaporation through the venting holes, the glass temperature of the wafer matrix rises and the stable structure is formed. The temperature of the wafer is coming up to 160–180°C, which is the temperature of the baking mould. Now, by Maillard reactions, the typical colour and flavour are developed. *See* Browning, Nonenzymatic

Overall baking times vary from 1.25 to 2.5 min, depending on wafer thickness and baking temperature.

During the manufacturing process, there is no substantial degradation of starch molecules compared to other bakery products such as extruded cereals. Therefore wafers have two unique textural properties:

1. Extreme crispness on biting and initial chewing.
2. Good mouth-feel during prolonged chewing and swallowing, owing to the absence of sticky, glutinous stimuli.

Release and Cooling (Fig. 1, process 4)

At one end of the oven, the plates open to release the baked sheets and spread fresh batter, and then reclose very quickly. The sheets are cooled to room temperature while passing through an arch-type sheet cooler.

Conditioning (Fig. 1, process 5)

After baking, the water content is below 1%; for this reason wafers absorb humidity very easily. Parallel to water uptake, the dimensions of the sheet increase by approximately 0.2% for every 1% of additional water. To compensate for the low water activity, humidity conditioning up to 3% or 4% water content is possible. It is recommended, especially if enrobed or chocolate-moulded wafer products are made, that this first dimension increase is anticipated, so that cracking of the coating during shelf life can be avoided.

Up to a water content of 5–6%, wafer sheets have the typical crisp texture, but higher water levels result in an inadequate, tough, or even soft and soggy texture.

Creaming and Book Building (Fig. 1, process 6)

The sheets then pass the creaming station, where a cream layer is applied to one side. Sugar and fat creams with different flavours (hazelnut, chocolate, caramel, milk, fruit) at temperatures of 30–40°C are used. Several creamed sheets, together with a non-creamed top sheet, form a so-called 'wafer book'.

Cooling and Cutting (Fig. 1, process 7)

The cooled wafer books are wire- or saw-cut into small biscuits.

Enrobing or Moulding, and Cooling (Fig. 1, processes 8 and 9)

The cut biscuits may be enrobed with chocolate, sometimes after the application of chopped nuts or crispies to the top wafer. Moulding in chocolate is another possibility. After a final cooling step, the biscuits are ready for packaging.

Packaging (Fig. 1, process 10)

The biscuits have to be packed tightly to protect against humidity, and also against oxygen and light, to ensure a shelf life of 6–9 months.

Manufacturing of Moulded Wafer Cones

The recipes for no- or low-sugar cones, sometimes known as 'cake cones', are similar to those for sheets (see Table 1). The so-called 'moulded sugar cones' have an intermediate sugar content, usually below 20 parts of sucrose to 100 parts of flour.

Cones, cups and fancy shapes can be produced by a technique using special cast-iron moulds. Holes for 4 to 6 cones are provided in each of these moulds, and 12 to 72 moulds are circulating in one oven.

The lower part of the mould is made of two symmetrical halves, which open for release of the baked cones. After their reclosure, they take up a fresh batter deposit and the core, the upper part of the mould, closes the mould for a new baking cycle.

Manufacturing of Rolled Wafer Cones
(see Table 2)

'Sugar cones' need a concentration of more than 25% sucrose or other sugars in the product. The cone shape is achieved by rolling the baked sheet while it is still hot.

Steps 1–3

According to the scheme in Table 2, steps 1–3 are very similar to the process for non-sugar wafers, with the exception that oval or round sheets are baked, and the baking plates are not closed by venting strips. Machines with up to 140 baking plates are available.

Step 4: Release and Forming

After the baking step, the sheet is automatically stripped off the plate and rolled immediately on tapered mandrels to form the finished cone. The molten sugar acts as a plasticizer. A series of rolling devices mounted on a round table is operating continuously: sheet removal, rolling, release, etc.

Steps 5–7: Cooling, Stacking, Packaging

The fresh cones pass through a cooling device where sugar recrystallization finishes to give the final strong and brittle texture. After that, the cones are stacked together automatically and packaged.

Alternatively, a combination with a paper cone is made, as this packaging material is typical for certain end products such as ice cream cones. In the ice cream plant, the wafer cones are sprayed inside with chocolate, filled and, finally, the paper cone is closed.

Manufacturing of Rolled Wafer Sticks

Another type of high-sugar wafer is the wafer stick, which is consumed directly or as a cream-filled, sometimes additionally enrobed biscuit.

In this rather new technique, a continuous wafer band is produced and rolled immediately, while hot to form an endless tube. The diameter and length of the sticks, as well as the number of the very thin wafer sheets forming the wall of the stick, can be adjusted individually.

Rolled wafer sticks are very tender and delicate products with a unique texture. Inside chocolate coating of the tubes or cream filling can be performed simultaneously with the tube-forming process.

Bibliography

Barron LF (1977) The expansion of wafer and its relation to the cracking of chocolate and 'baker's chocolate' coatings. *Journal of Food Technology* 12: 73–84.

Manley DJR (1983) *Technology of Biscuits, Crackers and Cookies.* pp 219–234. Chichester: Horwood (Ellis).

Negri G (1984) *Waffeln und Verfahren zu deren Herstellung.* European Patent 0 022.901.

Pritchard PE and Stevens DJ (1974) The influence of ingredients on the properties of wafer sheets. *Food Trade Review* 42(8): 9–15.

Seibel W, Menger A, Ludewig HG, Seiler K and Bretschneider F (1978) Standardisierung eines Backversuches für Flachwaffeln. *Getreide, Mehl und Brot* 32: 188–193.

Stevens DJ (1976) The role of starch in baked goods. Part 1. The structure of wafer biscuit sheets and its relation to composition. *Starch* 28: 25–29.

Wade P (1988) *Biscuits, Cookies and Crackers*, Vol. 1, pp 139–150. Essex: Elsevier Science Publishers.

K.F. Tiefenbacher
Franz Haas Waffelmaschinen, Vienna, Austria

Dietary Importance

Biscuits may be regarded as one of the earliest snack foods; their palatability and appeal makes them a ready-to-eat snack at any time of day – in the UK alone consumers spent over $£1 \times 10^{12}$ (1990) on them! Biscuits can also play a useful role as emergency foods and supplementary foods in famine or relief feeding. Although biscuits may be the oldest snack food, their place in the future seems well assured.

Whilst the terms 'biscuits', 'cookies' and 'crackers' are often used interchangeably, the word 'biscuit' is derived from the old French word *bescoit* meaning twice-baked. This refers to the former practice of first baking the dough in a hot oven, followed by baking in a cooler oven, thereby making the final product crisp and dry. Although the two-stage process is rarely used today, even as recently as the 1940s this method was used to make 'ship's biscuits'. The term 'cookie' appears to have originated from the Dutch word, *Koekje*, meaning 'small cake'. Products that we call biscuits in the UK are often cookies and crackers in USA. Despite their varied nomenclature these baked products share some common features. First, they are usually made of wheat flour. Second, they have a very low moisture content (2–5%). This low moisture content makes them microbiologically safe for protracted periods of time. If carefully wrapped and packaged, biscuits will not deteriorate and are usually free from microbial spoilage. Their low moisture content (Table 1) also affords another advantage – they are a concentrated source of energy.

The above features were well appreciated by voyagers and seafarers who routinely took biscuits as a part of their rations. Their taste and appeal made them a useful source of high-energy foods in times of emergency. In fact, it may be argued that many a voyage may not have been successfully accomplished without the use of biscuits as a source of energy. The importance of biscuits as a food item is well illustrated by examining the Navy rations in 1745 (Table 2). It is clear that biscuits were a key element in Naval rations.

Biscuit Formulation

The original ship's biscuit simply consisted of wheat bread that was sliced after baking and dried to a very low moisture content. Subsequently the ship's biscuit was made by mixing wheat flour with salt and water and baked to a 'state of immortal hardness' (Tannahill, 1988). Today, the term 'biscuit' covers a multitude of products, varying in composition, texture and shape. Some are sweet whilst others are salted or savoury. The ingredients used and the formulation will naturally influence the nutritional quality and composition of the biscuit.

Gross Composition of Biscuits

Whilst it is impossible to provide details of the chemical composition of all the available biscuits, some generalizations may be made. The chemical compositions of some biscuit classes are shown in Table 3.

Ingredients Used for Biscuit Manufacture

The final composition of the biscuit will depend on the ingredients used in biscuit manufacture. The ingredients used may be broadly classified as follows:

1. Flour
2. Fat
3. Sugar
4. Egg
5. Milk products
6. Leavening agents
7. Fruits and nuts
8. Colouring and flavouring.

Water should be included since, although not an ingredient, it is important in biscuit formation. This list is by no means complete or exhaustive, but it illustrates the range of raw materials used in biscuit manufacture.

Flour

Flour is a major component in most biscuit recipes. Although it is common to use wheat flour in biscuit manufacture, other flours have been used. These include

Table 1. Moisture content of biscuits compared to other bakery products

Food item	Moisture content (%)
Bread	30–40
Rolls	25–30
Cakes	15–30
Croissants	30
Biscuits, cookies	2–5
Wafers	1–2

Source: author's laboratory, Oxford Polytechnic, Oxford, UK.

Table 2. Navy rations in 1745

Food	Quantities per person per week
Cheese	12 oz (340 g)
Salt beef	4 lb (1·8 kg)
Salt pork	2 lb (0·9 kg)
Biscuits	7 lb (3·2 kg)
Oatmeal	2·5 lb (1·1 kg)
Butter	8 oz (227 g)
Beer	7 gal (32 l)

Adapted from Drummond JC and Wilbraham A (1957) *The Englishman's Food*. London: Jonathan Cape.

Dietary Importance

Table 3. Gross composition of various biscuit types (per 100 g)

Biscuit type	Moisture	Protein	Fat	Carbohydrate	Energy (kJ)	(kcal)
Crackers (e.g. cream crackers)	4·3	9·5	16·3	68·3	1857	440
Semisweet (e.g. tea biscuit 'Marie')	2·5	6·7	16·6	74·8	1925	457
Short sweet (e.g. digestive or shortbread)	2·6	6·2	23·4	62·2	1966	469
Wafers	2·3	4·7	21·0	72·0	2123	507
Crispbread (e.g. rye crisp)	6·4	9·4	2·1	70·6	1367	321

Adapted from Holland B, Unwin ID and Buss DH (1988) *Cereal and Cereal Products*. Cambridge: Royal Society of Chemistry.

triticale (grain developed by crossing wheat with rye) rye flour, corn, sorghum, cottonseed meal and soya meal.

When water is added to wheat flour the starch and protein absorb water to form a coherent mass called gluten. Gluten has a unique viscoelastic property which makes it ideally suited for the manufacture of biscuits. *See* Flour, Dietary Importance

Fat

A wide variety of fats and oils are used in biscuit manufacture. The commonly used oils (liquid at room temperature) are as follows:

- Soya bean
- Palm
- Palm kernel
- Sunflower
- Groundnut
- Rapeseed
- Cottonseed
- Coconut.

The commonly used fats (solid or semisolid at room temperature) are as follows:

- Butter
- Lard
- Tallow.

In addition to providing energy, fats are important in the manufacture of biscuits. They impart 'shortness' – the property that makes the biscuit 'crumbly', soft and appealing. *See* Fats, Requirements

Sugar

A selection of sugar products may be used in biscuits. These include white sugar, sugar syrup, molasses and brown sugar. Sugars are responsible for the following characteristics of the biscuit: sweetness, hardness, colour, and powers of preservation. *See* Sucrose, Dietary Importance

Eggs

Whilst eggs add to the nutritional quality of biscuits, their major contribution is to act as binding, leavening and emulsifying agents. *See* Eggs, Dietary Importance

Milk Products (Milk Powder)

Milk powder (which contains protein) combines with the gluten in wheat to produce a soft and moist product after baking. Milk protein also combines with reducing sugars to give colour and a 'browning' effect to biscuits and baked products. *See* Browning, Nonenzymatic

From a nutritional perspective, the factor most likely to influence the final nutritional quality of the biscuit is the type of flour, fat, sugar, eggs and milk powder used. *See* Milk, Dietary Importance

Influence of Baking on Nutritive Value

Whilst any nutritional change that occurs during baking must be kept in proper perspective, it is true that certain nutrients are lost or reduced during baking. Biscuits are baked to a much lower moisture content (Table 1) than other bakery products. This implies a much higher core temperature and the use of higher oven temperatures (250–300°C).

Changes in Protein Quality

Net protein utilization (NPU) is a measure of protein quality and is widely used to estimate the efficiency of protein utilization. Considerable changes in protein quality have been recorded during biscuit manufacture. Protein damage usually occurs when proteins are heated in the presence of reducing substances (found in sugars). The free amino groups of protein (usually the ε-amino group of lysine) reacts with carbonyl-containing compounds, resulting in a linkage that cannot be easily hydrolysed. This leads to a reduction in protein quality. For example, biscuits baked at 180°C for 13 min showed a fall in NPU of 70%. Paradoxically, supplementation of biscuits with milk protein (in order to make high-protein biscuits), especially with skimmed milk powder (which contains substantial amounts of lactose), resulted in considerable losses of lysine. This was largely attributable to lysine linking with lactose found in skimmed milk powder. In contrast, when casein was used as the protein source, there was much less protein damage resulting from lysine losses. The choice of protein source and duration of baking therefore have a strong influence on protein damage. In addition to protein source, the other factor that influences protein damage is the amount and type of sugars used. All reducing sugars have deleterious effects on lysine. Moreover, it has been shown that if the amount of sugar exceeds about 18% lysine losses become more significant.

Since biscuits today are rarely consumed as a source of protein in the adult diet, the nutritional changes discussed above are of little consequence. However, biscuits are an ideal vehicle for nutrient supplementation for children. In young children, biscuits can form a significant part of their diet. In this group, therefore, the nutrient losses discussed above must be considered in any dietary planning. *See* Protein, Quality; Protein, Requirements

Biscuits in Child Nutrition

The weaning period is a time when breast milk or formula milk is replaced with adult foods. The common weaning foods in many developing countries consist of soft gruels made from cereals or starchy tubers. These carbohydrate-rich gruels are high in water, and low in fat and other nutrients. Their energy density (kJ per g of food) is usually very low. The energy content of such food is so diluted (owing to the presence of water) that the child is unable (with his or her small stomach) to consume sufficient food to meet the need for growth and development. The result is undernutrition. As we have seen earlier, biscuits are an extremely rich package of energy. They are also ideally suited as a food for weaning children. They are palatable, pleasant to eat, and widely accepted by most cultures. Figure 1 shows the relationship between the energy density of food and the quantity of food that must be consumed in order to meet the energy requirement of a 1-year-old child (4·2 MJ, or 1000 kcal per day). If the child consumes cooked rice or tubers he or she needs to eat almost 1000–1500 g (1–1·5 kg) of food per day to meet the energy needs – an impossible task. Conversely, if the child is to eat biscuits, a meal containing 200–250 g of biscuits must be consumed daily to meet energy needs. This

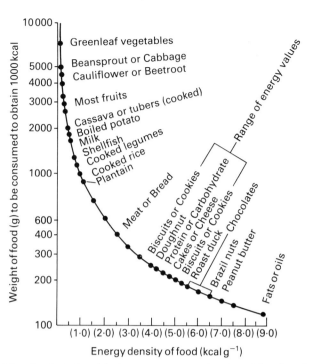

Fig. 1 Relationship between energy density of food and quantity of food that must be consumed in order to obtain 1000 kcal (4·2 MJ).

simple illustration shows, graphically, the importance of biscuits or biscuit-type products in infant nutrition. Biscuits are also a suitable vehicle for fortification with various vitamins and minerals. *See* Infants, Weaning

Role of Biscuits in Supplementary Feeding and Emergency Feeding

In general, the term 'supplementary feeding' is reserved for the process when extra food is given to vulnerable groups in adddition to their regular rations (which may be cereals) in a refugee camp, after an emergency or famine. *See* Food Aid for Emergencies; Refugees – Nutritional Management

Biscuits are an ideal source of food in these situations as they have the following attributes: (1) they require no further cooking before consumption (this may be a real problem in an emergency owing to scarcity of food, utensils, etc.); (2) they are highly palatable and acceptable in most instances; (3) they have a long storage life; (4) they provide a good source of energy; (5) they can be modified to suit specific nutritional needs of any target population; (6) they are produced in convenient bite-sized form. Biscuits have therefore become a popular food source in any emergency feeding programmes. In fact, between 1985 and 1986 over 6000 t of biscuits were distributed in Sudan and Ethiopia. The biscuits used for emergency feeding have a much higher protein and energy content than conventional biscuits (Table 3).

Dietary Importance

Table 4.   Nutritional composition of selected biscuits used in emergency feeding

	Protein (g)	Fat (g)	Carbohydrate (g)	Energy (kJ)	(kcal)
Australian Milk biscuit	20·0	20·0	50·0	1884	450
Biokost Prointact	20·0	16·0	53·0	1825	436
Calorie Mate	10·4	28·1	52·8	2114	505
Frukost Kex	10·0	14·0	70·0	1867	446
HGM HP biscuits	20·0	16·0	53·0	1825	436
Mellin biscotti	10·5	59·5	74·0	1771	423
Novofood	20·0	22·0	43·0	1884	450
Provita	15	18·0	55·0	1850	442

Source: manufacturers' information.

Table 5.   The vitamin and mineral content of biscuits used in emergency feeding (manufacturers' data per 100 g)

	Vitamins							Minerals			
	A (iu)[a]	D (iu)[b]	C (mg)	B_1 (mg)	B_2 (mg)	Nicotinic acid (mg)	B_6 (mg)	Folate (mg)	Iron (mg)	Calcium (mg)	Phosphorus (mg)
Australian HP	1000	—	62·5	2·7	4·0	27·5	—	—	25·0	1125	—
Calorie Mate	1139	95	31·0	0·5	0·7	—	1·30	—	—	—	—
Novofood	3300	300	62·2	10·0	—	—	5·1	0·1	22·2	581	387
Provita Plus	1560	160	17·0	0·8	0·8	6·5	0·8	0·27	4·2	360	360

Source: manufacturers' information.
[a] iu=0·3 μg retinol.
[b] iu=0·025 μg vitamin D_2.

Table 4 shows the composition of some biscuits used in emergency feeding. On certain occasions biscuits have served as the only source of food for over 2–3 months in some relief camps. Biscuits are also a valuable source of other micronutrients (Table 5). Biscuits are therefore a valuable food source in emergency situations and are likely to play an important role in future emergency feeding programmes.

Bibliography

Booth R G (1990) *Snack Foods*. New York: Van Nostrand Reinhold.
Tannahill R (1988) *Food in History*. London: Penguin.
Wade P (1988) *Biscuits, Cookies and Crackers*, vol. I. Essex: Elsevier Science Publishers.

C. J. K. Henry
Oxford Polytechnic, Oxford, UK

BLACKBERRIES AND RELATED FRUITS

Although in the same genus as raspberries, blackberries are often regarded by the food industry as the Cinderella of the soft fruits. Nevertheless, they have considerable potential, which is likely to be realized to an increasing extent as new and improved cultivars become available. This article first describes the main types of blackberries, their botanical structure and typical chemical content, including pigments. Some of the characteristics which determine fruit quality are discussed. It then discusses the problems of post-harvest storage and the various market outlets.

Types of Blackberries

The botanical classification of blackberries is complex, but from the food viewpoint it is useful to consider just three types: the traditional blackberries of Europe and eastern North America, the indigenous blackberries of western North America, and the blackberry–raspberry hybrids. World production is concentrated in a few areas, and there are low levels of production in most of the areas where raspberries are grown. One major production area is Washington and Oregon on the west coast of America, where cultivars of each type are grown but with a predominance of European forms; another is in New Zealand, where the boysenberry, a blackberry–raspberry hybrid, predominates, a third is in Arkansas, USA, where locally bred cultivars are grown. *See* Fruits of Temperate Climates, Commercial and Dietary Importance

The flavour usually associated with blackberries is that of the European type. The flavour of the western North American type is more intense, pleasantly acidic and has strong aromatic overtones. The Bedford Giant cultivar, important in the UK, is a blackberry–raspberry hybrid derived from a European blackberry and a red raspberry, while the loganberry, tayberry, boysenberry and youngberry are all hybrids derived from western North American blackberries and red raspberries. They have inherited the characteristic flavour of this type of blackberry. Of these hybrids, the loganberry and tayberry contain one third of raspberry germplasm and have purple fruits; the others contain a lower proportion and have black fruits. The Andean blackberry of South America, *Rubus glaucus*, is the only blackberry–raspberry hybrid to be derived from a black raspberry, which has undoubtedly contributed to its excellent flavour.

Until recently, the available cultivars of the western North America type have been low-yielding and not widely grown, but new cultivars, such as Silvan, Kotata and Waldo, are much improved in productivity and quality, and are providing new opportunities for blackberry production and usage, especially in Europe. Their excellent flavour and early cropping are so different from those of the European type that the two forms complement each other to provide a choice of flavour and a long season of production.

Fruit Structure

Blackberry fruits are aggregates of drupelets. A drupe fruit is one which develops entirely from a single ovary, and the aggregate of drupelets which makes a blackberry fruit is formed by the ripening together of some 50 to 100 ovaries from the same flower and adhering to a common receptacle: in a sense, each drupelet is a complete fruit in itself and a miniature homologue of such drupe fruits as the cherry or plum.

The cohesion of these drupelets depends on the entanglement of epidermal hairs, which are unicellular linear trichomes arising from surface cells. The hairs are abundant at the bases and sides of the drupelet, and shorter and less profuse over its dome; they are so tightly enmeshed that the drupelets cannot normally be separated without tearing the skin. A poor set of drupelets or poor cohesion between them causes 'crumbly fruit' and a serious loss of quality.

Internally, the soft part of the drupelet consists of thin-walled parenchymatous cells, radiating from the pyrene in the centre to a region of larger, oval-shaped cells which underlie the epidermis, and a slightly collenchymatous hypodermis of one to three cells. Fruits are succulent because the walls of the parenchyma are thin and the cells turgid: variations between cultivars in fruit firmness are influenced by variations in the frequency of cells of small diameter, tissue compactness and overall cell size, which influences the amount of supporting cell-wall. The strength of the epidermis and cuticle influences the 'skin' strength of the berry.

Pyrenes

In the centre of each drupelet is a pyrene (often erroneously referred to as the seed) with a hard endocarp enclosing one or two true seeds. The endocarp consists of two layers of elongated, parallel scleroid cells at right angles to each other and each several cells thick, the outer one forming the characteristic ridged pattern of the pyrene.

The large size of most blackberry pyrenes is one of the main reasons for the fact that relatively few blackberries are used for jam-making. Large pyrenes are also undesirable in fresh fruit. Blackberry cultivars show a wide range in this characteristic: surveys showed a range in pyrene weight, which is indicative of size, from 2·01 to 4·83 mg for American cultivars and from 2·10 to 6·10 mg for breeding material at the Scottish Crop Research Institute. The American cultivars Waldo and Kotata have individual pyrene weights of 2·18 and 2·41 mg respectively, and are examples of cultivars that have small pyrenes and are suitable for jam-making. However, small pyrenes are only advantageous if their small size is associated with good development of the soft tissues which surround them.

Another potentially important quality of the pyrenes is their tendancy to become 'blind' in jam. Nothing is known about this characteristic in blackberries, because few of them are used in jam-making. Blindness occurs during the storage of raspberry jam when a slow displacement of air from within the pyrenes allows the surrounding syrup to infiltrate and causes them to lose their opacity. They then appear to have merged with the surrounding jam, which acquires a dull appearance and gives the illusion of a low fruit content. The problem could appear if small-seeded blackberry cultivars become popular for jam-making. The rate at which the process proceeds would be expected to vary with cultivar, method of fruit storage and manufacturing procedure.

Fruit Ripening and Abscission

All the drupelets of a blackberry usually ripen together, but those at the top of the fruit may ripen relatively slowly to give a red tip to an otherwise black fruit, especially in large, elongated fruits. Ethylene production begins at a late stage of colour development in Maryland, USA, where the blackberries studied can therefore be described as 'climacteric' fruits. No ethylene production was detected in a study in Scotland, however. The difference between these two results may be attributable to the temperatures prevailing at ripening time, because blackberries ripen in mid-summer in Maryland and much later in Scotland, or to the different cultivars studied. It is interesting that, in the Scottish study, the behaviour of the blackberry–raspberry hybrids, tayberry and tummelberry, was intermediate between that of raspberries and blackberries, and was therefore closer to that described for blackberries in Maryland. For blackberries grown in the USA, the ethylene-releasing chemical 'Ethrel' has been used to hasten ripening for machine harvesting. *See* Ripening of Fruit

An abscission layer forms in the tissues as the fruit ripens. In blackberries it is a single layer at the base of the receptacle, which consequently separates from the plant with the fruit, in contrast to raspberries, in which a large number of abscission layers form, one at the point of attachment of each drupelet to the receptacle, which is therefore retained on the plant after fruit abscission. This is the most fundamental difference between blackberries and raspberries, and it leads to an interesting situation in blackberry–raspberry hybrids, which are heterozygous for both types of abscission. Dominance is not always complete, and the fruits of many hybrids do not abcise exactly like those of either parent, although most of them have the system of their blackberry parent. The tayberry, for example, has a poorly developed abscission layer, but the fruits separate like a blackberry, except that the point of separation is frequently proximal to the calyx, which is then retained on the fruit when it is picked.

This difference between blackberries and raspberries in their method of fruit abscission explains why the core of most blackberries is soft and palatable, while that of some blackberry–raspberry hybrids such as tayberry is less so: blackberry fruits have been selected for the edibility of their receptacles, which become the cores of the ripe fruits, whereas the receptacles of raspberries are always left on the plant and are never eaten. Fruits of the hybrids are intermediate and often have a central core which is less soft than that of the true blackberries.

Fruit Colour

The colour of blackberries results from the presence of anthocyanin pigments. The anthocyanin molecule consists of an aglycone with a varying number of sugar residues attached to the hydroxyl group, usually in the 3-position. Only two anthocyanins have been found in blackberries, which have a predominance of the monosaccharide form, cyanidin-3-glucoside, and a trace of the diglycoside cyanidin-3-rutinoside, in which an additional rhamnose sugar is present. This is a very small number of pigments for a *Rubus* fruit, and the presence of other anthocyanins indicates that a fruit has a hybrid origin. Thus the diglycoside cyanidin-3-sophoroside, which is a characteristic pigment of the red raspberry, occurs in the loganberry, boysenberry, youngberry and mertonberry and is consistent with these fruits being related to the red raspberry. Similarly, the occurrence in the Andean blackberry of the diglycoside cyanidin-3-sambubiose, which is a characteristic pigment of black raspberries, supports the hypothesis that this blackberry is related to the black raspberry. *See* Colours, Properties and Determination of Natural Pigments

The identity of the sugar residues attached to the aglycone part of the anthocyanin molecule is thus useful to complement taxonomic observations and establish the hybrid origin of some cultivars. However, there is no evidence to suggest that any particular glycoside should be preferred from the viewpoint of the quality of fruit colour.

The concentration of anthocyanins in blackberries is intermediate between those of red raspberries and black raspberries. For example, fruits of the cultivar, Ashton Cross, a typical nonhybrid blackberry, were found to contain 65·45 mg of cyanidin per 100 g of fruit (62·56 mg of cyanidin-3-glycoside and 2·89 mg of cyanidin-3-rutinoside), compared to 22·91 mg for a typical red raspberry and 253·77 mg for a typical black raspberry. Hence black raspberries and not blackberries are used as a source of this natural pigment.

The Expression of Fruit Colour

The colour of anthocyanin pigments is influenced by any chemicals that influence the pH of the solutions that contain them. The pigments are chemical indicators that are red in acid solutions, violet or purple in neutral solutions and blue in alkaline ones. This may explain why the colour of blackberries frequently changes from

Table 1. Typical sugar and acid contents (% w/w) of European blackberries and two blackberry–raspberry hybrids

	Sugars			Acids							
	Reducing	Sucrose	Total	pH	Typical ripe fruit	Range	Citric	Malic	Isocitric and lactone		Sugar:acid ratio
Blackberry	—	—	4·30	3·00	1·50	0·68–1·84	Trace	0·82	0·81		2·81
Boysenberry	4·20	1·14	5·34	2·91	1·51	—	1·24	0·21	0·06		3·5
Loganberry	—	—	3·40	2·90	2·63	1·02–3·12	2·10	0·53	—		1·3

Data from Green (1971).

black to red when the fruit is frozen: freezing causes widespread cellular disruption which possibly allows mixing of the cells' plasma and vacuolar contents and places the anthocyanins in a solution of lower pH than where they occur in nonfrozen fruits. However, thoroughly ripe blackberries are less prone to turn red when frozen than less ripe fruits, and a more likely explanation of the colour change is that many fruits are not fully ripe when picked. Anthocyanins develop first in cells near the surface of the fruit, where they are exposed to sunlight, so that slightly immature fruits cannot be recognized immediately. The immature fruits have a lower concentration of anthocyanins and the cell disruption following freezing allows the anthocyanins to spread within the tissues and become diluted by cytoplasmic sap: for these fruits this pigment dilution is probably sufficient in itself to cause the colour change. The problem is greater when fast freezing is used, and cultivars with purple-black fruits, such as Bedford Giant and Silvan, are more prone to it than cultivars with intensely black fruits. *See* Freezing, Structural and Flavour Changes

Fruit Chemistry

Blackberries contain about 14% solids, which are approximately equally divided between soluble and insoluble forms. The size of the pyrene and the relative development of the surrounding soft tissues influences the proportion of soluble to insoluble solids. Pectins are an important constituent of the soluble fraction and average 0·8% (w/w, expressed as calcium pectate) with a range of from 0·35% to 1·19%. Loganberries have a lower content. Protopectins form the intercellular cement and contribute towards the firmness of fruit texture, but they decrease with ripening owing to hydrolyses.

Flavour is determined by the content of sugar, acids and volatiles, all of which vary with cultivar and growing conditions. Flavour is not perceived as a number of separate characteristics but rather as an overall impression. It is therefore not strongly correlated with any one of these factors. Fruits of the western North American cultivars have a more aromatic flavour than those of the European types, and fruit grown in areas which have warm dry summers have more sugars and are more aromatic than fruit grown in wetter and milder regions. The ratio of sugars to acids plays a major part in determining flavour. *See* Sensory Evaluation, Taste

The main sugars are the reducing sugars, glucose and fructose, and there is a smaller amount of sucrose; these form the major soluble component of the juice. The main acids are malic acid and isocitric acid with its lactone; there is only a trace of citric acid (Table 1). In boysenberries the proportion of the different acids was found to change as ripening proceeded: the proportion of malic acid decreased while the proportion of citric and isocitric acids increased. A number of trace acids also occur, especially in blackberry–raspberry hybrids. *See* Acids, Natural Acids and Acidulants; Carbohydrates, Classification and Properties

The acids have a high buffering capacity, which maintains a stable pH close to 3·0. The best measurement of the amount of acid present is therefore titratable acidity. As fruit development proceeds, this quantity increases at first and then decreases as ripening starts. It is lower at high temperatures. The relationship between titratable acidity and ripeness is so close that it is the best quantitative measure of fruit ripeness and has been used to assess the ripeness of fruits harvested by machine.

Although a large number of volatile compounds that probably contribute to the flavour of *Rubus* fruits have been isolated and identified, blackberry fruits have received relatively little attention and no conclusions on the identity of the important components are available.

Blackberries are generally poor sources of vitamins but provide useful amounts of ascorbic acid and vitamin E. They also provide a useful source of fibre. Mineral content is also low, with a predominance of potassium and calcium, and there are low contents of proteins and polypeptides and traces or larger amounts of a number of amino acids (Table 2). *See* individual nutrients

Table 2. Typical vitamin, protein and mineral contents of European blackberries

	Content (mg per 100 g)
Vitamins	
Carotene	0·10–0·59
Thiamin	0·03
Riboflavin	0·34–0·038
Nicotinic acid	0·4
Ascorbic acid	20
Total nitrogen	181
Proteins	0·56
Amino acids	2·25
Minerals	
Ash	0·5
Phosphorus	23·8
Potassium	208·0
Sodium	3·7
Calcium	63·3
Magnesium	29·5
Iron	0·85
Copper	0·18
Sulphur	9·2
Chloride	22·1

Data from Green (1971).

Post-harvest Management

The commercial life of blackberries is short, partly because of the physiological activity of the fruit after harvest, and partly because of the common occurrence of infection by fruit-rotting pathogens, especially the ubiquitous *Botrytis cinerea*. This pathogen infects before fruit harvest, remains quiescent within the fruit until after harvest and then becomes aggressive and causes grey mould disease. *See* Spoilage, Moulds in Food Spoilage

The fungus can infect blackberries in various ways. It can probably infect at the flowering stage, as in raspberries; it can enter minute wounds in the fruit, and it can infect by the contact of diseased fruit. Its incidence can be reduced by sprays applied from flowering time until a short interval before harvest, and after harvest the development of the disease can be inhibited by rapid cooling within 3 h of picking. This also prolongs the fruits' shelf life by inhibiting physiological activity. It is done by placing the containers of fruit in a cold but humid airstream in a refrigerated store designed to lower the fruits' temperature from the field level of 20°C to 2°C in under 4 h.

Respiration is the physiological activity mostly responsible for reducing shelf life. Its rate is closely related to temperature within the range 0–16°C and rises very steeply at 21°C. These high rates of respiraton are associated with an increasingly high heat of respiration. It is thercfore rccommended that blackberries for fresh consumption should be stored at 0–0·5°C with a 90–95% relative humidity to avoid loss of moisture from dehydration.

Uses

Most blackberries are marketed as fresh fruit. Although consumers associate them with the autumn, it is interesting that Silvan, which ripens in midsummer, has also proved popular: clearly blackberries can compete with other soft fruits if they are of high quality. A high proportion of the crop is also marketed as individual quick-frozen fruit, mostly for use in the processing and catering industries for pie-fillings and flavourings, etc. Many of the boysenberries produced in New Zealand are exported in this way. Few blackberries are used for canning, and the large size of their pyrene ('seeds') limits the fruit's use for jam manufacture, although significant amounts of seed-free blackberry conserve are produced. The recent introduction of very highly flavoured cultivars with small seeds may change this. *See* Jams and Preserves, Chemistry of Manufacture

Blackberries and tayberries are used to a small extent in Europe for the production of liquors and wines, for which the tayberry is well suited because of its rich purple colour and excellent flavour. The Andean blackberry of Colombia has such a rich flavour which it is used to produce a popular breakfast fruit juice, but little blackberry juice is consumed elsewhere.

Bibliography

Green A (1971) Soft fruits. In: Hume AC (ed.) *The Biochemistry of Fruits and their Products*. London: Academic Press.

Jennings DL (1988) *Raspberries and Blackberries: their Breeding, Diseases and Growth*. London: Academic Press.

USDA (1984) *The Commercial Storage of Fruits, Vegetables, Flowers and Nursery Stock*. US Department of Agriculture, Agriculture Handbook 66. Washington, DC: US Government Printing Office.

D. L. Jennings
Otham, Maidstone, UK

BLUEBERRIES

See Fruits of Temperate Climates

BODY COMPOSITION

The assessment of nutritional status involves an understanding of the energy stores of the body. In developing countries, lack of food supply leads to wasting, whilst in developed countries obesity and cardiovascular disease are also important causes of illness. The prevention and management of these disorders requires techniques for measuring the extent of these changes in individuals and populations.

Elemental Composition of the Human Body

The human body is composed of many different elements. The International Commission on Radiation Protection (1975) compiled a list of the multitude of elements found in the body of the adult male. These data were based on the chemical analysis of human organs by several investigators, and represents the best estimate of total body content based on a wide review of the literature. Thirty-six elements have been listed as being present in the human body. Approximately eighteen to twenty of these elements have been shown to have a physiological function. Many factors will determine the amounts of a particular element in the body. Not only the health of the individual at the time of death, but also environmental exposure to an element, will contribute to individual differences. For example, exposure to compounds containing lead or mercury, or exposure to radiation fall-out leading to accumulation of caesium and strontium. Gender, age and size are also important determinants of the amount of differential elements in the body. Major element content is better correlated with lean weight than with total bodyweight, since adipose tissue is largely composed of neutral fat. Major element variation is relatively small for individuals of a given body size.

Models of Body Composition

Investigation into body composition began in the nineteenth century. Chemical analyses of fetus and adult cadavers were followed by the development of concepts of different functioning body compartments. In 1906, Adolf Magnus-Levy coined the term 'fat-free' mass (see Forbes, 1987). This was further refined in 1937, by Hastings and Eichelberger (see Forbes, 1987) who recognized that neutral fat does not bind water, nitrogen or electrolytes. It is now accepted practice in various body composition models to express body analyses in fat-free and fat mass terms. Several such models have been developed in order to better define and measure the different compartments that make up total body mass or weight.

The *two-compartment model* of body composition defines a lean compartment consisting of body cells and their surrounding extracellular water, plus the skeleton and connective tissue. Of course, the lean mass contains some lipid in the form of cell membranes, and is thus not truly fat-free. *See* Adipose Tissue, Structure and Function of White Adipose Tissue; Adipose Tissue, Structure and Function of Brown Adipose Tissue; Bone; Exercise, Muscle; Water, Physiology

In the healthy individual, the lean mass has a relatively constant composition, with a water content of 72–74%, an average density of $1 \cdot 1$ g cm^{-3} at 37°C, a potassium content of 60–70 mmol kg^{-1} in men and 50–60 mmol kg^{-1} in women, and a protein content of 20%.

The fat compartment varies considerably in healthy individuals, but it has a relatively constant density of $0 \cdot 9$ g cm^{-3} at 37°C, and a very small water and potassium content.

The *four-compartment model* which has been developed as techniques have become more sophisticated, involves measuring subcategories of the fat-free mass, i.e. protein content, skeletal mass and total body water, as well as the fat mass.

Glycogen stores and micronutrients (1–2% of bodyweight) are not included in this body composition model and need to be assessed separately where feasible.

Gender and Age Differences in Body Composition

Fetal growth rate reaches a maximum during the latter stages of pregnancy. Much of this growth is due to an increase in fat-free weight, consisting of water and protein as components of cell growth. Skeletal muscle contains about the same proportion of total body nitrogen, potassium and water in the newborn.

Growth velocity falls during infancy and childhood, reaching a nadir at about four years of age. A slow increase follows, culminating in the adolescent growth spurt. During this time there are differential rates of growth of different organs.

There is a small sex difference in lean body mass (LBM) throughout infancy and childhood, but in the adolescent period the rate of increase in growth to adult levels of the LBM in males is approximately twice as much as in females. The male adolescent increase in LBM is also of longer duration. This is a function of hormonal action which continues to be an important determinant of body composition throughout life, together with genetic, nutritional and activity influences.

Adult men have a greater LBM and less body fat then adult women. Women have approximately two thirds the LBM of their male counterparts, whilst also having a greater relative fat mass. In young adults, the gender difference in LBM is greater then the difference in stature and in bodyweight.

There is much less variability between LBM values in individuals matched for age and height, compared with the variability in body fat.

The skeletal mass continues to grow until the late third decade. In women, there is an oestrogen-withdrawal-related decline in bone density over the period of the menopause. *See* Osteoporosis

In old age, there is a decline in LBM, with a shift in body water towards the extracellular phase. Bone mass declines further in both sexes. Body fat content shows more variability than LBM, but generally increases with age, and accounts for most of the variance in weight.

Methods of Measuring Body Composition
(see Table 1)

Fat Compartment

Methods of measuring body composition in the fat compartment include anthropometry, bioelectrical impedance, heavy water (D_2O) dilution, and whole-body densitometry.

Anthropometry

Anthropometric techniques are readily portable and inexpensive. The equipment required includes a tape

Table 1. Summary of body composition measurement techniques

Model	Technique
Two-compartment[a]	
Fat mass	Anthropometry
Lean mass	Impedance
Four-compartment[b]	
Fat mass	Underwater weighing
	DEXA
	CT scan, MRI
Body water	
Intracellular	TBK
Extracellular	TBW − TBK
Total water (TBW)	Heavy water (D_2O)
Body protein	IVNAA nitrogen
Skeletal mass	DEXA

[a] The two-compartment techniques are portable and simple.
[b] The four-compartment techniques are laboratory-based and more invasive.
DEXA, dual-energy X ray absorptiometry; CT, computerized tomography; MRI, magnetic resonance imaging; TBW, total body water; IC, intracellular; TBK, total body potassium; D_2O, deuterium oxide; IVNAA, *in vivo* neutron activation analysis.

measure, height stick, scales and skin-fold callipers. Various formulae have been developed which allow the rapid calculation of different aspects of body composition, including percentage fat derived from triceps skin fold (Table 2), and the following anthropometric equations:

1. Body mass index (BMI) or Quetelet's index can be readily calculated from height and weight data: BMI = (weight in kg)/(height in m)^2.
2. Arm muscle circumference = mid-upper-arm circumference − (π × triceps skin fold).
3. Waist : hip ratio = (waist circumference)/(hip circumference).

Body mass index has a good correlation with body fatness, as measured by other techniques, and correlates well with morbidity and mortality in the obese individual.

Trunk circumferences define fat distribution. A waist : hip ratio > 0·95 (males) and > 0·85 (females) is consistent with abdominal obesity. As definitions of 'waist' and 'hip' have varied in the literature, it is important to have consistency in measurements in order to compare sets of data. The original Swedish observations of the risks and metabolic complications associated with abdominal obesity are reproducible whether the waist is taken as the smallest circumference or at the level of the umbilicus.

Table 2. Percentage fat derived from triceps skin fold

Triceps skin fold (mm)	Relative fat mass (%)									
	Males (years)					Females (years)				
	17–19	20–29	30–39	40–49	50+	17–19	20–29	30–39	40–49	50+
5	8·0	10·0	18·0	16·5	18·5	12·5	9·5	13·0	15·5	16·0
7	11·5	13·5	20·0	20·0	23·0	16·5	14·0	17·0	20·0	20·5
9	14·5	16·0	22·0	23·0	26·0	19·5	18·0	20·5	23·0	24·5
11	17·0	18·0	23·5	25·5	29·0	22·0	21·0	23·0	26·0	27·5
13	19·0	19·5	24·5	27·7	31·0	24·5	23·5	25·5	28·0	30·0
15	20·5	21·0	25·5	29·5	33·0	26·0	25·5	27·5	30·0	32·5
17	22·0	22·5	26·5	31·0	35·0	28·0	27·5	29·0	32·0	34·0
19	23·5	23·5	27·0	32·5	36·0	29·0	29·5	30·5	33·5	36·0
21	25·0	24·5	28·0	33·5	37·5	30·5	31·0	32·0	35·0	37·5
23	26·0	25·5	28·5	35·0	39·0	31·5	32·5	33·5	36·0	39·0
25	27·0	26·5	29·0	36·0	40·0	33·0	33·5	34·5	37·5	40·5
27	28·0	27·0	30·0	37·0	41·0	34·0	35·0	35·5	38·5	41·5
29	29·0	28·0	30·5	38·0	42·0	35·0	36·0	36·5	39·5	43·0
31	30·0	29·0	31·0	38·5	43·0	35·5	37·0	37·5	40·5	44·0
33	30·5	29·5	31·0	39·5	44·0	36·5	38·0	38·5	41·5	45·0
35	31·0	30·0	32·0	40·0	45·0	37·5	39·0	39·5	42·5	46·0
37	32·0	30·5	32·0	41·0	45·5	38·0	40·0	40·0	43·0	47·0
39	32·5	31·0	32·5	41·5	46·5	38·5	41·0	41·0	44·0	47·0
40	33·0	31·5	33·0	42·0	47·0	39·0	41·5	41·0	44·5	48·0

Sources: Durnin JVGA and Womersley J (1974).

Skin fold thicknesses have been used to measure body fat. This method assumes that subcutaneous fat measurements represent total body fat. Various sites can be assessed and equations applied to derive body density and hence subcutaneous fat mass. Durnin and Womersley (1974) developed the regression equation using four skin folds (biceps, triceps, subscapular and suprailiac), gender and age. Equations have been developed using multiple or single skin fold sites.

Precision of skin fold measurement depends on the skill of the operator as well as the character of the subcutaneous fat. In general, the error is 5%, although this can be higher in the very obese individual.

Arm Muscle Circumference Measurement of the mid-arm circumference has been used to approximate total body protein stores. The triceps skin fold has been used as a measure of total body subcutaneous fat (Table 3).

The arm muscle circumference (or 'arm muscle and bone circumference') can be derived from the arm circumference and the triceps skin fold, and it gives a good indication of protein stores. This correlation holds true particularly in under-developed countries, where populations tend to have little subcutaneous fat, and it can be a useful tool in diagnosis and monitoring of progress in the management of protein–energy malnutrition.

Bioelectrical Impedance

Application of a constant, low-level alternating current to the body, can be used principally to determine total body water (TBW) and, by regression analysis from other techniques, to determine fat mass and fat-free mass. Both resistance and reactance are measured.

Water and electrolyte distribution determine electrical conductance in the living organism. Virtually all the water and electrolytes in the body are found within the fat-free (lean) mass which represents a low-resistance pathway. Fat and bone are poor conductors. Reactance is the opposition to the flow of electrical current caused by capacitance. The cell membrane, by maintaining an osmotic gradient between extra- and intracellular compartments, serves as a capacitor. Reactance is a measure of the quantity of cell membrane capacitance and may give an indication of the quantity of the intracellular cell mass. Whereas fat and water offer resistance to an electric current, only cell membranes have reactance.

The measurement of total body impedance (resistance and reactance) is a vector sum of resistance and reactance in the limbs and torso, with the limbs making the major contribution.

Use of this method has been validated in healthy populations as a determinant of TBW and deduced lean and fat mass. In disease states such as renal failure and dehydration, metabolic function may alter the compartmentation of TBW and bioelectrical impedance may be less useful and less reproducible, with the literature reporting conflicting results.

Heavy Water (D₂O) Dilution

Water is not present in stored triglyceride and occupies a relatively fixed fraction of the fat-free mass. Estimation of TBW can therefore be used as an index of body composition. Several isotopes have been used, but deuterium oxide (D_2O, the naturally occurring non-radioactive isotope of water, containing hydrogen protons with two neutrons – heavy water – and present as 0·01% of naturally occurring water) is now seen as the 'gold standard' for measurement of TBW.

The technique involves the administration of a known quantity of D_2O, an equilibrium period, and a sampling period. It assumes that the D_2O has the same distribution volume as water and is exchanged by the body in a manner similar to water.

Sampling can be from either serum or saliva and whilst the analytical equipment is only suited to a laboratory, it enables collection of specimens in the field for later analysis.

A variety of analytical techniques have been used to measure D_2O, including mass spectrometry and Fourier Transform infrared spectroscopy.

Whole-body densitometry

Whole-body densitometry is the 'gold standard' for the measurement of *body fat*. The technique assumes that the body is composed of two distinct compartments (fat and fat-free, each of a known or assumed density) and that the relative amount of each can be determined by measurement of the whole-body density. *Underwater weighing* is the most widely used technique, based on Archimedes' principle which states that the volume of an object submerged in water is equal to the volume of water that the object displaced. The mass in air of the object and the mass in water of the object is then converted to a total body. *Body fat mass* can then be calculated using one of the empirical equations describing the relationship between fat content and body density.

Valuable body composition data can be obtained using underwater weighing, although there are several inherent disadvantages. Subjects must be accustomed to swimming and submersion in water and must be medically fit enough to endure such procedures. These caveats to its use exclude use of this technique in many hospitalized patients. The apparatus required is substantial in size, and thus only suited for use in large institutions. In addition, variation in bone density owing to ethnicity, gender or ageing is not taken into account in the constant used for non-fat density.

Fat-free Compartment

Methods of measuring body composition in the fat-free compartment include *in vivo* neutron activation analysis, total body potassium, and dual-energy X ray absorptiometry.

In Vivo *Neutron Activation Analysis*

In vivo neutron activation analysis (IVNAA) provides the only *in vivo* technique currently available to determine multi-elemental composition. Calcium, phosphorus, sodium and chloride content have been measured, but in current clinical practice only nitrogen is measured (from which total body protein is calculated).

Neutron activation involves delivery of a beam of neutrons to the subject. These neutrons are captured by the target atoms in the body, creating unstable isotopes; in the case of protein, the isotope formed is [15]nitrogen. The isotope reverts to a stable state by the emission of γ-rays of a characteristic energy, which can then be detected by the use of standard γ-spectrographic analysis. This method, targeting nitrogen, allows (1) the determination of total body nitrogen and, therefore, total body protein, which is the principal nitrogen-containing component of the body, and (2) the indirect determination of skeletal muscle mass, using the mathematical model derived by Burkinshaw *et al.* (1978).

Whilst IVNAA is a very useful tool for measurements of body composition, its development in only a few centres has limited the wider application of this methodology. In addition, concern has been expressed over the large expense of this technique. The American literature quotes costs as high as $400 000. Other units have been able to develop this methodology for less than $50 000 (Stroud DB *et al.* 1990).

Total Body Potassium

The naturally occurring radioactive isotope of potassium, ^{40}K, is present in a known, constant, very low percentage of total potassium. Since body potassium is essentially intracellular, and not present in stored fat, measurement of ^{40}K not only provides an estimate of total body potassium, but also allows estimation of body cell mass. If total body water is known (from deuterium dilution), extracellular water can be calculated.

The technique requires a highly shielded environment in which to detect the ^{40}K in the body, as ^{40}K also occurs in most environmental structures. In addition, the requirement for appropriate γ-ray detectors and corrections for factors such as body geometry make the technique expensive.

Dual-energy X Ray Absorptiometry

Dual-energy X ray absorptiometry (DEXA) is a recent addition to the body composition analysis field. It was originally developed to measure regional and total body bone mineral content, but it is also capable of measuring fat mass. It is more sensitive than dual-photon absorptiometry, which it has now replaced, and exposes the subject to substantially lower radiation doses than total body calcium measured by neutron activation analysis.

The DEXA technique exposes the subject to low-energy irradiation at two different energies. As there is differential absorption by tissues of different densities (bone, lean and fat tissues), values for bone mineral in the hip, spine, whole body or specialized regions, as well as values for fat or soft tissues, can be derived.

It is a sensitive technique for determining bone mineral content and densities, and has become the 'gold standard' for clinical and research work in osteoporosis.

A recent development in measurement of regional bone mineral density is the use of ultrasound for measuring os calcis bone density. This technique appears to be promising for use in assessing foot stress fractures in subjects involved in extensive physical training.

Other Techniques

Other techniques for measuring body composition include computerized tomography (CT) scanning and magnetic resonance imaging (MRI). These techniques have been used for accurate measurement of various body compartments. Whilst their clinical and research use is limited by expense, availability and patient exposure to ionizing radiation, much helpful information has been obtained from the research groups who have utilized such technology.

Error of the Methods

Each of the methods for measuring body composition has intrinsic and biological errors. In general, these are very comparable to the errors of biochemical methods commonly performed in hospital laboratories (Table 3).

Effect of Disease Processes on Human Body Composition

Obesity

The fat compartment – expressed as mass or percentage fat – has importance as an expression of adiposity. The association between increased adiposity and morbidity is well documented. The incidence of diabetes, hypertension, ischaemic heart disease and gall bladder disease is increased at higher levels of adiposity. *See* Obesity, Aetiology and Assessment; Obesity, Fat Distribution

Table 3.   Error of the methods

Method	Coefficient of variation (%)
Anthropometry	
Weight	$< 1^a$
Height	$< 1^a$
Skin folds	$3–5^b$
Circumferences	$\sim 2^a$
Bioelectrical impedance	$1–2^c$
Dual-energy X ray absorptiometry	
Bone density	$1–2^d$
Fat, lean	$3–4^e$
Deuterium dilution	$1–2^a$
In vivo neutron activation analysis	
Total body protein	4^a

[a] Unpublished data from the Body Composition Laboratory, Monash Medical Centre, Melbourne, Australia.
[b] Loman (1981).
[c] Lukaski *et al.* (1985).
[d] Mazess *et al.* (1989).
[e] Mazess *et al.* (1990).

Fat distribution is being increasingly recognized as a clinically relevant risk factor. Abdominal obesity, expressed as the waist:hip ratio, has been shown, independent of other factors, to represent an increased risk for morbidity and mortality. First described in the 1950s (Vague J, 1956), this association has been verified and strengthened by intense research interest in the last decade. The correlation is not just an epidemiological one: many metabolic abnormalities, such as insulin resistance, are associated with this condition.

With increasing adiposity, it is usual to find an increase in lean mass. This occurs because of the increased skeletal muscle mass required to carry the increased fat mass.

In obese people who have undergone repeated near-starvation dieting, there may be marked wasting of skeletal muscle, even in the presence of adiposity. Similarly, muscle wasting, or even marasmus, can occur in the obese person who has concomitant severe illness. For example, a chronic alcoholic with a poor quality of food intake, and liver impairment may be osese (excess fat stores) and also have skeletal muscle wasting.

Undernutrition

In global terms, undernutrition remains one of the greatest determinants of health status. The most common expressions of undernutrition are commonly known as kwashiorkor and marasmus. Intermediate forms are commonly seen. In marasmus, there is a wasting of total body protein without expansion of the TBW compartment. In kwashiorkor, there is an expansion of the extracellular component of TBW, giving rise to peripheral oedema and ascites. Exactly why undernutrition results in these two different forms remains unclear. *See* Kwashiorkor; Malnutrition, The Problem of Malnutrition; Marasmus

Both forms are associated with a reduction in the capacity of the cell-mediated immune system of the body, giving rise to an increased risk of infection. Where food intake is reduced, it is likely that other nutrient deficiencies, such as iron, folate or vitamin A deficiency, will be present and may mask the extent of the underlying body composition changes.

In developing countries, these forms of undernutrition usually arise from the combination of inadequate food resources and chronic infection. In malnutrition caused by inadequate food intake, many studies have shown an increase in the ratio of extracellular fluid (ECF) volume to TBW. Electrolyte abnormalities are common. Reduced levels of sodium, potassium and magnesium may be found. Protein stores, as measured by IVNAA and expressed as nitrogen index, are reduced.

In developed countries, these conditions are frequently seen in conjunction with malignancy, psychiatric conditions, organ failure and conditions in which self-feeding is difficult, e.g. stroke or arthritis. *See* Malnutrition, Malnutrition in Developed Countries

The wasting seen in many malignancies, even when nutritional intake and absorption is apparently adequate, may be caused by cytokines such as cachectin and tumour necrosis factor.

Visceral size may be better preserved in cancer patients, suggesting that loss of muscle accounts for the major proportion of weight loss. This may be the result of a difference in metabolic rate between malignancy and anorexia; the rate is often increased in patients with malignancy, but reduced in anorexia nervosa. *See* Anorexia Nervosa

In anorexia nervosa, many of the body composition changes seen are similar to those found in starved subjects. Total body nitrogen, total body potassium and blood volume are all reduced. Unlike primary starvation, ECF may be reduced by relatively greater amounts than the reduction in TBW owing to induced vomiting or purging. Interestingly, many patients with anorexia nervosa maintain normal levels of haemoglobin and serum albumin and rarely exhibit vitamin deficiencies or develop oedema.

Conclusion

An understanding of body composition and its measurement provides the clinician with further scientific data on which to base a nutritional assessment. Advances in this area are now available to provide accurate measurements which previously could only be estimated. Some of these techniques are easily applicable to office general practice or field studies, whilst others require more sophisticated equipment only available in specialized centres.

Body composition changes in health and disease help to explain the pathogenesis of illnesses which involve alteration in food intake or absorption and metabolic handling of macronutrients.

Bibliography

Alleyne GEO (1975) Mineral metabolism in protein-calorie malnutrition. In: Olsen RE (ed.) *Protein-Calorie Malnutrition*, pp 201–208. New York: Academic Press.

Brozek J, Grande F, Anderson JT and Keys A (1963) Densitometric analysis of body composition: revision of some quantitative assumptions. *Annals of the New York Academy of Sciences* 110: 113–140.

Burkinshaw L *et al.* (1978) *Assessment of the distribution of protein in the human by the* in vivo *neutron activation analysis*. International Symposium on Nuclear Activation Techniques in Life Sciences, SM227/39, pp 787–796.

Durnin JVGA and Womersley J (1974) Body fat assessed from body density and its estimation from skin fold thickness: measurements on 481 men and women aged from 16 to 72 years. *British Journal of Nutrition* 32: 77–97.

Forbes GB (1987) *Human Body Composition*, pp 2, 171. New York: Springer-Verlag.

Forbes GB (1990) Body composition. In: Brown M (ed.) *Present Knowledge in Nutrition* 6th edn. Washington, DC: International Life Sciences Institute.

Forbes GB, Kriepe RE, Lipinski BA and Hodgman CH (1984) Body composition changes during recovery from anorexia nervosa: comparison of two dietary regimes. *American Journal of Clinical Nutrition* 40: 1137–1145.

Fowler PA, Fuller MF, Glasby CA *et al.* Total and subcutaneous adipose tissue in women: the measurement of distribution and accurate prediction of quality by using magnetic resonance imaging. *American Journal of Clinical Nutrition* 54: 18–25.

Hastings AB and Eichelberger (1937) The exchange of salt and water between muscle and blood. *Journal of Biological Chemistry* 117: 73–93.

International Commission on Radiological Protection (1975) *Report of the Task Group on Reference Man*, No. 23. Oxford: Pergamon Press.

Jelliffe EPP and Jelliffe DB (1969) The arm circumference as a public health index of protein-calorie malnutrition of early childhood. *Journal of Tropical Paediatrics* 15: 179–192.

Kvist H, Choudury B, Grangard U, Tyler U and Sjostrom L (1988) Total and visceral adipose tissue volumes derived from measurements with computed tomography in adult men and women: predictive equations. *American Journal of Clinical Nutrition* 48: 1351–1361.

Lukaski HC (1987) Methods for the assessment of human body composition: traditional and new. *American Journal of Clinical Nutrition* 46: 537–556.

Lukaski HC and Johnson PE (1985) A simple, inexpensive method of determining total body water using a tracer dose of D_2O and infrared absorption of biological fluids. *American Journal of Clinical Nutrition* 41: 363–370.

Lukaski HC, Bolonchuk WW, Hall CB and Siders WA (1986) Validation of tetrapolar bioelectrical impedance method to assess human body composition. *Journal of Applied Physiology* 60: 1327–1332.

Mazess RB, Collick B, Trempe J, Barden HS and Hanson JA (1989) Performance evaluation of a dual-energy x-ray bone densitometer. *Calcified Tissue International* 44: 228–232.

Mazess RB, Barden HS, Bisek JP and Hanson J (1990) Dual energy X-ray absorptiometry for total body and regional bone mineral and soft tissue composition. *American Journal of Clinical Nutrition* 51: 1106–1112.

Mazess RB, Hanson JA, Trempe J and Bonnick SL (1991) *Ultrasound Measurement of the Os Calcis*. Proceedings of the 8th International Workshop on Bone Densitometry, 28 April, Bad Reichenhall, FRG.

Stroud DB, Borovnicar DJ, Lambert JR *et al.* (1990) Clinical studies of total body nitrogen in an Australian Hospital. In:

Yasumara S *et al.* (eds) *In vivo Body Composition Studies, Basic Life Sciences*, vol. 55, pp. 177–182. New York: Plenum Press.

Vague J (1956) The degree of masculine differentiation of obesities: a fact for determining predisposition to diabetes, atherosclerosis, gout, uric calculus disease. *American Journal of Clinical Nutrition* 4: 20–34.

Widdowson EM and Dickerson JWT (1964) Chemical composition of the body. In: Comari CL and Bronner F (eds) *Mineral Metabolism*, vol. 2, part A, pp 2–247. London: Academic Press.

*Julie Lustig, Mark L. Wahlqvist and Boyd J. G. Strauss
Monash Medical Centre, Melbourne, Australia*

BONE

Bone serves as a framework for the body and as a metabolic reserve of calcium and phosphate at times of mineral deficiency. It consists of cells from two distinct lineages, bone-forming osteoblasts and bone-resorbing osteoclasts, and the calcified extracellular matrix that these cells secrete and remodel.

Bone formation begins in the embryo, either via a cartilaginous intermediate, as in the case of the long bones, or via a membranous intermediate, as in the case of the flat bones of the skull. Continued production of cartilage at specialized sites on the long bones, termed growth plates, and the subsequent conversion of this cartilage into bone results in longitudinal postnatal growth. Skeletal growth and development is regulated by genetic, mechanical and hormonal mechanisms. In general, genetic influences dictate the basic structure of the skeleton, whilst responses to mechanical loading adjust the strength of particular bones to their functional environment. Simultaneously, hormonal mechanisms coordinate the movement of calcium and phosphate to and from the skeleton, thereby enabling bone to act as a reservoir of these minerals at times of calcium stress (e.g. pregnancy and lactation). At the cellular level, bone growth is coordinated by an array of interacting cytokines and growth factors which control bone cell division, maturation and activity. *See* Calcium, Physiology

Failure of the mechanisms controlling bone cell function, especially during bone turnover in adults, leads to bone loss and this can produce clinical osteoporosis. Other skeletal disease states result from nutritional deficiency, e.g. rickets, or from genetic defects, e.g. osteopetrosis or osteogenesis imperfecta. *See* Body Composition

Bone: Types, Composition and Structure

There are two types of bone in the skeleton – flat bones, e.g. the skull, and long bones, e.g. the femur. The principal anatomical features of a long bone are shown in Fig. 1.

Bone Matrix

Bone matrix is a composite material that derives its strength from a compression-resistant mineral phase and a tension-resistant network of collagen fibres. Bone's mineral phase – calcium hydroxyapatite, $Ca_{10}(PO_4)_6(OH)_2$ – is subdivided into a mosaic of tiny microcrystallites, thereby creating a large surface area for ion exchange and limiting the spread of cracks. Bone matrix also contains a number of specialized noncollagenous proteins, such as osteocalcin, osteonectin and osteopontin.

Macroscopic Architecture

Two types of internal bone architecture are visible to the naked eye. Cortical bone, the stronger but heavier of the two forms, comprises the outer wall of all bones and fulfils a mainly mechanical function (see insert, Fig. 1). It consists of parallel cylinders of matrix, (osteons), arranged along the load-bearing axis of the bone.

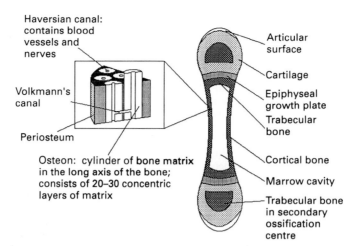

Fig. 1 The anatomy of a long bone, e.g. the femur. Inset shows an enlarged section of cortical bone.

Within each osteon the matrix is deposited in concentric layers, each 2–3 μm thick, with a predominant fibre direction (like multilayer plywood). The central canal of each osteon contains bone cells, blood vessels and nerves.

Trabecular bone, the second architectural form, is found at the ends of long bones and in the middle of the vertebrae. It consists of a latticework of bony struts, each 100–500 μm thick. Although weaker than cortical bone, it is more cellular and hence more metabolically active.

Bone Cells

Osteoblasts

Bone-forming cells are called osteoblasts. They are characterized by high levels of alkaline phosphatase, an enzyme required for matrix mineralization, and display structural features reflecting their intense secretory activity (e.g. prominent endoplasmic reticulum).

Osteoblasts are arranged as a closely packed layer of cells on growing bone surfaces, with each cell producing around three times its own volume of bone in about 3 days. Newly synthesized bone matrix is produced in an unmineralized form (termed osteoid), and consists of highly cross-linked collagen I fibres (which give the tissue its tensile strength), and a number of noncollagenous proteins such as osteocalcin. Osteoid is also rich in osteoblast-derived growth factors (insulin-like growth factor II, or IGFII, and transforming growth factor β), and these may regulate local bone turnover. Once formed, osteoid is mineralized. In cortical bone, crystal growth begins at sites along the collagen fibrils and is regulated by inhibitory molecules released by the osteoblasts.

Approximately 10–20% of osteoblasts become entombed in the matrix that they have produced and are termed osteocytes. They remain linked to the bone surface via long cell processes, and appear to respond to mechanical loading. Osteocytes may therefore be responsible for coupling of mechanical stimulation to bone growth.

Osteoblasts contribute to the control of bone resorption, responding to bone-resorbing signals by producing degradative enzymes and by releasing molecules that increase osteoclast activity and recruitment. Osteoblasts may therefore coordinate bone turnover by switching from bone formation to the control of bone resorption.

Origin of the Osteoblast

Osteoblasts are derived from stem cells located near bone surfaces. These 'stem-cells' can give rise to cartilage, fat and fibrous tissues in experimental systems, suggesting that osteoblasts form part of a superfamily of connective tissue cells.

The stem cells divide and mature into pre-osteoblasts, an intermediate cell type which displays some osteoblast-like features, e.g. type I collagen production, alkaline phosphatase and osteonectin mRNA (messenger ribonucleic acid), but which lack the intense alkaline phosphatase activity and highly developed endoplasmic reticulum of the mature cells.

Terminal differentiation into mature osteoblasts is associated with the cessation of cell division, the production of osteopontin and osteocalcin, and changes in both oncogene expression and nuclear protein–DNA (deoxyribonucleic acid) interactions. Further changes in regulatory nuclear proteins accompany the onset of mineralization.

Osteoclasts

Osteoclasts are large (3000–250 000 μm³), highly mobile, multinucleate cells (10–20 nuclei) which contribute to bone remodelling and calcium homoeostasis by resorbing bone. The osteoclast's resorptive apparatus consists of a central 'ruffled border', a highly folded region of cell membrane across which acid and degradative enzymes are extruded, and a peripheral 'clear zone', which seals the osteoclast onto the bone.

Osteoclasts dissolve bone mineral by secreting acid across their ruffled borders using proton-pumping ATPases. Acid production also requires carbonic anhydrase – an enzyme used for acid production by the stomach and which is absent in some forms of the lethal bone disease, osteopetrosis. The organic components of bone are degraded by lysosomal enzymes: one of these, acid phsophatase, is used as a marker for osteoclast activity.

Origin of the Osteoclast

Osteoclasts are descended from blood-cell-forming, interleukin-3-dependent stem cells located in the bone marrow and are therefore part of the same superfamily of cells as macrophages, lymphocytes and red blood cells. Partially differentiated, mononuclear pre-osteoclasts migrate via the circulation to resorption sites, where they proliferate and acquire differentiated features (e.g. acid phosphatase and calcitonin receptors), before fusing into multinucleate osteoclasts and beginning to resorb. *See* Cells

Regulation of Bone Cell Activity

Genetic and Mechanical

Whilst genetic influences dictate the basic structure of the skeleton, responses to mechanical loading adapt bone to its functional environment. In general, physical strain stimulates bone formation, whilst disuse (e.g. paralysis) results in bone loss. As a consequence, the cortical width of a professional tennis player's serving arm may be increased by 35% relative to his other arm. Such adaptation optimizes the balance between skeletal strength and weight.

Systemic Regulation of Serum Calcium: the Calciotropic Hormones, Parathyroid Hormone, Calcitonin and Dihydroxyvitamin D_3

Serum calcium is maintained within tight limits (2·2–2·6 mmol l^{-1}), a process necessary for the maintenance of many cellular activities including neuromuscular function.

Parathyroid hormone (PTH) releases calcium into the blood by mobilizing bone mineral at times of calcium shortage. It binds to receptors on pre-osteoblastic cells and signals the release of osteoclast activating factors. It also promotes calcium retention by the kidney and uptake from the gut.

Calcitonin is produced in response to a rise in serum calcium. It acts directly on osteoclasts and inhibits bone resorption. *See* Calcium, Physiology

Vitamin D metabolites regulate serum calcium and are essential for skeletal growth and development. The parent compound, vitamin D, is essentially inactive and requires two hydroxylation steps before gaining biological activity. The second of these hydroxylation steps is tightly regulated by PTH. Once formed, the most potent vitamin D metabolite, 1,25-dihydroxyvitamin D_3 ($1,25(OH)_2D_3$), increases intestinal calcium absorption and promotes bone-matrix mineralization. It also alters cell differentiation, influencing chondrocyte maturation within the growth plate and regulating gene expression in osteoblastic cells. *See* Cholecalciferol, Physiology

Systemic Hormones that Regulate Skeletal Growth or Function: Growth Hormone, Oestradiol and Vitamin A

Growth hormone stimulates bone growth by promoting cell division amongst the chondrocytes of the growth plate. It acts in part by stimulating IGFI production.

Whilst there is no doubt that the decreased levels of *oestradiol* that follow normal or artificially induced menopause lead to increased bone loss, oestradiol's role in skeletal biology remains obscure. The recent discovery of oestradiol receptors in osteoblasts suggests it may have a direct effect on osteoblastic cells.

Vitamin A is important for the maintenance of normal bone remodelling. It may also participate in the control of three-dimensional pattern formation during limb bud development. *See* Growth and Development; Retinol, Physiology

Local Regulation of Bone Cell Proliferation, Maturation and Function by Polypeptide Growth Factors

A variety of growth factors (e.g. fibroblast growth factor and IGFI) stimulate the division of pre-osteoblastic cells. Other signal molecules (e.g. transforming growth factor β) are associated with developmental events such as the formation of the vertebrae, jaws and palate. Osteoblasts produce many of these growth factors themselves and deposit them in their extracellular matrix, suggesting that they coordinate small groups of cells at specific locations. Osteoclast recruitment is regulated by a variety of blood cell growth factors, termed 'colony stimulating factors'. Several of these are produced by osteoblastic cells. Osteoblasts have also

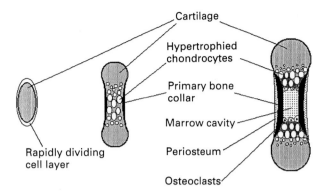

Fig. 2   The principal stages of embryonic long bone growth.

been shown to produce factors that stimulate mature osteoclasts to resorb.

Mechanisms of Bone Growth

Flat bones and long bones arise by two distinct mechanisms.

Growth of Long Bones (e.g. Femur): Endochondral Ossification

The principal stages of long bone growth are shown in Fig. 2. Long bones begin as cartilaginous regions in the early embryo. They grow as rapidly dividing peripheral cells add new chondrocytes to the outside of the structure and as older cells in the body of the cartilage divide, enlarge and secrete matrix (Fig. 2a).

The oldest chondrocytes (located in the middle) expand, calcify their matrix and are termed hypertrophic (Fig. 2b). Osteoblasts then secrete a bony layer around the midshaft of the cartilage, forming the 'primary bone collar'. This structure is extended and thickened by successive generations of osteoblasts.

Once established, the primary bone collar is penetrated at several points by osteoclasts (Fig. 2c). These rapidly erode the calcified cartilage of the interior to leave only a supportive framework inside the bone collar. As the peripheral bone gains in strength, osteoclasts remove this framework to leave the marrow cavity.

Continued Growth of Long Bones: the Growth Plate

Long bone growth continues at specialized 'epiphyseal growth plates' (Fig. 3). Proliferating chondrocytes at the top of the growth plate add new cells, whilst their more mature descendants secrete matrix and enlarge, thereby producing longitudinal growth. Ultimately, the chon-

drocytes hypertrophy and calcify their matrix. Osteoclasts present in the marrow cavity invade this calcified cartilage, destroying the horizontal septa separating the chondrocytes. This leaves vertical bars of calcified cartilage projecting into the marrow cavity and these act as a framework for subsequent bone deposition.

Complete calcification of the growth plate at the end of puberty marks the end of longitudinal growth.

Intramembranous Ossification (e.g. the Bones of the Cranium)

The flat bones of the skull begin as highly vascularized sheets of embryonic tissue. Undifferentiated cells within these sheets differentiate directly into osteoblasts and form a radiating network of bony spicules lying parallel to the surface of the brain. During growth, successive generations of osteoblasts add new bone to the outside and periphery of this structure, whilst osteoclasts resorb from the inner surface to maintain proportional thickness and shape.

Bone Atrophy: Hormonal Influences and the Effect of Age

Bones grow in size and strength until peak bone mass is attained around the age of 35. Peak mass varies between demographic subgroups (25–30% higher in males than females; 10% higher in blacks than whites), although there is a large variation within each group (one women in forty has a peak mass less than the average for women aged 65). Bone mass subsequently declines with age and as a result of a variety of factors that predispose an individual to bone loss. The observed bone mass of an individual over 35 therefore represents their peak bone mass, minus both the cumulative age-related bone loss and any losses resulting from disease or specific risk factors.

Bone Turnover and Age-related Bone Loss

Bone is continuously broken down and replaced throughout life, thereby mobilizing calcium for systemic needs and preventing the accumulation of old, fatigue-fractured material. Typically, 4% of cortical bone and 25% of trabecular bone is replaced each year.

Turnover begins with the recruitment of osteoclast precursors. These mature, fuse into multinucleate osteoclasts and resorb a depression 60 μm deep in the bone surface over a period of about 10 days. Osteoblasts, derived from undifferentiated cells located in the vicinity of the resorption site, then replace the resorbed material. The entire process lasts approximately 4 months.

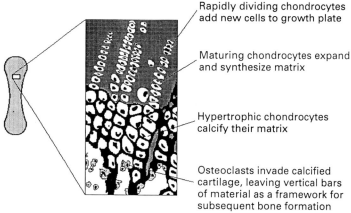

Rapidly dividing chondrocytes add new cells to growth plate

Maturing chondrocytes expand and synthesize matrix

Hypertrophic chondrocytes calcify their matrix

Osteoclasts invade calcified cartilage, leaving vertical bars of material as a framework for subsequent bone formation

Fig. 3 Continued longitudinal growth at the growth plate.

After the fourth decade of life, bone reformation fails to replace completely the resorbed bone, so that bone turnover produces a net bone loss. This so-called 'age-related bone loss' (0·3% and 1% of peak bone mass per year in males and females, respectively) occurs regardless of sex, physical activity, nutrition or socioeconomic status. Its rate depends upon the frequency of remodelling cycles and the imbalance between the amount of bone resorbed and replaced at each remodelling event.

Age-related bone loss therefore occurs more rapidly in trabecular bone (which turns over more rapidly), and is increased by factors that promote bone turnover (transient calcium deficiency). Risk factors or disease states associated with either low peak bone mass or increased rates of loss include small body size, nulliparity, inactivity, early natural menopause, anorexia, thyrotoxicosis and Cushing's syndrome.

Ultimately, the combination of reduced bone mass and disrupted trabecular architecture, (as individual bony struts are severed or removed from the lattice), leads to reduced bone strength and increased fracture risk.

Other Causes of Bone Loss: Hyperparathyroidism and Malignant Disease

Hyperparathyroidism is an endocrine disorder characterized by raised serum calcium and increased cortical bone loss. It is usually caused by a benign adenoma, which secretes excessive PTH, thereby increasing both bone resorption and calcium retention by the kidney. Pathological bone loss is also a feature of many malignant disease states. Bone destruction may result from osteoclast activation in the immediate vicinity of invading tumours or from the systemic effects of circulating factors released by the tumour cells.

Oestrogen

Sex hormone status and the pubertal growth spurt are important in determining bone mass at maturity. Con-versely, bone loss accelerates in the first years after the menopause as the skeleton adapts to declining oestrogen levels. In general, postmenopausal women who lose bone fastest have the lowest endogenous sex hormone levels. Although the skeletal role of oestrogens at the cellular level remains unclear, recent findings suggest that oestrogens may have a direct effect on osteoblastic cells.

Overview of Osteoporosis, Osteomalacia, Rickets and Osteopetrosis

Osteoporosis

Osteoporosis is the reduction of mineralized bone mass to the extent that fractures result from trivial trauma. It is the most common bone disease in Western societies where nutrition is adequate, and it has been estimated that 30% of all postmenopausal white women will sustain at least one osteoporotic fracture during life. The earliest fracture, generally occurring a decade after the menopause, is that of the distal radius (Colle's). Vertebral fractures tend to occur one decade later, and by 70, over 35% of white women will have sustained at least one such fracture. Many osteoporotic vertebral fractures heal readily and are asymptomatic, resulting only in height loss – so-called 'dowager's hump'. Hip fractures, which occur predominantly after the age of 75, are more serious, and incomplete healing and chronic pain mean that many hip fracture patients require prolonged institutional care.

Osteoporosis is less common amongst men (no increase in Colle's fracture, sevenfold fewer vertebral fractures), until cumulative age-related bone loss becomes significant.

Osteoporosis currently costs approximately £100 million in the UK, a cost that seems certain to increase as osteoporosis becomes more prevalent amongst an ageing and more sedentary population. *See* Osteoporosis

Osteomalacia and Rickets

Osteomalacia is a defect in bone mineralization resulting from either vitamin D deficiency or errors in the handling of this vitamin or its active metabolites. It results in bone pain, muscular weakness and increased fracture risk. Rickets is childhood osteomalacia and causes deformities in rapidly growing bones.

Vitamin D is mostly produced in the skin by sunlight irradiation of 7-dehydrocholesterol, although certain foods (e.g. fish oils) contain small amounts. Deficiency consequently results from either an inadequate exposure to sunlight (elderly or housebound individuals) or dietary lack of vitamin D. Treatment with vitamin D will usually cure these disorders.

Vitamin-D-resistant rickets is caused by an inherited defect in the cellular receptor for $1,25(OH)_2D_3$ that prevents cells from responding to vitamin D metabolites. The symptoms are similar to those of nutritional rickets but are associated with normal or elevated levels of $1,25(OH)_2D_3$. More rarely, errors in metabolism resulting genetic defects or disease prevent the production of the active vitamin D metabolites.

Osteopetrosis

Osteopetroses are a class of rare genetic disorders characterized by defective osteoclast function and a consequent failure of bone remodelling. Symptoms vary with severity but may include skeletal malformation with dense but fragile bones. Recurrent infection and spontaneous bleeding may result from the crowding out of the marrow cavity by unresorbed bone and mineralized cartilage.

Bibliography

Favus MJ (1990) *Primer on the Metabolic Bone Diseases and Disorders of Mineral Metabolism.* California: American Society for Bone and Mineral Research.
Goss RJ (1978) *The Physiology of Growth.* New York: Academic Press.
Ham AW (1969) *Histology* 6th edn. Philadelphia: Lippincott.
Riggs BL (1988) *Osteoporosis: Etiology, Diagnosis and Management.* New York: Raven Press.
Thomson BM and Loveridge N (1992) Bone growth. *The Control of Fat and Lean Deposition*, 51st University of Nottingham Easter School in Agricultural Science. Oxford: Butterworth Heinemann.
Vaughan JM (1970) *The Physiology of Bone.* Oxford: Clarendon Press.

B. M. Thomson
Rowett Research Institute, Aberdeen, UK

BORON

Boron is a light, nonmetallic element known to be essential for all vascular plants. Improvements in research technology have prompted renewed interest in determining the essentiality of boron for humans. Recent research findings show clearly that boron modifies, and possibly regulates, mineral and energy metabolism in humans and animals.

Biochemistry

Structure and Bonding

Boron, the fifth element in the periodic table, is the only nonmetal in group III. It has a ground state electronic configuration of $1s^22s^22p^1$ and is always trivalent. The element has an unusual chemistry as the result of its attempts to solve the problem of having fewer electrons (three) than atomic orbitals available for bonding (2s, $2p_x$, $2p_y$ and $2p_z$), a situation that is normally solved by metallic bonding. Because of the small size and high ionization energies of boron, the problem is solved by utilizing covalent bonding. In other words, simple electron loss to form a cation does not occur in boron chemistry; hybridization of the boron atomic orbitals to either the sp^2 or sp^3 configuration requires less energy.

Boron bonds with several elements to form either trigonal–planar (TP) or tetrahedral (TH) arrangements; the TP arrangement is preferred because it represents the stabilized mesomeric form. The TH arrangement arises from the tendency of boron to complete its outer shell of electrons to eight. Orthoboric acid, $B(OH)_3$, and the anionic borate, $B(OH)_4^-$, are examples of the TP and TH arrangements, respectively.

Boron does not occur free in geological formations nor binds directly to any element other than oxygen, with the possible exception of fluorine. The high affinity of boron for oxygen results in the biologically important borates and related oxo compounds. However, reactions between boron and other elements with electron pair donors would also be important in biological systems. Compounds with bonds between boron and sulphur, selenium, phosphorus, arsenic, antimony, carbon or nitrogen have been synthetically produced.

Boron Esters and Complexes

Partial esterification of boric acid yields many important boron esters characterized by the presence of the TP unit. At the same pH, the borate monoesters are easily hydrolysed whereas the diesters (structure **1**) are more stable. The ability of boron to form diesters is dependent upon the presence of hydroxyl groups in specific positions. Thus, because of the bond strain present in TP borate esters of 1,2-diols (structure **1**, $n=2$), only 1,3-diol (structure **1**, $n=3$) esters would be expected in aqueous solutions.

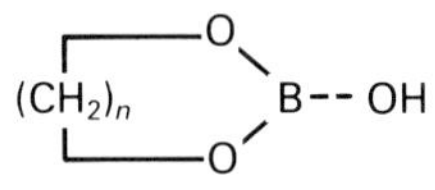

(1)

Several biologically important complexes are formed when boron links to four oxygen atoms (TH unit) contained by one or two biological ligands. Usually, the ligands contain adjacent hydroxyl groups in the *cis* position and reactivity generally increases with an increase in the number of those groups. Riboflavin and the pyridine nucleotides are examples of those ligands. The exact form of the complex varies according to pH and ligand:boron ratio (Structures **2–4**). The relevant

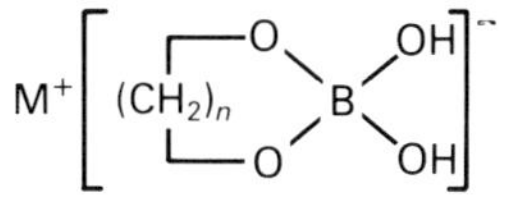

(2)

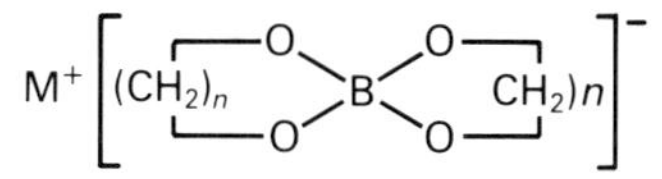

(3)

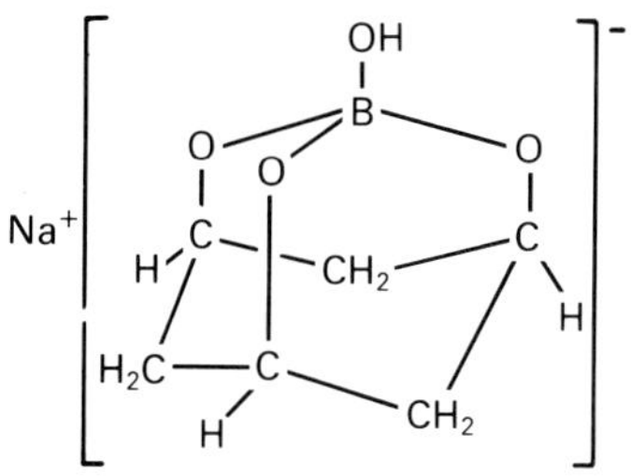

(4)

cisoid diol conformations are also present in several biologically important sugars and their derivatives (sugar alcohols, -onic and -uronic acids). Examples include mannose, ribose, galactose and fructose. The boration of dihydroxy ligands involves the uncharged $B(OH)_3$ and not the anion $B(OH)_4^-$. *See* Vitamin B_6, Properties and Determination; Riboflavin, Properties and Determination

A borate complex is sometimes formed without the presence of a *cisoid* diol group. For example, certain ring conformations in *trans*1,2-diols favour complex formation with boron. Also, hydroxyl groups arising from lactol formation (in glucose, α-D form only), hydration of carboxyl groups (in α-hydroxy, i.e. lactic and aromatic *o*-hydroxy acids, e.g. salicylic acid), or hydration of ketone groups (in benzil or alloxan) are reactive with $B(OH)_3$. A tridentate complex may be formed when a ligand contains three *cis*-oriented hydroxyl groups (structure **4**). A diborate complex of tridenate structure is also possible (not shown). Substitution of one or more of the hydroxyl groups coordinated with boron, or substitution of individual hydrogens in those hydroxyl groups, gives rise to many classes of cyclic coordination complexes.

Although attempts to isolate boron esters and complexes from biological systems have generally been unsuccessful, it is obvious that boron could react with a large number of substrate molecules, metabolites or enzymes. Four naturally occurring boron oxy compounds have been identified; they are all ionophoric macrodiolide antibiotics. Boromycin (structure **5**), synthesized by certain strains of *Streptomyces antibioticus*,

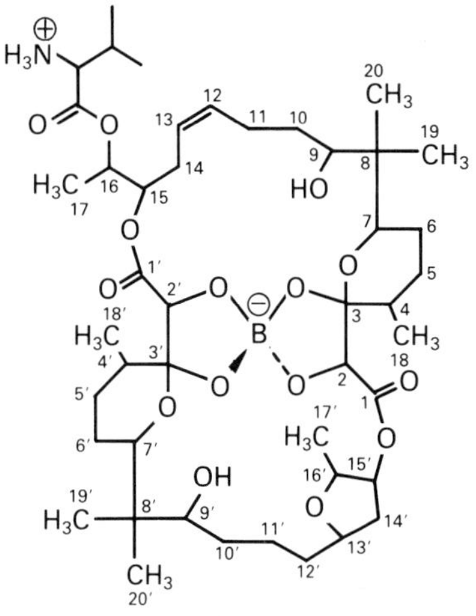

(5)

has the ability to encapsulate alkali metal cations and reduce the permeability barrier of the cytoplasmic membrane toward potassium ions. Structure **6** depicts aplasmomycin A ($R=R=H$), B ($R=COCH_3$, $R=H$) and C ($R=R=COCH_3$), which are closely related antibiotics isolated from strain SS-20 of *Streptomyces*

442 Boron

(6)

griseus obtained from a shallow sea sediment. The structures of all of these antibiotics show that boron is bound to four oxy groups.

Isotopes

Tracer studies for the determination of boron uptake and excretion in biological systems are hampered by the lack of usable radioisotopes: ^{8}B, ^{12}B and ^{13}B all have half-lives of less than 1 s. However, the two stable boron isotopes, ^{10}B and ^{11}B, are distributed equally in nature (19·8 and 80·2%, respectively). Attempts are being made to exploit this phenomenon for the determination of boron body pool size and distribution by isotopic dilution mass spectroscopy. ^{10}B has a very large cross-section for thermal neutron capture and this property has been used in neutron capture therapy (NCT) for inoperable brain tumours. During NCT, a boronated compound, preferentially bound to the tumour cells, is irradiated with thermal neutrons. Following neutron capture, the energy is released as a γ ray, α particle and lithium nucleus, the latter two travelling 9 and 5 μm, respectively. Thus, heavily ionizing radiation is deposited in single, targeted cells with mineral collateral damage. *See* Mass Spectrometry, Principles and Instrumentation

Occurrence in the Environment

Anthropomorphic Sources

Boron, in the form of borax, has been used since Egyptian and Roman times for the preparation of hard (borosilicate) glasses. At present, 30–35% of mined boron compounds are used in the manufacture of heat-resistant glasses (e.g. Pyrex), glass wool and fibreglass.

Boron is also used in the manufacture of detergents, soaps, cleaners, cosmetics (15–20%), porcelain enamels (15%), synthetic herbicides and fertilizers (10%), and for other unrelated processes including nuclear shielding, metallurgy, corrosion control, leather tanning, flame proofing and catalysis (30%).

Soil

Boron is not an abundant element but is universally distributed in soils. There are only a few commercially valuable geological deposits. These are located in areas of former volcanic activity and can be associated with the waters of former hot springs. Within geological boron deposits, the element is usually present as a borate mineral such as borax, $Na_2B_4O_5(OH_4 \cdot 8H_2O)$. The largest single natural deposit of boron is located at Boron, California.

The total boron content of soils is extremely variable (igneous rocks, 10 μg g^{-1}; marine shales, 300 μg g^{-1}; metamorphic rock, > 1000 μg g^{-1}) and depends upon the type of soil, the amount of rainfall, and the amount of soil organic matter. A 1956 survey of US soils indicated an average total boron content of 30 μg g^{-1}. The amount of soil boron available to plants is less than 5% of the total soil boron. To be available to plants, boron must be released from soil minerals, converted to an inorganic form (mineralized) from decomposed organic matter, or artificially added to soils (irrigation or fertilization), and subsequently distributed between the solid and liquid phases of the soil. Boron deficiency in plants is more common than deficiency of any other micronutrient because boron is easily leached out of soils by rainwater. Thus, plant boron deficiency is of concern in humid regions with light-textured, acid soil.

Water

The concentration of boron in seawater is 4·5 μg ml^{-1} (0·42 μmol ml^{-1}). Various analyses show that the concentration of boron in surface waters varies within and between countries (values in μg ml^{-1}; in parentheses, μmol ml^{-1}): UK, 0·046–0·822 (0·004–0·077); Italy, 0·400–1·00 (0·037–0·093); Sweden, 0·001–1·046 (0·00009–0·098); the FRG, 0·100–2·00 (0·009–0·187); the USA, 0·001–5 (0·00009–0·467). Shallow groundwater in the San Joaquin Valley region of California may have boron concentrations as high as 120 μg ml^{-1} (11·2 μmol ml^{-1}). Sewage effluent, which sometimes contains boron levels as high as 5 μg ml^{-1} (0·467 μmol ml^{-1}), can be an important source of boron, especially in areas where boron compounds are major constituents of detergent products. Waste water used for irrigation in the USA or Europe often contains boron concentrations between 0·13 (0·012) and 2·8 μg ml^{-1} (0·26 μmol ml^{-1}).

The US Department of the Interior has established 1 μg ml^{-1} (0·093 μmol ml^{-1}) as the upper limit for boron in public water supplies. If all beverages consumed contained that amount of boron, then calculations from beverage intake tables indicate that a 14–16 or 60–65-year-old US woman would consume 800 (74·7) or 1250 μg (117 μmol) boron per day, respectively, from beverages alone. Surface water samples from the Casa Diablo area in California contained 8·41 μg (0·784 μmol) of boron per millilitre; at that concentration, the beverage contribution could conceivably be 6860 (640) or 10 400 μg (971 mmol) boron per day for the same respective individuals.

Foods

Most reported values for the concentration of boron in foods are of questionable validity because of analytical insensitivity or inadvertently unsuitable sample preparation as discussed below. A recent survey (Table 1) indicates that the concentration of elemental boron in animal muscle and milk is essentially negligible. Salted meats or products with added plant matter, e.g. ice cream, contain measurable amounts of boron, but those amounts are considerably lower than those in many plants.

Vegetarians, compared to nonvegetarians, typically consume more boron because of their higher intake of fruits and vegetables. However, the source of plant foodstuffs is important when calculating individual boron intake because the concentration of boron in plants varies with soil type, length of exposure, rate of transpiration, and different agricultural practices. Furthermore, boron is unequally distributed within Angiospermae, the class of plants most often utilized in human and animal diets. For example, most species within the subclass Dicotyledoneae, which includes fruits, vegetables, tubers and legumes, have much higher concentrations of boron than do species in the subclass Monocotyledoneae, which includes the grasses, e.g. corn, rice and wheat (Table 1). The different content of boron in broccoli stalks and flowers illustrates the compartmentalization of the element even within the same species. Boron is also a significant contaminant or major ingredient of many nonfood, ingested, personal care products. *See* Vegetarian Diets

Diets representing the intake of 25–30-year-old adult US males were found recently to supply 1·52 mg of boron daily. The daily intake of boron often differs considerably between any two individuals because the concentration of boron in water varies considerably according to geographic source and invididual food preference also greatly influences daily intake of boron.

Table 1. Concentration of boron in selected foods (fresh wet weight)[a]

Food	μg per 100 g
Animal products	
Beef, round, ground, raw	≤1·5[b]
Chicken, breast, ground, raw	≤1·5
Ice cream, vanilla	19·2 + 3·0[c]
Milk, 2%	≤1·5
Cereal grain products	
Bread, white, enriched	20·2 + 7·0
Cookie, shortbread	≤1·5
Cornflakes, fortified	31·4 + 7·9
Rice, white, instant, prepared	≤1·5
Spaghetti, dry, enriched	≤1·5
Condiments	
Bouillon, beef, dry	126·4 + 60·9
Catsup	85·0 + 10·6
Confections	
Gelatin, raspberry, prepared	≤1·5
Jelly, grape	147·0 + 9·2
Sugar, white, granulated	≤1·5
Fruits and fruit beverages	
Apple juice, bottled, 100% natural	188 + 8
Apple sauce, bottled, 100% natural	283 + 12
Cherries, dark, unsweetened, frozen	147 + 24
Coffee, freeze-dried, reconstituted	4·8 + 1·7
Lemon juice, frozen, unsweetened	≤1·5
Orange juice, reconstituted from concentrate	41·0 + 1·4
Peaches, canned in water, drained	187 + 11
Pears, canned in water, drained	122 + 4
Pineapple juice, reconstituted from concentrate	26·8 + 11·2
Tuberized roots	
Carrots, canned in water, drained	75·0 + 5·9
Potatoes, sliced, canned, drained	17·2 + 6·5
Dicotyledon plant seeds, pods, stalks, bark and leaves	
Beans, green, frozen	46·1 + 13·3
Broccoli, flowers, frozen	185 + 40
Broccoli, stalks, frozen	88·9 + 3·9
Cinnamon, ground	1080 + 70
Lettuce, iceberg	≤1·5
Parsley flakes, dried	2690 + 180

[a] Data from Hunt CD, Shuler TR and Mullen LM (1991) Concentration of boron and other elements in human foods and personal care products. *Journal of the American Diabetic Association* 91: 558–568.
[b] Detection limit of analytical instrumentation (inductively coupled argon plasma emission spectroscopy).
[c] Mean ± standard deviation.

Chemical Properties of Boron Relevant to Foods

Boron Metabolism and Speciation in Foods and Water

In most natural freshwater systems, the predominant species of boron, regardless of its initial formulation, is undissociated boric acid. However, borate does form ion pairs with the cations present in natural waters with stability constants decreasing in the order $Mg^{2+} > Ca^{2+} > Sr^{2+} > Li^+ > Na^+$. Thus, in hard waters with relatively large amounts of calcium, formation of ion pairs between Ca^{2+} and $B(OH)_4^-$ may affect the speciation of boron.

The speciation of boron in foods has not been determined but is probably complex and dependent upon the nature of the integral ligands. If plant and animal boron absorption mechanisms are analogous, the organic forms of boron *per se* are probably unavailable to animals; the organic forms of boron in soil from decomposed organic matter are not immediately available to plants and can only be absorbed after subsequent mineralization. However, the strong association between polyhydroxyl ligands and boron is easily and rapidly reversed by dialysis, change in pH, heat or the excess addition of another low-molecular-weight polyhydroxyl ligand. Thus, within the intestinal tract, most ingested boron is probably converted to $B(OH)_3$, the normal end product of hydrolysis of most boron compounds. $B(OH)_3$ acts exclusively as a monobasic acid by hydroxyl ion acceptance rather than proton donation (eqn [1]). Therefore, at physiological concentrations of inorganic boron, essentially only the mononuclear species $B(OH)_3$ and $B(OH)_4^-$ are present and, within the normal pH range of the gut, $B(OH)_3$ would prevail as the dominant species (pH 1, $\sim 100\%$ $B(OH)_3$; pH 9·25, 50%; pH 11, $\sim 0\%$). Inorganic boron is absorbed well from the gastrointestinal tract and it is postulated that boron is absorbed and excreted mainly as undissociated $B(OH)_3$.

$$B(OH)_3 + 2H_2O \rightarrow H_3O^+ + B(OH)_4^- \quad pK_a = 9 \cdot 25 \ (25°C) \quad (1)$$

Homeostatic control of boron metabolism is suggested by the presence of significant amounts of boron in the faeces, the rapid urinary excretion of ingested inorganic boron compounds, and the lack of excessive accumulation of boron in tissues. Plasma boron concentrations were similar in cholecalciferol-deficient chicks fed 0·481 mg or less of boron per kilogram of feed whereas increased amounts of dietary boron elevated plasma boron concentrations progressively. Female rats consuming water high in boron (100 mg l^{-1}) for 21 days exhibited increased plasma boron concentrations although some type of homeostatic mechanism concurrently eliminated any excess of boron from the liver and

brain against their own concentration gradients. In cows, the percentage of filtered boron reabsorbed by the kidneys decreased significantly with increased boron intake.

Effects of Food Processing

Foods cooked in boiling water are quickly leached of boron. This loss could conceivably be further enhanced during pressure cooking with chlorinated or fluorinated water; boron–halogen compounds are extremely volatile at high temperatures.

Boron Nutrition

Plants

The vascular plants have acquired a unique requirement for boron. Boron seems to be involved in such diverse cellular processes as sugar biosynthesis and translocation, protein synthesis, nucleic acid metabolism, cell division and cell wall synthesis. The element may also interact with various hormones and phenolic compounds in the plant. Also, recent evidence suggests that boron is involved in plant cell wall membrane function. Thus, even though all vascular plants have an absolute requirement for boron, the primary role and mode of action of boron, if any, remain unknown.

Animals

Interest in boron in animal nutrition was renewed in the early 1980s when dietary boron was found to alleviate growth depression in cholecalciferol-deficient poultry. It is now established that physiological concentrations (no more than quantities ingested by vegetarians) of dietary boron affect mineral and energy metabolism in poultry, rats and humans. Those effects are more pronounced when a physiological stressor is present (e.g. cholecalciferol or magnesium deficiency, aluminium toxicity, streptozotocin injection or strenuous aerobic exercise). For example, dietary boron alleviated some of the symptoms of cholecalciferol deficiency in chicks (Fig. 1). The effect was modified by magnesium nutrition. Thus, in the cholecalciferol-deficient chick fed inadequate amounts of magnesium, boron (3 μg g^{-1} (0·28 μmol g^{-1}) enhanced growth but inhibited the initiation of cartilage calcification in the tibial epiphysial growth plate. Dietary boron had the opposite effects in the magnesium-adequate chick. Regardless of magnesium status, the boron supplement alleviated the cholecalciferol deficiency-induced distortion of the marrow sprouts in the same growth plate and increased the

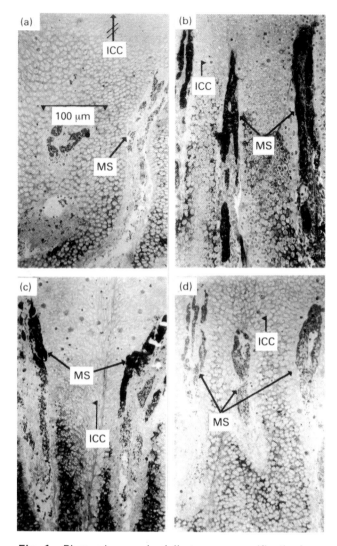

Fig. 1 Photomicrographs (all at same magnification) depicting marrow sprout (MS) orientation and initiation of cartilage calcification (ICC) in the chick proximal tibial epiphysial plate. ICC beyond a frame is denoted by slashed arrows. Boron supplementation corrected the cholecalciferol deficiency-induced disorientation of the MS (compare (a) and (b), and (c) and (d)). ICC is inhibited by boron in magnesium inadequacy (compare (a) and (c)), but enhanced in magnesium adequacy (compare (c) and (d)). Dietary supplements (milligrams per kilogram of diet): (a) B, 0; Mg, 300; (b) B, 3; Mg, 300; (c) B, 0; Mg, 500; (d) B, 3; Mg, 500. (Data from Hunt CD (1989) Dietary boron modified the effects of magnesium and molybdenum on mineral metabolism in the cholecalciferol-deficient chick. *Biological Trace Element Research* 22: 201–220.)

numbers of osteoclasts within the marrow sprouts. *See* Bone; Cholecalciferol, Physiology; Magnesium

Postmenopausal women fed a basal diet which supplied 0·25 mg (23 μmol) of boron per 2000 kcal exhibited decreased urinary loss of calcium and magnesium after a supplement of 3 mg (0·28 mmol) of boron per day was given for 48 days. The effect was more pronounced during concurrent magnesium inadequacy. Boron supplementation also affected indices of mineral metabolism in another human study described in the 'trace elements' article. *See* Biomineralization; Osteoporosis; Trace Elements

Several indices of energy metabolism, as measured in blood, are affected by boron. For example, physiological amounts of boron decreased glucose in chicks and humans, increased triglycerides in rats and humans, and decreased aspartate transaminase and creatine kinase activity in rats. Those affects could be mediated in part through the influence of boron on certain enzymes. Two classes of enzymes are competitively inhibited *in vitro* by borate or its derivatives. One class, the oxidoreductase enzymes which require pyridine or flavin nucleotides (e.g. aldehyde dehydrogenase, xanthine dehydrogenase or cytochrome-b_5 reductase) are inhibited as borate competes for the NAD, or flavin cofactor. Borate apparently complexes with the ribosyl *cis*-hydroxy groups of NAD. The other class forms transition state analogues with borate and boronic acid derivatives. The serine proteases (e.g. chymotrypsin) or glyceraldehyde-3-phosphate dehydrogenases are important examples. *See* Energy, Measurement of Food Energy; Enzymes, Functions and Characteristics; Glucose, Function and Metabolism; Triglycerides, Structures and Properties; Coenzymes

Because research findings show clearly that boron modifies mineral and energy metabolism, efforts are being made to demonstrate that boron deficiency reproducibly impairs a biological function from optimal to suboptimal. It is likely that boron is involved in a number of metabolic pathways because it has the ability to complex with a large number of compounds containing hydroxyl groups (e.g. several water-soluble vitamins, sugars and their derivatives, proteins, enzymes, hydroxylated steroids). In other words, it is possible that boron acts as an unobtrusive metabolic regulator by quenching the activity of some enzymes and/or stabilizing reactive compounds. *See* Ascorbic Acid, Properties and Determination; Vitamins, Overview

Toxicity

As with all other elements, boron produces toxicity in all tested biological organisms when excessive amounts are absorbed. Interestingly, boron becomes toxic to many plant species when soil solution boron concentrations are only slightly greater than those required for normal growth. However, tolerance to boron soil solution concentrations varies considerably among plant species. Borax was long used as a food preservative because it prevents rancidity in butter and meats. After Lister first used boric acid as an antiseptic in 1875, boric acid and/

or borax were used in a variety of pharmaceutical applications for many years. In lieu of antibiotics, the associated toxicity of boric acid, when used as an antiseptic on abraded epithelium (e.g. surgical wounds, abscesses, burns, diaper rash, and ulcers), was overlooked for many years even though signs of poisoning were reported soon after its introduction into clinical use. Boron is more of a bacteriostat than bacteriocide and as such is not sufficient for most modern usage.

The minimum lethal dose of boron for humans has not been established although single doses of 18–20 g in adults have been fatal. Signs of acute boron toxicity, regardless of route of administration, include nausea, vomiting, headache, diarrhoea, erythema, hypothermy, restlessness, weariness, desquamation, renal injury, and death from circulatory collapse and shock. Autopsy may reveal congestion and oedema of brain, myocardium, lungs and other organs, with fatty infiltration of the liver. Chronic boron toxicity symptoms include poor appetite, nausea, weight loss, decreased sexual activity, seminal volume, sperm count and motility, and increased seminal fructose. In one case, daily ingestion of 25 g of boric tartrate over a period of 20 years resulted in cachexia, dermatitis, alopecia, hypoplastic anaemia and gastric ulcer. At present, death from boron poisoning is exceptionally rare, probably because of the emphasis placed on maintaining electrolyte balance and supporting kidney function during the worst part of the illness. Depending upon blood boron concentrations, treatment ranges from observation to gastric lavage to dialysis.

Boron Analysis

Sample Digestion, Extraction, Isolation and Clean-up

Except for neutron activation analysis, all methods of boron analysis require dissolution of the sample. Thermal ionization mass spectrometry also requires a boron extraction step by ion exchange chromatography or distillation prior to analysis. Many boron compounds volatize at temperatures far below those required for most dry-ashing procedures; these include the extremely volatile boron halides. Bomb digestion technology prevents loss of volatized boron but typically introduces dilution of the digestate. Sequestration of boron during dry ashing with ashing agents (e.g. barium hydroxide or calcium oxide) is often unsuccessful as those agents usually contain concentrations of boron high enough to interfere with boron determination or leave unacceptable amounts of solid chemical residue in the final digestate. Alkali fusion methods for boron sequestration may cause damage to metal crucibles or loss of sample through splattering. The use of borosilicate glass

digestion vessels is unacceptable for obvious reasons but, surprisingly, is sometimes overlooked. The cost of boron-free digestion vessels such as pure metal (e.g. zirconium or platinum) or quartz crucibles is usually prohibitive. Most wet-ashing methods employ the use of either perchloric or hydrofluoric acid, both of which have extremely toxic and/or explosive qualities. Newer digestion procedures circumvent many of the problems associated with boron analysis. Samples are placed in Teflon tubes embedded in a hot sand bath (150°C) and subsequently are oxidized by high-purity nitric acid and hydrogen peroxide. The aqueous environment and low constant boiling point of nitric acid (120·5°C) minimizes boron volatilization.

Methods of Analysis

The difficult nature of boron analysis is exemplified by the fact that there is no reference biomaterial certified for boron by the US National Institute of Standards and Technology. Several common analytical methods and/or associated clean-up procedures are dependent upon the exact speciation of boron in a given sample, usually either $B(OH)_3$ or $B(OH)_4{}^-$. Inductively coupled argon plasma spectroscopy–mass spectrometry (ICP–MS) is one of the most sensitive (10 pg ml^{-1}) and accurate, although expensive, methods for the determination of boron in biomaterials. Boron colorimetric methods measure the visible absorbance peak of various boron complexes (e.g. methylene blue–tetrafluoroborate). These assays require that boron be present as undissociated $B(OH)_3$ because only that species complexes with a given assay ligand (e.g. curcumin, carminic acid, azomethine H). Also, various interferants (e.g. Cu^{2+}, Al^{3+}, Fe^{3+}, K^+, F^- or V^{5+}), when present, react with boron or with the free molecules of the ligand; additional clean-up procedures are required in those situations. Conductivity detection methods of boron polyol compounds after ion exclusion chromatographic separation are also dependent upon correct boron speciation. Atomic absorption spectrometry (AAS) requires that all the boron is converted to the elemental form. Certain boron compounds (e.g. the boron carbides) are stable to 3000°C, a temperature above that produced by a graphite furnace. Neutron activation (NA) of ^{10}B, followed by either mass spectrometry (NA–MS) or prompt γ ray spectrometry (NA–PGAA) is a very sensitive and nondestructive measure of boron concentration *per se*. However, this technology requires access to a working nuclear reactor and also assumes that the ^{10}B:^{11}B ratio in each sample is 'normal'.

Inductively coupled argon plasma atomic emission spectroscopy (ICP-AES) is relatively inexpensive, provides acceptable sensitivity (15 ng g^{-1}) for most biomaterials, and provides acceptable accuracy because most boron speciation problems are circumvented in both the clean-up and analytical phases of the procedure.

Bibliography

Green NN (1973) Boron. In: Bailar JC, Emeléus HJ, Nyholm R and Trotman-Dickenson AF (eds) *Comprehensive Inorganic Chemistry*, pp 665–991. Oxford: Pergamon Press.

Gupta UC, Jame YW, Campbell CA, Leyshon AJ and Nicholaichuk W (1985) Boron toxicity and deficiency: a review. *Canadian Journal of Soil Science* 65: 381–409.

Hunt CD and Shuler TR (1989) Open-vessel, wet-ash, low-temperature digestion of biological materials for inductively coupled argon plasma spectroscopy (ICAP) analysis of boron and other elements. *Journal of Micronutrient Analysis* 6: 161–174.

Johnson SL and Smith KW (1976) The interaction of borate and sulfite with pyridine nucleotides. *Biochemistry* 15: 553–559.

Nielsen FH, Hunt CD, Mullen LM and Hunt JR (1987) Effect of dietary boron on mineral, estrogen, and testosterone metabolism in postmenopausal women. *FASEB Journal* 1: 394–397.

Lovatt CJ and Dugger WM (1984) Boron. In: Frieden E (ed.) *Biochemistry of the Essential Ultratrace Elements*, pp 389–421. New York: Plenum Press.

Somers TC, White JD, Lee JJ, Keller PJ, Change C-J and Floss HG (1986) NMR analysis of boromycin sodium complex and sodium desvalinoboromycinate. *Journal of Organic Chemistry* 51: 464–471.

C. D. Hunt
Grand Forks Human Nutrition Research Center, Grand Forks, USA

BOTULISM

See Clostridium

BOURBON

See Whisky, Whiskey and Bourbon

BOVINE SPONGIFORM ENCEPHALOPATHY (BSE)

Bovine spongiform encephalopathy is a progressive, fatal, neurological disease of cattle which was first confirmed by brain histology in November 1986 in the UK. By June 1991, there were about 29 000 confirmed cases in the UK. The source of infection was meat and bone meal containing the causative agent incorporated into concentrate rations and fed largely to calves. Meat and bone meal is prepared from animal waste obtained largely from abattoirs and butcher's shops, by a heat process of industrial rendering and has been fed to farm animals over several decades without harmful effect. However, it appears that scrapie agent from sheep and, subsequently, the agent from cattle affected with BSE, escaped destruction by the rendering processes as a result of a change in a number of factors concerning the raw material and methods of processing. In particular, there was a sudden large reduction, in 1981/1982 onwards, in the amount of meat and bone meal produced by the hydrocarbon solvent extraction system. Thus increase in exposure of cattle in the period between 1981/1982 and July 1988 (when the feeding of ruminant protein to ruminants was banned) resulted in the appearance of clinical disease in 1985/1986. Between then and July 1988, recycling of infected cattle waste fuelled the epidemic.

The disease, which predominates in dairy rather than beef cattle because of the different methods of feeding calves, presents as progressive abnormalities of behaviour, sensation, posture and gait, with accompanying loss of weight and milk yield. The predominating neurological signs of BSE are apprehension, hyperaesthesia and gait ataxia. Insidious in their onset, neurological signs may increase in variety, and specific signs may worsen with time. The clinical course may run an unusually rapid progression of 2 weeks. More commonly, the course lasts several months and may rarely extend to over a year.

Initially, disease may be suspected because of changes in behaviour such as the animal becoming separated from the rest of the herd, being reluctant to enter the milking parlour, being unusually aggressive to herd mates and indulging in unprovoked kicking during milking. Hind limb hypermetria (exaggerated lifting of limbs), a trotting action when forcibly driven, difficulty in turning and a tendency to fall, with difficulty in rising, are also features. There is increased sensitivity to sound and touch, and ears may be moved constantly. There may be excessive licking of nostrils or flanks, or teeth grinding and low moaning sounds may be emitted. The head is often carried low with a vacant stare, the back arched and hind limbs widely separated. Some cows drink by lapping rather than sucking. The early signs should be differentiated from nervous ketosis or hypomagnesaemia by clinical biochemical methods. Gait ataxia becomes progressively worse, with lateral swaying prominent, and may lead finally to permanent recumbency, resulting in problems of welfare. However, most cases are now detected early in the clinical course and killed before such problems develop.

The lesions of the disease are restricted to the brain, which under the microscope shows vacuolar (spongy) change (Fig. 1) and neuronal vacuolation (Fig. 2) in the grey matter of specific sites, especially in the brain stem. Clinical diagnosis is confirmed postmortem by recognition of these changes in the fixed brain. There is a standardized method of diagnosis within the European Economic Community (EEC), and other countries too are adopting this method which was established first in the UK. Essentially, the brain, or if appropriate the hind brain, is removed from the skull, fixed in formalin, sliced and embedded in paraffin wax, from which sections are cut and then stained for microscopy.

There are other methods which can be used to detect affected animals and which are used more for research

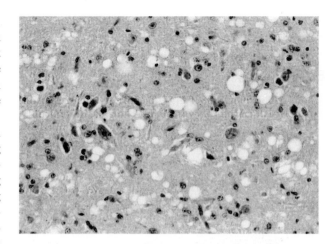

Fig. 1   Spongiform change of grey matter neuropil. Stain: haematoxylin–eosin (HE); ×134. (Crown Copyright, supplied with kind permission of Mr GAH Wells.)

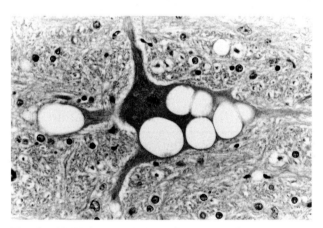

Fig. 2   Multiple vacuolation of a neuron. Stain: HE; ×208. (Crown Copyright, supplied with kind permission of Mr GAH Wells.)

purposes. These include immuno-blotting procedures to detect the abnormal form of host protein (PrP), which is found in the fresh unfixed brain of affected animals. Chemically produced aggregates of this protein, called scrapie-associated fibrils (Fig. 3), can be observed by electron microscopy following detergent extraction, proteinase K treatment and electron-dense staining of fresh unfixed brain tissue from specific sites. There is no test which can be used to detect infection of the live animal, although extensive research is continuing to develop such a test.

Bovine spongiform encephalopathy is a notifiable disease in the UK, EEC and some other European countries. Control of the notifiable disease is effected by compulsory slaughter and destruction of the carcass; in

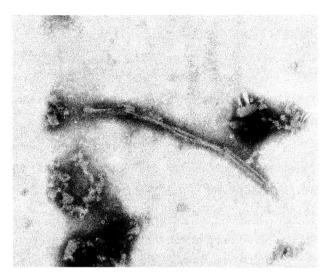

Fig. 3 Fibril (scrapie-associated fibril, SAF) in a brain extract from a cow affected by BSE; ×98 000. (Crown Copyright, supplied with kind permission of Mr AC Scott.)

the UK, in healthy animals over 6 months old, there is a ban on certain specified offals, or protein derived from them, for feeding to any animal or bird. These offals are brain, spinal cord, tonsil, thymus, spleen and intestine. Based on our knowledge of the comparable disease in sheep (scrapie), there is no detectable infectivity in milk or muscle (meat). As in scrapie, there is no evidence to suggest that BSE can be transmitted to humans by any means. Beef from healthy animals can be freely traded within the EEC subject to certain conditions. Live calves for veal can also be traded, provided that they are killed before they are 6 months old and are not the offspring of suspected or confirmed infected dams. *See* Beef

There has been no demonstrable transmission between cattle, each case having been the result of independent feed exposure. There is one exception, when one animal born after the feed ban (July 1988) and the offspring of an affected case had BSE confirmed in 1991. The source of infection is probably not food. However, a controlled experiment using 316 pairs of cattle from BSE-affected herds shows no case of BSE to date, despite some animals being over 3 years of age. One member of each pair is the offspring of a BSE case, the other a control. It is predicted that, as a result of the control measures introduced, and provided that no cattle-to-cattle transmission occurs, the monthly incidence figures will decline from 1992 onwards and BSE will become extinct in the UK before the end of the century.

The incidence of BSE is much lower in Northern Ireland, lower still in the Republic of Ireland, and sporadic in Switzerland and France where controls are in place. Two cases have occurred in Oman and one in the Falkland Islands, each of which was imported in the incubating stage from the UK.

Bibliography

Bradley R (1990) Bovine spongiform encephalopathy: the need for knowledge, balance, patience and action. (Editorial) *Journal of Pathology* 160: 283–285.

The Southwood Report (1989) *Report of the Working Party on Bovine Spongiform Encephalopathy*. London: Department of Health and Ministry of Agriculture, Fisheries and Food.

The Tyrrell Report (1989) *Consultative Committee on Research into Spongiform Encephalopathies. Interim Report*. London: MAFF Publications.

Wells GAH, Scott AC, Johnson CT *et al.* (1987) A novel progressive spongiform encephalopathy in cattle. *Veterinary Record* 121: 419–420.

Wells GAH, Wilesmith JW and McGill IS (1991) Review. Bovine spongiform encephalopathy: a neuropathological perspective. *Brain Pathology* 1: 69–78.

Wilesmith JW, Ryan JBM and Atkinson MJ (1991) Bovine spongiform encephalopathy. Epidemiological studies on the origin. *Veterinary Record* 128: 199–203.

Wilesmith JW, Wells GAH, Cranwell MP and Ryan JBM (1988) Bovine spongiform encephalopathy. Epidemiological studies. *Veterinary Record* 123: 638–644.

R. Bradley
Central Veterinary Laboratory, Weybridge, UK

BRANDY AND COGNAC

Contents

Brandy and its Manufacture*

Brandy is a distillate of fermented grape juice (wine) matured in wooden barrels. It is produced in a large number of countries in Europe (France, Spain, Portugal, Italy, the FRG, Cyprus and Russia), the USA, South America (Chile), Israel and South Africa. The most well-known production areas are undoubtedly Cognac and Armagnac in France. Therefore, these types of brandies and their production processes will be used to illustrate the manufacture of grape brandy.

Raw materials, vinification, distillation methods, maturation and blending are factors that determine the final quality of a brandy.

Method of Manufacture

Raw Materials

The raw material for the production of brandy is usually white grapes. Cognac and Armagnac consist of 80–90% of distillates which are produced from the Ugni Blanc grape. The popularity of that cultivar is based on its relatively high yield and its resistance against rot. The disadvantage of this cultivar, compared to traditional varieties such as Colombard and Folle Blanche, is its poor and relatively neutral aroma. This might partly be the effect of a lack of ripeness of the relatively late-ripening Ugni Blanc grapes.

Only grapes of a sound quality should be used for the production of brandies. The grapes are harvested mostly mechanically, and good logistics are essential in order to avoid oxidation of the harvested material.

Vinification

Depending on the vine growers opinion and expertise, different methods of vinification are applied. In some cases, dry yeasts are used to start the first fermentation of the season, but the application of selected yeast varieties is still limited and is only slowly increasing.

*The colour plate section for this article appears between p. 556 and p. 557.

This use of selected yeasts leads to a more constant quality level of product, and also limits the growth of undesirable microorganisms. The flavour of wines and distillates is strongly influenced by the type of yeast.

Wines for brandy production have not necessarily undergone malolactic fermentation, but it is generally recommended that wine should not be distilled while the malolactic fermentation is still proceeding. *See* Wines, Production of Table Wines

Distillation

The distillation process is one of the most important steps in the production of brandy, because here the composition of the aroma constituents is taking place.

Two types of distillation process are applicable to the production of brandy – batch and continuous.

Batch Distillation

In Cognac, the 'alambic charantais' process is applied. A schematic drawing of this distillation system is given in Fig. 1. The distillates are produced by a double distillation. First the wine is distilled to a raw distillate with an alcoholic strength of 26–32% (v/v). This product, called 'broullies' in Cognac, is subsequently distilled to a product of 67–72% (v/v). The distillation sequence involves the collection of a 'head', a 'heart' and a 'seconds' fraction, and quality of the distillate depends strongly on the skill and experience of the distiller. The 'seconds' fraction is recycled back into the process stream; depending on the procedure, it is added either to the wine or the 'brouillis' before distillation.

Continuous Distillation

In the production areas of Armagnac, continuous distillation is preferred to the batch system; about 90% of Armagnac is produced with the continuous still. In terms of energy and services, continuous distillation is more economic and faster than batch distillation. Distillates produced by means of continuous distillation are regarded as being richer in flavour than products from a pot still. A schematic drawing of an Armagnac still is presented in Fig. 2. Wines can be distilled with or

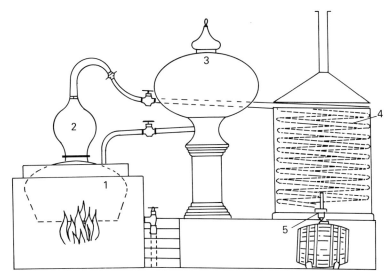

Fig. 1. Schematic drawing of a batch distillation system. Key: 1, boiler (chaudiere), (capacity—25 hl (for the first distillation, systems with a capacity of 120 hl are also employed); heating (direct heating with gas or wood); 2, helm (chapiteau); 3, preheater (rechauffe vin) (not included in all systems; wine can be heated to 40–50°C); 4, cooling system (serpentin) (the temperature varies in this system from 70–80°C in the top of the cooler to 10–20°C at the bottom); 5, effluent port (porte alcometre) (at this point the alcoholic strength of the distillate can be measured).

without their yeast deposit, but wines distilled with a certain amount of yeast contain higher amounts of volatiles, particularly ethyl esters of aliphatic acids. These components are released from the yeast cells, and while they give the product a heavy body, they do not provide it with a fresh or flower-like aroma.

Maturation

The maturation of the distillate in wooden barrels is an essential step in the production process of brandy. During maturation, the relatively sharp/raw odour and taste of fresh distillates are transformed into rounded, soft mellow flavours. The barrels used for the maturation of brandy are made of oak wood. In France, wood is taken from oaks grown in the Limousine and Troncais areas. The barrels have a volum of about 250 litres. Most brandies are matured for a period of 1–5 years, but some may be matured for several decades.

During the maturation period, compounds are extracted from the inner surface of the barrel. A number of substances, such as tannins, are extracted as such from the wood, but others are reaction and degradation products. The most important in this latter group of compounds are the phenolic aldehydes (e.g. vanillin, syringaldehyde, coniferaldehyde and sinapaldehyde) and their corresponding acids all being degradation products of ethanolysed lignin. They are regarded as the key components responsible for the mature character of brandy. The flavour of the mature product is strongly influenced by the age of the barrel, storage conditions (temperature, humidity), alcoholic strength of the distil-

late and, naturally, the period of maturation. *See* Phenolic Compounds; Tannins and Polyphenols

The mature character of brandy can also be increased by the application of wood extracts. Practice has shown that it is very difficult to produce a wood extract that provides a sensory character that is similar to that of a traditionally matured product. The problem in most cases is the balance between the direct extraction products and the degradation products. The application of wood extracts is very attractive from an economic point of view because it shortens the maturation period. This implies that less storage capacity is needed, and the loss of alcohol by evaporation (approximately 3% (v/v) per year) can be prevented. *See* Barrels

Composition of Brandy

Brandy is a product that contains a large number of volatile constituents. A complete review of these compounds and their concentration levels is presented in the compilation *Volatile Compounds in Foods, Qualitative and Quantitative Data* (see the Bibliography).

Defects

As mentioned earlier, brandy can be regarded as a product that has gone through a number of biochemical and physical steps from the grape in the vineyard to the bottle that is carefully opened in front of the fire place. During these steps, a number of factors can have a negative influence on the quality of the product. These

Brandy and its Manufacture

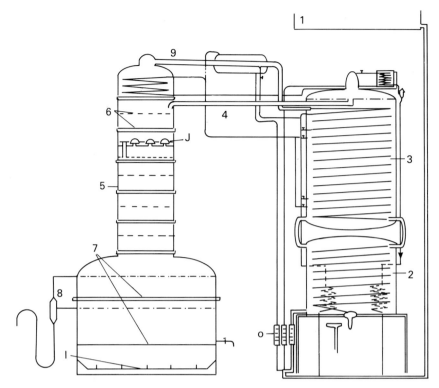

Fig. 2. Schematic drawing of an Armagnac still. Key: 1, wine container; 2, cooling; 3, wine preheater; 4, wine introduction into the column; 5, distillation column; 6, distillation plate; 7, heater; 8, exit residue; 9, vapour transfer pipe.

defects can be detected by means of sensory evaluation and confirmed by gas chromatographic analyses. The most important are discussed below.

Raw Materials

Oxidation and maderization of grapes can result in increased concentrations of acetaldehyde, acetal (both pungent odours) and 1-octen-3-ol (mushroom odour). The use of grapes that have been affected by *Botrytis cinerea* can result in loss of fruitiness, and camphor/phenol-like off-flavours. Furthermore, it can increase the concentration of sotolon (a lactone with a maderized flavour) and give the product a note of honey, sugar or caramel that is caused by 4,5-dimethyl-3-hydroxy-2(5H)-furanone.

Microbial

Infection with acetic acid bacteria can cause sourness as a result of increased acetic acid and ethyl acetate levels. Bacterial deterioration of the raw materials can result, furthermore, in increased levels of 1-butanol, 2-butanol, ethyl butanoate, acrolein and allyl alcohol. The last two components may cause a defect resulting in a 'burnt plastic' odour.

Distillative

Poor distillation may result in too much of the 'seconds' fraction in the main product, and consequently higher ethyl lactate and 2-phenylethanol concentrations, providing the brandy with an unpleasant heavy flavour. Furthermore, synthetic ester-like taints occur when too much 'heads' are included in the main fraction, resulting in increased aldehydes, higher alcohols and ethyl ester concentrations. *See* Chromatography, Gas Chromatography; Sensory Evaluation, Appearance; Sensory Evaluation, Taste

Types of Products

Brandy can be differentiated by origin and maturation period. Declarations as to origin are protected; for example, within the EEC, 44 geographical areas are officially defined. The maturation period in oak barrels can also be regarded as a quality parameter.

According to the regulations within the EEC, brandy has to be produced from a wine distillate with a maximum alcoholic strength of 94·8% (v/v); at least 50% of the alcohol in the end product has to originate from a wine distillate. The product has to be matured in oak barrels for at least 6 months, and with a maximum volume per cask of 1000 litres.

Brandy and its Manufacture

Local regulations regarding distillation procedures and maturation vary with country and region.

The actual quality and sensory profile/character of a product as sold on the market is strongly related to the origin and the applied regulations but, above all, it is related to the company marketing strategy and desired product image. *See* Sensory Evaluation, Descriptive Analysis

Bibliography

Maarse H and Visscher CA (1990) *Volatile Compounds in Food, Qualitative and Quantitative Data*, 6th edn. Zeist: TNO Biotechnology and Chemistry Institute.

F. van den Berg and H. Maarse
TNO Biotechnology and Chemistry Institute, Zeist, The Netherlands

Chemical Composition and Analysis of Cognac

Cognac is one of the most prestigious products in the world. It has received an 'Appellation d'Origine Contrôlée' or registered designation of origin and the term 'Cognac' must only be used for spirits from Cognac or the Charente region. It is subject to strict production regulations to guarantee origin and quality.

Cognac is characterized by a rich aroma and flavour which distinguishes it from other spirits distilled from wine, the production of which is not governed by such strict regulations.

Chemical Composition and Sources of Variations

The aroma of Cognac is the result of the characteristic aromas of many of its constituents, enhanced or modified by synergistic or masking effects. More than 500 substances have been detected in spirits; they belong to a large number of chemical classes: alcohols (ethanol, methanol, higher alcohols, etc.), aldehydes, esters, volatile acids (acetic acid, fatty acids, etc.), ketones, acetals, nitrogen-, oxygen- and sulphur-containing heterocyclic compounds, phenolic acids and aldehydes. These different aromatic constituents are contributed by:

- the grape (primary aromas);
- wine-making (fermentation aromas);
- distillation (specific aromas produced by the heating process);
- ageing (aromas imparted by the oak wood).

The main aim in the production of a spirit is to form pleasant, distinctive flavours and fragrances to be conveyed by the alcohol. *See* Wines, Production of Table Wines

The quality of a given Cognac depends on a number of factors:

(1) In the production process, variations can be due to:
- the weather conditions, which may vary from year to year causing differences in the chemical composition of the resulting wines and spirits;
- the diversity of grape producers;
- the different 'crus' or growth regions within the area of designated origin;
- the several hundred distillers;
- the several types of stills used with different distillation methods.
(2) In the ageing process, variations can be due to:
- the origin of the oak wood used for the barrels or casks;
- cask-making techniques;
- the layout and geographical location of the cellar (chai) where the spirits are aged;
- the length of the ageing period.

Variability of the Raw Material

The wines used in producing Cognac spirits are made essentially from the Ugni-blanc grape variety which produces wine with a relatively low alcohol content (generally 7–8% v/v) and fairly high acidity (6–12 g sulphuric acid per litre). This high degree of acidity ensures good conservation before distillation. Most of the constituents which make up a Cognac are present in the wine and lees used in the distillation.

Weather conditions are never the same from one year to the next. They determine the size of the grape harvest and the different qualities of wine produced by the vineyard. For example, the average alcoholic strength (v/v) of wines over the last 4 years in Cognac were:

- 1987, 7·5%;
- 1988, 9·6%
- 1989, 10·9%;
- 1990; 9·8%.

As a result, the chemical composition of the resulting spirits varies from year to year.

The figures below illustrate the diversity of the raw material obtained:

- the total area of the registered designation region is 80 000 ha, comprising six growth zones ('crus') within the designation region;
- the number of grape growers producing the white wine sold for Cognac is 13 000;
- the number of producers with vineyards larger than 3 ha is 8000;

Chemical Composition and Analysis of Cognac

454 Brandy and Cognac

454 Brandy and Cognac

454 Brandy and Cognac

Table 1. Variations in the concentration of wine constituents during storage for 5 months

Constituents		Variation (%)
Ethyl acetate		+24·1
Isoamyl acetate	1*	−55·7
Hexyl acetate	2*	−60·7
Phenylethyl acetate	3*	−62·1
Ethyl caproate	4*	−22·0
Ethyl caprylate	5*	−14·2
Ethyl caprate	6*	−18·9
Ethyl laurate	7*	−52·0
Total esters	1–7*	−25·8
Ethyl lactate		+49·1
Diethyl succinate		+226
Acetaldehyde (ethanal)		+117
Acetic acid		+18·8

* Organoleptically aromatic esters present in wine in low quantities. Ethyl acetate and ethyl lactate concentrations are much higher.

- the number of industrial-scale distillers is 150;
- the number of growers distilling on their own premises is 2500.

Cognac is an internationally recognized product, highly specific, and yet obtained from a number of different sources.

During the distillation period (about 5 months), the composition of the wines varies (see Table 1). The higher alcohol and polyol content does not change, but there is a significant decrease in the content of esters with aromatic properties of interest (isoamyl, hexyl and phenylethyl acetates, ethyl caproate, caprylate, caprate and laurate) and an increase in ethyl acetate, ethyl lactate, diethyl succinate, acetaldehyde (ethanal) and acetic acid. For this reason, the distillation is not performed in the same way in November, when the fermentation is completed, as in March.

Charente Distillation Method

The distillation period in Charente begins as soon as the alcohol fermentation ends (generally the beginning of November), and continues until March 31.

The Charente method of distillation is performed in two stages. From the first distillation stage the brouillis (27–30% (v/v) alcohol) is obtained; the second distillation stage yields the bonne chauffe (70% (v/v) alcohol). The purpose of this is threefold:

(1) To extract the volatile compounds contained in the wines used. Besides water and alcohol (ethanol), other compounds contribute more through their intense characteristics rather than their quantities; they represent 0·3–1% (v/v) of the alcohol.

(2) To select (rectification) from among the volatile substances present with the alcohol. Certain highly volatile products are undesirable at high doses (ethanal, ethyl acetate, acetal, etc.).
(3) To perform certain chemical transformations favourable to the quality of the spirit. The heating time has a decisive influence on the combination and decomposition of compounds.

This reactive function of the Charente pot still is the source of chemical reactions such as:

Esterification/hydrolysis:
$$\text{Acid} + \text{Alcohol} \rightleftharpoons \text{Ester} + \text{Water}$$
Acetal formation:
$$\text{Aldehyde} + \text{Alcohol} \rightleftharpoons \text{Acetal} + \text{Water}$$
Maillard reaction:
$$\text{Sugar} + \text{Amino acid} \rightarrow \text{Pyrazine, Furans (cocoa flavours)}$$
Strecker degradation:
$$\alpha\text{-Amino acid} \rightarrow \text{Aldehydes} \rightarrow \text{Acetals}$$

In order to prevent a coarse character appearing in the spirits, the wines are generally racked in order to leave only part of the lees. In keeping with tradition and local custom, the natural wine is distilled on fine lees. But of course, each firm gives its distillers specific instructions in order to obtain products in keeping with the distinctive types they each market. These instructions concern in particular the proportion of fine lees which must be kept in the wines used. Obviously, as a result there are considerable analytical differences among the various finished products. The presence of lees results in a greater quantity of aromatic esters which have a high sensory impact and produces spirits higher in floral aromas (Table 2). Care must be taken that the lees are of good quality, if not they are a major source of defects.

Given the very high number of chemical classes present in wines, all wine aromas which are volatile or carried over by water–alcohol vapours do not pass over with the same speed during distillation.

Obtaining a good quality spirit necessarily implies a harmonious balance of all the constituents: the distiller's entire art is required to achieve this balance.

Ageing Cognac

The Contribution to Product Diversity

Ageing is a basic factor in the quality of Cognacs; it is also the most costly. Cognac can be kept for many years in oak barrels; the longer the ageing, the more the intrinsic quality is enhanced. In order to maintain this quality, the producer is very careful in producing and ageing the product.

Ageing is an active process and there are several parameters that must be controlled:

Chemical Composition and Analysis of Cognac

Table 2. Effect of lees on ester contents (mg l^{-1} spirit at 70% vol.)

Constituents	Distillation With few lees	With lees
Ethyl caproate	6·76	8·3
Ethyl caprylate	8·95	23·6
Ethyl caprate	13·8	63·0
Ethyl laurate	12·45	36·2
Ethyl myristate	5·4	9·8
Ethyl palmitate	9·77	13·2
Ethyl palmitoleate	1·44	1·8
Ethyl stearate	0·59	0·61
Ethyl oleate	1·19	1·22
Ethyl linoleate	7·69	9·52
Ethyl linolenate	1·86	2·58
Isoamyl caprylate	0·42	2·48
Isoamyl caprate	1·67	5·76
Isoamyl laurate	0·78	1·83
2-Phenylethyl caprylate	Trace	1·20
2-Phenylethyl caprate	0·25	1·55
Total aromatic esters	73·02	182·65 (= +150%)

- the cellar or chai;
- the humidity;
- the temperature;
- the type of container used for ageing.

The cellar may have an earthen floor which provides good humidity, or it may be made of cement, in which case the humidity is lower The degree of humidity influences the evaporation rate. In a dry cellar, evaporation will mainly consist of water loss. In a very humid cellar, evaporation will mainly affect the alcoholic strength as alcohol is lost; Cognacs will then be smoother, mellower, and have a greater 'rancio' taste.

Differences in Cognac temperature from 7°C on average in winter to 22°C in summer are reasonable. This is one of the factors in the ability of a cellar to age spirits. Chemical reactions occurring during ageing depend on the temperature (esterification for example).

There are several types of containers. There are 1000–50 000 litre barrels (for delivery of Cognac and blends) and casks of 100, 270, 350, 400 and 550 litres (ageing). Currently, most casks are the 350 litre type manufactured by coopers (cask makers). The cask performs several functions during ageing. *See* Barrels

Quality Factors

The oak imparts aromatic elements to the Cognac in greater or lesser amounts according to:

- the choice of oak – coarse grain oak imparts tannins more easily than fine grain;
- the amount of time the staves are allowed to dry and their thickness;
- the method of heating when bending the staves to make the casks;
- the alcoholic strength of the spirits during ageing;
- the age of the cask or barrel;
- the grape production zone ('crus') and the distillation method.

Oak wood consists of cellulose (wood fibre), hemicelluloses, lignin and tannins. Tannins are highly soluble in spirits.

The first notable modification during ageing is the change in colour. This phenomenon is directly linked to the extraction and oxidation of tannins. As a direct result a young Cognac in a new cask will colour quickly, even excessively, if kept there for a long time, while a young Cognac in an old cask will change colour more slowly, remaining clear even after several years. Excess tannin (bitter taste) is often associated with a very high degree of extracted colour. *See* Tannins and Polyphenols

The aromatic aldehydes, mainly vanillin, appear when the lignin breaks down. They are produced by ageing and are very important for the bouquet of Cognac. Different types of casks result in substantial variations to their contents of these substances. These aldehydes, predominantly vanillin, contribute a vanilla note, which is not too heavy and is greatly appreciated.

The stave acts as a selective membrane enabling exchanges to take place between the Cognac within the cask and the air in the cellar by way of the evaporation of the most volatile and smallest molecules, a phenomenon which contributes to oxidation.

The quality of a Cognac's ageing is measured by its 'rancio taste' (hydrolyses of fatty acids esters together with oxidation and transformation into ketones). The formation of the rancio taste during ageing is accompanied by the continual extraction of tannins, slow oxidation and various chemical reactions. *See* Fatty Acids, Properties

The conditions necessary to make a good cask container are:

- the use of good-quality wood;
- the use of wood dried in the open air, exposed to inclement weather for at least 3 years;
- the careful preparation of a new cask and the judicious racking into older casks after proper storage of the recently distilled Cognac in new casks.

Important research work on the ageing of Cognac spirits has been a major contribution in identifying the molecules extracted from the oak by the spirits and to understanding the reaction mechanisms underlying the ageing process.

The development of gas–liquid chromatography

Chemical Composition and Analysis of Cognac

Table 3.   Effect of cask on a spirit aged 13 years

	Concentrations (mg l^{-1})	
Constituent	New cask	Old cask
Gallic acid	15·3	5·4
Vanillic acid	2·8	1·0
Syringic acid	7·0	2·2
5-Hydroxymethylfurfural	6·3	1·8
Furfural	21·3	10·8
5-Methylfurfural	1·6	0·2
Vanillin	8·8	2·9
Syringaldehyde	17·6	4·6
Coniferaldehyde	6·7	0·6
Sinapaldehyde	17·0	1·7

Table 4.   Effect of length of ageing period

	Concentrations (mg l^{-1})		
Constituent	0·7 years	5 years	13 years
Gallic acid	4·6	9·0	15·3
Vanillic acid	0·3	1·4	2·8
Syringic acid	0·6	2·6	7·0
5-Hydroxymethylfurfural	4·2	4·2	6·3
Furfural	26·8	24·7	21·3
5-Methylfurfural	1·5	1·4	1·6
Vanillin	0·9	4·4	8·8
Syringaldehyde	2·25	8·9	17·6
Coniferaldehyde	3·65	5·9	6·7
Sinapaldehyde	9·45	17·8	17·0

Table 5.   Main organoleptic characteristics of spirits from different Cognac crus

Crus	Sensory characteristics
Grande Champagne (GC)	Subtle fragrance, finish floral, fruity, persistent aromas, slightly viney
Petite Champagne (PC)	Elegant, added distinction with ageing, slightly heavier than GC, stronger alcoholic aroma, supple
Borderies	Discreet violet aroma, ages more rapidly than the GC and PC 'crus', floral aromas + vinosity, fine, elegant
Fins Bois	Powerful, rich and well balanced, vinous, fruity grapey aromas, heavier alcohol aromas
Bons Bois	Less elegant than Fins Bois, heavier, rough, less persistent aromas
Bois Ordinaires	Alcoholic aroma, heaviness, vinosity, rough

(GLC) and high-performance liquid chromatography (HPLC) techniques has enabled the analytical changes noted during ageing to be quantified with greater detail. Several aspects of variations observed in the ageing of Cognacs are shown in Tables 3 and 4 by way of example. The extraction of gallic acid is much greater in a cask made of coarse grain oak, 35·7 mg l^{-1} compared with 14·5 mg l^{-1} in a cask made of fine grain wood. In an old cask, the extration of phenolic compounds is less (Table 3), but the oxidation and exchange with the atmosphere continue to occur. *See* Pesticides and Herbicides, Types, Uses and Determination of Herbicides; Phenolic Compounds

Cognac is sold throughout the world mainly under commercial designations; among the ones currently in use are ☆☆☆, VSOP, Napoleon and X.O. These commercial qualities correspond to products of different ages. The price increases with age. These commercial products are obtained through blends (also called 'coupes') of different cognacs. Each dealer has his own blending technique and style. The blend of different Cognacs is above all a subjective choice. It enables representative product of constant and reproducible quality to be obtained. Blending is therefore an important step in the production of Cognac, since it is the key link between production and marketing.

Sensory Analysis

Cognac spirits are obtained from different 'crus' or growth zones within the area of designated origin: Grande Champagne, Petite Champagne, Borderies, Fins Bois, Bons Bois, Bois Ordinaires. They show major sensory differences (see Table 5). The blending of several crus influences the quality of the product. *See* Sensory Evaluation, Sensory Characteristics of Human Foods

During ageing the differences are increased both with regard to the quality of the flavours and the length of the ageing. A fins bois spirit is aged over a maximum period of 30 years, whereas a Grande Champagne spirit can be aged in casks over 60 years. *See* Flavour Compounds, Structures and Characteristics

Initial blending of new spirits provides more uniform batches.

Product Authenticity

The production of cognac spirits is subjected to very strict regulations with regard to both production and marketing. Regulations deriving from the Decrees of 15 May 1936 and 13 January 1938 are supplemented by genuine and consistent application of local custom for the area based on several parameters:

- the area of registered origin;
- the choice of grape varieties;
- the materials used in the wine-making;
- the distillation method;
- the containers for the spirits;
- the minimum period of ageing for each of the commercial designations.

Various governmental authorities are responsible for ensuring that these regulations are followed:

- the Institut National des Appellations d'Origines (INAO)
- the French internal revenue service (Direction Générale des Impôts, or DGI);
- the Directorate-General for Consumer Affairs, Competition and Fraud (Direction Générale de la Consommation, de la Concurrence et de la Répression des Fraudes, or DGCCRF).

The Bureau National Interprofessionnel du Cognac (BNIC) carries out inspections for age and issues certificates for age, designation of origin and analysis, certifying the authenticity of the products placed on the market.

Bibliography

Cantagrel R, Lurton L, Vidal JP and Galy B (1990) La distillation Charentaise pour l'obtention des eaux-de-vie de Cognac. *1er Symposium International, les Eaux-de-vie Traditionnelles d'Origine Viticole*, Bordeaux, 26–30 June.

Cantagrel R, Mazerolles G, Vidal JP, Lablanquie O and Boulesteix JM (1990) L'assemblage: une étape importante dans le processus d'élaboration des Cognacs. *1er Symposium International, les Eaux-de-vie Traditionnelles d'Origine Viticole*, Bordeaux, 26–30 June.

ter Heide R, de Valois PJ, Visser J, Jaegers PP and Timmer R (1978) Concentration and identification of trace constituents in alcoholic beverages. In: Charalambous G (ed.) *Analysis of Foods and Beverages. Headspace techniques*, pp 249–281. London: Academic Press.

Joseph E and Marche M (1972) Contribution à l'étude du vieillissement du Cognac. Identification de la scopolétine, de l'aesculine, de l'ombelliférone, de la β-méthyl ombelliférone, de l'aesculine et de la scopoline, hétérosides provenant du bois. *Connaissance de la Vigne et du Vin* 6(3): 1–58.

Lafon J (1971) Problèmes actuels de technologie et de vieillissement du Cognac et des eaux-de-vie de vin. *Bulletin de l'OIV*, No. 482, April, pp 339–355.

Lafon J, Couillaud P and Gay-Bellile F (1973) *Le Cognac, sa Distillation*. Paris: Editions J.B. Baillière.

Leaute R (1990) Distillation in alambic. *American Journal of Enology and Viticulture* 41(1): 90–103.

Puech JL, Leaute R, Clot G, Nomdedeu and Mondies H (1982) Etude de la lignine et de ses produits de dégradation dans les eaux-de-vie de Cognac. *Bulletin de liaison No. 11 du Groupe Polyphénols, Compte-rendu des Journées Internationales d'Etude et de l'Assemblé Générale Toulouse*, 29–30 September, 1 October, pp 605–611.

Puech JL, Leaute R, Clot G, Nomdedeu L and Mondies H (1984) Evolution de divers constituants volatils et phénoliques des eaux-de-vie de Cognac au cours du vieillissement. *Sciences des Aliments* 4(1): 65–80.

Puech JL (1986) Le vieillissement des eaux-de-vie. *Revue Française d'Oenologie* 103: 11–16.

R. Cantagrel and J.P. Vidal
Station Viticole du Bureau National Interprofessionnel du Cognac, Cognac, France

BRASSICAS

See Vegetables of Temperate Climates

BRAZIL NUTS

Brazil nuts are produced in the crown of one of the tallest trees of the Amazonian rainforest. An important dietary item of the indigenous Indian population, the Brazil nut later entered into commerce and is now a major export of the Amazonian countries, Bolivia, Brazil and Peru. The nuts are harvested from wild trees in the forest rather than from plantations. They are high in protein and oils and are also a useful source of thiamin (vitamin B$_1$). *See* Thiamin, Properties and Determination

Description and Taxonomy

The Brazil nut comes from the species *Bertholletia excelsa* Humb. & Bonpl., the only species in this genus of the Brazil nut family, Lecythidaceae. Several other species of the family have edible seeds, the best known being the sapucaia nut or monkey pot (*Lecythis pisonis* Cambess.). However, the sapucaia fruits open at matur-ity on the trees and the seeds are removed by bats, rendering large-scale harvesting almost impossible. The Brazil nuts are produced in large woody round fruits that are slightly larger than a baseball. These fruits, or pyxidia as they are termed, drop to the ground intact when they are mature, 14 months after flowering has taken place. Between 10 and 25 seeds, or nuts, as they are incorrectly called according to the botanical definition of a nut, are arranged like the segments of an orange inside the pyxidium. This explains their characteristic flattened triangular shape (Fig. 1). In nature a large terrestrial rodent, the agouti (*Dasyprocta*), gnaws open the pyxidium and buries the nuts in caches some distance from the parent tree; this is the means of seed dispersal for this species. Brazil nut gatherers go to the trees in January to March, when the fruits are falling and before the agoutis have removed all the nuts. The fruits are generally gathered in the morning because there is less danger of injury from fruit fall. The fruits weigh 0·5–2·5 kg and fall from a height of 40–50 m and injury and deaths have been reported of collectors who were struck by falling fruits. The gatherers open the pyxidia skilfully with machetes (see Fig. 2) and pour out the nuts into their baskets. They trade their harvest for goods, and the

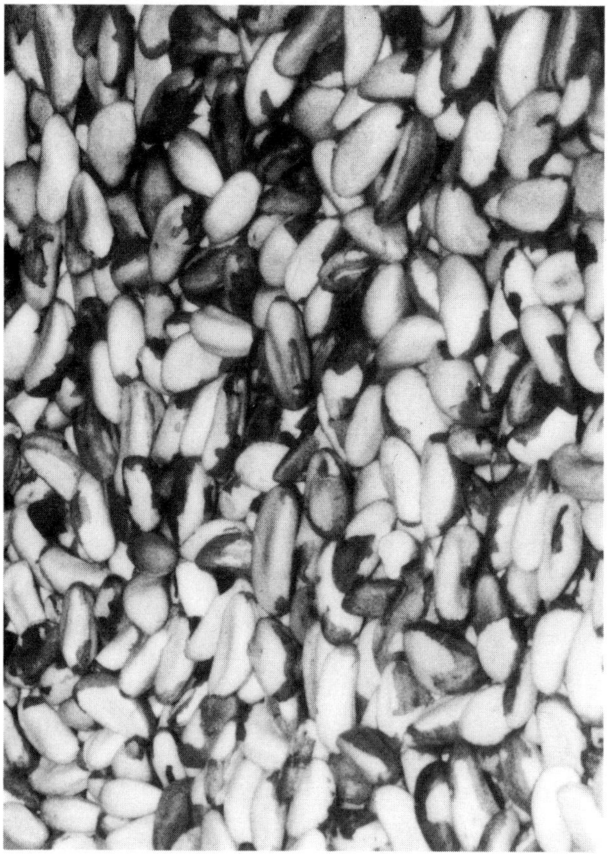

Fig. 1   Brazil nuts.

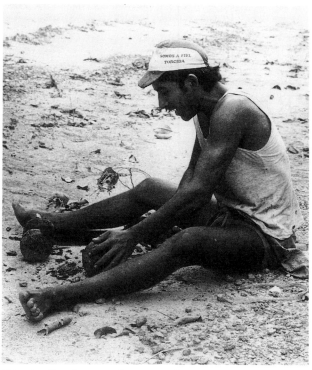

Fig. 2   Brazil nut gatherer opening nuts.

Table 1.   Chemical properties of Brazil nuts (percentage of total weight)

	Seeds from Peru (Sánchez, 1973)	Seeds from Brazil (Sánchez, 1973)	Seeds from Brazil (SUDAM, 1976)	Seeds from Brazil (Knuth 1939)
Oil	65·0	67·0	70·0	67·45
Protein	17·0	17·0	13·9	15·48
Ash	3·0	4·0	—	3·89
Crude fibre	0·9	—	—	3·21
Water	4·0	5·0	2·0	5·94
Carbohydrates	10·1	7·0	—	3·83
Ash/fibre/carbohydrates	—	—	14·1	—
	100·0	100·0	100·0	99·80

nuts are shipped to factories for processing. Before exportation they are pasteurized with steam to kill toxic fungi and, in many cases, they are also shelled and canned.

Distribution and Ecology

Brazil nuts grow in nonflooded rainforests of the Guianas and Amazonian Colombia, Venezuela, Peru, Bolivia and Brazil. They tend to grow in natural clusters or stands of 50–100 trees. These stands are known as *manchales* in Peru and *castanhais* in Brazil. Usually there are one or less trees per hectare, but stands of 15–20 trees per hectare have been reported in Madre de Dios, Peru. Some of the clustering may be the result of planting by Indians who formerly occupied the area. Brazil nuts grow in forests with an annual rainfall of 1400–2800 mm and do better where there is at least a short dry season. The trees are light demanding, i.e. they need gaps in the forest before they can grow up to adult size.

Flowering and Pollination

Flowering occurs in the dry season, which begins in September and can extend until February. The peak of flowering is September and October throughout most of central and eastern Amazonia, and slightly earlier to the west. After flowering and pollination, the fruits take approximately 14 months to mature and fall off in January and February.

   The flowers have a complicated androecium structure which forms a closed hood over the top of the flower. Nectar is produced inside the hood. Large bees are the only insects that have the strength to force open the flower to reach the nectar. As the bees force open the springed hood, their backs are forced against the pollen-

Table 2.   Principal amino acids of the Brazil nut (data from SUDAM, 1976)

	Amino acid content (mg per kg fresh wt.)
Lysine	4313
Threonine	3263
Valine	4888
Methionine	4088
Leucine	9250
Isoleucine	3450
Phenylalanine	4385
Tryptophane	1400

bearing stamens and the stigmatic surface where pollen is deposited. The bees therefore carry the pollen from flower to flower. Bees that have been found visiting Brazil nut flowers are from the genera *Bombus*, *Centris*, *Epicharis* and *Eulaema*. The Brazil nut is largely self-incompatible, i.e. the tree requires pollen from another tree in order for seed set to take place. Low seed set has been found in trees that are isolated in forest clearings and in areas of disturbance. The maintenance of the pollination system is essential for the production of Brazil nuts. Therefore plantations which are surrounded by forest where the pollinators thrive are much more likely to be productive than ones that cover larger open areas away from the forest.

Chemistry

The Brazil nut is rich in oil and protein (see Table 1). The oil extracted from the seed is bright yellow, nearly odourless and with a pleasant nutty taste. It has a specific gravity of 0·9165 at 15°C, solidifies at −4°C and does not become rancid easily. The first extraction of oil from the seeds yields an excellent cooking oil, and the

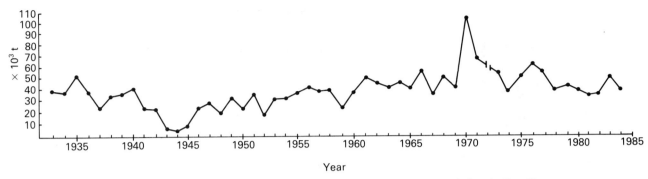

Fig. 3   Brazil nut seed production from 1933 to 1984 (data from the *Anuário Estatística do Brasil*).

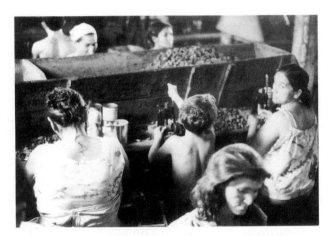

Fig. 4   Cracking Brazil nuts in a processing factory, Óbidos, Brazil.

second extraction produces an oil suitable for making soap and burning in lamps. Hence it furnished many of the needs of the Indian population of Amazonia. The residue left after pressing the seeds can be used as an animal feed. The average protein content of defatted Brazil nut flour is about 46% and it contains all the essential amino acids making both the nut and the flour highly nutritious. The principal amino acid content of the nuts is given in Table 2, which shows them to be rich in leucine. The nuts also contain vitamin A, vitamin B_1 (thiamin), vitamin B_2 (riboflavin) and niacin. It is a particularly good source of thiamin and niacin. *See* Amino Acids, Properties and Occurrence; Niacin, Properties and Determination; Retinol, Properties and Determination; Riboflavin, Properties and Determination; Thiamin, Physiology

Economic Botany

Until recently, Brazil nut seeds were second only to rubber as an export crop from Amazonian Brazil. The production from 1933 to 1986 has ranged from a low of 3557 t in 1944 to 104 487 t in 1970 (Fig. 3). The

production in 1986 was 36 136 t. The low of 1944 was caused by World War II. In the Department of Madre de Dios in Peru, 20% of the forests are rich in Brazil nuts and it is estimated that two thirds of the population are engaged in Brazil nut extraction and processing. Most of the seeds are exported to France, Great Britain, the USA and West Germany. Very little of the crop is consumed domestically in either Brazil or Peru. The nuts are exported intact or with the seed coat removed. In the latter case the seeds are soaked for 8–10 h in a tank of water, after which they are submerged in boiling water for 1–2 min. The seeds are dried to make the embryo shrink away from the seed coat; this facilitates the removal of the seed without breakage. Broken seeds have a lower export value and are often used locally for oil extraction and in the soap industry. The dried seeds are placed in a manual press and pressure is applied at both ends to crack open the seed coat (see Fig. 4). The seeds are canned for export. The Brazil nuts are eaten raw, roasted or are used in confectionery.

In addition to producing the nut, Brazil nut trees yield an excellent timber. Although it is against the law to fell Brazil nut trees in Brazil, there is still a clandestine market for its timber. The timber is also used in Peru. The fibrous bark of the tree is used for caulking boats and, in folk medicine, a bark tea is used as a cure for liver ailments. The empty fruit cases are used for fuel and for making a vast array of tourist souvenirs.

Bibliography

Knuth R (1939) Lecythidaceae. In: Engler A *Pflanzenreich IV*. 219a: 1–146.

Mori SA and Prance GT (1990) Taxonomy, ecology, and economic botany of the Brazil nut (*Bertholletia excelsa* Humb & Bonpl.: Lecythidaceae). *Advances in Economic Botany* 8: 130–150.

Mori SA and Prance GT (1990) Lecythidaceae – Part II. *Flora Neotropica Monograph* 21(II): 1–375.

Moritz A (1984) Estudos biológicos da castanha-do-Brasil (*Bertholletia excelsa* H.B.K.). EMBRAPA, Centro de Pesquisa Agropecuário do Trópico Umido *Documentos* 29: 1–82.

Müller CH (1981) Castanha-do-Brasil; estudos agronómicos.

EMBRAPA, Centro de Pesquisa Agropecuário do Trópico Umido *Miscelânea* 2: 1–25.

Nelson BW, Absy ML, Barbosa EM and Prance GT (1985) Observations on flower visitors to *Bertholletia excelsa* H.B.K. and *Couratari tenuicarpa* A.C.Sm. (Lecythidaceae). *Acta Amazônica* 15 (supplement 2): 225–234.

Sánchez JS (1973) Explotación y comercialización de la castaña en Madre de Dios. *Informe* No. 30, 84 pp. Lima, Peru: Ministerio de Agricultura, Dirección General de Forestal y Caza.

Souza AH (1963) Castanha-do-Pará; estudo botánico, químico e tecnológico. Edições S.I.A. *Estudos Técnicos* 23: 1–69.

SUDAM (Superintendência do Desenvolvimento da Amazonia) (1976) *Estudos e pesquisas sobre a castanha-do-Pará.* Belém, Brazil: Ministerio do Interior, Departamento de Recursos Naturais.

Vaz Pereira IC and Lima Costa SL (1981) *Bibliographia de Castanha-do-Pará* (Bertholletia excelsa H.B.K.). Belém, Brazil: EMBRAPA, Centro de Pesquisa Agropecuário do Trópico Umido.

Ghillean T. Prance
Royal Botanic Gardens, Kew, UK

BREAD

Contents

Dough Mixing and Testing Operations

The bakery industry has an important role to play in the economic development of a country, in fuller utilization of its wheat resources, and in building up the health of its people. Many attempts have been made to popularize bakery products, because these products are considered easy, convenient and rather inexpensive means of taking food in a hygienically prepared, ready-to-eat form. One of the most important operations in a bakery is the accurate and thorough mixing of ingredients. Mixing reduces nonuniformities of gradients in composition, properties or temperature of bulk materials or products in and out of a reactor, and was defined by Quillen as the 'intermingling of two or more dissimilar portions of a material, resulting in the attainment of a desired level of uniformity, either physical or chemical, in the final product'. This article discusses the purpose of kneading of dough, types of mixers for dough, dough mixing and dough development and empirical methods in physical dough testing.

Purpose of Dough Mixing

The dough is kneaded before it is allowed to ferment, and again before it is moulded into the desired shapes.

The purpose of kneading is to remove some of the excess carbon dioxide in order to prevent overstretching of the gluten strands, and to distribute the yeast cells throughout the dough. Kneading also tends to keep the dough at a uniform temperature. The dough is kneaded sufficiently when it has a smooth, 'satiny' surface, and small bubbles appear under the surface.

Types of Mixers for Dough

Mixers and kneaders are necessary for the proper blending or mixing of the various ingredients. Liquids can be easily blended using propeller-type agitators in a tank. For blending of premixes or preparation of adjuncts, ribbon blenders, twin-cone and V-shell blenders are usually employed when dry ingredients are to be mixed.

Dough mixing can be carried out using horizontal, vertical, reciprocating or continuous mixers as required. The horizontal type may have a fixed or tilting bowl, while the vertical mixer may be a planetary or fixed spindle type. The continuous mixers may be of the agitator-in-tube type, or the rotor and stator head type.

Horizontal Dough Mixers

These mixers can be used to mix various mixtures ranging in consistency from thin batters to tough doughs. They must be used when gluten development is desirable, e.g. in breadmaking. These mixers have a horizontal U-shaped bowl mounted on a rigid frame with a drive motor. Their capacities range from 10 kg upwards. Bowls are usually made of stainless steel or stainless-steel-clad mild steel. Bowls are sometimes provided with jackets for the circulation of cold or hot water.

High-speed mixers for gluten development usually contain a single axle on which two or more arms parallel to the front of the mixer are mounted. The limited clearance between the jacket wall and the agitator bars causes the dough to be repeatedly stretched and kneaded, resulting in quick gluten development. These mixers can usually be operated in two speed ranges, namely 30–60 and 40–80 rpm. In the slow-speed mixers, agitators of various forms, e.g. eight-arm, Z, etc., are employed on one or two axles.

The agitator configuration and its speed affects the action. Slow-speed Z or eight-arm mixers have a speed range of 14–60 rpm (25 rpm on an average).

The high-speed horizontal mixers are also called kneaders, and may contain bars projecting from the axle at right angles, while the bowl has radical bars intermeshing with axle bars. This construction gives very efficient dough kneading, and is particularly suitable for tough doughs.

The dough is discharged from these mixers by tilting the bowl so that the top is brought to a forward-facing position. In some models, the front of the bowl consists of a tightly fitting door which can be raised and lowered independently of the immobile section of the bowl, and the dough is discharged through this door. The bowl-tilting mechanism may be hand operated or it may be operated by a separate motor.

Vertical Mixers

Vertical mixers consist of a movable bowl or trough with one or two vertical shafts which may be stationary or may have planetary movement. The agitators themselves may be of various sizes and configurations. The most important design in the vertical mixer is the planetary mixer, which is particularly suitable for mixing batters or adjuncts such as icings. The agitator is called 'planetary' as it, apart from revolving around its own vertical axis at a relatively high speed, also moves in circles as it rotates around the bowl. This motion ensures 'beater' action throughout the bowl contents. The agitator may be provided with a variable-speed mechanism, and the bowl can be raised and lowered by a separate drive. The agitator may be of any of the various types available, e.g. simple, curved single-arm, wire meshing or paddle gate.

The hook-type agitator gives a good kneading action

to the dough, resulting in development of the gluten with a minimum of tearing. The wire-mesh-type agitator gives a good 'beater' action with maximum air incorporation. The paddle-type agitator ensures good mixing coupled with scraping of the bowl sides. Bowls are usually provided with covers to prevent splashing or dusting. Capacities range from 10 kg upwards.

Spindle-type mixers are used mainly for biscuit doughs. Their special advantage is with saltine doughs, in which case they are adapted for mixing in special mobile troughs used for fermentation. Thus, sponges and doughs need not be transferred in and out of the mixer between the various stages. The spindle speed is usually low, and spindles can be raised to allow the trough to be rolled into place under them. The mixer blades are so designed as to give a cutting action rather than a kneading or stretching action to the mix, thus a toughening effect on the cracker or biscuit doughs is avoided. *See* Biscuits, Cookies and Crackers, Methods of Manufacture

In reciprocating agitator or revolving bowl mixers, a pair of agitator arms travels through intersecting elliptical paths in a shallow, slowly revolving bowl. These mixers are useful for mixing temperature-sensitive doughs, and also where nuts and raisins in the mix are to be kept unbroken. Their output is usually low compared to horizontal mixers, and they are particularly suitable for pie doughs and puff pastry.

Dough Mixing and Dough Development

Dough Properties and Mixing Behaviour

Wheat flour doughs exhibit a wide range of properties when different flour samples are compared. Dough properties influence both the efficiency of throughput in the manufacturing plant, as well as the quality of the final baked product. In discussing the state of dough prior to baking, we need to differentiate between the contributions from the individual flour and those from the various treatments, which include added ingredients, mixing, and intermediate punching and moulding steps. Dough is a complex material from a rheological point of view. Knowledge about its structure comes from fundamental rheological studies, from standard physical dough testing, including mixing, and from microscopy.

Because of the trend towards greater use of baking processes involving intensive mixing and short fermentation times, much more attention has been given to basic studies of dough mixing in recent years. These studies have highlighted the sensitivity of dough structure to the conditions to which the dough has been subjected during its development. It is clear that meaningful interpretations of rheological measurements can

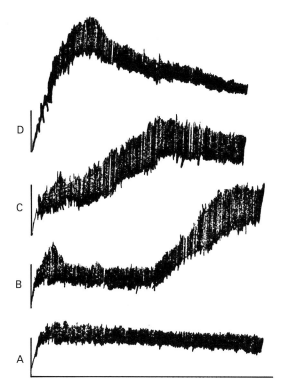

Fig. 1 Mixogram traces. The sequence from A through D may be used to represent either doughs of increasing mixing requirements mixed at a fixed intensity, one dough mixed at increasing intensities or one dough mixed at a fixed intensity but containing increasing additions of cysteine.

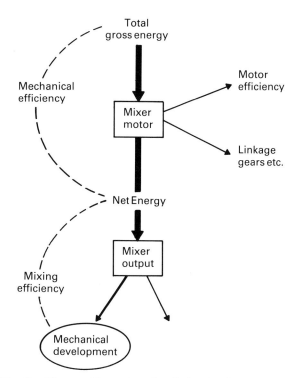

Fig. 2 Diagram illustrating the distinction between mechanical and mixing efficiencies. From Kilborn RH and Tipples KH (1972).

be made only if the state of dough development is well understood.

Factors affecting Dough Development

The first step in converting flour into bread is the mixing of flour, water and other additives. As mixing proceeds, the initially incoherent dough mass develops viscoelastic properties and finally acquires a sheen, this stage being termed 'clearing'. Prolonged mixing past this point causes the dough to lose its strength and become plastic and very sticky to the touch. If the torque on the pins, blades or arm of the mixer is monitored against time, the trace rises, reaches a maximum, and then falls steadily. This is illustrated in Fig. 1 for doughs mixed in a mixograph. Optimum bread-baking performance is usually achieved in a region at, or slightly past, the peak development point.

Critical Mixing Intensity and Critical Work Input

Two parameters are critical for optimum development and hence best performance. These are that (1) the mixing intensity must be above a minimum critical value, and (2) the total work imparted to the dough must be above a certain minimum value. Both parameters vary according to the flour used. Before discussing these requirements more fully, it is useful to consider the mechanical and mixing efficiencies of different dough mixers. The distinction between these two quantities is illustrated in Fig. 2. A percentage of the total energy consumed by the mixer motor is available for performing mechanical work on the dough. This is called the mechanical efficiency. However, not all of this energy is utilized for mechanical development of the dough but that portion which is utilized is denoted the 'mixing efficiency' of the mixer.

Mixing requirements of flours vary widely, and Fig. 1 illustrates the mixing behaviour of four flour types. The mixing curves are for doughs that have been mixed at a constant and moderate speed. Flour A has high mixing requirements, and the rate of mixing used is insufficient to develop the dough; such a dough would be a failure in a baking test. Flour B is a moderately strong flour that does develop at this mixing speed, although there is an initial induction period before the dough begins to exert any appreciable torque on the mixer. Flour C is of medium strength, and flour D is a comparatively weak flour that develops quickly. We may also make use of Fig. 1 to illustrate the effect of varying the mixing intensity (i.e. mixing speed) on the mixing curve of a given dough. At a low speed, the dough does not develop (trace A). As the mixing speed is increased the dough develops after a lag phase (trace B) and thereafter develops more easily (traces C and D). With increasing speed, and providing the amount of work applied to the dough is above a certain level (corresponding to a point at, or slightly past, the peak in the trace), the baked loaf volume increases up to a critical mixing speed, above which it plateaus.

For every dough there exists a critical mixing speed (which may vary for each mixer) below which dough handling properties and baked loaf characteristics are unsatisfactory. In addition, it is necessary to have imparted a minimum level of work input to the dough in order to bring it to an optimal developed state. If the mixing speed or work input level are below the critical values, unsatisfactory baking results are obtained. Baking results are less affected by exceeding the critical values than when these values are not reached. However, dough-handling properties deteriorate and doughs become sticky; weaker flours are more sensitive to overmixing.

Activated Dough Development

Because some flours have very long mixing requirements or have critical mixing speeds that exceed the capacity of many dough mixers, methods of overcoming these limitations have been devised. One method involves the addition of reducing agents, particularly sodium meta-bisulphite (SMS) and L-cysteine hydrochloride (cysteine), to doughs. Cysteine reduces the energy level required to achieve peak dough development, and also the critical mixing speed necessary to produce bread of satisfactory loaf volume. We may again make use of Fig. 1 to illustrate the effects of increasing additions of cysteine in altering the mixing characteristics of a strong dough. As the amount of added cysteine is increased, the nature of the mixing curve changes from A through D. Cysteine also increases slightly the rate of energy input at a given mixing speed and increases the tolerance to undermixing, i.e. enables satisfactory bread to be produced with energy levels less than those required to achieve peak dough development. There is an optimum level of cysteine addition, and too high a level causes deterioration of loaf characteristics.

Empirical Methods in Physical Dough Testing

A great variety of commercial testing instruments are used in routine physical tests on dough, either in quality control or research work. The deformation to which dough is subjected in these instruments is so complicated that it does not allow the evaluation of the properties of the material in simple physical terms. Though the results are evaluated more on an empirical basis than through

theoretical analysis, they provide valuable information on the baking characteristics of the tested material and are a useful tool.

Over the years, a physical testing system has been developed on the basis of the 'three-phase concept of breadbaking'. The system has been generally accepted and is used in many commercial milling and baking operations. It applies three principles of testing: dough mixing, dough stretching (load–extension) and viscosity measurements on buffered flour suspensions at elevated temperatures.

Mixing Tests

The two most common instruments used for testing wheat flour and wheat flour dough during the mixing operation are the Brabender farinograph and National Recording Dough Mixer (mixograph).

The Brabender farinograph is essentially a torque-measuring dough mixer which measures the plasticity and mobility of dough upon a relatively gentle mixing at constant temperature. The resistance of the dough to Z-shaped mixing blades is transmitted to a dynamometer connected to a mechanical recording system which records a curve (farinogram) on a kymograph chart. Farinograms provide information on optimum mixing time and dough stability on prolonged mixing (Fig. 3). Doughs are tested at a standard water content known as the 'farinograph water absorption' value. This value has to be determined by 'titration' of flour with water, and is the amount of water needed for a standard optimum consistency of the dough of 500 Brabender units (AACC, 1969). 'Farinograph water absorption', dough development time, and dough stability are useful parameters for the evaluation of the strength of a flour. In general, the higher the value of these parameters, the stronger the flour. To express the strength of a flour on the basis of farinograph data as a single score, the 'valorimetric value' may be determined by means of a special nomograph known as the valorimeter. The 'valorimeter value' is determined by the dough development time and the decreasing slope of the curve (degree of softening) – the higher the value, the stronger the flour.

The National Recording Dough Mixer is another widely used instrument for flour testing. Like the farinograph method, the mixograph method has become a standard physical dough test. The resistance offered by the dough to four vertical pins revolving around three stationary pins in a mixing bowl creates a force which deviates the mixing bowl from its original position. The torque is proportional to the shear strength and elasticity of the dough, and may be used as an index of the dough strength. Both Brabender farinographs and National Recording Dough Mixers may be

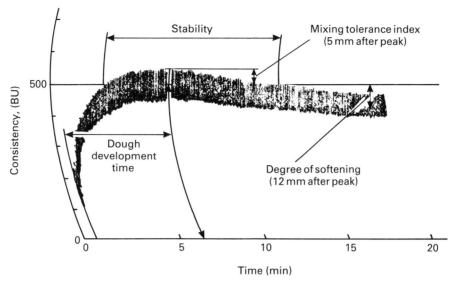

Fig. 3 Representative farinogram showing the most commonly measured parameters. BU, Brabender units are a measure of optimum consistency of the dough. From Bloksma AH (1971).

modified by replacing the mechanical recording device by an electronic strain gauge system. Electronic strain gauge recording offers several advantages: ease of calibration in terms of physical units, greater accuracy because of the elimination of friction from the torque-measuring system, a wide range of sensitivity, and a record on rectangular coordinates.

For testing the mixing characteristics of dough under conditions more closely related to those during mechanical development, a variant of the farinograph was developed. It is known under the name of the Brabender Do-Corder. It has a nearly closed mixing bowl with heavier mixing blades. The dough can be mixed at higher rates than in the standard farinograph. A more recent development is the Brabender resistograph. The instrument was developed to meet the needs of modern bread-baking technology in which high-speed mixers subject the dough to both kneading and stretching. The characteristics of doughs mixed under these conditions differ from those produced by conventional mixers, where mixing is accomplished more by pressure than stretching. The resistograph has a mixing head which combines blending with stretching, pressing and kneading. It imparts a high work input to the dough and can be used for the evaluation of dough response to high-speed mixing. Strong flours show a sharp increase in mixing resistance, and broadening and narrowing of the band. The resistograms of medium strength and weak flours are characterized by two pronounced maxima. The first is related to waterbonding and dough development and indicates the dough development time. The second measures the stickiness and extensibility at breakdown of the dough; the time to reach this point is most important in testing medium and weak flours. Both optimum and breaking points are reached when

the blades of the mixer are completely covered with dough.

Load–Extension Tests

Several commercial instruments are available for the routine testing of dough at large elongations. From the recorded curves, various characteristics, such as resistance to deformation, extensibility and energy needed to rupture the dough, can be computed. Among these instruments, the Brabender extensigraph is the most common one. It was developed about 1936 as a supplement to the farinograph, and has become particularly useful in the study of the effect of various chemical improvers on the rheological properties of dough. The extensigraph data (Fig. 4) reported for control purposes are usually the curve length in centimetres (extensibility), the curve height in extensigraph units either at the maximum or 5 cm from the start of the curve (resistance), the area under the curve in square centimetres (strength value), and the quotient of height over length – the greater this quotient the stronger the dough. Several attempts have been made to use the extensigraph for more fundamental studies, and to transform extensigraph data into rheological terms. The main problem in these transformations is the calculation of the actual cross-sectional area based on the 'effective mass' of the dough, i.e. the mass between the edges of the cradle supporting the dough. The effective mass progressively increases during stretching because some dough is pulled out from the cradle due to its resistance to extension. The effective mass and the actual cross-sectional area of the dough can be calculated from multiple regression equations. The coefficients in these

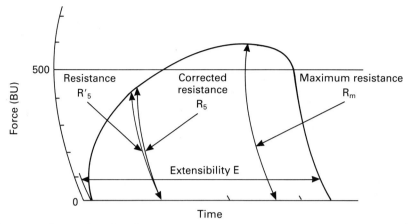

Fig. 4   Representative extensigram showing the most commonly measured parameters. From Bloksma AH (1971).

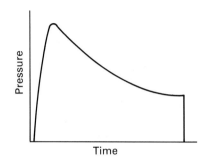

Fig. 5   Representative alveogram. From Bloksma AH (1971).

equations, however, change with the type of dough and have to be determined experimentally.

A higher sensitivity and wider applicability of the Brabender extensigraph may be achieved by replacing the mechanical recording device by an electronic strain gauge system.

Another load–extension meter used in cereal laboratories is the research extensometer (Halton extensigraph) designed by Halton and associates. While the actual extensometer works on a similar principle as the Brabender extensigraph, the required water content for dough preparation is measured on the principle of extrusion by means of a special water absorption meter which, together with a mixer/shaper, belongs to the three-unit extensometer. The interpretation of the curves is the same as with Brabender extensigrams. A great advantage of this instrument lies in its applicability to fermenting doughs.

The Chopin alveograph is more popular in Europe than in North America. The instrument consists of three parts: mixer, bubble blower and a recording manometer. The procedure involves using air pressure to blow a bubble from a disc of sheeted dough until it reaches its breaking point. A recording manometer records the pressure of the air in the bubble as a function of time. The manometer records a curve (Fig. 5) from

which three basic measurements are taken: the height and the length of the curve, and the area under the curve. The latter is proportional to the work of deformation.

Viscosity Measurements

The third step in the process of the physical testing of flour or dough, based on the 'three-phase concept of breadbaking', is the measurement of changes in flour paste viscosities at temperatures above the gelatinization temperature of starch present in flour. The data obtained by these measurements are not only related to the gelatinization characteristics of the crumb in the baking oven, but are also a good indicator of the diastatic activity of the flour. These measurements do not fall into the category of dough rheology, because all tests are done on flour slurries only. However, they help to evaluate factors which considerably affect the consistency of dough as well as the texture of bread crumb, its colour, general appearance and shelf-life. The most common instrument used for these tests is the Brabender amylograph. It is a torsion viscometer that provides a continuous record of changes in viscosity of the flour slurry at a uniform rate of temperature increase (decrease) of $1·5°C$ per minute under constant stirring. Although the instrument was originally developed for testing rye flour pastes, the amylographic method has become a standard method for controlling α-amylase activity in wheat flour (AACC, 1969)—the higher the activity, the lower the hot paste viscosity due to the liquefying effect of the enzyme. The effect of other amylolytic enzymes present is also reflected in the amylogram.

Bibliography

AACC (1969) *Approved Methods*, 8th edn. St Paul: American Association of Cereal Chemists.

Bloksma AH (1971) Rheology and chemistry of dough. In: *Wheat Chemistry and Technology*. St Paul: American Association of Cereal Chemists.

Chichester CO, Mrak EM and Schweigert BS (1984) Dough properties and mixing behaviour. In: *Advances in Food Research*, vol 29, pp 230–234. London: Academic Press.

De Man JM, Voisey PW, Rasper VF and Stanley DW (1975) Empirical methods in physical dough testing. In: *Rheology and Texture in Food Quality*, pp 310–323. Westport, CT: AVI.

Kilborn RH and Tipples KH (1972) Factors affecting mechanical dough development. I. Effect of mixing intensity and work input. *Cereal Chemistry* 49: 34–47.

Kilborn RH and Tipples KH (1973) Factors affecting mechanical dough development. IV. Effect of cysteine. *Cereal Chemistry* 50: 70–86.

Quillen CS (1954) Mixing – the universal operation. *Chemical Engineering* 61: 177–224.

Voisey PW and Kilborn RH (1974) An electronic recording Grain Research Laboratory mixer. *Cereal Chemistry* 51: 841–848.

S. D. Deshpande
Central Institute of Agricultural Engineering, Bhopal, India

Breadmaking Processes

Methods

All forms of breadmaking involve a certain number of separate operations, namely dough-making, dough development, scaling and shaping of the dough piece, and, finally, oven baking.

The traditional process of making leavened bread is thought to have originated with the ancient Egyptians, probably as long ago as 4000 BC. The first stage involves mixing the basic ingredients of flour, yeast, salt and water to form an apparently homogeneous mass, or dough. There then follows an extended period of 'panary fermentation' – where the dough, in bulk, is set aside in a warm place for from 3 to 18 or more hours to 'rise'. Often, the fermenting dough was 'knocked-back', or given a second short mixing at between one-half and two-thirds of the total fermentation time.

During the fermentation, not only does the dough 'rise' or increase in volume, but its physical nature changes such that it is more readily handled in the next stage – in which the dough is divided into pieces of the desired size and roughly moulded, generally into the shape of a ball.

The roughly moulded dough pieces are again allowed to rest for a period known as 'first proof', extending for from 10 to 30 min, and are then finally moulded into the final shape for baking and placed either in a tin or on a tray. The moulded dough is then allowed to continue fermentation for a further 45–60 min ('final proof')

before being transferred to the oven for baking for from 30 to 45 min, depending on the loaf size and oven temperature.

Until the later years of the 19th century the whole process was carried out by hand, in very much the same way as it is presumed to have occurred in ancient times. The process was then gradually adapted to mechanical handling with the design of mechanical dough mixers, dough dividers, dough moulders and mechanical transport of dough pieces through 'proving' chambers and ovens.

Until the development of mechanical handling, natural variations in the ingredients were balanced by adjustment of the handling procedures by the craftsman baker, such that acceptable bread could be produced from variable materials. However, attempts to link together mechanical handling procedures in a 'factory' bakery necessarily involved attempts to standardize the time-cycle of each stage of the overall process, and consequently to standardize, as far as is possible with natural materials, the properties of flour and yeast.

In the 19th century, bakers used brewer's yeast, culturally most suited to a watery medium rich in sugars, but subjected, in dough, to a situation where availability of both water and nutrients was restricted. A later improvement was to use distiller's yeast, which does not contain any residual bitter components from hops, but is still best suited to fermentation of a sugar-rich liquid medium. As a result of the demands of 'industrialized' baking, yeasts especially suited to panary fermentation were cultured industrially, and millers attempted to standardize their flour properties by wheat selection, changes in milling techniques, and the use of small quantities of chemical oxidizers for 'improving' and 'ageing' their flour. *See* Yeasts

In the late 20th century the major changes have been the extensive use, in both large and small bakeries, of mechanical dough development (the *Chorleywood bread process*), and the establishment of in-store bakeries in supermarkets and hypermarkets. While the mechanical developments in the late 19th and early 20th centuries, permitting the establishment of large and efficient plant bakeries, generally led to a fall in the number of small bakeries and to diminution in the number of bread types readily available to the public, the use of mechanical dough development has improved the working facilities and economic efficiency of the remaining small bakers – some of whom have also been involved in in-store developments in cooperation with supermarkets – and made possible the economic production of small runs of different bread types, resulting in renewed public interest in variety breads. Legislative control of additives in flour milling and baking has likewise become more thorough, such that the utilization of any chemical means of standardization is subject to extremely rigorous control. *See* Legislation, Additives

Traditional

Traditionally, dough is developed by yeast fermentation (*panary fermentation*, or *bulk fermentation*), allowing the yeasted dough to ferment for a period in which sugars in the dough are converted to carbon dioxide by the yeast, and for the dough to 'ripen', that is, develop the elastic properties necessary to enable it to be moulded to shape and to hold gas during the remainder of the baking process.

Straight-dough Process

In a typical procedure, the flour is mixed with the fat, and the required amount of water (usually about 55–57% of the flour weight) is adjusted to the temperature required to give a final dough temperature of about 27°C. The yeast and salt are separately mixed into some of the water, and then the yeast suspension, salt solution and remainder of the water are added to the mixed flour and fat and mixed and kneaded to make a 'clear' (i.e. apparently uniform) dough.

With hand mixing, the mixing meant extremely hard work, but insufficient mixing resulted in unsatisfactory bread. After 'throwing together' the solids and the water, it was necessary to cut the dough into comparatively small pieces, of say 20–25 kg, which could be kneaded on the table before finally combining the bulk together in the dough trough.

Slow-speed mechanical mixers generally produce a clear dough in about 15 min, and improved bread quality usually results from a slightly longer mixing time. *See* Bread, Dough Mixing and Testing Operations

After mixing, the dough is set aside at a temperature close to 27°C to ferment.

The amounts of yeast and salt used vary with the length of fermentation intended; for a 3 h process, 1% yeast and 2% salt (based on flour weight) are typical; for a longer process the yeast amount is reduced and the salt increased.

About from two-thirds to three-quarters of the time between dough-making and final scaling-off, the bulk dough is '*knocked-back*', that is, given a brief remixing, in order to bring about more vigorous fermentation or gas production by bringing yeast into contact with a fresh supply of sugar, to drive out stale gas and re-establish an even temperature throughout the dough.

The dough is then again set aside to rise for the remainder of the fermentation time, and is then divided into portions of the desired weight, roughly shaped and set aside to rest (*first proof*) for about 10–15 min, again at about 27°C.

At the end of the resting time, the dough pieces are finally moulded into the desired shape and placed in tins or on a baking tray for the *final proof* at a slightly higher temperature, usually at about 43°C, and high humidity

for from 45 to 60 min before baking in an oven at about 235°C for from 30 to 40 min, depending on loaf size.

Sponge and Dough Process

In the sponge and dough system, only part of the flour is mixed with all the yeast and part of the salt and sufficient water to give a slack (or soft) dough (known as the *sponge*). This sponge is allowed to ferment for some time (varying from only 1 h to overnight) before remixing with the remaining flour, salt and water to give the final dough, which is then given a short bulk fermentation before scaling or dividing, first and final proof and baking.

The sponge and dough system has been little used in England, but is the traditional process in both Scotland and the USA. It is claimed to produce bread of fuller flavour than the straight-dough system; it makes possible the use of some weaker flour in the final dough – strong flour only in the sponge stage with perhaps two-thirds strong flour, one-third weak flour in the final dough stage. In the past, the process had the advantage that it was suitable for use with a *barm* in place of pressed yeast.

No-time Doughs

Occasionally, in emergency conditions, bread may be made without bulk fermentation by using higher dough temperatures (between 30 and 32°C) and much higher than normal amounts of yeast – about 2·5% on a flour basis. The mixed dough is scaled immediately after mixing and given slightly longer than normal first and final proof times. The bread produced is not of a normal commercial standard; it has a coarse-grained and harsh crumb and stales rapidly.

Soda Bread

The traditional Irish home-baking process depends on the use of sodium bicarbonate and sour milk for gas production, and simply involves prolonged mixing and kneading, followed by a short rest period before baking.

Gas-injection Processes

Various patented procedures have been utilized from time to time in which carbon dioxide is injected into the dough and the dough is immediately divided, moulded and baked. In general these processes are more suited to the production of small goods, such as rolls and bun-rounds, rather than bread loaves.

Mechanical Dough Development

Mechanical development is the term applied to processes involving large, controlled work inputs at dough mixing which give rise to doughs which have physical properties akin to those developed after the hours of bulk fermentation in the traditional process, and are therefore suitable for almost immediate moulding and final proof.

The possibility of replacement of bulk fermentation by physical work was first proposed by Swanson and Working in 1926 (*Cereal Chemistry*, 1926; reprinted in *Cereal Foods World*, January 1990), but only became a practical possibility with the ready availability of small high-powered electric motors in the late 1940s and early 1950s.

The '*DoMaker process*', developed and patented in the USA, and involving the use of a pre-ferment in the dough mix, was introduced into the UK around 1953, but the type of bread produced found little favour with UK customers. A study of the factors involved in mechanical dough development was initiated at the newly formed British Baking Industries Research Association at Chorleywood, aimed at developing a straight-dough process suitable for producing British-type bread.

The resulting '*Chorleywood bread process*' involves the application of 11 watt-hours (40 kJ) of work, measured electrically, per kilogram of dough, with addition to the dough mix of both a fast-acting oxidizing improver (initially potassium iodate, now either 75 mg kg^{-1} of ascorbic acid or the equivalent amount of azodicarbonamide) and a small quantity (0.7% of the flour weight) of a high-melting fat. For success the work addition must be applied in a period of under 5 min and preferably within 2–3 min, so the process requires a very high-powered mixer, such as became available at that time in the form of the '*Tweedy*' mixer (originally developed for the plastics industry).

Commercial mixers are now readily available, provided with automatic electronic control of work input and suitable for mixes varying from 30 to 150 kg of flour. In large bakeries, such mixers can be linked to automatic feeders and weighing machines for flour, water and other ingredients such that dough mixes are produced at 3–5 min intervals, giving a semicontinuous feed to hoppers, producing a continuous feed to scaling, moulding, final proof, baking, cooling and, where applicable, slicing and wrapping. In small bakers, the speed of dough development permits rapid change between production of different bread varieties.

Activated Dough Development

An alternative to mechanical dough development, for use where powerful mechanical mixers are not available, is the so-called *activated dough development*, based on the combined use of a rapid-acting reducing agent, such as cysteine, and a slow-acting oxidizer, such as bromate

or ascorbic acid. Dough mixing is carried out in a slow mixer of conventional type, and subsequent dough handling then follows the same procedures as used following mechanical dough development. Evidently the reducing agent breaks bonds formed in the initial gluten formation when water is added to the flour; mixing distributes the gluten through the dough and the slow-acting oxidizer causes reformation of bonds in the gluten structure to establish an elastic three-dimensional network, such as is achieved after lengthy panary fermentation in the conventional process. In effect, the dough-softening action of the reducing agent drastically reduces the work input required for the production of a fully developed dough. *See* Oxidation of Food Components

The usual levels of additions are 35 mg kg^{-1} of L-cysteine hydrochloride (equivalent to 27 mg kg^{-1} of cysteine) plus 50 mg kg^{-1} of ascorbic acid both calculated on flour weight).

Microwave Baking

In principle, microwave baking is capable of greatly reducing baking time, and of permitting the use of flour which would, for oven baking, contain excessive amounts of α-amylase or be too low in protein content. Due to the short baking time (typically about 10 min for an 800 g loaf) and the fact that heat is generated internally rather than by heat transfer through the dough piece, gas retention is less dependent on gluten quantity and strength, and the length of time in the critical temperature range is insufficient for the production of unacceptable amounts of dextrins by amylase activity.

With microwave heating alone, no crust is produced, but combined microwave and radiant heating can produce acceptable loaves from flour having a protein content as low as 7.5%.

Ingredients

The main ingredients are flour, water, salt and yeast; minor ingredients may include malt flour, unprocessed soya bean flour, fat and 'yeast stimulants'; and, when using mechanical dough development, must include high-melting-point fat and 'improver'.

The UK Bread and Flour Regulations 1984 (SI 1984, No. 1304) permit the following ingredients to be used without their presence being indicated in the name of the bread if used in small quantities for technological purposes, or up to the maximum specified:

(1) Any bread (except wholemeal, for which the presence of the following ingredients shall be indicated) – milk and milk products, liquid or dried egg, wheat germ, rice

flour (maximum 20 g kg^{-1}), cracked oat grains, oatmeal or oat flour.

(2) Any bread – soya bean flour (maximum 50 g kg^{-1} for brown bread, maximum 20 g kg^{-1} for other bread), salt, vinegar, oils and fats, malt extract, malt flour, any soluble carbohydrate sweetening matter, prepared wheat gluten, poppy seeds, sesame seeds, caraway seeds, cracked wheat, cracked or kibbled malted wheat, flaked malted wheat, kibbled malted rye, cracked or kibbled malted barley, starch other than modified starch (maximum 225 mg kg^{-1}).

Any of these permitted ingredients may well be used, singly or in combination, in particular dough mixes for variety breads. The regulations also specify more specifically the requirements for specific bread types as follows.

Bread. A food of any size, shape or form which is usually known as bread, and consists of a dough made from flour and water, with or without other ingredients, which has been fermented by yeast or otherwise leavened and subsequently baked or partly baked. It does not include buns, bun loaves, chapatis, chollas, pitta bread, potato bread or bread specially prepared for coeliac sufferers.

Reserved Descriptions:

(1) Where all the flour is derived from wheat, the name of the bread shall include the following words*†:
- 'wholemeal' – all flour used is wholemeal;
- 'brown' – has a minimum fibre content (from wheat) of 0·6% (calculated on the dry matter of the bread) and includes flour other than wholemeal;
- 'wheat germ' – has a minimum added processed wheat germ content of 10% (calculated on the bread dry matter);
- 'white' – all bread other than wholemeal, brown or wheat germ;
- 'soda' – bread made using sodium hydrogencarbonate.

(2) Where the flour is derived from any cereal, the following shall be used*:
- 'Wholemeal' – made from the whole product derived from any cereal.

(3) Miscellaneous descriptions:
- 'Aerated' – bread, other than soda bread, in which the method of leavening is by the incorporation of air, carbon dioxide or nitrogen, either chemically or mechanically;
- 'partly baked' – bread requiring further cooking before consumption.

---

* No account shall be taken of any rice flour used (maximum 2% of the flour used), or any barley malt (small quantities for technological purposes).
† Not applicable to 'malt bread' or 'malt loaf'.

Breadmaking Processes

Flour

Flour for breadmaking is known generally as 'bakers' flour', and the highest quality as 'patents'. Quality in this connection refers to the physical and chemical properties of the dough, and its capacity to yield bold, well-aerated loaves with good colour and texture of crust and crumb. Baking quality depends on a number of factors, but the most important of these is the quantity and quality of the gluten that is formed on mixing with water. Gluten quantity and quality depends on protein content and composition, and baking quality is also largely affected by the water absorption capacity and diastatic activity of the flour. *See* Flour, Roller Milling Operations; Flour, Analysis of Wheat Flours

Of fundamental importance to the baker are *water absorption* and *physical dough characteristics*, with flour *colour* of subsidiary importance. These characteristics are dependent both of *wheat variety* and growth conditions, and on milling conditions, and quality assessment in chemical terms involves measurements of *moisture*, *protein* and *diastatic activity*.

The bakers' term '*water absorption*' means the water addition possible to produce a dough with properties suitable for the baking procedure in use. In general, a higher water absorption is desirable, giving a higher dough weight and hence yield of bread from a given flour weight.

The *moisture content* is governed by the moisture content of the wheat at commencement of milling and evaporative losses during milling, but is usually in the range 13–15%. Higher levels of moisture are undesirable if the flour is to be stored for any considerable length of time, but otherwise has no effect on baking quality except that increase in moisture content reduces water absorption at dough-making.

The *protein content* is a major determinant of baking quality; generally, the higher the protein content the better the baking quality. When flour and water are mixed together the protein forms a complex, known as *gluten*, the elastic properties of which are responsible for the moulding properties of the dough and its ability to retain the carbon dioxide produced by yeast fermentation during proof and to give a bold, well-risen loaf on baking.

Diastatic activity has both positive and negative connotations. Yeast activity during proof initially utilizes sugars naturally occurring in the flour, but these are insufficient in quantity for continuing yeast activity, which then depends on the diastatic production of maltose from *available starch* in the dough. However, excessive diastatic activity continuing during baking may produce dextrins from gelatinizing starch, resulting in a sticky crumb structure in the bread and difficulties in slicing.

The final quality assessment of flour is by test baking

under conditions approximating to the baking procedure for which the flour is intended, but predictive qualitative assessment from the miller's point of view involves determinations of moisture, protein, diastatic activity and colour combined with a rheological test of water absorption and physical dough characteristics. Commonly used commercial equipment for rheological examination of doughs include the *Simon Extensometer* and '*Water Absorption Meter*', the *Brabender Farinograph* and *Extensimeter*, and the *Chopin Alveographe*. *See* Flour, Dietary Importance

Water

For a simple flour/water dough, water of medium hardness generally gives the optimum physical properties, and very soft water tends to produce sticky doughs, but in practical breadmaking other ingredients are sufficient to ensure that any normal mains water is satisfactory.

The *amount* of water used is a critical determinant of the physical properties of the dough. The optimum water addition is known as the *water absorption* of the flour, and the *temperature* of the water is adjusted to produce the desired dough temperature.

Yeast

In former times yeast was added as a '*barm*' or preferment, in which malt and water were mashed together, then mixed with flour and 'scalded' with boiling water to gelatinize the starch and set aside to cool. A quantity of old barm, from a previous batch, was then added and the mixture allowed to ferment for 3 or 4 days before use. Pre-ferments of a similar nature, but based on the use of cultured baker's yeast, are still sometimes used to impart flavour to the loaf.

Baker's yeast comprises cultured varieties of *Saccharomyces cerevisiae* selected for optimum gas production in the comparatively nutrient-poor and semifluid conditions in dough. The yeast is obtainable either (and more generally as rectangular blocks of 1 kg nominal weight or as pelleted dried yeast.

The pressed yeast is added at dough-making without prior preparation; dried yeast requires to be mixed with a dilute sugar solution for a short while (say 30 min) before use and is, accordingly, regarded as 'for emergency use only', or for use in pre-ferments for speciality breads.

In the initial stage of dough fermentation, natural sugars in the flour provide the energy source for the yeast, which subsequently is provided by diastatically produced maltose. The change of energy source requires a metabolic adjustment by the yeast, which normally

results in a temporary hiatus in gas production. Recently selected yeast varieties adjust to the change in energy source very rapidly, with a scarcely perceptible variation in the rate of gas production.

Salt

Salt addition counteracts dough stickiness and improves bread flavour. With no salt addition doughs tend to be difficult to handle; with excessive salt addition fermentation is undesirably slowed. It is important that salt is never allowed to come into direct contact with the yeast.

Fat

In the traditional process, addition of fat to the dough has little or no effect on handling properties, but has a slight crumb-softening effect in the resulting bread, which therefore seems 'fresh' for slightly longer. In mechanically developed dough procedures, the addition of high-melting-point fat (melting point higher than the dough temperature during proof) has a marked improving effect on dough-handling properties, and is essential for acceptable loaf volume and crumb texture.

Minor Ingredients

Small quantities of unprocessed soya bean flour are often added in traditional recipes and are reputed to give improved crumb colour and texture, probably mainly as a result of lipoxygenase activity.

In mechanically developed doughs, marked improvement in loaf volume and crumb texture result from the addition of ascorbic acid or azodicarbonamide.

Flour Constituents

Moisture

The moisture content of flour is generally in the range 12·5–15% and variations within this range have no effect apart from a proportional decrease in water absorption as moisture content increases.

Protein

In both traditional and mechanically developed doughs, an increase in protein content is generally reflected in loaf volume, but the effect is also markedly dependent on protein quality, depending on wheat variety. In general, mechanically developed doughs produce similar loaf volumes from flours with protein levels approximately 1% less than required for the traditional process (e.g. 10% protein on 14·5% moisture basis in mechanical development as compared with 11% protein for the traditional process). *See* Protein, Interactions and Reactions Involved in Food Processing

Starch

During the proof stage of breadmaking, mechanically damaged starch grains (seen under visible light microscopy as 'ghost' grains with fainter than normal outlines and more readily stained with 0.35% congo red solution) provide the substrate for amylase activity to produce maltose – crucial for maintaining yeast activity and consequently gas production throughout the proof period. *See* Starch, Functional Properties

During baking, starch granules become partially gelatinized, and gelatinized grains are then subject to attack by α-amylase to produce sticky dextrins. Gelatinization commences at about 60°C, at which temperature α-amylase is still active, but beginning to be subject to heat denaturation, so the overall effect depends on the length of time that regions of the dough piece remain in the temperature range from about 60 to 80°C. This length of time is itself dependent on the rate of heat transfer to the dough piece in the oven (i.e. on oven temperature) and within the dough piece (i.e. on its size and shape). Heat transfer *within* the dough piece is comparatively slow, with a temperature of 95°C attained after some 25 min in the oven for a 450 g loaf. Consequently, the deleterious efects of α-amylase are more obvious in large loaves than in small goods.

As the baking process is completed, starch, both native and partially gelatinized, forms an intimate part, together with denatured gluten, of the crumb structure of the resulting bread, and it is the rate of physical changes taking place in the starch fraction during subsequent storage which plays a determinant part in the process known as staling.

Pentosans

Typical patents flour contains 2–3% of total pentosans, about half of which are soluble pentosans, which contribute largely to water absorption.

Lipids

The average fat content of flour is from 1 to 1·5%; stored flour is subject to deterioration as a result of the development of oxidative rancidity, particularly when stored at moisture contents less than about 12%.

Enzymes

α-Amylase

Flour contains a low level of fermentable sugars (about 0·5%), a level that is too low to support yeast activity throughout the proof period but is sufficient to produce adequate carbon dioxide for good-sized, well-aerated loaves. During dough fermentation, amylases produce maltose from 'available starch'. Granular starch is not susceptible to hydrolysis by amylases, but flour normally contains a proportion (usually 9–10% in a typical breadmaking flour) of starch granules which have been mechanically damaged during milling and provide 'available starch' for amylase activity. *See* Enzymes, Uses in Food Processing

During baking, the starch content of the dough undergoes partial gelatinization and, during the 2–3 min that the centre of the loaf is at 60–70°C, the partially gelatinized starch is subject to hydrolysis to dextrins by the indigenous α-amylase before this is inactivated by heat. (α-Amylase loses about 50% of its activity at 75°C.) Consequently, excessive α-amylase activity results in excessive dextrin production, producing sticky crumb in the resulting bread.

Amylase activity in the wheat grain increases by at least 1000-fold during germination – so that even incipient sprout renders wheat unsuitable for milling to breadmaking flour.

β-Amylase

The action of β-amylase produces maltose by complete hydrolysis of the amylose fraction of starch, and from the nonreducing chain ends of the amylopectin fraction. β-Amylase action is completely obstructed by a 1,6 linkage, and consequently the residues from its action on amylopectin are high-molecular-weight dextrins, sometimes referred to as *erythrodextrins*, which do not have the property of stickiness and have no deleterious effect on bread quality.

The starch in native starch granules is completely unavailable to β-amylase, and its seems probable that even its action on 'damaged starch' is mediated by accompanying α-amylase. From the breadmaking point of view, β-amylase activity in flour is never deficient – though its substrate (damaged or partially gelatinized starch) very well may be – and β-amylase activity (i.e. maltose production) can be increased by addition of a source of α-amylase (either fungal amylase or malt flour).

Proteinase

Small amounts of proteinase activity occur in most baking flours, small amounts occur in most commercially available sources of fungal amylase and rather larger amounts in malt flours.

The general effects of proteinase are to 'mellow' the dough, making it more readily moulded and worked by increasing gluten extensibility. Consequently, increased proteinase activity may be advantageous with very strong baking flours, but is not required with flours produced from grists containing high proportions of European wheats as is usual in this country.

Additives

Lipids

Loaf volume and crumb texture and grain are improved by the inclusion of high-melting point fat (i.e. melting point above proof temperature) in mechanically developed doughs. In particular, release of carbon dioxide from the loaf while the internal temperature is rising from 38 to 80°C is delayed, and the period of loaf expansion is correspondingly extended.

Surfactants

In both traditional and mechanically developed doughs, surfactants with an HLB (hydrophile–lypophile balance) between 6 and 14 find a place as crumb-softening and antistaling agents.

Permitted ingredients in this category to a total of 5000 mg kg^{-1} of bread weight, are: the mono- and diglycerides of fatty acids, their lactic acid, citric acid, and mono- and diacetyl esters (E471, E472(b), E472(c) and E472(e)); stearyl tartrate (E483); and sodium and calcium stearoyl-2-lactylates (E481 and E482).

Enzymes

α-Amylase

Supplementation with a source of α-amylase at an appropriate level is often necessary to ensure that sugar (maltose) production continues throughout the proof period. Whereas addition of either sucrose or glucose to provide nutrient for the yeast tends to give excessive initial production of carbon dioxide followed by a sharp fall in gas production, supplementation by α-amylase results in a continuous replacement of maltose as it is utilized by yeast and, therefore, a steady production of gas throughout the proof period.

Subsidiary advantages are that supplementation gives improved gas retention properties of the dough, due to the starch modification, improved crust colour (due to the Maillard reaction) and, possibly, improved flavour.

Supplementation may be in the form of malt (either malted barley or malted wheat) or as preparations of fungal or bacterial amylase. Malt has the advantage of adding flavour to the loaf, but the treatment level is critical. Excessive malt addition results in excessively sticky crumb and difficulties in slicing. *See* Malt, Chemistry of Malting

Fungal amylase preparations have the advantage over malt that fungal α-amylase is more heat-sensitive than malt α-amylase, such that overtreatment is unlikely. Small amounts of fungal α-amylase are often added to bakers' flours at the mill.

Bacterial α-amylase is much less heat-sensitive than either malt or fungal amylase and, therefore, can only be used in extremely small quantities without causing problems of sticky crumb. However, it is sometimes used in small amounts to retard staling as a result of increased starch modification.

Proteinase

Proteinase additions result in an increase in dough extensibility, and so can be used to mellow the dough resulting from excessively strong flour. Most commercial fungal α-amylase preparations contain small amounts of proteinase as an impurity.

Lipoxygenase

Additions of sources of lipoxygenases result in bleaching of carotenoid pigments to give a whiter and brighter crumb. Unprocessed soya bean flour at the level of 0·5–1·0% on a flour basis is used to provide lipoxygenase activity. The addition of soya bean flour also tends to give a finer crumb, better loaf volume and improved rheological properties to the dough.

Bread Problems

Weights and Measures

Bread is sold by weight, but dough is normally measured by volume, except in small-volume production, and in any case the weight of bread is less than the weight of dough because of moisture losses during baking and, to a much lesser extent, also to loss of weight due to conversion of solids to alcohol and carbon dioxide during fermentation. Furthermore, this loss of moisture continues during storage, to the time of sale and beyond. Loss of weight during baking is between 11 and 12%, depending on oven conditions and humidity in the prover and cooler, but reasonably reproducible over time for any particular bakery, and allowance for this loss must be made at scaling time. In addition, scaling variability must be allowed for – since weights and measures control concerns the average weight and variance of loaves leaving the bakery for sale.

Microbiological

Because of the slight acidity of dough and its heat treatment in the oven, bread is, when it emerges from the oven, free from vegetative organisms, although it may still contain viable bacterial spores. On cooling, and particularly on slicing, however, bread is readily contaminated with fungal spores from the atmosphere. The moist nature of the crumb means that it provides a good growth medium for such fungi, which may cause problems, particularly in warm weather conditions.

The most important preventative measures are those aimed at reducing the fungal spore load in the bakery atmosphere – such as by provision of filtered air and/or of ultraviolet lamps in the roof spaces – and frequent and efficient cleaning of slicing machines. Additional precautionary measures during warm weather conditions may usefully include the addition of permitted preservatives at dough-making, e.g. vinegar or dilute acetic acid, or sodium diacetate or sodium or calcium propionate. *See* Preservation of Food

Fungal

The main fungal species which grow on bread are *Penicillium glaucum* (greenish-blue), *Mucor mucedo* (white), and *Aspergillus niger* (black). Much less frequently pink or orange growths occur, which are usually caused by *Neurospora sitophila* or related species.

Bacterial

The main bacterial problem associated with bread is the development of 'ropy bread' – caused by the survival of spores of *Bacillus subtilis* var. *mesentericus*, a soil organism whose spores may be present in flour, spices and other ingredients used in the bakery, and which are capable of developing into vegetative organisms in the baked bread under warm storage conditions. The first indication of trouble is a very slight fruity smell (often described as reminiscent of pineapple) in the loaf. On subsequent warm storage, the odour rapidly develops, becoming more definitely unpleasant, and is associated with brown, soft and sticky spots showing in the crumb. Eventually the spots coalesce to form the sticky, stringy mass known as '*rope*'. *See* Spoilage, Bacterial Spoilage

Additional acidification of doughs during warm weather conditions is an effective measure of control, but any case of rope development requires to be countered by a thorough cleaning and sterilization of the bakery.

Of extremely rare occurrence is the development of 'bleeding bread', a condition involving the development of red spots, and eventually the semiliquefaction of affected portions of the crumb – due to the development of *Bacillus prodigiosus*, another soilborne, spore-forming organism.

Physical

Staling

Physical changes in bread commence immediately after baking; the crumb gradually loses its springiness, while the crust tends to lose its crispness. At the same time the loaf gradually loses moisture. To some degree these physical changes are due to moisture movement as crust and crumb, initially very different in moisture content, tend to equilibrate.

However, prevention of moisture loss does not prevent the onset of the physical changes which lead to an assessment of the loaf as 'stale'.

In the 1930s, Katz in the Netherlands showed that the development of staleness was associated with major changes in the starch fraction of the crumb. Katz demonstrated that these changes led to reduced swelling power of the crumb in water, a reduced content of soluble polysaccharides, and, more fundamentally, a change in the X ray diffraction pattern exhibited by the crumb. He also showed that the rate of these changes could be reduced by storage at above normal room temperature (were it not for the danger of rope and/or fungal development under such conditions). The changes in the starch fraction are also greatly reduced by freezing the bread, and substantially all staling ceases at temperatures below $-20°C$.

It was later shown that the rate of change is at a maximum at temperatures close to $0°C$ and at a minimum at about $55°C$. The change is partially reversible at higher temperatures, a feature well known in the improved acceptability of stale bread after toasting. This reversibility is also demonstrable by differential thermal analysis (DTA), when the DTA diagram of reheated stale breadcrumb resembles that of fresh bread.

Various emulsifier preparations are advocated for use as 'antistaling agents' in breadmaking, but it is probable that their function is truly as crumb softeners – the bread initially has a softer than normal crumb, so that a longer time passes before crumb hardness reaches the stage evaluated as 'stale', despite an unchanged rate for the physical changes occurring in the starch fraction. *See* Emulsifiers, Uses in Processed Foods

Bibliography

Fance WJ and Wragg BH (1968) *Up-to-Date Breadmaking*. London: McLaren and Sons.
Hoseney RC (1986) *Principles of Cereal Science and Technology*, St Paul: American Association of Cereal Chemists.
Kent NL (1983) *Technology of Cereals*, 3rd edn. London: Pergamon Press.
Kent-Jones DW and Amos AJ (1967) *Modern Cereal Chemistry*, 6th edn. London: Food Trade Press.
Kent-Jones DW and Mitchell EF (1962) *The Practice and*

Science of Breadmaking, 3rd edn. Liverpool: The Northern Publishing Company.

Lorenz KJ and Kulp K (eds) (1990) *Handbook of Cereal Science and Technology*, New York: Marcel Dekker.

Pomeranz Y (ed.) (1988) *Wheat: Chemistry and Technology*, 2nd edn, 2 vols. St Paul: American Association of Cereal Chemists.

E. C. Apling
Norwich, UK

Chemistry of Baking

Components of Wheat

Many of the components of wheat have a significant effect on the processing properties of wheat flour. Typical compositions for wheat and flour are shown in Table 1. Reactions and interactions of the components determine the milling quality, dough-mixing properties and breadmaking quality of wheat. Despite the extensive research effort put into the analysis of the components, little is still known about the ultimate effects of reactions and interactions. Furthermore, the effects strongly depend on the type of baking process and the bread formulation. Therefore, some elements of the chemistry of the baking process are still uncertain. In this article an overview will be given of the reactions and interactions of the components of wheat. *See* Wheat

Effects and Changes of Components

Proteins

Wheat flour contains 8–16% protein. The quantity and quality of protein determine the breadmaking quality to a large extent. The quantity of protein largely depends on conditions of cultivation, whereas protein quality predominantly has a genetic basis. Since over 140 different proteins or protein subunits are known to be present in wheat, the assessment of protein quality is extremely complex.

About 80–90% of the protein is insoluble in water and is called gluten. The other 10–20% soluble proteins of wheat flour consist of metabolic enzymes, α-amylase and protease inhibitors. Reports on their influence on dough-mixing properties and breadmaking quality are conflicting. Due to their unique viscoelastic, cohesive and gas-retaining properties it is the gluten proteins which are largely responsible for the breadmaking quality of wheat. *See* Protein, Chemistry

Gluten proteins are characterized by high glutamine (35–42%) and proline (13–20%) contents. They can be divided into two groups of proteins: gliadins and glutenins. The gliadins are globular proteins with a molecular weight between 30 and 75 kDa. They contain intramolecular disulphide bonds. Gliadins are soluble in 70% ethanol and can be separated according to their hydrophobicity into 60–70 peaks by reversed-phase high-performance liquid chromatography. Gliadins are considered to be responsible for the viscous properties of gluten. *See* Chromatography, High-performance Liquid Chromatography

Glutenins consist of longitudinally shaped subunits varying in molecular weight between 60 and 140 kDa. The subunits are cross-linked by intermolecular disulphide bonds to form aggregates larger than 2000 kDa, making the glutenins insoluble in water, 70% ethanol and only partially soluble in dilute acetic acid or sodium dodecyl sulphate (SDS) solutions. Upon reduction of their disulphide bonds, glutenins become completely soluble in dilute acetic acid or SDS. The amino-(N-) and carboxy-(C-) terminal ends of the glutenin subunits of high molecular weight (90–140 kDa) contain thiol groups. The high-molecular-weight glutenins are thought to form the structural backbone of the glutenin polymer to which low-molecular-weight glutenin subunits can become associated. Based on amino acid sequencing, the C- and N-terminal ends of the high-molecular-weight glutenin subunits are likely to have an α-helical structure (Fig. 1(a)). The central part of the glutenins consists of repetitive blocks of 6–15 amino acids (glycine, proline and glutamine). This results in a high content of β-turn structure, which is probably responsible for the elastic properties of the gluten. *See* Amino Acids, Properties and Occurrence

During mixing of the dough intermolecular disulphide bonds between the glutenin subunits are split and a thiol/disulphide bond interchange takes place. During proving, disulphide bonds are formed again. Not all disulphide bonds of the proteins are involved in the interchange (Fig. 2). Reduction of only a few essential

Table 1. Composition of wheat and patent flour

Component	Wheat (%, as is basis)	Patent flour (%, as is basis)
Protein	9–17	8–16
Soluble protein		10–20
Gliadin		40–50
Glutenin		40–45
Starch	57–65	65–71
NSPs[a]		2–3
Bran	10–15	
Lipids	2–3	1–2
Ash	1·6–1·8	0·4–0·6
Moisture	15–17	14–16

[a] NSPs, nonstarch polysaccharides.

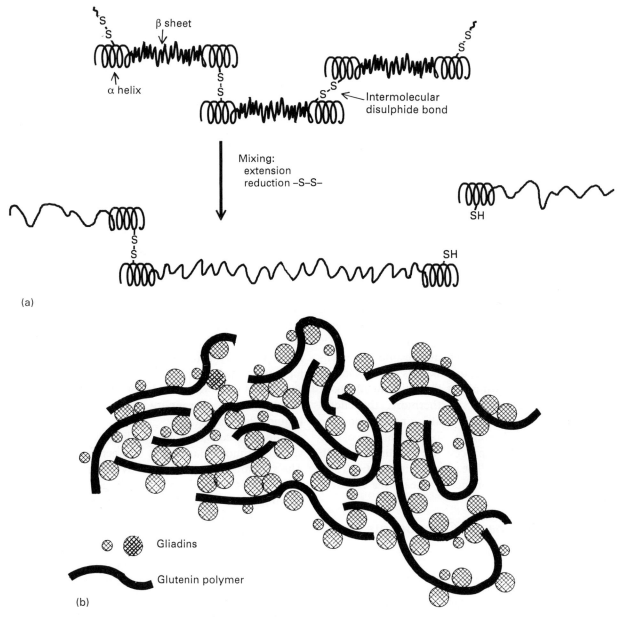

Fig. 1 Schematic presentation of (a) the structure of the glutenin polymer and of (b) the interaction of glutenins and gliadins.

disulphide bonds can have a large influence on dough properties. After breakdown of the glutenin matrix an optimum reformation is necessary for sufficient gas retention. Gliadins are seen as the plasticizers of the glutenins (Fig. 1(b)). They are probably also involved in this dynamic process, by means of hydrophilic and hydrophobic bonds.

During mixing small gas bubbles are introduced into the dough. During proving these gas cells expand and a foamy structure is formed. Gluten stabilizes this foam. During baking the proteins denature and the foam structure of dough is transformed into the open, spongy structure of bread. At 75°C the glutenins aggregate. Gliadins are more stable and denature at higher tem-

peratures. During thermosetting another thiol/disulphide interchange takes place by which the aggregation of the proteins is fixed. From 60°C onwards the viscosity increases sharply and carbon dioxide and ethanol escape from the gas cells. Finally, the increase in loaf volume in the oven is stopped.

Starch

Starch is the largest constituent of flour, but its role in the chemical reactions in dough and bread is less important compared to protein. Physicochemical changes are of importance, however.

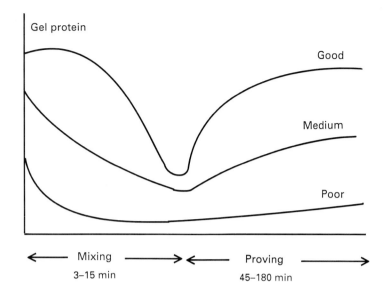

Fig. 2 Depolymerization of the glutenin polymer (gel proteins) during mixing and polymerization during the resting period of flours varying in breadmaking quality.

Bread wheat (*Triticum aestivum*) can be divided into hard- and soft-milling types. During milling, starch of the hard type is more damaged than starch from the soft type. Damaged starch absorbs more water than undamaged starch. Some degree of starch damage is necessary to increase the availability of carbohydrates by starch-degrading enzymes. Enzymes produce small fermentable sugars, necessary for the growth of yeast.

During baking, starch gelatinizes and more water is absorbed. The gelatinization reduces the availability of water for other components. The viscosity of the dough increases sharply and thermosetting of the dough starts. The gelatinized starch together with the denatured protein form a firm structure. Since dough contains less than 40% water, which is only partially in the free form, starch does not gelatinize completely. A few days after baking the partially gelatinized starch recrystallizes (retrogradation). This process is probably responsible for the increase in crumb firmness and staling of bread. *See* Starch, Structure, Properties and Determination

Minor Components

Nonstarch Polysaccharides

Although nonstarch polysaccharides (NSPs) are a minor component of flour (2–3%), they are able to bind 15–30% of the water in a dough. NSPs can be divided into a water-soluble and a water-insoluble fraction. Most of them are composed of a xylose chain with arabinose side-chains (arabinoxylan), but glucose and some mannose and galactose are also present. Ferulic acid (1–2% in the NSPs) can react by oxidative coupling with another ferulic acid molecule and probably also with certain amino acids. Thus, an NSP network can be formed or NSPs can react with proteins. This indicates that they can be involved in chemical reactions in a dough. Unfortunately, only ambiguous and conflicting information on this subject is available. *See* Carbohydrates, Classification and Properties

Whole meal contains about 15% bran, which consists largely of NSPs and lignin. The bran or bran fractions are not involved chemically in the breadmaking process. They are probably able to disrupt physically the membranes of gas cells in a dough.

Lipids

Wheat flour contains 1–2% lipids. Of the 40–50 different types present, triglycerides and digalactosyldiglyceride are the most abundant. Furthermore, lysophosphatidylcholine is found as a complex with starch. *See* Lipids, Classification; Triglycerides, Structures and Properties

Lipids have only a minor effect on dough-mixing properties, but have strong effects on the breadmaking process. The effects of lipids seem to depend largely on the type of process and the dough formula used. For US and Canadian wheat varieties high contents of free polar lipids (glycolipids and phospholipids) or low ratios of free nonpolar lipids to free polar lipids are correlated with loaf volume, whereas this has not been observed for Australian, French or UK wheats. *See* Phospholipids, Properties and Occurrence

Wheat germ contains a large proportion of polyunsaturated fatty acids. Whole meal often includes wheat germ. Too long a storage period causes rancidity of the flour, making it unsuitable for breadmaking.

Endogenous Enzymes

The most important endogenous enzyme in wheat is α-amylase. A certain amount of amylase is needed for the release of fermentable carbohydrates from damaged starch. Too large an amount of α-amylase, as found in wheat that has undergone preharvest sprouting, is detrimental. Excessive amylase action results in a large oven spring during baking but results in a coarse and open crumb structure. This makes sprout-damaged wheat unsuitable for bread production. Sprouting is a serious threat to wheat production in north-west Europe.

Of the other enzymes present in wheat (e.g. proteases, oxidases and ester hydrolases), the oxidases are the most important. They are probably involved in the oxidation–reduction reactions of the glutenin matrix in a dough.

Bread Improvers

The use of bread improvers is an old practice. Addition of yeast or sour dough is well known, and enzymes and improvers in the form of malt have been applied for a long time. In Europe, gluten, which is isolated on an industrial scale, is used to fortify wheat flour of medium quality or to improve the breadmaking quality of whole meal. *See* Malt, Malt Types and Products

Oxidizing and Reducing Agents

Since thiol groups play an important role in dough development, process tolerance and breadmaking quality, the use of oxidizing agents is widespread. Their mechanism of action is shown in eqn [1]. *See* Oxidation of Food Components

$$Ox_3^- + 2 \text{ protein—SH} \rightarrow \\ Ox_2^- + \text{Protein—SS—Protein} + H_2O \quad (1)$$

—SH, free thiol group
—SS—, disulphide bond

The halogenates potassium bromate and iodate have been widely used. Their use is more and more restricted by law. Thiol groups, which are formed upon mixing, are oxidized by bromate to disulphide bonds, thus cross-linking proteins to a large glutenin matrix. Potassium iodate works in a similar, but faster way.

L-Ascorbic acid is also used as an improving agent. In a dough, ascorbic acid is converted to dehydro-L-ascorbic acid. This is the active substance which oxidizes thiol groups to disulphide bonds. The overall effect on dough properties of ascorbic acid and the halogenates is different. There is not yet sufficient knowledge of the oxidation–reduction reactions in dough to explain these differences. *See* Ascorbic Acid, Properties and Determination

L-Cysteine can be used as a reducing agent together with oxidizing agents to regulate dough development. Cysteine addition results in a lower work input during mixing, but it can easily be overdosed.

Malt and Enzymes

In contrast to the enzymes from malt, food-grade enzymes from microorganisms have only recently been in use as a processing aid in the breadmaking industry. α-Amylases are used to improve the fermentation of yeast, to improve crust colour and – most importantly – to improve the shelf life of bread. Cellulases and hemicellulases are used to improve crumb structure and shelf life. Proteases can be used to improve mixing properties of a dough which is too tough, e.g. when gluten is added to flour. *See* Enzymes, Uses in Food Processing

Emulsifiers and Fats

A wide range of emulsifiers and fats are used in the baking process. Usually lard is used as fat. Some of the emulsifiers in use are: lecithin (E322), monoglycerides (E471), esters from monoglycerides and diacetyltartaric acid (DATEM; E472e) and sodium or calcium stearoyl-lactylate (E481 or E482). Lard and emulsifiers are added in 2% and 0·5% amounts or lower on a flour weight basis respectively. *See* Fats, Uses in the Food Industry

Most of the emulsifiers and fats have no effect on the rheological properties of a dough but improve the handling of a dough. They are able to increase loaf volume. Some emulsifiers and fats act as surface-active agents in stabilizing gas bubbles of a rising dough. They improve crumb structure, which results in a soft crumb and a longer shelf life. Furthermore, they can postpone the thermosetting in the oven and thus increase the oven spring.

Salt

Salt is added not only to improve the taste, but also to improve the dough properties. It has a stiffening effect and makes a dough less sticky. By reducing the electric double layer around flour particles, salt decreases the electrostatic repulsion between particles. The interaction between the particles is thus improved, which can explain the observed effects on dough properties.

Water

The amount of water is important during the whole baking process: it affects the rheological properties of dough, it determines the extent of starch gelatinization and protein denaturation and it is important for the firmness of the crumb after baking. The optimum amount of water varies among flours and is usually established with standard mixing equipment before baking.

Interactions

The process from mixing to baking and the use of additives is directed to obtain optimum interactions between the components. Therefore, it is not surprising that interactions play a central part in dough properties and breadmaking quality.

Protein–Protein

The interactions between gluten proteins have been already discussed. Strong interactions between the gluten proteins are possible by covalent (disulphide bonds), hydrogen (glutamine pairing), ionic and hydrophobic bonds.

Lipid–Protein

An increased lipid–protein interaction becomes evident after flour has been mixed with water, when lipids become less extractable with organic solvents. After isolation of gluten, most of the lipids appear to be firmly bound to the gluten.

Probably, gas cells formed by the protein starch matrix are stabilized by the surface-active properties of most lipids and emulsifiers.

Lipid–Starch

In contrast to many other starches, wheat starch contains lipids. The aliphatic chain of lysophosphatidylcholine is found in the helices of amylose or amylopectin of starch. This complex is disrupted at temperatures higher than 100°C. Also, some emulsifiers and some nonwheat lipids are able to form complexes with the helices. The helix is stabilized and, during heating, gelatinization is retarded. The thermosetting of a dough during baking is postponed and the increase in loaf volume continues for a longer time.

Starch–Protein

The partial gelatinization of starch during baking sets the structure of bread by stabilizing the gluten film around the gas cells.

Starch contains proteins, which are distinct from gluten proteins. The content of some of these proteins,

called friabilin, differs markedly between hard and soft wheats. Friabilin is thought to be involved in kernel hardness.

NSPs–Protein

Gluten proteins contain a small amount of NSPs. Some oxidizing agents (e.g. dehydroascorbic acid) are able to increase the amount of NSPs attached to the protein. The role of these NSPs on the protein is not completely clear. It is possible that they interfere with the formation of a glutenin matrix, since hydrolysis of NSPs by hemicellulases results in a finer crumb structure.

In conclusion, the complexity of the breadmaking process and the large number of physicochemical reactions make the chemistry of bread an intriguing and interesting topic.

Bibliography

Blanshard JMV, Frazier PJ and Galliard T (eds) (1985) *Chemistry and Physics of Baking. Materials, Processes and Products.* London: Royal Society of Chemistry.
Bushuk W and Tkachuk R (eds) (1990) *Gluten Proteins.* Proceedings of the 4th International Workshop on Gluten Proteins. St Paul, MN: American Association of Cereal Chemists.
Hamer RJ (1991) Enzymes in baking. In: Tucker GA and Woods LJ (eds) *Enzymes in Food Processing.* Glasgow: Blackie.
Lásztity R and Békés FF (eds) (1987) *Gluten Proteins.* Proceedings of the 3rd International Workshop on Gluten Proteins. Singapore: World Scientific.
Pomeranz Y (ed.) (1988) Wheat—Chemistry and Technology, 3rd edn, vols I and II. St Paul, MN: American Association of Cereal Chemists.

P. Weegels
TNO Biotechnology and Chemistry Institute, The Netherlands

Sourdough Bread

Sourdoughs are so called because the bread is leavened with a mixture of yeast(s) and lactic acid bacteria. It should be appreciated that a conventional yeast leaven will always contain some lactic acid bacteria, and that there will be a contribution to the final flavour which is attributable to them, but this will be minor and will certainly not result in an appreciate level of acidity in the final bread. In a true sourdough, on the other hand, the contribution of the lactic acid bacteria will always be detectable, at least to the experienced palate, and quite often the acidity is sufficient to be noticeable to the normal consumer. The sourdough way of making bread is of great antiquity, and many experts would agree that it is almost certainly the oldest way of leavening doughs, as a sour leaven will arise naturally if a mixture of flour and water is left in a warm place for a few hours; if this is used to inoculate a fresh flour/water mixture (dough), which is then allowed to ferment and used to inoculate a third portion of dough, and so forth, there will be a gradual evolution of a compatible mixture of yeast and *Lactobacillus* species. From the first mixing of flour and water, the developed sour ferment can be used to leaven a batch of bread dough, but as the sour is developed through succeeding generations, its quality and the consistency with which it leavens bread dough will improve, and the resulting bread will be more uniform. In some traditions the sour dough starter is thus maintained for a very long time, possibly centuries, while in other practices the sour starter is begun again every so often. *See* Leavening Agents; Lactic Acid Bacteria; Starter Cultures; Yeasts

Historical Background

Many people, especially in the USA, think first, or only, of the San Francisco area when sourdough breads are mentioned. These bakers trace their roots back to the days of the pioneers, when sourdough bread, pancakes, etc., were an essential part of life in the covered wagon trains. The same heritage is found in Alaska, where the pioneers and especially the gold-miners were called 'sourdoughs', as any reader of Jack London's stories will know. Dried yeast was not available at that time, so sourdough was the only way to have bread and other biologically leavened foods on the trail or in remote encampments.

This way of making bread, etc., would not have seemed particularly strange in those days as many of the settlers would know or have kinship with Europeans with traditions of making this type of bread.

This type of baking is still very widespread in Germany, Scandinavia, Eastern Europe, etc., but, perhaps surprisingly, French breads also quite often use this type of leaven. Even in Scotland there was a traditional way of making bread using a liquid leaven called a 'Parisian barm' which was still practised in some areas until quite well into this century, and one commercial bakery was still using a combination of Parisian barm and a final leavening with pressed yeast until a few years ago. Robert Service attached so much importance and familiarity to the word that one of his books of poems is called 'Songs of a Sourdough'.

Allied Products

Many products with a relationship to sourdough breads are produced in various parts of the world. Surplus

barm is used in making soups, e.g. in Poland. Kvass is a sharp, refreshing acidic drink found in Russia and much of Eastern Europe, which is traditionally made by toasting rye bread, crumbling it into water, then allowing a fermentation to take place, after which the golden-brown, sharp, slightly sparkling, rather nutty-tasting liquid is poured off and drunk. The brew is kept going by replenishing the mixture with fresh toast and water at intervals but, if a brew is to be started *de novo*, then fermentation is assured by inoculating with a portion of sourdough. The Italian festive cake called 'panettone' is properly made with a sourdough starter specially maintained for this purpose, and there are reputed to be a number of similar products in various parts of the world. There is also a link with products such as the Indian food called 'Idli', although it is a little tenuous as Idli is made from a mixture of black gram (a variety of mung bean) and rice, and the leavening action is due to gas produced by the heterofermentative lactic acid bacterium *Leuconostoc*. Another variation is found in the use of presoaking to prepare certain ingredients for use in specialist breads. In a particular case a bakery was using whole and kibbled (i.e. coarsely ground, crushed into large pieces or bruised) grains in breads such as the Vogel formula loaf and Turkestan-style bread. The whole and kibbled grains and coarse bran were mixed with water then left in the bakery overnight to soak up all the water that they could. Next morning this mixture was incorporated with the other ingredients to make the final dough, which was leavened with pressed yeast in the usual manner. The bakery had not appreciated that the overnight soaking in the warm environment of the bakery was having any particular effect, assuming that the only purpose of it was the one that they had originally intended, namely to ensure that the materials in question had imbibed all the water that they could, although the bakery workers had noticed that the vessels containing the materials had a sour aroma and a marked frothiness when uncovered in the morning. In fact there was a vigorous growth of lactic acid bacteria and some wild yeasts in the mixture overnight, and the acidity carried through to the finished bread, where it made an appreciable contribution to the flavour of the product.

Effects of Sour Fermentation on the Bread

Several effects are observed in addition to the obvious one of an acid note to the flavour. The dough proteins are particularly affected, with changes in elasticity and extensibility which may result in the dough becoming in effect stronger, thus improving the baking performance of weak flours, and it is thus clear why sourdough formulations are so often associated with rye breads, as rye flour is much weaker than the typical wheat flour. Rye flour also differs from wheat flour in that it

Sourdough Bread

possesses higher levels of α-amylase, so that if a rye-based dough is fermented at neutral pH, excessive breakdown of the starch is observed. At the lower pH associated with the sour dough process, the amylolytic activity is reduced to an acceptable level. *See* Rye

Sourdough fermentations result in an increased hydrolysis of phytate from the grain; two factors are probably at work here, the fact that these are rather slow fermentations, so allowing more time for the plant's phytases to effect hydrolysis, plus the lower pH, which is optimum for phytase activity. We have some evidence for both phytase and phosphatase activity in lactic acid bacteria isolated from such ferments (especially those from the 'presoaks' described in the previous section), but are not yet able to assess the significance of the results or the contribution which such activities (if confirmed by more detailed work) may make to the finished bread. The significance of phytase activity is that phytic acid is a powerful chelating agent for a number of nutritionally important metal ions, including calcium, copper, iron and zinc, so reducing the level of phytic acid will aid the absorption of these nutrients by the bread's consumer, which may be particularly important to those on vegetarian and 'macrobiotic' diets, although some authorities suggest that even the supposedly over-fed US consumer may be getting scarcely enough of these nutrients, and may even be nutritionally compromised for them. *See* Macrobiotic Diets; Phytic Acid, Nutritional Impact; Vegetarian Diets

The acids formed in the fermentation are principally lactic and acetic (ethanoic) acids and it is believed that their presence may contribute to the storage life of the bread by acting as mild antimicrobials, particularly effective against moulds, which are often the first agents of biodegradation of bread. There is also evidence that the acids are damaging to the spores of *Bacillus* species, bacteria often present in the ingredients used for breads, particularly the wholegrain and so-called 'organic' types of materials favoured by some makers of sourdough breads because of their association with particular lifestyles. There is also good evidence that the acidity, and possibly other factors associated with sourdough fermentations, increase the time between baking and the onset of evident staling of the loaf. *See* Bacillus, Occurrence; Organic Foods

Sourdough Bread Processes

From the foregoing, it will be clear that there are many variations on the theme of sourdough bread production, but in order to keep this discussion within reasonable bounds, it will be convenient to present two basic types, although bearing in mind that other approaches are not necessarily just variants on the processes described here as many of them have a quite clear identity, e.g. the Scottish 'Parisian barm' process mentioned above. However, the majority of the sourdough bread produced commercially can legitimately be regarded as variants on one or other of the two main types.

Rye Breads (particularly in Germany)

The work of the Detmold (Germany) group of Spicher and his colleagues over many years has provided a deep understanding of the sourdough breads of Germany. They report that several microbial species participate in the fermentations. From some sources it seems to be the practice to restart the German sour ferments fairly frequently, and this probably helps to bring about the diversity of species. On the other hand Spicher notes that 'The development of commercial sourdough starter cultures over several decades has led to a certain natural selection of organisms that predominate in the fermentation'. This observation is in agreement with the work of other investigators who have studied sourdoughs from various parts of the world. Spicher also reports that attempts to replace these natural associations of organisms with pure cultures, as has been done with success in the production of commercial pressed yeast for the baking industry, has not been possible. An opposite claim will be discussed later.

Among the processes in German practice according to Spicher are multistage, two-stage and single-stage sourdoughs. The last require the addition of yeast for good leavening, whereas the two-stage and multistage processes develop a yeast flora sufficient to leaven the dough fully. The single-stage processes are classified into the Detmold, Berlin and Manheim (salt–sour) methods. In the Detmold process the amount of starter and the temperature used for the fermentation are such that the process takes about 15–24 h. The temperature is in the range 20–28°C, with the amount of starter (as a proportion of the sourdough) ranging from 2% at 27–28°C to 20% at 20–23°C. The sourdough is made from a mixture of 55·6% rye flour and 44·4% water. When acidification is complete this sourdough is mixed with a mixture of wheat and rye flours and water plus the necessary yeast. Spicher quotes a typical mixture as 49·5 kg of sourdough, 42·5 kg of rye flour, 30·0 kg of wheat flour and 46·0 litres of water, giving a final proportion of 70% rye flour to 30% wheat flour. In the Berlin process the combination of a high temperature and a high addition of seed sour, plus a softer mixture, gives adequate acidification in only 3–4 h. Spicher quotes a typical mix for the souring stage of the Berlin process as 8·0 kg of seed sour, 40·0 kg of rye flour and 36·0 litres of water, giving a proportion of 52·6% flour to 47·4% water. The sourdough is mixed with 30·0 kg of rye flour, 30·0 kg of wheat flour and 32·0 litres of water, again giving a final ratio of 7:3 for rye to wheat flour. In the salt–sour process the fermentation to produce the sourdough is longer than in the preceding processes, about 48 h being typical, although the presence of the salt will permit times up to 80 h to be used without loss of quality. The mixture for the souring stage contains 5·0 kg of seed sour, 25·0 kg of rye flour and 25·0 litres of water, plus 500 g salt, and is fermented at an initial temperature of 30–35°C, dropping to 15–20°C during 48 h of fermentation. This dough is mixed with 45·0 kg of rye flour, 30·0 kg of wheat flour and 43·0 litres of water to give the final 7:3 ratio of rye to wheat flour. Because of the inhibitory effects of the salt, it is necessary to add 2·5–3·5% w/w of compressed yeast to the final dough mixture, as compared to the 1·0–1·5% used with the preceding processes.

In some other processes described by Spicher, and referred to above as multistage and two-stage, the sour is increased in volume by successive inoculation of larger mixes of rye flour and water, each stage used to inoculate the next. The processes seem to be rather more favourable to the growth of desirable types of wild yeast alongside the lactic acid bacteria (LAB), with the result that either less compressed yeast is added than in the single-stage processes, or that no added yeast at all is needed in some of the multistage processes.

In these multispecies fermentations the major LAB, according to a number of authors, are *Lactobacillus plantarum* (homofermentative), *L. brevis* and *L. fermentum* (both heterofermentative). From the hexose sugars available for fermentation homofermentative bacteria produce lactic acid only, or to such an overwhelming extent that other fermentation products are negligible in practice. Heterofermenters produce a mixture of products, including lactic and acetic acids, ethanol and carbon dioxide, the ratios of these products being influenced by various environmental factors. Other products exist of course, and some of these play a part in the flavours which are characteristic of lactic-fermented products. In addition, LAB can utilize various pentose sugars, with the production of equimolar amounts of lactic and acetic acids. However, it is the homo- or heterofermentative aspect of the fermentation which is important here. According to reports discussed by Oura *et al.* (1982) the best quality bread results when the three species of bacteria are all present. The heterofermenters are essential for development of the 'typical flavour of sour rye bread'. On the other hand the use of the heterofermenters alone gives a bread whose crumb lacks elasticity, but inclusion of the homofermentative *L. plantarum* restores this desirable attribute. The latter organism on its own gives the desired crumb characteristic but the bread lacks aroma. Thus, both types of organisms are essential for production of the finest quality of bread.

Spicher and his co-workers have reported that the yeasts found in sourdoughs used in the production of rye breads fall into four types; *Candida krusei, Saccharomyces cerevisiae, S. exiguus* and *Pichia saitoi*. Again the environmental conditions influence the distribution of yeast species in doughs. Interactions between the yeasts and LAB are complex, and they can stimulate, inhibit or be without influence, one upon another.

Lonner *et al.* (1986), in a study of a sourdough started spontaneously on Swedish rye meal, obtained a rather different result, with some similarities to the flora of the wheat sourdoughs to be discussed below in that the fermentation came to be dominated by only one species of yeast, although in association with three principal LAB isolates. The yeast was identified as *Saccharomyces delbrueckii*. The identities of the LAB were less certain, except that of *Pediococcus pentosaceus*; the other two dominant isolates were assigned as *Lactobacillus* sp. I and sp. II (probably *L. alimentarius*).

Wheat Sourdough Breads

The most important study of these products is that done on the San Francisco process by a group of workers from the US Department of Agriculture's Western Regional Research Laboratories, including Kline, Sugihara, Miller and McCready. They reported that the fermentation is dominated by just two microorganisms, *Lactobacillus sanfrancisco* and the yeast *Saccharomyces exiguus* (sometimes referred to as *Torulopsis holmii*), now reclassified as the new species *Candida milleri*. Thus, both of the dominant organisms are types first isolated from this fermentation, although both have since been reported from other bread fermentations, and also from other types of fermentation.

The most striking aspect of these studies is that the workers have been able to offer an explanation for the remarkable stability of the fermentation, characterized by a constant ratio of yeast to LAB cells of 1:100. The yeast, unlike the usual compressed baker's yeast (*S. cerevisiae*), cannot utilize maltose, whereas the LAB can utilize only this sugar, so, like Jack Sprat and his wife in the nursery rhyme, they live in perfect harmony because they do not compete for food. Indeed, they have a symbiosis, as the LAB utilizes maltose by the phosphorolytic route, so discarding one glucose molecule for every maltose used; the yeast assimilates the glucose, and there is evidence to suggest that the yeast liberates compounds which are stimulatory, or even essential, for the growth of the LAB, which is known to be exceptionally fastidious in its nutritional requirements. Growth of the LAB has been shown to be strongly stimulated by a small peptide which is present in freshly prepared yeast extract, and also to be somewhat stimulated by various minerals and vitamins present in the extract. The yeast also has the unusual property that it is exceptionally resistant to the antibiotic cycloheximide, which is used in media for enumerating LAB because of its ability to totally inhibit the growth of most yeasts. In collaborative studies of Polish bakeries with scientists at the Politechnika Lódzka and in an examination of a Polish–Jewish bakery in Glasgow, the presence of yeasts and LAB with characteristics similar to those described above has been demonstrated, and Magdalena Wlodarczyk has independently discovered the biochemical basis of the important symbiosis between the yeast and the LAB.

In the San Francisco process the starter is routinely rebuilt every 8 h, although it can be stored in the refrigerator for several days without evident deterioration. According to Sugihara the rebuilding is done by mixing 100 parts of developed sponge with 100 parts of high-gluten wheat flour and 46–52 parts of water (all by weight). From an initial pH of 4·4–4·5, it decreases to a final value of 3·8–3·9. To make bread, 20 parts of this starter sponge is mixed with 100 parts of what in the USA is called regular patent wheat flour, 60 parts water and 2 parts salt. From an initial pH of 5·2–5·3 the value drops during 7 h of proofing to a final value of 3·9, when it is ready for baking.

Pure Cultures in Sourdough Bread Making

Sugihara reports a French study in which pure cultures of a yeast (*Candida tropicalis*) and a LAB (*L. plantarum*) were inoculated into a mixture of 1 part wheat flour and 10 parts water plus nutrients, at equal numbers of each organism, then incubated at 30°C for 17 h, when the count of each organism had increased 100-fold. This was then used as an inoculum for breadmaking. Polish work has demonstrated that separately cultured *C. milleri* and *L. sanfrancisco* can be mixed in the bakery and used for the production of a starter which is reported to give results superior in flavour, general quality and consistent production characteristics to those obtained with their conventional starters; this technology is now being applied, together with improved designs of equipment for developing the sour, in bakeries in Lódź. These results are in marked contrast with the claims reported earlier in this review that pure cultures were not satisfactory for production of sourdough breads; this difference may relate to the type of bread which is being produced.

The Danish company Chr. Hansen's Laboratorium A/S is now offering a selection of freeze-dried starter cultures under the brand name 'Florapan'. Florapan L-22 is *Lactobacillus delbrueckii*, a homofermentative strain reported to give a 'mild and pleasant flavour' to the bread in which it is used. L-73 is also homofermentative (*L. plantarum*) but is reported to give the bread a 'piquant, spicy flavour'. Finally, L-62, the heterofermentative *L. brevis*, gives 'a penetrating but rounded

taste and a long shelf life of the bread'. The bacteria are particularly recommended for whole-grain flours because of their requirements for vitamins and minerals. It is recommended that a freshly inoculated dough be allowed to sour overnight before use, but that where a fully developed dough is added to a fresh dough at a ratio of up to 1 : 20, 8 h of development can be sufficient. The developed dough is then used at about 30–40% of the final mixture which includes baker's yeast. Their literature makes no comments on the crumb texture of the breads produced with the different bacteria, although it will be recalled that the German workers attached significance to this aspect, concluding that for the best combination of texture and flavour it is necessary to use a mixture of homo- and heterofermentative bacteria. So far as can be determined, no biochemical or other reason has been advanced for the claimed texture differences, so there would seem to be scope for some useful research here.

A combination of technical advances in our understanding of and capacity to control sourdough fermentations has made these processes more reliable on a commercial production scale. At the same time, an increased public interest in the more traditional and 'ethnic' types of foods has created an increasing demand for these breads. Further improvements in processes, products and marketing strategies are possible and can further increase the market penetration of these bread types.

Bibliography

Kent NL (1983) *Technology of Cereals*, 3rd edn. Oxford: Pergamon Press.

Lonner C, Welander T, Molin N, Dostalek M and Blickstad E (1986) The microflora in a sourdough started spontaneously on typical Swedish rye meal. *Food Microbiology* 3: 3–12.

Oura E, Suomalainen H and Viskari R (1982) Breadmaking. In: Rose AH (ed.) *Economic Microbiology*, vol. 7. *Fermented Foods*, pp 88–147. London: Academic Press.

Service R (1957) *Songs of a Sourdough*. London: Ernest Benn.

Spicher G and Pomeranz V (1985) Bread and other baked products. *Ullmann's Encyclopedia of Industrial Chemistry*, 5th edn, vol. A4, pp 331–389. Weinheim: VCH Verlagsgesellshaft.

Steinkraus KH (1983) *Handbook of Indigenous Fermented Foods*, pp 131–188. New York: Marcel Dekker.

Sugihara TF (1985) Microbiology of breadmaking. In: Wood BJB (ed.) *Microbiology of Fermented Foods*, vol. 1, pp 249–262. London: Elsevier.

Wlodarczyk M (1985) Associated cultures of lactic acid bacteria and yeasts in the industrial production of bread. *Acta Alimentaria Polonica* 11(3): 345–359.

Wlodarczyk M (1986) Characteristic of yeasts from spontaneously fermenting bread starters. *Acta Alimentaria Polonica* 12(2): 103–108.

Wood BJB, Cardenas OS, Yong FM and McNulty DW (1975) Lactobacilli in the production of soy sauce, sour dough and Parisian barm. In: Carr JG, Cutting CV and Whiting GC (eds) *Lactic Acid Bacteria in Beverages and Food*, pp 325–335. London: Academic Press.

BJB Wood
University of Strathclyde, Glasgow, UK

Dietary Importance

The History of Bread

The history of bread as we know it, i.e. made with yeast, does not begin until wheat began to be cultivated, for wheat is the only cereal containing proteins that enable the dough to 'rise' and entrap air bubbles during the process of fermentation. Archaeological explorers of Swiss Lake habitations dating back to 4000 BC discovered a 'cake' made from wheat flour which had been fermented but the history of bread begins before that time. The earliest origins appear to be in Mesopotamia, amongst the Natutians. Records show that it was made in Ancient Egypt, and it was later a familiar food among the Greeks and Romans. Bread made from wheat flour with yeast was characteristic of a high degree of civilization and culture. The rich ate wheaten bread, in contrast to the poorer people who consumed hard bread or porridge made from oats, barley or rye.

Throughout the Middle Ages wheat was the most important cereal used for breadmaking in the southern parts of Europe, and in the southern UK. In more northern countries, Scandinavia, The Netherlands, and the northern parts of Germany, a dark wholemeal rye loaf was the household bread.

From early times people began to separate the flour they obtained from the mill, for they found that the finer whiter parts made a lighter and softer loaf than the whole meal. White flour was one of the class distinctions in Roman times, and the kind of bread eaten was a mark of one's status, wealth and power. In Medieval and Tudor England also, white bread indicated wealth and substance. The finest flour was often baked into small rolls or 'manchets'. The larger white loaves were termed 'wastel bread', and the coarser browner breads were referred to as 'cheat breads'. The price of the different grades was regulated in the UK by the 'Assize of Bread'.

During the prosperous years at the beginning of the eighteenth century the labouring classes in the south and east of the UK began to eat white bread, and this increased the demand for it, even though it was more expensive. Towards the end of the eighteenth century the millers discovered that they could sell the offals to the manufacturers of ship's biscuits and horse owners, but they still charged a higher price for white flour than for wholemeal.

Although dark bread had been despised throughout history as the food of the poor, and the poor longed to eat white bread, there were always those who regarded bread made from the whole grain as more nourishing and health-giving. However, medical opinion was against this. Hippocrates (430 BC) taught that 'wholemeal bread clears out the gut and passes through as excrement; white bread is more nutritious'. Galen (*c.* 160 AD) believed that the nutritive value of bread varied inversely with the amount of bran in it because the greater the bulk of the stools made by a given amount of bread the less nutritious the bread was likely to be.

The nineteenth century brought developments in the milling industry. The introduction of silk bolting cloths and the replacement of the millstone by steel rollers made a great difference to the efficiency of the milling process. Moreover, the price of offals became high enough to allow the millers to reduce the price of white flour below that of wholemeal, and the public demand for white bread increased still further. The millers and bakers tried to make the flour whiter by adding various substances to it, one of them being chalk. This practice was forbidden in the UK by statute, but was reintroduced by statute during World War II as a means of increasing the calcium intake of the population. *See* Milling, Principles of Milling; Flour, Roller Milling Operations; Flour, Analysis of Wheat Flours; Rationing of Foods

However, the view that wholemeal bread was a symbol of all that was natural, vital and good spread widely among the intelligentsia under the teachings of Graham and Allinson. Chemical analysis of bread began in the early part of the nineteenth century, and the results showed that besides containing more indigestible cellulose, wholemeal flour contained more protein, fat and minerals than white flour. Liebig considered that, weight for weight, wholemeal flour was more nutritious. However, biologically minded scientists measured the amount of nutrients in the bread and other foods that people ate, and the amounts coming out in the faeces, and they found, as Hippocrates had stated 2000 years before, that the indigestible material of the branny parts of the wholemeal bread so increased the losses of nutrients in the stools that, weight for weight, the chemical advantages of wholemeal bread were more than counterbalanced by its physiological drawbacks. *See* Flour, Dietary Importance

Enrichment of Flour and Bread with Calcium

Studies were made during the early 1940s on the absorption of calcium by men and women when wholemeal or white bread formed a large part of their diet. The results showed that the human intestine absorbed calcium less well when large amounts of wholemeal

Table 1.   Major constituents of bread (per 100 g)

Bread type	Water (g)	Protein (g)	Fat (g)	Carbohydrate (g)	Dietary fibre (g)	Energy (kJ)
Made from wheat flour						
Wholemeal	38·3	9·2	2·5	41·6	7·4	903
'Brown'	39·5	8·5	2·0	44·3	5·9	916
Granary	35·4	9·3	2·7	46·3	6·5	987
Hovis	40·3	9·5	2·0	41·5	5·1	890
White	37·3	8·4	1·9	49·3	3·8	987
Made from rye flour						
Whole rye	37·4	8·3	1·7	45·8	5·8	920

Data from Holland B *et al.* (1991).

bread were eaten than when the diet contained large amounts of white bread. This was particularly evident when very little of the calcium-rich foods milk and cheese were consumed, and some individuals excreted more calcium in their faeces than they took in in their food. Wholemeal bread contains inositol hexaphosphoric acid or phytic acid, largely as its potassium salt, which forms insoluble salts with calcium in the intestine, so preventing calcium absorption. Phytate is present in the outer layers of the wheat grain, and white flour contains very little. In the UK, as the wartime rations provided little milk and cheese, and the National Loaf (85% extraction, i.e. the amount of flour produced expressed as a percentage of the whole grain) contained more phytate than white bread (which was no longer available), it was decided that by law flour should contain added calcium carbonate in a prescribed amount. Wholemeal flour was exempted from the legal requirement. This was in deference to the 'whole food' lobby, which opposed the addition of anything artificial to any item of their diet. *See* Calcium, Physiology; Food Fortification; Phytic Acid, Nutritional Impact

Calcium carbonate is still added to flour in the UK, even though there are unlimited supplies of milk and cheese. Wholemeal flour is still exempted from the regulation, and the flour and bread that need it most have never been enriched with calcium.

A study made on children aged 5–14 years in Germany after World War II compared the nutritive value of breads made from flours of different extraction and of breads made from white flour with added B vitamins and iron to equal the amounts in the higher extraction flours. The children were allowed their rations of meat, milk and cheese which provided only 8 g of protein from animal sources a day in addition to unlimited amounts of one of the five experimental breads, which the children ate in such large quantities to satisfy their appetites that it provided at least 75% of the energy value of the diet. Calcium carbonate was added

to all the experimental breads. The rest of the diet was made up of vegetables which were cooked and eaten as soups. The children were underheight and underweight at the outset and they were in poor physical condition. All grew at a rapid rate both in height and weight and improved physically during the 18 months of the study whatever bread they were eating – brown, white, or white enriched with B vitamins and iron. The synthetic nicotinic acid and riboflavin were absorbed more readily than the vitamins naturally present in wholemeal flour.

These results raised an important question: why were they so different from those on weanling rats which grew much better on diets made up with wholemeal flour compared with white? It was found that when diets made up to resemble the children's diets were fed to 3-week-old weanling rats, those eating wholemeal bread grew most rapidly. However, when the same diets were fed to 8-week-old rats, the type of bread in the diet made no difference to their rate of growth. The explanation lay in the amount of the amino acid lysine in the diet. Wholemeal flour contains a little more lysine than white. Weanling rats grow very rapidly and have a particularly high requirement for lysine. Older rats – and children – grow much more slowly and the amount of lysine in white bread, together with that in the rest of the diet, was sufficient.

It was later recommended that all flour should contain not less than 1·65 mg of iron, 0·24 mg of vitamin B_1 and 1·60 mg of nicotinic acid per 100 g, either present naturally in the wheat or added as supplement. Flour, other than wholemeal, must also contain 235–390 mg of calcium carbonate per 100 g. These regulations are still in force in the UK today.

Chemical Composition of Present-day Breads

Tables 1, 2 and 3 set out the chemical composition of six varieties of bread on sale in supermarkets and shops in

Table 2.   Vitamins of the B complex in bread (per 100 g)

Bread type	Thiamin (vitamin B₁) (mg)	Nicotinic acid (mg)	Riboflavin (vitamin B₂) (mg)	Vitamin B₆ (mg)	Folate (μg)
Made from wheat flour					
Wholemeal	0·34	4·1	0·09	0·12	39
'Brown'	0·27	2·5	0·09	0·13	40
Granary	0·30	3·0	0·11	0·17	90
Hovis	0·80	4·2	0·09	0·11	39
White	0·21	1·7	0·06	0·07	29
Made from rye flour					
Whole rye	0·29	2·32	0·05	0·07	24

Data from Holland *et al.* (1991).

Table 3.   Minerals in bread mg per 100 g

Bread type	Sodium	Potassium	Calcium	Magnesium	Phosphorus	Chloride	Iron	Copper	Zinc
Made from wheat flour									
Wholemeal	550	230	54	76	200	880	2·7	0·26	1·8
'Brown'	540	170	100	53	150	890	2·2	0·16	1·1
Granary	580	190	77	59	180	930	2·7	0·18	1·5
Hovis	600	200	120	56	190	900	3·7	0·24	2·1
White	520	110	110	24	91	820	1·6	0·19	0·6
Made from rye flour									
Whole rye	580	190	80	48	160	1410	2·5	0·18	1·3

Data from Holland *et al.* (1991).

1991. All of the wheaten breads are strikingly similar in content of major constituents (Table 1). The protein provides at least 15% of the total energy of the breads, which is in the same proportion as the contribution of all protein from all food to the energy value of the total diet. White bread has a little more carbohydrate and provides about 9% more energy, weight for weight, than wholemeal bread. The difference is accounted for largely by the greater amount of dietary fibre in wholemeal bread. This was regarded by Hippocrates and many others over the years as a disadvantage of wholemeal bread, but in recent years the positive advantages of dietary fibre have been recognized and intensively investigated. *See* Dietary Fibre, Physiological Effects; Dietary Fibre, Effects of Fibre on Absorption; Dietary Fibre, Fibre and Disease Prevention; *see also* individual nutrients

Table 2 shows the amounts of vitamins of the B complex in the breads. Bread contains more water than flour, and the legal requirements for bread corresponding to those shown above for flour are at least 0·175 mg of vitamin B₁ and 1·17 mg of nicotinic acid (niacin) per 100 g. All of the breads meet these requirements.

Table 3 gives information about minerals in bread. There are legal requirements for the amounts of calcium and iron in wheat flours. For bread these amount to 68·5–114 mg of calcium and 1·2 mg of iron per 100 g but, as already stated, wholemeal flour is exempt from the requirements for calcium, so that the amount in wholemeal bread represents that naturally present in the wheat. The other flours contain added calcium carbonate.

The sodium and chloride in bread are derived almost entirely from salt added during the baking process, and most breads contain about 1·5% added salt. This is added to improve flavour and is not subject to legal requirements. The other minerals are those naturally present in the wheat and the concentrations of all of them – potassium, magnesium, phosphorus, copper and zinc – are higher in wholemeal than in white bread.

Bread Consumption in the UK

The consumption of bread in the UK has been falling over the past 30 years as a wider variety of other foods

Table 4. Weight of bread (per person per week) purchased by households in 1990

Bread type	Weight	
	(g)	(oz)
Large, white, sliced loaves	278	9·82
Large, white, unsliced loaves	101	3·56
Small, white, sliced loaves	12	0·41
Small, white, unsliced loaves	27	0·96
Brown loaves	98	3·45
Wholemeal loaves	108	3·82
Vienna and French bread	15	0·53
Rolls	79	2·80
Malt and fruit bread	5	0·18

Data from MAFF (1991).

Table 5. Contributions (percentage of total intake) made by bread to the total nutrient intake

	White bread	Brown and wholemeal bread
Energy	7·2	3·4
Protein	7·6	4·3
Starch	20·4	9·0
Calcium	7·4	2·8
Iron	8·7	7·7
Thiamin	9·4	8·6
Nicotinic acid equivalents	5·2	2·6

Data from MAFF (1991).

have come on the market. When white bread became freely available in 1956 it immediately became the bread of choice and the mean amount of white bread eaten was 1200 g per person per week. Wholemeal and brown bread consumption amounted to about 85 g per person per week. By 1960 white bread consumption had fallen to 990 g, by 1970 to 900 g, by 1980 to 625 g, and by 1990 to 425 g per person per week. Over this period the consumption of brown and wholemeal bread has remained below 285 g per person per week. From the mid-1980s there has been a swing from white to high-extraction breads, and a rise in consumption of soft-grain breads because of increased awareness of the importance of dietary fibre among the general public.

These figures are for bread eaten at home, as measured by the National Food Survey (Ministry of Agriculture, Fisheries and Food). Much of this decrease in bread consumption has been offset by an increase in bread eaten outside the home. *See* Dietary Surveys, Surveys of National Food Intake

Table 4 shows that large sliced white loaves are the most popular type of bread in the UK at the present time. Table 5 shows the contribution of bread to the intake of some nutrients. White bread makes a greater contribution than brown because more is eaten, and, in the case of calcium, iron, thiamin and nicotinic acid, because white flour is enriched with these nutrients.

All bread is an important source of dietary fibre, resistant starch and complex carbohydrate. Current dietary recommendations in the UK are to increase consumption of fibre-rich carbohydrates to compensate for reduced fat intake. Nutritional labelling of bread enables consumers to make an informed choice when purchasing this staple food. *See* Legislation, Labelling Legislation; Starch, Resistant Starch

Bibliography

Chick H (1940) Nutritive value of white flour with vitamin B₁ added and of wholemeal flour. *Lancet* ii: 511–512.

Holland B, Welch AA, Unwin ID *et al.* (1991) *McCance and Widdowson's The Composition of Foods* 5th edn. London: Royal Society of Chemistry and Ministry of Agriculture, Fisheries and Food.

McCance RA and Widdowson EM (1942) Mineral metabolism of healthy adults on white and brown bread dietaries. *Journal of Physiology* 101: 44–85.

McCance RA and Widdowson EM (1956) *Breads White and Brown. Their Place in Thought and Social History.* London: Pitman Medical Publishing.

MAFF (1991) *Household Food Consumption and Expenditure, 1990.* London: Ministry of Agriculture, Fisheries and Food.

Spicer A (ed.) (1975) *Bread. Social, Nutritional and Agricultural Aspects of Wheaten Bread.* Essex: Elsevier Science Publishers.

Widdowson EM and McCance RA (1954) *Studies on the nutritive value of bread and on the effect of variations in the extraction rate of flour on the growth of undernourished children.* MRC Special Report Series No. 287. London: Her Majesty's Stationery Office.

Elsie M. Widdowson
Formerly of Department of Medicine, University of Cambridge, Cambridge, UK

BREADFRUIT

See Fruits of Tropical Climates

BREAKFAST – ROLE IN THE DIET

Breakfast is popularly referred to as the most important meal of the day. This is because of the long period since the previous meal – as the name implies – so that most individuals would not have eaten for the previous 10–15 hours, compared with the usual maximum of 4–5 hours before other meals.

This relatively prolonged fast results in a fall in several blood constituents to their minimum or 'fasting' levels. For example, blood glucose and insulin fall, while there may be an increase in β-hydroxybutyrate, lactate, free fatty acids and plasma glucagon. Indeed, for clinical purposes a number of blood parameters that rise after a meal are measured 'in the fasting state' which, in practice, is before breakfast.

Despite the term 'most important meal of the day', breakfast is usually the smallest meal, supplying around 15% of the day's energy intake compared with 30% each from the midday and evening meals and about 25% eaten between meals.

Before the twentieth century, developments in food technology, which have tended to internationalize eating habits, the composition of breakfast (as, indeed, the diet in general) was influenced by culture, tradition and habit. For example, the English breakfast was based on bacon and eggs, the Scots' breakfast included oatmeal porridge; in France, the 'small' breakfast, still known as the Continental breakfast, consisted of a croissant and coffee; German breakfast is associated with cold sausage, Dutch breakfast with cheese, and the older Australian breakfast with a large meal including meat and potatoes.

The British breakfast in the nineteenth century could be selected from fish, mutton chops and rump steak, sausages, bacon, ham and eggs together with muffins, toast and marmalade (Mrs Beeton). A similar choice was available at that time in the USA – meat and/or fried eggs, fried potatoes, toast, pie and coffee (WK Kellogg). In some countries coffee is regarded largely as a breakfast drink.

During the last 50 years or more there have been changes towards a smaller meal, based largely on ready-to-eat cereals with milk or fruit juice added. Toast and marmalade rather than other fruit preserves are generally regarded as foods particular to breakfast, and in recent years yoghurt has been included in Western breakfasts. *See* Cereals, Breakfast Cereals

Breakfast Habits

Despite the common regard of breakfast as an important meal, a large number of people in many countries do not eat breakfast, apart, sometimes, from a hot drink. Surveys have shown that 25% of children of various age groups in Germany skip breakfast, as do 21% of children in Canada, and 58% of women university students in Japan. In the UK this is the habit of 4% of the youngest schoolchildren, 6% of those of junior school age, 14% of seniors and 27% of adults.

Starting the day without breakfast is usually considered to be contrary to good nutrition but many of those who skip breakfast appear to do so because they feel unable to eat at that time. When breakfast time is at a later hour, as it usually is over weekends and at holiday time, many of the people who normally skip breakfast do eat the meal. There are also many people who do not eat breakfast at home but do so on arrival at work, or on the way to work after travelling from home – for some individuals there does appear to be a physiological barrier to eating early in the day.

Other reasons for skipping breakfast have been implicated, e.g. the morning rush or general lack of time (although ready-to-eat cereals should obviate this) and the domestic changes arising from the increased numbers of working mothers. On the other hand, some children refuse breakfast even when it is offered to them.

The availability of fast food outlets and coffee shops has led to increased numbers of people breakfasting away from home. One figure from the USA showed that there was a 32% increase in the numbers eating breakfast away from home between 1978 and 1982.

Another reason for skipping breakfast is the belief that this helps would-be slimmers to control their food intake but this may be counter-productive, as discussed below.

Effects of Omitting Breakfast

There are three areas of special interest: (1) whether lack of breakfast adversely affects physical and mental performance later in the morning; (2) whether it affects the total daily nutrient intake and thus nutritional status; (3) whether it assists in weight control.

There have been a number of investigations of the mental and physical effects of omitting breakfast but the results have been inconsistent, sometimes contradictory and no conclusions can be drawn. Many of these investigations concerned schoolchildren since any nutritional deprivation might adversely affect their mental and physical development, which might be more amenable to measurement than that in an adult. Some trials have attempted to compare classroom behaviour, such as attentiveness and general demeanour, as well as more specific measures such as school attendance and achievement, while others have compared the response to specific physical and mental tests of individuals before and after the midday meal when breakfast was eaten or omitted, or the performance of those who regularly ate or did not eat breakfast, or the effects of withdrawing breakfasts from those who habitually ate the meal. None of these tests has shown evidence of risk to performance through omitting the meal. *See* Children, Nutritional Requirements

Earlier reports consisted of unquantified subjective observations by teachers, indicating inattention thought to be due to lack of breakfast, and improvements when drinks and snacks were supplied. Some reports included tests of cognitive functions such as reaction time and problem-solving, measured in the late morning, which appeared to show a beneficial effect of breakfast. However, other tests of cognitive function, such as immediate recall of short-term memory tests and the ability to sustain attention, were shown by the same investigators to improve when breakfast was omitted (attributed to heightened arousal associated with a short fast).

Between 1949 and 1960 a series of investigations known as the Iowa Breakfast Studies used a range of physical tests – reaction time, choice reaction time, neuromuscular tremor, grip strength and work output – and 12 research papers compared breakfast and non-breakfast eating. However, the tests were carried out on small groups of subjects, 6–10 subjects of various age groups and the two sexes, and results were not consistent, some even contradictory, so that no conclusions can be drawn.

A series of large-scale trials was carried out on 487 children comparing their performances before and after lunch by assessment of visual acuity, attentiveness and vigilance through a series of short written tests. If those who skipped breakfast had been disadvantaged, then after lunch both eaters and noneaters of breakfast should be equalized. No differences were found. The same authors tested 105 pupils aged 16–17 years who habitually ate a substantial breakfast (average 2·1 MJ) in a crossover trial of those continuing with breakfast and those omitting breakfast. Pupils were tested for three successive days but no consistent ill-effects were reported when breakfast was omitted.

It is therefore impossible to confirm the view that omission or withdrawal of breakfast has a detrimental effect on the performance on schoolchildren. Few trials have been carried out on adults and these have been equally inconclusive.

Effect of Omission of Breakfast on Nutritional Status

There is no evidence that the omission of breakfast has any measurable detrimental effect on overall nutritional status, but there is evidence that the intake of nutrients may be reduced compared with those who do take breakfast.

Canadian and American studies have reported that breakfasts provide a higher ratio of nutrients to energy for calcium, iron and water-soluble vitamins compared with other meals for both children and adults. There was a reduction in daily nutrient intake in these respects since the shortfall resulting from the omission of breakfast was not compensated by the other meals. *See* Calcium, Physiology; Iron, Physiology; Vitamins, Overview

The Oslo Breakfast was introduced for schoolchildren in Norway in 1929 to supplement their nutrient intake and ensure that an adequate meal was eaten before the daily work started. It consisted of milk, rye-biscuit, brown bread, butter or vitaminized margarine, whey cheese, cod liver oil paste, carrot, apple and half an orange. No evaluation was carried out at the time but a later comparison of a group of children aged 5–16 years with others having milk only was said, in the opinions of nurses and teachers, to result in an improvement in general demeanour in the boys on the Oslo breakfast but not in the girls. Such an inconclusive report is typical of many unquantified observations that have been made in this area.

Effect on Slimming

As reported above, it has been shown that those who habitually go without breakfast eat less food overall and so have a lower intake of nutrients than those who regularly eat this meal. Evidence as regards slimming is not consistent with this observation since it has been observed that would-be slimmers who omit breakfast in an attempt to reduce their total energy intake tend to consume more at lunch and at other meals to compensate. However, there may well be a difference between those who habitually skip breakfast and those who change their habits and omit the meal. *See* Slimming, Slimming Diets

Other work has shown that there was increased bodyweight in those who ate only two or three meals a day compared with those who ate frequently, i.e. five or more meals a day. Hence the general advice to slimmers is not to omit breakfast.

Conclusion

It is clear that many people skip breakfast most or all days of the week without any measurable detriment to bodily function. While there are suggestions that missing breakfast might result in impaired glucose tolerance and elevated blood cholesterol levels, and that liver reserves of glycogen are depleted after a 12-hour fast, there is no clear evidence that those who habitually skip breakfast are at any nutritional risk compared with those who eat the regular three meals a day.

Bibliography

Chao ESM and Vanderkooy PS (1989) An overview of breakfast nutrition. *Journal of the Canadian Dietietic Association* 50: 225–228.

Dickie NH and Bender AE (1982a) Breakfast and Performance. *Human Nutrition. Applied Nutrition* 36A: 45–56.

Dickie NH and Bender AE (1982b) Breakfast and Performance in schoolchildren. *British Journal of Nutrition* 48: 483–496.

Hanes S, Vermeersch J and Gale S (1984) The national evaluation of school nutrition programs: program impact on dietary intake. *American Journal of Clinical Nutrition* 40: 390–413.

Health and Welfare Canada (1977) *Nutrition Canada; Food Consumption Patterns Report*. Ottawa: Bureau of Nutritional Sciences, Health Protection Branch.

Pollitt E, Gersovitz M and Gargiulo M (1978) Educational benefits of the United States school feeding program: a critical review of the literature. *American Journal of Public Health* 68: 477–481.

A. E. Bender
Leatherhead, Surrey, UK

BREAST CANCER AND DIET

Breast cancer is the most prevalent type of cancer in Western and other highly developed countries. In the USA and the UK, breast cancer is the single largest cause of death in women aged 35–54 years and the incidence in this age group is increasing. There are many influences implicated in the aetiology of human breast carcinoma. Heritage seems to play a major part since having a twin or other first-degree relative with breast cancer increases risk. Hormonal factors are also significant since early menarche, late menopause and nulliparity are associated with increased risk, whereas early first full-term pregnancy and increasing parity are associated with decreased risk. Since the 1960s, evidence suggesting that diet may also be a risk factor in breast cancer has accumulated; in particular, overnutrition and high-fat diets have been linked with higher prevalence and mortality rates. Evidence for an association with diet has been derived from both human epidemiological studies and an impressive array of experimental studies in laboratory animals. This article discusses the epidemiology of human breast cancer and evidence for the involvement of hormonal and dietary factors, as well as obesity, in the aetiology of this disease.

Epidemiology

The incidence of breast cancer varies greatly from one population to another throughout the world. In general, incidence is greatest in populations with the highest standard of living, e.g. northwest Europe and North America, where one woman in eleven develops breast cancer at some stage of life. Improvements in living standards, such as those which occurred in Japan between 1950 and 1975, are associated with increased incidence of this disease (Table 1). Changing incidence of breast cancer in migrant populations is also well documented. In the USA, first-generation Japanese migrants show higher rates of breast cancer than Japanese women in Japan, and second-generation migrants have rates approaching that of the indigenous

US population. Similar effects are seen in Polish migrants to the UK after World War II. These data suggest that environmental factors are important determinants of breast cancer incidence in different populations. Differences in dietary habits and intakes of major nutrients, particularly fat, have been suggested as the most likely cause of international differences in breast cancer incidence. *See* Cancer, Epidemiology

Risk Factors

Heredity

There are many risk factors implicated in the aetiology of human breast cancers. Heredity is an important factor since having a twin or first-degree relative with breast cancer substantially increases risk. Familial risk appears to be stronger for premenopausal than postmenopausal and for bilateral than unilateral forms of the disease. One estimate suggests that a woman with a first-degree relative with premenopausal bilateral breast cancer has an eightfold higher risk of developing the disease, although other studies suggest that familial history carries a lower risk than this.

Obesity

Obesity may be an important risk factor for some forms of breast cancer. An impressive number of case studies have demonstrated a positive relationship between obesity and risk of postmenopausal breast cancer. Only a few studies have shown no association, or a weak association when analysis is corrected for height. This relationship appears to operate solely for cancers presenting during the postmenopausal years, since an inverse association between weight and risk has been demonstrated for the premenopausal disease. Weight gain during adult life seems to be a more important risk factor for postmenopausal breast cancer than heavier bodyweight itself, since a number of recent studies have shown risk of breast cancer to be higher in women who

have a history of excessive weight gain (> 10 kg) during their adult years. Obesity also influences the progress and severity of the disease, since higher rates of recurrence and shorter survival times have been demonstrated in obese patients compared to those in lean patients. Poorer prognosis in obese women does not appear to be a consequence of delayed diagnosis in women with larger breasts; the effect remains even when stage at diagnosis is allowed for

Reproductive History

Menses, marital status and parity have been recognized as risk factors in breast cancer since the last century. Many case control studies have shown that early age at menarche is a risk factor and age of menarche is higher in countries where risk of breast cancer is low. Late menopause has also been shown in some studies to increase risk of postmenopausal breast cancer, but this is not a consistent finding in all studies. An association between parity and risk of breast cancer was first suggested by studies which showed higher risk of breast cancer in unmarried women than in married women. The effect of parity seems to depend not only on the number of births, but also their timing in relation to age at menstruation, and there may even be an effect of the sex of the first offspring. In general, delayed first pregnancy seems to increase risk, whilst an early first pregnancy may be protective. A number of studies have shown number of years between menarche and first pregnancy to be a significant risk variable, whilst others have shown that four or more births result in a consistent reduction of risk. Table 2 shows the relative risk factors for breast cancer found in one case control study. These data indicate that nulliparity and a positive family history increase risk of breast cancer to a similar degree. The mechanism by which differences in exposure to hormonally related events influence risk of breast cancer is not fully understood. There is an emerging view that an extended period of exposure to reproductive hormones resulting from early menarche or late menopause, uninterrupted by pregnancy and lactation, may be the common pathway through which these risk factors operate.

Table 1. Change in number of breast cancer deaths, 1950–1975, Japan

Year	Number of deaths per year
1950	1419
1955	1572
1960	1683
1965	1966
1970	2486
1975	3262

Table 2. Relative risk factors for breast cancer in a study of 40 000 women

Risk factor	Relative risk
Familial history	1·72
Nulliparous	1·74
Early menarche	1·45
High education	1·22
Breast-feeding	1·17
First delivery after age of 25	1·16

Influence of Hormones and Oral Contraceptives

The association between breast cancer risk and hormonally related events described above lends support to the view that hormones play a part in the aetiology of certain types of breast cancer. The hormones which have been most strongly implicated in the development of breast cancer are oestrogens and prolactin, although reduced exposure to progesterone has also been suggested to be a risk factor.

Oestrogens

Involvement of oestrogen in the development of breast cancer has been widely accepted since the nineteenth century, when ovariectomy was shown to be successful in inducing remission in some cases of premenopausal breast cancer. More recently, antioestrogen drugs have proved to be the most effective form of treatment for breast cancer in women with oestrogen-receptor-positive tumours. However, evidence for an involvement of excessive oestrogen secretion in the development of the disease remains equivocal. A minority of studies have shown evidence of higher total oestrogen levels in women at risk of familial breast cancer but most have not. Other studies have proposed that risk of breast cancer is inversely related to the ratio of oestriol to oestrone and oestradiol levels, since rodent studies suggested that the latter two oestrogens possess far greater carcinogenic potency than oestriol. This hypothesis is no longer widely accepted because although some population studies of Japanese, Chinese and North American women showed higher oestriol ratios in the low-risk populations, a number of case control studies found the opposite, namely higher oestriol ratios in women with breast cancer. Furthermore, recent carcinogen studies in rodents have demonstrated equal carcinogenic potencies of oestriol, oestrone and oestradiol. There is therefore limited evidence from studies of human populations to support the view that cancer patients are predisposed to the disease by virtue of their exposure to higher than normal circulating concentrations of oestrogens. It remains to be determined whether or not an extended duration of exposure, by virtue of early menarche, nulliparity or late menopause, plays a part in the aetiology of the disease. *See* Hormones, Steroid Hormones

Prolactin

The protective effect of early first full-term pregnancy against breast cancer has in part been attributed to the lower prolactin (PRL) levels reported in parous women.

However, the view that circulating concentrations of prolactin are raised in women at increased risk of cancer is not consistently supported by studies in these groups. Some have shown higher luteal-phase PRL in daughters of women with breast cancer and in women of families showing multiple cases of breast cancer, but others have shown no such differences, and one study demonstrated lower PRL in high-risk familial groups. There are a number of studies which have reported elevated PRL levels in patients with existing breast cancer, although the relevance of these studies to the aetiological role of PRL in breast cancer is debatable. In a comparison of women with early diagnosis of premenopausal cancer and those with benign conditions of the breast, PRL was found to be markedly elevated in the cancer group, with the most marked elevations seen in those individuals with invasive disease. Other studies have found exaggerated PRL responses to thyroid releasing hormone (TRH) stimulation in patients with breast cancer, whilst others have found elevated PRL only in cases with advanced disease. The difficulty with these retrospective studies is that PRL is known to be increased in response to various forms of stress, so that higher PRL in cases compared with controls may be the result of the stress of diagnosis and treatment. Furthermore, many recent studies, which have measured levels during the early stages of disease before treatment has begun, have failed to show elevated PRL in cases compared with controls.

In the studies described above, PRL has been measured by radioimmunoassay. An area of research interest at the present time is the possibility that variant forms of PRL, detectable only by bioassay, may be present at higher than normal concentrations in women with breast cancer and other benign breast conditions. These variant forms of PRL may be cleavage products of the parent molecule, but since they have been shown to possess mitogenic activity against breast tissue, the detection of these fragments at higher than normal concentrations in breast cancer cases may be significant.

Oral Contraceptives

Many studies have investigated effects of oral contraceptive (OC) usage on risk of breast cancer. A large majority have shown no association and some studies have shown decreased risk with OC use. However, a number have found some support for the theory that pre-existing subclinical breast cancer is promoted by OC usage after several months of use. Other studies have shown increased risk with OC use in nulliparous women, in women with a history of benign breast disease, and in those with a family history of breast cancer. In general, most studies suggest that if there is no incipient cancer present, the oral contraceptive pill does not increase risk of breast cancer and may even decrease it. *See* Oral Contraceptives and Essential Nutrients

Role of Dietary Factors – Fat, Sugar

A large number of international correlation studies have established a strong positive relationship between fat consumption per head of the population and mortality rates from breast cancer. Within-country studies of breast cancer incidence in different districts, or regions with different fat intakes, also point to a relationship between fat intake and breast cancer. Two studies which analysed nutrient intakes and mortality rates from breast cancer in the UK between the beginning of this century and 1975 showed the strongest associations were with per capita consumption of fat, sugar and animal protein and the incidence of breast cancer 10 years later. Although correlation studies strongly support a relationship between diet, particularly dietary fat content and risk of breast cancer, many case control studies conducted since the mid 1970s have failed to demonstrate increased risk of this disease in women with high fat intakes. Of eighteen studies reported since 1975, eight show a positive association between breast cancer and either saturated or total fat intake or meat intake, four show a suggestion of a positive effect, and six show no evidence for an effect of fat or any other dietary component. In particular, all the case control studies of fat and breast cancer conducted in the USA have failed to demonstrate any effect of diet in this disease. A study conducted in the USA in 1987 was of particular importance since this was a prospective study of diet and breast cancer and involved a study population of 90 000 women. At the first follow-up, 6 years after the initial dietary assessment, there was no evidence of higher rates of breast cancer in subjects with high fat intakes; on the contrary, there was a nonsignificant trend towards decreased risk with increasing fat intake.

The subject of the relationship between breast cancer and fat intake remains controversial, since negative findings have been reported more frequently in studies carried out in countries in which the range of fat intakes is relatively narrow in comparison to the international range of fat intakes. A recent study conducted in Italy, a country in which fat intakes vary between 22% and 45% (compared with 34–43% in the USA), demonstrated a positive association between both total fat and total energy intakes and risk of breast cancer. At the present time, definite conclusions cannot be drawn regarding the involvement of dietary fat in the aetiology of breast cancer because of conflicting evidence provided by these different studies. There is a need for between-country case control studies, which would enable the risk of breast cancer to be evaluated across a wider range of fat intakes than is possible in single-country studies.

Results from intervention trials of low-fat diets in women at risk of breast cancer, presently being conducted in Sweden and Canada, will of be of value in ascertaining the contribution made by diet to the aetiology of the disease.

Although dietary studies have generally failed to demonstrate clear-cut findings for an effect of fat in this disease, evidence that excess energy may be a factor in some human breast cancers is supported by the large number of studies which show higher risk of postmenopausal breast cancer in overweight and obese women. Obese subjects have a greater than normal capacity to convert androstenedione to oestrogen in adipose tissue, and obese women have been shown to possess reduced sex-hormone-binding globulin levels, so that increased synthesis and bioavailability of oestrogens are a likely consequence of greater adiposity. That the effect of obesity is mediated through oestrogen stimulation is suggested by a recent study which showed that advanced disease was more common in obese women than in those of normal weight, but only in those obese women who also had oestrogen-receptor-positive tumours. Excessive consumption of energy and accelerated growth during childhood, resulting in earlier age at menarche, could provide an additional mechanism by which nutrition may influence the prevalence of this disease. Thus, if there is an effect of fat in breast cancer, it may be mediated through higher intake of energy rather than through a specific effect of fat per se. If this were so, it might explain why some studies have also shown sugar and alcohol to be risk factors for this disease. In considering the effect of diet in this disease, some mention should be made of the findings from animal studies. A large number clearly show that both the amount and type of fat in the diet influence mammary tumorigenesis, with $n-6$ fatty acids stimulating it and $n-3$ fatty acids inhibiting it. At least some of the international variation in breast cancer incidence may be attributable to differences in fatty acid intakes in different countries. Fish eaters such as the populations of Iceland and Japan have the lowest rates of breast cancer world-wide, but further epidemiological studies of fatty acid intakes in different populations are required to determine whether or not the type as well as the amount of fat in the diet are important.

Role of Diet in Treatment and Prevention

Treatment

There is little evidence to suggest that diet has a part to play in the treatment of established breast cancer. Unlike many forms of cancer, excessive weight loss is not commonly seen until the very late stages of the disease when impaired appetite affects the patient's ability to eat. For this reason studies of specialized forms of nutritional support and effects of nutritional supplements have not been evaluated in this type of cancer. A few studies have investigated effects of low-fat or weight-reducing diets in patients with breast cancer and these have failed to show any effect of dietary therapy on survival times. Similarly, anecdotal reports of beneficial effects of high doses of vitamin C have not been supported by controlled studies in patients with breast cancer, although no large-scale placebo-controlled studies have been conducted. There is no evidence that vegetarian diets or diets high in dietary fibre have any effect on the progress of the disease. *See* Cancer, Diet in Cancer Treatment

Prevention

In 1982 the USA Committee on Diet, Nutrition and Cancer of the National Research Council (NRC) published interim dietary guidelines based on evidence from the literature for effects of specific dietary constituents in different forms of cancer. The committee considered the evidence for an effect of dietary fat in breast cancer to be particularly strong and recommended that, as a means of protecting against this disease, intakes should be reduced from their current high levels of around 40% energy as fat to 30% energy as fat. However, epidemiological studies carried out since this report was published have not consistently supported the earlier findings, so that specific dietary recommendations aimed at prevention of breast cancer are at the present time impossible to make with any degree of certainty. *See* Cancer, Diet in Cancer Prevention

Bibliography

Committee on Diet, Nutrition and Cancer, Assembly of Life Sciences, National Research Council (1982) *Diet, Nutrition and Cancer*, pp 1–16. Washington, DC: National Academy Press.

Helmrich SP, Shapiro S and Rosenberg L (1983) Risk factors for breast cancer. *American Journal of Epidemiology* 115: 241–245.

Moore DH, Moore II DH and Moore CT (1983) Breast carcinoma: etiological factors. *Advances in Cancer Research* 40: 189–253.

Williams CM and Dickerson JWT (1987) Dietary fat, hormones and breast cancer: the cell membrane as a possible site of interaction of these two risk factors. *European Journal of Surgical Oncology* 13: 89–104.

Christine M. Williams
University of Surrey, Guildford, UK

BREAST-FEEDING

See Infants

BROWNING

Contents

Nonenzymatic

The very complex reactions between reducing sugars and the free amino groups of amino acids or proteins are collectively known as nonenzymatic browning or the Maillard reaction. Accordingly, when reducing sugars react with amines, an extraordinarily complex mixture of compounds is obtained, which are present in widely ranging amounts. The product pattern is subject to large variations, depending on the reaction conditions. In particular, the reaction time, the temperature, the concentrations of the reactants and the pH play decisive roles. *See* Amines; Amino Acids, Properties and Occurrence

In foods it is essentially the monosaccharides glucose and fructose, and the disaccharides maltose and lactose, as well as in some cases (e.g. meat) reducing pentoses, that react with amino acids and/or proteins. Sugars linked glycosidically in glycoproteins, glycolipids, flavonoid compounds, or in disaccharides, such as sucrose, participate in nonenzymatic browning only after cleavage of the glycosidic bond. Hexuronic acids, insofar as they occur in the free form at all, behave in a similar manner to pentoses, i.e. in the course of nonenzymatic browning decarboxylation takes place. In certain cases (e.g. cheese), biogenic amines can react as the amino component. Ammonia constitutes a special case; it can be formed in small amounts from amino acids during nonenzymatic browning (Strecker degradation) and it is used in large amounts in the production of one type of caramel colour. In general, for nonenzymatic browning, primary amines are more important than secondary amines. Thus, in proteins, it is the primary amino group of the lysine side-chains that reacts predominantly and, wherever they occur in foods in the free form, primary amino acids take precedence. However, in cereals and in cereal products (malt, beer), considerable amounts of the secondary amino acid proline occur. Recently, it has been realized that nonenzymatic browning actually occurs in the human body. As a general rule, the longer the half-life of a protein, the larger the amount of its Maillard products found, i.e. important factors are the 'age' or persistence of the protein in the body and the glucose concentration, particularly in diabetics. Many of the symptoms developed by diabetics resemble those of premature ageing, which leads to the possibility that glucose, because of its reactivity towards proteins, is fundamentally involved in the normally slow progress of ageing. *See* Ageing – Nutritional Aspects; Beers, Ales and Stouts, Chemistry of Brewing; Caramel, Methods of Manufacture; Carbohydrates, Interactions with Other Food Components; Malt, Chemistry of Malting; Protein, Interactions and Reactions Involved in Food Processing

Chemistry

Although more than 75 years have passed since the first research on nonenzymatic browning, and although many results have been gathered in the meantime, it is still not possible to present a complete reaction scheme. In the reaction with reducing sugars, the amines act as bases or acids (depending on the prevailing pH) catalysing enolization, and as nucleophiles attacking carbonyl groups, etc.

Primary reaction products of glucose and fructose are the glycosylamines **1** and aminoketoses **2** or aminoaldoses **3**. (For simplification, open-chain structures are used. In fact, the sugars and many of their products exist mainly in their cyclic half-acetal or half-ketal form.) The relatively stable glycosylamines **1** are obtained from aromatic and heterocyclic amines (e.g. adenosine triphosphate). The glycosylamines of amino acids or aliphatic amines quickly rearrange into the aminoketoses **2** (Amadori rearrangement) or aminoaldoses **3** (Heyns rearrangement). Aminoketoses (or Amadori compounds) have been shown to be present, alongside other products, in heated and in stored foods, in dried fruit, in vegetable and milk products, as well as in soy sauce. They also occur in infusion solutions containing glucose and amino acids, intended for parenteral nutrition. They are present in the human body (in higher amounts in diabetics). The aminoaldoses **3** are not very stable and readily react further.

Deoxyosones **4–7** are formed as degradation products of the aminoketoses and aminoaldoses in the pH range 4–7. Desoxyosones can be described as intramolecular disproportionation products of sugars which undergo further reactions, markedly more rapidly than the original reactants. Products derived from the 3-deoxyosone **4** are the lactone **8**, the hydroxymethylfurfural **9** and the nitrogen-containing products **10–12**. The maltoxazine **12** is a major product when proline is heated with hexoses. In the formation of the pyrroles **13** and **14**, the participation of **4** can be assumed. Furthermore, the structures of the coloured compounds **15** and **16** reveal the participation of **4**. In caramelization reactions, i.e. heating of sugars to temperatures above 130°C in the absence of amines, the furane **9** is the main volatile compound.

To some extent, 1-deoxyosones are converted into

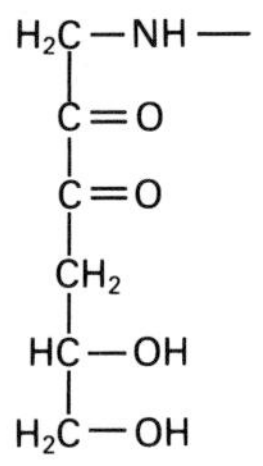

(7) 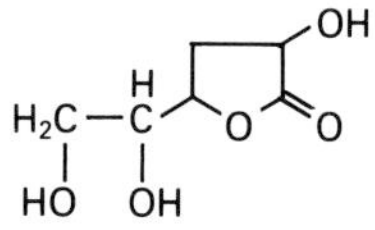 (8) 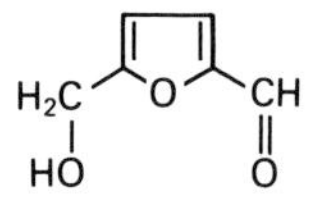 (9)

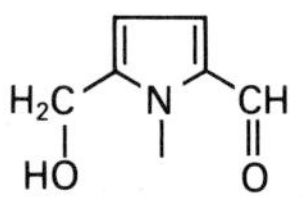

(10) 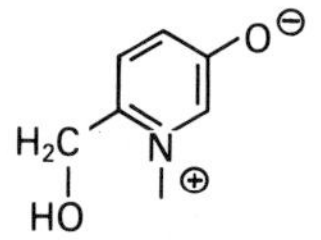 (11) 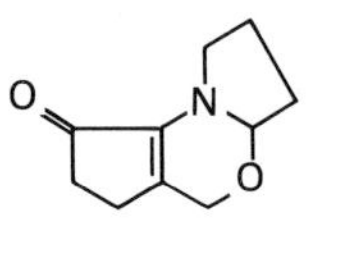 (12)

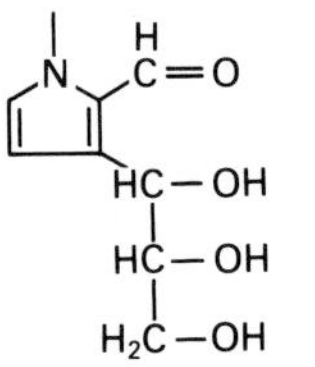

(13) 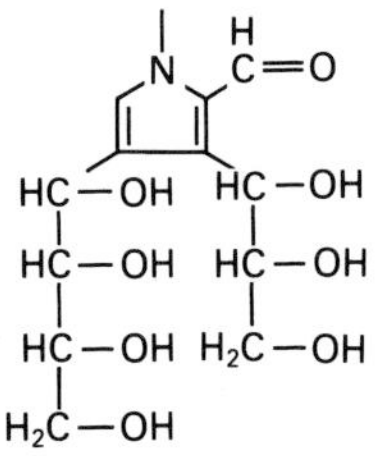 (14) 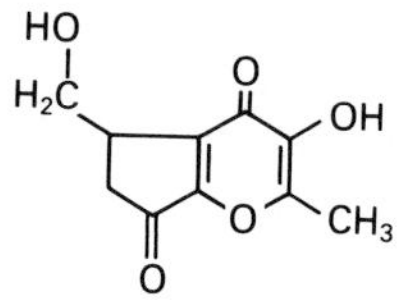 (15)

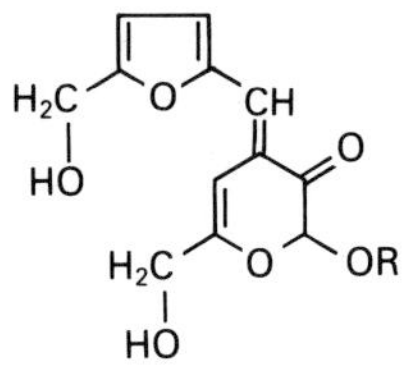

(16) 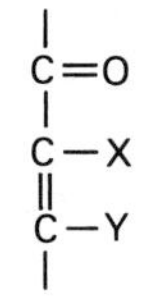 (17) (18)

X = Y = O—, N—

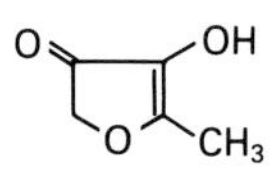

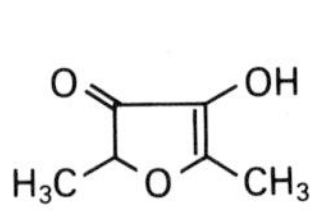

(19) 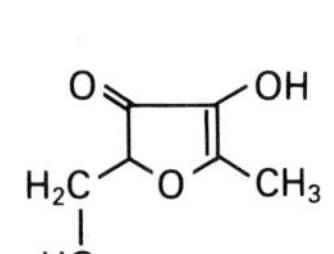 (20) 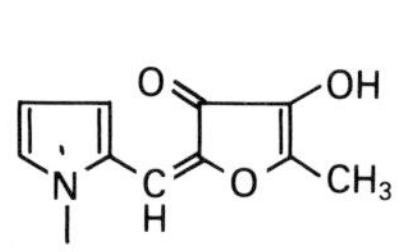 (21)

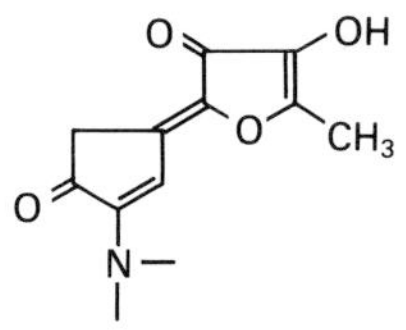

(22) 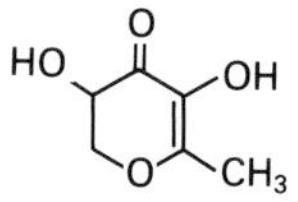 (23) 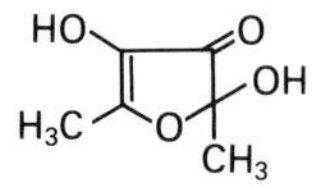 (24)

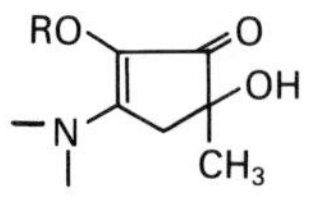

(25) 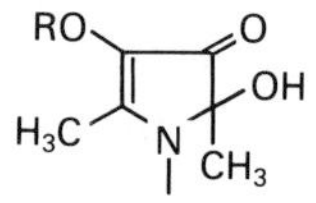 (26) 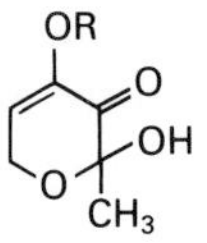 (27)

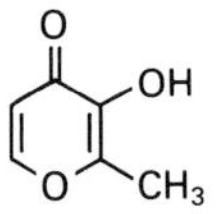

(28) 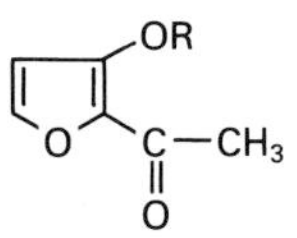 (29) 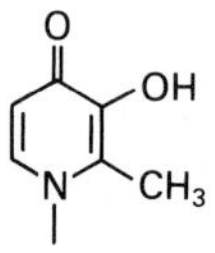 (30)

compounds with the general reductone structure 17. Cyclization, enolization and loss of water lead to a multitude of products. From pentoses, 6-deoxyhexoses (such as rhamnose), from hexoses, the furanones 18–20 are formed via the 1-deoxyosones. Compound 18 plays a crucial role in the browning of pentoses; from the coloured structures 21 and 22 the participation of 18 can be seen. The furanone 19 has a very low odour threshold and an aroma note (fruity/roast-caramel-like) that is

perceived as pleasant. It is now manufactured on a relatively large scale and is added to many products. The pyranone 23 can be used as a universal indicator substance for the occurrence of noneyzmatic browning since hexoses occur in virtually all foodstuffs. The hydroxyfuranone 24 readily undergoes further reactions and is therefore only found, if at all, in low concentrations in model systems or foodstuffs. In the presence of secondary amines, the so-called amino hexose reductones 25 (R = H) can be obtained in yields up to 30%. The pyrrolinones 26 (R = H) have been found in reaction mixtures of hexoses and primary amines. These compounds fluoresce strongly and, like the amino hexose reductones, possess antioxidant properties. From disaccharides, the cyclopentenones 25 and pyrrolinones 26 with R = α-glucose (α-Glc) and R = β-galactose (β-Gal) are formed where the galactosyl and glucosyl residues remain linked to the cyclic compounds.

The reactions of 1-deoxyosones derived from disaccharides differ in some respects from those of monosaccharides. Characteristic products are the compounds 27–34 (R = α-Glc, β-Gal). From the β-pyranone 27, maltol 28 and isomaltol 29 with the glycosidically bound galactosyl or glucosyl residue are formed. The main product in reaction mixtures of disaccharides with primary amines is the pyridone 30. Pyridones with this type of structure are known to bind metals such as iron and aluminium tightly. Further typical products of disaccharides in the presence of primary and secondary amines are the pyrrole 31, the cyclopentenone 32 and the furanes 33 and 34.

The concomitant formation of the furane 35, the

(31)   **(32)**   **(33)**

(34)   **(35)**   **(36)**

(37)   **(38)**   **(39)**   **(40)**

H₂N—CH—COOH
(CH₂)₄
NH
CH₂
COOH

(41)

H₃C—[X]—CHO

(42) X = O

(43) X = NH

(44)

pyrrole **36** and the pyridiniumbetaine **37** can be rationalized best as occurring via the 4-deoxyosone **6**.

Degradation of the 1-amino-1,4-dideoxyosone **7** leads to the aminoacetylfurane **38** and the aminoreductone **39**. The furane **38** is very reactive in the pH range 4–7 and is therefore involved in many browning reactions. The aminoreductone **39** has been isolated as its triacetyl derivative; there is some evidence that the precursor does not exist in the open-chain structure.

Sugars, and many of their degradation products, can undergo retroaldol-type reactions. Followed, in some cases, oxidation and/or dehydration. Some of the cleavage products are very reactive, readily undergoing condensation reactions. In the early phase of nonenzymatic browning, the C_2 fragments predominate, which have been formed from the aldose or the imine. Electron spin resonance (ESR) spectral data have provided evidence that the pyridinium radical **40** is formed intermediately. Retroaldol reactions of ketoses and aminoketoses lead to C_3 fragments.

Oxidative fragmentation reactions of deoxyosones are also known between the α-diketo function, leading to C_1 and C_5 fragments from the 3-deoxyosone **4**, and to C_2 and C_4 fragments from the 1-deoxyosone **5**. In model systems, formic acid, acetic acid and their derivatives (esters, amides), respectively, are often the main Maillard products. Carboxymethyllysine (**41**) formed in this way from the corresponding amino ketose can be detected in foodstuffs and also in the human body after hydrolysis of proteins. The decarboxylation of amino acids on heating with sugars has been known for many years. The decarboxylation is actually brought about by

reaction of the amino acids with α-dicarbonyl compounds (Strecker degradation). The significance of the Strecker degradation lies in the fact that the amino acids furnish ammonia and reactive aldehydes that can undergo, *inter alia*, condensation reactions. In addition to ammonia and the aldehyde from cysteine, hydrogen sulphide is produced, which is often involved in aroma formation. The Strecker degradation of amino acids brings about the reduction of the α-dicarbonyl compounds, mainly of the deoxyosones. Characteristic degradation products of the reduced 3-deoxyosones are compounds **42–44**.

If the reaction mixtures of sugars and amines are submitted to exclusion chromatography, fractions can be obtained with molecular weights of about 10 000 Da and even greater. So far, it has not yet proved possible to isolate homogeneous high-molecular-weight Maillard products. Very little is known about the structure of the high-molecular-weight substances, the so-called melanoidins. Some information has been gained from the interpretation of ^1H, ^{13}C and ^{15}N nuclear magnetic resonance (NMR) and ESR spectral data. The absorption of melanoidins in the ultraviolet and visible regions shows that condensation reactions have participated only to a limited extent in the linking of the monomers. Differently produced caramel colours have been differentiated by means of Curie point pyrolysis.

Significance of Nonenzymatic Browning for Foods

The great interest shown by the food industry in nonenzymatic browning largely stems from a desire to produce and control the characteristic aromas obtained on cooking, baking, roasting and grilling. With reaction mixtures of special amino acids and sugars, to some extent it is possible to create aromas similar to those produced by the foods. With the combined technique of gas chromatography–mass spectrometry, hundreds of volatile compounds have been isolated and identified from each model system and foodstuffs, respectively. At the moment the aromas of boiled or grilled meat, of roasted coffee, of chocolate and of bread cannot yet be satisfactorily reproduced by means of a single substance and one now suspects that this will never be the case. In general, reproduction of such aromas requires several

R = OH, R′ = CH₃
(45) R = H, R′ = CH₃
      R = R′ = H

(46) R = R′ = H
      R = H, R′ = CH₃
      R = OH, R′ = CH₃

(47) R = H
      R = CH₃

(50) R = CH—CH₂
             | |
            OH   OH

(51) R = H, CH₃

(48)

(49)

(52) R = H, CH₃

(53) R = H, CH₃

components, which need to be present in the correct proportions. Aroma dilution analysis will be very helpful to find the important impact substances. *See* Bread, Chemistry of Baking; Chromatography, Gas Chromatography; Cocoa, Chemistry of Processing; Coffee, Analysis of Coffee Products

When bread or meat is overheated on its surface during baking or roasting, respectively, the crust usually tastes bitter. The same effect is noted when wort boiling takes place at higher temperatures. Also, model mixtures of sugars and amino acids (especially proline) taste bitter when they have been heated under grilling conditions. A few bitter substances have been isolated from model systems (examples are compounds 45–47). *See* Flavour Compounds, Production Methods; Heat Treatment, Chemical and Microbiological Changes

Nonenzymatic browning contributes not only to desirable formation of colour (bread and meat crust, beer, coffee, etc.), but also to discoloration of foods, which is equivalent to a lowering of quality. The determination of the degree of browning (usually through absorbance at 420 nm) is often used analytically to assess the extent to which nonenzymatic browning has taken place. Since the concentrations of the sugar and amino components in foodstuffs are very variable, measurement of the colour intensity does not readily yield comparable results. The isolation and identification of coloured Maillard products has so far been achieved only with model systems. The structures of 15, 16, 21, 22, 48, 49 and 50 represent some coloured compounds from pentoses, hexoses and ascorbic acid. To react with amino acids, ascorbic acid has to be oxidized. With dehydroascorbic acid the Strecker degradation leads to the red compound 50. *See* Ascorbic Acid, Properties and Determination

It has been known for some time that beer is stabilized against oxidative changes through substances formed by nonenzymatic browning occurring during the kilning of germinated barley. Without at first knowing their structure, these substances were called reductones. More reductones are formed when milk is heated before the drying process. The resulting milk powder is more stable against oxidative degradation. Reductones 20, 23 and 24, and the aminoreductones 25, 26 and 39, structurally comparable with ascorbic acid, act as stabilizers.

Since the introduction of the Ames test for mutagenicity, a series of reaction mixtures, fractions and Maillard products has been subjected to such a test. At present, attention is focused on compounds 51–53; for some of these compounds, carcinogenicity, or at least a cocarcinogenic potential, has been established unequivocally. Rapid and definite detection of these compounds, which occur in some foodstuffs at the microgram per kilogram level or less, still presents certain problems.

The growth of animals fed with proteins that have been heated in the presence of sugars, may be retarded. Many such experiments have been carried out with milk proteins to study the reduction in nutritive value. It became apparent that reaction of the sugar with the ε-amino groups of lysine side-chains partly leads to the corresponding amino ketose which, after proteolysis of the protein in the alimentary canal, renders lysine no longer available to the organism. Therefore, in the production of milk powders and other products preferred in infant nutrition, particular attention must be paid to keeping damage of lysine to a minimum. Some Maillard products possess good complexing properties, which lead to increased heavy metal excretion via urine after parenteral or oral administration of such compounds. *See* Condensed Milk

There are situations where one wants to control nonenzymatic browning. If the Maillard reaction is to

$$
\begin{array}{c}
HC = O \\
| \\
C = O \\
| \\
CH_2 \\
| \\
HC - SO_3H \\
| \\
HC - OH \\
| \\
H_2C - OH
\end{array}
$$

(54)

be suppressed, this can be achieved by reducing the water activity. However, this method is not appropriate for all foodstuffs. The browning rate is reduced with decreasing pH values. It can be assumed that in acid and slightly acid solutions, retroaldol-type reactions are likely to play only a minor role. Retroaldol reactions lead to very reactive fragmentation products which are involved in the formation of coloured substances. It has long been known that sulphurous acid hinders nonenzymatic browning. One can assume that addition of sulphite to carbonyl groups or other activated carbon atoms occurs, blocking these functions which thus are no longer available for further reactions. One of the few products isolated and identified to date is the sulphonic acid **54**. The reaction of the acid with Maillard products is not always reversible, since part of the sulphite remains bound. There are reports that the Maillard reaction is also hindered by the addition of divalent sulphur derivatives, such as thioglycollic acid or cysteine. Sulphur (II) compounds are supposed to trap radicals formed in the Maillard reaction and to inactivate reactive carbonyl groups. Since addition of sulphur-containing compounds is expected to lead to large alterations in aroma in foods, their practical application is unlikely. Control of the nonenzymatic reaction *in vivo* has been tried by means of aminoguanidine. *See* Water Activity, Effect on Food Stability

Even 80 years after its discovery, nonenzymatic browning or the Maillard reaction, with its multitude of reaction pathways and products, is still only known in outline. In food chemistry, the objectives are for nonenzymatic browning to proceed in such a way that the formation of toxic substances and the reduction in nutritional value are suppressed, whilst, simultaneously, desirable components are formed in optimal amounts. *See* Antioxidants, Natural Antioxidants; Antioxidants, Synthetic Antioxidants; Storage Stability, Mechanisms of Degradation

Bibliography

Finot PA, Aeschbacher HU, Hurrell RF and Liardon R (1990) *The Maillard Reaction in Food Processing, Human Nutrition and Physiology.* Basel: Birkhäuser.
Ledl F and Schleicher E (1990) New aspects of the Maillard reaction in foods and in the human body. *Angewandte Chemie* 102: 597–626 (*Angewandte Chemie, International Edition in English* 29: 565–594).
Namiki M (1989). Chemistry of the Maillard reactions. *Advances in Food Research* 38: 115–184.
Paulsen H and Pflughaupt KW (1980) Glycosylamines. In: Pigman W and Horton D (eds) *The Carbohydrates: Chemistry and Biochemistry*, vol. IB, pp 881–927. New York: Academic Press.

F. Ledl†
Stuttgart University, Stuttgart, FRG

Enzymatic–Biochemical Aspects

The discoloration which occurs in plant material after cell disruption and which results in the formation of brown or sometimes yellow, black or pink pigments is mainly due to the process of enzymatic browning.

Cell disruption can be due either to mechanical injury or temperature changes which lead to physiological disorders or even cell death (e.g. for deep-frozen products). This loss of cell integrity results in the decompartmentation of phenolic substrates and enzymes and then, in the presence of molecular oxygen, the oxidative production of coloured quinones.

Brown pigmentation following this enzymatic reaction, and subsequent nonenzymatic reactions, is generally considered to be detrimental to food quality from both the organoleptic and nutritional points of view. The prevention of enzymatic browning has always been a challenge to food scientists owing to the losses of quality that it causes in many food products, e.g. fruits and vegetables during either storage or processing. It is only in a few exceptional cases that the enzymatic browning is desirable (prunes, dates, tea, tobacco, etc.).

With a better knowledge of the mechanism of browning reactions it will be possible to propose processes which avoid or at least minimize this discoloration and which can be adapted to each particular product. *See* Colours, Properties and Determination of Natural Pigments

Nomenclature

Two kinds of enzymes are able to act upon diphenols in the presence of molecular oxygen according to the reaction scheme shown in Fig. 1. Both have the trivial name polyphenol oxidase, but they are somewhat different in nature. The first class of enzymes, catechol oxidases (EC 1.10.3.1) catalyse two distinct reactions

---

† Deceased

(reactions (1) and (2) of Fig. 1), namely hydroxylation of monophenols into *o*-diphenols (cresolase activity) and oxidation of *o*-diphenols into *o*-quinones (catecholase activity). Both reactions consume oxygen and the overall stoichiometry is 1 mol of oxygen for 1 mol of monophenol, giving 1 mol of *o*-quinone. The second class, laccases (EC 1.10.3.2), oxidize *o*-diphenols as well as *p*-diphenols, forming their corresponding quinones (reaction (3) of Fig. 1). The stoichiometry is one atom of oxygen for 1 mol of diphenol giving 1 mol of quinone. The unique ability to oxidize *p*-diphenols can be used to distinguish the laccase activity from that of the first class of polyphenol oxidases. In all cases, the quinones formed are very reactive and, depending on the nature and the concentration of the reactive species in the medium, they can enter in numerous secondary nonenzymatic reactions which will be described later.

The nomenclature of these enzymes is somewhat confusing since, besides the two designated as EC 1.10.3.1 and 1.10.3.2, a third one, EC 1.14.18.1, exists. It is referred to as monophenol monooxygenase (tyrosinase) and corresponds to the same enzymes as EC 1.10.3.1 but which catalyse the hydroxylation of monophenols. For the sake of simplicity, we will use the general terms of polyphenol oxidase (PPO) for the first class (EC 1.10.3.1) and laccase for the second class (EC 1.10.3.2). *See* Enzymes, Functions and Characteristics

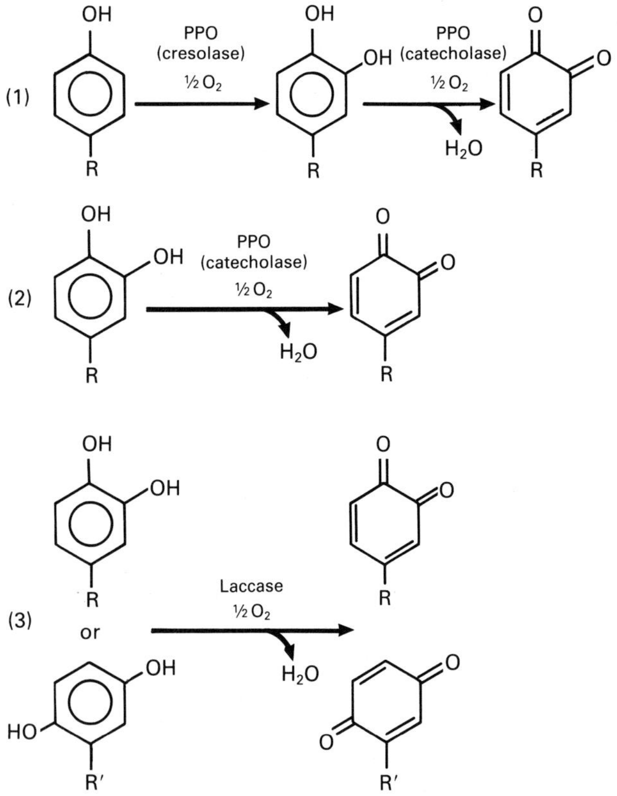

Fig. 1   Reactions catalysed by polyphenol oxidases.

Enzymatic–Biochemical Aspects

Enzymatic Browning Factors

The different factors of enzymatic browning are examined, including some minor ones which may, occasionally, play an important role, e.g. peroxidases.

Enzymes

Polyphenol Oxidases (EC 1.10.3.1)

PPOs are copper oxidoreductases exhibiting both cresolase and catecholase activities. However, many enzymatic preparations have a very low cresolase activity or none at all. It is difficult to be sure that the latter activity was originally absent in the plant or has not either been extracted or has been destroyed during extraction owing to its lability. Cresolase activity is very often lost during purification. Thus, in a preparation, the ratio of catecholase to cresolase activity (when the latter is present) can vary from 1 to more than 40.

PPO is present in a wide variety of plants. In a particular plant, PPO activity varies from one organ to another and varies inside an organ depending on the tissue considered. PPOs have been found in different cell fractions, in organelles (chloroplasts and, more precisely, in thylakoids, mitochondria, peroxisomes) where the enzymes are tightly bound to membranes and in the soluble fraction of the cell. The degree of binding to membranes varies with the tissue and its ontogenic state. Thus, the overall PPO activity is higher and mostly present in bound forms in young green fruits, whereas it generally decreases and the proportion of soluble forms increases in ripe fruits.

Extraction of the PPO activity from plant sources is complicated by the presence of endogenous phenolic substrates which are oxidized and then interact with proteins. Besides destroying activity, this may induce 'new' enzymatic forms corresponding to artefacts. As a consequence, this oxidation has to be prevented by adding a reducing agent (e.g. ascorbic acid or a thiol) and/or a phenol-complexing compound (e.g. polyamide, polyvinylpolypyrrolidone (PVPP) or polyethylene glycol) to the extracting solution. Solubilization after preparation of an acetone powder is a frequently used procedure. Detergents (Triton X100 or X114) are also used, but probably result in modifications of the enzyme structure and properties. Most of the purification procedures are based on fractional precipitation by ammonium sulphate followed by one or several chromatographic steps. Nevertheless, compared to the studies on fungi, there are only a few enzymes which have been completely purified and fully characterized from fruits. Molecular weights of PPOs range from 30 to 130 kDa. This wide range is mostly due to polymeric forms. However, part of this heterogeneity might also be the result of artefacts generated during the extraction procedure.

Most of the PPOs studied show an optimum activity between pH 4 and 7. However, there are often discrepancies in the published values for PPOs from the same source. In addition, several reports indicate differences in pH optimum depending on cultivars and maturity. These differences have been attributed to variations in the proportions of isoenzymes which have distinct pH optima. Moreover, pH optima were found to vary with the phenolic substrate used for several enzymatic preparations. The effect of temperature on PPO activity has been much less investigated than that of pH. The optimum temperature ranges from 15 to 40°C and depends on the same factors as does pH.

Laccases (EC 1.10.3.2)

The laccases catalyse the oxidation of o- and p-diphenols into their corresponding quinones according to reaction (3) in Fig. 1. They occur much less frequently in the plant kingdom than PPOs. Their presence has been mainly reported in many fungi and in species of the genus *Rhus* (e.g. the Japanese lacquer tree). They are almost absent from fruits and vegetables with the exception of certain peach cultivars and apricots. Nevertheless, the distinction between PPO and laccase activities is not always clear cut since the presence of endogenous phenols can induce the coupled oxidation of p-diphenols and therefore leads to a false conclusion on the presence of a laccase type of activity. Selective inhibitors can be used to ascertain the type of activity. Thus, cinnamic acid, salicylhydroxyamic acid, phenylhydrazine and carbon monoxide inhibit the PPO activity more specifically, whereas cetyl trimethyl ammonium bromide, a cationic detergent, is more specific for laccases.

Fungi laccases, which have been investigated most, are glycoproteins with a basic subunit consisting of a single polypeptide chain of 50–70 kDa containing a considerable amount of carbohydrate (10–45%) and four atoms of copper. The effect of pH on laccase activity is similar to that observed for PPO activity, i.e. an optimum pH which ranges between 4 and 7·5 and depends on the substrate being used.

Peroxidases (EC 1.11.1.7)

The peroxidases are enzymes whose primary function is to oxidize hydrogen donors at the expense of peroxides. They are highly specific for hydrogen peroxide, but they accept a wide range of hydrogen donors including polyphenols. The overall reaction catalysed is shown in eqn [1].

$$AH_2 + H_2O_2 \rightarrow A + 2H_2O \qquad (1)$$

Peroxidases are glycoproteins with a haematin compound as cofactor. Their molecular weights range between 30 and 55 kDa. Depending on the enzyme source, the isoenzyme considered and the donor substrate, the optimum activity is between pH 4 and 7. The higher thermostability of some isoenzymes is well known, and the residual peroxidase activity after blanching is often used as an index of thermal treatment.

The primary products of oxidized phenols are quinones similar to those obtained with PPOs and laccases. Although peroxidases are widely distributed, especially in plants, they generally appear to be little involved in enzymatic browning of fruits and vegetables following a mechanical stress. The explanation could be that the peroxidase activity is limited by the internal level of hydrogen peroxide. However, their involvement in slow processes such as internal browning during cold storage of fruits is possible.

Nevertheless, the direct involvement of peroxidase in browning remains questionnable, just as does that of laccase which may not be present in sound fruits and vegetables. Therefore, the following sections will be mainly devoted to PPO activity.

Substrates

Susceptibility to browning varies widely from one plant to another. This variation is linked to both quantitative and qualitative aspects of their phenolic content. Thus, browning after bruising of fruit cultivars with similar amounts of total phenolics can be either more or less intense. Among the wide variety of phenolic compounds found in fruits and vegetables, only a small number serve as direct substrates for PPO. Caffeic acid derivatives and monomeric flavan-3-ols (mainly (+)-(gallo)catechin and (−)-(gallo)epicatechin) appear often to be the best substrates. Other quantitatively important classes of phenols, namely anthocyannins, flavonols and condensed forms of flavan-3-ols (tannins), are weakly if not directly oxidized by PPO. The same holds for other less important classes of phenols (flavones, flavanones, flavononols, chalcones and dihydrochalcones). This restricted activity is probably related to the presence of a sugar moiety in many of these molecules which could cause steric hindrance since the aglycone forms are often good substrates of PPO. Nevertheless, phenolic compounds which are not direct substrates can actively participate in browning through coupled oxidation reactions. Thus, in model systems, it has been shown that the degradation of anthocyanins, procyanidins and flavonols by PPO is greatly accelerated in the presence of caffeic acid derivatives or catechins. The o-quinones enzymatically formed from either of the later compounds are able to promote co-oxidation reactions leading to both the degradation of the former compounds and the regeneration of good substrates for the enzymatic reaction. This degradation and the phenolic copolymerization resulting from nonenzymatic coupled

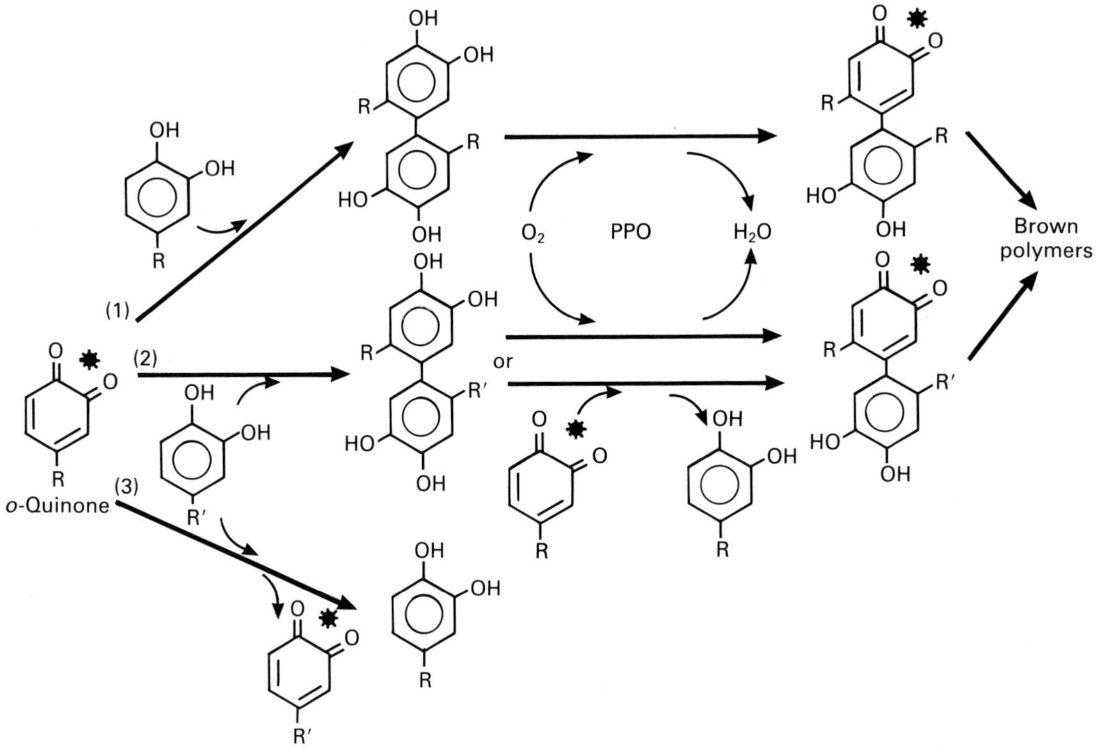

Fig. 2   Reactions of o-quinones with phenolic compounds. (All reactions are nonenzymatic except those with PPOs. Reactions (2) and (3) are able to regenerate the original phenol.) Products with differing colour intensities are indicated by asterisks.

Table 1. K_m (mM) and V_m values (are expressed as a percentage of the V_m of chlorogenic acid) of PPOs from different sources for three common natural substrates

	Apple		Grape		Pear		Peach	Apricot	Potato
	$V_m{}^a$	$K_m{}^a$	$V_m{}^b$	$K_m{}^c$	$V_m{}^b$	$K_m{}^c$	$V_m{}^b$	$K_m{}^c$	$K_m{}^c$
Chlorogenic acid	100	4·2	100	2·5	100	16·1	100	1·2	1·4
(+)-Catechin	58	6·2	64	1	60	2·1	373	0·74	—
Caffeic acid	8·1	0·14	69	5·5	43	—	61	0·5	2·4–2·9

Adapted from:
[a] Janovitz-Klapp A, Richard F, Goupy P and Nicolas J (1990) *Journal of Agricultural and Food Chemistry* 38: 1437–1441.
[b] See Macheix JJ *et al.* (1990).
[c] See Vamos-Vigyazo L (1981).

oxidations (reactions (2) and (3) of Fig. 2) lead to products which may be intensely brown.

Many studies have been devoted to the specificity of PPO towards phenolic substrates. Usually, the apparent K_m is higher than 1 mM, indicating a relatively low affinity. However, for a particular substrate, the K_m values can vary widely depending on the PPO source, and the same holds for the relative rate of oxidation among different phenolics (Table 1). It is often suggested

that the preferred substrate is the most abundant phenolic, although this is not always true.

By contrast, few studies have concerned oxygen, the other substrate. Steady-state kinetics carried out on PPO indicate that it probably follows an ordered Bi-Bi mechanism in which the oxygen binds first. The reported values for equilibrium constant are in the range 0·1–0·5 mM, corresponding to a rather low affinity for the oxygen (compared to, for example, cytochrome oxidase,

Table 2.   Molar extinction coefficients of quinones from different *o*-diphenolic substrates of PPOs

Substrate	Wavelength (nm)	Extinction coefficient	Substrate	Wavelength (nm)	Extinction coefficient
Pyrocatechol[a]	390	1417	3,4-Dihydroxyphenylacetic acid[a]	390	1311
4-t-Butylcatechol[a]	400	1150	4-Methylcatechol[a]	400	1400
L-DOPA[a]	480	3388	Hydrocaffeic acid[a]	412	1124
Chlorogenic acid[b]	420	2000	(+)-Catechin[b]	380	1200

Adapted from:
[a] Waite J.H. (1976) Calculating extinction coefficients for enzymatically produced *o*-quinones. *Analytical Biochemistry* 75: 211–218.
[b] Rouet-Mayer M.A., Ralambosoa J and Philippon J (1990) Roles of *o*-quinones and their polymers in the enzymic browning of apples. *Phytochemistry* 29: 435–440.

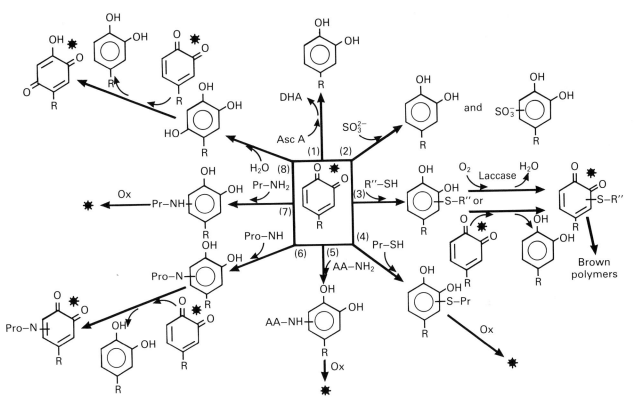

Fig. 3   Reactions of *o*-quinones with nonphenolic compounds. (All reactions are nonenzymatic except those with laccase. Reactions (1), (2), (3), (6) and (8) are able to regenerate the original phenol.) Products with differing colour intensities are indicated by asterisks. Ox, further oxidation reactions by oxygen or *o*-quinone; Pr-SH and Pr-NH₂, proteins; Pro-NH, Proline; AA-NH₂, amino acids; Asc A, ascorbic acid; DHA, dehydroascorbic acid; R″SH, small thiol compounds (e.g. cysteine and glutathione).

0·5–1 μM). *See* Oxidation of Food Components; Phenolic Compounds; Tannins and Polyphenols

Reaction Products

The primary products of enzymatic oxidation are *o*-quinones. These molecules have different spectral properties and their colour depends on the pH and the phenol from which they originate. The molar extinction coeffi-

cients at the maximum wavelengths are given for some of them in Table 2, and show a wide range of variation.

The colours are different from their precursors, since after oxidation catechin is bright yellow, chlorogenic acid is dull orange-yellow whereas DOPA is pink. Moreover, the *o*-quinones are reactive compounds as illustrated in Figs 2 and 3. Consider Fig. 2 for the reactions with phenolic compounds. *o*-Quinones can react with another phenol molecule, resulting in a dimer of the original phenol (reaction (1)). This dimer, having an o-diphenolic structure can be subject to reoxidation either enzymatically or by another o-quinone and gives larger oligomers with different colour intensities. The o-quinones can also react with a different phenol molecule, either leading to a copolymer (reaction (2)) or regenerating the original phenol and giving a different o-quinone (reaction (3) – coupled oxidation). In Fig. 3, corresponding to reactions with nonphenolic compounds, another coupled oxidation reaction is observed with ascorbic acid (reaction (1)), since the phenol is regenerated with the formation of dehydroascorbic acid. With sulphites colourless addition compounds are formed together with regenerated phenol (reaction (2)). The o-quinones can form addition compounds with thiol groups by nucleophilic substitution (reactions (3) and (4)). Cysteine, either free or bound in small peptides (e.g. glutathione) or in large proteins, gives colourless compounds. However, due to their o-diphenolic structures, these can be either oxidized by laccase or react with excess o-quinones (by a coupled oxidation mechanism) and form intensely coloured products. The same kind of addition reactions occur with amino groups (primary or secondary amines) although a little less readily (reactions (5)–(7)). Therefore, further subtitutions with other thiol or amino groups of proteins may occur, leading to intra- and intermolecular cross-links. Lastly, water slowly adds to the o-quinones to form triphenols which are readily oxidized by excess o-quinone (by a coupled oxidation mechanism), leading to the p-quinones (reaction (8)). *See* Amines; Ascorbic Acid, Properties and Determination

The reactivity (or in other terms the stability) of the o-quinones in these different cases is very variable. It depends strongly on the substituted nature of the parent phenol, and on the medium (composition, pH, temperature, etc.). Thus, in the same conditions, the o-quinones derived from 4-methylcatechol are more stable than those from chlorogenic acid which in turn are more stable than those from catechins. Obviously, the presence of reactive molecules, with amino or thiol groups, in the medium can greatly affect the stability of the o-quinones. Moreover, the reactivity with reducing compounds, namely those entering in coupled oxidation reactions, is under the control of the redox potentials of the systems involved. Thus, the o-quinones from chlorogenic acid are able to co-oxidize catechins into o-quinones of catechin and regenerate chlorogenic acid, whereas the reverse is not true.

Inhibition of Enzymatic Browning

Enzymatic browning is often an undesirable reaction and prevention of it is a major concern for food scientists. Therefore, a large part of the many studies devoted to enzymatic browning concern its control. This section gives only the physicochemical basis for the control of the reaction. The more applied view of this problem in food technology is described in the next article. The different ways of browning control can be divided in three classes, depending on whether they affect enzymes, substrates or reaction products. However, some inhibitors are able to act simultaneously on more than one of these factors.

Action on Enzymes

Firstly, heat treatment is often employed, and usually a short exposure to temperatures between 70 and 90°C is sufficient to inactivate PPOs. Since the optimum pH of most PPOs lies between pH 4 and 7 (see earlier) on the one hand, and the phenols are more readily oxidized when the pH increases on the other, acidification below pH 4 is often proposed, although PPOs are still active in some cases (grape, apple, etc.).

Besides these general treatments, more specific chemical inhibitors are known. PPOs having copper as a prosthetic group are inhibited by many metal-chelating agents such as cyanide, azide, diethyldithiocarbamate and ethylxanthate, although inhibition depends on the source of the PPO. Inhibition by halide ions observed in numerous cases is pH dependent, and increases when the pH decreases; it may be caused by the formation of a complex between the halide ion and copper which is enhanced by low pH values. Due to their structural resemblance to phenolic substrates, aromatic carboxylic compounds are usually found to be competitive inhibitors. As has been shown for apple PPOs, the inhibitory properties are highly dependent on structure (Table 3). Thus, for a particular substituent, inhibition decreases in the order cinnamic, benzoic, phenylpropionic and phenylacetic acid. In each series, inhibition was slightly enhanced by p-hydroxy substitution and greatly reduced by m-methoxy substitution. Moreover, the presence of a benzene nucleus is not an absolute structural requirement for the inhibitory effect since sorbic acid, an aliphatic carboxylic acid with two conjugated double bonds, is almost as effective as benzoic acid. In all cases, inhibition increases as pH decreases and it was shown that the unionized form of the carboxyl group is mainly responsible for inhibition.

Action on Substrates

Inhibition of enzymatic browning can also be obtained by removal of one of the two substrates (oxygen and phenolic compounds) from the reaction medium. Complete oxygen removal is the most satisfactory way to control the phenolic oxidation catalysed by PPOs. However, although this method may be applied to dead

Table 3. Inhibition constants of sodium halides and some carboxylic acids for apple PPOs at pH 4·5. All are competitive inhibitors with the exception of sodium chloride which is noncompetitive

	K_i (mM)		K_i (mM)		K_i (mM)		K_i (mM)
Sodium iodide	117	Benzoic	0·64	Cinnamic	0·092	Phenylacetic	13
Sodium bromide	106	p-Hydroxybenzoic	0·57	p-Coumaric	0·04	Phenylpropionic	1·4
Sodium chloride	20	Vanillic	10	Ferulic	0·29	p-Hydroxyphenylpropionic	1·1
Sodium fluoride	0·07	Syringic	34·5	Sinapic	15	Sorbic	0·51

Adapted from: Janovitz-Klapp A, Richard F, Goupy P and Nicolas J (1990) Inhibition studies on apple polyphenol oxidase. *Journal of Agricultural and Food Chemistry* 38: 926–931.

tissues, either by creating a physical barrier to oxygen diffusion or by vacuum infiltration (a more detailed description on this subject is given in the next article), it is inapplicable to living tissues due to the risk of metabolism deviations caused by anaerobic conditions. Concerning the phenolic substrates, two methods are available. The first one is the physical elimination by specific adsorbents. The most widely used, polyvinyl-pyrrolidone (PVP) and its insoluble form PVPP, are very effective in controlling enzymatic browning. Thus, PVP has also been shown to be a competitive inhibitor of PPOs. Other complexing agents of phenols can be used such as polyethylene glycol or polyamide. In the same way, borate acts by complexing the o-dihydroxy groups of phenolic substrates. Lastly, the inhibitory properties of β-cyclodextrins, recently observed for apple juice browning, are probably related to their abilities to form inclusion complexes with PPO substrates, although this assumption has not been confirmed. The second way of removing phenolic compounds is by their modification. This can be performed by two kinds of enzymes. The first modification is methylation of the o-diphenolic substrates of PPO by an O-methyltransferase (e.g. caffeic acid is converted to ferulic acid). Unfortunately, this elegant process is impeded by the high cost of the enzyme (S-adenosyl-methionine:catechol O-methyltransferase) and of one of its substrates (S-adenosylmethionine). The second modification is oxidative ring opening by protocate-chuate 3,4-dioxygenase. However, in addition to its cost, this enzyme has poor catalytic activities on chloro-genic acid and its derivatives.

Action on Reaction Products

Acting on reaction products is the third way of controlling enzymatic browning. o-Quinones are very reactive primary products (Figs 2 and 3) and, using chemical means, they can either be reduced back to o-diphenols or trapped as colourless addition compounds. However, secondary products resulting mainly from the oxidative polymerization of o-quinones often give highly coloured compounds which become less reactive as the browning reaction proceeds. Therefore, almost all the compounds listed in the section on reaction products which act on o-quinones, and more especially ascorbic acid, thiol compounds and sulphite derivatives, can be used for the control of enzymatic browning. However, their effectiveness in preventing browning is greatly reduced if their use is delayed until after the reaction has started.

Besides chemical means, brown pigments can be removed more or less completely by physical treatments such as ultrafiltration or use of resins in order to trap polymers of o-quinones. This can be an efficient method for the clarification of liquids such as fruit juices and wine.

Lastly, several studies have been devoted to the isolation of 'natural' inhibitors of enzymatic browning. Thus, low-molecular-weight compounds exhibiting inhibitory properties have been detected in cultures of *Penicillium expansum* and *Dactylium dendroides*. Recently, it has been shown that honey extracts contain substances which are able to inhibit the PPO activity. Nevertheless, in all cases, these inhibitory compounds have been only partially characterized and their exact mechanism of inhibition is not fully understood. *See* Antioxidants, Natural Antioxidants; Antioxidants, Synthetic Antioxidants

In recent years, considerable progress has been made in understanding PPOs and polyphenols of fruits and vegetables. However, many studies were restricted to model systems with an enzyme acting on one substrate only. There is a great need for studies on enzymatic action on mixtures of phenols on the one hand, and on nonenzymatic reactions that follow o-quinone formation on the other. These researches would give valuable information on the way that phenols affect both the enzymatic activity and the kind of brown pigments formed, and it would help in a better understanding of the relation between the extent of browning and the phenolic composition of fruit and vegetables.

Bibliography

Macheix JJ, Fleuriet A and Billot J (1990) *Fruit Phenolics.* Boca Raton: CRC Press.

Mayer AM (1987) Polyphenol oxidases in plants. Recent progress. *Phytochemistry* 26: 11–20.

Mayer AM and Harel E (1979) Polyphenol oxidases in plants. *Phytochemistry* 18: 193–215.

Vamos-Vigyazo L (1981) Polyphenol oxidase and peroxidase in fruits and vegetables. *CRC Critical Reviews in Food Science and Nutrition* 15: 49–127.

Marie-Aude Rouet-Mayer,
Centre National de la Recherche Scientifique, Meudon-Bellevue, France
Jean Philippon
Centre National du Machinisme Agricole du Génie Rural des Eaux et Forêts, Antony, France
Jacques Nicolas
Institut National de la Recherche Agronomique, Avignon, France

Enzymatic – Technical Aspects and Assays

Enzymatic browning affects numerous plant organs which are rich in oxidizable phenols, such as fruits, vegetables, aromatic plants and fungi. It occurs during various procedures used in the food industry: deep freezing, dehydrofreezing, freeze drying, hot air drying, etc. In practice, there are three approaches to prevention of this browning: varietal selection, physical methods and chemical inhibitors.

The various methods currently used or likely to be so in the future for prevention of browning are reviewed. Deep-frozen fruits and vegetables are considered in detail, since enzymatic browning is most difficult to resolve in these products. Also, the preventive methods used during industrial drying and freeze drying, and even canning and bottling, are in fact very similar.

A brief review is then given of the methods of measurement of browning and of the questions raised by objective assessment.

Practical Methods of Preventing Browning

Choice of Raw Material

Some plant tissues such as fruits or vegetables are less sensitive to browning than others. Most berries – raspberry, blackcurrant, redcurrant, bilberry – are virtually unaffected. Other species, however, quickly brown on freezing and thawing unless previously subject to antioxidant treatment. They are generally rich in total phenols and poor in ascorbic acid in cases of fruits with pips (apple, pear, quince), and stone fruits (apricots, peaches, plums).

The phenol content of fruits and vegetables varies naturally according to the degree of ripeness, the soil and climate, but also depends substantially on intraspecific genetic characteristics. The Sunbeam peach variety, for instance, which does not brown, contains 20 times less total phenols than the Elberta variety, which is sensitive to browning. This plainly illustrates the value of the development by genetic selection of new, low-phenol varieties. *See* Ascorbic Acid, Properties and Determination; Phenolic Compounds

Physical Methods of Prevention

Mechanical Factors

Browning is enhanced by wounding of plant tissue, notably during industrial processing. Upkeep of machine blades is important to ensure that fruits and vegetables are cut cleanly.

Effect of Temperature

Cold

A marked slowing in enzymatic browning is induced by a reduction in temperature. Nonetheless, colour change is still rapid at 0°C. This means that the most sensitive products are frozen by methods allowing the crystallization temperature of water to be reached as rapidly as possible. This is the case with mushrooms, for which cryogenic techniques are obligatory when they are frozen without prior antioxidant treatment. The same is true for peeled slices of white peach which brown during freezing if the cooling exceeds 10 min.

Once frozen, colour change is practically blocked at the temperature of commercial storage (-18°C). The value of Q_{10} is about 18 for halved, peeled yellow clingstone peaches. When the temperature rises, browning starts again, and will be more marked if the cellular structures of the plant organ have been severely damaged by freezing, chemical peeling, and slicing.

Heat

Heat treatment, or blanching, without doubt constitutes the simplest and most direct method of enzyme inactivation. It consists of brief immersion (from 1 to 6 min depending on size) of the produce in water, boiling syrup or steam at close to 100°C.

Catechol oxidases are inhibited above approximately 70°C. Their heat stability is closely pH dependent; it is maximal at about pH 6 and decreases very rapidly below and above this value.

In the deep freezing of foodstuffs, blanching is principally applied to vegetables that are eaten cooked (potatoes, salsify, asparagus, etc.), but it is also to stabilize frozen fruit purées, particularly of apricots. Blanching is little used with whole or sliced frozen fruits that are eaten raw, since it results in loss of firmness and in flavour changes which are unacceptable to the consumer. This is why blanching is used only for fruit with tissue sufficiently impermeable to oxygen to escape deep browning. Examples are apricot and peach, for which the brief surface treatment scarcely alters the organoleptic qualities. When blanching of pears and, particularly, apples (20–25% lacunae) is incomplete, marked deep browning occurs on thawing.

Protection from Oxygen

When plant organs cannot be blanched, protection from air constitutes another way of preventing browning. Prevention fails, however, as soon as the anoxic conditions no longer hold, and colour changes are even accelerated by the destruction of cell structures caused by freezing and thawing.

In the food industry, products are protected from oxygen using a variety of methods, either singly or combined.

Airtight Packages

These are indispensable for preventing the browning of sensitive fruits with active oxidase systems. In hermetically sealed metal cans, pitted cherries in syrup do not brown, even at −7°C, whereas spoilage occurs very rapidly if the container is not airtight. The differences between airtight and nonairtight packages increase as the temperature rises. Browning is also a function of the degree of can filling, and hence the quantity of residual air in the headspace.

Partial Vacuum

A partial vacuum of 380 torr is enough to block the browning of frozen peaches in syrup stored at −7°C. However, stronger vacuums should be avoided since, on thawing, raw fruit will have an unpleasant spongy consistency, and fruit packaged in syrup will tend to acquire an unwanted translucent appearance. *See* Chilled Storage, Packaging Under Vacuum

Oxygen-poor Atmospheres

Browning can also be avoided by keeping the foodstuff in oxygen-poor atmospheres.

This can be achieved chemically, or by use of an inert gas. The chemical approach involves the enzymatic oxidation of the sugar present in the medium (enzymatic deoxygenation), thus leading to the consumption of oxygen trapped within an airtight package. The sugar combines with oxygen under the effect of added glucose oxidase to give gluconic acid. This process has been shown to be effective in laboratory tests with peaches, but to our knowledge has not undergone industrial development.

The use of carbon dioxide or pure nitrogen atmospheres also effectively protects frozen fruits against enzymatic browning. Nitrogen, furthermore, affords better protection of the original flavour and aroma.

Sugaring of Fruits

In this process, fruit is immersed in a covering liquid, either of a chosen concentration of sugar syrup, or of the fruit's own juice drawn out by contact with dry sugar.

Sugar (generally sucrose) has several effects. It increases the osmotic pressure of the surrounding liquid, which contributes to the reduction in size of ice crystals on freezing, thereby protecting cellular structures. It also increases the viscosity of the medium, thus slowing the rate of enzymatic spoilage reactions. It may also have a slight inhibitory effect on the enzymes of browning when the syrup concentration exceeds 20% (w/w). *See* Sucrose, Properties and Determination

Sugar is also a well-known and valued enhancer of taste and aroma. It does, though, result in some dilution of aroma when used in the form of syrup. This defect is attenuated when sugar is added to fruit in the dry form, but severe changes in consistency result, thus harming the fruit's appearance. In addition, the exuded juice collects in the bottom of the package and only effectively protects part of the package contents.

In commercial practice, sugaring is only used with frozen fruits intended for the manufacture of juice, syrup, liqueur or purée: the concentrations used range from 1:9 to, more commonly, 1:4 (dry sugar:fruit).

Frozen fruits intended for direct consumption are frequently packaged under a covering syrup. The syrup concentrations are about 30–40° Brix for cherries, pears and plums, 40–50° Brix for bananas, apples and nectarines, and 40–60° Brix for strawberries, apricots and peaches. Nonetheless, syrup alone inadequately protects the most sensitive fruits, and an antioxidant is therefore incorporated. The most used antioxidant is ascorbic acid, and its derivatives, although other substances such as citric acid are employed, notably in the case of peeled, frozen bananas. The covering liquid comprises either a syrup of pure sucrose, or a mixture of sucrose and maize glucose. *See* Antioxidants, Natural Antioxidants; Antioxidants, Synthetic Antioxidants

Chemical Methods of Prevention

Numerous chemical compounds inhibit enzymatic browning. Of these, few combine effectiveness with recognized innocuousness, unaltered product flavour, and reasonable cost. The use of most of these compounds is banned by legislation.

In the case of plant foodstuffs, the legislation of most countries only permits ascorbic acid and its derivatives, sodium chloride and, within stricter limits, citric acid and sulphur dioxide (as well as its derivatives, sodium sulphite and sodium metabisulphite). *See* Legislation, Additives

Ascorbic Acid

Ascorbic acid, which with its first oxidation product dehydroascrobic acid, constitutes vitamin C, reduces *o*-quinones progressively as they are formed. Catechol oxidase, which indirectly controls the oxidation of ascorbic acid, is virtually unaffected during the reaction, as that browning begins as soon as the reductant has been consumed. *See* Ascorbic Acid, Properties and Determination

In practice, concentrations of 0·1–0·3% prove adequate when, as is often the case, the external conditions are unfavourable to browning, i.e. low temperature, acidic and poorly oxygenated medium.

Ascorbic acid is effective above all when thoroughly mixed in liquid or paste products (apple juice, purée). It is also used at concentrations of 0·2–0·25% in syrups covering frozen fruit to enhance the protective effect against enzymatic browning.

One of the drawbacks of ascorbic acid (apart from its relatively high cost) is that it is readily oxidized and rapidly disappears from the medium. To counter this rapid disappearance various derivatives have been proposed as substitutes, such as ascorbic acid-2-phosphate (AAP), or ascorbic acid-triphosphate (AATP). These compounds are not reducing agents, and therefore remain stable in the presence of oxygen, but they do hydrolyse progressively, releasing ascorbic acid under the action of the phosphatases present in the plant tissue. Such compounds are not, however, effective if the medium is too acid (e.g. apple juice, pH 3·7) since the activity of the phosphatases is then too low. They are effective, though, in solutions of soaked, sliced apples (0·8%) in cold storage.

Ascorbylpalmitate is a fat-soluble substance which over a long period is more effective than ascorbic acid in fruit juice when used at a concentration of 200 ppm. Its poor aqueous solubility, however, makes it ineffective in soaking solutions.

Sodium Chloride

Salt is frequently used in the food industry to slow microbial growth (bacteria, fungi), but it is inadequately protective at low concentrations and imparts an unwanted salty flavour at high concentrations. At a pH below 5·5, however, salt is a good inhibitor of enzymatic browning, hence the value of using it in conjunction with citric acid for neutral plant products, such as cultivated mushrooms. *See* Preservation of Food

Sodium chloride is sometimes used at low concentrations (1–2%) to afford temporary protection from surface browning of sliced, peeled apples intended for freezing, or to be sold as ready-to-use fresh foods. The soaking time is short, usually less than 1 min).

Used in combination with ascorbic acid, sodium chloride prolongs the duration of action of the acid.

Citric Acid

Oxidative enzyme activity is very pH dependent (see previous article). Highly acidic (pH < 2·5) or basic (pH > 10) media which result in protein denaturation destroy its activity. Although alkalization of the medium in which fruits are immersed is undesirable (spontaneous browning following nonenzymatic oxidation of *o*-diphenols), acidification can prove advantageous in certain circumstances. Apart from acetic acid used in vinegar production, citric acid is virtually the only substance authorized for this use. It is sometimes used in deep freezing and in fruit conserves in syrup; thus it is used to neutralize the rinsing water of halved, chemically peeled peaches, and at the same time to protect the fruit temporarily against enzymatic browning. The dose used is about 1% of the volume of water. *See* Acids, Natural Acids and Acidulants; Enzymes, Functions and Characteristics

Sulphur Dioxide and its Derivatives

Sulphur dioxide, which is an antiseptic widely used in foodstuffs, is by far the most effective of currently authorized chemical inhibitors of browning. It even acts at very low concentrations and is inexpensive. It can also be used with certain fruits to eliminate unwanted red pigmentation, as in the case of Bigarreau Napoléon cherries, used in confectionery, which must first be decolorized using sulphite to ensure that the pigment does not turn brown during heat treatment.

As an inhibitor of browning, sulphur dioxide has three actions: formation of colourless addition products with (coloured) *o*-quinones; reduction of *o*-quinones to their original *o*-diphenols (colourless); inhibition of catechol oxidase (see previous article). Sulphur dioxide also reacts with many other chemical constituents of plant tissues (notably ketones and aldehydes). The strength of the chemical bonds formed varies with the pH and the type of molecule involved. It would appear that such products are the cause of the abnormal flavours which sometimes develop when sulphur dioxide is used at too high a concentration and is not subsequently eliminated.

Sulphur dioxide can be used in the form of a gas or in aqueous solution as sodium sulphite or disulphite. As a disulphite, it acts less rapidly, but is more easily controlled and results in a few flavour changes.

Of deep-frozen products, apples and apricots are most suited to sulphur dioxide treatment. Fruit slices or halved fruits are soaked for 3–4 min in solutions containing 0·5–0·4% sulphur dioxide.

High doses are sometimes authorized and used to stabilize fruit pulp intended for the making of jams of standard quality (antiseptic action) and to clear fruits before drying (notably apricots). In this case, however, these semiprocessed products will lose most of the treatment compound during subsequent operations. Nevertheless, the tendency of national and international regulations is progressively to restrict the use of sulphur dioxide, or even to ban it altogether, since it has been shown on occasion to be implicated in severe disorders in asthmatics.

Assays for Evaluation of Browning

Accurate methods are required for the measurement of browning in tissue slices and extracts. This need is obvious when different cultivars are to be compared for susceptibility to browning or for evaluation of experimental treatments designed to control enzymatic browning.

Basically, two kinds of technique are available. The first uses absorbance measurements, usually in the 400 nm region, on solutions after extraction and purification of the brown pigments. The second uses tristimulus reflectance colorimetry and can be applied directly to cut surfaces or fruit purée. Although both methods are easy and rapid, they do have serious disadvantages. *See* Spectroscopy, Visible Spectroscopy and Colorimetry

Absorbance measurements evaluate only the soluble pigments. It is well known that, as the reaction proceeds, polymerization occurs (see preceding article) and the solubility of a large fraction of the brown pigments decreases. The insoluble entities are eliminated during the filtration and centrifugation steps in the purification process. Moreover, depending on the kind of pigments, which in turn depend on the original phenols and on their relative proportions, the wavelength of maximum absorbance ranges between 360 and 500 nm in the visible region. Therefore, absorbance measurements at a single wavelength are poorly correlated with the visual evaluation of browning.

Most of the data obtained in tristimulus reflectance colorimetry are now given as L (lightness), a (greenness

Table 1. Relations between the extent of browning, phenolic content, and PPO activity in different fruit species[a]

Species	Number of cultivars	Correlation with[b] Phenolics	PPO	Method used[c]
Apple	7	0	0	S ($A = 440$ nm)
	3	+	0	S ($A = 440$ nm)
	4	0	+	S ($A = 440$ nm)
	6–8	+		R (Tristimulus)
Avocado	3	0	+	Visual
	6	0	+	Visual
Banana	3–5	0	+	Visual
Eggplant	3		+	Visual
Grape	9 (red)	0	+	S ($A = 430$ nm)
	19 (white)	0	0	S ($A = 430$ nm)
Olive	6	+	+	R (545 nm)
	5		+	S ($A = 410$ nm)
	5	+	+	S ($A = 410$ nm)
	9	+		S ($A = 400$ nm)
Peach	6	+		S ($A = 395$ nm)
Pear	6	+		R (540 nm)

[a] Adapted from Macheix JJ *et al.* (1990).
[b] 0, no correlation; +, positive correlation.
[c] S, absorbance data; R, reflectance data. (Either at a single wavelength or tristimulus.)

or redness) and b (blueness or yellowness) values, or a combination of these factors. However, the values obtained are highly dependent on the method of measurement and on the state of the surface of the examined object. Thus, during browning, variations in tristimulus data are the result of both chemical and physical changes, the relative importance of the two processes being difficult to assess. Most authors use the decrease in lightness δL (i.e. the difference in L values before and after browning) to evaluate the extent of browning. Some authors have proposed a more sophisticated parameter, the colour difference δE, which can be calculated as

$$\delta E = \sqrt{[(\delta L)^2 + (\delta a)^2 (\delta b)^2]}. \quad (1)$$

This value gives the distance in colour space between two colours but not the direction in which they differ. Moreover, neither δL nor δE gives an idea of the resulting perceived colour.

In intervarietal comparisons, numerous authors have tried to correlate the extent of browning, measured by one of the above methods, with the phenolic content and/or the polyphenol oxidase (PPO) activity (Table 1). Clearly, there is no clear-cut relationship between browning and any of these chemical parameters for all fruits. Thus, depending on the fruit species, a correlation can be obtained with both the parameters, one of them, or neither. There are two potential explanations of these difficulties. Firstly, methods for evaluation of browning are only approximate and improved specificity is required. Secondly, the chemical parameters, and especially the total phenolic content, are probably not sufficient to explain the extent of browning. In the preceding article, it has been stressed that PPO has a wide specificity towards phenolic compounds, which are enzyme substrates to varying degrees. Moreover, the pigments resulting from these phenolics vary widely in colour intensity and hue. Thus, the relative balance among the different classes of phenols is probably fundamental in explaining the degree of browning. Lastly, additional factors may also be influential: some are chemical, such as the acidity and the concentration of reductants such as ascorbic acid, while others are physical, such as texture. The relative importance of each of these factors probably varies greatly from one species to another.

Enzymatic browning can be controlled by physical treatments, which are not applicable in all circumstances, and by the use of chemical compounds. Very few of the latter are presently available to prevent enzymatic browning in foodstuffs, and none is ideal.

Ascorbic acid is a good inhibitor of browning, but cannot always be used and is, moreover relatively expensive. Citric acid and sodium chloride have only a limited usefulness and are valuable principally as a complement to another treatment. Only sulphur dioxide is effective and inexpensive, but it has undesirable side effects and research is therefore necessary to find a suitable substitute.

Existing techniques for the measurement of browning provide useful information on differences in colour and colour density. However, these techniques give a very imperfect assessment of the degree of browning as noted by an observer. The main reason is that human ocular acuity in perception of a difference in hue or colour decreases sharply as the colour of the object darkens or tends towards saturation. Much more work will be necessary to establish for each product a strict correlation between instrumental measurements and consumer perception.

Bibliography

Clydesdale FM (1984) In: Gruenwedel DW and Whitaker JR (eds) *Color Measurement in Food Analysis: Principles and Techniques*, pp 95–150. New York: Marcel Dekker.

Macheix JJ, Fleuriet A and Billot J (1990) *Fruit Phenolics*. Boca Raton: CRC Press.

Philippon J, Rouet-Mayer MA, Gallet D and Herson A (1982) Précongélation des pêches entières à l'usage des conserveries de fruits au sirop. Conséquences des différentes étapes de la nouvelle filière technologique sur la qualité des fruits décongelés et sur celle du produit élaboré. *C.R. des Réunions des Commissions B2, C2, D1 de l'Institut International du Froid*, Sofia, pp 302–310.

Sapers GM, Hicks KB, Phillips JG, Garzarella L, Pondish DL, Matulaitis RM, McCormack TJ, Sondey SM, Seib PA and El-Atawy YS (1989) Control of enzymatic browning in apples with ascorbic acid derivatives, polyphenol oxidase inhibitors and complexing agents. *Journal of Food Science* 54: 997–1002, 1012.

Marie-Aude Rouet-Mayer
Centre National de la Recherche Scientifique, Meudon, France
Jean Philippon
Centre National du Machinisme Agricole, du Génie Rural, des Eaux et des Forêts, Antony, France
Jacques Nicolas
Institut National de la Recherche Agronomique, Avignon, France

Toxicology of Nonenzymatic Browning

Browning Reaction and Biological Effects

Reactions between reducing sugars and free amino groups in foods, without any catalytic involvement of enzymes, lead to nonenzymatic browning (Maillard reaction) causing a reduction in nutritive value and certain physiological and/or toxicological effects. The browning reaction develops during both home cooking and industrial processing of foods. Whilst contributing to an improvement of the organoleptic properties of foods, through aroma development, browning is often an undesirable side-effect of obligatory heat treatments applied for microbiological (sterilization and drying) or nutritional (cooking) reasons and for convenience (storage). Since the Maillard reaction occurs so frequently and Maillard reaction products are present in practically all meals, an understanding of its biological implications is of importance.

Because of the multiplicity of the food systems, the complexity of the chemical reactions and the large variety of heat treatments involved, any generalization on the biological outcome of nonenzymatic browning of foods is not easy. Nevertheless, a number of studies of model amino acid/protein and sugar reaction systems permits a classification of the biological outcome as (1) nutritional, (2) physiological and (3) toxic (including genotoxic) effects.

Nutritional Effects

The nutritional effects of the Maillard reaction in foods are due both to the chemical modification of essential nutrients which thereby become unavailable (direct effects) and to the presence of Maillard products which reduce the bioavailability and disturbs the metabolism of other nutrients (indirect effect).

Since it proceeds through many chemical routes and produces a large number of chemical species, the Maillard reaction has been divided for clarity and convenience into two distinct stages, 'early' and 'advanced', which are associated with different nutritional and physiological consequences (Fig. 1).

The 'Early' Maillard Reaction

This first stage involves the reaction between a free amino group and a reducing sugar to form, through the Amadori rearrangement, a stable deoxyketose addition compound, also called the Amadori compound. This is the obligatory step for the continuation of the reaction to the 'advanced' stage.

At this Amadori stage, nutritional damage has already been done. No enzyme in animal tissues can split these complexes to regenerate the amino compounds, which are nutritionally unavailable. In the case of amino acids, rat growth and metabolic studies have shown that

the Amadori compounds are biologically unavailable. Caecal and large intestinal microorganisms in experimental animals can liberate the complexed amino acids, but this occurs too late in the digestive/absorptive process for a significant *in vivo* utilization. The nutritional loss includes those free amino acids and peptides that have reactive α-amino groups, protein-bound lysine which has a reactive ε-amino group, and vitamins (thiamin, pyridoxine and folic acid).

In a model system representative of the 'early' stage, comprising milk powder stored at 60°C or lower for several weeks, the most quantitatively important nutrient which is damaged is lysine. This is due to its high level in milk protein compared to the other amino compounds and of the high reactivity of its ε-amino group (Table 1). Milk is one of the most sensitive foods to this reaction because of its high content of the reducing sugar lactose in addition to lysine. The most important negative consequence of the 'early' Maillard reaction is therefore the 'blockage' of lysine in milk-based products (infant formulae and weaning foods). Lysine is essential for growth and its requirement is high (103 mg kg^{-1} per day for babies as compared to 12 mg kg^{-1} per day for adults). The high, recommended

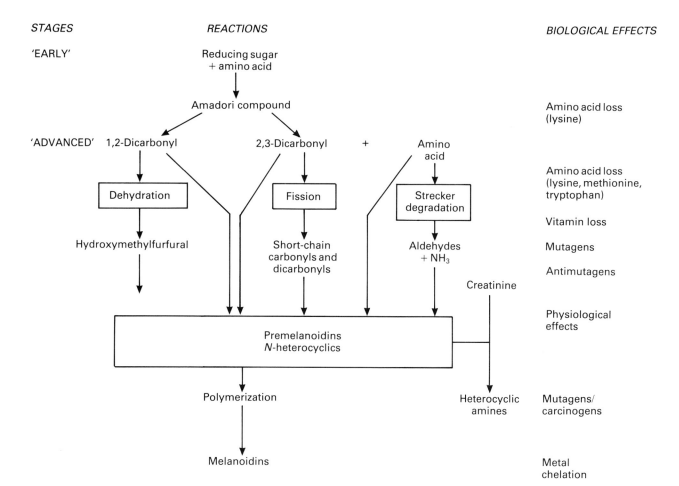

Fig. 1 Browning reaction. Chemical pathways and biological effects.

Table 1.   Nutritional effects of 'early' and 'advanced' Maillard reactions. Model system: dried milk powder

Maillard 'status' treatments	Percentage of original values of untreated sample							
	Reactive lysine	Lysine as Amadori compound	Lysine in 'advanced' Maillard products	Vitamin B_1	Pantothenic acid	Vitamin B_6	Folic acid	Vitamin B_{12}
'Early' 60°C, 4 weeks	74	26	0	81	90	84	29	100
'Advanced' 70°C, 4 weeks	17	14	69	5	7	18	3	31

	Reactive lysine	Nitrogen digestibility	Tryptophan		Methionine
			Chemical analysis	Bioavailability	
'Early' 50°C, 9 weeks	79	98	100	100	100
'Advanced' 60°C, 4 weeks	20	75	100	92	92

Table 2.   Lysine blockage in processed milk

Heat process	Percentage lysine as Amadori compound[a]
Freeze drying	0
Pasteurization	0
UHT sterilization	0–2
Spray drying	0–2
Spray-drying infant formula	5–10
HTST sterilization	5–10
Conventional sterilization	10–15
Roller drying	20–50

[a] According to the furosine method.

lysine level in baby formulae (minimum of 6·7 g per 100 g of protein, equal to the level in mother's milk) is reached using cow's milk which contains an excess of lysine of at least 20% compared to mother's milk.

Industrially treated milks contain a certain amount of such blocked lysine as its Amadori compound, the amount varying between 0 and 15% depending on the treatments applied (Table 2). Higher values are reached with the roller drying process, though this process is no longer used in the industrial-scale production of milk formulae.

Lysine bioavailability is also affected by the Maillard reaction in other heat-treated foods like bread, biscuits, pastas, etc., but the negative nutritional consequences are much lower than for milk-based infant formulae as these cereal foods are poor sources of lysine.

Quantification of Lysine Damage

Many biological and chemical methods have been developed to quantify available and reactive lysine respectively. Available lysine (= reactive lysine × digestibility) may be evaluated after enzymic hydrolysis, by microbiological tests and, in animals, by growth tests. Reactive lysine may be measured as ε-N-dinitrophenyl-lysine after derivatization with fluorodinitrobenzene, as homoarginine after derivatization with O-methylisourea, and as lysine after reduction of the Amadori compound with sodium borohydride. Reactive lysine can also be determined after conventional acid hydrolysis, by the furosine method. This method is based on the property of fructosyl-lysine to produce upon acid hydrolysis a new amino acid, i.e. furosine. The measurement of the furosine level allows quantification of the Amadori compound of lysine and calculation of the amount of reactive lysine.

The 'Advanced' Maillard Reaction

This stage of the reaction starts with the degradation of the sugar moiety of the Amadori compound involving dehydration, scission, oxidation and Strecker degradation, leading to the generation of new molecules (premelanoidins) contributing to aromas and flavours that vary in their characteristics according to the conditions employed. Some of these molecules are chemically more reactive than the initial sugar, e.g. α-dicarbonyls, reductones and aldehydes. They react not only with free amino groups still present in the food, but also with a

Toxicology of Nonenzymatic Browning

larger number of radical groups such as hydroxyl, amines, and other nitrogen containing molecules, vitamins and the side-chains of amino acids.

Polymerization of premelanoidins leads to the formation of the high molecular weight melanoidins, the reactions involved being responsible for the developments of pigments.

During the 'advanced' stage of the Maillard reaction, loss of lysine and of B vitamins in foods is accelerated. Other amino acids become less bioavailable because they are either chemically modified or a decrease in the total food nitrogen digestibility occurs. Lysine lost as new unavailable addition product(s) can be calculated by difference as 'lysine in advanced Maillard compound(s)' (Table 2). These addition products do not regenerate lysine on acid hydrolysis and their chemical structures are still unknown.

Indirect Effects

Associated with the presence of Maillard reaction products, a good example of an indirect negative nutritional effect of nonenzymatic browning is the reduction in protein digestibility. This is due to the inability of proteases and peptidases to hydrolyse the peptide bonds now containing modified amino acids. Feeding such a protein results in an increase in the amount of faecal nitrogen and a decrease in the bioavailability of the chemically unmodified amino acids. Another indirect effect is a modification of the metabolism (intestinal absorption, utilization and urinary excretion) of some minerals and trace elements (calcium, zinc, iron and copper). The increase in the urinary excretion of zinc, iron and copper in patients fed intravenously a sterilized aqueous solution of free amino acids and glucose, and the hyperzincuria observed in rats fed heated casein–glucose and casein–lactose mixtures, would be due to the chelating effect of Maillard reaction products. However, this increase in urinary zinc being a relatively minor route of excretion compared to faecal excretion, zinc retention and zinc status is not reduced in rats.

Physiological Effects

Many physiological changes in tissues of animals have been attributed to feeding Maillard reaction products. It has not always been easy, however, to distinguish between the changes that are directly due to the reduced nutritive value of the reacted protein and those that are probably induced by the Maillard components of the test protein in the diet. Furthermore, in many of these studies which corresponded to model systems, the reaction products tested were incorporated in the diets at such high levels that interpretation of observation has remained difficult.

Reduced growth rate and increased relative weight of liver, kidney and caecum have been noted in rats fed a severely reacted (brown), compared to an unreacted mixture, of egg protein and glucose. Parallel increases in values for blood glucose and urea nitrogen, and serum transaminases and alkaline phosphatase were also observed with the reacted mixture. The lower growth rate, attributable to the reduced nutritive value of the reacted egg protein may partly explain the above differences. Long-term rat feeding trials, designed to eliminate the influence of the nutritional factors through increased dietary protein level, improved protein quality and a lower, more realistic, level of incorporation of the reacted egg protein under test, showed less dramatic effects. Nevertheless, an apparent effect of the reacted brown Maillard compound was evident in the depressed growth rate, enlarged liver, spleen and caecum, lowered serum triglycerides, increased total iron and histopathologically observed fatty changes in the liver.

Activities of intestinal mucosal dissacharidases (lactase, sucrase and maltase) were also reduced in rats fed the reacted, brown egg protein, compared to those fed the unreacted material. Some improvement occurred on fortification of the diet with amino acids (apparently) destroyed during reaction, although a persistant decrease in the activity of these enzymes demonstrated a specific inhibitory effect of the Maillard compounds.

Diarrhoea is often observed in animals fed high levels of severely browned Maillard products. This is likely to be direct consequence of the increased amount of indigestible protein available for fermentation in the caecum, which is often found to be enlarged.

During the progress of the nonenzymatic browning reaction, additional glycosyl residues become fixed to specific milk proteins leading to an increase in their allergenicity. Using a skin reactivity test, a good correlation has been shown between the degree of browning and allergenic response of a modified bovine β-lactoglobulin. Whilst this may explain one of the mechanisms responsible for the enhancement of the allergenicity of a protein, it does not explain the 'how and why' of allergy to cow's milk protein.

Maillard reaction products of low molecular weight which are partially absorbed can affect the activity of detoxifying enzymes. Rats fed browned egg albumin exhibited increased hepatic benzo[a]pyrene hydroxylase activity and decreased colonic aminopyrine N-demethylase activity compared to animals fed nonbrowned egg albumin. This suggests that Maillard reaction products may modify the metabolism of endogenous substrates, exogenous drugs and other xenobiotics.

Dietary melanoidins appear to decrease plasma cholesterol in rats and to modify the composition of faecal, neutral steroids suggesting that melanoidins influence the intestinal metabolism of cholesterol.

Maillard reaction products also interact with the

microorganisms of the digestive tract. Thus they strongly inhibit the activity of glycosyl transferase of *Streptococcus mutans* which has an active role in the development of dental caries. This inhibition would hence reduce the adherence of this microorganism to the tooth surface. Also, in the gut, the microflora is able to regenerate the amino acids from their Amadori compound and oxidize the 'advanced' Maillard reaction products.

Toxicity

Studies of the toxicity of Maillard reaction products, both *in vitro* and *in vivo* are a recent development. This interest comes from the observation that Maillard reactions involving creatinine (a typical molecule of animal tissues) or protein pyrolysis represent a carcinogenic potential due to the formation of heterocyclic amines. In addition to these amines, there exist mutagenic products of the premelanoidin and melanoidin types resulting from heat-processed carbohydrate-rich foods such as bakery products, caramel, coffee and other milk and meat products.

Mutagenic/Carcinogenic Heterocyclic Amines

Using the short-term Ames' microbiological test, it has been possible to detect mutagenic activity in broiled fish and meat. A series of heterocyclic amines has been isolated from cooked foods and from protein and amino acid pyrolysates. Some of them, 2-amino-3-methylimidazo [4,5-*f*]quinoline (IQ), 2-amino-3,4-dimethylimidazo [4,5-*f*]quinoline (MeIQ), 2-amino-3-methylimidazo [4,5-*f*]quinoxaline (IQx), 2-amino-3,8-dimethyl-imidazo [4,5-*f*]quinoxaline (MeIQx), 2-amino-3,4,8-trimethyl-imidazo[4,5-*f*]quinoxaline (4,8-DiMeIQx) and 2-amino-1-methyl-6-phenylimidazo[4,5-*b*]pyridine (PhIP) possess an imidazole ring which is formed from creatinine. The remaining parts of the molecules (pyridines and pyrazines) are derived from Maillard reaction products formed by amino acids and sugars. Since creatinine is present only in animal protein sources, this class of substances is found only in these foods, albeit at low levels in the charred portions of broiled fish and the surface of grilled meat (PhIP 1 ppb; MeIQx 1 ppb) and in beef extracts (IQ 70 ppb; MeIQx 8–90 ppb).

The other heterocyclic amines detected in foods are pyrolysis products formed from tryptophan: 3-amino-1,4-dimethyl-5*H*-pyrido[4,5-*b*]indole (Trp-P-1), 3-amino-1-methyl-5*H*-pyrido[4,5-*b*]indole (Trp-P-2), from glutamic acid: 2-amino-6-methyldipyrido-[1,2-*a*:3',2'-*d*]imidazole (Glu-P-1), 2-aminodipyrido-[1,2-*a*:3',2'-*d*]imidazole (Glu-P-2), from phenylalanine: 2-amino-5-phenylpyridine (Phe-P-1), and from soya bean globulin: 2-amino-9*H*-pyrido[2,3-*b*]indole (AαC), 2-amino-3-methyl-9*H*-pyrido[2,3-*b*]indole (MeAαC). The

heterocyclic amines which are produced in very small amounts in foods have been found to be carcinogenic in rats and mice (Table 3). The major target organs are the small and large intestines, liver, lung and blood vessels.

Mutagenicity of Melanoidin Type Products

Heated mixtures of free amino acid or food proteins and sugars possess a weak mutagenic activity in the Ames test. This activity varies with the composition of the mixture and the conditions of the reaction. Generally, the mutagenic activity observed *in vitro* correlates quite well with the formation of brown pigments and with the presence of molecules with high antioxidant capacity.

The demonstration that carbonyl compounds can produce free radicals lends confirmation to the observation that the mutagenicity of the antioxidant fraction of the Maillard products is deactivated by catalases. This apparent contradiction suggests that, when applied at high concentration to *in vitro* tests, Maillard products can induce mutations due to an 'overpowering' of their pro-oxidant activity, a phenomenon already observed with other antioxidants, such as the antioxidant vitamins and phenolic compounds.

When considering model systems reflecting normal cooking conditions a relatively weak mutagenic activity was observed compared to that of heterocyclic amines. The typical mutagenic effects of this class of compounds reflect base pair, in contrast to frameshift mutations, as caused by heterocyclic amines. Furthermore, their mutagenic effect has been found to be effectively inactivated by the liver microsomal enzymes (S9 liver fraction), in contrast to heterocyclic amines which require S9 activation to mutagenic/carcinogenic species.

Examples of heated foods with such a weak mutagenic activity that is metabolically deactivated '*in vitro*' are some commercial caramel preparations (ammonia and sulphite/ammonia processes), hydroly ' plant proteins and roasted coffee. However, it has been confirmed in animal feeding studies that melanoidin containing foods such as roasted coffee and roasted cocoa are neither mutagenic nor carcinogenic. Moreover, tested *in vivo* under well controlled physiological conditions, Maillard reaction products with antioxidant activity are found to act as antimutagens and/or anticarcinogens.

Antioxidant and Antimutagenic Activity of Melanoidin Type Products

Many Maillard reaction products exhibit antioxidant properties which are utilized with success in different types of food. Such reaction products include premelanoidins which are rich in carbonyl compounds as well as melanoidins. The observed antioxidant property

Table 3. Mutagenic and carcinogenic effects of heterocyclic amines

Compound	Source	Mutagenicity Revertants (μg) TA 98	Carcinogenicity Species	Concentration (%)	Experimental period (weeks)	Target organs
Products formed from creatinine						
IQ	Broiled sardines	433 000	Rats	0·03	72	Liver, intestine, skin
			Mice	0·03	96	Liver, lung
MeIQ	Broiled sardines	661 000	Rats	0·03	40	Large intestine, mammary gland
			Mice	0·04	91	Liver, forestomach
MeIQx	Fried beef	145 000	Rats	0·04	61	Liver, skin
			Mice	0·06	84	Liver, lung
Pyrolysis products formed from tryptophan						
Trp-P-1	Tryptophan pyrolysate	39 000	Rats	0·02, 0·015	52	Liver
			Mice	0·02	89	Liver
Trp-P-2	Tryptophan pyrolysate	104 200	Mice	0·02	89	Liver
Pyrolysis products formed from glutamic acid						
Glu-P-1	Glutamic acid pyrolysate	49 000	Rats	0·05	67	Liver, small and large intestines
			Mice	0·05	68	Liver, blood vessels
Glu-P-2	Glutamic acid pyrolysate	1 900	Rats	0·05	104	Liver, small and large, intestines
			Mice	0·05	84	Liver, blood vessels

depends on the conditions of the reaction and on the amino acids. Thus, reaction mixtures containing histidine have been found to have the highest antioxidant activity. The mechanism itself of the antioxidant activity in food systems, involves both the reducing capacity of the carbonyl compounds in the premelanoidins and melanoidins, and the property of the melanoidin brown pigments to chelate pro-oxidant metals, copper and iron.

That Maillard reaction products possess antimutagenic and/or anticarcinogenic properties has been evidenced. Thus, such reaction products inhibit mutagenic activity of several food-borne heterocyclic amines and of aflatoxin B_1. Antimutagenic, and possible anticarcinogenic activities have been attributed to melanoidins and α-dicarbonyl compounds generated either during the aminocarbonyl or caramelization reactions. The scavenging of active oxygen by melanoidins, demonstrated by means of electron spin resonance, can explain their antimutagenic effects. The involvement of antioxidant reactions in the antimutagenicity of heat-reaction products suggests that these compounds might have anticarcinogenic properties which include inhibition of nitrosamine formation, scavenging of active oxygen involved in cancer initiation and promotion, and also change in the chemical structure of carcinogens during the browning process.

Nitrosamines of Amadori Compounds

Amadori compounds have been shown to be nitrosated to mutagenic N-nitroso derivatives. This has led to the postulation that such compounds, if present in human food or if formed in the stomach, will constitute a health hazard. However, heated foods rich in Maillard reaction products with antioxidant properties can both inhibit nitrosamine formation and reduce nitrosamine-induced carcinogenicity.

Bibliography

Eriksson C (ed.) (1981) The Maillard reaction in food. *Progress in Food and Nutritional Science* 5. Oxford: Pergamon Press.

Finot PA, Aeschbacher HU, Hurrell RF and Liardon R (eds) (1990) The Maillard reaction in food processing, human nutrition and physiology. *Advances in Life Sciences*. Basel: Birkhauser.

Friedman M (ed.) (1991) Nutritional and toxicological consequences of food processing. *Advances in Experimental Medicine and Biology* 289. New York: Plenum Press.

Lee TC, Pintauro SJ and Chichester CO (1982) Nutritional and toxicological effects of non-enzymic Maillard browning. *Diabetes* 31(Suppl. 3): 37–46.

P. A. Finot
Nestec, Nestlé Research Centre, Lausanne, Switzerland

BUCKWHEAT

Buckwheat is a crop commonly grown for its black or grey triangular seeds. It can also be grown as a green manure crop, a companion crop, a cover crop, a source of buckwheat honey, and as a pharmaceutical plant yielding rutin. Buckwheat belongs to the Polygonaceae family and is not a true cereal. Like cereals such as wheat, corn and rice, which belong to the grass family, the grain of buckwheat is a dry fruit.

Buckwheat is believed to have originated in central and northeastern Asia and was probably cultivated in China during the fifth and sixth centuries. It was introduced into Europe during the fourteenth and fifteenth centuries and into North America in the seventeenth century. World production of buckwheat peaked in the early nineteenth century, and has declined since then. During the past 10 years it has averaged about two million hectares, or about one million metric tons, with the USSR accounting for about 90% of the production. Other major producing countries are China, Japan, Poland, Canada, Brazil, the USA, South Africa and Australia.

Types and Cultivars

There are three known species of buckwheat: common buckwheat, *F. esculentum*; tartary buckwheat, *F. tataricum*; and perennial buckwheat, *F. cymosum*. Common buckwheat is also known as *F. saggitatum* and a form of tartary buckwheat may be called *F. kashmirianum*. The cytotaxonomy of buckwheat has not been thoroughly studied. It is generally believed, however, that perennial buckwheat, particularly the diploid type, is the ancestral form of both tartary and common buckwheat.

Tartary buckwheat is cultivated in the Himalaya region of India and China, in eastern Canada, and occasionally in mountain areas of the eastern USA. It is very frost resistant, and the seeds – and products made from them – are greenish in colour and somewhat bitter in taste. Used primarily as animal feed, or as a mixture of wheat and buckwheat flour, it may also be used as a source of rutin.

Common buckwheat is, by far, the most economically important species of buckwheat, accounting for over 90% of the world production. Many types, strains and cultivars of common buckwheat exist. There are late maturing and early maturing types, Japanese and European types, summer and autumn types. Within a given type there may be strains or varieties with tall or short plants, grey or black seeds, white or pink flowers.

Prior to 1950, producers of buckwheat planted unnamed strains of buckwheat harvested from their own fields or obtained from their neighbours or local stores. Named varieties developed through plant breeding were first released in the 1950s. Tokyo, the oldest of the named cultivars introduced into North America, was licensed by Agriculture Canada in 1955. Other cultivars licensed for production in Canada are Tempest, Mancan and Manor, all developed at the Agriculture Canada Research Station, Morden, Manitoba, since 1965. Mancan, which has large dark-brown seeds, is the Canadian cultivar preferred in the Japanese market because of its large seed, desirable flavour and colour, and high yield of groats in the milling process.

Cultivars licensed in the USA are Pennquad, released by the Pennsylvania Agricultural Experimental Station and the USDA (United States Department of Agriculture) in 1968, and Giant American, a Japanese-type cultivar apparently selected by a Minnesota farmer.

Cultivars developed in the USSR since the 1950s include Victoria, Galleya, Eneida, Podolyaka, Diadema, Aelita and Aestoria. Representative cultivars from other areas of the world include Pulawska, Emka and Hruszowska from Poland, Bednja 4n from Yugoslavia, and Botan-Soba, Shinano No. 1 and Kyushu-Akisoba from Japan.

Plant and Seed Morphology

Buckwheat is a broad-leaved, erect, herbaceous plant, which grows to a height of 0·70–1·5 m. It has a main stem and several branches, and reaches full maturity in less than 90 days. The stem is usually grooved, succulent, and hollow except for the nodes. Before maturity, the stems and branches are green to red in colour and after maturity they become brown. The plant has a shallow taproot, from which branched, lateral roots arise. Its root system is less extensive than that of the cereals and constitutes only 3–4% of the dry weight of the total plant.

Buckwheat has an indeterminate flowering habit. The flowers of common buckwheat are perfect but incomplete. They have no petals but the calyx is composed of five petal-like sepals that are usually white, but may also be pink or red. The flowers are arranged in dense clusters at the ends of branches or on short pedicels arising from the axils of the leaves. Common buckwheat has plants bearing one of two types of flowers. The pin-type flower has long styles, or female parts, and short stamens, or

Table 1. Proximate composition, on a dry weight basis (dwb), and selected mineral profile of three dehulled buckwheat cultivars

| | Cultivar | | |
Assay	Mancan (±SD)	Manor (±SD)	Tokyo (±SD)
Moisture (%)	16·2±0·9	10·1±0·2	10·9±0·1
Protein[a] (%)	14·2±0·6	14·6±0·3	11·9±0·4
Crude fibre (%)	1·57±0·30	1·21±0·03	1·57±0·10
Ash (%)	1·85±0·01	1·66±0·01	1·39±0·01
Lipids[b] (%)	2·6±0·3	2·2±0·3	2·1±0·2
Carbohydrates[c] (%)	79·8±1·6	80·3±0·8	83·0±1·1
K (%)	0·440±0·005	0·419±0·009	0·407±0·005
P (%)	0·359±0·018	0·347±0·003	0·262±0·016
Mg (%)	0·214±0·002	0·201±0·012	0·195±0·010
Ca (ppm)	180·5±7·4	180·5±10·6	220·5±6·5
Fe (ppm)	24·8±1·8	21·4±0·3	21·2±0·9
Zn (ppm)	23·4±0·4	22·0±1·6	22·8±1·1
Mn (ppm)	10·2±0·2	10·0±0·5	10·2±0·4
Cu (ppm)	4·6±0·3	3·7±0·1	4·3±0·2

[a] N×6·25;
[b] Soxhlet, petroleum ether for 8 h;
[c] by difference.
Data from Mazza G (1988) Lipid content and fatty acid composition of buckwheat seed. *Cereal Chemistry* 65: 122–126.

male parts, and the thrum-type has long styles and short pistils. The pistil consists of a one-celled superior ovary and a three-part style with knoblike stigmas and is surrounded by eight stamens. Nectar-secreting glands are located at the base of the ovary. The plants of common buckwheat are generally self-infertile, or self-fertilization is prevented by self-incompatibility. Seed production is usually dependent on cross-pollination between the pin and thrum flowers. Honey bees and leafcutter bees are effective pollinators. They increase seed set and seed yield.

The buckwheat kernel is a triangular, dry fruit (achene), 4–9 mm in length, consisting of a hull or pericarp, spermoderm, endosperm and embryo. Large seeds tend to be concave sided, and small seeds are usually convex sided. The hull may be glossy or gray, brown or black, and it may be solid or mottled. It may be either smooth or rough with lateral furrows. The hulls represent 17–26% (in tartary buckwheat 30–35%) of the kernel weight. Diploid varieties usually have less hull than tetraploids.

Structure of Kernel

Scanning electron microscopy of the buckwheat kernel has revealed that the hull, spermoderm, endosperm and embryo are each composed of several layers. For the hull, these are in order from the outside toward the inside: epicarp, fibre layers, parenchyma cells and endocarp. The spermoderm is composed of the outer epiderm, the spongy parenchyma and the inner epiderm. The endosperm is composed of an aleurone layer, 10–15 μm thick, and a subaleurone endosperm containing starch granules surrounded by a proteinaceous matrix. The embryo, with its two cotyledons, extends through the endosperm. The terminal parts of cotyledons are often parallel under the kernel surface.

Composition

Proximate composition and selected mineral profiles of Mancan, Manor and Tokyo buckwheat groats are shown in Table 1.

Carbohydrates

Starch is quantitatively the major component of buckwheat seed; the concentration varies with the method of extraction and between cultivars. In whole grain of common buckwheat, the starch content ranges from 59% to 70% of the dry matter. The chemical composition of starch isolated from buckwheat grains differs from the composition of cereal starches. The amylose content in buckwheat granules varies from 15% to 52% and its degree of polymerization varies from 12 to 45 glucose units. Buckwheat starch granules are irregular, 4–11 μm in size, with noticeable flat areas due to compact packing in the endosperm. The starch has a water binding capacity of 79–104%, a blue value of 0·35, a swelling power at 60°C of 2·35, a solubility at 60°C of 0·5%, an amylograph viscosity at 92°C of 640 BU (Brabender Units), an enzyme susceptibility (percentage of solubilized starch) of 2·63%, and an initial and final gelatinization temperature of 61·5°C and 76·0°C, respectively. *See* Starch, Structure, Properties and Determination

Buckwheat grains also contain 0·65–0·76% reducing sugars, 0·79–1·16% oligosaccharides and 0·1–0·2% nonstarchy polysaccharides. Among the low-molecular-weight sugars the major component is sucrose. There is a small amount of arabinose, xylose, glucose and probably the disaccharide melibiose. *See* Sucrose, Properties and Determination

Proteins

Protein content in buckwheat varies from 7% to 21%, depending on variety and environmental factors during growth. Most currently grown cultivars yield seeds with 11–15% protein. The major protein fractions are globulins which represent almost half of all proteins, and consist of 12 to 13 subunits with molecular weights between 17800 and 57000. Other known buckwheat protein fractions include albumins and prolamins. Older reports of gluten, or glutelin, being present in buckwheat seed have recently been discredited. The albumin fraction, with a molecular weight of 7000–8000, consists of at least 12 proteins. Prolamin has been fractioned into at least two peaks by gel filtration on Sephacryl S-200 and into three major and several minor components by SDS-PAGE (sodium dodecyl sulphate-polyacrylamide gel electrophoresis). *See* Protein, Chemistry

Buckwheat proteins are particularly rich in lysine. They contain less glutamic acid and proline, and more arginine, aspartic acid and tryptophan, than cereal proteins. Due to the high lysine content, buckwheat proteins have a higher biological value (BV) than the cereal proteins such as those of wheat, barley, rye and corn. Digestibility of buckwheat protein, however, is rather low and this is probably due to the high fibre content (17·8%) in buckwheat, which may be desirable in some parts of the world. Buckwheat fibre is free of phytic acid and is partially soluble. *See* Dietary Fibre, Properties and Sources

Lipids

Whole buckwheat seeds contain 1·5–3·7% total lipids. The highest concentration is in the embryo and the lowest in the hull, each containing 7–14% and 0·4–0·9%, respectively. Groats or dehulled seeds of Mancan, Tokyo and Manor buckwheat contain 2·1–2·6% total lipids (Table 1), of which 81–85% are neutral lipids, 8–11% phospholipids, and 3–5% glycolipids. The major fatty acids of buckwheat lipids are palmitic (16:0), oleic (18:1), linoleic (18:2), stearic (18:0), linolenic (18:3), arachidic (20:0), behenic (22:0), and lignoceric (24:0). Of these, the 16 and 18 carbon acids are commonly found in all cereals. The long-chain acids, arachidic, behenic and lignoceric, which represent, on average, 8% of the total acids in buckwheat, are only minor components or are not present in cereals. *See* Lipids, Classification; Phospholipids, Properties and Occurrence

Phenolic Compounds

The content of phenolics in hulls and groats of common buckwheat is 0·73% and 0·79%; that of tartary buckwheat is 1·87% and 1·52%, respectively. The three major classes of phenolics are flavonoids, phenolic acids and condensed tannins. Flavonoids are compounds that possess the same C_{15} (C_6–C_3–C_6) basic skeleton. The various classes differ in the oxidation level of the central pyran. Three of the numerous classes of flavonoids are found in buckwheat: flavonols, anthocyanins, and C-glycosyl-flavones. Rutin (quercetin 3-rutinoside), a well-known flavonol diglucoside used as a drug for treatment of vascular disorders caused by abnormally fragile or permeable capillaries, occurs in leaves, stems, flowers and fruit of buckwheat. Other reported flavonols are quercitin (quercitin 3-rhamnoside) and hyperin (quercetin 3-galactoside). At least three red pigments have been found in hypocotyls of buckwheat seedlings. One of these is cyanidin, the other two are presumed to be glycosides of cyanidin. C-Glycosylflavones present in buckwheat seedling cotyledons are vitexin, isovitexin, orientin and isoorientin. The phenolic acids of buckwheat seed are the hydroxybenzoic acids, syringic, p-hydroxy-benzoic, vanillic and p-coumaric acids. Also in buckwheat seed are soluble oligomeric condensed tannins, which, along with the phenolic acids, provide astringency and affect colour and nutritive value of buckwheat products. *See* Phenolic Compounds

Grading, Handling and Storage

Grading

In most countries, buckwheat grain is priced according to its physical condition in terms of size, soundness and general appearance. In Canada, buckwheat is marketed according to grades established under the Canada Grain Act. Grades are No. 1, No. 2 and No. 3 Canada, and

Table 2.   Primary grade determinants of buckwheat (Canada)

Grade	Minimum seed density (kg hl^{-1})	Degree of soundness	Maximum limits of foreign material (%)				
			Stones[a]	Ergot	*Sclerotinia*	Cereal grains	Total foreign material
No. 1	58·0	Well matured, cool and sweet	3	0·0	0·0	1·0%	1·0%
No. 2	55·0	Reasonably well matured, cool and sweet	3	0·05%	0·05%	2·5%	3·0%
No. 3	No minimum	May have a ground or grassy odour, but shall not be musty or sour	3	0·25%	0·25%	5·0%	5·0%

[a] Number of kernel size stones in 500 g.

Sample. Grade determinants are minimum test weight, degree of soundness and maximum limits of foreign material (Table 2). Grades No. 1 and 2 Canada must be free from objectionable odours; No. 3 Canada may have a ground or grassy odour, but shall not be musty or sour. Test weight, seed size and foreign material are determined on a dockage-free sample. Seed size is determined with a No. 8 slotted sieve (3·18 × 19·05 mm) and is added to and becomes part of the grade name, e.g. buckwheat, No. 1 Canada large. Foreign material refers to cereal grains (wheat, rye, barley, oats and triticale), weed seeds and other grains that are not readily removable by mechanical cleaners and may include peas, beans, corn and other domestic or wild weeds. Samples containing in excess of 5% are graded buckwheat, sample Canada (size) account admixture. Damaged seeds include frosted, mouldy, distinctly green or otherwise unsound and dehulled seeds.

In the USA, buckwheat is not marketed under official grades established by the USDA. However, some states (e.g. Minnesota) have Official Grain Standards that specify the use of Grades 1, 2, 3 and Sample. The grade determinants are similar to those of the Canadian grading system. The Soviet standards for food buckwheat are as follows: moisture, ≤14·5%; extraneous matter, ≤3% (including 0·2% mineral admixture of which 0·1% may be stones); pernicious admixtures, ≤0·2%; and spoiled grain, ≤0·5%. The Japanese Buckwheat Millers Association prefers buckwheat which has large and uniform seeds with black hulls and greenish groats.

Handling

The method of handling buckwheat varies among production areas. In most cases, however, losses and quality changes of the grain occur at various post-harvest stages. During harvest, shattering and losses due to germination, animals such as birds and rodents, and infection by moulds occur in all countries. Threshing is done with combines or by beating the dried plants against stones or wooden bars, or by trampling the plants under bullock feet, carts or tractor wheels. Transportation of grain from the field to the market results in losses and quality deterioration. Losses during transportation are mainly due to spillage. However, exposure of the grain to rain or frost during transit leads to spoilage due to infection by microorganisms. *See* Cereals, Handling of Grain for Storage

Storage

Like other grain crops, buckwheat is stored to ensure an even supply through time, to preserve the surplus grain for sale to deficit areas, and to be used as seed in the next planting season. Storage of the seeds may be at the farm, trader, market, government, retail or consumer levels. Storage containers range from sacks to straw huts and bulk storage bins. In developing countries, traditional storage methods include granaries of gunny, cotton or jute bags, and reed, bamboo or wood structures that are plastered with mud and cow dung. In North America, storage structures include metal, concrete or wooden bins at the farm level, elevators and annex at centralized receiving, storage and shipping points, and concrete silos at grain terminals. Bagged buckwheat is highly susceptible to attack by insects and rodents. Bulk storage in bins, elevators and silos is recommended. *See* Cereals, Bulk Storage of Grain

A moisture content of 16% or less is required for safe storage of buckwheat. If the seed requires drying, the maximum temperature of the drying air should not exceed 43°C. This temperature limit applies to seed for both seeding and processing. During storage at ambient temperature and relative humidity, the colour of the aleurone layer changes from a desirable light green to the undesirable reddish brown. This undesirable change can be reduced by storing the seed at a lower temperature and at a relative humidity below 45%. *See* Storage Stability, Parameters Affecting Storage Stability

Primary Processing

Primary processing of buckwheat includes cleaning, dehulling and milling. The aim of seed cleaning is to remove other plant parts, soil, stones, weed seeds, chaff, dust, seeds of other crops, metallic particles and small and immature buckwheat seeds. The extent and sophistication of the cleaning equipment depends largely on the size of the operation and the legal requirements for the finished product(s). Milling of buckwheat seed can be carried out by almost any equipment capable of milling cereal grains. Hammer mills, stone mills, pin mills, disk mills and roller mills have been used to mill buckwheat. Of these, stone mills and roller mills are used most extensively today.

The milling process may be of two types. In the first and most common type, the whole seeds are first dehulled and then milled. In the second type, the seeds are milled and then screened to remove the hulls. When dehulling and milling are separate operations, the seeds are segregated according to size and may be steamed and dried prior to dehulling. Dehulling is carried out by impact or abrasion against emery stones or steel, followed by air or screen separation of groats and hulls. A widely used buckwheat dehuller is built on the principle of stone-milling with emery stones set to crack the hull without breaking the groat. The effectiveness of this type of dehuller depends on the clearance between the seed cracking surfaces, and for any seed size there is an optimum setting. The ease of dehulling and percentage recovery of undamaged groats depends on variety and moisture content. From the dehuller, the groats go over sieves of different mesh for sizing into whole groats and two or more sizes of broken groats. Flour is produced by passing the groats through stone and/or roller grinders. *See* Flour, Roller Milling Operations

When buckwheat seed is to be processed only into flour, and production of groats is not a requirement, the seeds are ground on break rolls or stone mills and then screened to separate the coarse flour from the hulls. The coarse flour is further reduced by a series of size reduction rolls, each grinding operation followed by a sifting, in order to fractionate the mixture of particles according to their size. The flour yield ranges from 50% to 75% depending on the size, shape and condition of the seeds, and efficiency of the dehulling and milling operations.

End Products

Buckwheat flour is generally dark in colour due to the presence of hull fragments. In North America it is used primarily for making buckwheat pancakes, and is commonly marketed in the form of prepared mixes. These mixes generally contain buckwheat flour mixed with wheat, corn, rice, oat or soybean flours and a leavening agent. Buckwheat is also used with vegetables and spices in kasha and soup mixes, and with wheat, corn or rice in ready-to-eat breakfast products, porridge, bread and pasta products.

In Japan, buckwheat flour is used primarily for making *soba* or *sobakiri* (buckwheat noodles) and *Teuchi Soba* (hand-made buckwheat noodles). These products are prepared at *soba* shops or at home from a mixture of buckwheat and wheat flours. The wheat flour is used because of its binding properties and availability. *Soba* is made by hand or mechanically. In both methods, buckwheat and wheat flours are mixed with each other and then with water to form a stiff dough which is kneaded, rolled into a thin sheet (1·4 mm) with a rolling pin or by passing it between sheeting rolls and cut into long strips. The product may be cooked immediately, sold fresh, or dried. *See* Wheat

In Europe, most buckwheat is milled into groats, which are used in porridge, cabbage rolls or meat products (especially hamburger), or consumed with fresh or sour milk. Buckwheat groats with cottage cheese, sugar, peppermint and eggs is used as stuffing in a variety of dumplings. Buckwheat flour is used with wheat or rye flour and yeast to make fried speciality products such as bread, biscuits and other confectionaries. An extruded, ready-to-eat corn-buckwheat breakfast product of high nutritional value is being produced and marketed in western Europe. This product contains over 14% protein and 8% soluble fibre. Similar products have also been developed in Poland and the USSR.

In most countries, the quality of buckwheat end products is controlled by law. According to Canadian Government Specifications, buckwheat flour must have ≤1·5% ash, ≥1·1% protein nitrogen on a 14% moisture, and contain ≤12% moisture when delivered. Class B Pancake Mix should contain more than 40% and less than 50% buckwheat flour, with admixtures of 50% wheat, corn, rice or soya bean flour.

Bibliography

Campbell CG and Gubbels GH (1986) *Growing Buckwheat.* Agriculture Canada Research Branch, Technical Bulletin 1986–7E, 8 pp.
DeJong H (1972) Buckwheat. *Field Crops Abstracts* 25: 389–396.
Institute of Soil Science and Plant Cultivation (eds) (1986) *Buckwheat Research 1986*, Parts I, II and III. Pulawy, Poland: Laboratory of Science Publisher.
Kreft I, Javornik B and Dolisek B (eds) (1980) *Buckwheat*

genetics, plant breeding and utilization. Ljubljana, Yugoslavia: VTOZD za agronomijo Biotech. facultate.

Marshall HG and Pomeranz Y (1982) Buckwheat: description, breeding, production and utilization. In: Pomeranz Y (ed) *Cereals '78: Better Nutrition for the Worlds Millions*, pp 201–217. St. Paul, Minnesota: American Association of Cereal Chemists.

Nagatoma T and Adachi T (ed) (1983) *Buckwheat Research 1983*. Miyazaki, Japan: Kuroda-toshado Printing Co.

G. Mazza
Agriculture Canada Research Station, Morden, Canada

BUFFALO

Contents

Meat

The world population of buffaloes has been estimated as over 140 million head (FAO, 1988). Of these, 97% are found in Asia and the Pacific region, with India (75 million), China (21 million), Pakistan (14 million) and Thailand (6 million) producing most of the animals. About 98% of the buffaloes in the region are raised by small farmers owning not more than 2 ha of land and not more than five buffaloes. Historical evidence indicates that buffaloes (*Bubalus bubalis*) originated from Indo-Gangetic plains, thrived in Asia and acted as a symbol of life, religion and endurance. It has been suggested that water buffaloes were in the service of humans as early as 2500–2100 BC. The earliest record of buffaloes was found on a steatie-type seal discovered at Mohenjodaro and now at Lahore Museum (Pakistan). Another seal, depicting Lord Shiva, is in the New Delhi Museum. Buffaloes have been classified into two distinct classes: swamp buffaloes and river buffaloes.

Buffalo raising is mainly supportive to crop farming, especially rice cultivation. Swamp buffaloes, which are found in China, Thailand, the Philippines, Indonesia, Vietnam, Burma (Myamar) Laos, Sri Lanka, Kampuchea and Malaysia, are mainly used as draft animals for various farm operations. Very few swamp buffaloes are reared for milk since they only produce 1·0–1·5 litres of milk per day. In contrast, the riverine breeds of the Indian subcontinent are mainly raised for milk production since they yield 6–7 litres of milk daily.

The awareness of the potential of water buffaloes for meat has increased in recent years throughout the world due to the high content of lean meat. Buffalo meat is 25% higher in protein than beef and 50% lower in cholesterol. Most buffalo meat was, and still is, derived from old animals slaughtered at the end of their productive life. As a result, much of the buffalo meat sold is of poor quality, but, when buffaloes are properly reared and fed, their meat is tender and palatable. Instead of an every-day staple, however, today's buffalo meat comes packaged with a whole new image, namely that of a gourmet health food and a nostalgic 'slice' of the past. It is available in various North American towns and cities. *See* Meat, Dietary Importance

Nutrition

Buffaloes are mostly located in countries where land, cultivated forage crops and pastures are limited. Therefore, the animals are mainly raised on crop residues, sometimes supplemented with green fodder or by-products, available from the processing of cereal, grains, oil seeds, fruits and vegetables. Buffaloes ae known to be good converters of poor-quality roughage into milk and meat. They are reported to have a 5% higher digestibility of crude fibre than high-yielding cows and a 4–5% higher efficiency of utilization of metabolic energy for milk production. Buffaloes can gain as much as 1 kg in weight per day on good-quality roughage and concentrates.

The investigations carried out so far have amply confirmed that buffaloes digest feed more efficiently than cattle, particularly when feeds are fibrous and high in lignin and cellulose. The buffalo rumen is larger than that of cattle and exhibits slower movements and rate of digesta flow, resulting in a lower turnover rate and a longer retention time of feed compared to cattle. Thus, the feed consumed appears to be exposed for a longer period to microbial degradation. Microbial composition in the rumen of buffaloes always differs with the feeding regimen but the bacterial and protozoal count remains higher compared to cattle. The highest number

Table 1.   World distribution of cattle and buffaloes with slaughter rate and meat production in some Asian countries

Country	Cattle				Buffalo			
	Population (1000 head)	Slaughtered (1000 head)	Slaughter rate in % of population	Annual meat production (1000 tonnes)	Population (1000 head)	Slaughtered (1000 head)	Slaughter rate in % of population	Annual meat production (1000 tonnes)
World	1 268 934	229 938	18·1	46 072	129 283	7461	5·8	1006
Asia	368 738	23 503	6·4	2794	125 413	6435	5·1	857
Bangladesh	36 500	2300	6·3	129	1800	21	1·2	2
Burma	9550	660	6·9	79	2100	118	5·6	20
China	51 375	3219	6·3	283	19 547	1125	5·8	125
India	182 410	1115	0·6	89	64 500	980	1·5	135
Indonesia	6859	863	12·6	135	2424	221	9·1	35
Iran	8350	1870	22·4	108	230	66	28·7	10
Iraq	1500	320	21·3	35	145	20	13·8	3
Kampuchea	1500	135	9·0	16	685	53	7·7	8
Laos	615	78	12·7	9	1200	125	10·4	27
Malaysia	570	105	18·4	12	260	37	14·2	7
Nepal	7050	59	0·8	5	4500	175	3·9	23
Pakistan	16 549	1750	10·6	235	13 070	2450	18·7	245
Philippines	1900	541	28·5	72	2980	289	9·7	46
Sri Lanka	1750	200	11·4	13	900	—	—	—
Thailand	4800	762	15·4	152	6250	288	4·6	73
Vietnam	2150	512	23·8	64	2800	350	12·5	75

Source: data calculated from FAO (1985).

of ciliates, both entodiniomorphs and holotrichs, are observed on rations of high digestibility. Ruminal concentrations of ammonia nitrogen and volatile fatty acids, being higher in the buffalo, are indicative of higher proteolytic and cellulolytic activity in the rumen.

The rate of growth of buffalo calves responds differently to various feed combinations as well as management conditions. Dry matter consumption is least affected, even when feeds are fibrous and of low quality. On normal rations, dry matter intake varies from 2·5 to 3·0% of body weight. The consumption may increase on shifting the animal from a low to an optimum level of energy in the diet. A gain of 502 g per day in buffalo calves over a period of 18 months has been recorded. However, a much higher daily gain of over 1 kg in buffalo calves on rations consisting of 1·25 kg of concentrate and 1 kg of hay per 100 kg of body weight fed along with *ad lib* green fodder has also been reported. In other studies, a growth rate of 416 g per day in male Murrah calves fed on an *ad lib* urea–molasses liquid diet (2·5% urea in molasses) along with restricted intake of green fodder and a small quantity of fish meal has been observed. On normal and 40% higher digestible crude protein (DCP) levels, the observed body weight of female Murrah calves was 324 kg on normal and 342 kg when fed 40% higher DCP at 2 years of age. The time required for attaining slaughter weight is

significantly lower (301–314 days) in high-energy groups than in low-energy groups (315–418 days); daily gain was high (607 g) in high-protein and high-energy groups.

The conversion efficiency of metabolizable energy and DCP towards deposition is thought to be higher in younger (12 months) compared to older (19 months) groups of Murrah male buffalo calves.

Buffaloes are intolerant of direct sun and are readily susceptible to heat stress. Buffaloes possess certain characteristic physiological features associated with this intolerance such as lack of hair cover, few sweat glands, black pigmentation of skin, relatively low body temperature, wallowing behaviour and higher efficiency in oxygenation of the blood.

Slaughtering and Processing

The buffalo is an important source of meat in almost all Asian countries. The average extraction rate in cattle (6·4%) and buffaloes (5·1%) is almost the same in Asia (Table 1). The Asian figure comes to 5·1% despite the heavier hide and head of the buffalo.

The meat is highly perishable and heterogeneous and demands accurate grading, rapid and hygienic processing, and uncompromising quality control. There are some slaughterhouses which are exclusively designed for

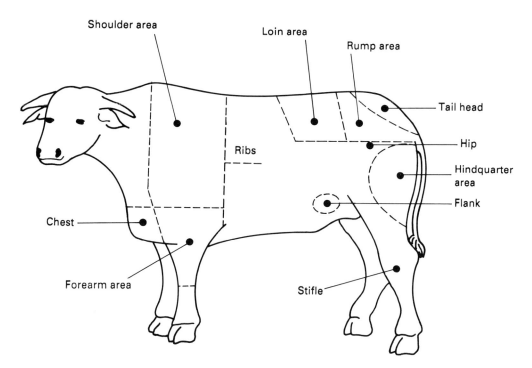

Fig. 1   Diagram showing the different regions of the buffalo body.

the slaughter of buffaloes. The *halal* method is generally followed in all abattoirs. In India, line slaughter is practiced; but in many places floor slaughtering is also prevalent. The animal is stunned by a suitable and appropriate device (electric current, carbon dioxide, captive bolt pistol, sledgehammer, etc.), rendering the animal unconscious and insensitive to pain. Immediately after stunning the blood pressure of the animal rises and its throat is cut with a sharp knife to facilitate total bleeding. Methods of slaughter also depend upon religious traditions and customs followed by different communities. Muslims follow the *Halal* method of slaughter where a prayer is said in the name of *Allah* at the time as the volar portion of the neck is cut. The Jewish community follows its own method called *Schechita*, according to which a Jewish priest slaughters the animals. The *jhatka* method is followed by certain Hindu communities. In this method the head of the animal is severed within a fraction of a second. With this last method, bleeding is not complete and this affects the keeping quality and shelf life of the meat. *See* Meat, Slaughter

After bleeding is complete, the hind legs are skinned to separate the tendons for hanging the carcass with the gambrells on a skid. The head and trotters are then removed, the carcass is flayed, the skin separated and the carcass thoroughly washed (Figs 1 and 2). In the dressing operation the carcass is opened and the abdominal organs are carefully removed without contaminating the carcass meat. Similarly, organs from the thoracic cavity are removed. Carcass and organs are

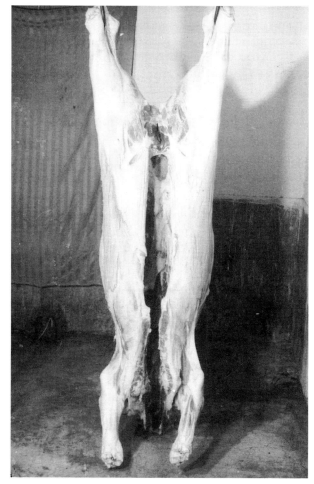

Fig. 2   Buffalo carcass following evisceration.

Meat

Table 2. Composition of fresh and cooked buffalo meat sausages

	Composition (%)	
	Fresh	Cooked
Moisture	61·85	55·95
Protein	13·05	14·97
Fat	20·51	23·72
Ash	2·62	1·83
Cooking loss		15·48

From Sharma N *et al.* (1982) *Indian Food Packer* 36: 50–52.

then thoroughly washed and post-mortem inspection is carried out by qualified staff. To prevent spoilage and to retain the original quality of the meat, the carcass is stored under refrigeration at a temperature ranging from 0 to −15°C. It is subjected to still lower temperature (−35°C or below) if it is to be frozen for carriage over longer distances. *See* Meat, Preservation

Important points to be observed during dressing of the carcass are:

(1) the whole carcass should be eviscerated within 1 h after bleeding;
(2) flaying, skinning and dressing should not be carried out on the floor;
(3) inflation of carcasses and lungs should be forbidden;
(4) when spraying of the carcass is practised, the pressure must not be such as to damage the meat or obliterate possible evidence of disease.

Buffalo Meat Products

Buffalo meat is used as a food item in a similar way to other meats such as beef (e.g. grilling, frying, etc.). In South Asia (Pacific region) meat curry is also prepared. Buffalo meat has very good emulsification and binding properties and is ideal for sausage making (Table 2). Buffalo meat has all the properties needed to prepare direct meat products such as *pastarma* and *gabrovi* in Bulgaria, and *biltong* in Nepal and Brazil. *See* Meat, Sausages and Comminuted Products

Common Asian uses of buffalo meat are described below.

Kababs. Also called seekh kababs, kababs are ready to eat meat products made from buffalo, sheep or goat meat. Minced buffalo meat, containing lean meat, fat, salt, spices, condiments, green curries, herbs, etc., in appropriate proportions, is moulded into hollow cylindrical structures around skewers; it is then grilled and smoked for 2–3 min.

Koftas and Tikkis. Carcass and/or offal meats are made into keema by chopping, salting and mincing. Keema and Bengal gram flour are then mixed in a ratio of 4:1. The material is cooked and ground into a paste, after which it is mixed with spices and green curries, and rolled into balls 3–4 cm in diameter or flattened to form round dishes for production in koftas or tikkis, respectively. These products are pan fried in oil and served hot. Shammi kabab is another name for tikki.

Bheja. The processed brain is called bheja. It is cooked in water for 5–8 min, after which the outer membrane is peeled off. It is then cut into small pieces and pan fried in oil with grated onion, chopped coriander leaves, salt and spice mixture to taste.

Curries. Carcass meat, offal meat (which are used as chunks or keema) and organ meat (e.g. liver, kidney, heart, tongue, ears, udder, etc.) can be made into curries either individually or in combination. The name of the curry will signify the kind of meat.

Corned Meat. The corning process consists of mixing cooked diced meat, minced raw meat, salt and other ingredients and canning.

Sausage. Sausages prepared from buffalo meat are highly acceptable due to their texture, juiciness, colour and flavour (Table 2).

Meat Quality

Buffaloes are lean animals. Although a layer of subcutaneous fat covers the carcass, it is usually thinner than that of comparably fed cattle. In general, the buffalo carcass has rounder ribs, a higher proportion of muscle and a lower proportion of bone and fat than beef. Buffalo meat is higher in protein content than the meat of other species. The amino acid composition, especially of critical amino acids of skeletal muscles, is higher than that of the ox. Philippine buffalo beef (carabeef) has more isoleucine, leucine, lysine, phenylalanine, tyrosine, threonine, valine and histidine but less tryptophan, cystine and methionine than beef. Except for cystine, the daily allowance recommended by the Food and Agriculture Organization can easily be met by carabeef as the principal source of protein. About 100 g of carabeef lean meat per head per day is enough to meet all the amino acids (except cystine) required for the body. Buffalo meat has about 44% more lysine than egg protein. Buffalo meat and beef are in many ways quite similar, e.g. muscle pH (5·4), shrinkage on chilling (2%), moisture (76·6%), protein (19%), and ash (1%). Buffalo fat, however, is always white and buffalo meat is darker in colour than beef because of more pigmentation and less intramuscular fat (2–3%), which leads to 'marbling', compared with beef (3–4% intramuscular fat). Based on

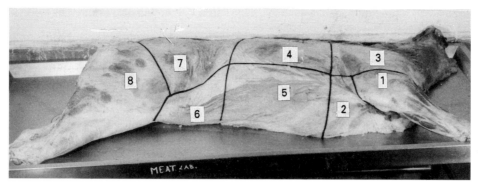

Fig. 3 Demarcations of various wholesale cuts: 1, shank; 2, brisket; 3, chuck; 4, rib; 5, plate; 6, flank; 7, loin; 8, round.

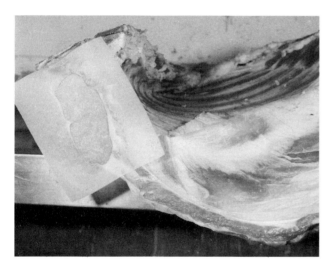

Fig. 4 Tracing of the eye muscle at the 12th rib for quality assessment.

Table 3. Carcass components of buffaloes slaughtered at different body weights

Slaughter body weight (kg)	Carcass weight (kg)	Dressing (%)	Meat (%)	Fat (%)	Bone (%)
161	83	51·4	66·8	9·7	23·5
258	139	53·9	67·5	12·7	19·8
356	193	62·8	66·7	12·9	19·7
446	239	53·6	69·0	13·1	17·9
260	141	55·5	67·0	12·0	18·0
300	151	51·0	70·0	6·0	19·0
480	277	59·7	66·0	17·0	14·0

visual colour scores for the eye muscle (longissimus dorsi) of market slaughtered buffaloes in India, the meat was classified into 35% light red, 47% red and 18% dark red. *See* Protein, Quality

The carcass is cut into eight major primal cuts (Fig. 3). For evaluating carcass quality, the eye muscle area at the 12th rib (Fig. 4) is one of the most important parameters. Buffalo meat, especially from older animals, is darker in colour than beef. The myoglobin content of the eye muscle from 3-year-old buffalo calves was noted to be 1·45%, compared to 0·46% for steers of the same age. The muscle fibre diameter of buffalo meat was found to be lower than that of beef up to 3 years of age. The stroma protein content was comparable and tenderness was more or less equal to beef. The hydroxyproline content of the eye muscle was 0·74% as compared to 0·65% in steers. However, connective tissue toughness increases in buffaloes at 4–5 years of age and, therefore, buffalo meat requires prolonged cooking at that age. The phosphorus, vitamin A and niacin contents were higher in beef than in carabeef.

The quality of meat depends upon both its physical structure and chemical characteristics, which further results in maximum desirability of appearance and cutability. Characteristics such as cooking loss, shear force, water-holding capacity, juiciness and tenderness of meat directly govern meat quality. Tenderness is not affected by dietary levels of protein but meat at early age is more tender. Some of the data regarding carcass components of buffaloes slaughtered at different body weights and ages are given in Tables 3 and 4. *See* Meat, Structure

Australian workers have observed a high proportion of muscle and a low proportion of fat in carcasses of buffalo calves ranging from 14 to 48 months in age.

A positive relationship has been observed between protein content and the amount of expressible fluid, since proteins are the principal water-binding constituents for meat. The higher the moisture:protein ratio the lower is the ability of muscles to retain available water. The approximate compositions of some commercial cuts and muscle tissues are given in Tables 5, 6 and 7.

Waste Utilization

The wastes (excluding meat, bone fat and hide) amount to 25% of the live weight. The list of various wastes

Meat

Table 4.   Meat quality of Murrah buffalo calves at different ages

	Age	
	12 months	19 months
Shearforce (kg cm^{-2})	3·5	4·2
Cooking loss (%)	34·7	34·4
Water-holding capacity (%)	21·7	21·4
Tenderness score	7·5	6·7
Juiciness score	6·4	6·5
Flavour score	6·5	6·7

From Sharma DD (1988).

Table 5.   Compositions of some commercial cuts of buffalo carcass

Cut	Fat (%)	Protein (%)	Ash (%)
Neck	2·72	18·22	0·98
Shoulder	2·45	18·89	1·00
Shank	2·73	19·90	0·94
Rib	1·87	19·99	0·92
Loin	2·78	19·66	1·00
Leg	2·77	19·74	1·00

From Sharma N et al. (1980).

Table 6.   Characteristics of muscle tissue

Character	Bulgarian buffalo	Murrah buffalo	Murrah × Bulgarian buffalo
Fat (%)	1·36	0·64	1·04
Myoglobin (%)	1·53	1·40	1·37
Oxyproline (%)	0·78	0·74	0·70
Muscle fibre diameter (μm)	58·83	57·14	56·67

From Ognjanovic A et al. (1970).

obtained from the buffalo meat industry and their uses are given in Table 8.

Blood

Blood has the potential for use as a human food of high protein content (80% on a dry matter basis) with excellent amino acid balance and nutritive value. The average yield of blood from buffaloes and cattle is about

Table 7.   Amino acid content in eye muscle

Amino acid	Bulgarian buffalo	Murrah buffalo	Murrah × Bulgarian buffalo
Lysine	1·800	2·162	1·722
Histidine	0·767	0·868	0·835
Arginine	1·218	1·435	1·422
Aspartic acid	2·555	2·518	2·625
Threonine	1·172	1·186	1·231
Serine	0·874	0·899	0·926
Glutamic acid	3·965	4·311	4·154
Proline	1·185	0·914	0·928
Glycine	1·066	1·053	1·051
Alanine	1·416	1·571	1·488
Cystine	0·363	0·523	0·544
Valine	1·318	1·370	1·355
Methionine	0·646	0·660	0·659
Isoleucine	1·227	1·159	1·233
Leucine	1·878	1·825	1·952
Tyrosine	0·816	0·871	0·894
Phenylalanine	0·904	0·955	0·960

Ognjanovic A et al. (1970).

Table 8.   Important biochemicals and pharmaceuticals obtained from wastes from the buffalo meat industry

By-products	Biochemical/pharmaceutical
Blood	Plasma, serum albumin, haematinics, blood-meal, etc.
Fibrin	Peptone, fibrin foam, fibrin powder, bioplast, etc.
Pancreas	Insulin, glucagon, pancreatin, trypsin and chymotrypsin
Lungs and intestinal mucosa	Heparin
Liver	Liver extract
Thyroid	Thyroxine
Pituitary	
Anterior	Follicle-stimulating hormone (FSH), luteinizing hormone (LH), adrenocorticotrophic hormone (ACTH), prolactin
Posterior	Oxytocin, vasopressin
Adrenals	Adrenaline
Testis	Hyaluronidase
Gall bladder	Bile, bile salts
Heart	Cardiolipins, cytochrome c
Spinal cord, brain	Cholesterol, lecithin
Bones	Gelatin, bone morphogenetic protein (BMP)
Hooves	Neats foot oil

Meat

Table 9. Yields of insulin obtained from the pancreas for different species

Species	Yield (mg kg^{-1})
Buffalo	326[a]
Sheep	140[b]
Goat	15·4[b]
Sheep:cattle (80:20)	20[a]
Sheep:cattle (65:35)	32·5[a]

[a] As crystalline insulin.
[b] As insulin hydrochloride.

10–12 kg per carcass. Appropriate methods of collection and preservation are very important factors for its further processing into biochemicals and pharmaceuticals.

Collection and Preservation

(1) For pharmaceutical use. Blood is collected with a trocar knife and cannula in a close container under strict hygienic conditions and chilled immediately. For plasma, anticoagulants such as sodium citrate and ethylenediaminetetra-acetic acid are added.
(2) For animal feed. Blood is collected in clean receptacles and treated with lime.
(3) For fertilizer. Spilt, soiled blood is collected in drums and preserved by adding 2% formalin or 2% lysol.

Glandular By-products

Glands are an important source of pharmaceuticals and biochemicals. Cardinal principles for harvesting glandular material for pharmaceutical use are outlined below:

(1) Glands must be collected from healthy animals within 10–20 min of slaughter.
(2) Glands are trimmed of connective tissues, fat and blood vessels, chilled immediately and frozen in solid carbon dioxide or freezing mixture (ice and sodium chloride).
(3) Glands are packed in thermocol boxes, labelled correctly and transported under chilled conditions.

Some of the commercially important products obtained from glands are described below.

Insulin

β Cells present in the pancreas contain insulin. The yields of insulin from the pancreas of different species are given in Table 9.

Heparin

This is a physiological anticoagulant used to prevent blood clotting during transfusion of blood and post-operative thrombi.

Liver Extract

Both aqueous and proteolysed liver extracts are used in the treatment of macrocytic anaemia. The appropriate antianaemia potency is expressed in terms of vitamin B_{12} content, and there should be at least 0·1 mg of vitamin B_{12} per millilitre of the extract. *See* Meat, Extracts

Bile Salts

From 100 kg of liquid bile, 18–19 kg of syrup with 20% moisture or 15 kg of powder containing 6% moisture can be obtained.

Thyroxine

The desiccated thyroid gland contains 0·17–0·23% iodine. Desiccated thyroid gland is used to treat myxoedema, cretinism, menstrual disturbances, sterility, abortions, psoriasis (a noncontagious skin disease marked by red scaly patches) of the skin and skin infections. A method for extraction of thyroxine from desiccated glands with a yield of 0·125% has been reported.

Pituitary Gland Hormones

The pituitary gland is a small bean-shaped, hazelnut-sized organ stituated in a bony cavity at the base of the brain. It weighs about 1–1·5 g in buffaloes. The anterior lobe of the pituitary gland produces FSH, LH growth hormone, thyroxine and ACTH, whereas the posterior lobe produces the hormones oxytocin and vasopressin.

Other By-products

Pepsin

About 200 g of lining obtained from each buffalo stomach will ultimately yield 7–8 g of crystalline pepsin. Pepsin is used for digestive disturbances and has some industrial use, mainly in breweries.

Cytochrome C

This is extracted from the heart, and has a diagnostic value in medicine and biochemical research.

Hyaluronidase

This enzyme is extracted commercially from ram orchids or bull testes. Hyaluronidase is also known as 'spreading factor', as it reduces viscosity by destroying tissue hyaluric acid. This permits greater spreading of material in the tissue. Hence, it is used as a diffusing agent in the administration of drugs and anaesthetics.

Cholesterol

The spinal cord and brain are rich sources of cholesterol. The buffalo spinal cord contains more cholesterol (7%) than sheep and goat spinal cord (5%). Cholesterol is used in the cosmetic industry and for the synthesis of testosterone.

Gelatin

Bones can be used for the manufacture of gelatin and bone morphogenetic protein (BMP), which are products of great commercial importance. Bones are also widely used for the manufacture of glue or as fertilizer. In the pharmaceutical industry, gelatin is used in making capsules, as a binder in tablets and as a plasma extender in blood transfusion. BMP is used for bone healing.

Hide

'Green' hides are transported to hide-processing premises where they are trimmed of fat, flesh and unwanted hide projection at the ears, anus, vulva and tail regions. They are preserved by salting or sun drying. As a rule, heavy hides are salted and light ones sun dried. Salt is applied on the flesh side at regular intervals and stocked on wooden planks. Sun drying is effected by pegging them to bamboo frames of 3×2 m in size and placing them obliquely under the shade with the hair side facing the sun. Salted and dried hides can be stored for up to 6 months before being sent to tanneries.

Casings

Casings are the submucosal coats of gastrointestinal tracts used as natural containers for meat products. Four varieties of casings are prepared from buffaloes: (1) weasands, (2) dry casings, (3) fat end and (4) bladders from the oesophagus, small intestine, rectal end of the gut and urinary bladder, respectively. The technique of processing includes steps such as flushing out the contents, turning (absent in bladders), fermenting and slimming (not applicable in weasands), inflating with air, sun drying, pressing, measuring and storage.

Tallow

Rendered animal fat is called tallow. It is mainly used for soap manufacture. However, the reprocessed and bleached tallow is sometimes used in confectionery.

Bones

The bones are obtained from a number of sources, such as rendered long bones from tallow-manufacturing units, scapula, ribs, skull, etc. from retaining stalls, and desert bones from animals which have died naturally. The bones are stored in the open and are exposed to heat, cold, rain and wind. Later, the bones are despatched to bone-crushing factories for further processing.

Production and Processing of Buffalo Meat for Export

Frozen buffalo meat is relatively well received due to its leanness, its guaranteed *halal* status, freedom from additives, customer-oriented packaging and a lower unit price. Rapid freezing technology using contact plate freezers is an advance over other practices prevalent in Australia and South America. *See* Freezing, Blast and Plate Freezing

The slaughterhouses are usually located in relatively disease-free areas. The slaughter operations are carried out separately under strict veterinary supervision. The carcasses, in the form of quarters, are packed neatly in high-density polythene bags and transported under chilled conditions to export processing units. The export material has to comply with the specifications of the importing countries in relation to meat handling/product packaging, labelling and prompt delivery and the operational standards have to be in line with current international code. Plant sanitation and hygiene must be of high order. The meat cutting, deboning, mincing, chilling, freezing and packing have to be by mechanical means and under strict sanitary conditions. The animals must be subjected to thorough ante- and post-mortem examination. The carcasses are deboned according to custom-designed primal cuts. The lean meat is packaged hygienically, quick frozen by contact plate freezing and packed in master cartons for shipping. The corned meat is manufactured in standard cans. The production of fresh and processed meats is subjected to regular in-plant quality tests, both chemical and microbiological.

Bacteriological Quality of Meat

Contamination may occur through the water used in the abattoir and meat-processing plant, equipment used for processing and personnel handling the product. The microbial flora consists of bacilli, micrococci, streptococci and staphylococci, *Escherichia coli* and other coliforms, pseudomonads, salmonellae, clostridia, yeasts, fungi, etc. The type of microflora depends upon the initial source of contamination of the carcass and additional contamination during subsequent handling of the meat. *See Bacillus*, Occurrence; *Clostridium*,

Occurrence of *Clostridium Perfringens*; *Clostridium*, Occurrence of *Clostridium Botulinum*; Enterobacteriaceae, Occurrence of *Escherichia Coli*; Spoilage, Moulds in Food Spoilage; Spoilage, Yeasts in Food Spoilage; *Staphylococcus*, Properties and Occurrence

The plate counts of meat processed in plants are reported to be around 10^5 organisms per gram. The lower number of organisms in meat processed in modern slaughterhouses could be attributed to the better hygienic handling during processing. Undesirable microbial contamination is possible at any stage if proper procedures are not followed. Certain strains of *E. coli* can cause enteric disease in humans, either by elaborating an enterotoxin or by penetrating the intestinal epethelium. Three interopathogenic isolates – namely O26, O27, and O28 – have been detected. *Staphylococcus aureus* has also been reported in most of dressed meat. *S. aureus* has been reported to be widely distributed in market meats. It has been confirmed that hygienic processing of meat improves the bacteriological quality of meat and reduces the incidence of food poisoning organisms.

Bibliography

Bailur DM (1989) Meat production and marketing. In: Bhat PN, Menon KKG and Srivastava HC (eds) *Animal Productivity*, pp 549–572. New Delhi: Oxford and IBH.

FAO (1985) *Production Year Book of the Food and Agriculture Organization of the United Nations*. Rome: Food and Agriculture Organization.

FAO (1988) FAO statistics of livestock population of the countries in Asia Pacific Region. *Asian Livestock* 13: 94.

Mudgal VD (1987) Prospects of buffalo as dairy animal in India. *Asian Livestock* 12: 28–32.

Ognjanovic A (1974) Meat and meat production. In: Cockrill WR (ed.) *The Husbandry and Health of the Domestic Buffalo*, p 387. Rome: Food and Agriculture Organization.

Ognjanovic A, Polikhronov D and Joksimovic J (1970) The possibility of improving the yield and quality of buffalo meat by crossing. *Proceedings of the 16th European Meeting of Meat Research Workers* September, Sofia, Bulgaria.

Oliveros BA, Ibarra PI, Arganosa FC, Hapitan, JE and del Rosario RR (1982) Studies on the utilization of meat byproducts. II. Selected physical and chemical characteristics of carabeef byproducts. *Philosophical Journal of Veterinary and Animal Science* 8: 8–19.

Punia BS, Sharma DD and Sinha RN (1981) Effect of level of concentrate in the diet on the microflora of buffalo rumen. *Indian Journal of Nutrition and Dietetics* 18: 218–223.

Ranjhan SK (1981) *Animal Nutrition in Tropics*, 2nd edn. New Delhi: Vikas.

Rumann H and Bryan FL (1979) *Food Borne Infections and Intoxications*. New York: Academic Press.

Sharma DD (1988) Nutritional aspect in relation to meat production from buffaloes. *Invited Papers and Special Lectures, Proceedings of the 2nd World Buffalo Congress*, New Delhi, India (ICAR), vol. II, part II, p 475–490.

Sharma DD, Sarma PA and Mudgal VD (1977) Utilization of feed nutrients by growing buffalo calves at various planes of nutrition. *Annual Report*. Karnal, India: National Dairy Research Institute.

Sharma N, Padda GS and Kondaiah N (1980) *Annual Scientific Report of the Division of Livestock Products Technology*, Izatnagar: Indian Veterinary Research Institute.

V.D. Mudgal
Project Directorate on Cattle, Meerut, India
D.D. Sharma
National Dairy Research Institute, Karnal, India

Milk

Production and Collection

In almost all the developing and developed dairying countries, production of buffalo milk is confined to rural areas, while demand is mostly from the urban populations. Hence buffalo milk has to be collected and transported from the production points in the rural areas to the processing and distribution points in cities. The common systems for collection of buffalo milk are as follows:

1. By cooperative organizations, which are formed by individual or collective milk societies. This system is favoured by producers as no profit-making middlemen are involved.
2. By contractors, who purchase the milk for a lump sum from producers. This results in less return for the producers.
3. By individual producers. This system is practical for those production points that are situated near the processing dairies.

Purchase

There are various methods for buying buffalo milk, used singly or in combination

1. Payment according to weight or volume (also known as a flat rate) saves time and is simple to calculate, but it encourages watering down or skimming. Payment by weight is preferred to payment by volume as the former is not affected by either foam or specific gravity.
2. Payment according to the fat content is practical and discourages adulteration with water. However, it does not prevent removal of the skim milk and it does not take into account the solids-not-fat content of the milk.
3. Payment according to use is a practice followed mainly for milk products.
4. Payment of premiums is usually confined to market

Table 1.   Compositional differences between cows' milk and buffalo milk

Type of Milk	Country	Composition (%)						
		Water	Total solids	Fat	Solids not fat	Protein	Lactose	Ash
Buffalo	USSR	82·00	18·00	8·00	10·00	4·32	4·96	0·84
Buffalo	Egypt	83·60	16·40	6·37	10·03	3·87	5·00	0·79
Buffalo	Italy	83·14	16·86	7·22	9·64	3·95	4·88	0·81
Buffalo	India	82·98	17·02	7·06	9·96	3·90	5·28	0·78
Cow	USA	86·61	13·39	4·14	9·25	3·58	4·96	0·71
Cow	India	86·07	13·93	4·90	9·43	3·42	4·91	0·70

Note: the casein content of buffalo milk is higher (3·00%) than that of cows' milk (2·65%).

milk. It is based on milk quality, as measured by sediment test, flavour score, and bacterial count (as measured by the methylene blue reduction test). This system encourages the production of high-grade milk.
5. Payment according to the cost of production, although rational, is complicated.

Composition

The macroconstituents of buffalo milk are water, fat, protein, lactose, and ash or mineral matter. The microconstituents include phospholipids, sterols, vitamins, enzymes, and pigments. The nutritionally important constituents are milk fat, casein and lactose. Several reports on the gross composition of milk from different breeds of buffaloes and from different regions have been published. Milk differs widely in composition. All milks contain the same constituents, but in varying amounts. Milk from individual buffaloes shows greater variation than mixed herd milk. The variation is always greater in small herds than in large ones. In general, milk fat shows the greatest daily variation, followed by protein, then ash and lactose. Several workers have reported that variation in composition is caused by factors such as season, stage of lactation, age of animal, region, and feed. In general, buffalo milk contains higher amounts of milk solids (i.e. fat, protein, lactose, minerals, solids not fat, and total solids) than cows' milk, as shown in Table 1. *See* Milk, Dietary Importance

Nutritional Significance

Buffalo milk has been of interest to nutritionists in their quest for better nutrition in the world. Milk is an almost ideal food, being of high nutritive value. It supplies body-building proteins, bone-forming minerals, health-giving vitamins, and energy-giving lactose and milk fat.

Besides supplying certain essential fatty acids, it contains the above nutrients in an easily digestible and assimilable form. All these properties make milk an almost ideal food for pregnant mothers, growing children, adolescents, adults, invalids, convalescents, and patients.

Proteins

Buffalo milk proteins are complete proteins of high quality, i.e. they contain all the essential amino acids in the proportions required by the body. The energy value of buffalo milk proteins is $17·2 \text{ J g}^{-1}$. *See* Protein, Quality

Minerals

Practically all the mineral elements found in milk are essential for nutrition. Milk is an excellent source of calcium and phosphorus, both of which, together with vitamin D, are essential for bone formation. Buffalo milk is rather low in iron, copper and iodine. *See* individual minerals

Vitamins

Buffalo milk is a good source of vitamin A (provided that the buffalo is fed sufficient green feed and fodder), vitamin D, thiamin, and riboflavin. However, buffalo milk is deficient in vitamin C. *See* individual vitamins

Fat

Buffalo milk fat plays a significant role in the nutritive value, flavour, and physical properties of the milk and its products. Besides serving as a rich source of energy, fat contains significant amounts of essential fatty acids. The most distinctive role which milk fat plays in dairy products concerns flavour. The energy value of buffalo milk fat is 39·1 J g⁻¹. *See* Essential Fatty Acids, Physiology

Lactose

The principal function of lactose is to supply energy. However, lactose also helps to establish a mildly acidic reaction in the intestine which checks the growth of proteolytic bacteria and facilitates assimilation of the milk. The energy value of lactose is $17·2$ J g^{-1}.

Energy Value

The energy value of buffalo milk varies with its composition. On average, buffalo milk provides 420 J per 100 g.

Processing of Liquid Milk

In India, where 50% of the world's buffalo population is concentrated, over 50% of the total milk production consists of buffalo milk. As it has a higher fat and total solids content, buffalo milk gives a greater output of milk products than cows' milk. However, owing to some basic differences in its physicochemical properties, the use of buffalo milk creates a few special problems during product manufacture and storage. Research into the technology of buffalo milk has spanned from the point of collection through various aspects of processing and packaging, to the quality of the products made. For liquid milk, the feasibility of preserving the milk with hydrogen peroxide, transportation by preconcentration, and the effects of homogenization and pasteurization have been studied.

Production of Processed Foods

The problems arising from the compositional and physicochemical characteristics of buffalo milk in the manufacture and storage of various products made from this raw material, together with their specific causes and suggested preventive measures, i.e. modified techniques, are summarized below.

Cheese

Owing to (1) differences in the micellar composition of milk protein, especially casein, and in the fatty-acid make-up of milk fat, and (2) the higher buffer value, calcium, casein and fat levels, buffalo milk behaves quite differently from cows' milk during both the manufacture and the curing of cheese. *See* Cheeses, Dietary Importance

The major problems faced by cheesemakers are as follows: slow ripening (i.e. acidity development) in milk; (2) faster rennet action (i.e. low rennetting time); (3) excessive syneresis (i.e. low retention of moisture); (4) slow cheddaring (i.e. mellowing of curd); (5) slow curing of cheese (i.e. slow proteolysis and lipolysis causes a delay in the development of the characteristic cheese flavour and body and texture); (6) slightly bitter taste in some cured cheese; and (7) hard body and texture in cured cheese. *See* Cheeses, Chemistry of Curd Manufacture

The suggested modified techniques include the following: (1) adjustment of casein:fat ratio to 0·70 (same as for cows' milk); (2) addition of more starter culture, i.e. 2·5% (for proper acidity development); (3) addition of less rennet (to ensure proper rennetting time and prevent the development of a bitter taste in cured cheese); (4) lower temperature and a longer heating period (to ensure proper development of acidity and greater retention of moisture); (5) piling cheeses in stacks of three during cheddaring (for greater retention of moisture); and (6) curing cheese first at a high temperature (10–12°C) for 2 months for rapid flavour development, and then at a low temperature (2°C) for desirable body and texture changes.

A method for quick curing cheddar-type cheese can be summarized as follows: buffalo milk is ripened to 0·18–0·19% acidity prior to rennetting; it is heated to a temperature of 42°C, and cheddared in whey up to 0·40–0·45% acidity (25–40 min); the milled curd is washed with 73°C water prior to hooping without cheesecloth. The cheese block is brined (18% pasteurized saline) for 15–30 days at 15°C, followed by warm water washing and turning the block every alternate day for a week. The paraffined cheese is stored at 15°C.

Yoghurt

Yoghurt can be prepared from buffalo milk. A heat treatment of 80–85°C for 30 min is sufficient for culturing yoghurt organisms (i.e. *Streptococcus thermophilus* and *Lactobacillus bulgaricus*) in buffalo milk at the rate of 1% each. Starters are mixed in the milk and incubated at 41–43°C until coagulation occurs.

On account of its higher total solids content, buffalo milk yoghurt scores higher in consistency, while cows' milk product scores better in flavour. It has been recommended that buffalo milk be reconstituted with 12–25% skim milk in the manufacture of yoghurt. *See* Yoghurt, The Product and its Manufacture; Yoghurt, Dietary Importance

Condensed Milks (Sweetened and Unsweetened)

Buffalo milk behaves quite differently from cows' milk, not only during production but also during the storage of condensed and evaporated milk. This is the result of (1) differences in micellar composition of milk proteins, especially casein, (2) higher levels of milk proteins (both casein and serum proteins), milk fat and milk sugar, and (3) higher calcium content and lower heat stability of milk. *See* Recombined and Filled Milks

The major problems faced by condensed milk manufacturers are as follows: (1) greater likelihood of undesirable gel formation during production of both condensed and evaporated milks; (2) greater incidence of age-thickening during storage of both condensed and evaporated milks; (3) greater possibility of the formation of hard, stony sugar crystals (sandiness) in sweetened condensed milk; and (4) a greater incidence of discoloration (browning) and cooked flavour development during storage of both condensed and evaporated milks.

The modified technique includes the following: (1) adjustment of the ratio of fat to solids not fat to $1:2.44$ (the same as for cows' milk); (2) addition of stabilizer (trisodium citrate or disodium phosphate) to correct the salt-balance ratio; (3) preheating of milk to $115–118°C/$ no hold, to ensure freedom from gelation in the resulting product; (4) for sweetened condensed milk only, the addition of sugar in the form of a 65–71% syrup to milk at the correct concentration (43–44 parts sugar to 31 parts milk solids) into the standardized milk and at the correct stage (towards the end of the condensing period); (5) cooling and crystallization of the product at the proper stage and in the correct manner (i.e. when total solids reach about 75%, condensing is stopped, and the product is cooled to $29.5°C$ and seeded with lactose by the standard technique used for cows' milk) for condensed milk; (6) storage at 5–8°C to ensure maximum shelf life and minimum browning and cooked flavour development; and (7) regular inversion of the canned product during storage to prevent sedimentation.

Microbiology of Buffalo Milk

Nearly all the changes that take place in the flavour and appearance of milk after it is drawn from the buffalo are the result of the activities of microorganisms. Of these, the most important in dairying are bacteria, moulds, yeasts and viruses – bacteria predominating. A few are desirable, while most cause undesirable changes. A relatively small proportion are disease-producing types, called 'pathogens'. There are several factors which influence microbiological quality of milk and milk products offered for sale. Each country has its own standards of microbiological control. These standards differ markedly. There are differences in general concepts of food hygiene, and differences in economic and technical advancements as applied to production, processing and distribution of foods.

Seasonal Variation

Seasonal changes are known to affect the bacteriological quality of buffalo milk and buffalo milk products. The seasonal incidence of psychrotrophs in can-collected milk was investigated in Canada.

The more rapid rate of growth of psychrotrophic populations in summer milk was probably due to the presence of more actively multiplying species or strains in the milk at this season. It has been observed that the bacteriological quality of farm milk supplies received at the Central Dairy, Stockholm, was not always of sufficiently high standard during July–September for the production of pasteurized milk of good keeping quality. A seasonal variation in the bacterial content of 194 milk samples from 35 grade-A bulk-tank milk supplies in Kansas was reported. Total colony counts at 35°C were, on average, highest in summer and lowest in spring; coliform colony counts were much higher in summer than in other seasons, but the average psychrotrophic colony counts (7°C for 7 days) were somewhat greater in winter than in other seasons, although the differences were not statistically significant.

Alternate-day Collected Milk

More recent appraisals of the bacteriological quality control of buffalo milk in refrigerated farm bulk tanks have been made. On the basis of preliminary trials in Norwegian farms, it was concluded that milk could be stored in refrigerated farm tanks for 4–5 days with little or no loss in bacteriological quality. It was further concluded that bulk-tank milk could be collected every 3–4 days by maintaining efficient cleaning and sterilization of dairy equipments and storing milk at 4°C.

Storage

Psychrotrophic microorganisms are reponsible for massive build-up of microbial counts during cold storage and are thus largely responsible for variations in bacteriological quality of buffalo milk and buffalo milk products offered for sale. The significance of the presence of these bacteria lies in (1) their ability to multiply in raw milk during refrigeration, (2) the possibility that organisms or their enzymes may produce taints or physical defects in raw milk prior to processing, some of which are not removed during pasteurization, and (3) the fact that although the vegetative cells of psychrotrophs are destroyed during pasteurization, some of their proteolytic or lipolytic enzymes are not inactivated by the heat treatment and thus may produce a defect in milk products during storage.

Contamination of Buffalo Milk

Sources of contamination include: interior of udder; exterior of the buffalo, particularly udder and flanks; barn air and dust; flies and other vermin; the milker; and utensils.

Bibliography

Bhanumurthi JL, Mathur BN, Trehan KS, Srinivasan MR and Samlilk O (1971) Problems in the use of buffalo milk in condensed milk manufacturing. *Food Industry Journal* 4(1): 3.

De S (1983) *Outlines of Dairy Technology*, pp 499–515. Delhi: Oxford University Press.

Kalra MA (1981) Variation in bacteriological quality of milk products offered for sale. *A Review of Progress of Research in Dairy Science during the Last Decade*, pp 120–135. New Delhi: Indian Dairy Association.

Singh RS and Ranganathan B (1981) Microbiological aspects of handling, processing and storage of milk and milk products. *A Review of Progress of Research in Dairy Science during the Last Decade*, pp 110–119. New Delhi: Indian Dairy Association.

C. D. Khedkar and G. D. Khedkar
Adarsha Education Society's College, Hingoli, India

BULIMIA NERVOSA

Definition

The symptom of bulimia refers specifically to binge eating, i.e. the consumption of a large amount of food in a discrete period of time. As an isolated symptom, bulimia may be present in a variety of medical conditions, such as the Prader–Willi syndrome and Parkinson's disease; furthermore, in conditions of experimental and clinical food deprivation, bulimia may follow abstinence from eating. Finally, isolated episodes of pleasurable binge eating among adolescents are relatively common.

The term bulimia nervosa (BN) refers to a distinct psychiatric disorder of eating behaviour which includes but is not limited to binge eating episodes. It is also characterized by distinct psychological preoccupations regarding fears of becoming fat that parallel concerns of its companion disorder anorexia nervosa (AN). Accompanying the episodes of binge eating, and fuelled by the fears of obesity, are feelings of loss of personal control and efforts to counter the effects of the ingested calories through a variety of purgative techniques. *See* Anorexia Nervosa

BN was formally described as an autonomous disorder in 1979 by Gerald Russell; the formal diagnostic criteria as defined by the American Psychiatric Association (1987) are listed below:

1.   Recurrent episodes of binge eating (rapid consumption of a large amount of food in a discrete period of time).

2.   A feeling of lack of control over eating behaviour during the eating binges.

3.   The person regularly engages in either self-induced vomiting, use of laxatives or diuretics, strict dieting or fasting, or vigorous exercise in order to prevent weight gain.

4.   A minimum average of two binge eating episodes a week for at least 3 months.

5.   Persistent overconcern with body shape and weight.

Prevalence

BN is largely but not exclusively a disorder of females, typically between the ages of 16 and 40. Refinement of the diagnostic criteria in 1987 to reflect severity through frequency of binge eating episodes has influenced studies of prevalence. Epidemiological surveys prior to 1987 focused on the symptom of bulimia without regard to frequency, and yielded prevalence rates of up to 20% among adolescent and young adult women. However, application of the 1987 diagnostic criteria for BN results in a prevalence of 1–3% among Western adolescent and young adult females.

Aetiology and Groups at Risk

The aetiology of BN is unknown; physiological, psychological and cultural cues have been invoked, as well as risk factors among these three domains. The commonest acute precipitant of binge eating *per se* is food restriction, whether experimental, or self imposed as in dieting or AN. This may result from adaptive physiological signals in the hypothalamus to ingest calories. At the same time, the cognitive consequences of having eaten when trying to abstain from food may provoke a transient relaxation of rules that results in a binge eating episode. Finally, the abundant and frequently instant availability of food in Western society may facilitate impulses to binge eat.

At the level of the individual, risk factors include dieting behaviour and weight preoccupation, particularly in the context of AN; up to 50% of patients with AN also exhibit BN. Premorbid obesity is a risk factor in the sense that these individuals are likely to be dieting and experiencing the prominent negative social attitudes to obesity. Impulsivity – as manifested by substance abuse, recurrent self-harm behaviour, intense and unstable interpersonal relationships, and an inability to tolerate mood states such as depression and boredom – may be an independent individual risk factor. This cluster of symptoms is often labelled borderline personality disorder. *See* Obesity, Aetiology and Assessment

At the familial level, psychiatric disorders such as depression, substance abuse, eating disorders and antisocial behaviour are overrepresented compared to control populations. It has been argued that BN may represent the cultural shaping of an underlying familial vulnerability to psychiatric disturbance. As with AN, families of individuals with BN may place undue emphasis on the importance of thinness. A study of twins with one BN proband shows an 83% concordance for monozygotic (identical) twins versus a 27% concordance for dizygotic (nonidentical) twins.

At the level of our society, the emergence of BN as an autonomous disorder in the final third of this century parallels the increased emphasis on thinness, dieting, and dieting disguised as fitness, as well as the mushrooming of technology that allows more widespread promulgation of social values. Many women with BN have 'failed' to achieve the weight loss requisite for a diagnosis of AN but share a set of beliefs and values seen commonly in AN. For others, BN represents only one expression of impulsive dyscontrol.

Psychopathology

A morbid fear of fatness is the overriding psychological preoccupation characteristic of BN. Psychometric assessment of eating attitudes parallels the results obtained in AN. It is important to recognize that in BN the act of binge eating seldom occurs in response to normative hunger. The extent to which it represents a physiological response to food deprivation usually reflects intensive dietary restriction for the purposes of weight loss. However, the subjective perception of binge eating falls typically into two categories: counterregulation and distraction. Counterregulation refers to the phenomenon whereby individuals who pursue dietary restraint find they have violated their self-imposed limits; their response is one of resignation to loss of control which then permits binge eating. In the case of BN, this permission to binge eat is facilitated and perpetuated by the availability of purging behaviours. Distraction refers to the role of binge eating in escaping from or quelling unpleasant or intolerable psychological states, such as depression, anger, boredom or conflict; indeed, some individuals describe their eating binges as automatic states where they dissociate, losing touch with all feelings. Drugs, alcohol, and nonlethal self-harm attempts may serve a similar function.

Clinical Features

As with AN, the commonest precipitant of BN is dieting behaviour. However, BN may emerge without the emaciation characteristic of AN. This may be especially true where women have been premorbidly overweight. Women with BN who have never had AN still experience up to a 30% fluctuation in adult bodyweight, compared to the 10% fluctuation among women without an eating disorder. Food that is usually avoided or assigned a negative moral value inevitably becomes food consumed during eating binges where dietary restraint is abandoned.

BN is typically a secretive behaviour. Eating binges often occur in the evening after a day of caloric restriction and/or psychological stressors as described above. Individuals may consume between 3000 and 6000 calories in an hour or less, and they describe their eating as rapid, often without savouring the taste, and with a sense of loss of control and an inability to stop. Macronutrient analysis of binge food indicates a predominance of carbohydrate, although perceived high-carbohydrate foods often have a significant fat content as well. A loss of the normal sense of satiety is evident from both subjective ratings and objective measures of the quantity of food consumed. Ironically, the aftermath of an episode of binge eating is often heightened dysphoria, weight concern and self-loathing, which then precipitates purging behaviour.

The commonest form of purgation is self-induced vomiting, with individuals using a finger or pen to stimulate an oropharyngeal vomiting reflex. The commonly available emetic, ipecac, has also been used for this purpose with catastrophic results: ipecac contains emetine, which is directly toxic to cardiac muscle. Other methods of counteracting the effects of ingested calories include laxative, diuretic, and diet pill abuse. These lead to a variety of physiological and psychological complications, including low serum and intracellular potassium levels from losses through vomiting and diuresis; this may precipitate cardiac arrhythmias. An associated state of metabolic alkalosis results from chloride losses through vomiting. Alternating diarrhoea and constipation may result from laxative abuse. Diet pills are typically amphetamine-like psychostimulants that not only suppress hunger but produce anxiety, insomnia, irritability and dependence. Less obvious forms of purgation include intensive exercise for the primary purpose of weight loss and severe dietary restriction after binges; this latter feature often serves to perpetuate the disorder.

There are few physical characteristics of BN that facilitate its diagnosis. However, two potential signs of the disorder are hypertrophy of the parotid salivary glands (likely secondary to overstimulation) and calluses or erosions on the dorsum of the hand (caused by friction against the incisor teeth while inducing vomiting). The acid content of vomitus has an erosive effect on dental enamel and may promote gum recession, leading at times to an initial diagnosis of BN by dentists. Feelings of depression and anxiety are common in BN; indeed, these women and their families are at higher than normal lifetime risk for the development of autonomous mood and anxiety disorders. However, when these symptoms coexist with BN, it is often difficult to separate them from other sequelae of the eating disorder.

Because BN is a disorder that generates secrecy, isolation and shame, affected individuals may wait months or years prior to seeking treatment. This contributes to the chronicity of the disorder.

Diagnosis

The diagnostic criteria of the American Psychiatric Association listed above reflect the confluence of behavioural and psychological features characteristic of BN. Earlier definitions of this disorder were less rigorous and included a wider range of eating disturbance without regard to issues of binge eating frequency or weight and shape concerns. This led to epidemiological overdiagnosis without regard to clinical severity. However, problems remain with respect to the definition of a binge eating episode. For some individuals, the sense of loss of control associated with eating 'banned' foods such as two biscuits or a piece of cake may constitute a qualitative binge, whereas there is consensus that eating more than is normal under the circumstances constitutes a quantitative binge. The accuracy of self-reported binge-eating quantities hampers research in BN.

The diagnosis of BN must be considered in the absence of disclosure by the individual where sequelae such as unexplained low serum potassium are evident.

BN may also contribute to disruption of normal menstrual function among women of a statistically normal bodyweight and may feature among the symptoms of women who experience premenstrual syndrome. *See* Menstrual Cycle and Premenstrual Syndrome – Nutritional Aspects

Treatment

The treatment of BN includes but is not limited to the re-establishment of normal eating behaviour, whether through education, psychotherapy or drug therapy. Unlike AN, individuals with BN are often eager to overcome their eating disturbance, although this is accompanied by a morbid fear of weight gain.

Treatment begins with a careful history which includes longitudinal weight history, including weight prior to the onset of dieting and desired weight; the discrepancy may reflect the conflict between culture and biology. The acute precipitants of binge eating states are identified and the non-binge meals are quantified. Methods of purgation and their potentially lethal complications are described. The associations between psychological states, eating behaviours, and weight and shape concerns may be facilitated by self-report diaries where individuals with BN discover these connections. Unlike AN, weight gain may not be a goal but weight stabilization may occur as a result of cessation of dieting and bulimic behaviours; typically, these individuals experience significant weight fluctuations.

An educational approach may include readings on cultural bias and bodyweight, the effect of dietary chaos and deprivation on physiological and psychological states as well as eating behaviour, and the biological regulation of bodyweight. Individual psychotherapy may explore the origins and extent of dysfunctional attitudes related to eating, weight and shape, as well as more global underlying disturbances related to self-esteem and self-appraisal. Often a specific meal plan may be prescribed, not to promote weight gain but to avoid long intervals of deprivation that may precipitate binge eating. Learning to tolerate feelings and impulses through understanding, or through learning more adaptive coping strategies, may also be useful.

The use of a wide range of antidepressant drugs has been studied since 1983. The evidence confirms that tricyclic antidepressants, monoamine-oxidase-inhibiting antidepressants, and novel antidepressants exert an antibulimic effect which is independent of their effect on mood. Their mechanism of action in BN is unclear but may relate to effects on neurotransmitters involved in hypothalamic regulation of appetitive behaviour. Extensive abnormalities of serotonin and noradrenaline have been documented in BN. The relative efficacies of antidepressant therapy, psychotherapy, or their combination, await elucidation.

Hospitalization is rarely necessary for individuals with BN. However, when the disorder is accompanied by suicidal tendency, serious electrolyte compromise, or coexistent diabetes mellitus, hospitalization may help in crisis resolution or metabolic stabilization.

Prognosis

The long-term prognosis of BN is unknown because of its relatively recent description. It is known that individuals with BN are vulnerable to mood, anxiety, and substance abuse disorders, as well as a general impairment in social adjustment. One follow-up study of four to six years indicated that two thirds of the treated sample recovered from BN; low self-esteem has been identified elsewhere as a poor prognostic factor of treatment.

Anorexia Nervosa

AN coexists with BN in up to 50% of cases of AN and clearly precedes BN in roughly 25% of cases of BN. While many psychological and behavioural features unite the disorders, studies of personality functioning have indicated a higher degree of impulsive features in the BN group. Archetypes of family functioning and premorbid obesity may also distinguish the disorders. However, to understand either disorder demands a comprehension of both disorders.

Adolescents

Surveys indicate that brief periods of dieting, episodes of binge eating, and experimentation with purgative techniques are common among adolescents – far more so than the clinical disorder BN. It remains to be seen whether primary prevention at the level of young adolescents regarding weight regulation and eating behaviour will reduce the emergence of BN characteristically at the end of adolescence.

Bibliography

American Psychiatric Association (1987) *Diagnostic and Statistical Manual of Mental Disorders*, 3rd edn. Washington DC: American Psychiatric Association.

Garner DM and Garfinkel PE (eds) (1985) *Handbook of Psychotherapy for Anorexia Nervosa and Bulimia*. New York: Guilford Press.

Hudson JI and Pope HG (eds) (1988) *The Psychobiology of Bulimia*. Washington DC: American Psychiatric Press.

Mitchell JE (1990) *Bulimia Nervosa*. Minneapolis: University of Minnesota Press.

Walsh BT (ed) (1988) *Eating Behaviour in Eating Disorders*. Washington DC: American Psychiatric Press.

David S. Goldbloom and Paul E. Garfinkel, University of Toronto, Toronto, Canada

BULK STORAGE

See Cereals and Controlled Atmosphere Storage

BURNS PATIENTS – NUTRITIONAL MANAGEMENT

Burns injury is the most severe form of trauma that humans can survive. One of the most important determinants of a successful outcome is maintenance of nutritional status. Achieving this goal, however, is hampered by both practical and metabolic complications in nutritional support, stemming from the extensive trauma. The ensuing article summarizes the metabolic responses and nutritional problems inherent in burns injury. Current guidelines for nutritional requirements and management of feeding are considered.

Hypermetabolism and Hypercatabolism following Burns Injury

Hypermetabolism following burns is multifactorial in origin. One factor which contributes to the raised metabolism is the increased latent heat of evaporation of water lost by evaporation from wound surfaces. Hypermetabolism also results from neuroendocrine stimuli that lead to hormonal changes which increase heat production directly and also indirectly by altering aspects of the metabolism, such as an increase in protein turnover, which obligate a massive increase in energy expenditure. *See* Energy, Energy Expenditure and Energy Balance; Protein, Synthesis and Turnover

Another factor contributing to the hypermetabolism is cytokine stimulation of energy expenditure. Cytokines cause an increase in heat production by acting directly on the temperature control centre within the brain. Cytokines may also exert an indirect effect on thermogenesis by increasing turnover of body protein. *See* Thermogenesis

The increased basal metabolic rate (BMR) observed in burns patients is of greater magnitude and duration than that observed following other forms of major injury, such as major surgery or sepsis. By 24 h following burns all patients have been shown to have a raised metabolic rate which reaches a peak a few days later. Duration of the increase in BMR depends on the severity of the burn. Patients with 50% body surface area burns may have BMR approaching twice the normal value. Raised energy expenditure persists until healing or skin grafting. Metabolic rate can be partly modified by the application of an occlusive dressing which reduces heat losses from the wound surface. Metabolic rate may also be reduced by raising the environmental temperature. Clinical studies have shown that increasing environmental temperature from 22°C to 32°C reduces metabolic rate by approximately one third. Despite intervention to minimize the increase in metabolic rate, for the majority of patients with extensive burns, BMR remains elevated and an increase in energy intake is required in order to maintain energy balance. It has long been recognized that in a state of energy imbalance, in which energy production exceeds energy input, body reserves will be utilized, resulting in clinical evidence of tissue wasting and weight loss. It is therefore not surprising that many investigators have observed weight loss following burns injury.

Hypercatabolism is caused by the neuroendocrine and cytokine responses which predispose to loss of both fat and lean body mass. A number of abnormalities in nutrient metabolism accompany the hypermetabolic state; these include hyperglycaemia and intolerance to glucose, increased ability to catabolize fat, but reduced gastric fat tolerance, and exacerbated protein loss. Hypermetabolism, hypercatabolism and abnormal nutrient metabolism all have important implications in terms of the nutritional management of the burns patient. The aim of nutritional support in the burns patient is to minimize the catabolic effects of trauma by counteracting the nutrient losses. *See* Glucose, Maintenance of Blood Glucose Level

Nutritional Requirements of Burned Patients

Energy Requirements

Metabolic energy expenditure and, hence, energy requirements of burns patients can be derived from indirect calorimetry measurements. However, this method is laborious and often impractical in the clinical setting.

There are many formulae from which energy requirements can be predicted. Such formulae can easily be applied to patients in the clinical setting. Formulae are usually based on bodyweight, burn surface area and predicted metabolic rate (using the Harris Benedict equation or those devised by Schofeild and Elia). Despite major deviations from normal conditions that define resting metabolic rate, metabolic energy expenditure and, hence, energy requirements are often expressed as multiples of predicted normal resting metabolic rate. For example, BMR multiplied by two is often used, but this overestimates energy requirements in patients with less than 30% burns. Various formulae used in calculating energy requirements of burns patients are presented in Table 1. The formulae do not take into account changes in metabolism which occur with healing (i.e. decreased energy expenditure). It has been suggested that energy intake should be decreased by 10% per week as the wound heals. However, it could be argued that, as the patient recovers mobility is increased, the energy for which would cancel out any decrease in metabolic rate that results from healing.

Protein

Protein requirement is increased following burns injury owing to an increase in protein turnover. Burns trauma results in protein being wasted and lost from the body in urine and in the burn wound exudate. Urine protein losses may amount to as much as 120–240 g per day. Approximately 0·2 g of nitrogen (1·25 g protein) per 1% burn are lost in wound exudate. Increased amounts of protein are required for healing processes.

Requirements for protein may be estimated on a basis of energy requirements: in adults, for every 420–504 kJ, 1 g of nitrogen (6·25 g protein) is usually provided. Alternatively, requirements may be calculated on a basis

Table 1.   Formulae used to estimate energy requirements of burns patients

Formula name	Energy requirement	Indications
Curreri formula	$(20 \times$ kg bw$) + (40 \times$ BSA$)$	For up to 50% burns in adults
Toronto formula	$4343 + (10 \cdot 5 \times$ BSA$) + (0 \cdot 23 \times$ Cl$) +$ $(0 \cdot 8 \times$ RMR$) + (114 \times$ T$) - (4 \cdot 5 \times$ PBD$)$	Adults
Cunningham	$2 \times$ RMR	Adults, $> 30\%$ BSAB
Cunningham	$1 \cdot 2 - 2 \cdot 0 \times$ RMR	Children
Hildreth and Caryajal	$(1800 \times$ BSA$) + (2000 \times$ BSAB$)$	Children
Curreri junior formula	RMR $+ (15 \times$ BSAB$)$	Children aged 0–1 years
	RMR $+ (25 \times$ BSAB$)$	Children aged 1–3 years
Bachelor formula	$(60 \times$ kg bw$) + 35 \times$ BSAB$)$	

BSA, body surface area (m^2); BSAB, body surface area burned (m^2); RMR, resting metabolic rate; Cl, kcals received in previous 24 h (1 kcal=4·2 kJ); T, temperature in °C; PBD, postburn days; bw, bodyweight.

Table 2.   Formulae used to estimate protein requirements of burns patients

Formula name	Equation	Indications
Cunningham	2·5 g per kg bw per 24 h	Children
Davies and Liljedahl	3·0 g per kg bw + 1·0 g per 1% BSAB	Children
Sutherland	1·0 g per kg bw + 3·0 g per 1% BSAB	Adult
Sutherland	3·0 g per kg bw + 1·0 g per 1% BSAB	Children

BSAB, body surface area burned (m^2); bw, bodyweight.

of bodyweight and/or percentage body surface area burned. In the case of the latter, the formulae presented in Table 2 have been used.

Protein requirement can also be estimated from protein balance determinations. Protein requirements are based on the amount of nitrogen (1 g nitrogen is equivalent to 6·25 g protein) lost to the urine and exudate in the previous 24 h. However, this method is laborious and exudate losses are difficult to measure accurately.

Protein provided should be of high biological value and should contain all the essential amino acids, balanced with nonessential amino acids. *See* Protein, Requirements

Vitamins and Minerals

There has been extensive research into energy and protein requirements following burns injury but less solid work on which to base guidelines for vitamin and mineral intakes. It is probable, however, that burns patients have an overall increased requirement for vitamins and minerals, which stems from the tissue injury and increase in metabolic processes. Studies indicate that several micronutrients are essential to maximize immune function and the wound healing

process. Vitamin and mineral supplementation is therefore a very important part of therapy; deficiencies lead to suboptimal clinical outcome. The fact that precise knowledge of the amounts of vitamins required during the recovery period does not yet exist may predispose to careless, inconsistent supplementation. Selective vitamin and mineral therapy is the goal of the future; meanwhile, balancing knowledge of function with evidence of toxicity is the most satisfactory approach. *See* Immunity and Nutrition

Vitamin A

Adequate vitamin A is required for optimum wound healing and epithelial integrity. Vitamin A is also involved in the immune response, which is vital for resistance to local and systemic infection following burns. Increased vitamin A levels have been reported in burns patients. Increased incidence of respiratory infections, prolonged healing and diarrhoea have been associated with suboptimal provision of vitamin A. Low circulating concentrations of vitamin A occur as a result of an increased rate of utilization coupled with a reduced synthesis of the carrier protein for vitamin A. Although dietary requirements are increased, the precise amounts are undefined. Intakes should be sufficient to prevent deficiency whilst avoiding the toxic effects of excess. A level of intake should be decided taking into account the UK estimated average requirement (EAR; 400 μg per day for adults) and the upper limit of intake to avoid toxic effects (7500 μg and 9000 μg for female and male adults respectively). *See* Retinol, Physiology

Vitamin D

Under normal circumstances, a major proportion of vitamin D is derived from the action of ultraviolet (UV) light on the skin, and dietary intake is not essential. Hospitalization, covered burns and reduced skin surface area limit UV-mediated vitamin D and necessitate the dietary provision of the vitamin.

The drug, cimetidine, often used in the treatment of burns patients, inhibits the hepatic hydroxylation of vitamin D. The requirement for vitamin D is therefore increased following burns. Excessively high intakes (50 μg or more per day) should be avoided in children. *See* Cholecalciferol, Physiology; Drug–Nutrient Interactions

Vitamin E

Low levels of vitamin E have been reported in burns patients, especially if inhalation injury has occurred. Vitamin E is an antioxidant, important in maintaining cell membrane stability. It also enhances the immune response. The integrity of the gut and, hence, the ability to tolerate gastric feeds are improved by vitamin E supplementation. Vitamin E stabilizes red blood cell membranes following burns, preventing their haemolysis and subsequent formation of free radicals. Supplementation may help to prevent the deterioration in lung function which follows thermal injury. Topically applied, vitamin E may also encourage wound healing. The requirement for vitamin E following burns injury may be greater than the average intake of a healthy person (c. 6 mg per day). Few adverse effects have been reported with megadoses of the vitamin (3200 mg per day). The content of polyunsaturated fats in formula feeds will also affect vitamin E requirement. *See* Tocopherols, Physiology

Vitamin K

Antibiotic therapy in burns patients may inhibit the synthesis of vitamin K in the gut, and supplementation may therefore be warranted.

Thiamin (Vitamin B₁)

Thiamin is required for the release of energy from carbohydrates. As energy requirement and, hence, carbohydrate intake are increased following burns, the requirement for thiamin will increase in concordance. Thiamin also functions in the synthesis of collagen, which further increases the requirement for this vitamin in the postburn period. In addition, urinary excretion may be increased. Supplements of 10 times normal intake have been recommended (c. 1 mg per 1000 kJ, or 10–20 mg per day). *See* Thiamin, Physiology

Riboflavin (Vitamin B₂)

Riboflavin functions in the healing process and, consequently, wound healing is impaired if there is a deficiency of this vitamin. Requirement for riboflavin is closely related to protein and energy needs. Flavin adenosine diribonucleotide (FAD), formed from riboflavin, takes part in energy formation from fats and protein. Urinary losses may be increased following burns. Supplementation is therefore indicated in burns patients. Intakes in the region of 10–20 mg per 24 h are thought to be sufficient. *See* Riboflavin, Physiology

Nicotinic Acid

Under normal circumstances, nicotinic acid is obtained from both the diet and from endogenous synthesis. Following burns, endogenous synthesis is diminished, a factor which in itself increases the dietary requirement. The metabolic processes in which nicotinic acid plays a crucial role further increases the demands for this vitamin. Nicotinic acid participates in protein and carbohydrate metabolism, fat synthesis and tissue respiration. The increase in utilization of nicotinic acid following burns is reflected in the increase in urinary excretion of metabolites of this vitamin, which persists for at least 2 months. Dietary allowances are largely related to energy requirements, which are increased in the postburn period. An intake of 150–200 mg per 24 h has been suggested for cases with extensive burns, which is approximately a 10-fold increase in intake. Prolonged supplementation into the convalescent period may be warranted in view of the persistent excretion of nicotinic acid metabolites.

There is some evidence that megadoses (2·0–3·6 mg) of nicotinic acid in the first 24 h following burns can minimize the formation of oedema. This practice, however, is not routinely recommended, as some patients may develop fatty livers with such high doses. *See* Niacin, Physiology

Pyridoxine (Vitamin B₆)

Pyridoxine functions in protein metabolism and is important for nucleic acid and protein synthesis, red blood cell formation and synthesis of several hormones. Low pyridoxine status has been found in children with burns. Stress may increase dietary needs and increase urinary losses. Requirements are increased with high protein intake. Intake should therefore be increased in proportion to the increase in protein intake. At least 15 μg per g protein should be provided in adults and 8–10 μg per g protein in infants under 1 year of age. *See* Vitamin B₆, Properties and Determination

Pantothenic Acid

Pantothenic acid functions in the metabolism of energy and is involved in anabolic and catabolic processes. Deficiency of pantothenic acid leads to decreased wound strength and also inhibits the stimulation of antibody producing cells. Demand for this vitamin is increased following burns owing to trauma-induced increase in energy metabolism. Pantothenic acid is synthesized by the gut microflora, which contributes a substantial proportion to total intake. Antibiotic therapy following burns reduces gut microbial pantothenic acid synthesis, and, an increase in intake may therefore be required to compensate for this. Supplements in excess of the UK average intake of 3–7 mg per day may be warranted. No evidence exists of a toxic effect of excess pantothenic acid. *See* Pantothenic Acid, Physiology

Folate

Folate is needed for growth and repair of damaged tissue, and for deoxyribonucleic acid and protein synthesis. There is an increased folate requirement in burns owing to increased utilization and excretion and reduced synthesis. Deficiency of folate predisposes to poor wound healing and depressed immune function. Intakes in excess of the UK reference nutrient intake (RNI) for folate are likely to be warranted in the recovery period following burns. *See* Folic Acid, Physiology

Biotin

Biotin is an important regulator in metabolism of proteins and fats; it is a component of many enzymes involved in these processes. Low serum levels have been found in children with burns; this may be caused by an increase in metabolism and excretion, and an increased requirement for tissue repair. Little is known of the requirements of this vitamin, but intakes up to 200 μg are known to be safe. *See* Biotin, Physiology

Vitamin C

Vitamin C functions in wound and skin healing, energy production and immune function. It also has an important function as a free radical scavenger, preventing tissue damage. Mild deficiency can occur in stressful situations, and this manifests as poor wound healing and an impaired immune response. In addition, vitamin C is lost from the burn wound exudate and urine. Owing to the important functions of vitamin C, patients with burns have increased requirements – 5–10-fold that of a healthy individual. *See* Ascorbic Acid, Physiology

Zinc

Zinc is involved in wound healing, and burns patients therefore have an increased requirement. Doses of over 50 mg per day should be avoided in case of interference with copper metabolism. *See* Zinc, Physiology

Iron

Although iron is important for maintaining haemoglobin levels following burns, therapeutic doses should not be given to a protein-depleted patient because availability of unbound iron will increase bacterial growth. *See* Iron, Physiology

Nutritional Management

When considering the patient with burns, there is a large gap between theoretical considerations on the one hand and practical provision of nutrients on the other. Feeding is often problematical. Nutritional guidelines, such as those outlined below, must be tempered with clinical judgement.

There are four steps to nutritional management of the burned patient:

1. Assessment of needs.
2. Method of feed delivery.
3. Formulation of a regime.
4. Evaluation and monitoring.

Assessment of Needs

Requirements for energy, protein and micronutrients are determined using information on age, sex, burn size, body size, and estimated or measured metabolic rate. Nutrient requirements may be re-assessed at intervals during the convalescent period.

Methods of Delivery

Oral Diet

In minor burns victims it may be feasible to provide the full nutritional requirement from normal food by providing high-protein, high-energy foods. Normal-sized meals may be fortified with protein and energy supplements.

When requirements cannot be met through consumption of a high-protein diet, e.g. when appetite is reduced or requirement is substantially increased, oral diet may be supplemented with between-meal sip feeds.

When an oral diet is being taken it is essential that food intake is recorded, especially in children, as food provided may be substantially greater than actual food consumed.

Tube Feeds

Adults with over 20–25% burns and children with over 15% burns are rarely well enough to be capable of voluntary intake to meet their needs. If a patient fails to meet total requirements orally they may be tube-fed nocturnally (e.g. 6 p.m. to 6 a.m.) in addition to their daytime food intake. If oral food plus nocturnal feeding fails to meet nutritional demands, or if the patient cannot tolerate oral food, continuous tube feeding is employed. Many commercially prepared, high-protein feeds are both convenient and safe to use.

The following guidelines for nasogastric tube feeding are useful. To avoid osmotic diuresis, abdominal cramps and vomiting, administration should be slow at first. Delivery rate for adults should commence at 20–50 ml h^{-1}, full strength, and be increased by 25 ml h^{-1} each day until the nutritional requirement is met. It is important to ensure an adequate fluid intake, either orally or via nasogastric tube, to compensate for exudate losses. The delivery rate for children should commence with 1–2 ml per kg bodyweight per hour, and be increased as tolerated until the nutritional requirement is met. Residual gastric volume should be monitored: if over 1·5 times the hourly delivery rate are aspirated, digestion is impaired, possibly owing to ileus.

Total Parenteral Nutrition

The parenteral route is used only as a last resort, if provision of sufficient nutrients by enteral feeding is impossible. Parenteral nutrition carries a risk of infection and metabolic derangement and is also expensive. Enteral feeding preserves gut integrity and helps minimize the metabolic response to trauma. In some patients, however, parenteral feeding provides the only option, if requirements are excessively high, or there is gastric intolerance owing to a prolonged ileus.

Formulation of a Regimen

Commercially prepared enteral formulae may be used in quantities to meet the calculated requirements. Alternatively, a modular feed may be compounded, tailored to the requirements of the individual patient. Energy requirement is met through a balance of carbohydrate (glucose and glucose polymers) and lipid (long-chain triglycerides) (LCT) or LCT plus medium-chain triglycerides (MCT). Carbohydrate usually provides approximately 40–50% of energy, and lipid provides up to 50%. Following trauma, metabolism is geared towards enhanced lipid utilization but low tolerance to lipid via the enteral route has been reported. Research into the optimum lipid content for an enteral formula for burns patients favours a low-fat formula. Low-fat (15% total energy) linolenic-restricted, ω3-enriched formulae have also been recommended, but such feeds would have to be specially prepared.

Parenteral feeds are formulated to meet energy and nitrogen requirements. Energy is provided from carbohydrate (in the form of glucose) and fat (LCT or LCT–MCT lipid emulsion). Parenteral lipid is tolerated well in adults: 35–40% of energy is usually provided as lipid. In infants, tolerance to lipid emulsions is reduced and lipid should be introduced cautiously. For example, delivery rate in infants commences at 0·5–1·0 g per kg body-weight per day and is increased by 0·5 g per kg per day up to a maximum of 4·0–5·0 g per kg per day.

Initiation of Nutritional Support – Benefits of Early Feeding

Traditionally, in patients with moderate to major burns, feeding commenced 48–72 h postburn, priority being given to fluid resuscitation and regaining haemodynamic stability in the first 48 h. Feeding usually waited until ileus was resolved and bowel sounds were present. However, postburn ileus only affects the stomach and it is now known to be possible, and beneficial, to initiate feeding immediately by the nasoduodenal route. A second large-bore tube may be simultaneously sited in the stomach, and when ileus has resolved feeding can be switched to the nasogastric route.

Early feeding overcomes some of the functional abnormalities associated with removal of enteral feeding, such as reduced concentration and activity of secretions (including sucrase, maltase, galactokinase, Na$^+$,K$^+$-ATPase, and gastric hormones – secretin and gastrin), decreased gut weight, decreased gut protein content and impairment of absorbable activity. When feeding into the jejunum, concentrations as low as 1·68 kJ ml^{-1} may be necessary to prevent abdominal discomfort. Although this may not provide much in terms of energy requirement, it will help to preserve gut integrity and function which will be beneficial for long-term feeding.

Feeding Problems

Although the hypermetabolic state associated with burns requires aggressive nutritional support, preferably via the enteral route, frequent surgical procedures interrupt feeding programmes and make it difficult to achieve targets. In addition, pulmonary complications may complicate nutrient delivery via the oral route.

Diarrhoea is a persistent complication and leads to poor nutritional status and disturbed fluid balance. Tube feeding hyperosmolality, antibiotics, low serum albumin, high-fat feeds, gut atrophy, and inadequate vitamin A may cause diarrhoea.

Use of antacids to reduce bleeding from the gut in burns increases the pH of the gut and interferes with digestion. Antibiotic therapy is frequently warranted to treat graft or systemic infections, but often results in diarrhoea. Low serum albumin causes low intravascular osmotic pressure, and nutrients are therefore less able to cross the gut. An association between lipid content of feed and diarrhoea in burns patients has been found. Immediate enteral feeding within 48 h has been shown to reduce diarrhoea, probably by minimizing gut atrophy. Vitamin-A-enriched formulae may also minimize diarrhoea. Owing to the belief that the hyperosmolar nature of the feed is a major cause of diarrhoea, it is widespread practice to use diluted formula in the case of diarrhoea. However, there are data to show that dietary tonicity is not related to diarrhoea. Feeding is now sometimes initiated on full-strength formula; improved formula composition should enable this to become more common. Choice of appropriate formula should be based on nutritional needs and not osmolality.

Hazards of overfeeding should be avoided. The aim is to provide adequate energy while minimizing the detrimental effects of overfeeding. Overfeeding glucose may lead to fatty infiltration of the liver and predisposes to pulmonary stress. Sufficient energy should be provided to maintain energy balance whilst avoiding respiratory and hepatic complications. Provision of nutrients at a modest level over a prolonged period may be more appropriate than short-term hyperalimentation during the acute phase following injury.

Evaluation and Monitoring

Monitoring and evaluating the efficacy of the nutritional regimen is a vital part of the nutritional management of the burns patient. Actual nutrient intakes achieved should be compared to theoretical requirements, to ensure the efficacy of the regime employed. Failure to provide the full requirement may warrant a different approach to nutrient delivery.

Anthropometric measurements can be used to assess and monitor nutritional status. Weight should be measured frequently and plotted on a weight chart. It is convenient to weigh patients at time of dressing changes, but this may not be possible for several days following grafting. Growth parameters (e.g. weight-for-age, height-for-age) should be monitored in children using percentile charts. *See* Nutritional Status, Anthropometry and Clinical Examination

The clinical record, such as rate of healing and incidence of infection, should also be considered when evaluating nutritional status.

Serum albumin is often monitored frequently in intensive burns patients, but this cannot be used as an index of nutritional status because of major fluid protein shifts, and protein loss through wound and multiple transfusions. Serum proteins with a short half-life are a more suitable means of monitoring visceral protein status – in conjunction with other indices. Urea nitrogen is not monitored routinely for the determination of nitrogen balance because unmeasured exudate loss leads

to false-positive factor. A correlation factor can be used but this is not entirely accurate. *See* Nutritional Status, Biochemical Tests for Vitamins and Minerals

Benefits in Aiding Recovery

Properly designed nutritional clinical trials during recovery from burns are lacking owing to practical and ethical constraints arising from the nature of the injury. However, most investigators have concluded that one of the major contributions to a successful outcome in the treatment of extensive burns is maintenance of good nutritional status, with a thorough approach to nutritional support. Wound healing, immune status, muscle strength and prognosis have been shown to be improved in well-nourished, compared to poorly nourished, traumatized patients. Skin grafts also take better in well-nourished patients.

Benefits of feeding are largely assessed in terms of weight loss and gain. Studies have shown that when nutrition is not carefully supervised weight loss can be substantial (up to 20% admission weight in 2 months); even patients with relatively minor burns suffer losses. Intensive nutritional support has been shown to result in weight gain in patients with minor burns, to prevent losses in those with moderate burns, and to minimize losses in patients with major burns.

Infection remains a major cause of mortality following thermal injury. Vitamins C and E improve immune status following burns, so that is is a fair assumption that supplementation with such vitamins may increase resistance to infection, thereby improving chances of survival. However, no properly controlled trial has yet been carried out to test this hypothesis.

Some clinical trials have been carried out to investigate the potential benefits of zinc supplementation on wound healing; these have shown that supplementation reduces healing time and time from grafting to complete epithelial cover. Zinc supplementation will also prevent anorexia and taste changes associated with deficiency.

Feeding studies in laboratory animals have shown that supplementation with vitamin A improves the rate of healing if deficiency previously existed. Riboflavin supplementation has also been shown to improve wound healing in rats.

Feeding high-protein formulae has been shown to help regain serum albumin concentrations and serum haemoglobin concentrations, reducing anaemia.

Bibliography

Davies JWT (1982) The metabolic responses. In: Davies JWT (ed.) *The Physiological Responses to Burning Injury*, pp 425–529. London: Academic Press.
Gottschlich MM and Warden GD (1990) Vitamin supplemen-

tation in the patient with burns. *Journal of Burn Care Rehabilitation* 11: 275–279.

Gottschlich MM, Warden GD, Michel M *et al.* (1988) Diarrhea in the tube fed burn patient: incidence, etiology, nutritional impact and prevention. *Journal of Parenteral and Enteral Nutrition* 12: 338–345.

O'Neil CE, Hutsler D and Hildreth MA (1989) Basic nutritional guidelines for pediatric burns patients. *Journal of Burn Care Rehabilitation* 10: 278–284.

Royle G and Burke JF (1987) Substrate requirements of burns patients. In: Grant A and Todd E (eds) *Enteral and Parenteral Nutrition, A Clinical Handbook* 2nd edn, pp 163–167. Oxford: Blackwell Scientific Publications.

Thomas B (1988) Catabolic states 'burn injury'. In: Thomas B (ed.) *Manual of Dietetic Practice*, pp 537–550. Oxford: Blackwell Scientific Publications.

Paula Jane Moynihan
University of Surrey, Guildford, UK

BUTTER

Contents

The Product and its Manufacture

Butter has long been recognized as a valuable food. Its method of manufacture has changed little over the years except in respect of the equipment used. The traditional craft methods have given away to large-scale sophisticated continuous production, but both can still be found.

In the process of buttermaking, cream is subjected to severe agitation. This 'churning', as it is called, causes concussion and friction of the fat globules to an extent that they are damaged and clump together. In simple terms it can be stated that the oil-in-water emulsion of cream changes to the water-in-oil emulsion of butter. Some of the fat globules from cream are found dispersed in a matrix of fat crystals and oil. *See* Colloids and Emulsions

Dirty equipment or unhygienic methods of production will produce a poor keeping quality and often a poor-flavoured butter. The commercial significance of this has long been recognized. Training in the form of dairy schools at institutes, such as that established at Reading, and itinerant classes organised by county councils, were an important means of education during the early part of the 20th century. These training courses emphasized cleanliness and explained the conditions necessary to achieve a good-quality butter from the milking cow to the handling and marketing of the finished product.

First-class quality butter can only be produced by attention to detail. The equipment used in the creameries of today makes a product of more uniform flavour and texture than the older craft methods. However, the quality may not necessarily be superior.

Economic forces are emphasizing the need to maximize efficiency in processing and production methods. These, combined with the decline in popularity of butter as a product, are causing milk fat to be increasingly seen as an ingredient rather than as an end product in its own right.

Types of Butter

Sweet cream:

(1) salted with a salt content normally about 2%, but can vary from 1·5 to 3%;
(2) unsalted.

Lactic:

(1) slightly salted with a salt content of approximately 1%;
(2) unsalted.

Whey, sometimes called 'farmhouse butter'. This is found in localized areas and is manufactured from whey cream – a by-product of cheesemaking. The salt content is about 2%. *See* Whey and Whey Powders, Production and Uses

Raw Materials

The quality and the handling of the raw material is of paramount importance in achieving a premium-quality end product.

Cream

The essential elements are:

(1) clean milk;
(2) efficient separation to a specific fat content;
(3) efficient pasteurization (heat treatment) and cooling;
(4) good temperature control during storage;
(5) care in the physical handling of the cream. *See* Cream, Types of Cream

Raw milk with a low microbiological content (of less than 20 000 organisms per millilitre) is now commonly obtained from UK herds. The quality schemes in operation within the UK have resulted in a general improvement of milk quality – a fact which is reflected in improved butter standards. *See* Milk, Processing of Liquid Milk

Each globule of milk fat is surrounded by a membrane, which consists mainly of phospholipids and protein, is on average 10 nm in thickness and sensitive to abrasion. The nature of the membrane alters slightly on cooling, part of it becoming solubilized.

Milk is separated into cream and skimmed milk by means of a centrifugal separator. At all stages in the handling of the milk and in the preparation of the cream, the utmost care is taken to avoid abrasion of the fat globule membrane by excessive pumping or turbulence. Separators are designed to cause as little damage as possible, while achieving a high degree of efficiency.

The optimum fat percentage of the cream, to obtain the maximum churning efficiency, needs to be adjusted according to the method and equipment used to make the butter. Traditional methods advise a fat content of 30–35%, a consistency which will run quickly off a Scotch hand. Modern continuous buttermakers normally operate at 40–44% butter fat for sweet cream and 38–40% butter fat for an acid or cultured cream.

It is usual to heat treat the cream after separation. This can be achieved on a small scale by heating in a vat to a temperature of not less than 63°C and holding the cream at that temperature for at least 30 min. This 'holder method' is slow and inefficient, as heating and cooling are carried out in the same vessel. It is only suitable for small quantities of cream.

For larger-scale production, cream is treated in a continuous plate heat exchanger (HTST) to a minimum of 72°C for 15 s. There is a danger of oxidative rancidity promoted by migration of copper from the serum to the fat globules. This increases with the higher processing temperatures and, for this reason, it is recommended that the cream used for buttermaking be processed at a maximum of 77°C for 15 s. However, in practice a temperature of 80°C and above is usual. Often the caramelized flavour obtained by heating to 85°C for 17 s is preferred. *See* Pasteurization, Principles

Vacreation is a form of heat treatment under vacuum, developed to remove feed and weed taints. It is a system commonly practised in New Zealand where the herds are pasture fed and taints can be easily passed into the butter. The heated cream is held in contact with steam under reduced pressure, then separated to allow volatile taints to be drawn off. This is a combined heating and flavour-stripping treatment. Evaporative cooling to approximately 60°C may also be used to adjust the fat content of the cream. The final cooling of the cream takes places in a plate heat exchanger. A milder, flavour-stripping method using vacuum treatment after an HTST process may also be used.

The cream used for buttermaking must be cooled and 'aged' to optimize the crystallization of the fat globules. The latent heat released will increase the temperature of the cream in the silo to 7–8°C from the initial cooled temperature of 5°C. Ageing, i.e. holding of the cream at a temperature of approximately 5°C for a minimum of 8 h, is essential to produce butter of the desired texture. Adequate temperature controls are key elements in successful buttermaking.

Both the rate of cooling and the temperature of holding play an important part in the size of the crystals, and in the proportion of solid-to-liquid fat achieved within the globules. Large silo tanks for storage are preferable to a series of small cream tanks. There is improved homogeneity, allowing the buttermaking equipment to operate with a more consistent product for a longer period.

Variable treatments to allow for seasonal compositional changes and to improve the spreadability of butter have not been entirely successful. The incorporation of vegetable oils with cream has overtaken these developments, although the resultant product is not butter.

Water

In a practical treatise issued to students at buttermaking classes in the 1920s, it was stated that 'if impure water be used, the bacteria introduced . . . . are a source of many troubles . . .'. That statement is as true today as it was then: water wherever used must of the highest possible microbiological quality.

Lactic Cultures

A soured or ripened cream is traditionally required to produce lactic butter. This is the preferred flavour in some countries. Although it is possible to allow milk or cream to sour naturally, it is neither advisable nor practical. A culture of lactic microorganisms – *Lactococcus lactis* subsp. *cremoris* (formerly *Streptococcus cremoris*), *Lactococcus lactis* subsp. *lactis* (*Streptococcus lactis*), *Lactococcus lactis* biovar. *diacetylactis* (*Strepto-*

coccus diacetylactis) – may be added to the cream to produce the desired flavour and aroma. The primary aroma producers are *L. lactis* biovar. *diacetylactis* and *Leuconostoc mesenteroides* subsp. *cremoris*. ***See*** Lactic Acid Bacteria

Salt

Salt adds flavour and also acts as a preservative in sweet cream butter. The latter is of less importance if good hygiene is observed. For short-term storage, bulk butter is stored at temperatures of −18°C whether it has added salt or not. Intervention (EEC subsidized) butter – for long-term storage – is unsalted and is stored at −25°C.

Only pure vacuum-dried salt (of at least BSI 998 (1969) or equivalent standard) should be used for butter.

Manufacturing Processes

Churn Method

A batch-type butter churn may vary in capacity from a few litres up to maximum of about 45 000 litres. These churns were originally made of wood (Fig. 1) but latterly of stainless steel.

After cleaning and disinfecting the churn, it must be specially prepared to prevent the butter from sticking to the surface. With wood this is achieved by scalding with boiling water and immediately cooling with chilled water. This treatment leaves a film of water on the surface of the wood and prevents the butter from adhering to it. All wooden equipment must be kept wet until used.

The surface of stainless steel equipment also requires special physical preparation. The detergents used in the cleaning of such equipment must contain silicates to maintain this special 'non-stick' surface. ***See*** Cleaning Procedures in the Factory, Types of Detergent; Cleaning Procedures in the Factory, Types of Disinfectant

Batch butter churns may be barrel or cone shaped with fixed or rotating internal 'workers'. As the churn is rotated the combined actions of rotating and beating cause the cream to break, forming the butter grains (fatty phase) and buttermilk (aqueous phase).

During the first few turns, gases, e.g. carbon dioxide from heterofermentative fermentation, may be liberated from the cream. In order to maintain an even pressure within the churn it is necessary to release these gases. This is done by depressing a small valve in the lid of the churn.

Each churn has an indicator glass – a small window through which it is possible to see what is happening inside the churn. When hand churning, the cream feels heavier when it begins to thicken. This takes about 15–

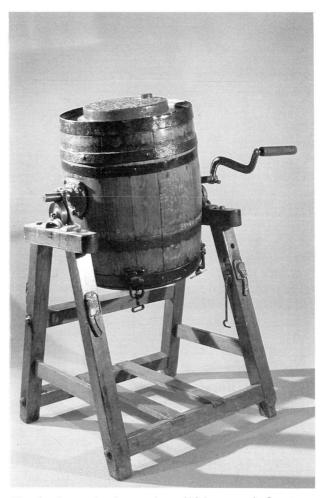

Fig. 1 A wooden butter churn (19th century). Courtesy of the National Dairy Council.

20 min from the beginning of churning. The cream breaks and forms small grains of butter which are clearly seen on the indicator glass. The actual size of the butter grains varies according to the type and size of the churn. It is essential not to allow them to grow and form lumps which will cause an uneven distribution of buttermilk.

For hand churning, the grains should be kept small, approximately 3 mm in diameter – traditionally stated as the size of wheat grains.

Chilled water at approximately 5°C is used to harden and control the size of these grains, as well as removing the traces of buttermilk. Washing reduces the yield, and is not necessary if the cream is of good quality and all the necessary hygienic precautions have been observed in the preparation of the butter churn. Traditionally, well-washed butter will have a longer shelf life than unwashed and overworked butter.

Salt may be added dry or in the form of brine as a final wash. The addition of brine (10% solution) to butter grains has been used to reduce the need for chilled water. This can be important during warm weather when there is a lack of chilled water. It will also prevent streakiness

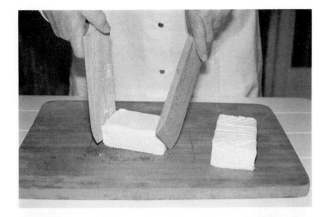

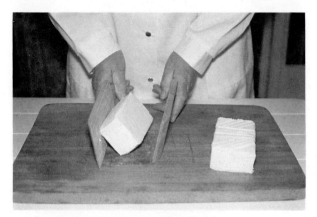

Fig. 2   Scotch hands. Courtesy of Joan Pozzoli.

due to uneven mixing of the salt. For dry salting, the calculated quantity is sprinkled onto the butter grains to give approximately 2% in the final product.

The butter grains are 'worked' to expel excess moisture, create an even, fine distribution of water droplets and produce a close textured, evenly coloured product. This may be carried out using the workers inside the churn or externally on a small scale, by using Scotch hands. These are made of grooved wood (or plastic), and are also used to shape and print attractive designs on the finished packs (Fig. 2).

During the period of working, drainage and addition of dry salt, samples are tested to determine the salt and moisture contents. The operator determines the 'end-point' of working when the moisture content is between 15·5 and 16% and by visual assessment of the butter. At this stage the butter is removed from the churn in readiness for packing.

The moisture content of butter must not exceed the legal maximum of 16%. Manufacturers attempt to be as near that limit as possible to ensure the maximum yield.

Cultured Butters

Traditionally, cream is inoculated with specific cultures of bacteria. The reduction in pH and development of flavours produce a lactic-flavoured end product. It is regarded by some as a more desirable product, i.e. a fuller flavoured butter. *See* Starter Cultures

This method of making butter requires starter culture facilities with the necessary laboratory controls, and additional equipment such as cream-ripening tanks as well as cooling and ageing facilities. There must also be a well-controlled programme of temperature controls and pH monitoring.

The cream is inoculated with approximately 1% of culture and incubated at 20–27°C to achieve a final pH of 5·3–4·7, depending on the preferred lactic flavour. The cream is then cooled to stop the fermentation and to attain the desired fat crystallization.

The method of manufacture on a batch basis is no different from that employed for sweet cream. The disadvantage of this traditional system is that the buttermilk has a lactic content which causes great problems in its disposal. The behaviour of the starter culture is not always consistent, and this can result in end product variations.

Because of the problems and expense of culturing cream and the disposal of 'lactic' buttermilk, several methods have been developed to make lactic or cultured butter from sweet cream.

The NIZO method developed in the mid-1970s consisted of churning sweet cream and adding a special mix containing cultured whey concentrate and bacterial culture after making the butter grains. This gave the major advantage of being able to manufacture from sweet cream, thus producing sweet cream buttermilk, which has a far greater commercial value than cultured cream buttermilk.

The need to maximize production efficiencies, combined with technological development, has resulted in there now being many methods of making lactic or cultured butters from sweet cream.

The indirect biological culturing system, as for example, described by Pasilac – Danish Turnkey Dairies Ltd, involves the addition of two types of prepared starter culture to the churn at the working stage. The combination of strong aroma-producing bacteria and the acidity of the culture mix results in the final pH and flavour of the butter conforming to that of traditional cultured butter.

The addition of a starter distillate provides an alternative method of flavouring butter without the need for culturing equipment.

Continuous Buttermaking

Continuous buttermaking equipment began to be widely used in the 1960s. The success of this equipment was such that, within a decade, most of the batch churns used in creamery manufacture had been superseded.

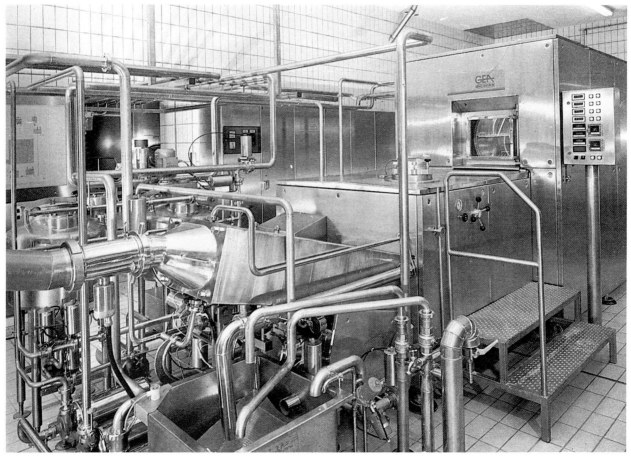

Fig. 3 A continuous buttermaker. Courtesy of Gea Ahlborn.

The initial advantages in hygiene, control of quality and process efficiency are being constantly improved.

Cream processing is an integral part of the whole buttermaking system. The preparation of the cream is similar to that for traditional manufacture. From the storage tanks it is pumped into the first stage of the buttermaker at a constant speed and temperature.

The capacity of continuous buttermakers varies from small units of $12 \, kg \, h^{-1}$ to more than 10 tonnes h^{-1} (Fig. 3). Although the design features vary, the basic principles remain the same.

The buttermaker consists of: (1) the beating and churning section; and (2) the working section.

The Beating and Churning Section

The beater operates within a cylindrical chamber. It is in this first chamber that the fat globule membrane is broken and the initial agglomeration takes place. The mixture of small butter grains and buttermilk is then transported from this beating chamber into the next unit, the churning chamber. This consists of a drum where the final churning takes place and in which there is a perforated filter – a separation drum – to separate the buttermilk from the butter granules.

Cooling may be effected by circulating chilled water in the walls of either churning chamber. In some machines, the first buttermilk is cooled and recirculated. It is in this particular section that the grains of butter are allowed to grow into the required size.

The speed of the beaters, the temperature of churning and the butterfat content of the cream will all vary slightly. An experienced buttermaker will adjust these parameters according to the season, the equipment, the texture and consistency of the resultant butter. A firmer fat and, therefore, firmer butter is obtained in winter than in summer. In addition, the temperature of the cream has to be maintained at a lower temperature, e.g. 5–7°C, in summer whereas it could be at 10°C in winter.

There is an observation window for the operators – similar to the sight glass of traditional equipment. The control panels may also have display screens, allowing operators to observe the processes inside the machine.

The Working Section

This is sometimes described as a 'cannon' due to its shape. Butter is conveyed by an Archimedean-type, screw-conveyor through aperture plates. The process of kneading or working of the butter influences the final

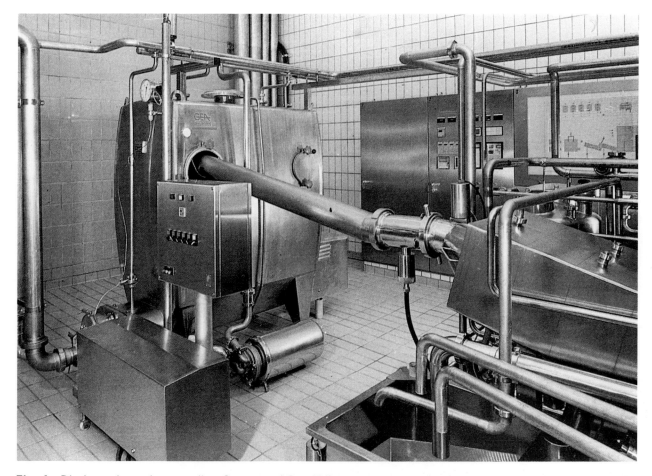

Fig. 4 Discharge into a butter trolley. Courtesy of Gea Ahlborn.

body and texture of the finished product. The moisture droplets must be fine and evently dispersed.

During this process of working, salt (if required) is added in the form of a 50% saturated slurry. Water may be added to adjust the final moisture content and, in the case of lactic butters, the mix of distilled flavour or concentrated bacterial cultures is added at this stage. The second part of the working section operates at a much higher speed to facilitate the mixing of the culture or salt.

The working sections are cooled with chilled water. The link between the first and second working sections operates under vacuum. This provides a controlled deaeration of the butter, so giving the end product a very close texture. The vacuum and auger speeds of the working section must be maintained to ensure a constant level of flow.

The body and texture of butter worked under vacuum is quite different from the open structure of traditionally worked butter. What was considered acceptable, or even desirable, in a premium product manufactured under traditional methods is no longer so.

Although there has been much technological advance, seasonal influences still affect process para-

meters, and an experienced operator remains of paramount importance.

To allow for the stoppages that must occur during normal production, a 'balance tank' (Fig. 4) is normally maintained between the buttermaker and packing equipment. This butter 'trolley', as it is known, is constructed of stainless steel and performs the essential task of maintaining the flow of butter both from the buttermaker and to the packing equipment.

Packing

Wholesale

The butter is packed in bulk or retail packs directly from the churn or from the trolley of a continuous buttermaker. Bulk butter is normally packed in 25 kg quantities in cardboard cartons. These can be lined with parchment paper, but coloured polythene, enabling the inner wrapper to be readily seen, is the preferred lining material.

The simplest form of bulk butter packer is the 'Vane' type packer – this is simply a hopper into which the butter is fed, either manually or pumped from the

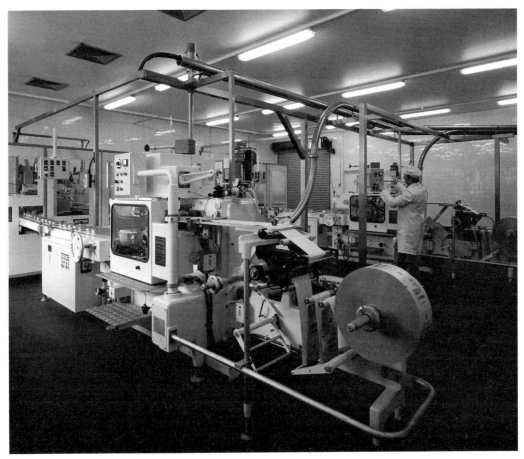

Fig. 5 Packing of retail butter. Courtesy of Whitland Creamery, Dairy Crest Foods.

buttermaker trolley. The butter is extruded by a screw-conveyor through a suitably sized nozzle into the lined carton when it is presented to the nozzle. When the carton is full, the flow of butter is stopped and the butter is 'cut', with a heated wire. The full carton is then removed and checked for weight, which is adjusted manually. The liner is closed, ensuring there is no exposed product, and the carton is sealed, coded and palletized. The normal quantity is 50 cases of 25 kg butter per pallet.

For large-scale production, automatic packers are normally an integral part of continuous buttermaking installations. The cardboard cartons are loaded flat and the inner wrap is polythene from a reel. The machine forms the carton, lines it and presents it for filling. Once full, the weight is checked and, if necessary, additions are made via an 'injection unit' which adds the required quantity of butter under the original surface.

On achieving the correct weight (25 kg), the liner is folded over the top surface, and the carton is closed, sealed and coded. This minimal exposure to the danger of possible contamination has contributed greatly to the extension of the keeping quality of butter. Automatic palletization is also a feature of some installations.

Retail

Butter is required to be sold in metric quantities. Most retail packs are in 250 or 500 g weights. The shape of the packs will vary from a brick of differing dimensions to rolls. They may be foil or parchment wrapped. Attractively designed plastic tubs holding 250 or 500 g are also available.

For retail packing (Fig. 5), the butter is formed in an appropriately shaped chamber on a rotating drum. This formed portion (roll or brick) is pushed out of the chamber into the waiting coded wrapper (parchment or foil), which is then folded. The portions are check weighed before passing onwards to an automatic case packer and palletizer. The butter at this stage is still very soft in consistency, and any mishandling is likely to deform the portion.

Catering butter portions are packed in foil or plastic tubs with foil lids. The machines developed to pack this size of butter portion must operate at maximum efficiency. The quality of the butter, in terms of body and texture, is of secondary importance. The butter is extruded into the partly folded foil held within a shaped chamber, and the folding is then completed. Alterna-

The Product and its Manufacture

tively, the butter is discharged into a plastic tub before sealing.

Larger catering packs, e.g. 2 kg plastic tubs, are filled by extrusion before the lid is applied.

Reworked Butter

When there is insufficient cream for the direct packing of retail packs, i.e. fresh butter from the buttermaker, it is necessary to rework bulk butter, i.e. wholesale (25 kg) stored blocks. This butter, which has been stored at either −18 or −25°C, must be attempered, i.e. brought to a temperature suitable for packing.

Attemperation traditionally involves placing bulk butter in a store at 5–8°C for a period to attain that temperature. The use of microwave tunnel heaters has reduced the space and time necessary, and is a far more efficient way of attemperation than the traditional method. Blocks of butter may be brought up to blending temperature within hours, then blended and standardized on a batch or continuous basis to the required salt and moisture contents for packing.

Product Evaluation

Notwithstanding the aesthetic requirements of packaging and any legal requirements, the most important quality parameters of butter are its taste and keeping quality.

The modern continuous machines and their associated equipment are normally cleaned in place. Close collaboration between the design engineers, the operators and the quality controllers is necessary to ensure effective cleaning. *See* Plant Design, Basic Principles; Plant Design, Designing for Hygienic Operation; Plant Design, Process Control and Automation

Attention to detail, monitoring the critical aspects of the process, whether it be batch or continuous, is essential. Only thus can good quality butter be produced. It is, however, normal to sample the finished product to confirm that the desired microbiological, chemical and organoleptic qualities have been achieved.

Microbiological

The standards set for bulk butter by the Intervention Board for Agricultural Produce is as follows:

Total viable count	Target < 1000, maximum 5000
Coliforms	Absence in 0·1 gm^{-1}
Yeasts and moulds	Less than 10 g^{-1}

These standards may not always be attainable. Each manufacturer and customer will have their own quality parameters as dictated by circumstances and perceived quality standards.

Chemical

The UK Butter Regulatons (Statutory Instrument 1966/1074) state that butter must contain at least 80% milk fat, not more than 2% milk solids other than fat and not more than 16% water. Only if the salt content exceeds 3% may the level of fat be reduced to 78%.

Constant monitoring of the moisture and salt levels – where appropriate – is carried out during processing. On-line automatic devices are available which link the machine controls to the moisture and salt determinations. These have not yet proven themselves, and most manufacturers continue the practice of laboratory analysis.

Organoleptic Grading

The grading of butter involves much more than the tasting of the product. First it must be carried out by a trained person. Grading normally takes place at not less than 48 h after manufacture – a period necessary to allow the butter to 'cool' and 'settle'. The temperature of the butter at grading should be in the region of 10°C. *See* Sensory Evaluation, Sensory Characteristics of Human Foods; Sensory Evaluation, Practical Considerations

A sample of the bulk butter is taken using a special instrument called a butter iron. With this, a representative sample is obtained. For retail portions, the brick or roll is cut half way down, and the lower half is broken apart.

The qualities measured at grading are:

(1) Flavour and Aroma. These are judged by the smell and taste. A portion of the butter should be tasted but not swallowed. *See* Sensory Evaluation, Aroma; Sensory Evaluation, Taste

(2) Body and Texture. A premium butter should have a close body and waxy texture. The appearance of the butter on the iron will provide the experienced butter grader with much information. A portion of the plug is broken off to enable the texture to be examined, and a section is cut to observe the cut surface. Each parameter has a described optimum. *See* Sensory Evaluation, Texture

(3) Appearance and Finish. Evenness of colour and absence of mottling, giving what is termed a clean bright butter, is the requirement for good-quality butter. The packs, whether they be bulk or retail, should be well presented with no exposed butter. *See* Sensory Evaluation, Appearance

(4) Absence of Free Moisture. Traditionally made butter had a very open texture and free moisture was a

frequent fault. With the advent of the vacuum section in continuous buttermakers, this particular characteristic or fault is now rarely seen. If moisture is present, it will be seen as droplets on the cut surface.

Each of these attributes is given a score, dependent on the perceived relative importance of the characteristic. Varying pointing systems are used, e.g. the Creamery Proprietors Association grading system allocates points as follows:

	Maximum points
Flavour and aroma	50
Body and texture	20
Colour and appearance	20
Absence of free moisture	10
Total	100

The butter is placed in a grade appropriate to the total points, e.g. 'extra selected' has not less than 93 points including not less than 47 points for flavour and aroma. *See* Sensory Evaluation, Sensory Rating and Scoring Methods

Defects

Defects which arise in the finished product can normally be attributed to problems arising from two main areas: (1) the quality of the original milk or cream and its handling; (2) manufacturing defects; or a combination of both.

Taints and poor microbiological quality will give rise to off-flavours. A reduced shelf life and physical defects can be caused by poor hygiene, temperature abuse, the use of inappropriate pumps and overagitation.

Cream received from other sources, e.g. accommodation cream, can give rise to numerous problems unless the receiving plant can be absolutely sure of the conditions under which it was produced and handled. The practice of transporting cream to central butter-making units is not conducive to the production of the best-quality butter, nor is it the most efficient operation.

Operating faults, such as an imbalance between the speed of the first section of the buttermaker and too slow a cream flow, will cause the grains to be too large. Consequently, the buttermilk drains poorly and the result will be a streaky, weak-bodied butter with free moisture.

Underchurning, with too high a cream flow and too slow a churn speed, results in small grains and incomplete separation of the fat and aqueous phases. This gives a butter with a very high moisture content and a pale colour.

Overworking due to, for example, too much product in the working section, excessive conveyor speed or apertures too restricted, will give a weak-bodied, lifeless and sticky butter, difficult to handle and likely to lose points at grading.

An open-textured butter with uneven salt and moisture distribution may be caused by too slow an auger speed, inadequate vacuum or too little product in the working section, or insufficient restriction at the adjustable apertures.

A mottled butter with excess moisture or excess salt can be the result of an inaccurate salt:water ratio in the slurry, or an improperly mixed slurry.

Packed butters held under chilled conditions have a finite life. Defects can develop on exposure to light, and taints are easily absorbed if butter is stored near strong flavours or smells. Foil-wrapped retail packs stored under the recommended chilled conditions should retain their premium quality for 2 months, whereas parchment-wrapped butters will develop surface faults after some 4–6 weeks.

Bibliography

Murphy MF (1990) In: Robinson RK (ed.) *Dairy Microbiology*, 2nd edn, vol. II. London: Elsevier.

Rajah KK and Burgess KJ (eds) (1991) *Milk Fat, Production, Technology and Utilization*. Huntingdon: Society of Dairy Technology.

Romney AJD (ed.) (1990) *CIP: Cleaning in Place*, 2nd edn. Huntingdon: Society of Dairy Technology.

Rothwell J (ed.) (1988) *Cream Procesing Manual*, 2nd edn. Huntingdon: Society of Dairy Technology.

Wilbey RA (1986) In: Robinson RK (ed.) *Modern Dairy Technology*, vol. I. London: Elsevier.

Wilbey RA (1991) In: Russell JB and Pritchard L (eds) *Analysis of Oilseeds Fats and Fatty Foods*. London: Elsevier.

Eurwen Richards
Wembley, UK

Properties and Analysis

In the manufacture of butter, cream is churned to bring about a phase inversion and then worked to give a product having a continuous fat phase and a disperse phase containing water and globular fat. The properties of butter are determined both by its chemical composition and by the physical treatments applied throughout its manufacture. This article reviews the physical properties and chemical composition of butter, what factors affect these properties and how they may be determined.

Physical Changes During Churning

The first stage of the physical transformation of cream into butter occurs during the ageing or tempering of the cream prior to churning. During this period, milk fat crystallizes and the fat globule membrane is weakened. The churning process is based on the incorporation of air into cream to create a foam and is achieved by vigorous agitation. Fat globule membranes already weakened by cold ageing are further damaged by the mechanical stresses applied and liquid fat escapes. This brings about collapse of the foam and clumping of the fat globules to produce butter granules which are then worked together to form butter. Some globular fat will be found in the final product, but this will depend on the prechurning cream tempering treatment and the severity of the working conditions before and after processing. *See* Cream, Types of Cream

Butter Microstructure

The microstructure of butter and the influence of processing factors on it have been studied using freeze–fracture techniques in association with electron microscopy (Fig. 1). These have shown how cream tempering conditions can influence the milk fat crystallization pattern within the globules and hence their process stability and, ultimately, product firmness. The cold–warm–cold cream tempering procedure which was developed to improve winter butter spreadability results in globules with a thick surface shell of solid fat and crystal aggregates of varying shapes and sizes in the liquid fat in the interior. This type of cream globule can withstand mechanical stress during churning and consequently gives a softer butter with a higher proportion of globular fat than is obtained from a low-temperature cream treatment. Electron microscopic studies have also

shown how intensive mechanical working during processing destroys fat globules, resulting in a highly homogeneous butter structure with a more crystalline interglobular phase and consequently a firmer butter.

Chemical Changes During Churning

Butter is basically a concentration of milk fat along with some water and milk solids not fat (MSNF). The composition of the fat in butter reflects that of the original milk fat although there is some loss of phospholipid, sterols and free fatty acids, particularly volatile fatty acids, into the buttermilk during separation and churning. Greater change occurs in the physical state of milk fat during churning than in the chemical nature of its constituents. However, the combination of agitation of the milk during milking and extended holding of the milk on the farm and at the factory before pasteurization lead also to an increase in concentration of free fatty acids and consequently lipolysed flavour in the product. The increase in lipolysis is probably due to increased accessibility of the fat to lipolytic enzymes because of damage or loss of the protective milk fat globule membrane. Lipolysed flavour may increase in stored butter due to the preferential release of short-chain fatty acids by enzymes with a high specificity for these acids (elaborated by psychrotrophic bacteria). In sweet cream butter, in particular unsalted butter, the primary cause of flavour impairment is lipolytic rancidity. Thus, good manufacturing practice both at the farm and the factory is necessary to prevent high free fatty acid levels in the final product. *See* Fatty Acids, Properties; Milk, Dietary Importance

Chemical and Physical Properties of Butter

Chemical Composition and Analysis

The composition of butter is described in the food regulations of most countries. Typically, butter contains 80–84% milk fat, 15·3–15·9% water, about 1% milk solids other than fat (casein, lactose and minerals) and 0·03–1·8% salt. Milk fat is the only fat permitted and it must be as secreted by the cow, with nothing added or removed from it during processing. A maximum water content (16%) is usually stated as it is important for good keeping properties of the product. Butter may be salted or unsalted, but may not contain any added antioxidants. In some countries natural colouring agents such as annatto, turmeric, carotene or curcumin are permitted. Neutralizing salts and lactic acid cultures are allowed for the manufacture of ripened or lactic butters. *See* Colours, Properties and Determination of Natural Pigments; Lactic Acid Bacteria

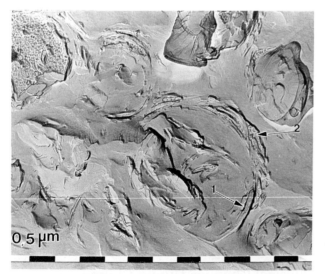

0.5 μm

Fig. 1 A scanning electron micrograph of a cross-fractured butter globule showing fat crystals orientated parallel to the droplet surface (arrow 1) and traces of remaining water around the droplet (arrow 2). From Juriaanse AC and Heertje I (1988).

Properties and Analysis

Table 1. Chemical constants for milk fat

Chemical constant	Value
Saponification value	220–240
SV = mg KOH needed to saponify 1 g of fat	
Iodine value	26–42
IV = g of iodine reacted with 100 g of fat	
Reichert–Meissl number	20–35
RMW = ml of 0·1 N alkali needed to neutralize water-soluble volatile fatty acids distilled from 5 g of saponified fat	
Polenske number	1·0–3·3
PN = ml of 0·1 N alkali needed to neutralize the water-insoluble volatile fatty acids distilled from 5 g of saponified fat	
Kirschner number	18–30
KN = ml of 0·1 N alkali needed to neutralize the water-soluble volatile fatty acids distilled from 5 g of saponified fat and which form soluble silver salts	

Data reprinted with permission of John Wiley and Sons. From Walstra P and Jenness R (1984).

Table 2. Fatty acid composition of milk fat triacyglycerols

Fatty acid	g per 100 g fatty acid		Class
4:0	3·3	4·9	Saturated short chain
6:0	1·6		
8:0	1·3	7·4	Saturated medium chain
10:0	3·0		
12:0	3·1		
14:0	9·5	50·4	Saturated long chain
16:0	26·3		
18:0	14·6		
16:1	2·3	32·1	Mono-unsaturated
18:1	29·8		
18:2	2·4	3·2	Polyunsaturated
18:3	0·8		

Data from Gurr MI (1989)

Analytical methods for butter are included in the inventory prepared by the International Dairy Federation (IDF), the Association of Official Analytical Chemists (AOAC) and the International Standards Organization (ISO) on methods of analysis for milk and milk products. Apart from standard methods of analysis of butter components (moisture, fat, solids not fat, and salt) other analytical methods are catalogued, including methods to characterize milk fat, to determine the presence of a foreign fat and to detect rancidity in butter.

Not surprisingly, many of the analyses for butter are concerned with the composition and properties of its fat. Some chemical constants for milk fat are summarized in Table 1. Milk fat contains a comparatively high proportion of water-soluble volatile fatty acids, in particular butyric acid. The presence of these is the basis of both traditional (Reichert–Meissl, Kirschner) and modern (chromatography) tests to detect the presence of adulterating fat. Iodine value (a measure of unsaturation) is a useful identifier of summer or winter butter but it has commercial value too. Continental buttermakers apply the appropriate cream-tempering treatment, the Alnarp process, to produce harder or softer butter on the basis of cream iodine value.

Although more than 450 fatty acids have been identified in milk fat, only twelve of these (Table 2) play a significant role in determining its physical and chemi-cal properties. For detailed information on the composition of milk fat it is necessary to use chromatographic techniques. Fatty acid profiles of milk fat are obtained by first preparing the more volatile fatty acid methyl esters and then separating these by gas–liquid chromatography (GLC) using a packed or capillary column and a flame ionization detector. A triacylglycerol (triglyceride) fingerprint of the fat may also be obtained using capillary column GLC, with resolution on the basis of carbon number and degree of unsaturation possible. Rapidly developing high-performance liquid chromatography (HPLC) techniques have found application for milk triacylglycerol separation while a combination of techniques, e.g. silver nitrate thin-layer chromatography (TLC), and high-temperature GLC, can provide more detailed informaton on the molecular structure of milk fat. *See* Chromatography, High-performance Liquid Chromatography; Chromatography, Gas Chromatography; Phospholipids, Determination; Triglycerides, Characterization and Determination

Factors Influencing Chemical Composition

The fatty acids in milk fat may be divided into those synthesized *de novo* in the mammary gland, C_4–C_{14} and a proportion of C_{16} acids, and those taken up by the gland from the circulating blood, a proportion of C_{16} and the longer-chain C_{18} acids. The principal factors influencing the relative contributions of fatty acids from these two sources are stage of lactation and diet. Changes in the shorter-chain acids, C_4–C_{14}, can be accounted for mainly by stage of lactation while those of the longer-chain acids, $C_{16:0}$, $C_{18:0}$ and $C_{18:1}$, are diet related. Summer grazing of fresh pasture leads to a softer milk fat with a decrease in $C_{16:0}$ and an increase in $C_{18:0}$ and $C_{18:1}$ acids, while the reverse occurs during winter feeding of concentrates and silage.

Table 3. Physical constants of milk fat

Physical constant	Value
Refractive index (40°C)	1·4524–1·4561
Specific gravity (37·8°C)	0·910–0·913
Melting interval	28–33°C
Solidification interval	24–19°C

Data from Egan M *et al.* (1981).

Supplementation of the cows' diet with fats or oils to increase energy input can also affect fatty acid composition. Generally, such a diet will tend to increase the yields of fatty acids $C_{18:0}$ and $C_{18:1}$ while decreasing the yields of the shorter-chain acids C_6–C_{16}. If the supplemented fat is presented in a protected form, then it can pass through the rumen without being subjected to ruminal lipolysis or biohydrogenation and the resulting milk fat composition will reflect that of the supplement. Protected fats also allow rumen metabolic activity to proceed unimpaired by the adverse effect of large amounts of fat. This technology has been used to produce butter with higher levels of $C_{18:2}$ fatty acids and greatly improved spreadability. However, the increase in polyunsaturated fatty acid levels greatly enhances the oxidative susceptibility of milk fat, leads to too soft a product and oiling off at 21°C. An alternative approach has been based on exploiting the $C_{18:0}$ to $C_{18:1}$ conversion which occurs during milk fat biosynthesis by the action of desaturase enzymes in the cow's intestine and mammary gland. The diet must supply a high proportion of C_{18} fatty acids (e.g. rapeseed or soya beans) in order to optimize the desaturating activity of the bovine tissue. The resulting milk fat has increased levels of $C_{18:1}$ (oleic) acid and decreased levels of $C_{16:0}$ (palmitic) acid. Mono-unsaturated acids are less susceptible to oxidative reactions than polyunsaturated acids and the increased content of oleic acid in butter greatly enhances its spreadability at low temperatures.

Physical Properties

Physical Constants

Values for physical constants of milk fat are presented in Table 3. The refractive index for milk fat at 40°C was once a valuable indication of its purity, but nowadays many fats used in the margarine industry will give similar figures. The specific gravity of milk fat may be measured at different temperatures, although the difference in specific gravity between milk fat and other fats is greatest around 40°C.

Milk fat melts and solidifies over a temperature range, so rather than having a melting or solidification point it has a melting and solidification interval (Table 3).

Ideally these points should coincide, but the dependence of the solidification interval on rate of cooling and the influence of previous thermal history on melting interval, as well as the dissolution rather than melting of fat crystals during heating, means that they rarely do so. Further information on the melting behaviour of milk fat may be obtained using differential scanning calorimetry. This analysis is based on the thermal transitions that occur in a substance during heating and cooling.

The solid fat content in milk fat over a range of temperatures may be measured by nuclear magnetic resonance (NMR). This technique operates on the principle that protons placed in a strong magnetic field can, under certain circumstances, absorb energy from electromagnetic waves. This absorption, termed nuclear magnetic resonance, depends on the physical state of the protons and allows determination of the solid fat content (% SFC). The method was previously only applied to butter for research purposes but is now a regular quality control test for the new dairy spreads whose physical properties at refrigerator temperatures are an important selling point. *See* Spectroscopy, Nuclear Magnetic Resonance

Rheology

Butter may be described as a plastic fat and depicted for rheological purposes by the Bingham model which describes ideal plastic behaviour. In rheological terms a plastic material flows when a stress greater than a limiting value (yield value) acts on it. Various instrumental techniques to evaluate butter firmness were examined by the International Dairy Federation (IDF), who recommended the cone penetrometer as easy, quick and cheap to use and with acceptable reproducibility. The IDF method relates penetration depth (p) to apparent yield stress (AYS) by the equation $AYS = gW/\pi p^2 \tan^2$ (cone angle $\div 2$), where W is the cone mass and g the acceleration due to gravity. For more detailed information on the textural characteristics of butter, a two-bite compression test using the Instron Universal Testing Equipment can be carried out. This provides a texture profile from which such properties as fracturability, hardness, cohesiveness and springiness can be measured.

Factors Influencing Butter Consistency

A number of factors influence butter consistency, not all within the control of the manufacturers. The proportion of solid fat in butter is highly correlated with product firmness and is strongly influenced by the cows' diet. Feeding is responsible for the difference in firmness between summer and winter butters and can be directly related to the change in fatty acid composition of the milk fat, which is largely due to the changeover from summer grazing to winter silage and concentrates.

Properties and Analysis

The number and size of fat crystals also affect consistency and are determined by crystallization temperature and rate during cream ageing. Slow or stepwise cooling promotes the formation of fewer, larger crystals and a lower solid fat content which favour a softer fat.

Plastic fats like butter possess a three-dimensional crystal network held together by reversible weak van der Waals attractive bonds and irreversible stronger bonds formed where crystals have grown together. During mechanical working of butter, such as the microfixing of bulk butter prior to printing, the butter hardness is reduced; although the butter increases in firmness again over several weeks it will not reach its original value. Work softening may be explained by the breaking of the bonds in the crystal network, while the reformation of reversible bonds into a new network structure is responsible for the gradual increase in hardness. This property of work softening has been made use of by butter manufacturers to produce an easier spreading butter. Recovery of hardness during storage, a factor accentuated by temperature fluctuations, means such a product requires careful control during marketing.

Nutritional Properties of Butter

Butter, along with other fat-containing dairy products, contributes just under one-quarter of dietary lipid in the UK. Much interest has centred on dietary lipid in relation to coronary heart disease (CHD) and atherosclerosis. Two inversely-related cholesterol-containing blood lipid fractions, low-density lipoprotein (LDL) and high-density lipoprotein (HDL), have an important influence on these diseases. High concentrations of plasma LDL generally indicate increased risk of CHD with dietary saturated fats tending to increase LDL concentrations and polyunsaturated fats tending to decrease them. Milk fat, although containing about 30% oleic acid ($C_{18:1}$), is defined as a saturated fat, probably because of the low levels of polyunsaturated fatty acids present. Butter itself has been shown to cause elevated LDL levels and this has been linked not only to its content of saturated fatty acids but also to their esterified configuration. However, there is now evidence that *cis* mono-unsaturated fatty acids, far from occupying a neutral position in the diet and CHD, actually lower LDL concentrations while maintaining beneficial HDL levels. Indeed, high levels of polyunsaturated fatty acids in the diet may be detrimental to health, increasing the incidence of some forms of cancer. Consequently, the new 'monobutters' containing elevated levels of mono-unsaturated fatty acids (mostly oleic acid) will be attractive to consumers not only for improved spreadability but also for health reasons. *See* Cholesterol, Role of Cholesterol in Heart Disease; Fatty Acids, Dietary Importance; Lipoproteins

Government recommendations for a healthy diet have included a reduction in total fat intake, particularly saturated fat. However, the balance of nutrients and fat types must also be considered. Milk fat is an important source of fat-soluble vitamins, especially vitamin A, and provides small but useful amounts of vitamin D to diets of children, pregnant and lactating women, whose requirements are particularly high. *See* Cholecalciferol, Physiology; Retinol, Physiology

Dietary lipids, of the correct balance, are essential for our health but, in general, food will only be eaten if it is palatable. Milk fat contributes not only a pleasant flavour and aroma, but also an attractive texture and mouth feel.

Additives and Contaminants

Certain additives such as salt, natural colouring agents, lactic cultures and neutralizing salts may be permitted in butter but these vary from country to country. However, butter may also contain very low concentrations of other components, called contaminants. Although contaminants are primarily synthetic chemicals, they also include microbial toxins, endogenous plant toxicants, heavy metals and radionuclides. *See* Contamination, Types and Causes

Chemicals such as the organochlorine-type pesticides and polychlorinated biphenyls have been scrutinized as they are lipophilic and tend to accumulate in the fat. However, levels of these chemicals detected in butter are below limits set in most countries and there is legislation in place governing their use. Organophosphates and carbamates are also widely used as pesticides but, as they are not lipophilic and are readily broken down by the cow, they give less cause for concern.

The risk of contamination of milk by such substances as detergents, disinfectants and plasticizers (from packing materials and pipelines) may be minimized by good production practice both on the farm and at the factory. Antibiotics in milk can have a detrimental effect on the manufacture of cultured products and their use on farms is governed by legislation. Strict control of feed manufacture should avoid mould growth and the possibility of mycotoxin production and contamination of the milk. *See* Antibiotics and Drugs, Uses in Food Production; Mycotoxins, Occurrence and Determination

There is little heavy metal contamination of butter through the feed, the cow acting as an effective filter. However, some contamination with copper and iron from dairy equipment can occur during and after milking; these metals act as pro-oxidants and the manufacturing treatments which are applied to butter make its component fat phase particularly susceptible. *See* Heavy Metal Toxicology

There is little cause for concern over radionuclide levels in milk. Nevertheless, since the Chernobyl reactor incident in May 1986 and the associated increase in radioactive fallout over Europe and Scandinavia, considerable monitoring of agricultural produce has taken place. The isotopes concerned were iodine-131, caesium-134 and caesium-137. Although iodine-131 has a short half-life of 8 days, iodine accumulates in the thyroid gland and high concentrations can be reached. Milk tested was found to contain all three radioactive isotopes of concern but butter had very low counts, with the isotopes being located in the serum rather than the fat phase. *See* Radioactivity in Food

Dairy Spreads

Traditional table spread products such as butter and margarine now compete with new dairy spreads which currently hold over 20% of the market. These newer blended spreads have improved spreadability over butter, are more competitively priced and appeal to the health lobby with their increased levels of unsaturated fatty acids and, in some instances, lower fat contents.

The simplest type of dairy spread may be obtained by blending cream or butter with a liquid vegetable oil such as soya bean oil. The mixture of cream and vegetable oil may be churned in a batch or continuous buttermaker, but if oil is added to butter itself, high shear rates are required to ensure good mixing. Increasing the level of oil to improve spreadability at low temperatures results in oiling off and loss of body at higher temperatures. This can be avoided by imitating margarine manufacturers and including a proportion of saturated fat to maintain body and aid emulsion stability. Typically, such a product would contain a vegetable oil such as soya bean oil, a partially hydrogenated oil and cream and may be manufactured in a continuous buttermaker or by using a scraped-surface heat exchanger. The fat content of these two types of dairy spreads is usually in the region of 73–80%.

The third type of dairy spread available is the 'low-fat' product. In low-fat spreads the aqueous phase makes up about 52–75% of the product compared with a maximum of 16% in butter. The fat phase is composed of vegetable oils, hydrogenated vegetable oils and, possibly, milk fat with sodium caseinate or a buttermilk protein concentrate added for both flavour and water-binding/emulsification purposes. The early low-fat products contained milk fat as the principal fat but both financial and consistency considerations have led to the development of products having no or very low levels of milk fat and depending on the milk protein for flavour. One particular problem arises with these products due to the use of milk protein. As the fat content is lowered the water-in-oil emulsion becomes less stable and milk protein, when added to products with fat levels of about 40%, tends to promote an oil-in-water emulsion. This problem may be overcome by increasing the milk protein level (and increasing the cost), modifying their properties by heat treatment and by carefully selecting the emulsifer and stabilizer levels needed to maintain a stable emulsion. This type of product, which most closely resembles margarines, is manufactured using margarine technology in a scraped-surface cooler to bring about crystallization mainly in the β' form. During manufacture, it is critical to the keeping properties of the product that good moisture distribution with large numbers of discrete moisture droplets and an absence of channelling is achieved. All three types of dairy spreads require packaging in tubs as the traditional foil laminate or parchment wrapping provides inadequate support. Because of increased levels of unsaturated fats and an increased level of aqueous phase (which results in a larger size of moisture droplet) the products should all be stored at low temperatures to preserve chemical and microbiological quality. *See* Emulsifiers, Uses in Processed Foods; Stabilizers, Types and Function

Bibliography

De Man JM (1976) In: De Man JM, Voisey PW, Rasper VF and Stanley DW (eds) *Rheology and Texture in Food Quality*, pp 355–381. Westport, CT: AVI.

Egan M, Kirk RS and Sawyer R (eds) (1981) *Pearson's Chemical Analysis of Foods*, 8th edn, pp 474–487. Edinburgh: Churchill Livingstone.

Gurr MI (1989) In: Cambie RC (ed.) *Fats for the Future*, 41–61. Chichester: Ellis Horwood.

Hawke JC and Taylor MW (1983) In: Fox, PF (ed.) *Lipids. Developments in Dairy Chemistry*, vol. 2, pp 37–81. Barking: Applied Science.

IDF (1981) *Evaluation of the Firmness of Butter. International Dairy Federation Bulletin Document*, No. 135. Brussels: International Dairy Federation.

IDF (1990) *Inventory of IDF/ISO/AOAC Adopted Methods of Analysis of Milk and Milk Products*, 3rd edn. *International Dairy Federation Bulletin*, No. 248. Brussels: International Dairy Federation.

Juriaanse AC and Heertje I (1988) Microstructure of shortenings, margarine and butter – a review. *Food Microstructure* 7: 181–188.

Keogh MK, Quigley T, Connolly JF and Phelan JA (1988) Anhydrous milk fat. 4. Low fat spreads. *Irish Journal of Food Science and Technology* 12: 53–75.

Murphy JJ and Connolly JF (1991) Supplementing cows with full fat rapeseed (FFR) at pasture – effects on production and the chemical and physical properties of milk fat. Paper presented at the 42nd Annual Meeting of the European Association of Animal Production, Berlin, 1991.

Walstra P and Jenness R (1984) *Dairy Chemistry and Physics*, pp 377–457. Chichester: Wiley.

Wilbey RA (1986) In: Robinson RK (ed.) *Advances in Milk Processing. Modern Dairy Technology*, vol. 1, pp 92–129. Barking: Elsevier.

A. M. Fearon
The Queen's University of Belfast, Belfast, UK

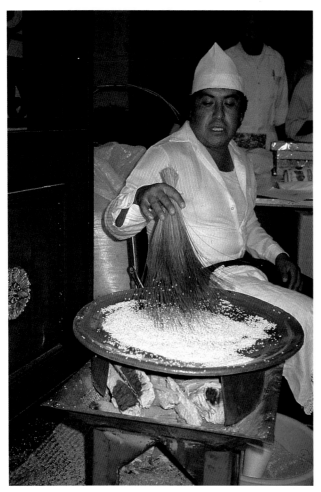

Plate 1 Amaranth: popping in Mexico.

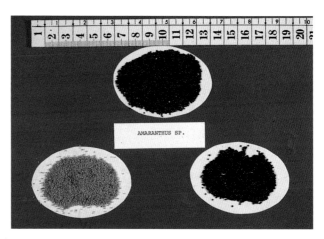

Plate 2 Amaranth: picture of grain.

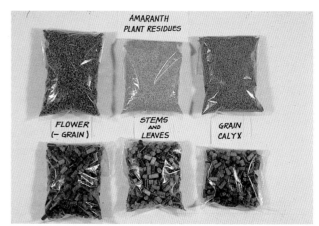

Plate 3 Amaranth: products for animal feed. (Upper) ground material and (lower) pelleted material.

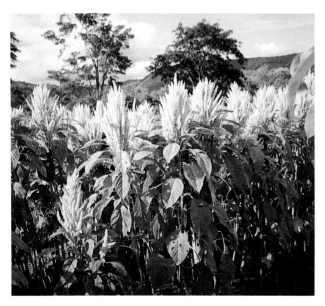

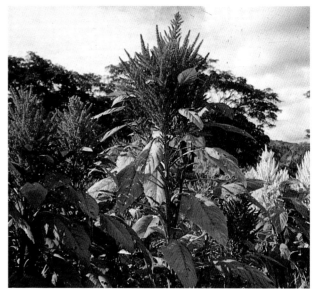

Plate 4 Amaranth: plants growing in different experimental plots.

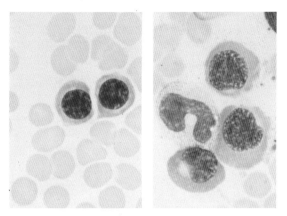

Plate 5 Two erythroblasts from a normal bone marrow (left) compared with three megaloblasts from a patient with severe pernicious anaemia (right). The fourth nucleated cell accompanying the megaloblasts is a metamyelocyte.

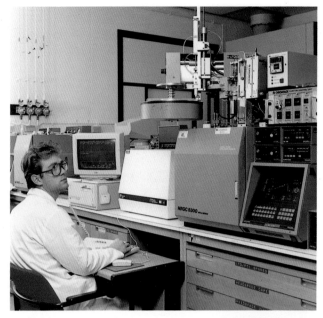

Plate 6 Analysis of food carried out at the Laboratory of the Government Chemist at Teddington, UK.

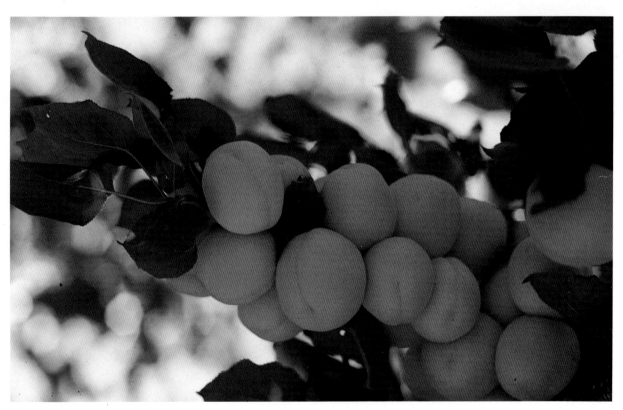

Plate 7 Apricots.

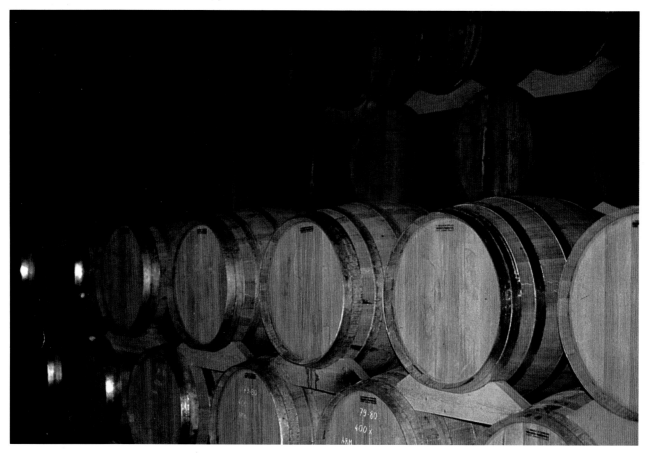

Plate 8 Ageing spirits in oak barrels (Puech, INRA, Montpellier, France).

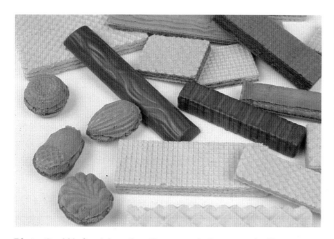

Plate 9 Wafer biscuits. Creamed, flat and hollow wafers, partially enrobed or moulded in chocolate.

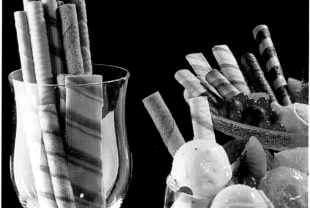

Plate 10 Rolled wafer sticks in different shapes and colours.

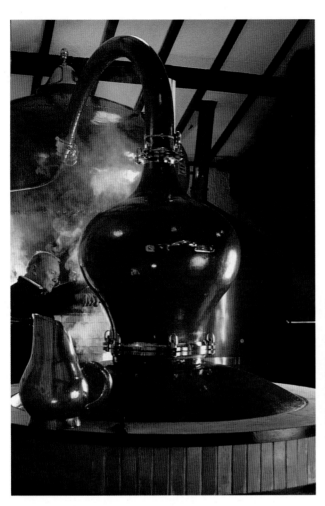

Plate 11 (left) A pot still of the type employed for the production of brandy by the batch process.

Plate 12 (below) Food products which contain casein or casein derivatives.

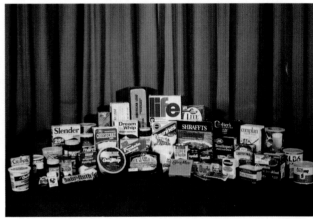

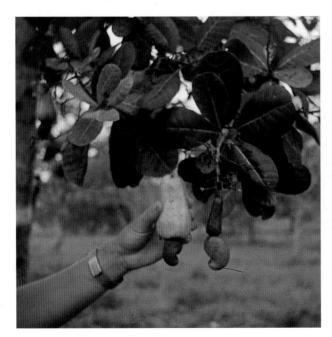

Plate 13 Immature and mature cashews hang side-by-side. The fleshy stalk is slender at first, enlarges to form the cashew apple just before the nut is mature and ready to fall with apple attached.

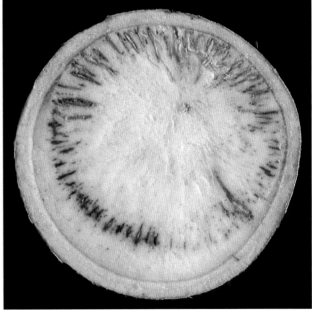

Plate 14 Transverse section through cassava root showing symptoms of physiological deterioration, 3 days after harvest.

CABBAGE

See Vegetables of Temperate Climates

CADMIUM

Contents

Properties and Determination
Toxicology

Properties and Determination

Cadmium is the 48th element in the periodic table, with an atomic weight of 112·4. Cadmium metal is generally described as bluish or silver white in colour, and as being relatively soft, ductile and malleable. Cadmium is one of the rarer elements in the earth's crust, but it is fairly widely distributed and is found in shales and igneous rocks, coal, sandstones, limestone, lake and oceanic sediments, soils, etc. Cadmium metal has been produced in large amounts by the USA, the USSR, Japan and Canada. Production figures vary from year to year and depend primarily on zinc requirements.

Cadmium has a number of important industrial applications: electroplating, alloys and solders, pigments, stabilizers for polyvinyl chloride, batteries, photovoltaic cells, etc. Most of the uses of cadmium are 'dissipative', the products using it being widely distributed in the environment and hard to recycle.

Though cadmium has come into widespread use only fairly recently, it is quite likely that for many centuries this highly toxic metal has caused incidents of food poisoning. After mercury and lead, cadmium can probably be considered next in importance as an environmental pollutant. Its sources are many and include smelting and plating operations, lithography, engraving, soldering and welding. Cadmium is found in nature in very small amounts associated with lead, copper and, particularly, zinc ores, probably owing to its chemical similarity. Other sources of cadmium include dust and fumes from the mining and refining of metals, miscellaneous industrial sources, as an impurity in fertilizers, petrol, oil, coal, organic waste products, and cigarette smoke.

Occurrence in Foods

In order to understand the biological effects of cadmium in foods, it is necessary to have some idea of the distribution and occurrence of cadmium in air, water and soil. Furthermore, it is essential to try to determine how cadmium normally moves from one sector to another and to explore the way in which human activities may influence these processes. The importance of atmospheric cadmium in relation to its potential effects on humans lies not so much in its direct inhalation as in its possible contribution to soil, water and vegetation through either dry or wet deposition and, ultimately, to food. In this respect, the solubility, pH and chemical nature of the deposited fraction may be essential factors for controlling concentrations in food.

Cadmium in Air

Cadmium is universally present in the atmosphere in amounts varying from 1 ng m^{-3} or less in rural or uncontaminated areas to 10–50 ng m^{-3} in congested urban areas. The principal sources of cadmium in the atmosphere are thought to have resulted from emissions from smelters, reprocessing of various cadmium-containing metals, burning of plastics or power generation from coal.

In areas around cadmium-emitting factories, cadmium concentrations in air are several hundred times greater than those in noncontaminated areas. The compounds of cadmium which exist in the atmosphere are not known with any certainty but it can be assumed that they are nonvolatile and that they are present in the particulate phase. Some of the probable forms are the oxide, sulphide, sulphate, chlorides and other more complex ions or compounds.

The mean cadmium value is $0.01\ \mu g\ m^{-3}$ in urban areas and below $0.003\ \mu g\ m^{-3}$ in nonurban areas. There is no definite relation of cadmium levels to the size of cities; some small but highly industrialized cities have levels which are greater than those of some very large metropolitan areas.

Cadmium in Water

The cadmium content of water is extremely low. The occurrence in drinking water has of course been of special interest since this directly affects human intake. Cadmium levels in water, in the absence of contamination, are seldom above $1\ \mu g\ l^{-1}$. Contamination may occur as a result of the use of galvanized pipes and cisterns. Cadmium-containing solders in water heaters and other fittings can be another cause. Pollution of water due to the use of cadmium-rich sewage sludge for agricultural purposes has been reported on a number of occasions. The mean concentration of cadmium in rainwater is $0.001\ \mu g\ ml^{-1}$ in clean areas and $0.0037\ \mu g\ ml^{-1}$ in contaminated areas.

Cadmium in Soils

Agricultural soils receive inputs of cadmium from soil supplements, such as phosphate fertilizers and sewage sludge, and from atmospheric deposition. Although the significance of sewage sludge as a source of cadmium contamination of soil is well established, European soil inventory studies indicate that, on a national basis, phosphate fertilizer and atmospheric inputs are the greatest sources of cadmium addition to soils. Levels in soils vary widely from about $0.06\ mg\ kg^{-1}$ in virgin soil to several hundred times this level in the vicinity of some smelters.

Cadmium in Plants

Some species of plants have an ability to concentrate cadmium at levels that are sometimes much greater than those in the immediate environment. The ratio of cadmium concentration in plants to that in the corresponding soil has been reported to be about 10:1. The average cadmium content of terrestrial plants is about $0.6\ mg\ kg^{-1}$, although there is obviously a very wide variation even in uncontaminated areas. The range of values in species growing in clean areas is of the order of $0.01-10\ mg\ kg^{-1}$ or more, but most plants contain below $1\ mg\ kg^{-1}$. Certain mushrooms contain about 10 times this level. Variations in species are very great even in plants growing in the same area, and there is also variation in different parts of the same plant. There seems to be good evidence that plants generally show increased tissue cadmium levels in response to an increase in the environment from normal sources or from soil, water or air contamination.

Plants undoubtedly absorb cadmium from the soil through their roots. This absorption is influenced by, among other factors, the pH of the soil and the organic matter content. The cadmium concentration in plants appears to be inversely related to the amount of organic matter in the soil. A large amount of organic matter in the soil limits the availability of cadmium to plants. Organic soils form the strongest metal complexes and hence retain the metal more firmly. An increased accumulation of cadmium by plants fertilized with superphosphate which contains cadmium as an impurity has been reported. However, it has been proved that the aerial zone of plants is the most important entry point for cadmium.

Contamination of Food During Processing

The processing of vegetables prior to canning can modify the initial content of cadmium. It has been proved that, after washing, the amount of cadmium slightly decreases. Blanching has an influence on the decrease of cadmium to varying degrees. These decreases are probably caused by cadmium being extracted during washing prior to blanching and/or during the thermal processing where cadmium is extracted into the brine.

Cadmium contamination occurs as a result of its use to plate small pieces of equipment. Cadmium is readily soluble in weak acid solutions, and its use in food-processing plants should be confined to parts which do not come directly into contact with food.

Another source of cadmium contamination is the utilization of ceramic and enamelled utensils. Some glazed pottery, especially of the craft and home-made kind, is capable of releasing toxic amounts of cadmium and other metals into food.

Enamelled kitchenware can also be a source of cadmium contamination of food, especially those made by unknown manufacturers which have bright colours, indicating the possible use of cadmium pigments.

Another domestic source of cadmium contamination is the decoration and printing applied to glass tumblers and other containers.

Furthermore, the spices, condiments, colourings, preservatives, etc., which are added to foodstuffs may contain cadmium and be a vehicle of contamination.

Cadmium Levels in Foods

Except where there has been pollution, cadmium is normally found at a fairly low concentration in food-

Table 1. Cadmium levels (μg g^{-1}) in some foods

Sample/site	Cd level	Sample/site	Cd level
Apples/Australia	0·002–0·019[a]	Lettuce/FRG	0·031–0·198[e]
Apples/FRG	0·009[b]	Liver (beef)/Switzerland	0·11[b]
Asparagus/Spain	0·022[c]	Liver paté (pork)/Spain	0·120[c]
Beer/Belgium	0·004[d]	Oyster/USA	0·20–2·10[b]
Bread/Australia	0·002–0·043[a]	Oyster/New Zealand	0·20–2·10[e]
Cabbage/Australia	0·002–0·026[a]	Oyster/UK	3·50–29·70[h]
Cauliflower/Spain	0·009[c]	Potatoes/UK	0·150[i]
Chicken/New Zealand	0·03–0·10[e]	Potatoes/Australia	0·002–0·051[a]
Cod/UK	0·16[f]	Pork/New Zealand	0·03–0·10[e]
Crayfish/Spain	0·032[g]	Prawns/UK	0·40[b]
Eggs/Belgium	0·002–0·066[d]	Prawns/Australia	0·017–0·913[a]
Fish/Australia	0·05[a]	Rice/Belgium	0·045[d]
Flour/Belgium	0·147[d]	Rice/USA	0·040[b]
Flour/UK	0·070[b]	Sausage/Spain	0·036[j]
Flour/USA	0·070[b]	Shellfish/Belgium	0·016–0·53[d]
Kidney (sheep)/Australia	0·013–2·000[a]	Spice/Belgium	0·120[d]
Kidney (beef)/UK	0·50[b]	Spinach/FRG	0·055–0·063[e]
Lettuce/Spain	0·010[c]	Wheat/USA	0·050[b]

Data from: [a]Reilly C (1991);
[b]Nordberg GF (1974) Health hazards of environmental cadmium pollution. *Ambio* 3: 55–56;
[c]Zurera-Cosano G, Moreno-Rojas R, Pozo-Lora R and Rincon-Leon F (1989) Mineral elements in canned Spanish liver pate. *Food Chemistry* 32: 217–222;
[c]Zurera-Cosano G, Moreno-Rojas R and Amaro-Lopez M. (1990) Cadmium and lead distribution in fresh asparagus. *Food Additives and Contaminants* 7: 381–385;
[d]Fouassin A and Fondu M (1980) Evaluation de la teneur moyenne en plomb et en cadmium de la ration alimentaire en Belgique. *Archives Belges de Médecine Sociale, Hygiène, Médecine du Travail et Médecine Légale* 38: 453–467;
[e]Förstner U (1980) Anthropogenic compounds. In: (Hutzinger O, ed) *The Handbook of Environmental Chemistry*, Vol 3, part A, pp. 59–107. Heidelberg: Springer-Verlag;
[f]Orlando CP, de Renzi GP, Baston W, Franco Y, Perdelli F and Coppola R (1983) Indagine sulla concentrazione ambientale de alcuni metalli pesanti in una zona industriale della Liguria. *Inquinamento* 1: 33–37;
[g]Rincón-León F, Zurera-Cosano G and Pozo-Lora R (1988) Lead and cadmium concentrations in red crayfish (*Procambarus clarkii, G.*) in the Guadalquivir river marshes (Spain). *Archives of Environmental Contamination and Toxicology* 17: 251–256;
[h]Bland S, Ackroyd DR, Marsh JG and Millward GE (1982) Heavy metal content of oysters from the Lynher estuary UK. *Science of Total Environment* 22: 235–241;
[i]Sherlock JC (1984) Cadmium in foods and the diet. *Experientia* 40: 152–165;
[j]Ybañez N, Montoro R, Catalá R and Flores J (1982) Conetenido en cadmiu, plomo y cobre de productos carnicos. *Revista de Agroquimica y Teconologia de Alimentos* 22: 419–425.

stuffs. However, a wide range of concentrations has been reported by different workers (Table 1). Some of these results possibly reflect defective analytical techniques rather than absolute values. Certain fish and shellfish, however, possess protein inducers (metallothioneins) and are able to concentrate cadmium at levels 100 times higher than those in the aquatic environment in which they live. *See* Fish, Spoilage; Shellfish, Contamination and Spoilage of Molluscs and Crustacea

Analysis of Foods for Cadmium

For trace element analysis, the steps necessary include the initial collection of the bulk sample, storage and handling, homogenization, analytical subsampling, analytical sample preparation, digestion or destruction of the organic matrix, and obtaining the analytical response in the appropriate instrumentation.

For cadmium analysis, a most important aspect is the avoidance of airborne particulate contamination. The low level of cadmium in foods and the ubiquitous presence of significant levels of this element in some reagents, containers and air make it necessary for the analyst to evaluate and eliminate all potential sources of contamination at each stage of the analysis.

Sample Preparation

Prior to the destruction of the organic matter, the sample should be subjected to drying and grinding in order to remove water from the product without reducing its dry matter content. Normally, the moisture is removed and the analytical result expressed on a dry weight basis. However, for nutritional purposes, it is common practice to express the concentration on a fresh weight basis (i.e. wet weight basis).

The drying procedure recommended by the Association of Official Analytical Chemists (AOAC) is vacuum oven drying at 100 mmHg pressure and at a temperature of 70°C.

Table 2. Comparison of wet oxidation and dry ashing techniques

Wet oxidation	Dry ashing
Faster	Rather slow
Temperature lower, less volatilization and retention	Temperature higher, more volatilization and retention
Generally less sensitive to nature of sample	Generally more sensitive to nature of sample
Relatively more supervision	Relatively less supervision
Reagent blank larger	Reagent blank smaller
Inconvenient for large samples	Large samples easily handled

From Gorsuch TT (1976) In: *Accuracy in Trace Analysis: Sampling, Sample Handling and Analysis*, National Bureau of Standards Publication No. 422, pp 491–508. Washington, DC: National Bureau of Standards.

Table 3. AOAC procedure for destroying organic matter by dry ashing

(1) Weight 1 g of sample, dry and grind into a glazed, high-form porcelain crucible
(2) Ash for 2 h at 500°C, and allow to cool
(3) Wet ash with 10 drops water and carefully add 3–4 ml of nitric acid (1:1)
(4) Evaporate excess nitric acid on a hot plate set at 100–120°C
(5) Return crucible to furnace and ash for an additional 1 h at 500°C
(6) Cool crucible and dissolve ash in 10 ml of hydrochloric acid (1:1)
(7) Transfer quantitatively to a 50 ml volumetric flask

From Horwitz, W (ed) (1980) *Official Methods of Analysis of the Association of Official Analytical Chemists*, 13th edn, section 3.007, p. 31. Washington DC: Association of Official Analytical Chemists.

The primary objective of grinding a sample is to homogenize it and, at the same time, reduce it to a suitable physical consistency so that it can be easily measured or weighed. A number of grinding procedures can be employed, but in any case reducing the sample to a finer particle size is desirable if the subsample chosen for analysis is to be less than 1·0 g. With all grinding procedures, contamination and segregation are potential sources of error.

Once the sample has been reduced to a usable form, it should be stored in an air-tight container in the dark at a reduced temperature.

Organic Matter Destruction

This is probably still the weakest link in the determination of the elemental content of biological substances. The two most common decomposition procedures are wet oxidation and dry ashing. The latter is frequently criticized for several reasons. For instance, elemental loss by volatilization can occur. Wet ashing, on the other hand, is a longer more tedious procedure with a greater potential for sample contamination and danger to the analyst. The advantages and disadvantages of both techniques are shown in Table 2.

Numerous wet oxidation procedures have been proposed but they all fit basically into three categories of digestion mixtures: (1) nitric and sulphuric acids, (2) sulphuric acid and hydrogen peroxide and (3) mixtures containing perchloric acid. Contrary to popular belief, volatilization can occur with wet oxidation if the temperature of the digestion vessel is greater than 250°C. Wet digestion under pressure is also a suitable procedure for the destruction of organic matter. With the utilization of a microwave oven, the digestion time is considerably reduced.

Dry ashing procedures are accomplished by high-temperature oxidation. The critical requirements are (1) the nature of the ashing vessel, (2) position in the muffle furnace, (3) ashing temperature and (4) time.

Silica is probably one of the best materials for the ashing vessel, although glass beakers and well-glazed porcelain crucibles are also suitable.

A critical initial requirement is to keep the temperature sufficiently low to prevent flaming or burning.

One of the procedures most commonly used for destroying organic matter by dry ashing is shown in Table 3.

The addition of 1:1 dilute sulphuric acid to food materials prior to dry ashing eliminates losses of cadmium, although losses due to volatilization are possible as well as lack of recovery due to the formation of insoluble silicates.

Both techniques, wet oxidation and dry ashing, give reasonably comparable results and, in many instances, it is the analyst who makes the difference whichever technique is employed. However, wet digestion is recommended, using sulphuric acid and hydrogen peroxide: dry ashing can result in low recoveries since cadmium is volatile at temperatures over 500°C, temperatures of below 450°C being more appropriate.

The digestions obtained using the procedures described above are not usually used directly since interference effects from other substances present in the solution may cause problems, especially if determinations are to be carried out at levels approaching the limits of detection. A pretreatment of the sample in order to concentrate cadmium with respect to competing substances is necessary. This may be achieved by chelation, followed by solvent extraction of the chelated cadmium into an organic phase. The compounds used most commonly as ligands are dithiocarbamates such as ammonium pyrrolidine dithiocarbamate (APDC), diphenyl thiocarbazone (dithiozone), and others. They vary in their selectivity and are usually very dependent on the pH at which extraction is carried out. For cadmium the optimum pH is 3–4. The organic solvent used most is methyl isobutyl ketone (MIBK).

Ion exchange resins (Amberlite LA-2) are being extensively used in removing interfering metals from solutions in preparation for final analysis.

Methods

Analysts nowadays have a number of techniques to choose from when making an elementary assay. The choice to be made depends on a number of factors such as accuracy, precision, detection limit, sensitivity, the user's experience, performance with standard samples and safety considerations. However, it may be the more practical considerations of instrument availability, cost and sample form and quantity that become the governing factors rather than the choice being based on the above criteria. The analyst's skill, past experience or lack of experience may dictate the selection of the analytical technique chosen. Personal preference may equally be a significant factor in this decision. *See* Heavy Metal Toxicology

Atomic Absorption Spectrophotometry (AAS)

This is the most popular method for metal determination in general and the most widely used technique for analyses of trace elements in foods. The popularity of this method arises from its analytical specificity, good detection limits, excellent precision and relatively low cost.

The AAS instrument consists of a light source (a hollow cathode lamp), an atomization source, and a dispersion/detection device. Three types of atomizers are commonly used: flame, graphite furnace, and chemical vaporization.

Air–acetylene is the most commonly used gas mixture, producing a flame of about 2400°C, but is not totally interference free. The use of chelating agents such as APDC and an organic solvent such as MIBK are also effective in reducing interference effects. Background correction is essential for cadmium determination. This can usually be done with a deuterium lamp. The Zeeman method is one of the most effective techniques for background correction.

Flameless AAS, using electrothermal atomization techniques, has been developed in recent years in order to avoid problems associated with the flame. Flameless AAS allows an estimation of as little as 5 μg kg^{-1}, but chemical interference, especially from sodium salts, may result in inaccuracies.

Flame and flameless AAS have one serious limitation since only one element can be determined at a time, requiring additional set-up and analysis time if assay for more than one element is desired. Flameless AAS will continue to be a major analytical technique for those elements, such as cadmium, and samples where ultra-trace concentrations are to be determined and/or sample volume is limited. However, inductively coupled plasma atomic emission spectrometry (ICP-AES) is beginning to be used preferentially due to the possibility of quantifying all the metals present, hence reducing analysis times and avoiding problems of interference.

Electrochemical Methods

The electrochemical methods are polarographic, both direct and alternating current, and anodic or cathodic stripping voltametry and polarography. Both techniques rely on the fact that different metals require the application of different electrical potentials before they are deposited from solution on to the cathode. The polarographic methods are suitable for dilute solutions with sensitivities of 10^{-6} to 10^{-9} mol l^{-1}. Anodic or cathodic stripping voltametry is even more sensitive than usual polarography. After the cadmium ions have been preconcentrated from the solution and amalgamated into a stationary hanging mercury drop electrode, the process is reversed by using a more negative potential than the reduction potential of cadmium. Cadmium is oxidized and stripped anodically, using a slowly increasing positive potential. The measured current recorded during the stripping step is a direct linear function of the bulk concentration of cadmium.

Bibliography

Friberg L, Piscator M, Nordberg GR and Kjellström T (1974) *Cadmium in the Environment*. Cleveland: CRC Press.

Gilbert J (ed.) (1984) *Analysis of Food Contaminants*. Barking: Elsevier.

King RD (ed.) (1978) *Developments in Food Analysis Techniques*, vol. 1. Barking: Applied Science.

King RD (ed.) (1984) *Developments in Food Analysis Techniques*, vol. 3. Barking: Elsevier.

Reilly C (1991) *Metal Contamination of Food*, 2nd edn. London: Elsevier.

Waldron HA (ed.) (1980) *Metals in the Environment*. London: Academic Press.

G. Zurera-Cosano
Universidad de Cordoba, Cordoba, Spain

Toxicology

The industrial extraction of the nutritionally nonessential metal, cadmium, has increased significantly over the past 50 years. Cadmium is used in electroplating, welding and soldering operations, and in the manufacture of batteries, plastics and pigments. This has led to an increasing prevalence of cadmium in the environment. The quantities of cadmium derived from natural sources are small, and the concentrations of the metal in unpolluted soils are normally $< 1\ \mu g$ per g. Soils may be contaminated by the deposition of cadmium from the atmosphere in the vicinity of mining and smelting operations, the discharge of cadmium-containing waste materials, and the application of water, fertilizers (e.g. municipal sewage sludge, superphosphate) and pesticides which contain cadmium. Thus all food crops contain at least trace concentrations of cadmium, whilst elevated concentrations have also been measured in certain edible marine organisms such as oysters, scallops and mussels. The hazardous nature of cadmium to human health is a result of its long-term persistence in the environment, its rapid uptake and accumulation by food crops, its inherent high toxicity and its efficient retention and accumulation in the body throughout life. This article reviews the current state of knowledge of the toxicology of cadmium.

Pharmacokinetics

Absorption

The gastrointestinal absorption of cadmium in man is 2–8% of the amount ingested. It is not under homeostatic control. The actual bioavailability is determined by physiological variables such as age, sex, dietary status, and the composition and concentration of gastrointestinal secretions. Young children can be considered at special risk of intoxication, whilst cadmium may be more toxic for females than for males. Cadmium absorption may also be enhanced by diets low or deficient in iron, zinc, calcium, phosphorus or selenium. The interaction of these factors in the human body is complex and difficult to predict. It is generally assumed that the bioavailability of cadmium remains essentially constant with time and over a typical range of dietary intakes. See Bioavailability of Nutrients

The pulmonary absorption of cadmium is probably slightly greater than that of gastrointestinal absorption. On the basis of animal experimental data, 20–30% of the cadmium in inhaled air is deposited in the human lung. Assuming that about 60% of the deposited cadmium is absorbed, the pulmonary bioavailability is in the order of 12–18% of the amount of inhaled cadmium. The absorption of cadmium through the skin is negligible in comparison with that through the gastrointestinal tract.

Distribution

About 90% of the cadmium in the blood is localized in the red cells, and the remainder is associated mainly with high-molecular-weight proteins in the plasma. Cadmium concentrations in whole blood are normally below 10 μg per litre, and are usually higher in smokers than in non-smokers. About 10% of the cadmium entering the systemic circulation is apparently available for early excretion with a half-life of 1·5 days. The half-life in the blood is estimated to be 150 days.

The cadmium is transported to the tissues, in many of which (e.g. liver, kidneys, stomach, small intestine, spleen, pancreas and testes) it induces the synthesis of metallothionein, a cysteine-rich protein (molecular weight 6000–10 000) in which the cadmium ion is bound to the apoprotein by mercaptide bonds. Metallothionein regulates the metabolism of zinc and copper by providing a temporary storage mechanism and by preventing toxic interactions if the tolerable physiological limits are exceeded. The induction of metallothionein synthesis by cadmium is an extension of this normal homeostatic function of the protein. Thus, whilst chronic exposure leads to progressive accumulation of cadmium in the kidneys and liver, toxicity is normally avoided because most of the cadmium is bound to metallothionein. See Copper, Physiology; Zinc, Physiology

Small amounts of metallothionein are constantly transported from the liver to the kidneys by the blood. The metallothionein is filtered into the urine and reabsorbed into the proximal tubular cells where it is degraded into peptides and amino acids. Free ionic cadmium released within the cells then initiates the synthesis of further metallothionein.

The progressive accumulation of cadmium in the body continues until about 55 years of age. The body burden is 5–40 mg in unexposed European and American adults. It has been estimated that, of the cadmium which enters the systemic circulation, about 20%, 30% and 10% is deposited in the liver, kidneys and bone respectively. The kidney has the highest concentration of cadmium. The concentration in the renal cortex (15–50 μg per g wet weight at 40–50 years of age) is higher than in the whole kidney. In some populations in Japan concentrations in the range 60–120 μg per g have been observed. From 50–60 years of age the kidney cadmium concentration declines progressively, possibly as a result of dietary changes, reductions in renal efficiency or the development of kidney dysfunction. If renal damage occurs, the urinary excretion of cadmium increases in parallel with the decrease in kidney cadmium concentration. In unexposed adults liver cadmium concentrations range from about 0·5 to 5 μg per g. Cadmium is relatively uniformly distributed throughout the other organs and tissues, with an estimated mean concentration of about 0·4 μg per g. Typical concentrations in human milk range from 2 to 10 μg per litre. The placental transfer of cadmium is limited, although placental cadmium concentrations are higher in smokers than in nonsmokers. *See* Kidney, Structure and Function

Excretion

Cadmium is eliminated from the body mainly in the faeces because of the low bioavailability of ingested cadmium. About 0·005–0·01% of the body burden ($<2 \mu g$) per day is excreted in the urine. On a group basis, urinary excretion is proportional to the body burden and increases up to 50–60 years of age, after which it may decline slowly. Excretion in hair, sweat and saliva occurs but is not significant in comparison with that in faeces and urine. The biological half-life is in the range 10 to 50 years.

Toxicology

Acute Toxicity

The ingestion of food and beverages contaminated with cadmium, the use of cadmium-plated cooking utensils, and the storage of acid juice in cadmium-containing earthenware can cause gastrointestinal toxicity. Reports of such food poisoning have been rare in recent years. Acute oral intoxication has also been observed in workers exposed to cadmium dust who eat with dirty hands. The initial symptoms are immediate nausea, and vomiting which is normally so violent that little of the cadmium is absorbed and fatal poisoning does not result. Additional important symptoms may include salivation, abdominal pain, diarrhoea and headache.

The treatment of acute cadmium poisoning involves the induction of vomiting to decontaminate the gastrointestinal tract, and the intravenous injection of calcium disodium edetate to chelate the cadmium and promote its excretion. Recent studies in rodents have shown that meso-2,3-dimercaptosuccinic acid given by mouth can inhibit the gastrointestinal absorption of ingested cadmium.

Chronic Toxicity

The kidney is the critical organ in poisoning resulting from long-term excessive environmental and occupational exposure to cadmium. Kidney dysfunction, including an increased incidence of β_2-microglobulinuria, proteinuria, glucosuria and aminoaciduria, has been observed amongst inhabitants of certain cadmium-polluted areas of Japan and Belgium. In cadmium-exposed workers the urinary excretion of low-molecular-weight proteins (molecular weight $<40\,000$, in particular β_2-microglobulin, retinol-binding protein, lysosome, ribonuclease, light-chain immunoglobulins, carbonic anhydrase, α_1-microglobulin, and urinary protein 1) may be markedly increased. This is often accompanied by an increased excretion of high-molecular-weight proteins such as albumin, transferrin and immunoglobulin G. As the kidney dysfunction progresses, moderate increases in the urinary excretion of amino acids, glucose, minerals such as calcium and phosphorus, and enzymes (e.g. β-galactosidase, β-N-acetylglucosaminidase and alkaline phosphatase) may also be observed. Once an increased proteinuria has occurred it is normally irreversible, although there is evidence that a slight proteinuria, detectable only by β_2-microglobulinuria, may be reversible. A reduction in glomerular filtration rate has also been detected in some cadmium-exposed people.

At the end of World War II, an endemic bone disease occurred in the Zinzu river basin of Toyama prefecture in Japan. This syndrome, called itai-itai disease, was characterized, in addition to renal dysfunction, by a painful type of bone disease consisting of osteomalacia and osteoporosis with multiple pseudofractures. Bone lesions have also been observed in cadmium workers, but usually as a late manifestation of severe chronic cadmium poisoning.

Respiratory toxicity has been described in workers subject to excessive exposure to cadmium dust and fumes. The effects normally involve bronchitis, which may lead to a mild form of obstructive lung disease with functional impairment.

The use of chelation therapy in cases of chronic cadmium poisoning is complicated by the high affinity of metallothionein for cadmium. Currently it is recommended only that the patient should be removed from the source of the poisoning. Considerable progress has been made recently in the development of compounds such as dithiocarbamate derivatives as chelating agents for chronic cadmium poisoning. It may be possible, in the near future, to give serious consideration to the use of some of these compounds in cases of cadmium intoxication.

Carcinogenicity

Cadmium compounds can produce local sarcomas in rats and interstitial tumours in the testes of rats and mice, and there is limited epidemiological evidence that workers who inhale cadmium oxide may have an increased risk of prostatic cancer. The International Agency for Research on Cancer has therefore classified cadmium as probably carcinogenic for humans. However, there is no evidence that exposure to cadmium at normal dietary levels is carcinogenic in man. *See* Carcinogens, Carcinogenic Substances in Food

Cardiotoxicity

Animal studies have produced good evidence that chronic exposure to cadmium, at dose levels within the normal dietary range of intake, can produce hypertension, but epidemiological investigations have failed to demonstrate a clear relationship between cadmium exposure and hypertension. Further studies are needed to assess the cardiotoxic effects of chronic cadmium exposure in humans.

Mutagenicity

There is no evidence that cadmium is mutagenic at normal dietary levels. Studies on itai-itai patients exposed to elevated dietary levels of cadmium have yielded conflicting evidence of the existence of chromosomal aberrations. The presence of chromosomal anomalies in the blood lymphocytes of cadmium workers has been observed, but the influence of exposure to other metals and to environmental mutagens is uncertain. *See* Mutagens

Teratogenicity

Cadmium is nontoxic to the developing conceptus at normal dietary intake levels. A reduction in the birth-weight of newborn infants of women occupationally exposed to cadmium has been observed, and high doses of cadmium compounds can induce teratogenic effects in experimental animals.

Mode of Action

The concentration of metallothionein-bound cadmium increases in proportion to the total kidney concentration of cadmium. Free cadmium ions, released by the degradation of metallothionein, initiate the synthesis of new metallothionein which binds the cadmium, thereby protecting the particulate components and other cytosolic proteins of the tubular cell from the toxic action of the free cadmium ions. It has yet to be established whether the onset of renal damage is coincident with a critical concentration of non-metallothionein-bound cadmium or whether the capacity of metallothionein synthesis is limited.

The toxic effect of cadmium on the kidney is identified as tubular proteinuria on the basis that (1) the majority of the proteins in the urine have molecular weights less than that of albumin, and (2) although, quantitatively, the high-molecular-weight proteins (albumin) are the most important components, the concentration of low-molecular-weight proteins (β_2-microglobulin) is increased proportionally much more. The increased urinary concentration of β_2-microglobulin is caused by a cadmium-induced defect in the tubular reabsorption of low-molecular-weight proteins. It has also been suggested that cadmium may stimulate the synthesis of β_2-microglobulin, and that the increased urinary levels may reflect increased serum levels of this protein. Increased urinary concentrations of high-molecular-weight proteins, in the absence of low-molecular-weight proteins, probably reflect an alteration in glomerular function. In the case of mixed-type proteinuria, high-molecular-weight proteins may be filtered at the glomerulus and then incompletely reabsorbed in the proximal tubules. Alternatively, high-molecular-weight proteins may be released from the kidneys into the urine. A third possibility is that cadmium might interact directly with components of the glomerulus to increase glomerular permeability.

The close epidemiological association between cadmium exposure and itai-itai disease, the accumulation of cadmium in the tissues of itai-itai patients, and the finding of osteomalacia in cadmium-exposed workers indicate that cadmium was a necessary factor in the aetiology of itai-itai disease. Since the disease mainly affected aged women who had had several children and had suffered from calcium and phosphorus deficiency, it is now considered that this severe bone disease resulted from the combination of various nutritional deficiencies with an exceptionally high intake of cadmium. It has been suggested that cadmium-induced renal tubular dysfunction may have led to increased urinary excretion of calcium and phosphorus. Another possibility is that cadmium-induced inhibition of the activation of vitamin D in the kidney may have led to decreased synthesis of calcium-binding protein in the intestinal mucosa and decreased intestinal absorption of calcium. A third possibility is that cadmium may have inhibited calcium-dependent ATPase (adenosine 5′ triphosphatase) and calcium-binding protein in the intestinal mucosa, leading to a decrease in intestinal calcium absorption. Finally, it has also been suggested that cadmium may have had a direct toxic action on bone tissue. *See* Calcium, Physiology

Toxic Levels in Humans

About 3 mg of cadmium can be ingested by an adult without causing adverse effects. The ingestion of drinks containing cadmium at concentrations above 15 mg per litre may cause symptoms of food poisoning. Lethal doses range from 350 to 8900 mg. Whole blood cadmium concentration is the best measure of recent exposure. Concentrations above 10 μg per litre indicate that significant exposure has occurred.

The critical concentration of cadmium in the renal

Table 1 Daily intake and systemic absorption of cadmium

		μg of cadmium per day	
Source of intake	Fractional absorption	Typical intake	Amount absorbed
Food	0·05	20–100	1–5
Water	0·05	<2–12[a]	<0·1–0·6
Smoking	0·15	2–4[b]	0·3–0·6
Air	0·15	0·02–1[c]	0·003–0·15

[a] Based on the consumption of 2 litres of liquid per day.
[b] Based on the smoking of 20 cigarettes per day.
[c] Based on the inhalation of 20 m^3 of air per day, and cadmium air concentrations of 0·001–0·005 μg m^{-3} and 0·003–0·05 μg m^{-3} in uncontaminated rural and urban areas respectively.

cortex, corresponding to a 10% incidence of proteinuria in an exposed population, is about 200 μg per g with a range of about 100–300 μg per g. For long-term, low-level exposure, urine cadmium concentration best reflects the total body burden. In unexposed populations urinary excretion of cadmium is 0·5–1 μg per g of creatinine. In cadmium-exposed populations, renal dysfunction is usually present when the urinary cadmium concentration exceeds 10 μg per g of creatinine. The onset of low-molecular-weight proteinuria is normally detected by an increase in the urinary excretion of β_2-microglobulin which, in unexposed people, is normally about 100 μg per day.

The critical body burden is about 180 mg. A daily oral intake of 2–4 μg cadmium per kg of bodyweight is required to reach the critical concentration of about 200 μg per g in the renal cortex at 50 years of age. In 1972 an FAO/WHO (Food and Agriculture Organization/ World Health Organization) Expert Committee proposed a level of 1 μg of cadmium per kg of bodyweight as the provisional tolerable daily intake of cadmium in food. The US EPA (Environmental Protection Agency) and the WHO recommend a maximum permissible concentration of cadmium in drinking water of 10 μg per litre to protect human health.

Range of Dietary Intakes

The major source of exposure to cadmium is the ingestion of food (Table 1). Grains (wheat and rice), potatoes, and marine molluscs and crustaceans (mussels, scallops and oysters) are the principal sources of the metal. Cadmium concentrations in food stuffs normally range up to about 100 μg per kg wet weight; they vary substantially among species, and are dependent upon the cadmium concentration in the soil. The average diet contains about 20 μg of cadmium per kg wet weight.

Dietary intake varies with preference and local environmental cadmium levels. The average daily intake in uncontaminated areas is 20–100 μg. Although daily intakes of 600–2000 μg have been reported in certain areas of Japan, diets containing in excess of 100–200 μg of cadmium per day are uncommon unless local contamination is present. Other minor sources of cadmium for the general population include drinking water, cigarette smoking and air (Table 1). The contribution of air-borne cadmium to the daily intake may be much greater in people who live near cadmium-emitting sources where the cadmium concentration in the ambient air may be up to 0·6 μg m^{-3}, or who are occupationally exposed to dust and fumes containing cadmium at concentrations up to and exceeding the WHO recommended exposure limit of 20 μg m^{-3}.

Incidences of Cadmium Toxicity and Scares

The major incident of poisoning from environmental exposure to cadmium occurred in the Zinzu river basin of Japan at the end of World War II. The people had been exposed to cadmium from contamination of water and rice by discharges from a zinc mine located 50 km upstream. In May 1968, itai-itai disease was acknowledged as a pollution-related disease by the Japan Ministry of Health and Welfare. In March 1983, 116 cases had been officially recognized. Increased incidences of β_2-microglobulinuria were also found in other cadmium-polluted areas of Japan, but no cases of itai-itai disease are known.

In 1975, following the death of cattle in the vicinity of a non-ferrous smelting factory near Freiberg, West Germany, it was discovered that the land was contaminated with cadmium. The health effects of this pollution on the inhabitants of Freiberg are unknown.

In 1979, a high degree of soil contamination by cadmium was discovered in Shipham, a village in Somerset, England. The cadmium originated from the wastes of old mining operations. High levels of cadmium were found in vegetables grown in the village, and the inhabitants were advised not to use these as food. A health study failed to reveal any adverse effects from the contamination of the soil by cadmium.

In 1980, it was discovered that elderly women living in Liège, Belgium, an area known to be polluted by cadmium emissions from non-ferrous metal smelters, had higher body burdens of cadmium and an increased incidence of tubular proteinuria than women of the same age in other areas.

Bibliography

Foulkes EC (ed.) (1986) *Handbook of Experimental Pharmacology, Cadmium*. Berlin: Springer-Verlag.

Friberg L, Kjellstrom T, Nordberg G and Piscator M (1979) Cadmium. In: Friberg L, Nordberg GF and Vouk VB (eds) *Handbook on the Toxicology of Metals*, pp 351–381. Amsterdam: Elsevier Biomedical Press.

Jones MM and Cherian MG (1990) The search for chelate antagonists for chronic cadmium intoxication. *Toxicology* 62: 1–25.

Kagi JHR and Kojima Y (eds) (1987) Metallothionein II: Proceedings of the Second International Meeting on Metallothionein and Other Low Molecular Weight Metal Binding Proteins, Zurich, August 21–24, 1985. *Experentia Supplementum* vol. 52. Basel: Birkhauser Verlag.

Mislin H and Ravera O (eds) (1986) Cadmium in the environment. *Experentia Supplementum* vol. 50. Basel: Birkhauser Verlag.

Richard Mason
University of Otago, Dunedin, New Zealand

CAFFEINE

During the period 1820–1827, three white crystalline substances called 'caffein' or 'coffein', 'guaranin' and 'thein' were isolated from green coffee beans, guarana and tea, respectively. These substances were shown in 1838–1840 to be identical. Later, caffeine was also discovered in maté prepared from *Ilex paraguariensis* and kola nuts. Since then, caffeine has been shown to be a natural constituent of more than 60 plant species.

Two other related compounds, theophylline and theobromine, have also been isolated from tea and cocoa beans, respectively (Fig. 1). By the end of the 19th century, all of these methylated xanthines had been synthesized. Caffeine, both natural and synthetic, has been used as a flavouring agent in food and beverages and as well as an active component of a variety of over-the-counter pharmaceutical products and drugs.

In addition to natural caffeine obtained by the industrial decaffeination process, caffeine can also be obtained by the methylation of theobromine and also by total chemical synthesis using dimethylcarbamide and malonic acid. *See* Cocoa, Chemistry of Processing; Coffee, Green Coffee; Tea, Chemistry

Chemistry

Caffeine (M_r 194·19) is also called, more systematically, 1,3,7-trimethylxanthine, 1,3,7-trimethyl-2,6-dioxopurine or 3,7-dihydro-1,3,7-trimethyl-1H-purine-2,6-dione and has been referred to as a purine alkaloid. *See* Alkaloids, Properties and Determination

Caffeine is odourless and has a characteristic bitter taste. It is a white powder (density ($d^{18}/_4$) 1·23) moderately soluble in organic solvents and water. However, its solubility in water is considerably increased at higher temperatures (1% (w/v) at 15°C and 10% at 60°C). Its melting point is 234–239°C and the temperature of sublimation at atmospheric pressure is 178°C. Caffeine is a very weak base, reacting with acids to yield readily hydrolysed salts and relatively stable in dilute acids and

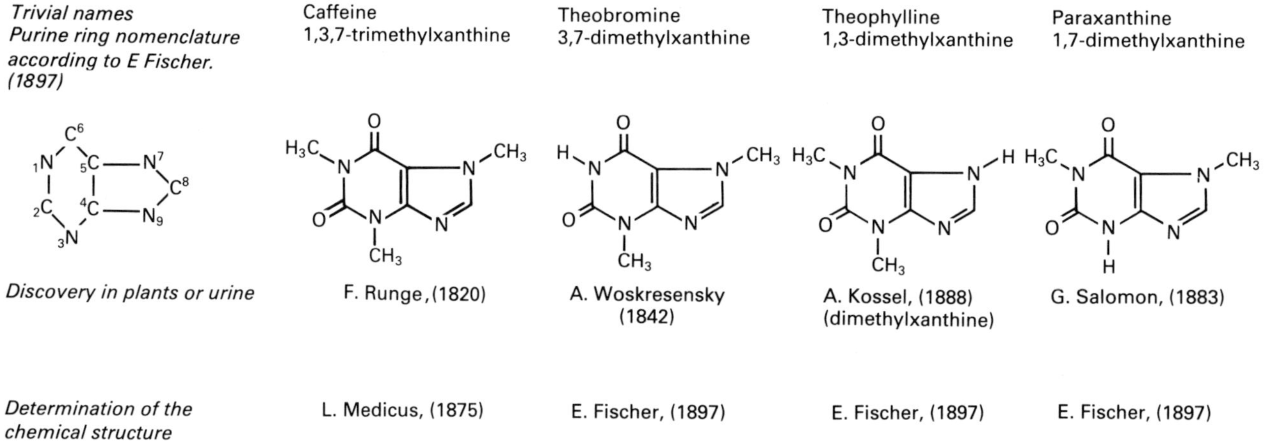

Trivial names Purine ring nomenclature according to E Fischer. (1897)	Caffeine 1,3,7-trimethylxanthine	Theobromine 3,7-dimethylxanthine	Theophylline 1,3-dimethylxanthine	Paraxanthine 1,7-dimethylxanthine
Discovery in plants or urine	F. Runge, (1820)	A. Woskresensky (1842)	A. Kossel, (1888) (dimethylxanthine)	G. Salomon, (1883)
Determination of the chemical structure	L. Medicus, (1875)	E. Fischer, (1897)	E. Fischer, (1897)	E. Fischer, (1897)

Fig. 1 Caffeine and related compounds: nomenclature, discovery and chemical structure (Arnaud MJ, 1987).

Caffeine

alkali. Caffeine forms unstable salts with acids and is decomposed by strong solutions of caustic alkali.

In aqueous solution, caffeine is nonionized at physiological pH. Dimers as well as polymers have been described. The solubility of caffeine in water is increased by the formation of benzoate, cinnamate, citrate and salicylate complexes. In plants, chlorogenic acid, coumarin, isoeugenol, indolacetic acid and anthocyanidin have been shown to complex with caffeine.

Caffeine exhibits an ultraviolet absorption spectrum with a maximum at 274 nm and an absorption coefficient of 9700 in aqueous solution.

Upon crystallization from water, silky needles are obtained containing 6·9% water (a 4/5 hydrate).

Determination

Caffeine has been traditionally determined in foods by ultraviolet spectrophotometry of an organic solvent extract, after suitable clean-up by column chromatography. Such methods tend to be laborious and may be subject to interference from other ultraviolet-absorbing compounds. More recently, high-performance liquid chromatography (HPLC) has been more extensively used. This technique, often in conjunction with solid phase extraction, can provide accurate data for the determination of caffeine in foods and physiological samples. These methods are discussed in more detail in the article on coffee. *See* Chromatography, High-performance Liquid Chromatography; Coffee, Analysis of Coffee Products; Tea, Analysis and Tasting

Absorption, Distribution and Elimination

Following oral ingestion, caffeine is rapidly and virtually completely absorbed from the gastrointestinal tract into the bloodstream. Mean plasma concentrations of 8–10 mg l^{-1} are observed following oral or intravenous doses of 5–8 mg kg^{-1}. The plasma kinetics of caffeine can be influenced by a number of factors, including the total dose of caffeine, the presence of food in the stomach and low pH values of drinks, which can modify gastric emptying. Caffeine enters the intracellular tissue water and is found in all body fluids: cerebrospinal fluid, saliva, bile, semen, breast milk and umbilical cord blood. The fraction of caffeine bound to plasma protein varies from 10 to 30%.

There is no blood–brain barrier and no placental barrier limiting the passage of caffeine through tissues. Therefore, from mother to fetus and to the embryo, an equilibrium can be continuously maintained.

The elimination of caffeine is impaired in neonates because of their immature metabolizing hepatic enzyme systems. For example, plasma half-lives of 65–103 h in the neonate have been reported, compared to 3–6 h in the adult and the elderly.

Cigarette smoking increases the elimination of caffeine whereas decreases have been observed during late pregnancy or with the use of oral contraceptives and in patients with liver diseases. Drug interactions leading to impaired caffeine elimination are frequently reported.

There is no accumulation of caffeine or its metabolites in the body and less than 2% of the caffeine is excreted unchanged in the urine. Some rate-limiting steps in caffeine metabolism, particularly demethylation into paraxanthine, may explain the dose-dependent pharmacokinetics in humans.

Important kinetic differences and variations in the quantitative as well as qualitative metabolic profiles have been shown between species, thus making extrapolation from one species to another very difficult. All of the metabolic transformations include multiple and separate pathways with demethylation to dimethyl- and monomethylxanthines, formation of dimethyl- and monomethylurates and ring opening yielding substituted diaminouracils (Fig. 2).

The reverse biotransformation of theophylline back to caffeine is demonstrated not only in infant but also in adult subjects.

From these metabolic studies, an isotopic caffeine breath test has been developed which detects impaired liver function using the quantitative formation of labelled carbon dioxide as an index. From the urinary excretion of an acetylated uracil metabolite (AFMU), human acetylator phenotype can be easily identified and the analysis of the ratio of the urinary concentrations of other metabolites represents sensitive tests to determine the hepatic enzymatic activities of xanthine oxidase and microsomal 3-methyl demethylation, 7-methyl demethylation and 8-hydroxylation. Faecal excretion is a minor elimination route with recovery of only 2–5% of the ingested dose.

Physiological and Pharmacological Properties

As the physiological and pharmacological properties of caffeine represent the cumulative effects of not only the parent compound but also its metabolites, it is quite possible that effects attributed to caffeine *per se* are in fact mediated by one or more of its metabolites. It must also be noted that most of the knowledge about caffeine's effects has been derived from acute administration to fasted subjects submitted to a period of caffeine abstinence in order to ensure low plasma caffeine concentrations. It is thus difficult from this type of protocol to extrapolate these results to the usual pattern of caffeine consumption in which most people consume caffeine at different intervals throughout the

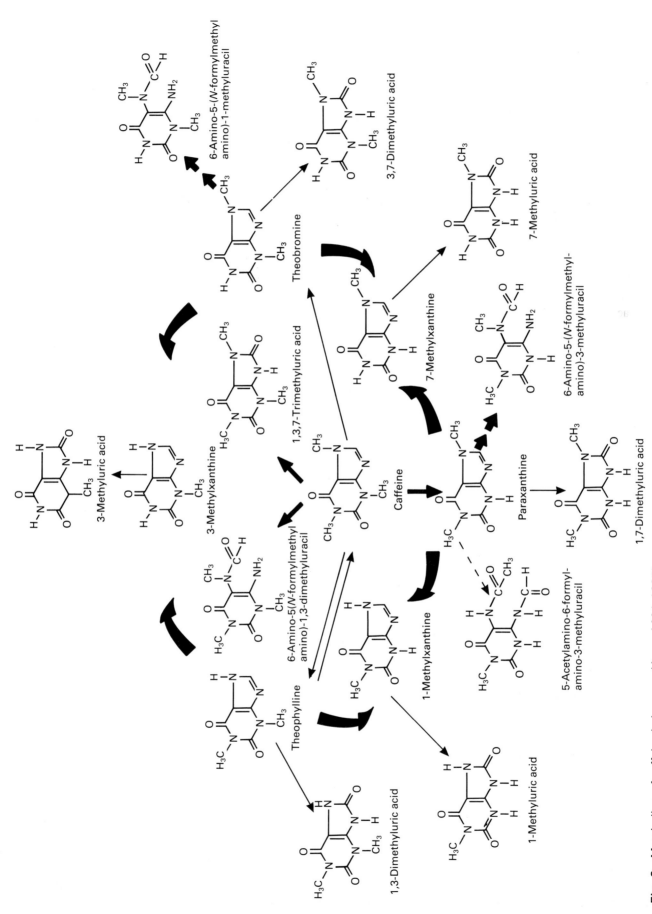

Fig. 2 Metabolism of caffeine in humans (Arnaud MJ, 1987).

day and over periods of years. *See* Coffee, Physiological Effects

Effects on the Central Nervous System

Animal experiments have shown caffeine-mediated effects at the neuroendocrine level such as increased serum corticosterone and β-endorphin, and decreased serum growth hormone and thyrotropin, but it is expected that habitual human consumption has only marginal or inconsistent neuroendocrine effects. Caffeine is described as a central nervous system (CNS) stimulant and the increased formation and release of neurotransmitters such as catecholamines, serotonin, γ-aminobutyric acid (GABA), norepinephrine and acetylcholine have been reported.

Behavioural effects can be observed in humans after an acute dose of $1-5\,\mathrm{mg\,kg^{-1}}$ of caffeine. In these studies, the subjects felt more alert and active with an increased vigilance and clarity of mind. It was claimed that they would be better able to cope with their jobs when bored or fatigued.

A dose-dependent delay in sleep onset is found as well as a decrease in total sleep time and an impairment of sleep quality characterized by an increased number of spontaneous awakings and body movements.

The observation that sensitive subjects are more likely to have trembling hands is considered to be a CNS effect and not a direct effect on muscle. Caffeine doses higher than $15\,\mathrm{mg\,kg^{-1}}$ induce headaches, jitteriness, nervousness, restlessness, irritability, tinnitus, muscle twitchings and palpitations. These symptoms of chronic excessive caffeine intake are part of the criteria used in making the diagnosis of caffeinism.

With $100-200\,\mathrm{mg\,kg^{-1}}$ doses mild delirium appears followed by seizures and death. While tolerance with low doses led to a pleasant stimulation, alertness and performance benefits, on withdrawal, headache, drowsiness, fatigue and anxiety were reported.

Effects on the Cardiovascular System

Caffeine produces a direct stimulation of myocardial tissue leading to an increase in rate and force of contraction. This direct cardiac effect can be inhibited by a depressant effect on the heart via medullary vagal stimulation. These two opposing effects may explain why bradycardia, tachycardia or no change can be observed in individuals receiving similar doses of caffeine.

The traditional clinical view that caffeine induces arrhythmias in humans has not been confirmed by controlled experimental studies.

Caffeine decreases peripheral resistance by direct vasodilatation and increases blood flow to a small extent. This effect results from the relaxation of smooth muscle of blood vessels. For coronary arteries, vasodilatation is also observed *in vitro* but the effects of caffeine in human coronary arteries *in vivo* remains unknown. Different effects of caffeine on circulation can be observed in different vascular beds and, for example, the treatment of migraine headaches by caffeine is mediated through the vasoconstriction of cerebral arteries. It has also been shown that caffeine is capable of attenuating postprandial hypotension in patients with autonomic failure.

The observed cardiovascular effects consist of an increase by 5–10% and for 1–3 h of both mean systolic and diastolic blood pressures. The heart rate is decreased by 5–10% during the first hour followed then by an increase above baseline during the next 2 h. These effects are not detectable in regular coffee drinkers, suggesting that a complete tolerance can be developed. The tolerance to chronic caffeine intake can explain contradictory results reported in the literature.

Epidemiological studies designed to establish a relationship between caffeine intake and the incidences of myocardial infarction, mortality from ischaemic heart disease or cerebrovascular accidents have given conflicting results and have failed to establish a significant correlation.

Effects on Renal Functions

The administration in humans of a single dose of $4\,\mathrm{mg\,kg^{-1}}$ caffeine increases the urinary excretion of sodium, potassium, chloride and urine volume. The mechanism of this mild diuresis is due to an increase in renal blood flow, an increased glomerular filtration and to a decrease in tubular reabsorption of sodium ions. *See* Kidney, Structure and Function

Tolerance to the diuretic action of caffeine was demonstrated more than 50 years ago and was shown to develop on chronic caffeine intake so that the clinical significance of hypokalaemia and calciuria is difficult to evaluate.

Effects on the Respiratory System

In caffeine-naive subjects, a dose of $4\,\mathrm{mg\,kg^{-1}}$ caffeine increases the mean respiratory rate. This effect is not found in chronic caffeine ingestion. Several mechanisms have been suggested such as an increase in pulmonary blood flow, and increased supply of air to the lungs by the relaxation of bronchiolar and alveolar smooth muscle, an increase in sensitivity of the medullary respiratory centre to carbon dioxide, a stimulation of central respiratory drive, an improved skeletal muscle contraction and an increase in cardiac output.

At higher doses (7 mg kg^{-1}), caffeine ingested by trained volunteers alters ventilatory and gas exchange kinetics during exercise, leading to a transient reduction in body carbon dioxide stores.

Effects on Muscles

Caffeine has been shown to have a bronchial and smooth muscle relaxant effect and to improve skeletal muscle contractility. Significant increases in hand tremor and forearm extensor electromyogram were observed in human subjects after the ingestion of 6 mg kg^{-1} of caffeine. This effect is more likely due to a CNS stimulatory effect than to a direct action on the muscle fibres. Skeletal muscle fatigue can be reversed by high concentrations of caffeine obtained only *in vitro* but not *in vivo*. *See* Exercise, Muscle

Effects on the Gastrointestinal System

Caffeine relaxes smooth muscle of the biliary and gastrointestinal tracts and has a weak effect on peristalsis. However, high doses can produce biphasic responses with an initial contraction followed by relaxation. Caffeine seems to have no effect on the lower oesophageal sphincter. The increase in both gastric and pepsin secretions is linearly related to the plasma levels obtained after the administration of a dose from 4 up to 8 mg kg^{-1}. In the small intestine, caffeine modifies the fluid exchange from a net absorption to a net excretion of water and sodium.

The role of caffeine in the pathogenesis of peptic ulcer and gastrointestinal complaints remains unclear and no association can be found from clinical and epidemiological studies.

Effects on Energy Metabolism

Acute administration of caffeine produces a 5–25% increase in the basal metabolic rate. Inactive subjects exhibit a greater increase in resting metabolic rate than do exercise-trained subjects. It is concluded that endurance training seems to result in a reduced thermogenic response to a caffeine challenge.

These modifications of energy metabolism were associated with significant increases in serum free fatty acids concentrations while inconsistent findings were reported for blood glucose levels. The lipolytic effect is generally explained by the inhibition of phosphodiesterase, the release of catecholamine or adenosine receptor antagonism. The increased availability of free fatty acids and their oxidation may have a glycogen-sparing effect. The current hypothesis to explain the enhanced endurance performance capacity is based on these data. However, this effect may be suppressed by the simultaneous ingestion of a high-carbohydrate meal, which is a common practice prior to competition. *See* Energy, Energy Expenditure and Energy Balance

In spite of the controversy among scientists concerning the ergogenic potential of caffeine on sport performance, it is accepted that caffeine will not improve performance during short-term high-intensity work, while an increase both in the work output and endurance in long-term exercise is expected.

On the assumption that caffeine may enhance athletic performance, the International Olympic Committee (IOC) defines an acceptable upper concentration limit of 12 mg l^{-1} in urine samples above which the athlete is disqualified.

Safety and Toxicology

The acute oral LD$_{50}$ (dose sufficient to kill one-half of the population of tested subjects) of caffeine is over 200 mg kg^{-1} in rats, 230 mg kg^{-1} in hamsters and in guinea-pigs, 246 mg kg^{-1} in rabbits and 127 mg kg^{-1} in mice. The sensitivity of rats to the lethal effects of caffeine increased with age and higher toxicity is observed in male than in female rats.

Vomiting, abdominal pain, photophobia, palpitations, muscle twitching, convulsions, miosis and unconsciousness were described in several reports of nonfatal caffeine poisonings in children who ingested 80 mg kg^{-1} caffeine. Several fatal accidental caffeine poisonings reported cold chills, stomach cramps, tetanic spasms and cyanosis. The likely lethal dose in adult humans has been estimated to be about 10 g, which corresponds roughly to 150–200 mg kg^{-1}. With daily doses of 110 mg kg^{-1} given via intragastric cannula to female rats over 100 days, hypertrophy of organs such as salivary gland, liver, heart and kidneys were reported. Caffeine also induced thymic and testicular atrophy. Developmental and reproductive toxicity was associated at high, single, daily doses of caffeine. A no-effect level for teratogenicity is 40 mg kg^{-1} caffeine per day in the rat although delayed sternebral ossification can be observed at lower doses. This effect has been shown to be reversed in the postnatal period. Available epidemiological evidence suggests that maternal caffeine consumption does not cause morphological malformation in the fetus.

High daily levels given as divided doses in rats were less toxic than when given as a single dose. In that case, reduced fetal body weight was the only effect observed.

Caffeine at high concentration levels has mutagenic effects in bacteria and fungi and causes chromosomal damage '*in vitro*'. It is, however, agreed that caffeine is not mutagenic in higher animals.

An epidemiological study showed no chromosomal aberrations in lymphocytes of normal, caffeine-exposed people and other studies reported an increased frequency of micronucleated blood cells and the absence of mutagenic compounds in their urine.

In long-term studies, caffeine was shown to have no carcinogenic potential in rodents. Caffeine has not been classified as carcinogenic either in animals or in humans by the International Agency for Research on Cancer (IARC).

Therapeutic Uses

The most extensively investigated and most firmly established clinical application of caffeine is the control of neonatal apnoea in premature infants. The respirogenic properties of theophylline was first reported and caffeine is increasingly being used for this purpose as a substitute for theophylline because of its wider therapeutic index. For infants of 2·5 kg body weight, the therapeutic loading doses varied from 5 to 30 mg kg^{-1}, followed by a maintenance dose of 3 mg kg^{-1} per day. Plasma caffeine levels must be controlled carefully to reach 10–20 mg l^{-1}.

Because of the bronchial muscle relaxant effect, caffeine is used in chronic obstructive pulmonary disease and for the treatment of asthma.

The use of caffeine in the treatment of children with minimal brain dysfunction, to increase the duration of electroconvulsive therapy-induced seizure, for allergic rhinitis as well as atopic dermatitis have also been described.

Recently, caffeine has been used as a diagnostic test for malignant hyperthermia and in the diagnosis of neuroleptic malignant syndrome, a complication of neuroleptic therapy.

Caffeine is found in many drug preparations, both those sold by prescription and over-the-counter. Caffeine is present in drugs used as stimulants, pain relievers, diuretics and cold remedies. When used as an analgesic adjuvant, the potency of the analgesic drug is significantly enhanced by the addition of caffeine.

Although caffeine was shown to promote thermogenesis in humans, its use is no longer allowed as an ingredient of weight-control products in the US market because long-term clinical studies demonstrate that it does not help those wishing to lose weight. *See* Thermogenesis

Biochemical Mechanisms of Action

The physiological and pharmacological properties of caffeine cannot be explained by a single biochemical mechanism. Three principal hypotheses have been investigated to explain the diverse actions of caffeine.

The first biochemical effect described was the inhibition of phosphodiesterase, the enzyme that catalyses the breakdown of cyclic adenosine 3′,5′-phosphate (cAMP). Caffeine was shown to increase cAMP concentrations in various tissues. This inhibition appears at large concentrations (millimolar range) and would be of limited importance when explaining the physiological effects of caffeine at levels at which it is normally consumed.

Calcium translocation is the second mechanism frequently suggested from experiments using skeletal muscles. However, high concentrations of caffeine are also necessary to modify intracellular calcium ion storage.

In the plasma, increased levels of β-endorphin, epinephrine, norepinephrine, corticosterone, ACTH, renin, angiotensin I and decreased levels of growth hormone, thyroxine, triiodothyronine and thyrotropin were reported with high caffeine doses. The mechanisms responsible for these various effects are largely unknown and the mediation of adenosine receptors is suggested.

The antagonism of benzodiazepine at the receptor level is observed at lower caffeine concentrations (0·5–0·7 mM) than those required for phosphodiesterase inhibition.

The third mechanism, the antagonism of the endogenous adenosine, is presently the most plausible mode of action because caffeine at micromolar levels exerts its antagonism either at the A_1 or A_2 adenosine receptors. Tolerance has been tentatively correlated with the action of caffeine at the receptor level, by the adaptation of the density of the receptors.

Adenosine receptor antagonism appears to be the mechanism which explains most of the effects of caffeine: CNS activity, intestinal peristalsis, respiration, blood pressure, lipolysis, catecholamine release and renin release. However, some effects, like opiate antagonism or effects which are similar to adenosine, must be mediated by other mechanisms such as the potentiation by caffeine of inhibitors of prostaglandin synthesis.

Bibliography

Anon (1991) *IARC Monographs on the Evaluation of Carcinogenic Risks to Humans: Coffee, Tea, Mate, Methylxanthines and Methylglyoxal*, vol. 51. Lyon: World Health Organization – International Agency for Research on Cancer.

Arnaud MJ (1987) The pharmacology of caffeine. *Progress in Drug Research* 31: 273–313.

Clarke RJ and Macrae R (eds) (1988) Physiology. *Coffee*, vol. 3. London: Elsevier.

Dews PB (ed.) (1984) *Caffeine*. Berlin: Springer-Verlag.

James JE (1991) *Caffeine and Health*. London: Academic Press.

Maurice J. Arnaud
Nestec Ltd, Lausanne, Switzerland

CAKES

Contents

Nature of Cakes

Classification

Generally speaking, the confectionery industry derives its name from the single component always present in its many final products, i.e. sugar. Other ingredients, although influencing many specific products (e.g. cacao in chocolate, flour in biscuits), do not have the same intrinsic possibility of characterizing the industry, but only the specific subcategories; neither can the various processes used by industry be taken as the basis for a general definition.

In terms of their composition, and on the basis of specific working processes, the confectionery products can be classified as follows:

1. Oven-baked products (cakes and biscuits).
2. Chocolate-based products (chocolate, toffees, etc.).
3. Sugar-based products (sweets, jellies, jams, nougats, etc.).
4. Milk-based products (ice creams, puddings, etc.).
See Biscuits, Cookies and Crackers, Nature of the Products; Ice Cream, Methods of Manufacture; Jams and Preserves, Chemistry of Manufacture

Definition

Many definitions of cakes have been reported in the literature by various authors, and they have used a multiplicity of key words, such as principal components, technological processes, external characteristics, and functional and rheological properties.

The most acceptable, basic definition of a cake is 'an edible, (un)leavened, baked, sweet flour confectionery, often enriched with other minor compounds for appearance, typically round and flat in shape'. This definition, although not exhaustive, allows cakes to be easily distinguished from several other sweet food items which are commonly used as desserts (pastries, biscuits, cookies, crème caramels, etc.).

Types of Cakes on the Market

The following approaches can be used for classifying cakes.

Ingredients Characterizing the Base Formulation

- Wheat flour, oat flour, starches (essentially in the flour:water ratio); Fig. 1 shows how Bennion and Bamford (1973) used this ratio to classify cakes among various confectionery items.
- Sugars (sucrose, glucose, isoglucose, honey).
- Fats or shortenings, e.g. in butter cakes, short cakes.
- Fruit (both fresh and dried, candied or jellied), e.g. in plumcake, strudel, fruitcake, nutcake, Genoa cake.
- Eggs, e.g. in sponge cake, angel cake, meringue, beignet.
- Others (presence of specific local liquors and spices), e.g. in rum cake, ginger cake, honey cake.

Elements Characterizing the Final Appearance

This classification covers sponge cake, angel cake, layer cake, pound cake, chiffon cake, torte, pie, etc.

Name

Classification by name covers morning (coffee) cakes, Danish pastry, pancakes, party torte, Christmas pie, Madeira cake, birthday cake, tennis cake, wedding cake, etc.

Technology of Production

In addition to classifications based on different kinds of mixing, forming and baking, cakes are chiefly identified as follows:

- Yeast-leavened cakes (fruit bread, brioche, Danish pastry, baba, savarin, sponge cake).
- Chemically leavened cakes by gaseous development from baking powders, including carbonates, ammonia, acetone (doughnut, loaf cake, angel cake, layer cake, scones) and ethanol (plumcake). Gaseous development can derive from decomposition as a result of heating, or from an acid–base reaction.

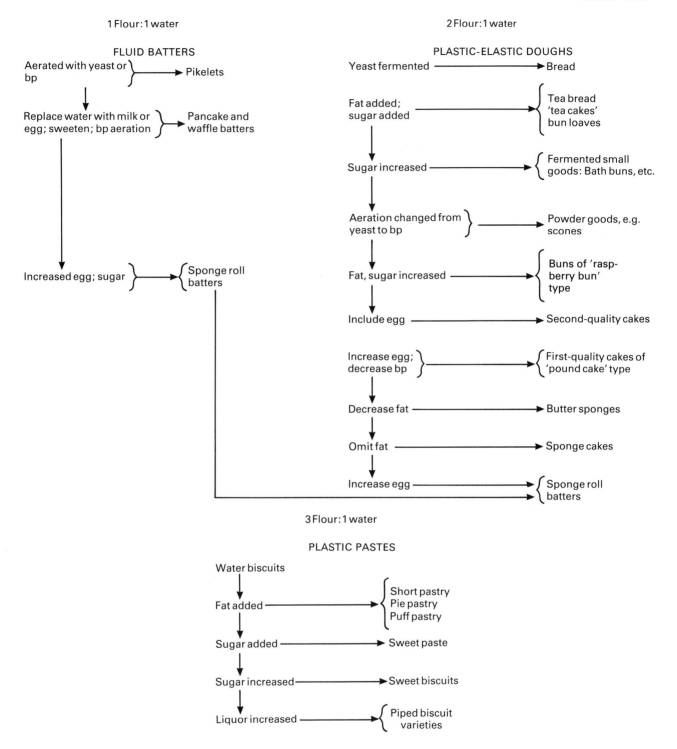

1 Flour:1 water

FLUID BATTERS

Aerated with yeast or bp ⟩ → Pikelets

Replace water with milk or egg; sweeten; bp aeration ⟩ → Pancake and waffle batters

Increased egg; sugar ⟩ → Sponge roll batters

2 Flour:1 water

PLASTIC-ELASTIC DOUGHS

Yeast fermented —————→ Bread

Fat added; sugar added ————— Tea bread 'tea cakes' bun loaves

Sugar increased ————— Fermented small goods: Bath buns, etc.

Aeration changed from yeast to bp ⟩ → Powder goods, e.g. scones

Fat, sugar increased ————— Buns of 'raspberry bun' type

Include egg —————→ Second-quality cakes

Increase egg; decrease bp ⟩ → First-quality cakes of 'pound cake' type

Decrease fat —————→ Butter sponges

Omit fat —————→ Sponge cakes

Increase egg —————→ Sponge roll batters

3 Flour:1 water

PLASTIC PASTES

Water biscuits

Fat added ————— Short pastry Pie pastry Puff pastry

Sugar added —————→ Sweet paste

Sugar increased —————→ Sweet biscuits

Liquor increased ————— Piped biscuit varieties

Fig. 1 Confectionery product classification in relation to different flour and water mixtures. bp, Baking powder. Data from Butterworth and Davlin, as reported by Bennion EB and Bamford GST (1973).

- Air-leavened cakes (short or puff paste, sponge cake, angel food cake, pound cake, chiffon cake, Swiss roll).
- Unleavened cakes (wafer, pie crust, fruit pie dough, fried pie, puff pastry). *See* Pastry Products, Types and Production

Important Features of the Basic Raw Materials

The system which we have chosen for classifying the raw materials used in the confectionery industry takes into account, in order of priority, the various properties of

Nature of Cakes

Table 1. Composition (g per 100 g of product) and energy value of some products in the confectionery industry

Products	Water	Lipids	Soluble carbohydrates	Proteins	Available carbohydrates	Energy (per 100 g) kcal	MJ
Flour-based							
Leavened							
Panettone (Italian Christmas cake)	27·0	10·7	22·9	6·4	56·5	334	1·40
Chocolate cake	28·0	17·5	27·6	4·9	36·8	377	1·58
Toast (bread)	2·0	5·2	4·5	10·9	84·9	409	1·72
Brioche	20·0	18·3	10·6	7·2	58·4	412	1·73
Swiss roll	14·0	15·1	45·7	6·2	67·6	414	1·74
Unleavened							
Pie	18·0	17·7	32·6	5·3	60·6	408	1·71
Wafer	4·0	15·0	48·3	7·1	73·5	439	1·84
Cocoa-based							
Chocolate spread	0·8	32·4	58·1	6·9	58·1	537	2·26
Bitter chocolate bar	1·1	34·0	56·7	5·8	56·7	564	2·37
Milk chocolate bar	2·0	37·6	50·8	8·9	50·8	564	2·37
Sugar-based							
Cherry marmalade	33·0	tr	62·3	0·6	62·3	236	0·99
Orange marmalade	28·0	0·1	69·5	0·1	69·5	261	1·10
Chewing gum	3·5	—	70·0	—	70·0	262	1·10
Marzipan	30·0	5·8	32·5	11·2	55·4	304	1·28
Almond nougat	7·0	26·8	52·0	10·8	52·0	479	2·01
Milk-based							
Fruit yoghurt	81·0	3·3	12·6	2·8	12·6	88	0·37
Vanilla ice cream	60·6	13·7	20·7	4·2	20·7	218	0·92
Chocolate ice cream	56·0	23·6	25·8	5·2	25·8	240	1·01

Data from Fantozzi P (1992).
tr, trace; —, not detectable.

the individual components and their functions during the various technological processes. The energy value and the nutritional composition of some confectionery products, as described in Table 1, are of secondary importance according to such a classification.

The main raw materials used in cake making, in relationship to their specific function(s), are reported in detail below and are listed in decreasing order of importance.

Water

Water is used only as a moistening agent in mixing in order to obtain the desired texture (gluten development, starch gelation, etc.). Knowledge of the water activity in the product is very important because it affects the organoleptic characteristics (flavour, taste, etc.) of the product as well as the shelf life owing to its effect on

staling, i.e. starch retrogradation, fat hydrolysis and peroxidation, as well as microbial activity. *See* Water Activity, Effect on Food Stability

Water content of the initial cake recipe (i.e. the quantity of ingredients used for making a specific cake) is of fundamental importance for the secondary classification of the cake, as already shown in Fig. 1. Some cakes, however, are made from recipes in which water is replaced by eggs or milk.

Flours (wheat, oat, corn, rye, soy, barley – as malt – potato, etc.)

Flour composition (starch, sugars, proteins, fat and minerals) varies significantly in relation to the plant source and percentage of germ and/or bran still present (i.e. whole-bran flour). *See* Flour, Dietary Importance

Present market trends, greatly influenced by the growing attention to the value of fibre, have given

Nature of Cakes

increasing importance to the use of whole-grain flours in the confectionery industry (particularly in biscuits, but also in cakes). *See* Dietary Fibre, Fibre and Disease Prevention

Flours are used essentially for their specific ability to perform the following functions:

1. Give consistency to the final product, owing to the presence of starch.
2. Create a proper internal, aerated, sponge-like structure which is then stabilized during the baking phase, owing to the presence of a gluten network which confers viscoelastic properties on the dough.
3. Contribute to the formation of specific flavours during baking.

Natural Sweeteners

Crystals

Sucrose, produced from cane or beet sugar, is also available in other forms (granulated, castor, syrup), each of which, owing to different amounts of impurities, can significantly influence the final product. The main reason for the presence of sucrose in the product is to give a sweet taste; at the same time and as a result of caramelization at high temperature, it can affect some fundamental organoleptic characteristics, such as colour and flavour. *See* Caramel, Properties and Analysis; Sucrose, Dietary Importance

Dextrose (crystallized glucose) is also widely used as an ingredient.

Syrups

Glucose, different starch syrups used for their content of glucose, fructose, maltose and other polymers, such as dextrans, are obtained from corn, potato, wheat starches, malt, etc. They are primarily used in confectionery products with a sugar base, because of their ease of measuring in mixing, and their various sweetening abilities, compared to that of sucrose (sucrose, 1; fructose, 1·5; glucose, 0·5; maltose, 0·5; invert sugar, 0·85). *See* Carbohydrates, Sensory Properties; Fructose

These sugars are also able to produce the amino-sugar reaction, influencing colour and flavour, while dextrins play a very important role as moisteners. *See* Browning, Nonenzymatic

Others

Honey and lactose are used as natural sweeteners. Sorbitol, mannitol and glycerol are sweetening polyalcohols with other peculiar functional properties such as water retention and wettability.

Artificial Sweeteners

Artificial sweeteners are used essentially in dietetic, hypoenergetic products as a substitute for natural sweeteners. The most frequently utilized is saccharin and its salts, while many others are available even if sparingly utilized in cakemaking (cyclamates, thaumarin, etc.). *See* Cyclamates; Saccharin; Sweeteners – Intense

Proteins (from eggs, milk and milk derivatives)

Proteins are very important for structure, palatability, fat retention, and foaming (e.g. in cheese pie, beignet, meringue). *See* Protein, Functional Properties

Colloids, Gellifiers and Emulsifiers

Many substances can be included in this vast category: the previously mentioned proteins, gums, pectins, starches, lecithins. *See* Gums, Nutritional Role of Guar Gum; Pectin, Food Uses; Starch, Modified Starches

They play an important role in the functional properties of various products, owing to their ability to gel a fluid, absorb water and vary viscosity, as well as their plasticity, emulsifying capacity, foam formation, structure formation, etc., both in the cake preparation and in its final use, i.e. toppings, fillings, icings. *See* Colloids and Emulsions; Emulsifiers, Organic Emulsifiers

Fats or Shortenings

In some types of cakes, fats and shortenings are the fundamental ingredients. They are numerous and their use affects the final characteristics of the product. The main ones are butter, milk cream, margarines, palm oil, coconut and palm-kernel, butters, hydrogenated fats, and cocoa butter. *See* Fats, Uses in the Food Industry

Their action is complex:

1. The majority of the lipid compounds used have a high melting point, and hence act as texturing agents and possess characteristics of contractability on cooling and, therefore, high covering capacity in toppings.
2. If used in fillings and, mainly, in toppings, those with a low melting point are chosen for their ability to increase creaming and plasticity. These properties are related to the maintenance of the plastic state.
3. From the organoleptic point of view, some have no influence, while others (cocoa butter, butter) have their own flavour characteristics. All, however, are important vehicles and enhancers of aromatic substances.

Milk

Used as whole, skimmed, condensed and dried as well as its fractions (whey proteins, casein), milk has the following functions:

1. Moistening agent. When used in the liquid form, it can be added to the dough as a substitute for water.
2. Emulsifying agent, owing to its fat and protein content.
3. Jellying agent, owing to its protein content, primarily casein, and serum albumin.
4. Flavouring agent, for the secondary products formed during the Maillard reaction, starting with sugars (lactose) and protein and/or amino acids. *See* Casein and Caseinates, Uses in the Food Industry; Whey and Whey Powders, Production and Uses

Leavening Agents

Leavening agents are used for their lifting capacity, which is achieved by means of different gases or the formation of carbon dioxide of biological (yeast) or chemical (baking powders) origin. *See* Leavening Agents

Gas

Gases used include air (injection, whipping, overrun), water vapour (during baking), and ethanol (from fermentation or added as an ingredient).

Carbon Dioxide

Yeast is generally *Saccharomyces cerevisiae*, in the dried or fresh compressed state. *See* Yeasts

Baking powders, according to the USA federal government definition, consist of 'the mixture of an acid reacting material (tartaric acid or its acid salts, acid salts of phosphoric acid, compounds of aluminium, any combination of the foregoing) and sodium bicarbonate'. They are used essentially to allow speed and continuity in the process of production, and differ from products fermented with yeasts which require a certain amount of time to undergo the proper metabolic activity.

Acidulants, with the role of freeing the carbon dioxide in the chemically leavened cakes, can be organic, glucono-δ-lactone) or inorganic (acid potassium or sodium phosphate, acid sodium pyrophosphate). *See* Acids, Natural Acids and Acidulants

Acids are also used in order to improve the gellifying properties of the pectin, because of their acidifying action.

Cacao Products

Cacao products are chocolate, cocoa powders (at different grades of defatting) and cocoa butter. They are used because of their influence on the organoleptic characteristics (colour, flavour, aroma) of the product and because of their functional properties, which essentially depend on the amount of fat (chocolate and cocoa butter). *See* Cocoa, Production, Products and Uses

Essential Oils, Essences and Spices

Used because of their characteristic flavour, essential oils, essences and spices are obtained, respectively, as follows: by pressure or distillation in a vapour current from plants, fruit or fruit parts; by shredding roots, fruit, seeds, etc., in particular alcoholic solvents; by drying and pulverizing specific aromatic parts of plants. *See* Essential Oils, Properties and Uses

Preserves (Jams, Jellies and Marmalades) and Dehydrated Fruits

Preserves and dehydrated fruits are used for (1) their sweetening, colouring and aromatic properties, and (2) some specific functional properties in toppings (e.g. jellifying ability).

The addition of fruit to cakes should be carefully controlled because it adds extra moisture. Because of this, the use of dehydrated fruit, as well as the use of fruit prepared via nonconventional systems (osmotic dehydration) or mild technologies (dehydrofreezing), are to be studied.

Similarly, a fruit-based topping, primarily in pies, should have a barrier between it and the cake, in order to avoid excessive rehydration with consequent softening and loss of consistency.

Dried Fruit and Nuts

Traditionally, dried fruit and nuts are used for their specific organoleptic characteristics (flavour, taste, consistency), as well as on the grounds that they do not contribute additional moisture to the cake. The main types are almonds, hazel nuts, raisins, walnuts, figs and dates.

Basic Formulations

The main ingredients in a basic cake formula are flour, sugar, colloids (from eggs, milk, fruit and/or animal or vegetable gums), fat or shortening, water, and leavening agent (biological or chemical).

These ingredients, when used in different proportions based upon their specific properties, will give rise to the large and varied cake world. The most important effects of ingredients on the final cake can be recognized as follows:

1. Strengthening, attributed to flours and colloids.
2. Structural, owing to flours and colloids.
3. Lifting, owing to sugars, fats, colloids, leavening agents.
4. Toppings, produced by colloids, water, sugars.
5. Carrying, owing to water, milk.

Fance, in 1960, reported a practical application of the basic formulation rules for cakemaking:

1. The flour:egg weight ratio should not exceed 1:1 (dry-weight basis).
2. The weight of fats should not exceed the weight of eggs.
3. The weight of fats should not exceed that of the sugars.
4. The weight of sugars should not exceed the total liquid.
5. Leavening agents are used for the final adjustment.

Bibliography

Bennion EB and Bamford GST (1973) *The Technology of Cake Making*. London: Leonard Hill Books.
Fance WJ (1960) *The Student's Technology of Breadmaking and Flour Confectionery*. London: Routledge.
Fantozzi P (1992) L'industria dolciaria. *Nuovo Manuale dell'Agronomo*. Roma: REDA (Ramo Editoriale degli Agricoltori). In press.
Kiger JL and Kiger JG (1968) *Techniques Modernes de la Biscuiterie- Patisserie- Boulangerie*, vol. 1. Paris: Dunod.
Matz SA (1989a) *Bakery Technology*. Essex: Elsevier Science Publishers.
Matz SA (1989b) *Formulas and Processes for Bakers*. Essex: Elsevier Science Publishers.
Matz SA (1989c) *Equipment for Bakers*. Essex: Elsevier Science Publishers.
Wade P (1988) *Biscuits, Cookies and Crackers*, vol. 1. Essex: Elsevier Science Publishers.

P. Fantozzi
Instituto di Industrie Agrarie, Perugia, Italy
A. Sensidoni
Instituto di Industrie Agrarie, Perugia, Italy

Methods of Manufacture

In cake manufacture, the processing techniques at the industrial level may allow totally innovative products to be obtained as substitutes for home-made goods, or they may preserve and recreate the image of traditional and country-style products, both tendencies being very important in marketing.

The high level of quality control in industrial production requires extensive knowledge of the specific roles of both the raw materials and the process.

Furthermore, mastery and control of packaging, storage and distribution are fundamental for obtaining a satisfactory shelf life for the industrial product.

Production of Mixes, Including Plant and Processes

Raw Materials

The raw materials should first be acquired, received, analysed and stored at the manufacturing plant. Each of these preliminary operations requires a coding system and precise observance of the mandatory specifications, in order to ensure that all of the qualitative, analytical and normal characteristics of the basic raw materials, which are fundamental to successful technological processing, are up to production standard. For example, the aim of raw material storage is to allow for its later use, but without any modification of the composition and qualitative and organoleptic characteristics. It is, therefore, important to avoid every possible alteration, or physical, chemical or biological contamination, of the crude product, regardless of whether it is loose or packaged. Proper storage, therefore, must include control of temperature, amount of oxygen, light, moisture and microorganisms, which are specific for each case. *See* Storage Stability, Parameters Affecting Storage Stability

Once this preliminary operation has been satisfactorily completed, the raw materials can be mixed, in the right quantities, and according to specific procedures, in order to follow the recipes specified by the industry for each type of cake.

Raw Material Movement, Weighing and Mixing

In the formulation of cakes, the first step is transport of the raw materials (liquid or solid) to be weighed and mixed. These operations can be done in a discontinuous (manual or automatic) or continuous way, according to the volume needed and the size of the plant.

The entire cycle of continuous operations can be managed by computers, with 'on-line' control. Depending on the use, there are specific instruments on the market for both solids and liquids, and whose functioning (by weight, volume, or viscosity measure) varies according to the rheological characteristics of the ingredient.

It is important to note that the transport and continuous weighing of solids (flour, sugar, etc.) is more difficult than for liquids, on account of the multiplicity of variables connected with solids (moisture content, blend, reduction rate, composition and the physical characteristics of the 'flow' and the conveyors). On the other hand, mixing of liquids, especially those with high viscosity, with other products causes more difficult technical problems than with solids.

Obtaining mixes at the industrial level should take into account savings in labour and time. As a general rule, it is advisable to always plan the preparation of large batches of mixes, especially when each single mix is made up of numerous minor ingredients.

Mixing is a combined operation which is not only the simple mechanical union of different components, but also allows ingredients (mainly gluten) to be melted and oriented by compression, shearing, stretching and stirring, as well as giving plasticity and creating the network of the dough. *See* Bread, Dough Mixing and Testing Operations

It is recommended that, initially, the manufacturer should plan the premixing of solids, and then complete the formulation with the successive addition of ingredients which act as carrier liquids (water, milk, shortening, etc.). This general practice is subject to notable exceptions in the case of the mixing of ingredients for obtaining leavened products. In this case, it is necessary to take into account the rheological characteristics (Newtonian, pseudoplastic, thixotropic, dilatant or rheopectic) of the liquids mixed with the solids in order to obtain a dough in which the physicochemical properties are most suitable for the technology.

Once the requested mix is obtained, it is necessary to produce a well-creamed and plastified dough, because these characteristics are fundamental for uniformity of heat transfer and product deformation during baking, and for final product structure.

The major role in this operation is played by the flour proteins (gliadins and glutenins) and, as a function of their ratio, they develop gluten during mixing. Gluten-rich flours will produce a hard dough, ready for biological leavening. Gluten-poor flours will produce a short dough, generally used for chemically leavened products with higher solid/liquid ratios. *See* Flour, Analysis of Wheat Flours; Flour, Dietary Importance

For baked products, there are many mixers available in different sizes, power and working capacities and principles of operation. They may be classified as continuous or batch.

Although they have different advantages and disadvantages, batch mixers are the most widely used.

Mixers may be divided into two categories (vertical and horizontal) in relation to the positioning in space of the mixing arms (beaters) inside the bowl.

Vertical Mixers

(1) One-beater mixer: the movement inside the bowl is generally double, i.e. an axial rotation of the beater itself and a circular (planetary) revolution around the bowl.
(2) Multiple beater mixer: the beaters rotate axially and separately inside the bowl, influencing reciprocally the mixing action.

The beaters used in vertical mixers can be of different shapes (spiral, hook, sigmoid, blade-like) and can rotate at different speeds. Bowls can also rotate in opposition to the beater(s), Bowls are cylindrical in shape, vertical and open at the top to allow the beater unit entrance.

Horizontal Mixers

The bowl (cylindrical or U-shaped) is positioned horizontally. Generally, it is stationary, but may rotate for discharge of the dough. The beater, single or multiple, moves inside the bowl at various speeds for mixing. If single, the beater may be inclined in relation to the axis of the bowl. Some mixers possess 'braker' blades on the inner surface of the bowl, in order to enhance the mixing action of the beaters.

Dividing, Rounding and Sheeting

After mixing, the dough is submitted to the following further operations:

(1) Dividing – in order to separate the dough by cutting it into regular pieces of similar weight.
(2) Rounding – in order to (a) rearrange the cut dough into a regular shape, and (b) to avoid the loss of gases by diffusion.
(3) Sheeting – in order to create a sheet of dough, when needed.

Commercial Techniques for Baking

Fermentation and Proving Rooms

The dough, correctly divided, rounded and, if needed, sheeted, is put, in sequence, into the fermentation and proving rooms, which require optimal temperature and relative humidity for the fermentation activity of the microorganisms used (25–38°C, 75–80% relative humidity).

The purpose of fermentation is to cause the following changes:

(1) formation of carbon dioxide, ethanol and an aerated, sponge-like structure;
(2) formation of flavours and flavour precursors.

Forming

This occurs when the fermenting dough is placed in a suitable container. The product can rise, taking the form of the container, except for the top.

Matz SA (1989) describes in detail all the forming equipment commercially available and their specific features, and takes into account that they differ when

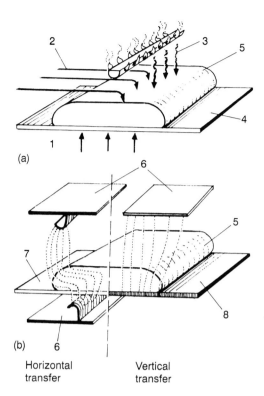

Fig. 1. Heat transfer in ovens: (a) traditional oven (b) radiation oven (microwave). Key: 1, heat transfer by conduction; 2, heat transfer by convection; 3, heat transfer by radiation; 4, metal oven plate; 5, dough; 6, high-frequency metal electrodes; 7, plastic oven plate; 8, metal oven plate acting as high-frequency electrode.

utilized for bread, cakes or cookies. According to him, cake-forming equipment can be classified as follows:

(1) drum moulders;
(2) cross-grain moulders;
(3) reversed sheeting moulders;
(4) twist bread moulders;
(5) extrusion moulders;
(6) rotary moulders.

Baking Equipment

The baking operation can be considered fundamental in cake making, and the oven used definitely affects the final product.

The choice of heating system (direct or indirect), or energy source (steam, fuel, electricity) and of heat transfer (conduction, convection or radiation), as shown in Fig. 1, is fundamental, and is also based on the specific variables of the cake (size, shape, recipe) and its container.

For example, it is important to note that, in the case of radiation ovens (infrared and microwave), the electromagnetic waves should preferably pass through the product horizontally, for better homogeneity of heating (Fig. 1(b)).

Furthermore, all cakes should be baked with respect to specific time/temperature ratios. Therefore, the need for careful control of these parameters is obvious in order to control the following modifications, which take place during baking:

(1) evolution and expansion of gases (carbon dioxide or air);
(2) structure formation by coagulation of gluten and other proteins (i.e. eggs) and starch gelatinization;
(3) partial dehydration due to water evaporation;
(4) development of flavours;
(5) changes in colour due to Maillard browning reactions between milk, gluten and egg proteins with reducing sugars, as well as other chemical (colour and flavour) changes;
(6) crust formation due to surface dehydration, and darkening due to Maillard browning reactions and sugar caramelization. *See* Browning, Nonenzymatic

Ovens can be classified as batch and continuous. Deck, rack and revolving ovens are based on a batch system, while tray and band ovens are based on a continuous system. Figure 2 shows a schematic drawing of a batch rack oven, while Fig. 3 shows the final part of a modular continuous band oven. The band oven generally consists of (1) entrance of product, (2) preheating, (3) heating, (4) cooling, (5) cutting and (6) delivery.

Special Techniques for Cake Decoration

Once produced and properly cooled, the exterior appearance of the cake needs to be completed, using a series of different components which determine its final look, contribute to its identification and correspond to the type of cake.

From a classification point of view, the methods used for applying the decorative items can be subdivided as follows:

● topping – covering the top of the cake with different decorative items;
● dusting – application of small quantities of edible powders or granules to the top of the cake;
● coating – application of an edible liquid layer (e.g. honey, caramel, whipped cream, yolk or egg white) to the surface of the cake to protect and decorate it;
● enrobing – fat-based, moisture-free coating;
● glazing – coating the cake with thin transparent layers of sugar/gelatine-rich liquid preparations;
● icing – coating the cake (1) with thick, opaque layers of sugar/gelatine-rich liquid preparation (water icing) or (2) with thick sugar/fat-rich, semisolid-plastic materials (cream icing);
● filling – injection of fat/sugar preparations into the cake.

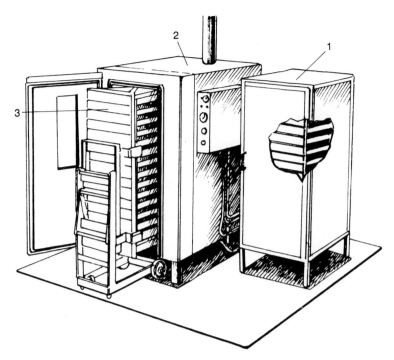

Fig. 2. Schematic drawing of a discontinuous rack oven. Key: 1, fermentation room; 2, oven; 3, rack of plates.

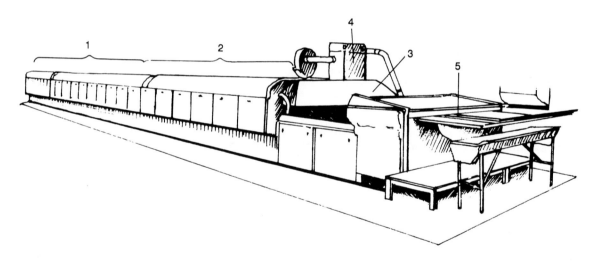

Fig. 3. Schematic drawing of a continuous band oven. Key: 1, heating section; 2, cooling section; 3, cutting section; 4, cooling air conveyor; 5, delivery section.

Commercial Techniques and Requirements of Cakes for Freezing, Canning, Slicing, Wrapping and Packing.

Packaging, by creating a barrier between the product and the external environment, is the final operation in cake making, and has the following functions:

(1) to preserve the qualitative and organoleptic characteristics;
(2) to inhibit entrance of pollutants or external contaminants (moulds, microorganisms, oxygen, water, light, heat);
(3) to inhibit the loss of volatile compounds from the product (flavours, moisture, gases);
(4) to protect the product from mechanical damage;
(5) to allow the product, if desired, to be sold in portions;
(6) to supply consumer information (legal labelling, storage conditions and shelf life, composition); *See* Legislation, Labelling Legislation
(7) to facilitate the storage classification, movement, inventory and identification of the product by use of a bar code.

Furthermore, packaging allows the marketing of the following frozen products:

Methods of Manufacture

(1) Cakes with a cream or ice cream base, by significantly increasing their shelf life to months; if these products were refrigerated without packaging they would only have a very short shelf life (1 or 2 days).

(2) Particular mixes (puff pastry, croissant base, pie and torte bases) which need further operations before consumption (generally defrosting and cooking, or cooking without previous defrosting, in an oven). It is well known that, in oven-baked products (e.g. bread), freezing plays an important role as it slows down staling.

In order to lengthen the shelf life of the cake, special methods have been experimented with, e.g. packaging under vacuum and modified atmosphere packaging (MAP) using nitrogen or carbon dioxide. It is also possible to place ethanol in the cake container as a microbial and aromatic stabilizer. *See* Chilled Storage, Use of Modified Atmosphere Packaging; Chilled Storage, Effect of Modified Atmosphere Packaging on Food Quality; Chilled Storage, Packaging Under Vacuum

Bibliography

Almond N (1988) *Biscuits, Cookies and Crackers*, vol. 2. London: Elsevier.

Bennion EB, Stewart J and Bamford GST (1966) *Cake Making*. London: Leonard Hill Books.

Fantozzi P (1992) *L'Industria Dolciaria. Nuovo Manuale dell'Agronomo*. Rome: REDA (Ramo Editoriale degli Agricoltozi).

Kiger JL and Kiger JG (1968) *Techniques Modernes de la Biscuiterie – Patisserie – Boulangerie*, vol. 2. Paris: Dunod.

Manley DJR (1983) *Technology of Biscuits, Crackers and Cookies*. Chichester: Ellis Horwood.

Matz SA (1960) *Bakery. Technology and Engineering*. Westport, CT: AVI.

Matz SA (1968) *Cookie and Cracker Technology*. Westport, CT: AVI.

Matz SA (1989) *Equipment for Bakers*. London: Elsevier.

P. Fantozzi
Universita Degli Studi di Perugia, Perugia, Italy
A. Sensidoni
Universita Degli Studi di Perugia, Perugia, Italy

Chemistry of Baking

This article considers typical cake formulae and ingredient functionality. Cakes include: foam types, such as angel food and sponge; pound cakes; shortened cakes; and high-ratio or box cakes. Their principal ingredients include wheat flour, sugar, shortening, eggs, chemical leavening agents, milk and salt.

Chemical and physical changes during mixing and baking are described together with mechanisms for flavour development and the role of additives.

Principal Ingredients in Cake Batter

Flour is the most important ingredient in cakes. Cake flour is usually milled from a soft wheat with low protein and ash (mineral) contents and has a fine particle size. The flour is normally treated with chlorine gas in the USA, which causes hydrolytic depolymerization of the starch molecules, increasing the hydration capacity of the flour. The flour must develop a mellow gluten during mixing, with no tough properties, but it must have the strength to assure a fine foam structure. A protein content of $8·5 \pm 0·5\%$ is the optimum, with $0·36 \pm 0·04\%$ ash content, a pH of $4·7 \pm 0·2$, and an average particle size of $10 \pm 0·5 \ \mu m$. *See* Flour, Roller Milling Operations; Flour, Analysis of Wheat Flours; Flour, Dietary Importance

Shortening has three basic functions. First, it entraps air during the creaming process to aid in proper aeration, or leavening, of the batter and the finished cake. Second, it coats the protein and starch particles, disrupting the continuity of the gluten and starch structure to tenderize the cake crumb. Third, it contributes desirable moisture and softness. However, a satisfactory cell structure can be made in foam-type cakes without shortening. *See* Fats, Uses in the Food Industry; Vegetable Oils, Applications

Eggs affect structure, volume, tenderness and eating properties. They perform a binding action, and their rich protein content and ability to whip into a foam are important to cake structure. The aerated structure carries the other ingredients, because the egg proteins help the gluten form a complex network for structural support. As the cake bakes, the egg protein coagulates, contributing to crumb rigidity. *See* Eggs, Dietary Importance

Eggs also have a tenderizing action, because the yolks are high in lipids and lecithin, which act as emulsifying agents. They also act as leaveners by entrapping air bubbles which, when heated, expand to increase volume by retaining leavening gases. Eggs add a mild but distinctive flavour and increase the nutritive value.

Chemical leavening agents are added to aerate the batter and to make a light, tender, porous product. A porous batter (before baking) ensures good volume, uniform cell structure, bright crumb colour, and soft texture and improves the eating quality. Sodium bicarbonate plus an acidic agent (see Table 1), usually the salt

Table 1. Acidic agents used in leavening

Acid	Formula	Neutralization value
Monocalcium phosphate (MCP)	$Ca(H_2PO_4)_2 \cdot H_2O$	80
Anhydrous monocalcium phosphate (AMCP)	$Ca(H_2PO_4)_2$	83·5
Sodium acid pyrophosphate (SAPP)	$Na_2H_2P_2O_7$	72
Sodium aluminum phosphate (SALP)	$NaH_{14}Al_3(PO_4)_8 \cdot 4H_2O$	100
Monopotassium tartrate (cream of tartar)	$KHC_4H_4O_6$	45
Sodium aluminum sulphate (SAS)	$Al_2(SO_4)_3 \cdot Na_2SO_4$	100
Dicalcium phosphate dihydrate (DCP)	$CaHPO_4 \cdot 2H_2O$	33
Glucono-δ-lactone (GDL)	$C_5H_{10}O_6$	50

of a weak acid, are the most common leaveners. *See* Leavening Agents

Baking powders are a combination of sodium bicarbonate and one of the agents in Table 1 or some other acidic components. A diluent of starch or flour is usually added to standardize the baking powder. Baking powder should yield not less than 12% by weight of available carbon dioxide.

Baking powders are classified by their reaction rates as fast, slow, or double-acting. The fast-acting types release almost all of their gas in the first few moments after contact with liquid. The dough or batter must expand quite readily. If too much carbon dioxide is lost before the batter is set, the volume decreases significantly.

The slow-acting powders require oven heat to release their gas. Double-acting types react partially at low temperatures, but need heat to complete the reaction. These powders produce a smooth-flowing batter.

The neutralization value (NV) gives the proper balance of the acidic and alkaline agents. The NV indicates the amount of sodium bicarbonate required to release all the carbon dioxide gas from 100 units of the acid.

Milk is included in some shortened cake formulae. Its lactose and proteins aid browning. Milk also stabilizes the foam and contributes to cake structure.

Sugar plays different roles. It contributes a desirable sweet taste and acts as a moistener, if it is added as a liquid sugar or syrup, but, in its crystalline form, it acts as a drier and aids in air incorporation into fats as they are creamed. Cake volume generally increases as sugar granulation becomes finer.

Finally, salt is added as a flavour enhancer.

Formula balance is important to produce a well-aerated cake with good crumb texture and eating properties. Foam-type cakes with little or no shortening include angel food and sponge. Egg whites whipped into a foam, sugar and flour are the primary ingredients in an angel cake, often in a ratio of 42:42:15, respectively. Small amounts of salt, cream of tartar, and flavouring are also added to the formula. The weight of sugar in the

Table 2. Angel food cake formula

Ingredient	Baker's %[a]
Flour	100
Sugar	280
Egg white	280
Salt	4
Cream of tartar	4
Vanilla	5

[a] Baker's % based on 100 parts flour.

Table 3. Sponge cake formula

Ingredient	Baker's %[a]
Flour	100
Sugar	95
Corn syrup	12
Eggs	105
Water	12
Vanilla	3
Baking powder	1·5
Salt	0·75

[a] Baker's % based on 100 parts flour.

formula is usually equal to the weight of egg whites, and the flour is about one-third the weight of the sugar. A typical angel food cake formula is given in Table 2.

Sponge cakes use whole egg instead of just the whites. To dilute the toughening effect of the whole eggs, more sugar may be added as a tenderizer. The amount of sugar should about equal the amount of whole eggs. Also, the total liquid (whole eggs and milk or water) should be about 25% greater than the weight of sugar. The weight of sugar should exceed that of flour, and the eggs plus flour should be greater than the sugar plus liquids other than eggs. A typical sponge cake formula is listed in Table 3.

Table 4. Commercial pound cake formula

Ingredient	Baker's %[a]
Flour	100
Sugar	100
Shortening	50
Whole eggs	50
Milk	50
Vanilla	2
Salt	1·5

[a] Baker's % based on 100 parts flour.

Table 5. Ordinary yellow cake formula

Ingredient	Baker's %[a]
Flour	100
Sugar	85[b]
Shortening	45
Whole eggs	50
Milk	50
Baking powder	2·5
Salt	2
Flavour	1·5

[a] Baker's % based on 100 parts flour.
[b] In the USA, sugar would run to 120 or more.

One of the oldest cake formulae, better known as the pound cake, contained equal amounts (originally, 1 lb each) of flour, butter, eggs and sugar. However, the large amounts of butter and eggs make the cake expensive to produce, so commercial bakers developed a formula to produce a lighter cake with better eating qualities (Table 4).

Shortened cakes also have a formula that has been modified from the pound cake (Table 5).

White shortened cakes would use egg whites but no yolks. Chocolate shortened cakes contain more sugar, frequently with the flour reduced by the amount of cocoa powder added.

Finally, the high-ratio cake formulae, otherwise known as box cake mixes, were invented to produce a light tender cake for the busy housewife. The single-stage mixing batter is richer and more fluid. They are called high-ratio because the sugar weight exceeds the flour weight and may reach 140%. An emulsified fat is essential to facilitate air incorporation into the batter's aqueous phase.

Chemical and Physical Changes during Mixing

Mixing plays an important role in the production of quality cakes. The objectives of mixing are to disperse all the ingredients as efficiently as possible and to incorporate air into the mix. Air incorporation happens in two stages: a period of rapid incorporation in the form of large bubbles, followed by a stabilizing period when the bubbles are reduced in size. There are several methods for mixing cake batters.

In the creaming, or conventional, method, the fat and sugar are mixed until thoroughly blended and the mixture is aerated. Large amounts of air are incorporated into the fat phase and form small cells throughout the batter. The more the fat–sugar mixture is creamed, the more air is incorporated into the batter. Sugar crystals and air bubbles are suspended in the fat.

The eggs are then added, and the batter beaten until fluffy and is well aerated. The dry ingredients are then added. Fat coats the flour and sugar, delaying their hydration and solubilization, and there is little gluten development.

The conventional sponge method is related to foam-type cakes. The egg whites are whipped to a foam with some sugar for stability. The flour and other dry ingredients are then gently folded in. The egg protein matrix, with its air incorporation, forms the structure of the cake as it bakes.

The muffin mix method blends the eggs and milk with melted fat. This combination is then blended briefly with the dry ingredients. The batter tends to be thin and produces a cake with a coarse crumb and lower volume that tends to stale rapidly.

The pastry-blend method blends the fat and flour until it is fluffy. Then the sugar, salt, baking powder and half of the milk are combined with the fat–flour mixture. This is followed by the egg and the remainder of the milk. This method produces a cake with a fine texture and grain because of the good fat dispersion.

Finally, the single-stage mixing method is used with the high-ratio or box cake mixes. All the ingredients are placed in a container and mixed for a selected amount of time. This gives a fine textured cake for home or retail baking, but it is not stable enough to ship in the wholesale trade.

Chemical and Physical Changes during Baking

Air bubbles, creamed in the fat, are released into the aqueous phase, even before the fat is melted by the time the temperature reaches 40°C. More carbon dioxide is liberated from the baking powder and collects in air bubbles. As the batter heats, the batter is set in motion

Chemistry of Baking

by convection currents, because the batter next to the sides and the bottom of the pan heats first, and that in the centre of the cake heats last.

Heat enlarges the gas cells more rapidly at about 80°C. The liberation of carbon dioxide and the expansion of the gas cells as they are heated causes the cake to rise. Steam also forms, contributing to the leavening action. Emulsifiers improve the elasticity of the protein film around the gas bubbles. Polyvalent ions supplied by the milk, eggs, flour and leaveners also contribute to batter stability.

The pressure inside the gas cells causes their expansion. The resistance to this expansion is caused by coagulation of the protein and starch gelatinization. The timing must be just right for the protein film to expand with the expanding gases, just before it coagulates and the gelatinizing starch takes up water to set the batter. Major swelling of the starch granules occurs just before the batter sets. Then, air cells, without destruction, exude leavening gases to break the emulsion, and part of the fat appears on the cake crumb surface.

As the batter is heated, its viscosity initially decreases. As the starch gelatinizes, the starch granules go from inert bodies to a form that can bind several times their own weight of water. This increases the batter viscosity, giving it a solid appearance and setting the cake. The sugar and some emulsifiers in the formula control the temperature at which the starch gelatinizes. The cake normally sets into a solid system well below the boiling point of water.

Moisture evaporates from the cake surface during baking, keeping it cool. However, near the end, the surface gets hot enough to brown. The richer the cake, (higher sugar and fat contents), the lower the temperature at which it should be baked. The baking time should be as short as possible, however, to avoid a cake with too much colour or too thick a crust.

Role of Additives

The first additive is actually added to the cake flour itself. In the USA, chlorine gas is added to soft wheat flour made especially for cakes at a rate of 0·5–2·5 oz per 100 lb (0·3 to 1·5 g per kilogram) of flour. This lowers the pH and improves the flour's ability to carry the extra sugar in a high-ratio cake. It improves the baking performance by increasing the volume, improving the symmetry, and improving grain and texture. A flour with a pH range of 4·5–4·8 gives the best results.

Overchlorinated cake flour will cause the batter to set up around the sides of the pan before full expansion has been reached. The centre continues to rise, and the result is a cake with a strong peak. If the flour is underchlorinated, the leavening gases escape and the centre of the cake falls upon cooling.

Emulsifiers promote air incorporation in the form of fine bubbles and disperse the shortening into small-sized particles. They exhibit a unique interfacial behaviour at the oil/water surface. When their concentration exceeds the solubility limit, they form an interfacial membrane whose hydrophilic portions extend into the aqueous phase. The membrane surrounds the dispersed oil and prevents the emulsion from breaking. Hydrogenated shortenings typically contain approximately 3% emulsifiers, often glycerol monostearate with some distearate, though many others, including blends, are now used. *See* Emulsifiers, Uses in Processed Foods

Antioxidants are sometimes added to cake mixes. All fats are subject to oxidative and hydrolytic rancidity, which causes objectionable odours and flavours, but antioxidants retard the development of oxidative rancidity during storage. Four compounds commonly used as antioxidants are butylated hydroxyanisole (BHA), butylated hydroxytoluene (BHT), t-butyl hydroquinone (TBHQ) and propyl gallate. Citric and phosphoric acids aid the antioxidants. The levels used are limited by law, economics and functionality, but vary with the additive. *See* Antioxidants, Synthetic Antioxidants

Colour additives are used in many baked products, including cakes and their icings. This gives the perception of a richer or higher quality product or gives the product a more traditional appearance that consumers expect. There are two types of colour additives, certified and uncertified. The certified colours are synthetic and regulated quite strictly, whereas the uncertified usually come from natural sources. The certified colours used in the USA include FD&C Blue No. 1, FD&C Red No. 3, FD&C Yellow No. 5 and FD&C Red No. 40. Uncertified colour additives include annatto extract, β-carotene, beet powder, β-apo-8-carotenal, the xanthins, caramel, carmine, carrot oil, cochineal extract, toasted partially defatted cottonseed flour, fruit and vegetable juices, paprika and paprika oleoresin, riboflavin, saffron, titanium dioxide, turmeric and turmeric oleoresin. *See* Colours, Properties and Determination of Natural Pigments; Colours, Properties and Determination of Synthetic Pigments

Many flavouring agents are used in cake batters. Spices are processed from different parts of aromatic plants including fruits, barks or seeds. Some commonly used spices include allspice, anise, caraway seed, cardamon, cinnamon, cloves, coriander seed, fennel seed, ginger, mace, nutmeg, poppy seed, saffron and sesame seed. Some of these act both as flavouring and colouring agents. They are used in cakes, as well as in icings and fillings.

Cakes are also flavoured with extracts, a solution in ethanol or propylene glycol of the sapid and odorous principles derived from an aromatic plant or parts of the plant. Vanilla, the flavouring extracted from the dried vanilla bean, is commonly used in cakes.

Chemistry of Baking

Chocolate and cocoa from the cacao tree bean are also popular flavouring agents. However, they can also add to the bulk of the cake, up to 10% of the total weight of the formula, because they often replace flour. *See* Cocoa, Production, Products and Uses

Bibliography

Bennion EB and Bamford GST (1986) *The Technology of Cake Making*. Glasgow: Blackie.

Bennion M (1980) *The Science of Food*. San Francisco: Harper and Row.

Blanshard JMV, Frazier PJ and Galliard T (1986) *Chemistry and Physics of Baking. Special Publication*, No. 56. London: The Royal Society of Chemistry.

Charley H (1982) *Food Science*, 2nd edn. New York: Macmillan.

Hoseney RC (1986) *Principles of Cereal Science and Technology*. St Paul, MN: American Association of Cereal Chemists.

Pyler EJ (1988) *Baking Science and Technology*. Merriam, KS: Sosland.

Stauffer CE (1990) *Functional Additives for Bakery Foods*. New York: Van Nostrand Reinhold.

Sultan WJ (1990) *Practical Baking*, 5th edn. New York: Van Nostrand Reinhold.

K.D. Seitz and C.E. Walker
Kansas State University, Manhattan, USA

CALCIUM

Contents

Properties and Determination

Calcium is an alkaline earth metal which is essential for plant and animal life. This article discusses the occurrence of calcium in foods, the influence of processing on calcium content, and methods for determination of calcium in foods.

Occurrence in Foods

Calcium is the fifth most abundant element in the earth's crust. It is an essential nutrient for plant and animal life and is required for cell elongation and division. Most human populations derive more than 50% of their calcium consumption from milk and dairy products, and milk and milk by-products contribute 75% of the calcium in Western diets. Green leafy vegetables rank next to dairy products as good sources of calcium (Table 1). Meat and grains are poor sources, though fish (particularly crab and shrimp) contains more calcium than meat. Often, breads and cereals are enriched with calcium and are, therefore, better sources than they would naturally be. Dried beans are fair calcium sources.

Speciation

Calcium in the earth's crust is found in the silicate, carbonate, sulphate, phosphate and fluoride forms. Feldspars and amphiboles are calcium silicates, whose distribution is widespread. In mammals, most calcium is found in bones and teeth in the forms of calcium phosphate, carbonate and fluoride. In plants, more calcium is found in older leaves than in younger leaves due to minimal transportation of calcium in the phloem. Calcium uptake is through the apoplastic pathway and is a predominantly passive process; it is translocated preferentially towards the shoot apex in the xylem, and translocation is controlled mainly by transpiration rate.

Plant calcium levels usually range from 5 to 30 g kg^{-1} on a dry weight basis. Most plant calcium is present in the cell walls in the form of calcium pectate in the middle lamella; this acts as a cementing substance between plant cells. Excesses of oxalic and other organic acids may appear in cell vacuoles as crystalline calcium salts, e.g. calcium oxalates, carbonates and phosphates. Free Ca^{2+} exists in the apparent free space as a physiological ion. The Ca^{2+} ion adsorbs to xylem walls and saturates the apoplasm. The divalent ionic form can be adsorbed to carboxylic, phosphorylic and phenolic hydroxyl groups. In seeds, calcium is found primarily as phytic acid.

Chemical Properties

Calcium is an alkaline earth metal. Alkaline earths are good conductors of heat and electricity and have a great

Table 1. Occurrence of calcium in food

Food	Calcium concentration (g kg^{-1})[a]
Dairy	
Milk[b]	1·19
Meat	
Beef, fresh[d]	0·09
Lamb, fresh[d]	0·09
Pork, fresh[b]	0·07
Chicken, fresh[d]	0·14
Turkey, fresh[d]	0·23
Egg[b]	0·56
Fish	
Clams, breaded and fried[c]	0·18
Crab, baked[c]	3·81
Oysters, breaded and fried[c]	0·20
Scallops, breaded and fried[c]	0·13
Shrimp, breaded and fried[c]	0·51
Fish fillet, breaded and fried[c]	0·18
Fruits	
Oranges[b]	0·41
Apples, dry weight basis[d]	0·19
Apricots, dry weight basis[d]	0·86
Figs, dry weight basis[d]	1·86
Peaches, dry weight basis[d]	0·44
Tomatoes, dry weight basis[d]	1·19
Vegetables	
Cabbage, dry weight basis[d]	3·94
Carrots, dry weight basis[d]	2·46
Onions, dry weight basis[d]	1·68
Potatoes, dry weight basis[d]	0·25
Sweet potatoes, dry weight basis[d]	0·75
Mustard greens[b]	1·38
Broccoli[b]	0·87
Green beans[b]	0·51
Lima beans[b]	0·20
Grains	
Oatmeal[b]	0·09
Corn meal[d]	0·10
Brown rice, dry weight basis[d]	0·14
Polished rice, dry weight basis[d]	0·08
Cereal, corn flakes[d]	0·08
Cereal, shredded wheat[d]	0·51
Cereal, puffed rice[d]	0·07
Bread, white, enriched[b]	0·86
Bread, whole wheat[b]	0·86
Beverages	
Beer[c]	0·05
Cola[c]	0·03
Coffee[c]	0·02
Tea[c]	0
Orange juice[c]	0·09
Hot chocolate[c]	0·47

[a] Concentrations are reported for food as is, unless otherwise stated.
[b] Data from Gebhardt SE and Matthews RH (1991) *Nutritive Value of Foods*. US Department of Agriculture, Home and Garden Bulletin No. 72.
[c] Data from Dickey E and Weihrauch JL (1988) *Composition of Foods: Fast foods*. US Department of Agriculture, Human Nutrition Information Service, Agriculture Handbook, No. 8–21.
[d] Data from Harris RS and von Loesecke H (1971).

Properties and Determination

affinity for oxygen. There are two electrons in the outermost energy level, and, therefore, calcium forms compounds in which it has an oxidation state of $+2$. The doubly charged ion interacts strongly with water to form a tightly hydrated ion. Many calcium compounds (e.g. fluorspar, calcium carbonate) are very insoluble, but there are exceptions (e.g. calcium chloride and calcium nitrate).

Elimination/Concentration in Processing

Dairy Products

The milk-processing method used has a large influence on the calcium content of dairy products. Lactic acid cheeses (e.g. cottage cheese, cream cheese) are poor sources of calcium, but processing involving rennet coagulation (e.g. Cheddar cheese) results in cheeses which are good calcium sources. Cheddar cheese retains 61% of the calcium content of raw milk, brick cheese retains 58% and blue cheese retains 46%. Cheddar cheese is a hard-pressed cheese and losses of calcium are small during making and ripening. Stilton cheese (an unpressed cheese) has a constantly increasing percentage calcium loss during ageing which is correlated to the titratable acidity in the whey. Stilton cheese retains only 6–8% of the calcium content of raw milk; 40% is left in the new curd, 28% within 2 weeks after hooping, and 10–15% by the time of ripening. *See* Cheeses, Dietary Importance; Dairy Products – Dietary Importance; Milk, Dietary Importance

Cottage and cream cheeses have less than 10% of the calcium concentration found in cheddar cheese (Table 2). Low-fat milk has a slightly higher calcium content than whole milk, and cream has a lower calcium content than whole milk. Consequently, ice cream also has a lower calcium concentration than ice milk. Ice cream sundaes and milk shakes have slightly lower calcium contents than ice cream. *See* Ice Cream, Dietary Importance

Meat

Fresh meat is quite low in calcium (0·06–0·13 g kg^{-1}), with a few exceptions, e.g. pork heart which contains 0·35 g kg^{-1}. Processing meat increases the calcium content in some cases. For example, luncheon meat and dried beef have about double the calcium content of fresh meat. Canned meat, particularly corned beef and beef liver, has calcium contents ranging from 0·29–0·40 g kg^{-1}. *See* Meat, Dietary Importance

Vegetables

The calcium content changes in some vegetables as the plant matures. For example, the calcium content increases with maturity in snap beans, but does not change

Table 2. Influence of milk processing and preparation on calcium content

Food	Calcium concentration (g kg^{-1})[a]
Milk[b]	1·19
Low-fat milk, 2%[c]	1·22
Light cream[b]	0·93
Ice cream[b]	1·33
Ice milk[c]	1·49
Ice cream sundae	
Caramel[c]	1·22
Hot fudge[c]	1·31
Strawberry[c]	1·05
Milk shakes	
Chocolate[c]	1·13
Strawberry[c]	1·13
Vanilla[c]	1·22
Cheddar cheese[b]	7·29
Cottage cheese[b]	0·61
Cream cheese[b]	0·61

[a] Concentrations are reported for food as is.
[b] Data from Gebhardt SE and Matthews RH (1991) *Nutritive Value of Foods.* US Department of Agriculture, Home and Garden Bulletin No. 72.
[c] Data from Dickey LE and Weihrauch JL (1988) *Composition of Foods: Fast foods.* United States Department of Agriculture, Human Nutrition Information Service, Agriculture Handbook, No. 8–21.

Table 3. Influence of potato processing and preparation on calcium

Food	Calcium concentration (g kg^{-1})[a]
Baked potato[b]	0·09
With sour cream and chives[c]	0·35
With cheese sauce[c]	1·05
With cheese sauce and bacon[c]	1·03
With cheese sauce and broccoli[c]	0·99
With cheese sauce and chili[c]	1·04
Mashed potato[c]	0·21
Dehydrated potato[d]	0·25
Potato crisps[c]	0·24
Potato salad[c]	0·14
French fried potatoes	
Fried in beef tallow[c]	0·16
Fried in vegetable oil[c]	0·16
Hash browned potatoes[c]	0·10

[a] Concentrations are reported for food as is.
[b] Data from Gebhardt SE and Matthews RH (1991) *Nutritive Value of Foods.* US Department of Agriculture, Home and Garden Bulletin No. 72.
[c] Data from Dickey LE and Weihrauch JL (1988) *Composition of Foods: Fast Foods.* United States Department of Agriculture, Human Nutrition Information Service, Agriculture Handbook, No. 8–21.
[d] Data from Harris RS and von Loesecke H (1971)

for turnip greens. Baking, pickling, frying, roasting and steaming have no significant effect on the calcium content, but boiling extracts calcium from vegetables. Boiling extracts 12% of the original calcium from beans, 20% from carrots and 20% from cabbage. Pressure cooking cabbage, on the other hand, decreases the calcium content only by 9%. When vegetables are covered by water, up to 25% of the calcium can leach out of the vegetables into the water. *See* Cooking, Domestic Techniques; Vegetables of Temperate Climates, Commercial and Dietary Importance; Vegetables of Tropical Climates, Commercial and Dietary Importance

Processing and preparation of potatoes have a large effect on the calcium content (Table 3). Mashed potatoes have higher calcium concentration than baked potatoes, probably due to milk and butter addition to the potatoes. Potato crisps (chips in the USA) have more calcium than French fried potatoes, and frying in beef tallow or vegetable oil does not influence calcium content of French fried potatoes. Putting cheese sauce on a baked potato increases the calcium concentration 10-fold. *See* Potatoes and Related Crops, Processing Potato Tubers

Cereals

Milling of wheat into flour decreases the calcium concentration by 50%. Oats and oatmeal have higher

calcium contents than other processed foods since only the fibrous hull and adhering portion of the oat grain are removed. The germ and bran remain. Many cereal products, particularly infant cereals, are enriched with calcium in order to supplement the naturally low calcium levels in cereal grains, which are even lower after milling. *See* Cereals, Contribution to the Diet

Sample Preparation and Extraction

Preparation

Food samples should be rinsed with distilled water to remove foreign material, but excessive washing should be prevented, due to the potential for calcium removal in the wash water. The sample must be ground in a meat chopper or blender three times and mixed well in order to achieve as homogeneous a sample as possible. Predrying, for 24 h at 70°C, prior to ashing, is recommended to prevent burning. Leafy vegetables should be dried for 24 h at 70°C before grinding; after grinding with a Wiley mill, the sample should be passed through a 40 mesh screen, prior to ashing.

Ashing

Dry ashing is the process of ignition of samples at a very high temperature. The resulting ash is then dissolved in dilute acid. One gram of a sample is weighed into a porcelain crucible, and ashed for 4 h at 500°C in a muffle furnace. After cooling, the ash is wetted with several drops of water, 10 ml of 3 N HCl is added and the whole is heated to a slow boil on a hot plate. The dissolved ash is filtered through a filter paper (prewashed with 3 N HCl) into a volumetric flask, the crucible is rinsed with 10 ml of 3 N HCl and the solution transferred to the filter. The filter is rinsed with distilled water, and the solution is diluted to volume with water.

If a muffle furnace is unavailable, wet ashing can be utilized. However, this method is not recommended for samples high in oils, due to the hazardous nature of perchloric acid. An acid mixture is prepared of two parts concentrated nitric acid to one part concentrated perchloric acid. A 0·5 g sample is weighed into a 50 ml test tube, 5 ml of acid mixture is added, and the whole transferred to a block digestor. The sample is heated at 60°C for 15 min or until the reaction has subsided. The heat is increased to 120°C and the sample is digested for about 75 min, until it clears. The digest is cooled and diluted to volume with distilled water.

Analysis of Extracts

Atomic Absorption Spectroscopy

Atomic absorption spectroscopy is the most convenient and widely used method for calcium determination. Absorption is the process by which atoms in the ground state absorb energy, at different wavelengths characteristic for each element. Chemical interferences (by formation of calcium compounds) may be overcome by diluting samples 1:100 with a 2500 mg l^{-1} lanthanum solution (117 g of La$_2$O$_3$ in 500 ml of concentrated HCl, diluted to 40 litres with distilled water). The recommendations for calcium determination on a Perkin Elmer 2100 atomic absorption spectrometer are a wavelength of 424 nm, slit setting of 0·7 and a current of 20 mA. Standard solutions with a matrix similar to sample solutions must be used; the calcium absorption-to-concentration relationship is linear to 5·0 mg l^{-1}. The detection limit for calcium by flame atomic absorption is <0·0005 mg l^{-1}, and for furnace atomic absorption the detection limit is 0·00005 mg l^{-1}.

Titrimetry

There are many titrimetric procedures which can be used for the determination of calcium when an atomic absorption unit is unavailable. One of these methods is described here. Ethylenediaminetetraacetic acid (EDTA) titrimetry can be utilized to measure calcium and magnesium simultaneously or individually. EDTA, potassium cyanide, hydroxylamine hydrochloride and potassium ferrocyanide are used to chelate or precipitate ions (Fe, Mn, Cu, Zn, Ni, Al) which interfere in the analysis. To determine the calcium content, an aliquot containing 1–2 mg of calcium is placed in a 250 ml Erlenmeyer flask, and distilled water added to obtain a total volume of 150 ml. Ten drops each of KCN (1 g in 100 ml), NH$_2$OH·HCl (5 g in 100 ml), K$_4$Fe(CN)$_6$ (4 g of K$_4$Fe(CN)$_6$·3H$_2$O in 100 ml) and triethanolamine are added, followed by enough 10% NaOH (about 1 ml) to raise the pH to 12 or slightly higher. Five drops of Calcon indicator (20 mg of Calcon in 50 ml of methanol) are added, and the solution titrated from red to blue with standardized EDTA disodium. Calcon indicator must be made fresh weekly.

To prepare the EDTA disodium, 2 g of EDTA disodium and 0·039 g of MgCl$_2$·6H$_2$O are dissolved in distilled water and diluted to 1 litre. To prepare the buffer solution, 67·5 g of NH$_4$Cl is dissolved in 200 ml of water, 570 ml of concentrated NH$_4$OH is added, and the solution diluted to 1 litre. To prepare the standard calcium solution (0·5 mM), 0·5004 g of reagent-grade CaCO$_3$ (dried at 150°C) are dissolved in 5 ml of 6 N HCl and diluted to 1 litre. To standardize the EDTA solution, three 5 ml aliquots of standard calcium solution are pipetted into three 250 ml Erlenmeyer flasks, and each diluted with 150 ml of distilled water. Fifteen mls of buffer solution and ten drops each of KCN, NH$_2$OH·HCl, K$_4$Fe(CN)$_6$ and triethanolamine are added, and enough 10% NaOH (about 1 ml) is added to raise the pH to 12 or slightly higher. Five drops of Calcon indicator are added and the solution titrated from red to blue with standardized EDTA disodium. Three distilled water blanks are titrated to check for contamination.

Examples

Milk

Milk samples should be frozen prior to and thawed immediately preceding calcium analysis. Gaines TP *et al.* (1990) describe a method for calcium determination in milk. Samples are mixed thoroughly with a vortex mixer. A 1 ml aliquot is pipetted into a 30 ml high-form porcelain crucible to prevent splattering. Samples are ashed in a muffle furnace at 550°C for 1 h. After cooling, 10 drops of water are added, followed by 10 ml of 3 M HCl. Samples are heated to a gentle boil on a hot plate, then filtered into a 100 ml volumetric flask. The crucible is rinsed into the filter with 10 ml of 3 M HCl, and the filter rinsed with deionized water. Filtrate is brought to volume with water, and the samples are shaken thoroughly.

A 1 ml aliquot of the filtrate is diluted to 10 ml with

2500 mg l^{-1} lanthanum solution (made using La_2O_3), and samples are analysed for calcium using an atomic absorption spectrophotometer. Calcium standards used contain 0·5, 1·0 and 2·0 mg l^{-1} calcium.

Potato

Kratzke MG and Palta JP (1986) describe a procedure for the analysis of calcium in potatoes. Potato tubers are rinsed in distilled water and stored at 4°C. The potatoes are peeled in 1 mm layers to collect the surface 3 mm (the surface and medullary tissues) of the tubers. Samples are dried in an oven at 60°C, ground to pass a 20-mesh screen, and ashed at 450°C. The ash is dissolved in 2 N HCl, and this solution diluted 1:10 with $LaCl_3$ solution. The calcium concentration is determined by atomic absorption spectroscopy.

Bibliography

American Meat Institute Foundation (1960) *The Science of Meat and Meat Products*. San Francisco: Freeman.

Gaines TP and Mitchell G (1979) *Chemical Methods for Soil and Plant Analysis. Agronomy Handbook*, No. 1. Tifton: University of Georgia, Coastal Plain Experiment Station.

Gaines TP, West JW and McAllister JF (1990) Determination of calcium and phosphorus in milk. *Journal of the Science of Food and Agriculture* 51: 207–213.

Harris RS and von Loesecke H (eds) (1971) *Nutritional Evaluation of Food Processing*. Westport, CT: AVI.

Kratzke MG and Palta JP (1986) Calcium accumulation in potato tubers: role of the basal roots. *HortScience* 21(4): 1022–1024.

Lanyon LE and Heald WR (1982) Magnesium, calcium, strontium, and barium. In: Page AL (ed.) *Methods of Soil Analysis. Part 2. Chemical and Microbiological Properties*, 2nd edn, pp 247–262. Madison: American Society of Agronomy.

Mengel K and Kirkby EA (1978) *Principles of Plant Nutrition*. Bern: Der Bund.

Williams S (1984) *Official Methods of Analysis of the Association of Official Analytical Chemists*, 14th edn. Arlington: Association of Official Analytical Chemists.

Jessica G. Davis-Carter
University of Georgia, Tifton, USA

Physiology

Calcium is the most abundant mineral in the body, making up about 2% of bodyweight. It fulfils important structural and metabolic roles. Calcium is a major constituent of the mineral salt, hydroxyapatite, which provides strength and resilience to bones. In addition, calcium acts as an important intracellular signal, triggering many metabolic functions within cells in response to the actions of a number of hormones. Calcium is also necessary for the blood clotting mechanisms.

The concentration of plasma-ionized calcium is maintained within narrow limits by the concerted action of three hormones which control calcium absorption, excretion and uptake by bone. This article will review the role of calcium in the body, the physiological mechanisms that regulate plasma concentration, calcium requirements, and the current intakes of different groups of the population.

Factors Affecting Calcium Bioavailability

Calcium bioavailability is a measure of the amount of calcium from different foods and diets that can be utilized by the body for normal metabolic functions. Calcium is absorbed in the small intestine. At low intakes this is mainly by an active, vitamin-D-dependent mechanism. As intakes increase, this mechanism becomes saturated and additional calcium is absorbed by diffusion. On average, about 30% of calcium ingested is absorbed, i.e. about 250 mg per person per day, but this is affected by several dietary and physiological factors. *See* Bioavailability of Nutrients; Cholecalciferol, Physiology

Physiological Factors

The efficiency of calcium absorption is greater during periods of growth, in pregnancy and in lactation. Vitamin D status and age also affect the efficiency of absorption. *See* Growth and Development; Lactation

Dietary Factors

Dietary factors that affect calcium bioavailability include the chemical form and solubility of the calcium and the presence of inhibitors in the food or diet. Substances that form insoluble complexes with calcium in the intestine, such as phytate, oxalate and uronic acid and some nonstarch polysaccharides (NSP), have all been reported to reduce calcium bioavailability. Fermentable NSP are unlikely to affect net absorption since the calcium is released on fermentation and may then be absorbed in the colon. The presence of these inhibitors in foods such as cereals and vegetables reduces the bioavailability not only of the calcium present in them but also of the calcium present in other foods consumed with them.

High levels of protein in the diet increase calcium absorption but also lead to an increase in urinary excretion, so that the net result is a decrease in calcium bioavailability.

Calcium in milk is generally considered to be more available than that in cereals and vegetables. This could be the result of either the absence of inhibitors or the presence of absorption promotors in milk.

Calcium Excretion

The major route of excretion of absorbed calcium is the kidney. There is considerable variation in the amount of calcium excreted in the urine each day by healthy men and women. The variation is related to differences in age, sex, body size, dietary intake of calcium and of other food components (e.g. protein) that either affect absorption from the intestine, or its handling by the kidney. A small amount of calcium (about 60 mg per day) is lost with hair, sweat and skin and some is secreted into the small intestine and lost in the faeces.

Plasma Homeostasis

Despite the considerable variation in intake, absorption and excretion of calcium, the concentration of ionized calcium in the plasma remains remarkably constant ($1 \cdot 2$ mmol l^{-1}). Calcium circulates in the plasma in three forms: bound to plasma proteins (about 45%), in complexes with citrate, phosphate or bicarbonate (about 10%), and as free calcium ions (about 45%). The free ionized form is the biologically important form and its concentration is closely regulated through the integrated actions of three hormones (parathyroid hormone, vitamin D and calcitonin) which either increase or decrease the plasma concentration, in response to either decreases or increases in the plasma concentration of ionized calcium (see Fig. 1). The secretion of these hormones is controlled by the plasma concentration of ionized calcium so that a negative feedback system is formed.

Factors Influencing Calcium Homeostasis

Parathyroid Hormone

The most important hormone controlling plasma ionized calcium is parathyroid hormone (PTH). It acts mainly by controlling the amount of calcium excreted by the kidney. PTH increases reabsorption of calcium from the kidney tubule and thus decreases calcium excretion. It has no direct effect on the absorption of calcium from the intestine but it promotes the conversion of vitamin D to 1,25-(OH)$_2$ vitamin D (the active form of vitamin D) in the kidney, which does have a direct effect in the small intestine. *See* Hormones, Thyroid Hormones

Vitamin D

In man, vitamin D is derived from two main sources: the skin, where cholecalciferol is formed by the action of

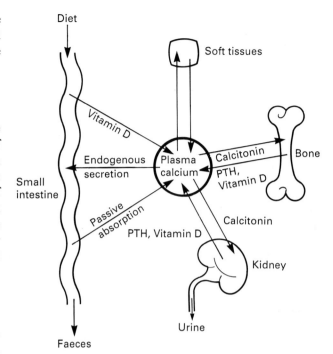

Fig. 1   Factors influencing calcium homeostasis.

ultraviolet light on 7-dehydrocholesterol; and the diet, in the form of ergocalciferol. In the UK the dermal source is the more important. Subgroups of the adult population who get little sunshine, or who are confined indoors, are vulnerable to vitamin D deficiency.

Both cholecalciferol and ergocalciferol are converted, in the liver, to the storage form, 25-(OH) vitamin D. This circulates in the plasma and is converted in the kidney to the active form, 1,25-(OH)$_2$ vitamin D, under closely controlled conditions.

1,25-(OH)$_2$ Vitamin D promotes the active absorption of calcium from the small intestine, and enhances reabsorption of calcium in the kidney. The plasma concentration of 1,25-(OH)$_2$ vitamin D decreases in response to increases in dietary calcium.

Calcitonin

In contrast to PTH and vitamin D, calcitonin decreases the concentration of plasma ionized calcium. Its secretion is stimulated by increases in plasma calcium. Calcitonin inhibits the release of calcium from bone. It also acts on the kidney to promote the urinary excretion of calcium.

Functions of Calcium

Growth

Measurements of Calcium Accretion

About 99% of calcium in the body is found in the bones, all of which must be provided by the diet, though the calcium requirements for growth have not yet been adequately determined. There are several techniques for measuring the amount of calcium in individual bones at different ages, but results obtained from the various methods do not correlate particularly well. *See* Bone

The total calcium content of the body has been estimated to increase from about 28 g (8 g per kg of bodyweight) at birth to around 1000 g (19 g per kg) at maturity. This indicates an average requirement of 143 mg a day over 18 years. Growth rate is not constant, however, and net calcium requirements will, at times, be greater or less than this. A recently developed technique, using neutron activation analysis, enables total body calcium to be measured in living persons and could yield valuable new data on calcium requirements for growth.

Rates of Growth

The maximal growth rate (i.e. rate of increase in height) occurs soon after birth and then decelerates to a rate less than one third of the first year values by age 10 in girls and age 12 in boys. This is followed by another period of accelerated growth rate, the so called prepubertal growth spurt. The maximum growth rate achieved at this stage is attained at about age 12 in girls and about age 14 in boys, and is not as high as growth rates during infancy. Growth rates then reduce again until adult stature is attained, when growth stops. It has been estimated that calcium requirements for growth vary more than fivefold, from about 70 mg per day during periods of slow growth to 375 mg per day during periods of fast growth. The efficiency of absorption of calcium increases during periods of rapid growth. During the first year it may be as high as 66% in breast-fed infants. The dietary requirements of calcium, therefore, will not vary by as much as fivefold. *See* Infants, Nutritional Requirements

Skeletal Homeostasis

Bone is a specialized form of connective tissue containing cells and collagen fibres impregnated with a crystalline mineral salt, similar to hydroxyapatite ($3Ca_3[PO_4]_2Ca[OH]_2$). Bone tissue is found in two forms:

1. Compact, or cortical, bone forms the outer part of bones, in particular the shafts of the long bones.
2. Trabecular bone forms the meshwork in the inner parts of the long bones, the vertebrae and the pelvis.

All bones contain both compact and trabecular bone, although the proportion of each varies in different bones.

Bone tissue is constantly being remodelled, with bone continually being removed and reformed. This takes place at centres of cellular activity called basic remodell-

ing units. Once a basic remodelling unit has been activated it proceeds in a predetermined way. The factors which influence the number of units initiated have no effect on the lifespan of pre-existing units, although the relative amounts of bone formed or eroded at each unit can be modified. The highest rates of bone loss occur when a large number of basic remodelling units have been initiated and when more bone is eroded than is reformed at each unit.

Bone formation is stimulated by growth and exercise, and inhibited by immobility, undernutrition and glucocorticosteroids. Bone erosion is stimulated by PTH and immobility, and inhibited by calcitonin. Bone metabolism is affected by many other hormones, such as oestrogens, androgens, growth hormone and thyroid hormone.

Bone Loss

Factors Affecting Bone Loss

Mineral continues to be deposited for about 10 years or so after growth has ceased, and peak bone mass (PBM) is not reached until the third decade of life. The final amount of bone accumulated at maturity varies among individuals and is governed by genetic and environmental factors.

From about the age of 30 or so, both mineral and matrix are removed from the inner surface of the bone more rapidly than new bone is added to the outer surface; this is a normal part of the ageing process. As a consequence, the cortex of the long bones becomes thinner and more liable to fracture. In women at the time of the menopause, or in women who are amenorrhoeic (e.g. as a result of intensive exercise), oestrogen deficiency leads to an increase in bone turnover and to an imbalance between bone formation and bone resorption at each remodelling unit. This results in a net loss of bone. These accelerated rates of bone loss last for about 5 years following the menopause. Because trabecular bone is more active than compact bone, the effects of oestrogen deficiency are more commonly seen in bones with a higher proportion of trabecular bone, such as the vertebrae. *See* Osteoporosis

Does Extra Calcium Reduce Bone Loss?

A daily supply of calcium is important throughout life. The value of extra dietary calcium in the prevention of bone loss is uncertain. The accelerated bone loss after the menopause is due to increased bone turnover and an imbalance between bone formation and bone resorption as a result of oestrogen deficiency. It cannot be prevented by extra calcium alone. However, extra calcium might reduce the dose of oestrogen necessary to prevent bone loss.

In the elderly population, where calcium absorption may be impaired due to reduced renal function with a consequent reduction in vitamin D activation, extra calcium might be of benefit in reducing the age-related loss of compact bone.

Regulatory Role of Calcium

In addition to its structural role in the skeleton, calcium has an important regulatory role. This can be divided into two categories:

1.   Passive – calcium acts as a cofactor for many enzymes and is an important component of the blood clotting mechanism.
2.   Active – changes in calcium concentration inside cells, in response to a physiological stimulus such as a hormone or neurotransmitter, can act as an intracellular signal. This triggers events such as cell aggregation, muscle contraction and cell movement, muscle protein degradation, secretion, transformation and cell division.

The concentration of free calcium inside the cell is about 10 000 times less than that outside. A small increase in the permeability of the cell membrane to calcium, or a small release of calcium from an internal store, causes a rise in the intracellular calcium concentration which may stimulate a response. An excessive increase, however, may injure the cell. The low intracellular concentration of calcium is maintained by a pump which removes calcium from the cell. Necrotic cells contain between 10 and 100 times the normal concentration of calcium but whether this is a cause or a consequence of cell death is uncertain.

Calcium and Hypertension

A number of epidemiological studies, showing that calcium intake is lower in hypertensive patients than in normal controls, have given rise to the suggestion that low dietary calcium can predispose to high blood pressure. All the studies were cross-sectional in design and most of the studies relied on 24-hour dietary recall. Some of the studies were not controlled adequately and others found negative correlations with other nutrients as well. The epidemiological evidence that a low calcium intake leads to hypertension is therefore inconclusive. *See* Hypertension, Physiology

Other authors have suggested that abnormalities in calcium metabolism may be involved in hypertension. Some studies have reported that plasma ionized calcium is low or 'modestly decreased' in hypertension. Others have not been able to confirm these findings or have found it to be raised.

Urinary calcium levels are also increased, as are blood levels of PTH. Abnormalities in intracellular calcium have also been reported. Some of these changes are present before the blood pressure rises, which implies that they may be part of the more fundamental disturbances of membrane structure and function that occur in hypertension.

Early dietary intervention studies suggested that oral calcium supplements could lead to a fall in blood pressure but three out of five recent double-blind randomized studies have failed to confirm this finding. It may be that the effects are small and take time to develop or only affect a susceptible subgroup of the population, but it seems unlikely that increasing calcium intake has any effect on the blood pressure of those with hypertension or normal blood pressure.

Hypercalcaemia

Body calcium is under such close homeostatic control that an excessive accumulation in blood or tissues from overconsumption is virtually unknown. Hypercalcaemia usually occurs as a result of failure of control mechanisms, either generally or locally. The increased concentration of circulatory calcium results in calcium salt deposition in many tissues, including the heart and the kidneys.

Hypercalcaemia of infants was reported in the 1950s as a result of excessive vitamin D in infant foods. Calcification of the heart and kidneys, mental retardation, brain damage and death were reported in a number of infants.

Hypocalcaemia

About half the calcium in the blood is bound to the plasma protein, albumin. If plasma albumin is low, this value is also low. The action of PTH and vitamin D ensures that plasma ionized calcium concentration does not fall far below its normal value. Hypocalcaemia may occur, however, as a result of PTH deficiency after thyroid surgery, or vitamin D deficiency leading to reduced absorption of calcium. It is a feature of rickets and osteomalacia.

Hypocalcaemia leads to increased excitability of nerve and muscle cells. This causes numbness, and tingling and twitching, especially in the hands, feet and face.

Calcium Requirements and Reference Nutrient Intakes (RNIs)

Calcium Balance Studies

Calcium balance studies in adults have produced figures for the dietary requirement of calcium ranging from

200 mg per day to 975 mg per day. The lowest value was found in 10 Peruvian men and it is doubtful whether such results are relevant in Britain. The highest value was obtained when the absorption of calcium was unaccountably low. The average of 212 balance studies was 578 mg per day and a calcium intake of 900 mg per day was needed to prevent negative balance in 95% of subjects.

However, many assumptions have to be made if balance studies are to be used as a method for assessing requirements. For example:

1. Endogenous secretion of calcium into the gut is assumed to be constant but there are few measurements to support this.
2. Losses of calcium in the urine and faeces are assumed to be constant but in fact they are affected considerably by other components in the diet, such as protein, phytate, and nonstarch polysaccharides.
3. Individual variation in adaptation to different intakes is not taken into account. Most balance studies have not continued for long enough to be able to judge whether or not adaptation has occurred.

Setting the RNI

The current RNI for calcium in the UK is 500 mg per day for a nonpregnant, nonlactating adult. Throughout the world, values of RNI range from 450 mg per day in India to 1200 mg per day in the USA for the 11–24 age group. *See* Dietary Requirements of Adults

Average calcium intakes in the UK are 937 mg per day for men and 726 mg per day for women. Figures from the National Food Survey show that there has been a steady decline in calcium intake over the last 20 years from 1037 mg per day in 1960 to 840 mg per day in 1989 (average of men, women and children). This is mainly due to the fall in consumption of milk and bread, which provide the major dietary supply.

Vegans, who do not consume milk or milk products and who often prefer (unfortified) wholemeal bread, have lower calcium intakes and consume an average of 537 mg of calcium per day, mainly from vegetable sources. This may not be absorbed as well as calcium from dairy products because of the presence of inhibitors in wholemeal bread and some vegetables. *See* Vegan Diets

A recent survey of British schoolchildren (aged 10–15 years) showed that the intakes of some girls who consumed very little milk or cereal products were less than 300 mg per day. This is less than the Lower Reference Nutrient Intake (LRNI) of 480 mg per day for this age group. If this represents the habitual dietary intake of these girls it is probable that they are getting insufficient calcium. *See* Children, Nutritional Requirements

Setting the RNI is a matter of critical judgement involving scientific and other considerations. More firmly based recommendations cannot be made until further research has been done in the following areas: the influence of calcium in early life on the attainment of peak bone mass; on the range of abilities of individuals to adapt to different calcium intakes at different ages; on the relationship between dietary calcium and blood pressure in normal diets; and on the interactions between calcium and other nutrients that might limit or enhance the absorption and utilization of those nutrients or of calcium itself.

Bibliography

Allen LH (1982) Calcium bioavailability and absorption: a review. *American Journal of Clinical Nutrition* 35: 783–808.

British Nutrition Foundation (1989) *Task Force Report on Calcium*. London: British Nutrition Foundation.

Kanis JA and Passmore R (1989) Calcium supplementation of the diet (I and II). *British Medical Journal* 298: 137–140, 205–208.

Kolata G (1984) Does a lack of calcium cause hypertension? *Science* 225: 705–706.

Nordin BEC (1976) *Calcium, Phosphate and Magnesium Metabolism*. London: Churchill Livingstone.

Nordin BEC (1988) *Calcium in Human Biology*. Berlin: Springer-Verlag.

A. Halliday
Nutrition Scientist, British Nutrition Foundation, London, UK

CALORIFIC VALUES

See Energy

CAMPYLOBACTER

Contents

Properties and Occurrence

It was not until the late 1970s that campylobacters were recognised as a leading cause of acute infective diarrhoea. The discovery came late because conventional methods of culture did not cater for the special gaseous requirements of campylobacters (they are strictly microaerophilic), nor did they allow the isolation of these fastidious bacteria from among normal faecal flora. Butzler, a Belgian medical microbiologist, was instrumental in developing appropriate methods and recognizing the importance of these bacteria as human pathogens. In many countries, campylobacters are the most frequently identified enteric pathogens, exceeding even salmonellae.

Classification

Campylobacters are small, spirally curved, flagellated gram-negative bacteria that were formerly classified in the genus *Vibrio*. Together with *Arcobacter*, *Helicobacter*, and *Wolinella* they are known to form a phylogenetic group distantly related to other eubacteria. Several species are associated with human disease, but only *Campylobacter jejuni* and *C. coli* are of major importance as causes of campylobacter enteritis. *C. lari*, '*C. upsaliensis*' and *C. hyointestinalis* are occasionally isolated from patients with diarrhoea, but their pathogenic status is less clear-cut and they are not necessarily foodborne. *C. fetus*, the type species of the genus, is a rare cause of systemic campylobacteriosis in people with immune deficiency (see p. 000). Although *C. fetus* infection has been attributed to eating raw lambs' liver, its rarity and low virulence make it of small concern to the food microbiologist. Henceforth in this article the term 'campylobacters' refers to the two species *C. jejuni* and *C. coli*.

Occurrence in the Environment

C. jejuni and *C. coli* live mainly as commensals in the intestinal tract of a wide variety of warm-blooded animals, particularly birds (Table 1). Carriage rates in wild animals are generally lower than in birds, but a rate of 24% has been found in urban rats (*Rattus norvegicus*). Campylobacters have been found in various zoo animals, including an occasional reptile. Domestic and food-producing animals are commonly colonized and constitute the main source of human infection. Poultry are a particularly important source. Colonization rates of 50–100% are commonplace in broiler chickens, turkeys and ducks, whose caecal contents may have campylobacter counts as high as 10^8 per gram. *See* Poultry, Chicken; Poultry, Ducks and Geese; Poultry, Turkey

C. jejuni is the predominant species, except in pigs, which seem to be the natural hosts of *C. coli*. Horses are seldom colonized. Although carriage rates vary widely, average figures compiled from numerous surveys give an idea of the prevalence of these bacteria in food-producing animals (Tables 2 and 3). In general, immature animals have higher carriage rates than adult ones.

The faecal shedding of campylobacters by wild and domestic animals results in contamination of virtually all surface water, even in remote areas. Campylobacters are present in sewage and survive, though do not grow, in sea as well as fresh water. Surface water is probably the chief vehicle of infection for farm animals, and drinking untreated water carries a high risk of infection for human beings.

Table 1. Occurrence of campylobacters (*C. jejuni* and *C. coli*) in wild birds. The data are given as mean percentage positive with the number of surveys from which the data were extracted in parentheses

Crows (*Corvidae*)	60 (3)
Starling (*Sturnus vulgaris*)	47 (2)
Gulls (*Larus* spp.)	34 (6)
Ducks and geese (*Anatidae*)	27 (6)
Pigeons (mainly urban)	25 (6)
Sparrows	14 (4)

Also isolated from waders (*Charadriidae*, *Haematopodidae*, *Scolopacidae*), owls (*Strigidae*), puffin (*Fratula arctica*), sandhill crane (*Grus canadensis*)

Table 2. Occurrence of campylobacters in poultry. The data are given as mean percentage positive with the number of studies from which the data are extracted in parentheses

Product	Carcase ready for packing at processing plant	Retailed product	
		Fresh	Frozen
Broiler chickens	58 (20)	59 (17)	43 (6)
Chicken livers	76 (3)	48 (3)	9 (2)
Turkeys	48 (7)	22 (3)	56 (1)
Ducks	52 (4)	—	—
Geese	—	38 (1)	—
Game birds	—	14 (2)	—

Occurrence in Foods

Given such high intestinal carriage rates in food-producing animals it is not surprising that their products are often contaminated. Table 2 shows the occurrence of campylobacters in eviscerated dressed poultry at the end of the processing line and at the point of retail sale. Table 3 shows the same data for red meats and other foods.

Milk is also a major potential vehicle of infection. The average isolation rate from bulked raw milk (over 6400 samples) in 10 surveys carried out in the UK, USA and The Netherlands was 2·5%. Figures in the region of 6% were obtained in the more recent surveys in which more sensitive methods were used. Mean campylobacter counts of 16 ± 30 per 100 ml were recorded in the positive samples. *See* Milk, Processing of Liquid Milk

Growth Factors and Properties

Campylobacters are strictly microaerophilic bacteria that require oxygen for growth, yet are poisoned by concentrations much above 10%. They also have a narrow growth temperature range. *C. jejuni*, *C. coli* and *C. lari* are thermophilic relative to other campylobacters: their optimum growth temperature is 42–43°C and their minimum is about 30°C.

Campylobacters are more sensitive to physical and chemical agents than enterobacteria such as *Escherichia coli*. Dense saline suspensions (10^{10} cfu ml^{-1}; cfu, colony-forming unit) dried on hard surfaces survive for only 2–10 h at 37°C, though suspensions in broth or skimmed milk dried and held at 4°C survive for several weeks. Campylobacters have a pH growth range of 6·0–8·0, but they are inactivated below pH 5·5 or above pH 9·0. Hypochlorites, phenols, iodophors and quaternary ammonium compounds kill campylobacters within 1 min at standard working dilutions. *See* Enterobacteriaceae, Food Poisoning by *Escherichia Coli*

These factors combine to prevent their multiplication in food under usual circumstances, unlike salmonellae and other enterobacteria. Indeed, they tend to die in food stored at ambient temperatures, owing to overgrowth by other bacteria. Their survival is prolonged by refrigeration.

Food Poisoning From Campylobacters

Incidence

The proportion of campylobacter infections attributable to the consumption of food is not precisely known, but it is believed to be high. A few infections are acquired through direct contact with infected animals or their products. These are mostly occupational, e.g. in workers in poultry-processing plants, but some arise through contact with domestic pets, notably puppies and kittens that are themselves suffering from campylobacter diarrhoea. Animal contact is more important in developing countries, where transmission rates are far higher than in developed countries. In such areas the disease is mainly confined to young children through the early acquisition of immunity.

As diagnosis depends on the identification of campylobacters in patients' faeces – a precise diagnosis cannot be made clinically – a measurement of incidence depends on laboratory reports. This in turn is dependent on the availability and use of medical and laboratory services, which are highly variable. Prospective surveillance has provided annual incidences ranging from 60/100 000 in the USA to 87/100 000 in the UK. True incidences are estimated to be at least 10 times those gleaned from laboratory reports. For example, analysis of a waterborne outbreak in the USA suggested that the national incidence was about 1000/100 000; and a survey of patients attending a general practice surgery in England indicated an incidence of 1100/100 000. The cost in terms of health care and lost productivity has been measured at £273 per case in the UK in 1991, so campylobacter enteritis is clearly an expensive disease and a major burden on society.

Foods Implicated in Campylobacter Enteritis

The sporadic nature of most infections makes it difficult to identify food sources. Outbreaks, which provide good opportunities to pinpoint sources, are uncommon and mainly caused by the consumption of untreated water or raw milk (see below). Assessments depend on several types of data:

(1) Identification of foods that are regularly contaminated with campylobacters (Tables 2 and 3), and a comparison of the strains found in those foods with

Table 3. Occurrence of campylobacters in red meats, their source animals, and miscellaneous foods. The data are given as mean percentage positive with the number of studies from which the data were extracted in parentheses

Product	Source animal	Carcass before chilling	Retailed product	
			Fresh	Frozen
Cattle/beef	21 (12)	12 (3)	3·5 (9)	0 (1)
Sheep/lamb	22 (8)	15 (3)	5·8 (5)	2·0 (1)
Pigs/pork	82 (14)	31 (6)	3·4 (9)	0 (1)
Miscellaneous red meats	—	—	1·3 (1)	—
Offal[a]	—	—	22 (8)	1·8 (3)
Cooked meats	—	—	2·3 (1)	—
Seafood, including oysters (*Crassostrea commercialis*)	—	—	14 (2)	—
Mushrooms (PVC wrapped)	—	—	1·5 (1)	—

[a] Mostly liver, kidney and heart from cattle, sheep and pigs.

Table 4. Foods other than milk implicated in 20 outbreaks of campylobacter enteritis. The number of outbreaks for each food are given in parentheses

Chicken		Turkey		Red meat		Eggs	Sea food	Foods believed to have been cross-contaminated in the kitchen	
								Food	Suspected source
Undercooked	(3)	Processed and		Raw beef		Frozen (1)	Raw clam	Salads	Chicken (3)
Casseroled	(1)	sliced	(1)	hamburgers	(1)		salad (1)	Sausage	Dirty slicer (1)
Fondued (liver)	(1)	Boned, stuffed		Raw beef and/or				Boiled egg	Undetermined (1)
Unspecified	(1)	and rolled	(1)	raw egg	(1)			salad with	
				Beef in cabbage				mayonnaise	
				stew	(1)			Cake icing	Undetermined (1)
				Vinegared pork	(1)				
Totals	6		2		4	1	1		6

strains found in patients. For example, strain identification tells us that pigs are a relatively minor source of campylobacter enteritis, as almost all strains in pigs are *C. coli*, yet in most regions *C. coli* accounts for only about 5% of human infection. The common serotypes of *C. jejuni* found in man are well represented in poultry, cattle and sheep. In the UK, about 70% of the strains most commonly isolated from patients are also found in chickens. *See* Essential Oils, Isolation and Production; Pork

(2) Identification of foods that have been implicated in outbreaks of campylobacter enteritis. These foods are listed in Table 4, from which it can be seen that poultry feature prominently. Most foodborne outbreaks arise in institutions (Table 5).

(3) Identification of foods that are statistically associated with infection in case–control studies. Such

studies provide two valuable indices: the relative risk of consuming or handling a food (usually expressed as the odds ratio); and the aetiological fraction, i.e. the proportion of infections attributable to that food. Table 6 shows the foods or activities that have been associated with a risk of acquiring campylobacter infection. Again the consumption of chickens, especially if they are undercooked, stands out as a prominent risk factor.

(4) Observation of the effects of eliminating or reducing campylobacters from a food on the incidence of infection in the community that consumes that food. In a UK study, the control of *C. jejuni* serotype P4:L1 in a heavily colonized chicken farm was followed by a fall in the proportion of human infections with this serotype from over 30% to 5% in the community supplied with the chickens.

Properties and Occurrence

Table 5. Places where foodborne oubreaks of campylobacter enteritis arose (excluding milkborne outbreaks)

Place	Number of outbreaks
Institution (residential and nonresidential schools, colleges, military barracks)	29
Restaurant or other public catering establishment	10
Outdoor camps	2
General community	2
Total	43

Table 6. Food other than milk implicated in sporadic campylobacter enteritis as determined by case–control studies

Food	Number of studies	Odds ratio	Proportion of cases attributable to food
Chicken (any)	6	2·4–5·2	48% (1 study)
Chicken (raw/undercooked)	3	6·3–9·0	
Game hens	1	3·3	
Turkey sandwiches	1	1·7	
Raw/rare fish	1	4·0	
Raw/rare shellfish	1	1·5	
Mushrooms	1	1·5	
Paté (unspecified)	1	—	
Sliced beef	1	—	

Poultry

Although the sources of foodborne campylobacter infection are many and varied, poultry stand out as being the most important, especially broiler chickens on account of the vast numbers consumed. The best estimate we have of their contribution (in the USA) is about one-half of the human cases of campylobacter enteritis.

Milk and Dairy Products

The distribution of inadequately pasteurized milk was responsible for the largest outbreak of campylobacter enteritis on record. In 1979, in England, an estimated 3500 people, mostly primary school children, were affected over a period of 3 weeks. In the 10 years since 1978, some 50 milkborne outbreaks were reported in the UK and 26 in the USA affecting over 7600 people. The average attack rate in exposed persons in 14 outbreaks

in which data were available was 54% (range 24–79%). In the USA, milkborne outbreaks accounted for 50% of all reported foodborne campylobacter outbreaks. Roughly one-half of the milkborne outbreaks arose in the general community, 20% in schools or other institutions, 17% on school visits to farms (all in the USA) and 8% in holiday or rural camps. In all but two instances the implicated milk was drunk raw; in the two exceptions the milk was distributed as pasteurized, but there had been unnoticed processing failures. It is notable that four of 10 people who drank their raw milk in coffee became infected.

The consumption of raw milk has also shown up as an infection risk in case–control studies on sporadic cases, even in places where the sale of raw milk is prohibited. In one study in the USA the relative risk was 9·3 and, in another, 23% of all cases were attributed to this activity. These are probably unusually high figures which reflect the easy availability of raw milk in rural farming communities. There is evidence that the higher incidences of campylobacter enteritis generally found in rural areas relative to urban ones is due to raw milk consumption rather than contact with farm animals.

Most milkborne infections are associated with cows' milk, but raw goats' milk has also been implicated.

Cheese

A soft cheese made from unpasteurized sheep's milk was incriminated in an outbreak of campylobacter enteritis in Czechoslovakia, and there is a single instance of infection associated with home-made ricotta cheese prepared from unpasteurized goats' milk.

Introduction of Campylobacters into Food

Contamination of Meat at Slaughter

The contamination of animal carcasses with intestinal contents at slaughter and the persistence of the bacteria in raw meat is the most important source of campylobacters in food. Because it is inextricably bound with processing methods it is considered below in the section on the effects of food processing on campylobacters. ***See*** Meat, Slaughter

Contamination of Milk from Milk-producing Animals

At any one time an average of about 25% of milking cows excrete campylobacters in their faeces. Carriage in individual animals is variable and several strains may circulate in a herd over a period. Some degree of faecal contamination is unavoidable even in well-run milking parlours, and several outbreaks have been caused by drinking top-grade certified milk in the USA. With sensitive methods of detection campylobacters have been isolated from 6% of bulked raw milk samples in the UK. In general, campylobacter-positive samples have high counts of *E. coli*, but occasionally campylobacters have been found without *E. coli*, possibly through excretion from the udder. Campylobacter mastitis has been produced experimentally and occasionally reported as a natural infection. Many organisms may be excreted from an infected quarter before the milk appears obviously granular.

Campylobacters have also been found in goats' milk and it must be assumed that they could be present in the milk of any animal that carries campylobacters in their gut.

Contamination of Milk by Wild Birds

In the UK, where it is common practice for fresh milk to be delivered to the doorstep in metal-foil-topped bottles, magpies (*Pica pica*) and jackdaws (*Corvus monedula*) have developed the habit of pecking through the foil tops and contaminating the contents. This is a seasonal activity when the birds are raising fledglings (April to June), which is also a time when they frequently probe cow dung for invertebrates. The habit is geographically variable; in areas of highest prevalence case–control studies have shown it to account for a high proportion of campylobacter infections at that time of year.

Contamination of Foods with Untreated Water

The contamination of foods with untreated water is probably an important mode of transmission in developing countries. In developed countries, such contamination seems to be limited to seafoods, which are known to be a risk food when eaten raw (Tables 4 and 6). A study in Australia showed that Sydney Rock Oysters (*Crassostrea commercialis*) allowed to feed in waters containing about 10^4 cfu campylobacters per millilitre concentrated them to 10^2–10^3 cfu per gram in their tissues within 1 h, but they were effectively cleared by depuration for 48 h. Campylobacters were found to survive for several months in frozen oysters and for 8–14 days in refrigerated oysters. *See* Shellfish, Contamination and Spoilage of Molluscs and Crustacea

Cross-contamination in the Kitchen

Items of food, such as raw poultry that are heavily contaminated with campylobacters, provide a reservoir of bacteria in the kitchen from which other foods can become contaminated. This may come about through direct contact (e.g. from the dripping juices from a thawing chicken), via common utensils and surfaces such as chopping boards, and by the hands of kitchen staff. The contamination of food from domestic animals is believed to play a major role in the transmission of infection in developing countries.

Insects

Theoretically, insects could be passive vectors of infection via food. Campylobacters have been isolated from houseflies (e.g. 2·4% of flies caught in houses and gardens in the UK) and cockroaches, but substantial contamination has only been found in the close vicinity of chicken sheds and piggeries. Campylobacters failed to survive for more than 2 days in flies artificially fed with campylobacter broth cultures. *See* Insect Pests, Problems Caused by Insects and Mites

Eggs

There is no vertical transmission to eggs from laying hens, but shell eggs may become externally contaminated with campylobacters from chicken excreta and may thus be a source of contamination for other foods, Campylobacters do not penetrate the shell and membranes into the egg contents.

Fate of Campylobacters During Food Processing

Animal Slaughter and Meat Processing

Contamination of animal carcasses with intestinal contents during slaughter and preparation is universal and to some degree unavoidable. Fortunately, in the case of large animals (cattle, sheep, pigs) conventional forced-air evaporative chilling with frequent mechanical spraying greatly reduces the numbers of live campylobacters remaining on the surfaces of carcasses, mainly through the effect of drying. Cooling without mechanical assistance causes only about a 50% reduction in campylobacter counts.

Broiler chickens and other poultry pose a greater problem, owing to the high degree of mechanization required for processing birds at rates that satisfy public demand. Two stages of processing are particularly problematic:

(1) Mechanical defeathering, which is preceded by immersion in hot water ('scalding') to facilitate plucking. 'Hard scalding' at temperatures above 58°C causes a reduction in bacterial counts, but 'soft scalding' at 50–52°C, used for birds that are to be sold fresh, has little effect; thus, leakage of intestinal contents, which is common, results in gross cross-contamination.

(2) Mechanical evisceration, which often results in the rupture of the gut of birds that are not of consistent size. Again, widespread cross-contamination is the inevitable consequence; birds that are initially clean may become contaminated during processing. Contamination can be reduced, but not eliminated, by chilling in well-designed reverse-flow systems containing chlorinated water (10 ppm chlorine). Uneviscerated ('New York dressed') birds are the most heavily contaminated; campylobacter counts of up to $2·4 \times 10^7$ per chicken have been recorded. Frozen birds are least contaminated owing to the damaging effect on the bacteria of freezing and thawing.

Effects of Storage

Campylobacter counts decline on stored meat by 1–2 $\log_{10}$ at 4°C and 2–5 $\log_{10}$ at 23°C over 2 weeks, but much depends on the particular campylobacter strain and the type of meat – minced beef, for example, is unusually protective. Reduced conditions, such as are present in vacuum-packed meats, are also protective. Freezing and thawing causes a 1–2 $\log_{10}$ reduction in campylobacter counts, but at -20°C counts fall very slowly. *See* Storage Stability, Mechanisms of Degradation

Salting

C. jejuni and *C. coli* do not grow in the presence of salt at concentrations greater than 1·5%. They can survive for 3–5 days at room temperature in 4·5% sodium chloride and for 3 weeks at 4°C in 6·5% sodium chloride, albeit with a several $\log_{10}$ fall in viable counts. Campylobacters can survive on washed pig intestines after overnight salting.

Acidification

Campylobacters cannot grow at pH values of 5·5 or less and are inactivated at pH 5·0 or below.

Irradiation

Campylobacters are more sensitive than *E. coli* to γ and ultraviolet irradiation. The largest D_{10} value for *C. jejuni* in one study was 320 Gy of ionizing radiation. *See* Irradiation of Foods, Basic Principles

Survival in Milk and Dairy Products

Most campylobacter strains are recoverable from raw milk held at 4°C for 7 days if the initial concentration is heavy, e.g. 10^7 cells ml^{-1}. Inactivation of strains parallels a rise in the aerobic plate count and fall in pH. Thus, survival in raw milk is about half that in sterilized milk. The lactoperoxidase system may also reduce survival in milk. Survival becomes progressively shorter as the temperature is increased, so that at 20°C it is only 1–2 days. Campylobacters are readily destroyed by conventional pasteurization and give D values of 1 min or less at 60°C in raw, pasteurized or skimmed cows' milk.

In one study, campylobacters were not recovered from cheddar cheese curd after 30 days of curing, or from whey or curd of cottage cheese after cooking for 30 min at 55°C. In another study no strain survived for more than 25 min in yoghurt. *See* Yoghurt, The Product and its Manufacture

Survival in Other Foods

Egg

Campylobacters can grow in egg yolk and yolk–albumen melanges, but albumen alone is toxic. The major factor in the sensitivity of egg white is apparently conalbumen.

Spices

The spices oregano, sage and ground cloves are mildly inhibitory to *C. jejuni*, but not sufficiently to reduce numbers in refrigerated food.

Bibliography

Blaser MJ, Taylor DN and Feldman RA (1983) Epidemiology of *Campylobacter jejuni* infections. *Epidemiologic Reviews* 5: 157–176.

Finch MJ and Blake PA (1985) Foodborne outbreaks of campylobacteriosis: the United States experience, 1980–1982. *American Journal of Epidemiology* 122: 262–268.

Skirrow MB (1987) A demographic survey of campylobacter, salmonella and shigella infections in England. A Public Health Laboratory Service survey. *Epidemiology and Infection* 99: 647–657.

Skirrow MB (1990) *Campylobacter, Helicobacter* and other motile curved Gram-negative rods. In: Parker MT and Collier LH (eds) *Topley and Wilson's Principles of Bacteriology, Virology and Immunity*, 8th edn, vol. 2, pp 531–549. London: Edward Arnold.

Skirrow MB (1990) *Campylobacter* and *Helicobacter* infections of man and animals. In: Parker MT and Collier LH (eds) *Topley and Wilson's Principles of Bacteriology, Virology and Immunity*, 8th edn, vol. 3, pp 531–545. London: Edward Arnold.

Tauxe RV, Hargrett-Bean N, Patton CM and Wachsmuth IK (1988) *Campylobacter* isolates in the United States, 1982–1986. *Morbidity and Mortality Weekly Report* 37: 1–13.

M. B. Skirrow
Public Health Laboratory, Gloucester, UK

Detection

The conventional means of detecting campylobacters is by isolation in culture. Direct detection by immunological and DNA probe techniques are being developed, but are not yet sufficiently advanced to be of practical value. Campylobacters have specific growth requirements which are now considered.

Principles of Campylobacter Cultivation

The failure of traditional cultural methods to provide the conditions necessary for the growth of campylobacters was the main reason why their role in human disease remained hidden for so long. The main peculiarity of campylobacters is that they are strictly microaerophilic and require specially prepared atmospheres for satisfactory growth. Specific selection, either by means of selective media or filtration, are essential for their isolation from faeces or other specimens containing mixed organisms. Moreover, they only grow well on supplemented media, and *Campylobacter jejuni*, *C. coli* and *C. lari* – the so-called thermophilic group that cause campylobacter enteritis – have an optimum growth temperature of 42–43°C.

Oxygen Sensitivity

Oxygen sensitivity is the most critical factor in the cultivation of campylobacters. Campylobacters have a respiratory type of metabolism based on the Krebs cycle, so oxygen is necessary for growth; yet oxygen at atmospheric pressures is toxic. This toxicity is due to superoxides and free radicals that form in unsupplemented media exposed to air. Campylobacters are especially vulnerable to these compounds despite being able to produce superoxide dismutase and catalase. They are most vulnerable in the resting phase; once they have started to grow they become more oxygen-tolerant, probably owing to the production of nicotinamide adenine dinucleotide (NAD) or nicotinamide adenine dinucleotide phosphate (NADP), which form a physiological barrier that protects oxygen-sensitive enzymes. The practical points that arise from this are twofold:

(1) Heavy inocula are required to initiate growth on unsupplemented media. Large populations usually have a few bacteria that are able to start growing and thereby create conditions suitable for other cells to grow. The result of seeding campylobacters on most unsupplemented media is either confluent growth or none at all.

(2) The key supplements for growing campylobacters are agents that neutralize superoxides and free radicals; any nutrient value they have is incidental. Blood, haemin, haematin, activated charcoal, dihydroxyphenyl and iron compounds are examples of such agents. A simple and widely used supplement is the triple combination of ferrous sulphate, sodium metabisulphite and sodium pyruvate, each at a final concentration of 0·02% (FBP).

Detection in Food by Culture

Growing campylobacters from food is more difficult than growing them from the faeces of a patient with campylobacter enteritis, as there are usually far fewer organisms present. For faecal specimens direct plate culture is normally adequate – indeed, organisms may be so plentiful that a presumptive diagnosis can be made by direct microscopy – but, for food, selective enrichment cultures are essential. Possible exceptions are raw poultry products, which are often so heavily contaminated that enrichment is not critical.

The principle of the enrichment method is to incubate the food (after 'stomaching' or other treatment to break it down) in a selective broth for 24–48 h and then to subculture it on a selective agar for the isolation and identification of individual colonies. A pre-enrichment stage is necessary for organisms that have been subjected to heat or cold stress (see below). As the treatment the foods have received is not always known, there is much to be said for including pre-enrichment routinely.

When properly carried out, cultural methods are able to detect 1 campylobacter colony-forming unit (cfu) in 20 g of food that contains at least 10^6 g^{-1} of other bacteria.

Specimen Handling and Transport

The correct handling and preservation of specimens is crucial for food specimens; incorrect handling negates the value of sensitive isolation procedures. The three most important factors are refrigeration (as near to 4°C as possible), exclusion of oxygen and prevention of drying. Oxygen may be excluded by gassing with 100% nitrogen, but this is not always practicable. Provided specimens are not unduly large, they can be placed in a semisolid transport medium, such as Cary–Blair medium (0·16% agar), or directly into a campylobacter-selective broth, each containing either FBP or sodium bisulphite 0·01%. The choice of medium may be critical, and it is often better to use a highly selective formulation (see below), as campylobacters do not compete well with other microorganisms. This will be influenced by the nature of the sample, the physical state of the target organisms, and the time likely to elapse before cultures are set up.

Milk and liquid foods should be held refrigerated after adding sodium bisulphite 0·01% and either sodium thioglycollate 0·15% or 100% nitrogen. Under these conditions there is little loss of viability over several days, but the sooner specimens are cultured the better.

Pre-enrichment and Enrichment

Campylobacters that have been frozen, chilled (4°C) or subjected to mild heating become sublethally injured. This is manifested by increased susceptibility to antibiotics (notably rifampicin and polymyxin), deoxycholate, oxygen radicals and high incubation temperatures. This is thought to be due to damage to the outer membrane and it can reduce significantly the efficacy of detection by culture. The principal controlling factor is increased sensitivity to raised incubation temperatures and it is important to allow the organisms time to recover. This can be achieved by preincubation at 37°C in either basal or selective broth for a minimum of 4 h. For convenience in the laboratory, the preincubation period can be extended to 18 h with no loss of sensitivity and, with samples such as water, where the target population may be severely injured, sensitivity is in fact increased. For most samples the convenience of preincubation directly in antibiotic-containing selective broth outweighs the slight advantage of using base medium. The preincubation broth should be at about room temperature when inoculated and, if the volume is large, incubation is best done in a water bath.

With clinical specimens the choice of selective media may not influence significantly isolation rates. This is not the case with food and environmental samples and it is important to choose a medium which is able to suppress the growth of competing flora adequately, particularly *Pseudomonas* and *Proteus* species. The formula for EX1 (Exeter) broth (Table 1) is highly selective for campylobacters and is recommended.

Various protocols have been laid down for incubation procedures. In general, maximum sensitivity can be attained by a period of preincubation at 37°C for 18 h followed by enrichment at 42–43°C for 30 h. This latter period can be extended for a further 24 h, and with some lightly contaminated samples the use of this protocol has been shown to improve isolation rates. The sensitivities of the various protocols have not been compared but, in general, as large a volume of broth as is practicable should be used in order to accommodate as much of the sample as possible; a minimum of 25 g in 225 ml of broth is recommended.

For liquid samples such as milk, it may be convenient to add the sample to an equal volume of double-strength medium. For maximum sensitivity, however, it is necessary to examine large volumes (around 200 ml) and this can present problems. Alternative methods of testing

Table 1. Formula for EX1 (Exeter) campylobacter-selective enrichment broth (and agar)

Nutrient broth[a]	1 litre
Sodium metabisulphite	0·2 g
Sodium pyruvate	0·2 g
Ferrous sulphate (7 H_2O)	0·2 g
Colistin sodium sulphomethate	4 mg
Rifampicin	10 mg
Trimethoprim	10 mg
Cefoperazone	15 mg
Amphotericin	2 mg
Lysed horse blood	50 ml
(New Zealand agar	15 g)[b]

[a] Nutrient Broth No. 2 (CM67, Oxoid Ltd, Basingstoke, UK) in original formula.
[b] Only for solid plating medium.

large volumes are to culture gauze or cotton wool pads through which the milk has been filtered, or to culture heavily centrifuged deposits.

Fluid cultures can be incubated in closed containers, and this is generally acceptable. Slight increases in sensitivity can be attained by the use of Erlenmeyer flasks with stoppered side-arms, so that air can be partially extracted and replaced with a mixture of 10% carbon dioxide, 10% hydrogen and 80% nitrogen. Best results are obtained if there is a constant flow of gas mixture with agitation of the broth.

Subculture to Agar Plates

Mature enrichment cultures are subcultured on a campylobacter-selective agar. There are numerous formulae, but either Preston or EX1 agars are recommended. EX1, which is highly selective, may have advantages. Hydrogen peroxide and other potentially toxic oxygen metabolites can accumulate in agar even if the plates are stored in the dark under refrigeration. It has been shown that these compounds act synergically with antibiotics, such as rifampicin, to inhibit campylobacter growth. Thus, for maximum sensitivity it is important to use fresh plates and include FBP supplement in the agar even if blood is also included. Plates are incubated at 42–43°C in a microaerobic atmosphere containing 5–10% oxygen and preferably some hydrogen. If cylinder gasses are available, the easiest method is to extract two-thirds of the air from a closed container, such as an anaerobic jar (without catalyst), and replace with a mixture of 10% carbon dioxide, 10% hydrogen and 80% nitrogen. If there is no cylinder gas, an anaerobic-type gas-generating envelope can be used, and the jar partially evacuated after closure. Alternatively, special gas-generating envelopes for campylobacters are commercially available for use in jars with a catalyst.

Table 2. Basic differential characters of campylobacters likely to be found in food

Species	Growth at 25°C	Hippurate hydrolysis	Indoxyl acetate hydrolysis	Sensitivities Nalidixic acid	Cephalothin
C. jejuni	−	+	+	S	R
C. coli	−	−	+	S	R
C. lari	−	−	−	R	R
C. fetus	+	−	−	R	S

−, negative; +, positive; R, resistant (no zone of inhibition to 30 μg disc); S, sensitive (any zone of inhibition to 30 μg disc).

Growth is usually visible after 24 h, but occasional strains do not appear until incubation has been maintained for 48 h.

Identification

Campylobacter colonies are typically flat, effuse and wet-looking. Identity is confirmed by a positive oxidase reaction and the presence of characteristic motile, spiral or S-shaped Gram-negative organisms in wet preparations and Gram-stained smears. Additional basic identification tests are shown in Table 2.

Typing

Serotyping on the basis of heat-stable lipopolysaccharide antigens (Penner system) and heat-labile flagellar and outer-membrane protein antigens (Lior system) is a valuable tool in epidemiological investigations. There are well over 100 designated serotypes and certainly many more to be identified. The discriminatory power of serotyping can be enhanced by the parallel use of biotyping and/or phage typing. Typing facilities are available only at reference laboratories.

Detection in Food by Noncultural Methods

Although cultural methods are the only practicable ones currently available for detecting campylobacters in food, direct methods are being developed. Latex agglutination and enzyme linked immunosorbent assay (ELISA) are immunological methods that make use of high-affinity monoclonal antibodies, but there is greater potential in DNA probe technology. At present these methods lack adequate sensitivity for direct detection in clinical or food samples, but they can be used to identify campylobacters in cultures, though there are much simpler ways of doing this. DNA probes can be too specific in that they detect only some C. jejuni or C. coli strains. A single probe that would detect all strains of both species, but not any other organism, would be ideal. It is probably only a matter of time before probes of adequate sensitivity will be produced, possibly by use of the polymerase chain reaction. *See* Immunoassays, Radioimmunoassay and Enzyme Immunoassay

Faecal Indicator Bacteria and Campylobacters

It will be evident from the foregoing account that the culture of campylobacters from food is time consuming and costly, especially if regular monitoring is undertaken. Campylobacters are rarely found in the absence of faecal bacteria, so for processed foods it is reasonable to screen for the latter rather than look for campylobacters. Most raw meats have faecal coliforms on them, and it must be assumed they also have campylobacters, regardless of culture results. In short, it pays to think carefully about the value of screening for campylobacters before undertaking a monitoring programme; it could be unproductive and uneconomic.

Detection in Suspected Food Poisoning

Outbreaks of campylobacter enteritis usually come to light through the recognition of a sudden excess of campylobacter isolations in a clinical laboratory, or less often by the recognition of an excess of diarrhoea in a community. Either way the laboratory plays a key role, as the infection cannot be diagnosed clinically. Unfortunately, outbreak investigations are hampered by the long time that elapses between food consumption and awareness of an outbreak: the average incubation period is 3 days; people tend not to seek medical attention until they have been ill for several days; sampling, testing and reporting may take 2–3 days; and several more days may pass before someone realizes that cases are epidemiologically connected. Thus, the investigation may only start 2 weeks or more after ingestion of the food, long after suspect items have been discarded. Even if foods are available, the vulnerability of campylobacters mitigates against their survival in detectable numbers. *See* Food Poisoning, Tracing Origins and Testing

For the above reasons reliance must usually be placed on statistical associations of infection with foods eaten. Such evidence can be powerful and incriminate beyond all reasonable doubt that a particular food was the vehicle of infection. Protocols for investigating such outbreaks can be complex and require close cooperation between community doctors, public health workers, microbiologists, veterinarians and food producers. The prime essential is to have all efforts directed and coordinated by one person.

Bibliography

Barrow GI and Feltham RKA (1991) *Cowan and Steel's Manual for the Identification of Medical bacteria.* Cambridge: Cambridge University Press.
Doyle MP (1984) *Campylobacter* in foods. In: Butzler J-P (ed.) *Campylobacter Infection in Man and Animals*, pp 163–180. Boca Raton: CRC Press.
Griffiths PL and Park RWA (1990) Campylobacters associated with human diarrhoeal disease. *Journal of Applied Bacteriology* 69: 281–301.
Humphrey TJ and Muscat I (1989) Incubation temperature and the isolation of *Campylobacter jejuni* from food, milk or water. *Letters in Applied Microbiology* 9: 137–139.
Public Health Laboratory Service Campylobacter Working Group (1985) Guidelines for the investigation of suspected milkborne outbreaks of campylobacter enteritis. *PHLS Microbiology Digest* 2: 6–10.

M. B. Skirrow
Public Health Laboratory, Gloucester, UK

Campylobacteriosis

Campylobacteriosis in human beings is virtually synonymous with campylobacter enteritis, which is a major cause of acute diarrhoeal illness and is the main topic of this article. But before describing the disease, brief mention must be made of an uncommon low-grade septicaemic form of infection known as systemic campylobacteriosis. It is classically caused by *Campylobacter fetus*, but it may also be caused by other campylobacters, including *C. jejuni* and *C. coli*. Only patients with immune deficiency or some underlying chronic disease are prone to this sort of infection. It is often associated with focal infection, such as endocarditis, cellulitis or, rarely, meningitis. Invasion is thought to arise from intestinal colonization, and some patients have diarrhoea. Although *C. fetus* infection has been ascribed to eating raw meat, systemic campylobacteriosis accounts for only a tiny proportion of foodborne campylobacter infection.

Clinical Features

Campylobacter enteritis is an acute self-limiting diarrhoeal disease clinically indistinguishable from salmonella enteritis, although minor differences become apparent when groups of patients are compared.

Infection can be established with as few as 500–800 organisms. The average incubation period is 3 days (range, 1–7 days). In most patients the illness starts with abdominal pain and diarrhoea, but in about one-third of cases there is an influenza-like prodrome of malaise, headache and fever, sometimes with rigors, for a period ranging from a few hours to a day or so before the onset of gastrointestinal symptoms. Profuse diarrhoea lasts for 2–3 days and is invariably accompanied by abdominal pain, which is sometimes severe enough to simulate acute appendicitis and result in admission to hospital; some patients undergo surgery as a result. A few patients, usually children, have abdominal pain without diarrhoea. Surveys of patients affected in community outbreaks show that, on average, about 50% have fever, 8% rigors, 10% frank blood in their stools, but only 16% vomit, even though nausea is common.

After a few days the diarrhoea eases and about 80% of patients recover within a week, irrespective of any treatment they may receive. Minor relapses have been reported in about 20% of patients after a day or two without diarrhoea.

Young and middle-aged adults seem to be most severely affected by the infection. Unlike salmonellosis, campylobacter enteritis in infants is often mild and, although infection in old people tends to be more invasive, it is seldom dangerous. Death is extremely uncommon and virtually limited to frail patients debilitated from other causes.

Complications

Apart from simulated appendicitis, acute complications are rare. Among those described are intestinal haemorrhage, haemolytic uraemic syndrome, and septic abortion, but there are only a handful of reports of the first two in the world literature, and less than 20 reports of abortion. More important are two late complications that may arise 1–2 weeks after onset of illness:

(1) Reactive (aseptic) arthritis affects an estimated 1% of patients. It is benign, but can cause painful debility lasting for several months. Clinically, it is the same as the reactive arthritis that sometimes follows other forms of acute bacterial enteritis.

(2) Guillain–Barré syndrome, an acute polyneuropathy, is a more serious complication, causing paralysis that is not always resolved completely. Severely affected patients may require nursing on a ventilator for respiratory paralysis. Surveys have shown that 14–30% of Guillain–Barré patients have evidence of recent campylobacter infection but, fortunately, it is an uncommon condition and only a tiny proportion of campylobacter enteritis patients develop it.

Convalescent Excretion

Excretion of campylobacters in faeces falls off exponentially after illness. About 50% of patients are culture-negative after 3 weeks, and virtually all are negative after 3 months. Long-term carriage is unknown except in patients with major immune deficiency. Spread of infection from a healthy excreter with formed stools is a remote risk and the suspension of an excreting food handler from work is rarely justified.

Site of Infection

Any part of the intestinal tract may be affected. Infection probably starts in the jejunum and then extends to the ileum and eventually to the colon and rectum. In some patients infection is predominantly colitic and may mimic acute ulcerative colitis. Campylobacters tend to be invasive. The high fever with rigors, dizziness and occasional delirium seen in some patients early in the illness strongly suggest bacteraemia, and occasionally campylobacters are isolated from blood cultures. Regional lymph nodes are often enlarged and inflamed, again suggesting invasion. A cholera-like enterotoxin is produced by most strains, which probably accounts for the watery diarrhoea suffered by most patients. Campylobacters also produce at least one cytotoxin, but their role is not clear.

The histopathology of the intestinal mucosa is that of acute inflammation and is of a pattern indistinguishable from that seen in salmonella, shigella, or other acute bacterial infections of the gut. *See Shigella*

Treatment and Course of Illness

As campylobacter enteritis is a self-limiting disease that resolves spontaneously, treatment is primarily symptomatic and supportive. The most important element, as with all forms of acute diarrhoea, is to correct dehydration and electrolyte loss, particularly in infants and old people, who are least able to do this on their own.

Antimicrobial therapy has a place in severely affected patients. In such cases, which usually arise in hospital, ciprofloxacin or an equivalent quinolone drug would be appropriate before a bacteriological diagnosis had been made. If it is known that the patient has a campylobacter infection, erythromycin is the agent of choice. Several trials of erythrocmycin in campylobacter enteritis failed to show a shortening of the period of illness, although campylobacters disappeared from the faeces within 2 days of starting treatment. The problem with these studies was that, by the time treatment was started, patients had already been ill for 5–6 days and were on the point of getting better anyway. In a study in Peru, in which treatment was started empirically when patients with symptoms – mostly children – were first seen, erythromycin was effective. A 5 day course in standard dosage is adequate.

Erythromycin resistance has been reported at varying rates according to geographic location. In developed countries it ranges from about 1–5% of strains, but higher rates have been found in some developing countries, notably 65% in Thailand. Erythromycin resistance is much more common in *C. coli* than *C. jejuni*, and it has been suggested that this is due to the use of tylosin, a similar macrolide antibiotic, in pig rearing. The use of ciprofloxacin, which is highly effective against normally sensitive strains, is currently being severely compromised, owing to the rapid emergence of resistance, almost certainly through the widespread use of quinolones in poultry.

Immunity

Circulating antibodies are produced within a few days of the onset of illness and for a time patients are refractory to reinfection with the same strain. People regularly exposed to infection develop solid immunity. Children in developing countries become immune within the first 2 years or so of life, and occupationally exposed groups in developed countries have evidence of immunity. For example, in a milkborne outbreak of campylobacter enteritis in the USA, 76% of people exposed for the first time were ill, whereas no person who habitually drank raw milk became ill. In the UK significant amounts of antibody were found in 18% of veterinary assistants, 36% of cattle abattoir workers and 27–68% of workers in poultry-processing plants, compared with 2–5% in nonexposed adults. Infection with one or two strains is probably sufficient to give broad immunity, but it is not known how long immunity lasts. There are several records of patients who had two attacks of campylobacter enteritis many months apart; in each case the second attack was with a different strain. Regular exposure is probably necessary for maintenance of immunity, but firm evidence for this is lacking.

Prevention

Most of the measures appropriate for the prevention of gastrointestinal infections in general apply to campylobacter enteritis. These include the treatment and safe disposal of sewage, the provision of purified and bacteriologically safe water, the pasteurization or equivalent heat treatment of milk, and the general hygienic processing and handling of food. An important aspect of the prevention of campylobacter infection is the interruption of transmission from food-producing animals, particularly poultry, to the final food product.

Sewage Disposal

Campylobacters are capable of surviving for several weeks in cold water, including sea water. Organisms may also be capable of forming viable but nonculturable forms, which are alleged to be more resistant than vegetative forms and to survive for several months in water. The potential role of such dormant cells in the epidemiology of campylobacters has yet to be established. The discharge of untreated sewage helps to maintain the campylobacter population in the environment, but conventional sewage treatment is effective in eliminating campylobacters. In one study over 78% were removed after primary sedimentation, and less than 0·1% remained in the final effluent.

Water Purification

Conventional treatments are fully adequate for removing campylobacters, which are generally more sensitive to chlorine and other disinfecting agents than *Escherichia coli*. Contact with monochloramine $1 \cdot 0$ mg l^{-1} for 15 min, or free chlorine $0 \cdot 1$ mg l^{-1} for 5 min causes more than 99% inactivation.

Major community outbreaks of campylobacter enteritis have been caused by the distribution of unchlorinated or inadequately chlorinated water, which serves to emphasize the importance of proper treatment. This applies equally to remote lakes and surface waters, which become contaminated from wild birds and other animals. A number of outbreaks have arisen as a result of the failure of outdated, overloaded or inadequately maintained water works or distribution systems. *See* Water Supplies, Water Treatment

Heat Treatment of Milk

Pasteurization and other orthodox treatment processes are fully effective in destroying campylobacters. Despite this, milkborne outbreaks of infection regularly occur, even where it is illegal to sell raw milk to the public. Some of the largest outbreaks of campylobacter enteritis on record have been milkborne, a few of them from ostensibly pasteurized milk. Thus, although compulsory pasteurization is a highly desirable goal, it is unlikely to eliminate all risks of milkborne infection. Bad design, malfunctioning of machinery or those running the machinery, and the difficulty of designing satisfactory small pasteurizing units at reasonable cost are all factors that need attention in order to minimize risks. Electricity supply failures putting pasteurizing machinery out of action and bad weather preventing the delivery of milk to central pasteurizing plants have also been precipitating factors in outbreaks of milkborne infection.

Food Hygiene

Measures taken to maintain good hygiene and food-handling practice in restaurants and other catering establishments are fundamental to the prevention of campylobacter enteritis. Much infection is believed to be transmitted through the cross-contamination of cooked or ready-to-eat foods from raw poultry and other raw meats. The separation of raw from cooked foods and the use of dedicated equipment for each, such as chopping boards, mixers, knives and other utensils, is the single most important principle to be observed. If raw meats cannot be stored separately they should always be placed on a bottom shelf so they cannot drip juices on to other foods.

Raw poultry should be handled as little as possible and washing carcasses only spreads organisms around work areas. The discipline of washing hands after touching raw meats of any sort should be rigorously observed. It has been shown that campylobacters can be isolated from the flesh of chicken carcasses even when the surface has been disinfected by immersion in boiling water. Chicken muscle affords the organism some protection from the effects of heat and is a possible explanation for the implication of barbecued chicken in outbreaks of campylobacter enteritis. It is thus especially important that chicken and other poultry meat are properly cooked. *See* Poultry, Chicken

Control of Campylobacters in Source Animals

Elimination of campylobacters in food-producing animals is clearly impracticable, owing to the wide natural distribution of the organisms. Yet there are possible measures for reducing colonization in farm animals, especially in poultry, which have by far the highest colonization rates.

The epidemiology of campylobacter colonization in broiler chickens differs from that of salmonellae in that there is a delay of 2 weeks or more in the appearance of the organism in the growing flock. This suggests that an environmental threshold of contamination needs to be exceeded before the birds acquire the organism. It is probable that broiler chickens acquire campylobacters from the environment either within or outside of the broiler house. Thus, there is the possibility of extending the campylobacter-free period by improving hygienic practice among broiler house attendants and proofing houses against intrusion by birds and rodents.

Evidence is also accumulating that water may be a major source of the organism in broiler houses. Many houses are served by unchlorinated private borehole supplies. Even if the houses are on mains supplies campylobacters can become established in distribution systems beyond header tanks. Experimental interventions, in which header tanks and distribution pipework have been thoroughly cleaned and disinfected, have been followed by dramatic falls in colonization rates in the broilers. However, such measures are difficult to sustain under agricultural conditions and further research is needed. It might be possible to reduce campylobacter colonization by manipulating the intestinal flora of the chickens (competitive exclusion).

Reduction in colonization would probably be sufficient to prevent transmission from chickens. The logistics, precise methods and costs of such measures have yet to be worked out, but they offer considerable hope for a substantial reduction in broiler contamination. The problems of controlling cross-contamination during mechanical processing are discussed elsewhere. Terminal irradiation of dressed poultry eliminates campylobacters, but there are problems with this, not least public acceptability. *See* Irradiation of Foods, Basic Principles

Waste Disposal from Poultry Farms

An added advantage of controlling campylobacter colonization of poultry is that fewer bacteria would be returned to the environment and to surface waters. Heavily colonized flocks have a prodigious output of campylobacters that are likely to be recycled in farm stock via surface water and wild and feral animals that are closely associated with farms, such as magpies, jackdaws, rooks, starlings, sparrows, rats and mice. Cattle with access to surface water are commonly colonized, whereas those with access only to mains water have been found to be free of campylobacters.

Public Education

It has been said that if everyone handled their foods properly, foodborne campylobacter enteritis would virtually disappear. This is probably true, but it is an unrealistic expectation. Yet much could be done to educate the public towards this end and there is every reason to pursue such a policy, for it would help the control of other infections such as salmonellosis and listeriosis, as well as campylobacter enteritis. The presence of these organisms in food will probably persist for some time. Television is the most influential medium and a substantial impact could be made by broadcasting high-quality entertaining yet informative spot 'advertisements'. The understandable fears of the poultry and retail industries could be allayed by inviting their participation and ensuring that the content of the spots was sensibly balanced. With appropriate professional skills, it could even be turned to their advantage. Public money used to fund such a venture should be amply offset by the savings from infections prevented.

Bibliography

Humphrey TJ (1989) Salmonella, campylobacter and poultry: possible control measures. *Abstracts on Hygiene and communicable diseases* 64: R1–R8.
Skirrow MB (1984) *Campylobacter* infections of man. In: Easmon CSF and Jeljaszevicz J (eds) *Medical Microbiology*, vol. 4, pp 105–141. London: Academic Press.

M. B. Skirrow
Public Health Laboratory, Gloucester, UK

CANCER

Contents

Epidemiology

Approaches to Identifying Causes of Cancer in Populations

Evidence relating dietary factors and cancer in humans can be obtained from a variety of sources. Mutagenicity tests are useful but are not comprehensive because many compounds that influence carcinogenicity are not mutagenic. These substances may act by modifying the permeability of cells to carcinogens, inducing cell proliferation, influencing tumour immunity, altering hormonal balance, or other mechanisms. They can be studied in animal tumour models that are responsive to dietary manipulation, but the doses customarily used and metabolic differences among species preclude the direct extrapolation of results to humans. The quantification of a risk between a nutritional factor and cancer requires direct evidence from human beings. The study designs used in investigating dietary factors and cancer in humans, including a discussion of their relative strengths and limitations, are discussed in this article. *See* Epidemiology; Mutagens

Descriptive Studies

International Correlation Studies

'Ecological' or 'correlation' studies compare disease rates in populations with the population per capita consumption of specific dietary factors. Comparing per capita meat intake and incidence of colon cancer, Armstrong and Doll (1975) observed correlations of 0·85 for men and 0·89 for women. Correlation studies have several strengths, the most important being that the contrasts in dietary intake are very large. For example, the range of fat intake within a population tends to be small compared to differences among different populations. In addition, the average diets of persons residing in a country tend to be more stable over time than individuals' diets within a population. Finally, the number of total cancers is very large and thus provides statistically stable estimates.

While ecological studies have provided leads regarding diet and cancer, limitations have prevented these studies from surpassing the level of hypothesis generation. The primary limitation of this study design is that many potential differences other than the dietary factor under consideration may vary among populations. For example, the correlation between gross national product and colon cancer mortality is 0·77 for men and 0·69 for women; because many factors are correlated with industrialization, it is difficult to implicate meat eating as the primary factor in the aetiology of colon cancer. Moreover, correlation studies generally use disappearance data as a measure of dietary intake. Disappearance data include foods lost to wastage and animal feed and do not directly measure human intake. Similarly, the quality of cancer incidence data varies among countries. Statistical adjustment for potentially confounding factors and more uniform collection of data may aid in interpreting results from these studies.

Special-exposure Groups

Groups within populations that have atypical dietary patterns may provide important information in the diet–cancer relation. These groups are often defined by ethnic or religious characteristics and offer many of the advantages of correlation studies. In addition, if the special-exposure group lives in the same general area as the comparison group, the number of alternative explanations for any observations may be reduced. Seventh Day Adventists, a largely vegetarian group, have been used in studies of meat eating and cancer. Findings based on special-exposure groups are subject to the same limitations as ecological studies. For example, lower rates of colon cancer have been observed among Seventh Day Adventists, supporting the hypothesis that meat is related to colon cancer. However, this group is also characterized by other lifestyle variables, such as low rates of smoking and alcohol intake, which could also modify rates of colon cancer. *See* Colon, Cancer of the Colon

Migrant Studies and Secular Trends

Migrant studies are useful in addressing the possibility that correlations observed in ecological studies are due to genetic differences. For most cancers, migrating groups take on the rate of cancer of the new country. For example, while Japan has low rates of cancers of the breast, colon and prostate, the rate of these cancers among Japanese migrants to the USA increases toward the higher US rates. The increase in rate of breast cancer among migrants occurs primarily in later generations, suggesting that the causal factors operate early in life. Major changes in the rate of a disease within a population over time also provide evidence that nongenetic factors play an important role in the aetiology of cancer. Limitations of these studies are similar to those for correlation studies. *See* Breast Cancer and Diet

Evidence from Descriptive Studies

Based largely on descriptive studies, Doll and Peto (1981) have estimated that 35% of cancers in the USA may be attributable to dietary factors, but this estimate could be as low as 10% or as high as 70%. The evidence that dietary factors influence the development of cancer is based on the marked variation in the rates of most cancers among countries. The variation in rates cannot be attributed solely to genetic factors because rates of specific cancers increase in populations migrating from low- to high-incidence areas and change within the same population over time. In the USA and other Western countries, the cancer sites most likely to be influenced by dietary factors are colon, breast and prostate. The potential scope of dietary factors that may influence cancer risk is illustrated in Table 1. While descriptive studies provide a rich source of hypotheses, more definitive evidence is required from analytical epidemiology.

Analytical Epidemiological Studies

Intervention Studies or Controlled Trials

Intervention studies provide the most rigorous test of a hypothesis. In a randomized control trial, individuals are assigned randomly by the investigator either to an experimental or a control group. If the sample size is sufficient, after randomization the groups are identical in all respects except for the experimental treatment; hence any difference in outcomes between groups can be attributed to the treatment. To reduce the likelihood of bias, the trial should be conducted as a double-blind experiment, i.e. neither the subjects nor the investigators know to which treatment a subject is allocated.

Double-blind randomized trials may be feasible for

Table 1. Examples of suspected dietary factors influencing cancer risk

Dietary factor	Site of cancer
Increase risk	
Overnutrition	Endometrium, gall bladder, breast
Alcohol	Liver, oesophagus, larynx, pharynx, breast
Beer	Rectum
Fat (especially saturated)	Colorectum, breast, prostate
Red meat	Colorectum
Salt	Gastric, nasopharyngeal
Heterocyclic amines (from cooked meat)	Colorectum
Decrease Risk	
Fibre	Colorectum, breast
Vitamins A, C, E	Many sites
Protease inhibitors	Colorectum
Calcium, vitamin D	Colorectum

minor components of diet that may prevent cancer. For example, there is currently a randomized intervention study testing the hypothesis that β-carotene, administered in a capsule, reduces the risk of cancer. However, whether it is feasible to conduct trials that involve a major change in diet, such as a significant reduction in total fat intake, remains uncertain because of the length of time to observe an influence on cancer. Specifically, it is unclear whether a high degree of compliance to a major dietary change over a period of years or decades can be achieved in a large group of people.

Because of practical or ethical reasons, it will not be possible to test all hypotheses by controlled trials. In these situations, it is likely that case-control and cohort studies will provide the most direct evidence of the dietary-factor–cancer relation.

Case-control and Cohort Studies

Case-control and cohort studies can potentially avoid many of the limitations of ecological studies. In these study designs, information on exposure and outcome is collected on an individual basis. Confounding by other variables can be controlled either in the design (by matching or restricting individuals on the basis of potentially confounding factors), or in the analysis (by multivariate statistical techniques) if information on confounders is collected.

In cohort studies, information is collected from healthy participants who are then followed to determine disease rates according to levels of dietary factors. At the end of follow-up, the disease frequency within a cohort may be measured as either a cumulative incidence rate, i.e. the number of cases divided by the entire base population, or incidence density rate, i.e. the number of cases divided by the person-time of follow-up*. The rate ratio, or relative risk, is the rate of disease (cumulative incidence rate or incidence density rate) in the exposed (e.g. those with a high intake of dietary fat) divided by the rate of disease in the unexposed (e.g. those on a low-fat diet). For example, a relative risk of two implies that the exposed group has twice the rate of disease relative to the unexposed group.

In case-control studies, information is obtained from diseased participants and compared to information provided by disease-free controls. The cases are selected from a defined population, such as individuals living in a particular region during a specified period. Each time someone in the population develops the disease during the specified period, this individual joins the case series. Conceptually, controls should be a random sample of all the individuals who, if they had developed the disease, would have joined the case series under the specified study parameters of time and place. For example, if the case series is derived from a specified region during 1986–1988, the controls should be a random sample of all individuals who lived in that region during the years 1986–1988. Cumulative incidence rates or incidence density rates requires information on the entire population at risk and cannot be calculated in case-control studies. However, the rate ratio or relative risk can be estimated by a measure that is easily calculated from case-control studies, the odds ratio.

Relative to cohort studies, case-control studies are quick and less expensive to conduct because they require many fewer subjects. Case-control studies are well suited to the study of rare diseases. In cohort studies, tens of thousands of individuals must be followed to study the most common cancers; it may not be feasible to study rarer cancers through cohort designs unless subjects from several large cohorts are pooled for analysis.

Although more efficient, case-control studies generally have greater potential for bias than cohort studies. In a cohort study, the exposure of interest, such as a dietary factor, is measured before the onset of disease. In a case-control study, the exposure is assessed in individuals who already know whether they have the disease. In addition, the interviewer may also be aware of the case-control status of the subject. It is unclear if knowledge of health status influences a subject's response. The potential of bias appears especially plausible for the recall of diet, which is inherently prone to errors of memory. Evidence indicates that an indi-

vidual's recall of remote diet is influenced by the present diet. In cohort studies, the subjects do not know if they will eventually be a case or noncase by the end of the follow-up period hence recall bias is unlikely.

Bias can be introduced in case-control studies by the selection of an inappropriate control series. Although, in principle, the controls should be a random sample of the entire population at risk, the selection of such a group may not always be practical. For convenience, controls are often selected from patients hospitalized with another disease, with the assumption that the exposure of interest is unrelated with this condition. In other words, the diet of the selected control group should be representative of that of the population at risk. This assumption is questionable because diet may be related to many medical conditions. In practice, our limited knowledge of dietary factors and most diseases hinders the interpretation of case-control studies using hospitalized patients as controls.

In some case-control studies, investigators attempt to sample persons from the general population. Unfortunately, typically only 60% or 70% of eligible population controls complete the interview. If the diets of the participants are different from those who do not participate, selection bias will be introduced. Because the degree of health consciousness is probably related to diet and the willingness to participate in a health study, bias from nonresponse is a distinct possibility. In general, the lower the response rate in a study, the greater the potential for this kind of bias.

Important Issues in the Study of Diet

The epidemiological study of nutrition and cancer has special complexities that merit discussion. In most populations, the range of diet is relatively limited. For example, in most populations where foods high in fat are readily available, few individuals consume significantly less than 30% of energy from fat. Hence it may be difficult to study the impact of reducing fat intake to less than 30% of total energy intake. However, some individuals of even a relatively homogeneous population may have very different dietary patterns. For example, in a cohort of 52 000 male health professionals in the USA, the intake of dietary fat was quite varied and a contrast of diet from 25% to 40% of total energy from fat was possible.

Accurate measure of long-term dietary intake is crucial in a study of cancer because most neoplasms have a long induction period (the time from an exposure to the development of cancer). Thus short-term methods of dietary assessment such as diet records and 24-h recalls are usually insufficient. These short-term methods are especially inappropriate in case-control studies because they measure current diet and individuals may

* Person-time of follow-up; total follow-up time accumulated by all members of the population.

change their diet after the diagnosis of cancer. Studies have established that the most feasible method of assessing long-term intakes in large numbers of individuals is the food frequency questionnaire which measures usual frequency of a selected list of foods. In case-control studies, the usual intake prior to the diagnosis of cancer is assessed. *See* Dietary Surveys, Surveys of Food Intakes in Groups and Individuals

In order to measure diet accurately, the food items must represent the major source of the nutrients of interest within the study population. The precision of dietary questionnaires varies among nutrients depending on the consistency of the concentration of a nutrient in a given food. For example, cholesterol intake is generally measured adequately by questionnaires because the concentration of cholesterol is relatively constant in a given food item. Selenium levels in foods, on the other hand, vary widely depending on the selenium content of the soil. Thus alternative methods, such as measuring serum selenium levels, must be used to estimate selenium intake in individuals.

Food frequency questionnaires provide rankings of individuals by level of intake of a nutrient but generally do not quantify actual intake. A dietary questionnaire may effectively distinguish between individuals with a low and a high fat intake in a given population but does not necessarily provide a precise assessment of the absolute fat intake. This is not a major hindrance to epidemiological analyses, which are usually based on comparing categories of intake (such as high, medium and low). In large studies based on dietary questionnaires, more precise quantification of intake may be achieved by having a random sample of the participants provide a more comprehensive assessment of intake, such as multiple weeks of dietary records. For example, the study could be comprised of tens of thousands of individuals, while only several hundred participants are necessary for the comprehensive assessment of diet. This additional information will help to estimate true dose-response relationships between a nutrient and diet expressed in absolute intake (such as grams per day).

Despite significant improvements in the assessment of diet by questionnaires, there will always be an appreciable degree of error. If there is systematic error between cases and controls, such as the general over-reporting of intake of a nutrient by cases, then false conclusions may be drawn from a study. Random error between cases and noncases will cause an underestimation of the strength of a true relation between a dietary factor and cancer. The magnitude of measurement error of a questionnaire can be estimated in a sample of participants who, in addition to the questionnaire, provide a more precise measure of intake. Statistical techniques can then be used to quantify the influence of measurement error on epidemiological measures such as relative risk.

Bibliography

Armstrong B and Doll R (1975) Environmental factors and cancer incidence and mortality in different countries, with special reference to dietary practices. *International Journal of Cancer* 15: 617–631.

Doll R and Peto R (1981) The causes of cancer: quantitative estimates of avoidable risks in the United States today. *Journal of the National Cancer Institute* 66: 1191–1308.

Hennekens CH and Buring JE (1987) *Epidemiology in Medicine.* Boston: Little, Brown.

Schottenfeld D and Fraumeni JF (eds) (1982) *Cancer Epidemiology and Prevention.* Philadelphia: WB Saunders.

Willett WC (1989) *Nutritional Epidemiology.* New York: Oxford University Press.

Edward Giovannucci and Graham A. Colditz
Harvard University, Boston, USA

Carcinogens in the Diet

It has become increasingly clear in recent decades that food can have a substantial effect on cancer risk. This conclusion is based on the results of both human population studies and animal studies. Presently available evidence indicates that dietary fat may be a risk factor for cancer and that fresh fruits and vegetables may have a protective effect. In addition, the human diet contains specific carcinogenic substances, most, but not all of which are present at such low levels that their effects on human cancer rates, if any, are likely to be small. This article summarizes current information on carcinogens in the diet that are (1) naturally occurring components of food, (2) produced by the processing of food, or (3) added intentionally to food. Carcinogenic contaminants of food, including mycotoxins and pesticides, are discussed elsewhere. *See* Carcinogens, Carcinogenic Substances in Food; Carcinogens, Carcinogenicity Tests; Fatty Acids, Dietary Importance; Contamination, Types and Causes; Mycotoxins, Occurrence and Determination

Naturally Occurring Components of Foods

Bracken Fern

The toxic effects of bracken fern on livestock have been observed for a century or more. Bracken fern is not only toxic, but also carcinogenic when fed to rats and other experimental animals at high levels. Both the toxicity and the carcinogenicity are attributed to the same chemical constituent, ptaquiloside (Fig. 1).

Young bracken fronds in the fiddlehead or crosier stage are used as a salad green in some countries, including Japan. In Japan, bracken fern is boiled or pickled before eating to remove the astringent taste; this reduces but does not eliminate its carcinogenicity. Milk from cattle that were fed bracken fern was found to be carcinogenic to rats. This raises the possibility that there may be a risk associated with the drinking of milk in areas where dried bracken fern is used for bedding in winter or where range-fed cattle may consume bracken fern; this occurs, for example, in Turkey and Bulgaria.

Pyrrolizidine Alkaloids

Pyrrolizidine alkaloids occur in a variety of plants used as food and herbal medicines in many parts of the world, particularly in Africa and Asia. The first natural substances shown to cause liver tumours were pyrrolizidine alkaloids from plants. Among the pyrrolizidine-alkaloid-containing plants used by humans are *Petasites japonicus* Maxim (a kind of coltsfoot), which is used as a food and herbal remedy in Japan, and *Symphytum officinale* L. (comfrey), which is widely used as a medicinal herb, salad ingredient, or a 'tea'. Both of these plants have been shown to be carcinogenic when fed to rats. Senkirkine (Fig. 1), which is found in *P. japonicus* M., induced liver tumours when injected intraperitoneally into male rats, as did symphytine (Fig. 1), extracted from roots of comfrey (*S. officinale*). Both alkaloids can also induce mutations in the bacterium *Salmonella typhimurium*; this is an indication of their ability to react with deoxyribonucleic acid (DNA) and may be relevant to the mechanism of their carcinogenicity. *See* Alkaloids, Toxicology

Mate

Mate (pronounced 'mah-tay') is a beverage which is widely consumed in southern Brazil and Paraguay, Uruguay and northern Argentina. It is made by brewing the toasted, dried and aged leaves of a particular type of tree, *Ilex paraguariensis*, which is indigenous to this area. Several studies have compared mate consumption among patients with cancers of the oesophagus, larynx, oral cavity or pharynx with that of comparable individuals who did not have these cancers. Taken as a whole, these studies indicate that consumption of hot mate is probably carcinogenic to the upper gastrointesti-

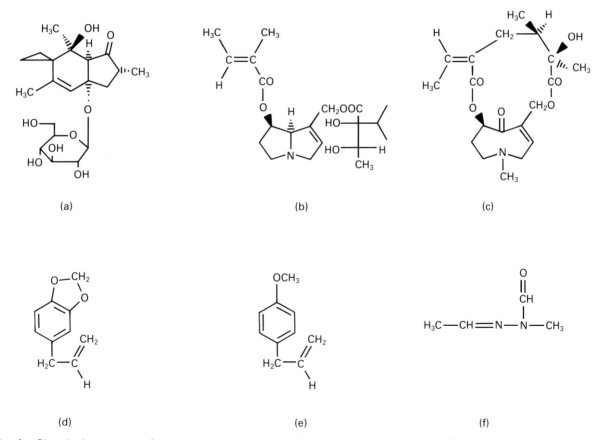

Fig. 1 Chemical structures of some naturally occurring dietary carcinogens: (a) ptaquiloside, the carcinogenic constituent of bracken fern; (b) symphytine and (c) senkirkine, two pyrrolizidine alkaloids; (d) safrole and (e) estragole, two alkenylbenzene carcinogens found in foods; and (f) gyromitrin, a toxic and carcinogenic compound found in the false morel mushroom, *Gyromitra esculanta*.

nal tract. There is currently no way of knowing to what extent the chemicals present in the mate contribute to its apparent carcinogenicity and to what extent the high temperature of the consumed beverage is the problem. Experiments on the carcinogenicity of mate on animals might help to resolve this question, but unfortunately no such experiments have been reported.

Coffee

The many studies on the possible association between coffee consumption and cancer in people have given conflicting results. Overall, the evidence suggests that coffee consumption may increase the risk of bladder cancer in humans, but this conclusion is by no means definitive because of the possible failure to account properly for other factors that can affect cancer rates. Some studies, but not others, have linked high levels of coffee consumption to cancer of the pancreas, but again the positive findings may result from methodological problems. Unfortunately, currently available studies on the carcinogenicity of coffee to experimental animals do little to shed light on the issue owing to the inadequacy of these studies. Caffeine, which is found in tea, cola drinks and cocoa as well as coffee, has not been found to be carcinogenic when tested in animals. *See* Caffeine; Coffee, Physiological Effects

Alkenylbenzenes and Benzene

Several alkenylbenzene compounds have been shown to induce liver tumours in experimental animals. One of these compounds, safrole (Fig. 1), constitutes 80–90% of the volatile oil of sassafras, and is also present at much lower concentrations in certain spices and flavouring ingredients such as sweet basil, cananga oil, nutmeg, pepper, tamarind, and ylang ylang oil. As a result of the carcinogenicity of safrole, the US Food and Drug Administration (FDA) prohibited the use of safrole or sassafras oil in food, which resulted in the cessation of its use as the principal flavouring ingredient in root beer. Furthermore, sassafras extracts or leaves can only be sold in the USA if the safrole has been removed from them.

Another carcinogenic alkenylbenzene related in chemical structure to safrole is estragole (Fig. 1; also called methylchavicol), which is found in tarragon, sweet basil, anise, West Indian bay, fennel, chervil and marjoram. The level of estragole from these sources in a typical diet is very low and the resulting risk is, at most, vanishingly small.

Benzene is a well-established human and animal carcinogen, inducing leukaemia in occupationally exposed workers and several types of cancer in benzene-treated rodents. Traces of benzene have been detected among the volatile components of a variety of foods, including oat groats, processed pork and ham, cooked meats and baked potatoes, and in the aromas of coffee and cocoa.

Mushrooms and Hydrazine Derivatives

Gyromitra esculanta is one of the mushrooms known as false morels. It is harvested and eaten by many people in northern Europe and also in the USA, although it is poisonous, even fatal, unless properly dried and boiled. The principal poisonous ingredient is gyromitrin (Fig. 1), which is carcinogenic to animals and which can give rise to the carcinogen methylhydrazine under acidic conditions, such as exist in the stomach. Both methylhydrazine and another carcinogen, N-methyl-N-formylhydrazine, appear to form during the preparation of false morel for consumption. In fact, cooking must be performed in an open vessel to permit escape of methylhydrazine; otherwise, poisoning can occur.

The widely available edible mushroom cultivated in countries with a temperate climate is *Agaricus bisporus*. The principal hydrazine derivative in *A. bisporus*, agaritine, has not been shown to be carcinogenic, but there are reports of carcinogenicity for some hydrazine derivatives related to compounds that have been identified in this mushroom. When uncooked *A. bisporus* was fed to mice as their only food for three days per week throughout their lifetimes, tumours developed in several organs. No adequate study has yet been performed on the carcinogenicity of cooked mushrooms, and cooking may inactivate carcinogens that may be present. Additional studies are needed to determine the significance of the results with uncooked *A. bisporus* and the hydrazine derivatives.

Carcinogens Produced by the Processing of Food

Alcoholic Beverages

Alcoholic beverages probably constitute the most widely consumed class of substances for which human carcinogenicity is definitively established. The most clearly affected sites are the mouth, pharynx, larynx, oesophagus and liver. Smoking of tobacco and consumption of alcohol, each of which are carcinogenic independently, appear to have a far greater than additive effect in inducing human cancer at these sites, excluding the liver. There are also studies implying that alcoholic beverages increase the risk of breast cancer, but the data in this regard are not nearly as definitive as for the other sites mentioned. *See* Breast Cancer and Diet; Oesophageal Cancer

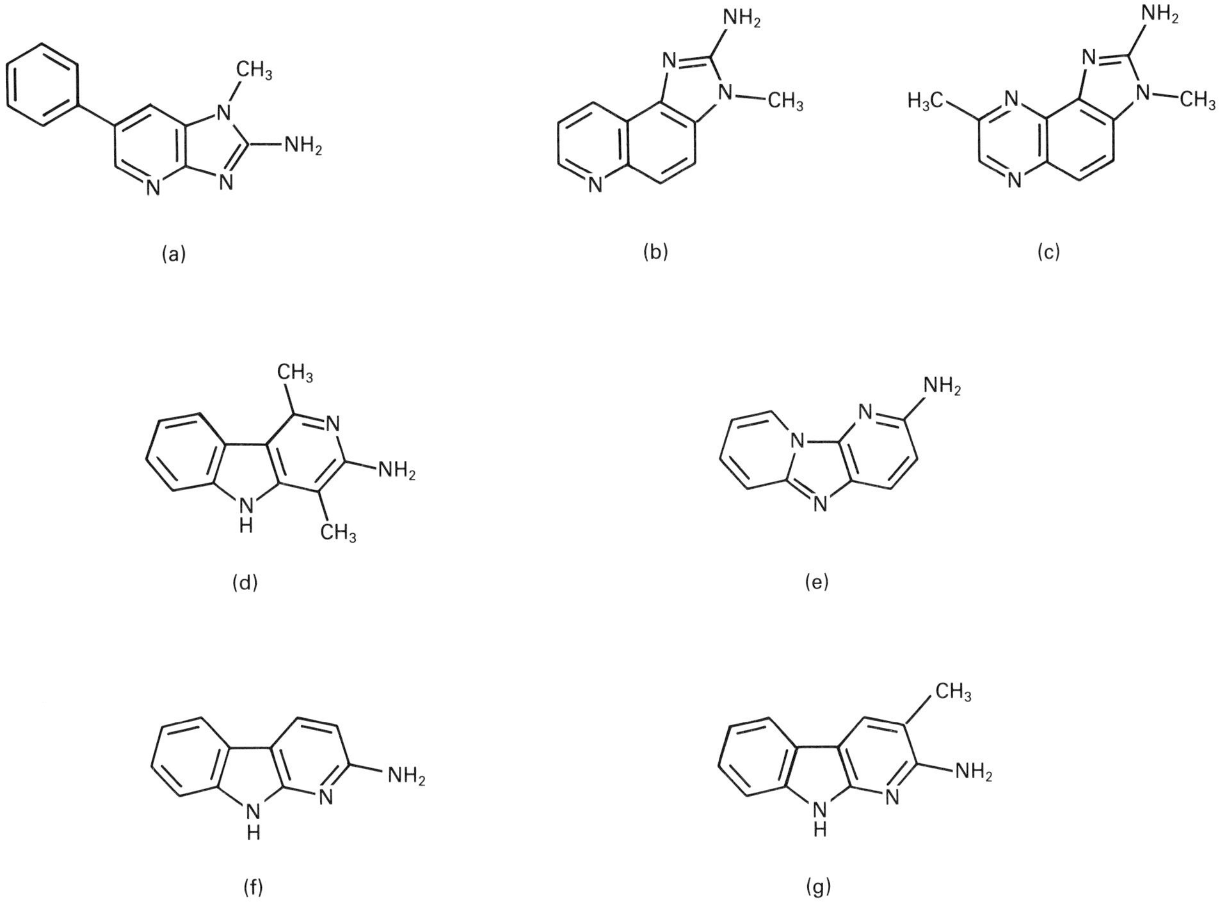

Fig. 2 Chemical structures of some cooking-induced heterocyclic amine carcinogens. Their commonly used short names are (a) PhIP, (b) IQ, (c) 8-MeIQx, (d) Trp-P-1, (e) Glu-P-2, (f) A-α-C, and (g) MeA-α-C.

It is not clear which components of the alcoholic beverages are responsible for the human cancers. Animal experiments have failed to show that ethanol (alcohol) itself is carcinogenic, although the major metabolite of ethanol, i.e. acetaldehyde, induces respiratory tract tumours when inhaled by experimental animals. Alcoholic beverages contain numerous chemicals that may contribute to the carcinogenicity of the beverages, including traces of acetaldehyde, N-nitroso compounds (including N-nitrosodimethylamine), and urethan (ethyl carbamate). Urethan has been found in the highest concentrations in 'stone fruit' (i.e. cherry, plum, apricot, etc.), brandies, sake and rice wine; at lower levels in various other types of distilled spirits and wines; and at even lower levels in beer. Urethan is also found in other fermented food products such as soya sauce, bread, yoghurt and some cheeses. The carcinogenic risks from urethan appear to be extremely low, and are probably negligible, but may be somewhat increased among those who frequently consume alcoholic beverages with the highest levels of this carcinogen. *See* Alcohol, Metabolism, Toxicology and Beneficial Effects; Alcohol, Alcohol Consumption; Smoking, Diet and Health

Carcinogens Produced by Cooking

Under most circumstances, the cooking of meat, fish or eggs results in the formation, at very low concentrations, of a group of heterocyclic amines that are very potent mutagens when tested on bacteria. A few of these mutagens, all of which are carcinogenic when fed to experimental animals, are shown in Fig. 2 with their commonly used abbreviated names.

The formation of mutagenic activity has been observed in beef, pork, ham, bacon, lamb, chicken, fish and eggs after broiling (grilling), frying and barbecuing. Other high-protein foods, such as tofu, beans and cheese, gave little or no mutagenic activity when cooked under similar conditions. Beef extract is also mutagenic. *See* Browning, Nonenzymatic

While the cooking-induced mutagens that have been isolated are extraordinarily potent mutagens when tested on bacteria, these chemicals tend to be only moderately potent as carcinogens. The fact that the mutagens are found in foods in the parts per thousand million range, and the fact that their carcinogenic potency, in animals at least, does not seem to be particularly great, are factors that minimize the anticipated risk from these substances. However, exposure to them occurs each time a person eats cooked meat or fish, and such exposure often occurs at a high frequency over the lifetime of the individual. While it is possible to reduce the level of carcinogenic heterocyclic amines by reducing the temperature or time of cooking, the reduction in carcinogenic risk thus effected must be weighed against the very real possibility of increased risk from bacterial or parasitic infection from undercooked meat or fish. Recent reports concerning the isolation of an anticarcinogen from fried ground beef also imply that caution is necessary before recommending any reduction in the degree of cooking. Microwave cooking without surface browning apparently does not result in the formation of heterocyclic amine mutagens or carcinogens. *See* Mutagens

Another class of chemicals that contains a number of carcinogens, the polynuclear aromatic hydrocarbons, are also introduced into food when meat or fish are grilled, but not when cooking is performed by the lower-temperature processes of frying, roasting or microwave cooking. The pyrolysis of fat dripping onto the heat source appears to be a major source of this class of carcinogens. Benzo[a]pyrene and other polynuclear aromatic hydrocarbon carcinogens appear to be relatively weak carcinogens when administered orally to experimental animals, but much more potent when applied to the skin. Whether this is also true for humans is unknown, and the risks associated with these carcinogens are difficult to evaluate. *See* Polycyclic Aromatic Hydrocarbons

Salting of fish

The salting of fish in southeastern China is carried out for several days using sea salt, followed by drying in direct sunlight. Sometimes the fish is permitted to soften by decomposition. Several studies have found that the consumption of such salted fish contributes to the high incidence of cancer of the nasal passages and pharynx (nasopharyngeal carcinoma) among Chinese people in southeastern China, Hong Kong and Malaysia. Nasopharyngeal carcinoma is rare in most populations, but accounts for about 15% of all cancer deaths among males in Guangdong Province, China. Feeding of salted fish to children and to babies during weaning seems to be a particularly strong risk factor.

The conclusions of these population studies have been confirmed by animal studies in which feeding of Cantonese-style salted fish to rats resulted in the induction of nasopharyngeal carcinomas. *N*-Nitroso compounds formed as a result of the salting process may be responsible for the carcinogenicity of the salted fish. Nitrate, which contaminates the salt used to prepare the fish, can be reduced to nitrite during the processing, and

the nitrite can react with amines in the fish to form *N*-nitroso compounds. Since salted fish consumption appears to account for most of the nasopharyngeal carcinoma cases among Chinese populations, it must be considered to be a very high risk factor when consumed regularly, particularly by children and infants.

Chemicals Added to Foods

Saccharin

Saccharin has been used as a non-nutritive sweetening agent since 1907, and its safety has been a subject of debate by scientists and public health officials from that time. Experiments conducted in the 1970s and 1980s have demonstrated that high levels of sodium saccharin in the diets of rats resulted in the appearance of tumours of the urinary bladder. In spite of this, the controversy concerning the safety of saccharin continues. *See* Saccharin

Studies on human populations have failed to show any association between bladder cancer incidence and the consumption of saccharin or other artificial sweeteners, but such studies have limited ability to detect such associations, even if they exist. The fact that saccharin is generally not mutagenic, or is very marginally mutagenic, in a variety of test systems may imply that saccharin does not interact with DNA and, therefore, that it may not pose a significant carcinogenic risk at the usually consumed human doses, which are far below the doses fed to the rats in the positive carcinogenicity studies. Saccharin continues to be widely used in food products around the world.

Cyclamates

Other widely used non-nutritive sweeteners include sodium cyclamate and calcium cyclamate. In a study performed in the 1970s, rats that were fed high doses of a mixture of sodium cyclamate and saccharin had an increased incidence of bladder tumours. Some additional studies reported that rats receiving sodium cyclamate alone developed bladder tumours, but the results were not statistically significant. Based on these findings, cyclamates were banned in some countries, including the UK and the USA. However, many consider the experimental reports of carcinogenicity to be of questionable value and cyclamates continue to be approved for use in many countries. As mentioned above, there are no data from human populations indicating that consumption of non-nutritive sweeteners are associated with increased cancer risk, although such studies are, by their very nature, insensitive. *See* Cyclamates

Carcinogens in the Diet

Nitrate and Nitrite

Sodium nitrate and sodium nitrite are used as preservative agents in cured meats, such as bacon, sausage and ham, and in some cheeses. While neither salt has been shown to be carcinogenic, there is some concern because nitrite can react with (nitrosate) amines present in food to form *N*-nitroso compounds, many of which are carcinogens; this reaction can occur under the acid conditions in the stomach. Since nitrate can be converted to nitrite either in a food product or in the mouth or gastrointestinal tract, both nitrate and nitrite must be considered together in assessing any possible hazard. *See* Curing; Nitrosamines

There are dietary sources of nitrate and nitrite other than cured meats, including vegetables and some drinking waters. Over the past few decades, the levels of nitrate and nitrite in cured meats have been reduced considerably, and the potential for formation of *N*-nitroso compounds has been further mitigated by the addition to cured meats of antioxidants such as ascorbic acid, which inhibit the nitrosation of amines.

The addition of nitrate and nitrite to food is only one of many sources of *N*-nitroso compounds to which humans are exposed; salt-preserved fish and smoked foods are among the other sources of *N*-nitroso compounds in the human diet. While there are some data indicating that nasopharyngeal, oesophageal and stomach cancer are more common in populations that consume high levels of nitrate or certain types of preserved meat or fish, the specific role of *N*-nitroso compounds or of added nitrate or nitrite in human cancer remains to be clarified. It is possible that the presence of inhibitors of nitrosation in fresh fruits and vegetables is a factor in explaining why consumption of these foods appears to have a protective effect against cancer in human populations. *See* Stomach Cancer

BHA

The antioxidant butylated hydroxyanisole (BHA) has been used since 1947 to prevent rancidity in edible fats and oils and in fat-containing foods. Experiments performed since 1982 have shown that BHA in the diet can cause tumours of the forestomach in rats and hamsters. However, the relevance of this finding has been questioned because humans do not possess a forestomach, nor do their stomachs contain the type of tissue (squamous epithelium) found in the rodent forestomach. Although humans have squamous epithelium at other sites along the digestive tract, no tumours have been noted in such sites in experimental animals. The possibility that BHA may be a carcinogenic hazard at normal human dietary levels, which are much lower than the experimental tumour-inducing levels, has also

been questioned on the grounds that it is not mutagenic in a variety of test systems. Because of the questions that have been raised concerning the relevance of the experimental forestomach tumours induced by BHA to human exposure at low dietary levels, and the effectiveness of BHA as an antioxidant in fatty foods, it continues to be approved for use in many countries around the world. *See* Dietary Fibre, Properties and Sources; Food Additives, Safety

Bibliography

Aeschbacher H-U (ed.) (1991) Potential carcinogens in the diet. *Mutation Research* special issue, vol. 259, nos 3 and 4.

Hayatsu H (ed.) (1991) *Mutagens in Food: Detection and Prevention*. Boca Raton, Florida: CRC Press.

Hirono I (ed.) (1987) *Bioactive Molecules*, vol. 2. *Naturally Occurring Carcinogens of Plant Origin*. Amsterdam: Elsevier Science Publishers BV.

IARC Monographs on the Evaluation of Carcinogenic Risks to Humans: vol. 22, *Some Non-Nutritive Sweetening Agents* (1980); vol. 31, *Some Food Additives, Feed Additives, and Naturally Occurring Substances* (1983); vol. 40, *Some Naturally Occurring and Synthetic Food Components, Furocoumarins, and Ultraviolet Radiation* (1986); vol. 44, *Alcohol Drinking* (1988); vol. 51, *Coffee, Tea, Mate, Methylxanthines, and Methylglyoxal* (1991) Lyon: International Agency for Research on Cancer.

National Research Council (1989) *Diet and Health: Implications for Reducing Chronic Disease Risk*. Washington, DC: National Academy Press.

Pariza MW, Aeschbacher H-U, Felton JS and Sato S (eds) (1990) *Progress in Clinical and Biological Research*, vol. 347. *Mutagens and Carcinogens in the Diet*. New York: Wiley-Liss.

Weisburger EK (1987) Carcinogenic natural products in the environment. In Mehlman M (ed.) *Advances in Modern Environmental Toxicology*, vol. X, pp 243–266.

*Michael J. Prival**
Food and Drug Administration, Washington, DC, USA

Diet in Cancer Prevention

Over the past 20 years evidence has accumulated from human epidemiological studies and experimental studies in animals to suggest that certain components of the diet may have protective effects against some forms of cancer. This article reviews the evidence for antitumorigenic effects of dietary fibre and of the antioxidant nutrients β-carotene and vitamin A. Some discussion of the other antioxidant nutrients, notably vitamins E and C and the trace element selenium, is also included.

---

* This article was written by Michael J. Prival in his private capacity. No official support or endorsement by the FDA is intended or should be inferred.

Mechanisms put forward to explain inhibition of tumorigenesis by these dietary constituents are discussed.

Dietary Inhibitors of Carcinogenesis; Implications for Cancer Prevention

Marked international variations in incidence and mortality rates for different forms of cancer and the change in incidence observed in migrant populations demonstrate the relative importance of environmental and genetic factors in the aetiology of human cancer. Some estimates suggest that 80–90% of human cancers are environmental in origin and that diet may be responsible for at least 35% of the international variation in cancer mortality.

There are a number of ways in which diet may affect cancer incidence and these can be divided into causative and protective factors (Table 1). Natural carcinogens in food and those produced during cooking and storage, have the potential to cause cancer in humans but evidence available at the present time suggests that the elimination of these chemicals from foods would have an insignificant effect on the incidence of cancer. Other dietary manipulations, such as reductions in energy, fat and alcohol in populations with high levels of intake, may be of benefit in preventing some types of cancer, but in practice would be difficult to achieve. Increased consumption of protective agents may be of more practical importance than elimination or reduction of causative agents. Epidemiological cross-cultural studies conducted in the 1970s suggested protective effects of dietary fibre against colon cancer, and of vitamins C and A (or its precursors found in fruit and vegetables), against gastric and lung cancers respectively. Since that time, experimental studies in animals and case-control and cohort studies of human populations have not consistently supported the early evidence for the protective effects of high-fibre diets against colon cancer. However, the case for protective effects of the antioxi-

dant nutrients, including β-carotene and vitamins C and A, has strengthened considerably and there is now a strong basis for the belief that dietary antioxidants may have a role in the prevention of carcinogenesis. Further studies are required before dietary guidelines, based on the potential of these agents to prevent cancer, can be given to the population.

Evidence for a Role of Dietary Fibre

The majority of research studies on dietary fibre and cancer have focused on colon cancer. Rates of colon cancer are extremely high in most Westernized countries, including the USA, UK and Australia, and epidemiological studies suggest that environmental factors, notably diet, are of particular importance in determining incidence of this disease. Correlation studies provide the strongest evidence for protective effects of dietary fibre against development of colon cancer. Some 86% of international, within-country and metabolic correlation studies have shown a lower incidence of colon cancer in populations with high intakes of dietary fibre. The weakness of such studies is that different populations may differ in many factors, including other dietary variables which may be strongly correlated with dietary fibre, and these factors may be responsible for the observed relationship. A majority of case-control studies which have compared fibre intakes of subjects with colon cancer and age-matched control subjects, have shown lower intakes of fibre in cases than in controls. However, in 9 of the 16 studies which showed apparently beneficial effects of high-fibre diets, vegetables were found to be the protective fibre-containing food, so that an ingredient of vegetables other than fibre may be the protective agent. Thus, in correlation and analytical (case-control) epidemiology studies of dietary fibre and colon cancer, the problem of highly correlated dietary variables makes it difficult to state with certainty that the relationships observed are causal

Table 1. Causative and preventative food factors in cancer

Causative factors	Preventative factors
Chemicals	*Antioxidants*
Naturally occurring	Vitamins E, C, A and β-carotene
Heat products	Trace elements Se, Zn, Cu, Mn
Additives	Non-nutrient – e.g. phenols
Contaminants	
Excess nutrients	*Dietary fibre*
Energy	Soluble fibres – e.g. guar, pectin
Fat	Insoluble fibres – e.g. cellulose, wheat bran
Alcohol	

in origin. Randomized, prospective intervention trials of fibre-enriched diets in high-risk populations (individuals with adenomatous polyps), initiated in the 1990s, may help to clarify the role of dietary fibre in reducing risk of colon cancer in human populations. *See* Colon, Cancer of the Colon

Animal feeding studies allow the effects of fibre on the incidence of experimental tumours to be investigated by means of prospective, controlled experiments. They also allow the effects of different types of fibres, soluble and insoluble, to be studied. Most experiments conducted in animals for effects of soluble fibre on tumour incidence do not provide support for protective effects of this type of fibre against tumour development. Soluble fibres such as pectins, guar, agar and carrageenan are ineffective at tumour prevention and at high dose levels can even enhance tumour development. The majority of animal studies designed to investigate effects of insoluble fibres such as cellulose and wheat bran fibre on colon tumour incidence have also largely failed to demonstrate antitumorigenic properties of this type of fibre. Approximately 25% of the studies have shown decreased tumour incidence in animals fed fibre-containing diets, but most have shown no effect and a small number have shown increased tumour incidence with high-fibre diets. Definite conclusions regarding effects of insoluble fibres on colon tumour incidence cannot be drawn from the studies conducted to date owing to the variable experimental conditions which have been used. Further studies are required in which the type of fibre employed, the content and nature of dietary fat and the carcinogen used to initiate tumour development are defined, so that dose–response effects of dietary fibre and tumour incidence can be studied. *See* Dietary Fibre, Fibre and Disease Prevention

Evidence for a Role of Carotenoids and Vitamin A

Prospective and retrospective dietary studies of human populations have consistently shown protective effects of vegetables, fruits and carotenoids against lung cancer. These dietary studies are supported by prospective studies which show low levels of β-carotene in serum or plasma of individuals who subsequently develop lung cancer. The concordance of the dietary and blood data strongly support the view that the protective agent against lung cancer is indeed carotene, but studies carried out to date have not adequately addressed the possibility that other components of fruits and vegetables, such as vitamin C and dietary fibre, may also contribute to this protection. Also not fully addressed is the protective role of dietary carotenoids other than β-carotene, such as lycopene and lutein. Five to ten distinct carotenoids have been identified in human

serum and these may also modulate carcinogenesis. Not all studies have controlled for the effects of smoking; this is an important limitation since smokers appear to have lower intakes of dietary carotenoids and smoking may deplete circulating β-carotene concentrations. *See* Carotenoids, Physiology; Smoking, Diet and Health

Evidence for a protective role for vitamin A against lung cancer is not as strong as that for β-carotene. Strongest evidence for protective actions of vitamin A against lung cancer come from prospective studies which show lower serum retinol levels in lung cancer cases than in controls, but low levels seem to be restricted to individuals diagnosed within a year of blood collection and thus appear to be a consequence, rather than a cause, of cancer. In most Western diets conversion of carotenoids to vitamin A contributes only 25% of dietary vitamin A. Since evidence for anticarcinogenic effects is stronger for carotenoids than for vitamin A it appears that, in lung cancer, the protective effects of carotenoids are independent of their role as a dietary precursor of vitamin A. However, in oral cancers vitamin A seems to be the protective agent since low concentrations of the vitamin are observed in betel nut chewers with precancerous lesions (leucoplakia), and supplements of vitamin A have been shown to be more potent in reversing leucoplakia than supplements of β-carotene. *See* Retinol, Physiology

Evidence for a protective effect of carotene against cancers at sites other than the lung is less convincing because of fewer studies and inconsistency in results. Furthermore, in these studies there is less evidence that carotene is the sole protective agent since low intakes of vitamin C, riboflavin, and vitamin A were all associated with increased risk. *See* Riboflavin, Physiology

Evidence for a Role of other Antioxidant Nutrients

A number of micronutrients participate in the antioxidant defence mechanisms which protect against adverse effects of free radical species generated as a natural consequence of cellular oxidative processes. These include the minerals selenium, copper, zinc and manganese, and vitamins C, E and A and the carotenoids. Inadequacies in this system arising as a result of dietary lack of some of these nutrients, alone or in combination, have been implicated in the causation of certain forms of cancer. Evidence for protective effects of the carotenoids and vitamin A has been presented above, although it is by no means certain that the protective effects described can be solely attributed to the antioxidant properties of these compounds. There is little evidence that dietary lack of the micronutrients manganese, copper or zinc play a part in the aetiology of cancer. However, both animal and human studies suggest that protection against certain types of cancer may be afforded by increased intake of selenium. Cross-cultural and analytical studies of diet, and prospective studies of blood selenium levels have shown higher risk of certain cancers, particularly cancers of the oral cavity, in individuals with low selenium status. Protective effects against cancer, of selenium at high levels of intake, have been observed in many animal studies but the levels required to produce protection are far greater than those needed by glutathione peroxidase, an antioxidant selenoenzyme, so that the relevance of these findings to human cancers is debatable. *See* Selenium, Physiology

Vitamin E functions as an important antioxidant in mammalian cell membranes, protecting membrane phospholipid polyunsaturated fatty acids (PUFAs) against lipoperoxidation. However, evidence for a protective role of this vitamin against cancer is more consistently found in animal studies than in studies of human populations. Experimental animal studies have shown inhibitory effects of vitamin E against oral and skin cancers, with variable findings in the case of mammary and colon cancers. Inconsistent findings have been observed in studies of the relationship between vitamin E status and cancer in human populations, which may in part be due to inadequacies in the collection and analysis of blood samples. As in the case of vitamin A, one prospective study demonstrated low levels of vitamin E only in cases diagnosed within one year of blood collection, suggesting that low status was a consequence rather than a cause of the disease. In a more recent study subjects with low levels of vitamin E had a 1·5-fold risk of cancer compared with those with a higher level. Furthermore, in women, a stronger association was seen in those individuals who also had low levels of selenium, a finding which is consistent with observations made in experimental tumour studies in animals. *See* Tocopherols, Physiology

In view of the important role of vitamin C in free-radical scavenging and in protection against lipid peroxidation, it is not surprising that many epidemiological studies have concerned themselves with the potential protective effects, against cancer, of this vitamin. Of 75 case-control and prospective studies of vitamin C or fruit consumption and cancer, 72% have demonstrated significant protection by high levels of intake or high blood concentrations of this vitamin. The evidence is particularly strong for cancers of the oral cavity, oesophagus, stomach, pancreas and rectum. Other than the gastrointestinal tract there is also evidence for protective effects of vitamin C against cervical, breast and lung cancers. As with other nutrients these studies do not allow definite conclusions to be drawn regarding the specific antitumorigenic role of this nutrient alone since the intake of vitamin C is highly correlated with other nutrients, including dietary fibre, vitamin A and carotenoids. Studies of blood

vitamin C levels in relation to cancer risk are lacking, largely because of the instability of this vitamin in stored blood samples. *See* Breast Cancer and Diet; Ascorbic Acid, Physiology

Dietary Recommendations

Since the early 1980s a number of national reports on diet and health have included the recommendation that for optimal health, including prevention of cancer, intake of fruits, vegetables and cereal products should be increased. More recent reports have concentrated on the specific health benefits of β-carotene and other antioxidant nutrients. In 1989 the US National Academy of Sciences stated explicitly 'every day eat five or more servings of a combination of vegetables and fruits, especially green and yellow vegetables and citrus fruits'. However, reports on recommended intakes of individual nutrients have generally been unable to advise increased intake of specific nutrients on the basis of their protective effects against cancer. In the recent report on recommended intakes of various nutrients for the UK population (*Dietary Reference Values for Food Energy and Nutrients for the United Kingdom*, 1991), evidence for protective effects, against some cancers, of the antioxidant nutrients vitamin E and β-carotene were considered to be strong but insufficient to allow recommendations for increased intake of these nutrients at the present time. Recommendation for increased intake of dietary fibre was made on the basis of likely benefit from increases in average stool weight. Evidence for protective effects of dietary fibre against colon cancer were thought to be confounded by other dietary variables and no recommendations were made for increased intake of this dietary constituent alone as a means of protection against this type of cancer.

Protective Mechanisms in the Body against Carcinogens and Tumour Formation

Dietary Fibre

A number of mechanisms have been put forward to explain the proposed protective effects of dietary fibre against colorectal cancer; these are summarized in Table 2. There is good evidence that insoluble fibres, including cellulose and wheat bran, cause stool bulking with dilution of colonic contents and increased transit time. These effects may be beneficial by reducing the concentration of potentially harmful substrates such as steroids and bile acids. However, evidence that high-fibre diets produce changes in bacterial metabolism, or in the physicochemical conditions in the colon, that could reduce the carcinogenic potency of these substrates is

Table 2. Proposed mechanisms by which dietary fibre may prevent colorectal carcinogenesis

Proposed mechanism	Evidence in humans
Increased stool bulking causes dilution of faecal contents	Yes
Increased transit time reduces time of contact with colonic contents	Yes
Change in type of bacterial flora reduces metabolism of potential carcinogens	No
Change in physicochemical conditions (reduced pH) reduces harmful substrates	No

not provided by studies carried out to date. Some studies suggest that the increase in bacterial metabolism brought about by the consumption of soluble fibres may have harmful effects, and further studies are required to distinguish the effects on colonic metabolism of soluble and insoluble dietary fibres.

Antioxidants

Excessive production of free-radical species, including the superoxide anion and the hydroxyl radical, have been implicated in the aetiology of cancer. Singlet oxygen which is not a free radical, but another highly reactive oxygen species, may also be important. The antioxidant nutrients are thought to protect against cancer by preventing excess generation of, and damage by, free radicals and singlet oxygen. These reactive species can attack organic macromolecules, including enzymes and membrane phospholipid PUFAs. The latter can result in the generation of peroxyl radicals and lipid hydroperoxides, setting up a chain reaction which, if unchecked, will lead to membrane damage and loss of membrane integrity (Fig. 1). Membrane damage may make the cell more susceptible to toxic and carcinogenic agents and free radicals may also cause activation of potentially carcinogenic compounds. Direct damage to DNA caused by superoxide anions and hydroxyl radicals produced within the nucleus may also occur, although the evidence for this is sparse. Antioxidant nutrients protect the cell against free-radical-induced damage by their participation in a complex network of enzymatic and nonenzymatic reactions. The enzyme system includes the mitochondrial and cytoplasmic superoxide dismutase enzymes which contain manganese (mitochondria) and copper (cytoplasm), also catalase, and the selenium-containing enzyme glutathione peroxidase. Vitamin E protects membrane phospholipid PUFAs by donating the hydrogen atom necessary to quench lipid peroxyl radicals generated as a consequence of hydroxyl radical attack on the unsaturated carbon chain of PUFAs. Vitamin C regenerates vitamin E from vitamin E radicals formed by the above reaction and thereby acts as a buffer against depletion of the

primary defence mechanism. Vitamin A and β-carotene also have radical-quenching properties but the potent quenching properties of β-carotene against singlet oxygen may be a more important determinant of its protective actions against lung cancer. Because of the multilevel nature of this defence system it is unlikely that inadequacies will arise as a result of deficiency of a single

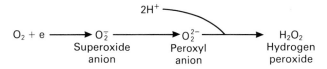

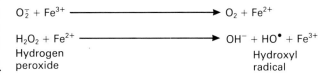

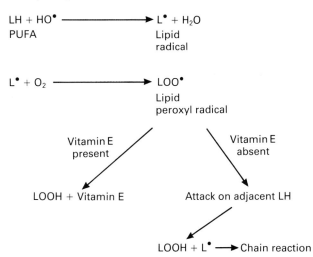

Fig. 1 Formation of superoxide anion, hydroxyl radicals, and lipid peroxyl radicals.

nutrient. This possibility is supported by evidence from both animal and epidemiological studies which show highest tumour rates and increased cancer incidence when two or more dietary antioxidants are lacking. Interaction between micronutrient antioxidants in protection against cancer is likely to provide an active area of research in future years. *See* Antioxidants, Role of Antioxidant Nutrients in Defence Systems

Bibliography

Department of Health (1991) *Dietary Reference Values for Food Energy and Nutrients for the United Kingdom.* Report on Health and Social Subjects 41. London: Her Majesty's Stationery Office.

Ito N and Hirose M (1987) The role of antioxidants in chemical carcinogenesis. *Gann* 78: 1011–1026.

Kritchevsky D, Bonfield C and Anderson JW (eds) (1990) *Dietary Fibre. Chemistry, Physiology and Health Effects.* New York: Plenum Press.

Slater TS and Block G (eds) (1990) Antioxidant vitamins and β-carotene in disease prevention. Proceedings of a conference held in London 2–4 October 1989. *American Journal of Clinical Nutrition* 53: 189S–396S.

Williams CM and Dickerson JWT (1990) Nutrition and cancer – some biochemical mechanisms. *Nutrition Research Reviews* 3: 75–100.

Williams DE, Dashwood RM, Hendricks JD and Bailey GS (1989) Anticarcinogen and tumour promoters in foods In: Taylor SL and Scanlan RA (eds) *Food Toxicology*, pp 101–150. New York: Marcel Dekker.

Christine M. Williams
University of Surrey, Guildford, UK

Diet in Cancer Treatment

It is possible that 40% of patients hospitalized for the treatment of cancer are malnourished. In some patients, weight loss maybe the first indication of the presence of a tumour. This is particularly true in persons with gastrointestinal cancer in whom protein–energy malnutrition (PEM) may develop somewhat insidiously owing to a decrease in food intake which may be denied by the patient. Protein–energy malnutrition is associated with a poor prognosis, reduced response to antineoplastic treatment, prolonged or enhanced morbidity of therapeutic side-effects, and a reduced quality of life. The nutritional problems of cancer patients may be complex in their aetiology, resulting in part from the effects of the disease and exacerbated by the effects of treatment. Nutritional management of these problems requires an understanding of their aetiology, and the application of knowledge, skill and psychological understanding.

Physiological Effects of Malignancy

The PEM of the cancer patient may develop into the syndrome known as 'cancer cachexia', which is characterized clinically by emaciation, debilitation and inanition associated with anorexia, early satiety, anaemia and muscle weakness. These changes result from profound alterations in host metabolism.

Anorexia

The factors responsible for anorexia in the cancer patient may be psychological, physical and metabolic. Moreover, the anorexia may be one of three types:

1.   *Transient* anorexia is caused by emotional distress such as during a diagnostic work-up, or when recurrence or metastases are diagnosed or when pain or discouragement are experienced.
2.   *Iatrogenic* anorexia is related to treatment by surgery, the result of radiation sickness, or a side-effect of chemotherapy.
3.   *Pathological* anorexia is related to the disease, particularly gastrointestinal or bronchial cancers, or part of the anorexia–cachexia syndrome of advanced disease.

The importance of psychological factors may decrease with the progress of the disease as physical factors become more prominent; nonetheless, they may make a substantial contribution to appetite failure. Feelings of worthlessness, loss of self-esteem, pessimism, guilt and suicidal ideas may be experienced. Anorexia and cachexia may be the physical result of the patients' own beliefs and attitudes towards their disease and its treatment. Patients may become quite unable to overcome a sense of fear and hopelessness leading to withdrawal.

Disturbances in the sense of taste often accompany cancer. The incidence of such abnormalities is directly proportional to the tumour burden, being most common in those whose tumours are most extensive. There is some evidence that taste changes are inversely proportional to energy intake, and that they become less obvious when the energy intake is raised. Taste changes can have important consequences for the feeding of cancer patients. Reduced threshold for bitter taste (as determined with urea) results in beef and pork becoming less acceptable, poultry and fish rather intermediate, and cheese and eggs pleasurable. Taste abnormalities vary between patients and this is one aspect of the condition which needs to be individually assessed.

Taste changes may result in food aversions, but aversions may also develop in patients who do not have disturbances in taste. There is some evidence that food aversions may be associated, or learned, by the association of certain foods with side-effects of drug treatment. Whatever the mechanisms by which they develop, aversions to foods may be persistent, lasting for several months, and ignoring them will have a definite effect on food intake.

Cachexia

The cause of cancer cachexia is at present unknown. It seems doubtful that it is simply an extreme form of malnutrition. Not all forms of cancer result in the development of the syndrome. Whilst it possesses some features which are similar to those of starvation, there are some important differences. Thus, after a period of starvation, the appetite of a healthy individual remains good, whereas that of the cancer patient is generally poor. Metabolically, the cachectic patient is unable to adapt to a reduced food intake. It is possible that some tumours produce 'toxic' substances, so-called 'toxohormones', which are able to change cellular enzyme systems. Such changes may be the first phase which is followed by secondary effects such as lesions in the mouth or intestinal obstruction. The effects of radiation or chemotherapy on gastrointestinal functions combine with the direct effect of the tumour to produce a state of malnutrition which includes deficiencies of energy and protein, vitamins and minerals. At this stage the condition is reversible if the patient is given appropriate nutritional support. The third phase is characterized by marked negative energy and protein balance with low serum albumin, weight loss and a reduced white cell count, and is more difficult to manage.

Attention has recently focused on a substance called 'cachectin' or 'tumour necrosis factor', produced by macrophages as a mediator or cause of the enzyme changes which occur in the development of cancer cachexia. It seems that cachectin may therefore be involved in the wasting that occurs in chronic invasive states. From a practical standpoint it would seem more profitable to try to prevent malnutrition and cachexia than to rehabilitate a severely malnourished patient. The key to this prevention may lie in the further understanding of the complex metabolic changes that characterize the cancer patient, and particularly those in carbohydrate, protein and fat metabolism.

Energy Expenditure and Glucose Metabolism

In some cancer patients the resting metabolic energy expenditure (RMEE) is raised. Since this rise is unlikely to be accompanied by a corresponding rise in energy intake, it will contribute to the patients' weight loss. Two hypotheses have been put forward to account for the rise in RMEE. First, the metabolic activity of malignant tissue is continuous, in contrast to the diurnal periodicity of normal tissues, thus increasing energy expenditure. Second, alterations in pathways of intermediary metabolism could result in selective removal of nutrients by the tumour, thus forcing other tissues in the host to use more energy-expensive pathways.

Altered glucose metabolism in the patient who is losing weight is the result of glucose intolerance, changed β-cell function and decreased sensitivity and responsiveness to insulin. The causes of these changes are not clear but it seems likely that decreased food intake, protein loss and hormone changes contribute, as do specific characteristics of the tumour. Increased glucose turnover is a composite of increased Cori cycle activity (80%), glucose oxidation (15%) and lipid synthesis, ketone formation, etc. (5%). *See* Glucose, Function and Metabolism

Protein Metabolism

Muscle wasting is clear evidence of altered protein metabolism. Most studies on this subject have been performed using experimental animals but insofar as similar studies have been carried out in patients, they have confirmed those in animals. Cancer increases whole-body protein turnover, with an increased rate of protein synthesis in the liver, but a decreased rate of synthesis in skeletal muscle with a simultaneous increase in skeletal muscle protein degradation. It is likely that a number of factors affect protein metabolism in the cancer patient, e.g. tumour specificity, the staging of the tumour, age, sex and previous nutritional condition of the patient. *See* Protein, Synthesis and Turnover; Protein, Digestion and Absorption of Protein and Nitrogen Balance

The biggest challenge in the nutritional management of a patient with cancer is to reverse the changes in protein metabolism which result in the severe muscle wasting so characteristic of cachexia.

Hypoalbuminaemia is common in cancer patients and is often interpreted as evidence of malnutrition. However, this is only so if the other causes have been eliminated. These other causes are decreased synthesis, increased plasma volume and passage of protein-rich fluid into the gut, i.e. protein-losing enteropathy.

Fat Metabolism

Loss of subcutaneous fat is an obvious feature of cancer cachexia. Patients with progressive disease metabolize more fat than those with non-progressive disease. If a rise in plasma-free fatty acids (FFA) can be taken as an index of the mobilization of fat stores, then a significant increase has been found to correlate with the clinical activity of a tumour. However, these findings have not

Table 1. Vitamin abnormalities in the cancer patient

Abnormality	Percentage affected
Abnormal leucocyte ascorbic acid	71
Anaemia	49
Thiamin (vitamin B_1)	37
Abnormal folic acid	23
Vitamin A	15
Carotene	15

From Holmes S and Dickerson JWT (1987).

been confirmed. There does seem to be a failure of normal homeostatic mechanisms, possibly owing to insulin resistance, because glucose does not depress FFA oxidation to the same degree in cancer patients as it does in control subjects.

Whatever their cause, loss of body fat, inappropriate energy consumption, and loss of lean body mass can only contribute to a negative energy balance and continuing weight loss. *See* Fats, Digestion, Absorption and Transport; Fatty Acids, Metabolism

Vitamins

Patients with malignant disease are likely to suffer some degree of vitamin deficiency (Table 1) which may affect their continuing resistance to the disease and determine their response to treatment. Poor food intake and abnormal losses through the alimentary and renal tracts, possibly coupled with increased requirements which may be drug-induced, contribute to vitamin deficiencies. In the case of vitamin A, low plasma retinol values may be a consequence of the effect of PEM on the synthesis of the carrier protein, retinol-binding protein (RBP). *See* Retinol, Physiology

Effects of Antineoplastic Treatment on Nutritional Status

Surgery

The neuroendocrine response to surgery, consequent upon the production of cytokines by macrophages, results in a sequence of metabolic changes, particularly in energy, protein, water and electrolyte metabolism (see *Bibliography* for specific references). The extent of these changes, their duration, and the period of convalescence are directly proportional to the severity of the surgery. This is important for the patient with cancer in whom surgery may need to be extensive in order to remove all

cancerous tissue. Moreover, surgery is the treatment of choice for cancers of the alimentary tract and may have direct nutritional consequences (Table 2) which will be superimposed on the general 'metabolic response to injury' experienced by all surgical patients. Nutritional management of these patients requires careful attention to specific problems, possibly over an extended period of time. *See* Surgery, Nutrition in Elective and Emergency Surgery

Radiation Therapy

The purpose of radiation therapy is to kill cells and the effects may be dramatic. As the cells are destroyed toxic waste products are liberated, causing an inflammatory response with consequent oedema. Cells may be lost from tissue surfaces which then become ulcerated and clinically the patient shows symptoms such as mucositis and stomatitis, nausea, vomiting, cystitis or diarrhoea. Irradiation may have both immediate and late effects on tissues and hence on nutritional status. Normal and tumour cells are affected in similar ways and cell death may be immediate, delayed or 'natural':

1. *Immediate* cell death is the result of irreversible damage to DNA; this mechanism is responsible for the immediate side-effects.
2. *Delayed* cell death occurs after mutation of DNA; limited functions usually continue until the M phase in the multiplication process, when the cells are unable to divide; this mechanism is responsible for late effects.
3. '*Natural*' cell death involves the formation of giant (sterile) cells which function but cannot divide.

Nutritional consequences of radiation therapy in different regions of the body are shown in Table 3. Some of these symptoms may be severely disabling, even life-threatening, and occur in patients whose nutritional status is already compromised. Food intake is substantially reduced and malabsorption resulting from treatment of tumours in or near the gastrointestinal tract may be very difficult to control. The severity of these problems means that aggressive nutritional support is an essential adjunct to radiation therapy in order to prevent deterioration of nutritional status and to allow compensatory hyperplasia of undamaged bowel.

Chemotherapy

Anticancer drugs have profound cytotoxic effects and since they cannot discriminate between 'normal' and 'cancer' cells they may seriously affect 'normal' tissues. Contributions to host malnutrition may be by both direct and indirect mechanisms that cause many symptoms (Holmes S, 1990):

- Nausea and vomiting
- Anorexia
- Taste changes
- Changes in the sense of smell
- Xerostomia
- Mucositis and stomatitis
- Dental problems
- Oesophagitis, pharyngitis, dysphagia
- Oesophageal stricture, fistulae obstruction
- Diarrhoea
- Malabsorption
- Dyspnoea
- Fatigue, malaise, lethargy, depression
- Weight loss

Current medical practice is to administer drugs cyclically in multiple combinations, sometimes called 'cocktails'. This increases the possibility of 'killing' cancer cells at different stages of cell multiplication, but it can increase both the range and severity of side-effects. Different anticancer drugs cause a slightly different pattern of side-effects, but the general effect is to reduce food intake and since this may occur over prolonged periods it will lead to weight loss and debility.

Indirect effects of chemotherapy that may contribute to a reduced food intake include moniliasis or candidiasis. These are particularly common in patients with leukaemia and lymphoma and affect the oral cavity, pharynx or oesophagus, causing a sore, painful mouth, odynophagia and dysphagia.

Nutritional Management of Cancer Patients

The feeding of cancer patients should be seen as part of their total care. Provision of food for these patients requires the following:

1. *Understanding*. Carers and providers should appreciate the clinical problems and difficulties experienced by individual patients so that the 'diet', whether oral, enteral or parenteral, is suited to the patients' needs including the effects of the anticancer treatment.
2. *Flexibility*. Dietary provision must be flexible, with menus to cater for a wide range of needs with respect both to the nature of the food and the timing of its availability.
3. *Psychological importance*. The provider should be sensitive to the psychological condition of patients and the importance of food to them. This involves the way in which food is provided, as well as its nature. Food can be a 'messenger' between the carer and the patient.

Oral food is always the first choice and considerable skill may be needed to obtain an appropriate intake. Detailed suggestions for dealing with specific problems are given in some of the works quoted in the *Bibliogra-*

Table 2. Possible nutritional effects of gastrointestinal surgery

Surgical procedure	Possible effects
Resection of the oropharyngeal region	Chewing or swallowing difficulties
	Prolonged dependence on tube feeding
Oesophagectomy	Gastric stasis ⎫
Oesophageal reconstruction	Reduced acid secretion ⎬ Secondary to cutting the vagus nerve
	Fat malabsorption
	Diarrhoea
Gastric resection (partial or total)	'Dumping syndrome'
	Malabsorption
	Reduced acid secretion
	Reduced absorption of vitamin B_{12}
	Low blood glucose level
Small intestine	
Duodenum	Reduced secretion of pancreatic juice and bile
Jejunum	Reduced efficiency of absorption
Ileum	Reduced absorption of bile salts
	Reduced absorption of vitamin B_{12}
	Increased urinary excretion of oxalate
Massive resection	Severe malabsorption
	Malnutrition
	Metabolic acidosis
Colon	Fluid and electrolyte imbalance
Removal of pancreas	Reduced secretion of pancreatic enzymes
	Reduced secretion of insulin – diabetes mellitus

From Holmes S and Dickerson JWT (1987).

Diet in Cancer Treatment

Table 3. Effects of radiation therapy with nutritional implications

	Immediate effects	Late effects
Oropharyngeal region	Loss of taste	Altered taste
	Decreased saliva	Decreased saliva
	Odynophagia	
	Damage to teeth	Poor dentition
	Stomatitis or mucositis	Mandibular necrosis
Lower neck or mediastinum	Oesophagitis	Ulceration
	Dysphagia	
	Fibrosis	Stenosis or stricture
	Oesophageal stricture	
Abdomen or pelvis	Acute bowel damage (enteritis)	Chronic bowel damage
	Diarrhoea	Diarrhoea
	Malabsorption	Malabsorption
	Obstruction	Fistulae formation

From Holmes S and Dickerson JWT (1987).

phy. Practical suggestions for increasing energy and protein intakes (from Dickerson JWT and Williams CW, 1988) are as follows:

1. Plan a definite eating schedule and then adhere to it. Do not omit meals or between-meals snacks.
2. Add cereal with banana or other fruit, sugar, and cream to the breakfast menu.
3. Butter toast or bread when it is hot because more butter can be used.
4. Use jam, marmalade or cheese with toast or bread.
5. Add cream to milk beverages.
6. Add skim milk powder to milk, soups, pudding, mashed potatoes, etc.
7. Add ice cream or whipped cream to desserts (cake and ice cream, apple pie with whipped cream, etc.)
8. Use mayonnaise, salad dressing, butter or margarine with sandwiches, salads and vegetables.
9. Serve thickened gravy with meat and potatoes.
10. Have bacon, ham or sausages with eggs at breakfast.
11. Add eggs to beverages or recipes to increase the protein.
12. Use milk instead of water to prepared canned condensed cream soups.

Oral food can be supplemented with 'sip' feeds. These may be home-made, milk- and egg-based, or commercially available complete feeds such as Ensure, Clinifeed or Fortisip. If elemental feeds such as Flexical or Vivonex are needed due to malabsorption, they should never be given orally because of their taste.

Patients with inadequate oral intake should be fed through a fine-bore tube (1–2 mm diameter) inserted nasogastrically, or directly into the stomach or intestine. Feeds used as sip feeds should be introduced from a reservoir either by gravity or with a pump.

If the gastrointestinal tract cannot be used, or if the patient cannot tolerate a tube, complete nutrition can be given parenterally through a central vein. Parenteral feeds contain energy (usually fat and glucose), amino acids, vitamins and minerals. Parenteral feeding can be dangerous, is very expensive, and requires expert supervision.

Therapeutic Role of Vitamins

Cancer patients are at risk of vitamin deficiencies. If present they should be countered with supplements. It has been claimed that vitamin C in doses of up to 10 g (or more) daily can have an anticancer effect. There is no evidence from properly conducted trials to support such claims. Drug cocktails containing 5-fluorouracil increase the requirement for vitamin B_1. There is currently interest in the possibility that antioxidant vitamins, particularly vitamin E and β-carotene may prevent cancer. Synthetic retinoids (compounds with vitamin-A-like action) are currently being tested for direct antitumour action against specific tumours. *See* Antioxidants, Role of Antioxidant Nutrients in Defence Systems; Ascorbic Acid, Physiology; Nutritional Status, Importance of Measuring Nutritional Status; Nutritional Status, Anthropometry and Clinical Examination; Nutritional Status, Biochemical Tests for Vitamins and Minerals; Nutritional Status, Functional Tests; Thiamin, Physiology

Bibliography

Dickerson JWT and Williams CW (1988) Nutrition and cancer. In: Dickerson JWT and Lee HA (eds) *Nutrition in* the Clinical Management of Disease 2nd edn, pp 350–373. London: Edward Arnold.

Holmes S (1988) Radiotherapy. London: Austin Cornish Publishers.

Holmes S (1990) Cancer Chemotherapy. London: Austin Cornish Publishers.

Holmes S and Dickerson JWT (1987) Malignant disease: nutritional implications of disease and treatment. Cancer and Metastasis Reviews 6: 357–381.

J. W. T. Dickerson
University of Surrey, Guildford, UK

CANDIES

See Sweets and Candies

CANNING

Contents

Principles

Canning is the general term applied to the process of packaging a food in a container and subjecting it to a thermal process for the purpose of extending its useful life. An optimal thermal process will destroy pathogenic (disease-causing) bacteria, kill or control spoilage organisms present and have minimal impact on the nutritional and physical qualities of the food. Although we think of canning in terms of steel or possibly aluminium cans, the principles apply equally well to a variety of food containers, such as glass jars, plastic and foil-laminated pouches, semirigid plastic trays or bowls, as well as metal cans of any one of several shapes including cylindrical, oval, oblong or rectangular. The concept of aseptic packaging (sterilizing the food and the container prior to filling and sealing) also follows the same principles. *See* Spoilage, Bacterial Spoilage

Basic Concepts

In 1810, Nicolas Appert presented the first methods on the thermal treatment of food. His method of preserva-tion was primarily aimed at the elimination of the use of large quantities of sugar, salt and vinegar as preserving agents because they distracted from the natural flavour and quality of the food. His methods developed over the years into procedures that not only prevented the large economic loss associated with microbial spoilage, but also destroyed the microorganisms that are capable of causing illness, or even death, in humans.

The extent of the thermal process ranges from a pasteurization process, designed to kill pathogenic microorganisms and extend product life under refrigerated storage, to sterilization for indefinite product life at ambient temperatures. Thermal processing temperatures range from below 100°C to as high as 150°C. Whereas the principles of thermal process design are the same for these extremes, the concepts for process establishment that will follow are those for the sterilization of foods known as low-acid canned foods (LACFs), packaged in hermetically sealed containers. Low-acid foods have a pH greater than 4·6 and a water activity greater than 0·85; this combination is capable of supporting the growth of *Clostridium botulinum*, a bacterium that produces an exotoxin which is one of the most deadly neuroparalytic toxins known. *C. botulinum*

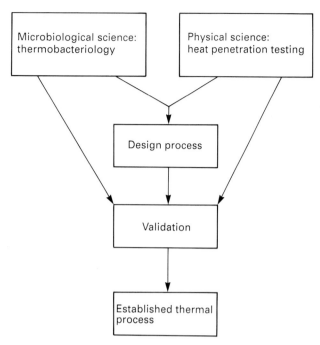

Fig. 1 Establishment of the thermal process.

is ubiquitous; it occurs in both cultivated and forest soils, in sediments of streams, lakes and coastal waters, in the intestinal tracts of fish and mammals, in the gills and viscera of crabs and other shellfish. For many years, canning industry laboratories have devoted much attention to *C. botulinum* and have found that at a pH of less than 4·6 it will not grow and produce toxin. At a pH above 4·6 *C. botulinum* will multiply and produce toxin in a favourable medium. Examples of foods with a pH greater than 4·6 are vegetables, fresh meats and seafood. Tomatoes normally have a pH that is less than 4·6 and require a less severe heat treatment (pasteurization) to achieve preservation. *See Clostridium*, Occurrence of *Clostridium Botulinum*; Heat Treatment, Chemical and Microbiological Changes; Metals Used in the Food Industry; Sterilization of Foods

Water activity (a_w) is a measure of the amount of available water in the food. The a_w of fresh fruits, vegetables and meats is normally greater than 0·85. Dried fruits, honey and salami have insufficient water content to support the growth of most hazardous microorganisms and thus do not require a sterilization process to produce a shelf-stable product. *See* Water Activity, Principles and Measurement

Establishment of the Thermal Process

The establishment of the thermal process for sterilization of canned food results from a successful marriage of microbiological science and physical science, specifically thermobacteriology and heat penetration testing, their validation and iteration, as shown diagrammatically in Fig. 1.

Thermobacteriology

Thermobacteriology is the science which studies the potential microbiological contaminants in foods, the relationship between temperature and time levels required to destroy them, and the influence of the food itself on the destruction rates.

There are three microbiological parameters which are involved in all process establishment work, namely D_T, z, and F. These variables define the thermal resistance of bacteria and indicate how much of an effect a particular thermal process is likely to have. The D_T value, which is defined graphically in Fig. 2a, is the time in minutes at constant temperature (T) to inactivate 90% (one log reduction) of the target organisms present in a food. The D_T value is also known as the 'death rate constant' or 'decimal reduction time'.

Thermal resistance or thermal destruction tests (TDTs) that measure D_T are conducted using small food samples inoculated with known levels of microorganisms. The samples, contained in specially designed, low-profile TDT cans or glass tubes, are heated in chambers capable of rapidly heating the sample to a precise temperature, holding for a precise time period, and rapidly cooling to sublethal temperatures. Common heating devices are the TDT retort and the thermoresistometer.

A plot of the thermal resistance (or survival) data must approximate a straight line on semilogarithmic graph paper (as in Fig. 2a) for the D_T value to be meaningful. Each TDT curve is unique for the microbial spore crop, food medium and exposure temperature. The D_T value describes the effect on the population of organisms of exposure at a constant temperature for a precise time period, without influence of a heating (come-up) or cooling period effect.

The $D_{121·1}$ value for *C. botulinum* is normally taken as 0·2 min. This is based on thermal resistance studies conducted in the early 1920s on spores harvested from the most heat-resistant strains known. These studies demonstrated that, by extrapolation from the semilogarithmic survival curve, it was necessary to heat a spore suspension in phosphate buffer for 2·78 min at 121·1°C to reduce the survival population from about 10^{11} spores per unit to less than one spore per unit (12-log reduction). Later, a correction in the come-up time resulted in a reduction of the heating time to 2·45 min to achieve the same lethal effect; hence the $D_{121·1}$ value of 0·2 min.

The time–temperature data in Fig. 3 (see *Thermal Process Calculations*, below) are typical of the way in which cans of food heat, and illustrate that food in containers does not heat (or cool) instantly. To be efficient in the thermal process design, we must take advantage of the microbial kill at each step along the thermal process path. The thermal resistance curve, Fig. 2b, is the vehicle that makes this possible. A series of

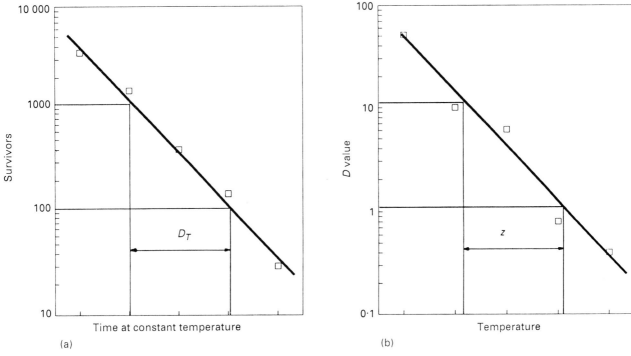

Fig. 2 Graphical representations of D_T and z values. (*a*) D value: time required at temperature to reduce survivors by 90%. (*b*) z value: temperature change which influences destruction by a factor of 10.

TDT tests are conducted to determine the effect of different temperatures (D_T values) on the thermal resistance of an organism. By plotting the measured D_T values on a logarithmic scale against temperature on a linear scale (Fig. 2b), a thermal resistance curve is constructed. The thermal resistance curve relates time for a one-log kill with the kill temperature. From this plot, the z value can be obtained; it is the inverse slope of the curve and represents the number of degrees of temperature required for the curve to traverse one log cycle. In other words, the z value denotes the number of degrees of temperature required to effect a 10-fold change in time to achieve the same lethal effect. A higher z value means that a greater change in process temperature is required for the same change in the destruction rate of an organism. The z value is a means to quantify the death rate of a microorganism with respect to the effect of changes in temperature during a thermal process.

A range of z values from 7°C to 12°C have been measured over the years for *C. botulinum*. These differences are attributed to the spore type (strain), heating system, test substrate and method of calculation. Much effort has been expended on determining the appropriate z value for LACF process establishment. Consensus would lead to the singular conclusion that use of a single z value of 10°C – which has been in general use for 30–50 years – is still the best recommendation for calculating LACF sterilization processes that are to be safe from a public health standpoint. It is possible that

this choice was fortuitous; on the other hand, it may have been the purposeful result of research by the canning industry pioneers of the 1920s and 1930s. *See* Consumer Protection Legislation

Lethality

Containers of food do not heat instantaneously, and since all temperatures (above a minimum value) have a lethal effect and contribute to the destruction of microorganisms, a mechanism to determine the relative effect of a changing temperature while the food is heated and cooled during thermal processing is necessary. The z value is the parameter that allows us to calculate the lethal effect of various temperatures on the destruction of microorganisms. The lethal rate (L) describes, through use of the z value, the relative effect of temperature on microbial destruction with respect to the effect of a certain reference temperature (T_{REF}). In descriptive terms, L is the equivalent time in minutes at the reference temperature per minute at temperature T:

$$L = 10^{(T - T_{\text{REF}})/z} \qquad (1)$$

Table 1 shows lethal rates at five temperatures for *C. botulinum* assuming a reference temperature of 121·1°C and a z value of 10°C, and times required at each temperature for a 12-log spore reduction. If the initial *C. botulinum* population per container (N_0) is 10^3 and we desire a final probability (N_F) of 10^{-9}, then a 12-log

Table 1. Lethal rates and times required at selected temperatures for the destruction of *C. botulinum* (reference temperature, 121·1°C; z, 10°C)

Temperature, T (°C)	Lethal rate (min at 121·1°C/min at T)	Time $(F_T)^a$ required for a 12-log spore reduction
101·1	0·01	4 h
111·1	0·1	24 min
121·1	1	2·4 min
131·1	10	15 s
141·1	100	1·5 s

^{a} $F_T = D_T Y_n$ where $D_{121·1} = 0·2$ and Y_n is the spore log reduction (log N_0 − log N_F) where N_o and N_F are 10^3 and 10^{-9}, respectively.

spore reduction is required. The difference in each temperature in Table 1 is one z value (10°C), which illustrates that changing the exposure or processing temperature by one z value will require a 10-fold change in processing time.

Sterilization Value

The parameter which accumulates the lethal effect as a function of time (t) during the thermal process is the sterilization value, defined as

$$F_{T_{REF}}^z = \int_0^t 10^{(T - T_{REF})/z} dt \qquad (2)$$

In terms of lethal rate, L (eqn [1]),

$$F_{T_{REF}}^z = \Sigma L \Delta t \qquad (3)$$

When temperature (T) characterizes the slowest-heating zone in the container of food and when the reference temperature and z value are 121·1°C and 10°C, respectively, then the sterilization value is known as the F_0 value for the thermal process. The F_0 value is specific for the food, container, processing conditions, processing system and thermal process (processing time, temperature and other physical factors affecting the process). The F_0 value is the equivalent value of the process in terms of minutes at 121·1°C as if no time is involved in heating to 121·1°C and cooling to sublethal temperatures. An F_0 value of 3·0 min ($z = 10$°C) is generally accepted as a realistic, minimum botulinum thermal process that will produce LACFs that are safe from a public health standpoint.

Commercial Sterility

Commercial sterility of food means the condition achieved by application of heat which renders such food free of viable forms of those microorganisms which have public health significance, as well as any microorganisms of nonhealth significance capable of reproducing in the food under normal nonrefrigerated conditions of storage and distribution.

Several additional considerations go into the decision as to the design F_0 for commercial sterility which could be as much as 20 F_0 units higher than the minimum *C. botulinum* public health thermal process. These considerations include the following: initial bacterial level of the food product; physical parameters of the food itself (style, consistency, particle size, liquid : solid ratio, etc.); food container; processing system (still, hydrostatic, continuous agitating, retorts etc.); conditions of storage and distribution; natural or added ingredients that prevent spoilage; economics and the general experience of the food processor. As examples, foods that will be distributed to a high temperature geographical area may require an F_0 of 15–20 min to afford the same protection from economic loss due to spoilage as an F_0 of 5–7 min would afford for a moderate temperature area. An F_0 of 8–12 min is recommended for products heated with induced agitation.

With regard to the initial bacterial level of the food, it is important to note that the same thermal process (F_0) does not guarantee the same degree of processing. The F_0 value is a measure of processing conditions necessary to affect the level of *C. botulinum* spores by a certain number of log reductions, such as 12 $D_{121·1}$ values. The higher the initial spore concentration, the higher the spore concentration after processing for a process delivering the same F_0 value.

There is a potential hazard in expressing process requirements as '12*D*', in that only the spore-log reduction is specified. A spore-log reduction of 12 will yield a probability of a spore surviving of 10^{-9} (one spore per 10^9 containers) only when the initial spore contamination level is 10^3. To provide all consumers of canned food with equal protection, regardless of the initial numbers of *C. botulinum* spores, the heat process F_0 value should always satisfy a constant, agreed end-point value of probability of a surviving spore.

Heat Penetration Testing

The purpose of the heat penetration (HP) test is to determine accurately the temperature of the slowest-heating zone in the food container during thermal processing. The results of the HP test are experimentally determined time–temperature relationships describing the heating and cooling of the product. These data are derived from tests which duplicate commercial processing with a high degree of reliability. The HP data are normally collected in the laboratory because of the complexity of heat transfer through products in containers, especially products that heat by natural or forced convection, and interaction with the processing system. The HP test provides the temperature history of the product during the process which, when combined with the thermal resistance information for the organism of concern (the required F_0 value), allows us to calculate the length (process time) of the thermal process at the specified retort temperature.

The factors which affect the HP results are numerous and tend to be more complex as the food product, package and processing systems (retorts or autoclaves) become more complex. The following factors must be considered by the HP technician during the conduct of a HP test because they may influence the resulting heating and cooling temperature profiles:

- Processing (retort) temperature
- Processing time
- Initial temperature and temperature distribution within the container
- Size and shape of container
- Container orientation and distribution within retort
- Agitation of containers during processing*
- Container fill and headspace*
- Product formulation and preparation procedures*
- Proportion of solids to liquid*
- Size, shape, arrangement and composition of food particles
- Consistency of product*
- Product drained weight after processing
- Style of container (plastic or metal; rigid, semirigid or flexible)
- Vacuum or air remaining in container
- Temperature distribution (uniformity) in processing vessel
- Operating conditions during processing (come-up time, sequence of events, controller function, reel rotation, etc.)*
- Location and type of temperature sensor in container
- Ability of test retort to duplicate commercial conditions*

Every thermal process will have factors that are critical for delivery of the design F_0. For example, the critical factors of retorting systems that are designed to agitate the contents of the container during processing to increase the rate of heat penetration will differ from those of a still retorting system for the same product. It is the responsibility of the person establishing a thermal process to understand all the factors that may influence the way in which the product heats and cools. It has been repeatedly observed that the HP testing programme must continue until all parameters are fully understood.

*Particularly significant when processing with agitation.

Only accurate and applicable HP factors are meaningful for thermal process establishment.

The instrument of choice for measuring food temperature during HP testing has historically been the thermocouple (TC) with recording potentiometer. Normally, nonprojecting-style TC receptacles are attached to the container and hard-wired to the potentiometer. The TCs are placed to measure the temperature at the slowest-heating zone within the container; this is determined a priori by auxiliary testing. Since the objective of the HP test is to obtain accurate time–temperature data, care must be exercised in the selection and use of the TC. For products that have considerable natural or induced convection, such as whole-kernel corn in brine, a TC of small diameter is used in order to avoid interfering with product movement. For conduction-heating foods that remain motionless during processing, such as a viscous stew, the TC material is selected to have thermal properties similar to the food in order to avoid conducting heat to or from the TC junction. If the TC and/or container are not adequately grounded, especially in water processes, stray voltages may cause large temperature errors.

In recent years, temperature measuring devices have been modernized to include resistance temperature devices (RTDs) and miniature telemetry or recording systems. These systems have allowed HP testing in systems that were previously not possible since they have removed the requirement of direct wiring to the container.

The accuracy of the measuring instrument is extremely important. A consistent $0.5°C$ difference in temperature measurement results in a 10% difference in F_0. For minimally processed foods, this could result in severe underprocessing and survival of numerous pathogenic or spoilage organisms.

Thermal Process Calculations

The methods for calculating the sterilization value (F_0) from the HP and TDT data can be classified as either 'general' or 'formula'. The two methods use similar principles but the procedures are distinctly different.

The general method is essentially a graphical or numerical integration of eqn [2], using the time–temperature data obtained during the HP test. It is the most accurate and simplest method to determine the F_0 delivered by the thermal process. The disadvantage is that the method affords little or no ability (1) to change the process time, heating parameters or initial product temperature and predict their influence on F_0, or (2) to use F_0 as an input to predict process time. An example of calculating F_0 using the general method is given in Table 2. In this example, eqn [3] is numerically integrated using typical time–temperature data at 2-minute intervals

Table 2. Example calculation of the sterilization value by the general method (reference temperature, 121·1°C; z, 10°C)

Time[a] t (min)	Temperature[a] T (°C)	Lethal rate, L (eqn [1])	Lethality, $(L \times \Delta t)$	Cumulative lethality, F_0 (eqn [3])
0[b]	58·0	0·00	0·00	0·00
2	81·0	0·00	0·00	0·00
4	96·0	0·00	0·01	0·01
6	104·0	0·02	0·04	0·05
8	109·0	0·06	0·12	0·17
10	114·0	0·19	0·39	0·56
12	116·0	0·31	0·62	1·18
14	118·5	0·55	1·10	2·28
16	119·8	0·74	1·48	3·76
18	120·7	0·91	1·82	5·58
20	121·6	1·12	2·24	7·83
22[c]	120·1	0·79	1·59	9·42
24	114·0	0·19	0·39	9·81
26	100·0	0·01	0·02	9·82
28	79·0	0·00	0·00	9·82
30	60·0	0·00	0·00	9·8

[a] During heat penetration test.
[b] Begin heating.
[c] Begin cooling.

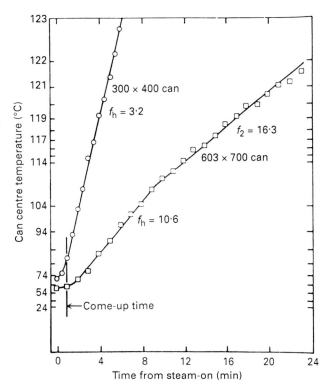

Fig. 3 Typical simple and broken heat penetration curves. Tests were for two can sizes of mushrooms in brine, heated simulating the FMC sterilmatic continuous agitating retort. Can sizes are American designations: 603×700 implies an outside diameter of 6 3/16 inches and an overall height of 7 inches. From Berry MR and Bradshaw JG (1982) Heat penetration for sliced mushrooms in brine processed in still and agitating retorts with comparisons to spore count reduction. *Journal of Food Science* 47: 1699.

from a HP test. The resulting F_0 for the combined heating and cooling phases is 9·8 min at 121·1°C. In the general method, improved accuracy may be achieved by reducing the time interval for the HP data.

The various formula methods are mostly iterations and improvements of the formula method first proposed by CO Ball in 1923. The HP data are first plotted on semilogarithmic paper as either simple- or broken-heating curves, as shown in Fig. 3. The shapes of the respective heating curves are defined in terms of parameters commonly known as HP factors: a heating lag factor (j); a temperature response parameter which is a function of the slope of the heating curve (f_h) and the second slope and break point (f_2 and X_{bh}) when the heating curve has a change of slope and can be represented by two straight-line segments.

The simple (single, straight-line) heating curve normally occurs for food products heating by conduction, or by forced convection induced by mechanical agitation of the container. Broken-heating curves normally occur for products heating by natural convection in still retorts and for products that undergo a change in their thermophysical properties during processing (such as a rapid increase in viscosity as temperature increases).

In the formula methods, a series of mathematical expressions describe the temperature of the food in terms of the HP factors for the heating, cooling and transitional phases of the processing cycle. When the expressions are substituted into eqn [2], a direct mathe-

matical solution is not possible. F_0 values are calculated by either numerical procedures that use high-speed computing equipment or by classical 'cookbook' procedures using supplemental tabulated data. The versatility of the formula method makes it possible to vary the heating time, process temperature, design F_0, and even can size, using the same HP data, and to determine the influence of each of these factors on the thermal process delivered to the product.

Sterilization values calculated from the original Ball formula method are reported to be conservative. Numerous investigators have offered modifications which have improved the method, resulting in F_0 values nearer those calculated by the general method.

Process Validation

The F_0 which results from the process establishment procedure is simply a calculated value or prediction of the reduction in microorganisms which occurs when the process is used for commercial production of canned foods. The final step in the process establishment procedure is the validation or confirmation of the design process to provide assurance that the HP studies accurately reflect commercial conditions.

Process validation is normally performed using microbial techniques involving the inoculation of calibrated bacterial spores into the cans before the containers are sealed and processed. After the process, the cans are incubated and observed for evidence of spoilage after a certain period. Another approach involves aseptic sampling of each container after processing, and placing the food into selected growth media in order to determine whether or not any bacteria survived the process. It is impossible to measure the design level of sterilization processes (about 10^{-9} spores for *C. botulinum* or 10^{-6} for nonpathogenic organisms) using the organism for which the process is intended to destroy.

The bacteria used in biovalidation have a heat resistance higher than *C. botulinum* and are typically spore-forming, putrefactive mesophiles or thermophiles. A commonly used organism is PA3679, which is nontoxic and, therefore, safe for use in food plants and not hazardous to microbiologists conducting the validation tests.

Experience in commercial processing indicates that the microbial kill measured by biological methods does not always agree with the measurements of physical parameters (HP and TDT). This is why each process must be validated biologically. If the bacterial spores have been adequately calibrated, they give an indication of the actual killing power of the thermal process as delivered by the commercial processing equipment. A common biological validation is to carry out an inoculated pack in which 10 000 resistant PA3679 spores ($D_{121.1}$ of between 1·0 and 1·5 in phosphate buffer) are added to each container of product before processing. After processing, inoculated containers are incubated. An acceptable process should produce a greater than 5-log reduction in PA3679. The test must be carried out with good technique and appropriate controls. If the validation tests do not agree with the physical process design, there is an indication that the critical processing parameters were not adequately understood and the differences should be resolved.

Bibliography

Ball CO and Olson FCW (1957) *Sterilization in Food Technology*. New York: McGraw-Hill.
Goldblith SA, Joslyn MA and Nickerson JTR (1961) *An Introduction to the Thermal Processing of Foods*. Westport, Connecticut: AVI Publishing.
Joslyn MA and Heid JL (1967) *Fundamentals of Food Processing Operations*. Westport, Connecticut: AVI Publishing.
Lopez A (1987) *A Complete Course in Canning* 12th edn. Baltimore, Maryland: The Canning Trade, Inc.
National Food Processors Association (formerly National Canners Association) (1968) *Laboratory Manual for Food Canners and Processors*. Westport, Connecticut: AVI Publishing
Pflug IJ (ed.) (1988) *Selected Papers on the Microbiology and Engineering of Sterilization Processes* 5th edn. Minneapolis: Environmental Sterilization Laboratory.
Pflug IJ (1990) *Microbiology and Engineering of Sterilization Processes* 7th edn. Minneapolis: Environmental Sterilization Laboratory.
Stumbo CR (1973) *Thermobacteriology in Food Processing* 2nd edn. New York: Academic Press.

M. R. Berry Jr
Cincinnati, USA
I. J. Pflug
University of Minnesota, Minneapolis, USA

Cans and Their Manufacture

History of the Can

The Origins

Throughout human history, food preservation has been essential to survival. The storage of foods started with the traditional preservation methods like sun drying, salting, smoking and pickling. These methods alone, however, could not give a balanced diet with preserved foods. In the 18th century, industrialization, the increase in urban populations and long sea voyages of discovery all gave incentives for improvements in food preservation.

Various attempts at preserving cooked foods in jars were recorded, but the greatest contribution to the establishment of the canning industry was made by Nicolas Appert, a confectioner from Châlons-sur-Marne in France (Fig. 1). He carried out his experiments in Paris between 1780 and 1795, at which time he started to supply the French navy with his new preserved foods and by 1809 had set up a factory in Massy. A year later his book *L'Art de Conserver pendant plusieurs années toutes les Substances Animales et Végétales* was published. It described his process of putting food into bottles which were carefully corked, sealed and then heated in boiling water, and gave recipes for a wide range of individual food products. *See* Preservation of Food

Tins and Sea Travel

Three months after the publication of Appert's book, Peter Durand published a patent identical in parts to

L'Art de Conserver. It has been suggested that this was plagiarism, but he did make one important addition – he included tinned iron canisters amongst the possible containers.

Soon after this, Britain's first cannery was established by Donkin, Hall and Gamble. These cans were made from three pieces of tin-plated iron, the body made from one piece, bent round into a cylinder and the edges soldered together. The ends were made of tinplate discs, and the flanged edges of these discs soldered onto the body.

One end-disc was made with a half-inch hole to top up the brine or gravy and, after filling, a small cap was then soldered over the hole. This cap had a small vent hole which was soldered after heat processing, so allowing relief of the steam pressure during the process.

Bryan Donkin's design of the can remained largely unchanged for almost a century. Tin canisters (shortened to 'tins' or 'cans') had advantages over glass bottles: they were lighter, more easily sealed and less prone to damage during transport and storage.

The early development of cans and canned foods is very much linked to sea travel and exploration. Sir Edward Parry and Sir John Ross both used Donkin, Hall and Gamble's products on their expeditions, and canned foods gained acceptance as food stores for naval and merchant ships.

In 1819 an English immigrant, William Underwood, opened the first cannery in the USA using glass containers and, about the same time, Thomas Kensett also set up a plant, going into partnership with Ezra Daggett who was granted the first US patent for canning in metal containers.

Acceptance of canned provisions was a little slower in France than in Britain, and this is thought to be due to the persistence of Appert with glass containers rather than metal cans; Appert, however, was using cans by 1817.

During the early part of the 19th century, canned foods still did not reach the general public. Large can sizes, difficulty of opening (a hammer and chisel had to be used!), high prices because of the laborious canning process and the fact that a good tinsmith could manufacture only 10 cans a day by hand, all went against general distribution.

Technical Innovation and Commercial Advancement

Technical innovation in the mid-19th century included the invention of a machine for stamping out can bodies and machinery to automate the soldering process for can ends. In addition, pressure processing introduced by Albert Fryer in Britain and Andrew Shriver in the USA during the 1870s, meant that heating and cooling times could be significantly reduced.

The most significant development to influence the development of the can occurred in the late 19th century. W. R. Lake, Max Ams and Julius Brenzinger all played a part in the invention of the process of double seaming a can end coated at the periphery with a gasket.

In 1904 Ams, Cobb and Bogle formed the Sanitary Can Company, and the new double-seamed can became known as the 'sanitary can' in the USA and as the 'open-top' can in UK, but these cans took many years to achieve predominance. These processes opened the way to high-speed manufacture and the expansion of the can and canned food production in the USA.

In 1903 J. J. Carnaud in France joined forces with Les Forges de Basse-Indre to become the number one French can and tinplate manufacturer. A company founded in the 1850s by W. B. Williamson of Worcester installed, in 1927, a Max Ams line which revolutionized can making in the UK. Williamson was one of the companies which became part of Metal Box Ltd, which merged with Carnaud in 1989 to become Europe's premier can maker: CMB Packaging SA.

After the 1920s, canned food lost its military image and became fully accepted as part of the national diet, and the industry steadily progressed and increased efficiency.

Over the years the thickness of the tinplate used gradually diminished, but the next major change was during the 1970s with the introduction of both three-piece welded cans (described below) and two-piece cans (a drawn can with a loose end) and the use of ends with easy open features.

Materials used in Can Manufacture

Both steel and aluminium are used in container manufacture. In the development from the fully soldered cans

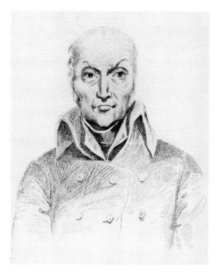

Fig. 1   Nicolas Appert, 1750–1841.

Cans and Their Manufacture

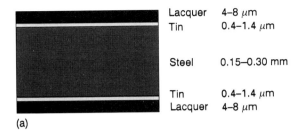

Lacquer	4–8 μm
Tin	0.4–1.4 μm
Steel	0.15–0.30 mm
Tin	0.4–1.4 μm
Lacquer	4–8 μm

(a)

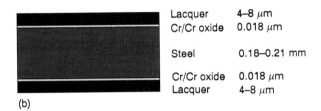

Lacquer	4–8 μm
Cr/Cr oxide	0.018 μm
Steel	0.18–0.21 mm
Cr/Cr oxide	0.018 μm
Lacquer	4–8 μm

(b)

Fig. 2 Typical structure of can-making materials: (a) tin-plate; (b) tin-free steel.

of Donkin to open-top soldered and welded cans, tinned steel has been the most widely used material. This is not only because it lends itself to the process of three-piece can making, which is by far the most common method of manufacture, but also because of performance and cost factors.

In recent years tin-free steel (TFS) has become widely used for end manufacture because it avoids the use of costly tin. Figure 2 shows the typical structure of both tinplate and TFS.

Lacquer is added for the protection of tinplate for certain can applications, but it is always widely used with TFS to avoid tool wear on component formation and double seaming, as the plain chrome/chrome oxide coating would be too abrasive.

The Steel Base

The steel base that makes up the largest proportion of the plate is typically a low-carbon steel continuously cast and hot rolled into strip. It is then reduced in thickness by a number of cold reduction processes.

Heating or annealing of the steel to around 600°C, either in continuous or batch furnaces, takes place to produce the required temper, followed by a further cold reduction to achieve the required surface finish, thickness and temper.

Finishing of the plate is either carried out by electrolytic tinning in the case of tinplate, or electrolytic deposition of chrome/chrome oxide in the case of TFS. Following this, the tinplate is treated with a chromate passivation process and finally oil is applied to both types of plate.

The Type of Plate and its Application

The requirements for different tin coating thicknesses depend on a number of factors: whether the surface is the internal or external surface of the can, if a lacquer coating is used and the type of product and processing conditions. Typically, coatings vary from 2·8 to 15·1 g m^{-2}.

The mechanical properties and thickness of the plate will depend on the application: two-piece or three-piece cans or ends.

Aluminium is not used for three-piece food cans, but it is used for certain shallow drawn, round or oblong cans and easy-open ends.

The Construction of Three-piece Cans

In Europe by far the most common manufacturing method for three-piece cans is by resistance welding of the side seam. Soldering of the side seam is still in use for some applications, but is gradually being phased out as welded cans have significant technical advantages. There is also limited use of cemented side seam cans principally in Japan.

Three-piece Welded Can Manufacture

The main steps in the manufacture of three-piece welded cans are shown in Fig. 3. Tinplate is used in the manufacture of can bodies mainly because of welding difficulties with other materials. The plate is usually supplied in stacks or stillages of cut rectangular sheet which may be used plain or lacquered or printed before can manufacture according to the requirements of the product or can filler.

At the start of the production line the individual sheets are automatically destacked from the stillage and are cut into smaller rectangles or body blanks on the slitter. The slitter carries out the cutting operations in two directions by use of two banks of shear rollers.

The Bodymaker

Body blanks are then transferred to the bodymaker, which carries out the forming and welding operation. These machines typically operate at 150–800 containers per minute for open-top cans.

The first operation of the bodymaker is to flex and roll the body blanks into a cylinder shape and overlap the edges at the side seam (where the weld will be formed) by about 0·5 mm. During the welding operation, the overlapped edges of the cylinder are compressed between two opposing welding rolls or electrodes which carry the welding wire that passes, simultaneously, a

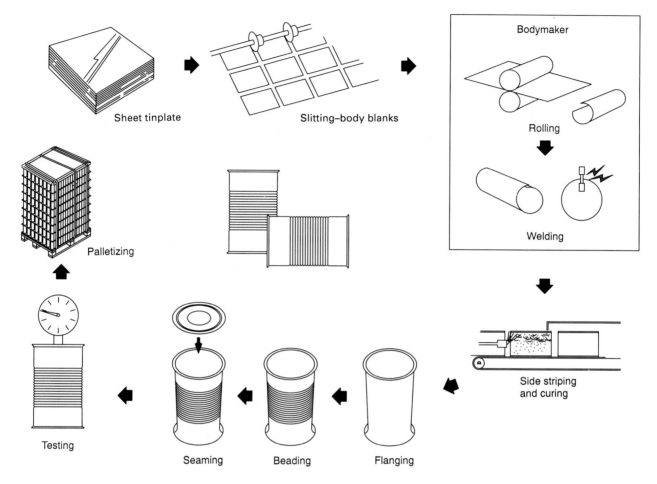

Fig. 3 Three-piece-can manufacture.

pulsed welding current through the overlap. The action of the pressure and the pulses of current fuses the two edges together and compresses the overlap.

The inner welding arm needs to carry cooling water, be robust enough to support the welding roll, conduct the welding current and carry the side stripe supply (see below). In order to do this, there is a necessary limit of a minimum diameter of 45 mm for resistance-welded cans.

During the welding process, if the weld is subsequently to be protected by either an internal or an external side stripe, an atmosphere of nitrogen gas is supplied to shroud the weld and prevent brittle oxides forming on its surface.

Following welding, a side stripe may be applied, and this is done either by spraying or roller coating a liquid lacquer onto the joint, or by electrostatic powder coating. All three methods are followed by a heat-curing process.

Subsequent Operations

Having produced a cylinder of steel, flanging of the edges is now carried out either by means of a die process or by spinning. This causes a rounded flange to be formed at either end of the can so that the container can later be double seamed. In some cases, food cans may also be necked in at this stage so that smaller diameter ends can be used, and this helps can stacking by nesting one end into another.

To allow for a reduction in body plate materials whilst retaining the 'hoop strength' or panelling resistance, most cans (apart from very short ones) are beaded. These are formed on a beader by a die process. The important factors relating to the improvement of panelling resistance are the depth, radius and the number of beads used.

Related to panelling resistance is axial strength or resistance to top load pressure. This is another critical feature limiting can design features, such as necking, beading and bodywall thickness.

After this, the flanged and beaded cylinder is double seamed with one end. The manufacture of ends and the double-seaming process are described later.

Following double seaming, the can will normally be pressure tested on a wheel tester to check for leakage. The accuracy of the manufacturing process is vital to the integrity and success of the can. This final testing process

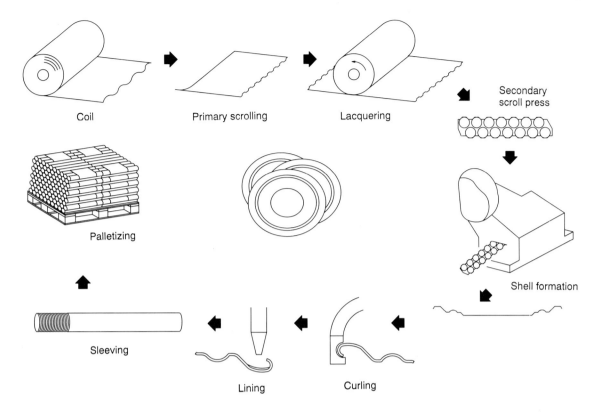

Fig. 4 Can-end manufacture.

is done in addition to stringent quality control procedures which apply to all stages of can production, and ensures the quality of the final product.

At this stage, a complete open-top container has been produced, and all that remains is to package it in a way suitable for delivery to the can filler. This is normally done by palletization. Rows of cans are packed onto a pallet board with layer pads of cardboard in between the layers for protection of the flanges. These may then either be overwrapped with cardboard or compression packed (as in Fig. 3) A description of warehousing and distribution is given later.

Choice of Three- or Two-piece Cans

The choice will depend on a number of factors such as the product to be packed, the quantity of cans to be produced, the range of size of the cans and the availability and price of raw materials.

In general terms, welded lines have a lower capital cost and higher versatility as they can accommodate size changes more easily.

Can Ends – Design and Manufacture

End Design

During the processing of canned foods, the contents expand and exert a pressure on the end. The material

used and the design of the end must allow for this, so that the end survives the heat process without permanent distortion or peaking. The most important factors are:

(1) gauge and temper of the end-plate;
(2) design features of the end, e.g. countersink radius and expansion bead profile (related to peaking resistance), bulge pressure (the more bulge, the greater the pressure relief) and the 'flip' characteristics of the end (the need to return to a normal, slightly concave position after processing);
(3) lacquer requirements, e.g. product resistance and toolability;
(4) process factors, e.g. product type, headspace level, vacuum level, occluded gases and processing temperature and pressure.

These factors, plus the ability to be double seamed, have to be carefully considered in the design of can ends.

End Manufacture

The main steps in the manufacture of can ends are shown in Fig. 4. Plate for the manufacture of ends, commonly TFS, is usually supplied on coils. This enables the sheets to be cut on a primary scroll line to produce sheets with scroll edges.

Because ends are produced in a staggered or scroll pattern (see secondary scroll image Fig. 4), this ensures minimal wastage of tinplate during the end stamping process.

Following primary scrolling, the end-plate is normally lacquered and may be printed before end manufacture.

After lacquering, the plate is cut into strips in a secondary scroll or scroll shear operation. Plate may be waxed at this stage as a lubricant for the end-forming operations. The strips are then fed into the press which will normally punch out a number of end shells in each operation.

The edge of the end is then curled by rotation between two curling rails, this rolls the edge of the metal enabling subsequent double seaming to take place. After curling, a liquid sealing compound is applied to the seaming panel of the end. This sealing or lining compound is a mixture of synthetic and natural rubbers in either a water or solvent base. If the compound applied is water based, oven or hot-air drying is necessary.

As with can bodies, the accuracy of the manufacturing process is vital to the integrity and success of the can. Visual and vision inspection systems and stringent quality-control procedures ensure the quality of the final product.

At this stage the can end is now complete, and all that remains is to accumulate the cans into 'sticks' and pack into paper sleeves. These are then palletized as illustrated in Fig. 4 with paper interleaving and stretch-wrapping to hold the sleeves together and to protect the ends.

Double Seaming

A double seam is defined as the formation of a hermetic seal by interlocking the edges of the end seaming panel and the body flange. The seal is produced in two operations and is therefore referred to as a double seam. As it prevents the entry of microorganisms into the sterilized can, it is crucial to the success of the canning operation. Details of the dimensional terminology used and the two forming operations are illustrated in Fig. 5.

Double-seam Formation

The seam is formed on closing machines or double seamers and essentially the same process is involved whether applying the 'fixed' end at the can manufacturer or 'loose' end at the can filler. Most double seamers accomplish the two forming operations with seaming rolls. The can body and end are clamped on a seaming chuck by a load applied vertically to the base plate or lifter of the seamer.

During the first operation, the end-seaming panel and the body flange are rolled together into the correct interlock position. This first operation determines seam dimensional quality and is the critical forming step.

The second operation finishes the seam by ironing it and compressing it to the correct tightness.

Double Seamers and Target Setting

Double seamers have a variety of designs. They may be single- or multihead with stationary or driven chucks and lifters, and a variety of seaming speeds (2–2000 cans per minute). In the can-filling plant, they may also be used to condition the headspace (the space between the product surface and can end) by using steam flow, cold vacuum or undercover gassing, depending on the product being packed.

In the adjustment of a double seam, the following need to be set correctly and checked:

(1) first and second operation roll profiles;
(2) chuck and roll type and specification;
(3) base load;
(4) pin height (distance between baseplate and chuck).

Having established these basic settings, the first-operation seam is set to target for seam thickness and countersink depth. Following this, the second operation is set to produce the correct final seam dimensions. This process, known as 'target setting', is crucial to obtaining satisfactory double seam formation.

Double-seam Evaluation

This involves three basic procedures:

(1) visual examination for obvious defects;
(2) sectioning;
(3) complete tear down.

Many dimensional targets, derived from either sectioning or complete tear down, may be quoted, e.g. seam length, seam thickness and body hooks. These dimensions are measured in the computation of the *Critical Seam Parameters* which are the features or dimensions to which a double seam must conform to be satisfactory:

- *Correct tightness rating*: the compressive tightness of the finished double seam measured by rating the extent of wrinkling present on the end hook
- *Correct actual overlap* of end and body hook.
- Correct embedding of the body hook into the lining compound at the bottom of the internal seam – *body hook butting*.
- Freedom from obvious *visual defects*.

Measurements are usually the average of results from two opposite positions on the can seam.

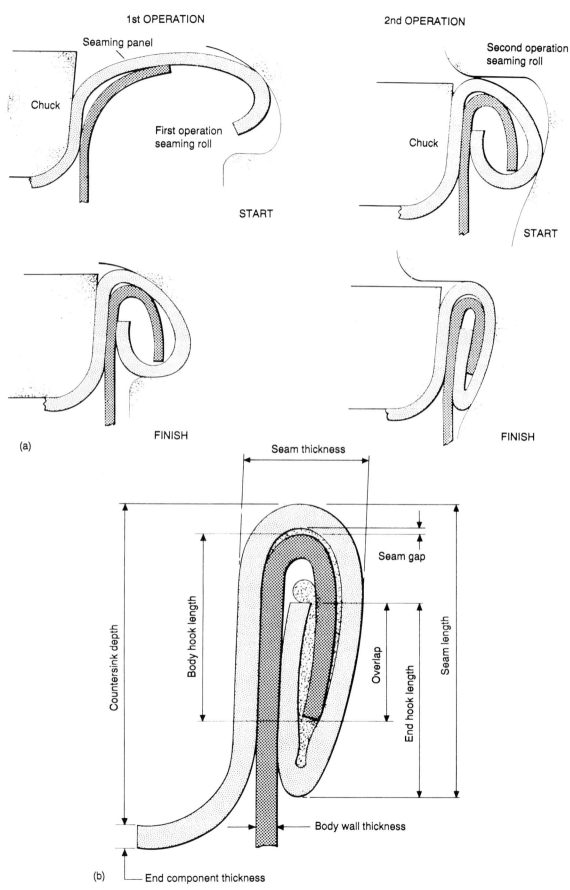

1st OPERATION

2nd OPERATION

Seaming panel

Second operation
seaming roll

Chuck

First operation
seaming roll

Chuck

START

START

FINISH

FINISH

(a)

Seam thickness

Seam gap

Countersink depth

Body hook length

Overlap

End hook length

Seam length

Body wall thickness

(b)

End component thickness

Fig. 5   (a) Double-seam formation. (b) Dimensional terminology of double seams.

Table 1.   Some common can sizes

UK trade name	Continental trade name	Size in.	mm[a]	Capacity (ml)
—	$\frac{1}{4}$ l US	—	65×71	212
Picnic	—	211×301	65×78	235
A1	Soup can	211×400	$65 \times 100/2$	315
U8	—	300×207	73×62	230
—	$\frac{1}{4}$ l medium	—	73×58	212
14Z	—	300×402	73×105	400
ET	$\frac{1}{2}$ l tall	—	$73 \times 109/10$	425
UT	—	300×408	73×115	445
A2	No. 2	307×408	$83 \times 114/5$	580
A2$\frac{1}{2}$	1/1 l tall	401×411	99×119	850
A10	3 l	603×700	$153 \times 151/2$	3100
—	5 l	603×904	153×235	4100

[a] Height dimensions may vary depending on the point at which the measurement is made and the nearest whole millimetre.

Types of double-seam profiles and dimensions may vary according to the type of container, the materials used and the type of product (food or beverage). Information on the frequency of evaluation and the standards to be applied are available from the can manufacturer who validates specifications by leakage and microbiological challenge testing.

Can Distribution and Can Sizes

Distribution

Palletized ends and bodies are usually stored in a warehouse after manufacture. Good warehouse practice applies to protect the finished cans from damage and corrosion.

Pallets are normally distributed on curtain-sided trailers which are easily loaded and unloaded by conventional forklift trucks.

Can Sizes

These vary world-wide from country to country according to market requirements for the products. In continental Europe, and increasingly in the UK, dimensions are described in millimetres (diameter followed by height). In the USA and the UK, each dimension is described by three digits. The first represents the whole inches and the next two fractions of an inch in sixteenths; again the values are diameter followed by height. So a 211×400 can is $2\frac{11}{16}$ in. in diameter and 4 in. tall (or 65×102 mm). Some common can sizes are listed in Table 1.

Bibliography

Anonymous (n.d.) *A History of Canned Foods*. Reading: Metal Box plc.
Anonymous (1978) *Double Seam Manual*. Reading: Metal Box.
Rees JAG and Bettison J (eds) (1991) *Processing and Packaging of Heat Preserved Foods*. Glasgow: Blackie.
Thorne S (1986) *The History of Food Preservation*. Kirkby Longside: The Parthenon Publishing Group.

David North
CMB Packaging Technology, Wantage, UK
Pierre Sirbat
CMB Alimentaire, Paris, France

Recent Developments in Can Design

Technical developments in metal can design and manufacture have been particularly marked during the last decade. Dramatic improvements have been made, from can design and protection, to easier ways of can opening. New materials have also appeared in answer to specific requirements from the market place. Some of these steps in the evolution of metal cans are described.

Can Lacquering and Printing

While metal cans produced in the early 1900s were made with plain tinplate, a move towards lacquered plate then took place as the industry progressed and the range of products increased. About 1914 the first 'off-set' machines, previously used in the paper industry, were used to decorate tinplate sheets (these are described later).

Today, a large proportion of food cans and ends have an internal, and sometimes an external, protective coating or lacquer. In the case of processed food cans, these coating materials must be able to withstand the high temperature and pressure conditions of sterilization in water and steam without losing adhesion to the metal base whilst, at the same time, maintaining their resistance to the product.

Coatings and Lacquers

Coatings and lacquers are complex blends of resins in a mixture of solvents with additives designed to give specific performance features.

Protective lacquers for metal containers and closures are known by the principal resin or resin combination, or by their basic formulation. Examples are: oleoresinous, vinyl, phenolic, epoxy, epoxyphenolic, polyester phenolic, organosol, solvent and water based. Whether protective or decorative, lacquers are normally applied as liquids; the solvent phase is usually organic, but can also be water and organic cosolvent for certain applications. These materials may be applied either before or after fabrication of the container, depending on the method of manufacture, by roller coaster or by spraying.

Coating and Lacquer Application and Stoving

The technique for application of the coating varies according to the type of can construction:

(1) Roller coating of lacquers onto tinplate sheet is achieved by a series of rollers which pick up and distribute lacquer across an application roll which then, in turn, applies the coating to one surface of the metal passing through the machine. A similar approach can also be used for metal sheet printing (see Fig. 1). Three-piece cans, some two-piece cans and can ends are lacquered in this way.
(2) Spray lacquers are used for two-piece drawn and wall ironed cans, one or two coats of lacquer may be applied under controlled conditions to produce a continuous and consistent coating with maximum coverage of the metal.
(3) As an alternative to liquid lacquers, surface coatings can be applied as powders and subsequently fused onto the surface. Two-piece cans or three-piece can bodies may be coated in this way, but the most common current use of this method is side-seam protection for three-piece cans.

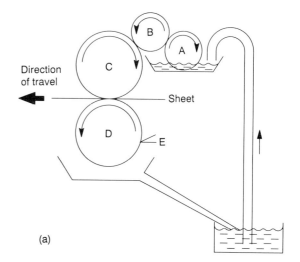

(a)

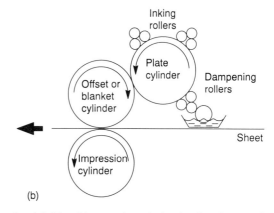

(b)

Fig. 1 (a) Metal lacquering: A, feed roller; B, transfer roller; C, application roller; D, pressure roller; E, scraper. (b) Metal printing.

After applying the lacquer, it is necessary to give a full stoving in order to dry and heat polymerize (cure) the lacquer, and to achieve the required chemical and physical resistance of the lacquer film, varnish or pigmented coating. Depending on the resin used, there is an appropriate critical curing temperature, normally in the region 185–195°C for most lacquers.

Most ovens are of the continuous or conveyor type; they consist of a series of individual metal frames or wickets mounted on a chain. The coated metal sheets are transferred from the coater onto the wickets and transported through the heating chamber at a suitable speed to give the required time/temperature combination.

Typical stoving schedules give an approximately 10 min exposure at the required peak metal temperature out of a total time in the oven of 14–15 min.

Curing of the lacquers is controlled by strictly monitoring and maintaining stoving temperatures, and by quality-control checks on the lacquered plate to evaluate chemical and mechanical properties.

Recent Developments in Can Design

Recent Developments in Lacquering and Printing

Environmental Issues

Many of the developments in this area have been related to the reduction of volatile organic compound (VOC) emission. Water has been introduced as a base for some lacquer systems instead of organic solvents. These have been particularly successful in spray applications for two-piece cans where the surface to be coated is particularly suitable for water-based lacquers.

Similarly, ultraviolet (UV) curing has been developed for solvent-free varnishes and inks. Currently, most UV units are used for inks and external varnish applications.

The advantages of UV curing, in addition to that of less VOC emission, are increased line speeds and energy and space saving.

Recently, the use of polyvinylchloride (PVC) has come under close scrutiny in many countries because of effluent by-products. The can-coating industry is seeking wherever possible to substitute PVC with other resins in lacquers and coatings.

Plastic Lamination of Metal

An alternative to lacquering is the plastic lamination of the metal base by a preformed polymer film. This can be achieved by adhesive or heat bonding of the polymer to the base.

There are a number of commercially available systems and the Metpolam system produced by CMB Packaging S.A. is one example. This process uses a continuous heat-bonding system which coats both sides of a metal coil, either steel or aluminium, depending on the application. It has extremely low VOC emission, is PVC free, enjoys low application energy consumption, improved container performance and a cleaner, more modern image. This method is currently used for 'easy open ends', aerosol components and food trays.

Other Lacquering and Printing Developments

The production of high-quality print on two-piece beverage cans has always been difficult as the production constraints mean that only one print operation is possible. The 'reprotherm' multicolour printing process overcomes this difficulty by applying a high-quality design to a paper surface, and this design is then transferred to the can surface by a process of heat transfer. This approach has been used in the UK on premium branded beer cans.

Colour matching for tinplate print has traditionally been done by eye, an unreliable and time-consuming process. Recently, computerized colour matching, to the exact customer specification, has meant that the correct mix of standard colours is provided by the computer to ensure accurate colour matching.

Two-piece Cans

Two-piece cans are so called as they are made from two distinct components. The body and bottom end are formed by drawing a single piece of metal and onto this a separate end is seamed after filling. The advantages of this type of can are: lower per unit cost, reduced raw materials usage in manufacture, simpler design (fewer seams or joints), and product differentiation on the supermarket shelf.

As a process it has less flexibility than three-piece can manufacture and the capital cost of the manufacturing equipment is usually higher. It is used where large numbers of a small variety of can sizes and specifications is required, e.g. beverage cans.

There are two common methods for the manufacture of two-piece cans: single- and multistage drawing, which includes draw–redraw (DRD), and drawn and wall ironed (DWI), sometimes also referred to as drawn and ironed (D & I).

Single and Multi-stage Drawing

Drawing is a well-known technique which has been used for many years in different industrial fields, and which consists of mechanically deforming a flat metal plate into a cup, giving a reduction of the blank disc diameter at essentially constant metal thickness.

This manufacturing technology has been used for many years for the production of fish and pâté cans, and more recently for metal trays; it can be used for either round, rectangular or oval cans. The relatively low height of these cans makes it possible to produce the can body in a single-stroke or a single-draw operation. If a deeper can is required it is necessary to adopt a multistage drawing operation or DRD. There are some limits to the draw ratio for round-can bodies according to their height (H) and diameter (D):

- single draw $H/D \leqslant 0.7$;
- draw and one redraw $0.7 < H/D \leqslant 1.4$;
- draw and two redraws $1.4 < H/D \leqslant 1.8$.

Multistage Drawing

The first stage in this process is the same as for the single-draw operation. It involves cutting a circular blank from the metal sheet; a cup is then drawn from this disc on the first press (Fig. 2; steps 1 and 2). Further operations

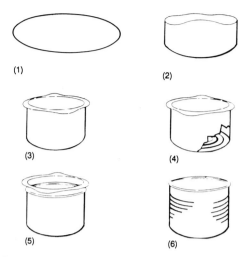

Fig. 2   Draw–redraw (DRD) can manufacture.

include base forming, flange forming and beading (Fig. 2; steps 4, 5 and 6).

These cans have been used successfully in a variety of European markets, including baby food, vegetables and pet food.

Production speeds are normally higher with DRD than for three-piece containers, and line outputs of around 1000 cans per minute are achieved.

Lacquers for Drawn Containers

Drawn containers are normally manufactured from lacquered plate. Great care is necessary in the selection of lacquers as they must:

(1) provide a lubricated surface to aid the drawing process – this is achieved by incorporating appropriate food contact lubricants in the lacquer;
(2) be highly flexible so they are not damaged during metal deformation and do not lose their adhesion to the metal base;
(3) be compatible with the products to be packed and prevent chemical reaction between the product and the container.

Drawn and Wall Ironed Cans

This technique, developed in the USA during the early 1960s, is now mainly used for tinplate or aluminium beverage cans. There are, however, also many lines producing containers for the canning of processed food. This method of manufacture is similar to that of DRD described above, except that the walls of the redrawn cup are stretched and thinned by ironing.

The cup formed during the first draw is placed on a punch and forced through a series of ironing dies or rings where the gap between the punch and the die is less than the thickness of the metal. In the DWI bodymaker, there are a series of three or four dies with progressively smaller gaps which reduce the body wall thickness by up to 75%.

Because of the nature of the ironing process, cans must be lacquered after formation.

The typical can-making steps are:

- circular blank cutting;
- cup drawing;
- redraw;
- multistage ironing;
- trimming of body;
- washing;
- external protection;
- internal protection;
- beading/necking/flanging;
- optical testing of each can for integrity.

In addition, beverage cans are normally decorated after manufacture, whereas food cans are normally paper labelled.

DWI manufacturing line speeds are typically 800–1600 cans per minute.

Comparison of DWI and DRD Cans

When deciding on whether to use the DWI or DRD manufacturing processes the following factors should be considered:

- cost advantages of wall thinning in DWI;
- the wall strength required by the can filler and the distribution network;
- the height of can (DWI is better for taller cans and DRD is better for shorter cans);
- for steel-based containers DWI requires the use of tinplate, whilst DRD can use both tinplate and tin-free steel;
- the capital cost of DWI equipment is usually higher.

Special Cans: Trays and Shaped Cans

Manufacturers have developed a number of cans for special applications and for a variety of reasons varying from trying to achieve better organoleptic quality of the food to enhancing the attractiveness of the metal can and achieving product differentiation.

Some examples of these cans are illustrated in Fig. 3, and examples of both two- and three-piece containers are discussed below.

Trays

The term 'tray' is usually applied to containers in which the depth is very much lower than the other dimensions.

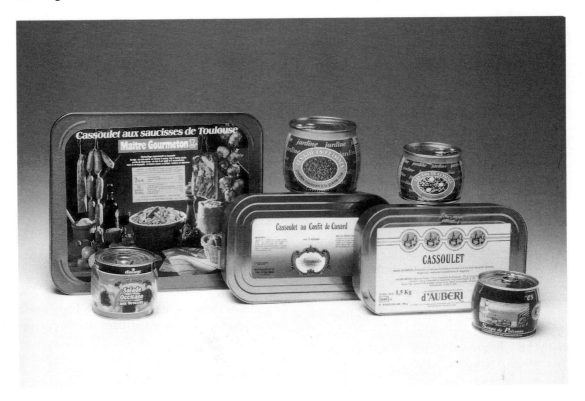

Fig. 3 Examples of trays and shaped cans.

Trays for food products currently on the market have generally been rectangular rather than round. Trays are mostly used for ready-made meal products which benefit from a shorter process; faster heat penetration is achieved during sterilization as trays have a shallower profile than most cans. As a result of this reduced heat process, trays have greater potential for improved organoleptic quality.

There are two main categories of metal tray:

- rigid trays, made from steel or aluminium (metal thicknesses of 0·20–0·30 mm);
- semirigid trays, always made of aluminium (thickness of the body and ends is 0·05–0·20 mm).

Trays are normally drawn containers and, like the round two-piece cans, they are always internally and externally protected by lacquers with a film weight which can vary from 5 to 20 g m^{-2}; for example, on double-seamed, rigid trays.

In the case of semirigid trays, the internal coating is usually a polymer (e.g. polypropylene) to allow for heat sealing of the tray and to protect the aluminium beneath it from the products. The weight of these internal films may be up to 50 g m^{-2}.

Different tray sizes are available, from single-portion retail sizes of 100–325 g to larger trays for institutional or catering use (1·5–3 litres).

Shaped Cans

After more than 30 years of container development based mainly on material reductions and process/productivity improvements, can manufacturers and fillers have now started to look at container differentiation and special designs. Cans are produced to fit new customer requirements of greater attractiveness of the pack, especially for new, high-quality products.

Since 1985, new can shapes have become commercially available, changing the traditional image of round metal cans. Irregular shapes, for example 'barrels', 'bowls' and 'pots', are obtained by mechanically expanding the welded body of three-piece cans. (These cans are also illustrated in Fig. 3.) Tailor-made can designs are available to can fillers who would like to differentiate their newly developed products from others on the market.

Easy-open Ends

The first canned foods were only used by explorers and troops who could tolerate the difficulties of opening the cans. The extension of canned foods to a wider domestic market led to new developments in the technology of can opening. A progressive standardization of can sizes, the reduction of can-material thickness and the intro-

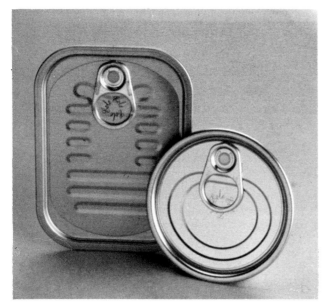

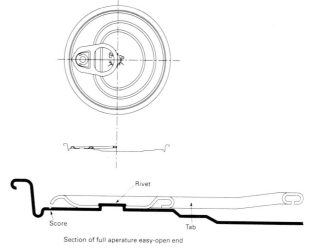

Rivet

Score

Tab

Section of full aperature easy-open end

Fig. 4 Easy-open can ends.

duction of double-seamed cans allowed a change from can openers which just cut a hole in the tinplate of one can end to openers that cut and removed the entire end panel.

At the beginning of the 20th century, the first easy-open ends appeared making the use of a can opener unnecessary. It took many years for these to be both perfected and accepted, but they are now increasingly being used for a wide range of canned products.

Design, Manufacture and Use

Made from aluminium or steel (tinplate or tin-free steel), these ends can be either full aperture, easy opening for food cans, or the familiar pouring aperture of beverage can ends.

The opening feature for food ends is achieved by means of a score line alongside the double seam and a tab which is lifted and then pulled back to allow the removal of the central panel of the end (see Fig. 4).

The manufacture of this type of end is a very precise operation. Easy-open ends are produced on special press equipment which, in addition to the normal end stamping process which produces the so-called 'shell', has three additional operations: tab manufacture, tab attachment, and rivet formation and scoring. The tab is manufactured from a separate strip of material and is attached to the end by a rivet formation and heading operation (see in Fig. 4).

The scoring operation cuts a V shape in the metal so that metal fracture is initiated from the score when the tab is lifted and pulled. The score can be either external or internal. The lacquer in the scored area may require repair coating, and this is usually achieved by either spraying lacquer, oil or by electrophoretic lacquer application.

Due to the mechanical deformation of the lacquered plate during the production of the score and the rivet, it is necessary to use lacquers with good flexibility and adhesion. The lacquers used may include a range of polymer types such as epoxyphenolics, generally associated with aluminium easy-open ends in contact with non-aggressive foodstuffs, or multilayer systems involving organosol lacquers used on either steel or aluminium ends with more aggressive products. A wide range of easy-open ends sizes are available and, in Europe, the most common are 65, 73, 83 and 99 mm.

Over the last 5 years, a great deal of development has been taking place to improve the ease of opening of steel easy-open ends. These ends are now easier for the consumer to open without compromising the physical performance required for processed cans (see Fig. 4).

Plastic Cans – Metal Can Alternatives

The replacement of the metal can by a more 'modern' pack has been widely researched during the last 30 years.

The Retort Pouch

In the 1970s in Europe and the USA, it was the retort pouch, so dominant in the Japanese processed-food industry, that attracted most attention. The pack is usually manufactured from a flexible laminate of polyester, aluminium foil and polyethylene or polypropylene and heat sealed along its edges.

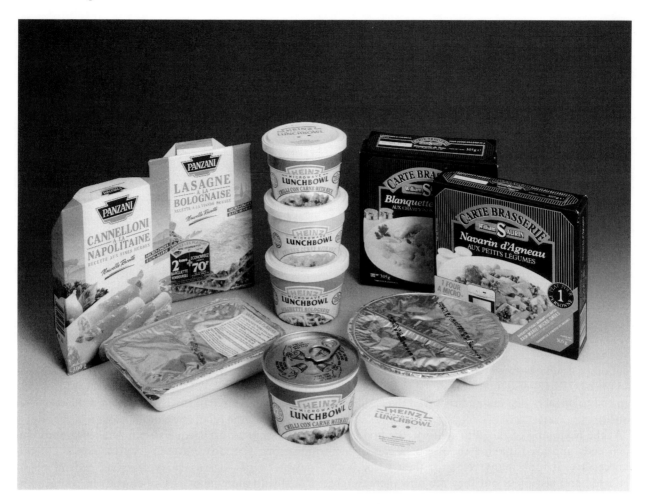

Fig. 5 Plastic cans.

The use of this pouch for some products, e.g. potato rösti, has been, and still is, very successful, as is its use for military rations. Most European ventures, however, did not achieve commercial success, which has been attributed by some to the slow and costly filling and sealing operations and to the lack of acceptance of such packaging by European and North American consumers.

Plastic Cans, Trays and Bowls

A changing lifestyle, a demand for new, high quality, convenience snack meals, and the commercial success of the microwave oven has led to the development of a container that acts both as primary packaging and a vessel to eat from. During the last 5–10 years, the use of retortable plastic packaging for food has increased for the reasons given above, and is considered by many to be still in its infancy. *See* Cooking, Domestic Use of Microwave Ovens; Snack Foods, Range on the Market

Materials and Manufacture

For ambient shelf-stable food products, any polymers used must be both thermally stable, strong and have suitable oxygen-barrier properties. This is normally achieved by using a multilayer structure. The most commonly used structural polymer is polypropylene with ethylvinyl alcohol (EVOH) or polyvinylidene chloride (PVDC) as the barrier layer, sandwiched between the structural polymer. Adhesives are used to tie the layers together, and usually trimmings or reclaim are regranulated and used as a discrete layer in the structure. Sheet is usually coextruded and thermoforming of the containers may take place directly afterwards, or reels of the material may be used to feed a form/fill/seal machine at the filler plant. Examples of containers and their outer packaging are shown in Fig. 5.

Container Closing

Plastic containers may be heat sealed or double seamed with metal ends. Square trays are commonly heat sealed

Recent Developments in Can Design

with metal foil or foil-free lidding which must provide an hermetic seal and be easy to open by the customer. Air in the headspace of the pack may be removed either by vacuum or steam, or the atmosphere may be conditioned with an inert gas during the closing operation.

Distribution

As the container is more susceptible to distribution damage, secondary packaging, such as an overcarton or overcap, is used to protect the lid of the container. This may have a secondary use as a splash guard during microwave reheating.

Summary

The use of modern metal cans manufactured with the latest technology to the highest quality will not on its own assure product quality and safety to the final consumer.

Good manufacturing guidelines for all the processes involved in container raw material selection, can manufacture, can filling, processing and distribution are developed in partnerships between the manufacturers involved, research and trade associations, and universities. These partnerships ensure that all aspects of container manufacturing, filling and distribution are interlinked, and means that the consumer obtains the best safety and quality in canned foods.

Bibliography

Anonymous (n.d.) *A History of Canned Foods.* Reading: Metal Box.

Pilley KP (1968) *Lacquers, Varnishes & Coatings for Food and Drink Cans and for the Metal Decorating Industry.* Birmingham: Holden Surface Coatings.

Rees JAG and Bettison J (eds) (1991) *Processing and Packaging of Heat Preserved Foods.* Glasgow: Blackie & Son Ltd.

Sirbat P (1989) *L'emballage des denrées alimentaires de grande consommation. Les barquettes métalliques et plastiques stérilisables.* Technique & Documentation. Paris: Lavoisier.

Vaher JP (1989) *L'emballage des denrées alimentaires de grande consommation. Les boîtes embouties-réembouties et embouties-étirées.* Technique & Documentation. Paris: Lavoisier.

Pierre Sirbat
CMB Alimentaire, Paris, France
David North
CMB Packaging Technology, Wantage, UK

Food Handling

There is a large variety of affordable, canned foods available on supermarket shelves. These foods comprise the full range of the food groups which include meat, fruit, vegetables, cereals and dairy products. Preparation methods and canning technology vary depending upon the product. Vegetables and fruits are canned directly after harvest and require washing, blanching and sometimes peeling before canning. Meat, once it is butchered, is cut into chunks or minced, while cereals are often used as the ground flour.

Farm produce is generally seasonal and is only available for a matter of weeks each year. Canneries require enough produce during this short time to maintain stock in the supermarket from season to season. This means the scale of operation is in tonnes per hour for sometimes 24 h per day to process enough product while it is available. Mechanical handling and processing systems are essential under these conditions.

Preparation of Vegetables

Vegetables are normally mechanically harvested. Mechanical harvesters do not distinguish between the wanted vegetable material and other extraneous plant material and soil. Some of this is removed by fans and belts on the harvester before the crop is transported to the cannery. Cannery cleaning operations must be very thorough to removed the unwanted material and wash the vegetable.

Cleaning

The preparation of vegetables harvested from under the ground, such as carrots and potatoes, requires the removal of adhering soil and stones. Several systems are available to remove the soil, and they start with dry brushing or soaking to remove the bulk of the dirt, followed by washing. Washing involves wet scrubbing with rotary brushes or rubber fingers, followed by rinsing in a rod washer. In the rod washer, the vegetables are tumbled in a cylinder made from steel rods while being washed by water sprays from inside the cylinder. These vegetables are usually peeled in a subsequent operation which ensures a clean product.

Legumes, such as green peas and beans, are mechanically harvested and transported in bulk ready for canning to the processing plant. Specialized equipment is used, for example, to carry out operations such as husking corn and breaking up clusters of green beans. Dry cleaning with air blowers to remove extraneous leaf material from this type of vegetable is followed by washing in tanks which removes mud balls and stones. Some systems use froth flotation cleaners to remove small pieces of vegetable material. A final rinse with water follows the cleaning treatment to remove the last of the soil.

Leaf vegetables, such as spinach, are difficult to clean

as extraneous material lodges between the leaves. Leaves are cleaned by floating them in tanks of water where the water is agitated with air or water injection. This separates the leaves and removes the soil.

Inspection of the washed vegetable by instruments, such as colour sorters or electronic sorters, at this stage will remove any remaining unwanted material. Manual inspection is still carried out where the removal of specific material cannot be achieved mechanically.

Peeling

Vegetable peeling may be by mechanical cutting or abrasion, by the use of high-pressure steam, or by chemical treatment. Abrasion peeling uses carborundum covered rollers or disks which come in contact with the skin of the tumbled vegetable. The abraded skin is removed with water sprays. To remove material from depressions in the vegetable, some of the flesh of the vegetable is also removed with abrasion and, as such, gives the lowest yield of the three methods.

Vegetables are steam peeled by holding them for a short time in high-pressure steam. This super heats a layer of tissue under the skin. When the pressure is suddenly released the tissue explosively boils releasing the skin from intimate contact with the vegetable. Typical conditions for steam peeling are 17 atmospheres steam pressure for about 30 s. The skin is washed from the vegetable. This system is the most efficient in removing the skin and in yield of peeled vegetable.

A hot lye (sodium hydroxide) solution is used for chemically peeling vegetables and some fruits. It is important that the vegetable is thoroughly washed after peeling to remove all traces of the lye. The treatment varies depending upon the skin to be removed, but a boiling solution of 10% lye will remove most skins in less than 1 min. The skin is removed by rotating brushes or rubber fingers and water sprays. Caustic waste, both liquid and solid, has to be neutralized with acid before disposal which increases the cost of peeling.

Slicing and Dicing

Cutting operations are used to supply the required size of vegetable for canning. Asparagus spears are sawn to the correct length for the can, and carrot and potato are sliced or diced to give an attractive piece of canned vegetable. Canned food in which the particles are of uniform size generally has a superior appearance to that with large variations in particle size. Some dicers are designed to give an irregular-shaped dice so the product looks home-made. The size and shape of the canned vegetable depends upon the style of pack that the market requires.

Preparation of Fruit

Washing

Generally fruit is more easily damaged than vegetables. Therefore, fruit is washed by submersion in tanks of water, which is agitated, followed by water sprays on the elevators as the fruit is removed from the tank. Rod washers may be used with fruit, such as citrus, which are not easily damaged.

Peeling and Pitting

Pome and some stone fruit require peeling and pitting before canning. Pitting is a mechanical operation, and each type of fruit has specialized equipment designed for pit removal. Mechanical apple and pear peelers remove the core section and skin before halving the fruit. Stone fruit that is peeled for canning is usually chemically peeled with lye followed by washing. Other fruit with stems, such as cherries, are rolled over sets of small rotating rollers which pick up the stems and remove them.

Blanching

Blanching is a heat treatment in a near-boiling water or steam followed by rapid cooling given to vegetables and some fruit. Blanching removes gases from within the tissue and softens the product. Blanching makes the product easier to fill into the can and to obtain the correct fill weight. The removal of the gas also reduces the oxidation of the product, maintains the vacuum in the can and prevents excessive can corrosion.

Blanching gives the product another washing treatment and inactivates enzymes which may cause deterioration of the food. Enzyme inactivation is not as important for canned foods as it is for frozen foods, as canned foods receive a far greater heat treatment during thermal processing of the can. It can be important if there is a long delay between filling the can and retorting. Typical blanch times in near boiling water are 60–90 s for small objects, such as green peas and diced carrot, and up to 3 min for larger pieces.

Preparation of Juices

Juices are the liquid which may be squeezed from fruits and vegetables. The major methods of extracting juices are to apply a force to the whole or pulped material followed by screening out pulp from the resultant liquid. This can be carried out continuously in screw presses and belt presses, and there are many different types of batch presses. Citrus fruit is reamed on mechanical reamers or crushed in such a way as to remove the edible portion from the skin. Unwanted material is removed from the juice in paddle or brush finishers, or in some cases small screw presses. These machines push the juice through a screen while separating and removing the pulp which is too large to pass through the screen.

Citrus juice is pasteurized, which is a heat treatment of 95°C, immediately after extraction to inactivate pectinase which will cause the cloud in the juice to 'fall'. The cloud in the juice is held by naturally occurring pectin which, when attacked by pectinase, allows the juice to separate into a clear serum and a solid deposit. Conversely pectinase may be added to other juices, such as apple juice, to manufacture a clear juice. If the juice is not hot-filled it will receive another heat treatment during the canning process.

Meat Preparation

Meat preparation, after slaughter and deboning, mainly consists of removing unwanted tissue such as fat, skin and visible arteries. Meat shrinks by about 30% when it is cooked, so for formulated products using meat it is usually precooked before filling into the cans. Some meat products are corned, which means they are cooked with a cure containing salt and nitrite. Nitrite causes the meat to turn a characteristic pink colour during heating and, because of its antimicrobial action, permits for a less severe heat treatment during retorting. *See* Curing; Meat, Slaughter

Fish such as tuna are cleaned and then steamed to allow for the easy removal of skin and bones. The steamed fillets are filled into a machine which shapes and cuts them to the can size before filling into the can. Other fish are cut to size and filled raw. Fish are canned with brine or oil or, in some cases, a formulated sauce. *See* Fish, Processing

Preparation of Formulated Products

There is an infinite variety of formulated products from meat stews to dairy desserts, and beverages such as beer that are canned. Most of these products are cooked or blended or brewed prior to filling. Those that are cooked in the preparation stage are filled into the can hot.

Carbonated products, such as beer and sparkling fruit juices, are filled at temperatures just above freezing to maintain the carbonation. Soft drinks, although they are often packed in metal cans, are not 'canned products' as preservatives are used to maintain their microbiological stability. *See* Preservation of Food

Cans

Cans are delivered to the factory on pallets. The pallets are automatically unloaded into the can race system.

This delivers the correct size can to the can filler. Canning lines operate between 200 and 2000 cans per minute, so this system must work effectively. Cans may be contaminated so they are thoroughly washed prior to filling.

Filling

There are many types of machines used to fill cans, and the type employed depends, of course, on the product to be filled. Volumetric piston fillers can be used with liquid products and liquid products with entrained solids, such as mushrooms in butter sauce. A turntable is used containing several filling 'heads' so that several cans are filled sequentially as the turntable rotates; filler speed depends upon the number of heads. A slow filler might have 12 heads with high-speed fillers have up to 72 heads.

Tumble fillers are used to fill solid materials, such as vegetable pieces, into cans. The washed cans move through a large rotating drum containing the pieces of product. The product falls into the can and excess is removed by tilting and shaking the can at the exit of the filler. Other volumetric fillers wipe the solid products into pockets on a turntable and the products are then dumped by gravity into the can.

Hand filling is used for products that are difficult to fill by machine. The filling of asparagus into cans can be carried out by machine but, in some cases the tips are damaged, so some processors prefer hand filling.

Some products are canned with syrup or brine. This is a separate operation to filling the solid food. It may take place before or after the filling of the solids. Some solid products may have pockets of air held between the pieces and, in these cases, the liquid is added prior to filling the solids so the liquid will fill these spaces. Sometimes the cans are topped up after the solids are filled.

A headspace must be left in the top of the can after filling. This small space is evacuated on closing, but is important to the integrity of the can. An overfilled can prevents the expansion of the product during the thermal process which may result in permanent damage to the can end. Also the thermal characteristics of the can change, which may invalidate the calculated thermal process.

Exhausting

Oxgyen remaining in the headspace of cans accelerates corrosion of the tin plate in the headspace area. To prevent this occurring, the volume of gas between the product and the lid of the can (known as the headspace) must contain a partial vacuum.

The conventional system of exhausting the cans is to clinch the lid on the can. Clinching is a partial, first operation seaming roll which holds the lid loosely on the can. Exhausting is carried out by passing the filled cans with clinched lids through a steam-filled compartment for several minutes to heat the can contents and displace the air in the can with steam. This is immediately followed by the completion of the seaming operation.

Another method of exhausting is by filling the product hot into the can followed by hot brining or syruping which has the same effect as steam exhausting. This is followed by 'steam flow closing'. Steam is injected between the can and the lid as they come together in the can closer. This displaces the air in the headspace region. When the steam condenses a vacuum is formed in the headspace of the can.

Alternatively, mechanical vacuum pumps can be used to reduce the air in the headspace of the can. This can be done during filling, as fruit may be vacuum syruped by pulling a vacuum on the can and air is replaced by the incoming syrup. Some closers have a vacuum chamber in which the can is seamed. This is common in meat and fish canning, where the canning lines are slowed by the relatively slow operation of the vacuum closer.

Acid products, such as fruit juices, jams, pickles and chutneys, may be filled into the can at near boiling temperatures. The cans are seamed, inverted to sterilize the lid and then cooled. This is called the hot-fill process. The vacuum results from the shrinkage of the product on cooling and the displacement of air by the steam from the hot product.

Can Closing or Seaming

The modern can closer also has a turntable similar to the filler where the cans are fed into a closing 'station'. The lid is aligned over the can and the baseplate of the station raises the can and lid to engage the top chuck. The seaming rollers then roll around the seam to form the seal. The rollers retract, the baseplate is lowered and the closed can exits from the closer. Closers with four to six stations are common.

The seaming operation is carried out by two rolling operations. The first operation roller bends the two flanges together, and the second operation roller flattens them to form a seal. The seal is ensured by a thin layer of mastic-like material deposited in the flange of the can end called 'compound'.

Rates of can seaming depend more on the speed of the filler than that of the can closer. Beverages which are easy to fill can be closed at speeds of 2000 cans per minute. New fillers for semisolid foods, such as pet food, allow closer speeds of about 1300 cans per minute and vegetables are often closed at 500 cans per minute.

Thermal Processing

There are two important factors in canning which make the food safe for long-term storage. Food is sealed to prevent recontamination, and it is heated to inactivate microbes which spoil the food. The seaming operation on the can hermetically seals the food, and the thermal process provides the sterilization step.

Products which have a pH of less than 4·5 are called 'acid foods' and can be thermally processed at temperatures less than 100°C, which is called a pasteurization process. Those with a pH above 4·5 are called 'low-acid foods' and must be thermally processed at temperatures between 110 and 125°C in a retort or pressure vessel.

The details of thermal processing and cooling can be found in the Principles of Canning.

Postprocessing Operation

Cans exiting from water cooling operations are wet with chlorinated water and must be dried before they can be handled safely. Some canners label the cans directly after processing and other palletize the cans for storage before labelling. Lithographed cans do not require further labelling.

Can stores should be maintained at a temperature designed to prevent water vapour condensation which could rust the outside of the cans. The temperature must, however, not be too high as this can, on very rare occasions, promote the growth of heat-resistant thermophilic bacterial spores which may have survived the thermal process.

Cans are held by the canner in store until an incubation period has passed. This provides added protection for the customers as it ensures that only safe wholesome food is placed in the marketplace. All cans are packed in cardboard outers to prevent damage to the cans during transport and handling, and also as a convenient package for the supermarket.

Storage of Canned Food in the Home

Canned food should be stored in a dry cupboard. Most canned food is safe for at least 2 years, but care should be taken to use the oldest cans first. Stock rotation is important at home as well as in the supermarket.

Bibliography

Arthey D and Dennis C (1991) *Vegetable Processing*. Glasgow: Blackie.
Hersom AC and Hulland ED (1980) *Canned foods – Thermal Processing and Microbiology*, 7th edn. Edinburgh: Churchill Livingstone.

Food Handling

Lopez A (1987) *A Complete Course in Canning*, 12th edn. Baltimore: The Canning Trade Inc.

Peter Rutledge
CSIRO Food Processing, North Ryde, Australia

Quality Changes During Canning

Canned foods are a significant component of the diet of most individuals living in developed countries, offering food in a convenient form with year-round availability. The canning process relies on heat treatment for the destruction of microorganisms and preservation of the food, which is then generally considered to have an indefinite microbiological shelf life provided that pack integrity is maintained. The extent of the thermal processing, in terms of both temperature and duration of the treatment, is dependent upon the chemical and physical composition of the product. Both physical and chemical changes occur during processing and, to a lesser extent, during storage, and it is these which determine product quality in terms of its organoleptic properties and nutrient content. These changes, which can be either desirable or undesirable, are influenced by the time and temperature of the process, the composition and properties of the food, and the canning medium. *See* Heat Treatment, Chemical and Microbiological Changes; Storage Stability, Mechanisms of Degradation

This article will consider the changes that can occur during canning and their effect on the quality of the product.

Changes in the Sensory Properties of Foods

The sensory properties of a food – flavour, colour and texture – can all be affected by thermal processing. Changes in these properties may be in the form of either direct effects of heat on food constituents (e.g. starch gelatinization, protein denaturation, and cell separation; see Table 1), or heat-induced reactions such as the Maillard reaction. Significant changes in all three sensory properties can also be brought about by oxidation reactions, which can occur not only during processing but also on subsequent storage of the canned product. *See* Browning, Nonenzymatic; Protein, Interactions and Reactions Involved in Food Processing; Starch, Structure, Properties and Determination

Flavour Changes

The flavour of food can be retained, modified or, occasionally, significantly changed during heat process-

Table 1. The effect of heat processing on sensory quality

Chemical or physical reactions or changes occurring	Impact on sensory attribute
Texture	
Cell membrane damage	Loss of crispness
Cell separation	Loss of firmness
Protein denaturation	Gelling, firming
Starch gelatinization	Gelling
Colour	
Natural pigment breakdown	Bleaching
	Loss of colour
Maillard reactions	Browning
Others, e.g. vitamin C	Discoloration
Flavour	
Volatile loss (scalping oxidation)	Loss of flavour
Volatile formation	
Maillard	Roasted flavour, bitterness
Oxidation	Rancidity
Pyrazines	Roasted flavour

ing, with most of the changes occurring in the volatile flavour components.

Lipid Oxidation

Lipids occur in almost all foodstuffs, and lipid oxidation can therefore occur during canning of most foods. Saturated fatty acids are relatively stable at the temperatures used in standard canning operations, but unsaturated fats are degraded, under the conditions of oxygen and heat, to a large number of volatile compounds, which give rise to both desirable and undesirable flavours. *See* Fatty Acids, Properties; Oxidation of Food Components

The first stage of the oxidation reaction involves uptake of oxygen in the presence of catalysts, such as transition metals and haemoproteins, and is initiated by heat or light. Highly reactive hydroperoxides are formed and these undergo secondary reactions, giving rise to a complex mixture of low-molecular-weight compounds, including aldehydes, ketones, alcohols, acids, alkanes, alkenes and alkynes. A certain level of volatile compounds is generally considered necessary to give characteristic odour and flavour properties to many foods; however, since many of the volatile compounds give rise to typical rancid or stale off-flavours, an ideal balance needs to be achieved in the food.

Maillard Reaction

In foodstuffs, Maillard reactions normally occur between reducing sugars and amino acids or proteins. A very important aspect of the Maillard reaction in food preparation is the production of flavours and aromas. The rate of Maillard reaction increases with temperature, although pH and water content also influence the reaction. Water is essential for the Maillard reaction to occur, with the maximum reaction rate at about 30% moisture level; alkaline pH and the presence of phosphate citrate buffers also accelerate the reaction. The Maillard reaction can be split into three main stages.

The first stage is a condensation reaction between the carbonyl group of a reducing carbohydrate and the free amino group of an amino acid or protein, followed by rearrangement of the resulting glycosylamines into Amadori compounds. These early Maillard reactions can lead to losses in protein quality but do not give rise to flavours in the food.

The second stage involves the advanced Maillard reactions – many complex reactions and pathways that are beyond the scope of this text. It is these reactions which give rise to the many compounds responsible for the flavours and off-flavours in foods. The flavours produced by Maillard reaction can be classified into four main groups: nitrogen heterocyclics and cyclic enolenes, which give characteristic flavours to heated foods, and monocarbonyls and polycarbonyls, which include more volatile supplementary flavours not necessarily associated with product characteristics.

The final stage of the Maillard reaction is the polymerization of the highly reactive compounds formed in the second stage, which results in the formation of brown melanoidin pigments.

Most Maillard reaction products contribute highly desirable flavours to heated foods such as bread, toast, cereal products, meat, etc. These flavours are often described as baked, nutty, roasted, caramel and burnt aromas, but even these can be considered to be off-flavours in certain foods (e.g. the burnt caramel taste in heat-processed milk).

Taints

Other types of off-flavour in canned foods can be caused by contamination of the product leading to an undesirable taint. The range of tainting compounds is enormous, but one particularly unpleasant taint that has been found in a range of foods is the 'catty taint'. This is caused by a heat-dependent reaction between natural-sulphur-containing compounds of the food and unsaturated ketones, such as mesityl oxide, which are widespread in many solvent-based products.

Catty taint has occurred in processed meat products when the meat was stored in a cold store painted with a material containing mesityl oxide as a solvent contaminant; it has also occurred in ox tongues which had been hung on hooks coated with a protective oil, and in pork packed in cans where the side-seam lacquer had been dissolved in an impure solvent. Catty taint has also been

a problem in canned rice pudding where the dye used for printing on the rice sacks contained traces of mesityl oxide, which was picked up by the rice and reacted with the trace amounts of hydrogen sulphide in the milk during processing.

Texture

Canning can bring about both desirable and undesirable changes in texture of foods, through starch gelatinization, protein denaturation, and pectin changes.

Starch Gelatinization

Starch gelatinization commences at a range of temperatures dependent on the type of starch, i.e. proportions of amylose and amylopectin present, and the availability of water. These two components of starch behave differently on canning, with amylose giving an opaque solution that sets to a firm gel on cooling, and with amylopectin forming a translucent paste that remains fluid when cooled. The swelling of the starch granules during canning or other heat processes causes cellular disruption which, together with the starch gelatinization, gives a softening in texture and increased palatability to the product. During canning of vegetables, starch can often be leached into the brine, making it viscous or turbid, e.g. in mature canned peas.

Pectin Changes

Canning of plant materials can lead to loss of semipermeability of cell membranes, and solubilization and breakdown of pectic substances in the cell walls and middle lamellae. The resultant cell separation results in loss of crispness and a softening of the product. This is generally a desirable effect, improving the palatability of foods, but overprocessing can lead to excessive softening of fruits and vegetables. High-temperature processing of certain fruits can lead to an intentional firmness in the product caused by cross-linking of pectins, e.g. in apples and cherries.

Protein Denaturation

Application of heat through the canning process brings about changes in the tertiary structure of proteins, often followed by denaturation which leads to changes in texture. The hydrogen bonds maintaining the secondary and higher structure of the protein rupture and form into a predominantly random coil configuraton, which affects solubility, elasticity and flexibility of the proteins. The sarcoplasmic and myofibrillar proteins in meat coagulate during heat processing, resulting in a firming of the texture, while the collagen proteins become more soluble, softening up as they take up water. The resultant texture of canned meat is similar to that of cooked products. *See* Protein, Chemistry

Colour

Colour changes during canning can be brought about by breakdown of natural pigments, by the production of colours as a result of oxidation reactions, by the Maillard reaction, and by interactions between product constituents, e.g. metals and polyphenolic compounds.

Chlorophyll

Chlorophyll pigments are present in all green vegetables, but canning leads to breakdown with the associated colour change from bright green to olive green or brown. The chlorophyll is converted to pheophytin by the loss of magnesium ions (Mg^{2+}), with heat and low pH during processing greatly accelerating this change. The addition of alkaline salts in the canning liquor to maintain a pH of 6·2–7·0, and high-temperature, short-time (HTST) processing have both been used in canning to reduce chlorophyll degradation. *See* Chlorophyll

Haem Pigments

The red coloration in meat is caused by two haem pigments, haemoglobin in the blood and myoglobin in the muscle tissue; as most of the blood is removed after slaughter, the main pigment is myoglobin. Canning causes oxidation of myoglobin to produce ferrihaemochromagen which gives rise to the typical colour of cooked red meats. It is this reaction which is also the main cause of colour change on canning of dark-fleshed fish, e.g. tuna and mackerel. Overheating during canning can cause a green discoloration as a result of a reaction of myoglobin with hydrogen sulphide, produced from severe protein denaturation, such as that caused by microbial spoilage.

Carotenoids

Carotenoids are fat-soluble, highly unsaturated, red, orange or yellow pigments which are susceptible to oxidation and isomerization under the conditions of heat and low pH, such as those used in the canning process. *See* Carotenoids, Properties and Determination

Carotenoids are generally found complexed with either proteins or fatty acids, which protect them from oxidation, and it is the breakdown of these complexes during processing that leads to degradation of the carotenoids, resulting in blanching or discoloration of the product.

In crustaceans, the denaturation of carotenoprotein on heating releases the carotenoid astaxanthin which causes a change in colour from natural blue-grey to pinky red. Two types of isomerization, *cis-trans* and epoxide, can also occur, and these give rise to a slight lightening in colour.

Anthocyanins

Anthocyanins are water-soluble, red-violet pigments which can take part in a wide range of reactions during canning. A combination of heat and oxygen can lead to the hydrolysis of the glycosidic bonds, resulting in loss of colour and the formation of yellow or brown precipitates; however, low pH gives rise to greater colour stability. Aldehydes, produced by the breakdown of sugars during canning, and ascorbic acid both accelerate the breakdown of the anthocyanins. These colour losses are a particular problem in canned red fruits, e.g. strawberries. *See* Colours, Properties and Determination of Natural Pigments

Anthocyanins can also be produced on thermal processing from leucoanthocyanidins, giving rise to defects such as red gooseberries and dark broad beans. Leucoanthocyanidin and leucoanthocyanin can also form metal complexes with tin and iron from the can, causing pink discoloration, especially in pears and peaches, and 'blueing' of red fruits. Canning of asparagus in lacquered cans can also cause a dark discoloration resulting from the formation of a complex between rutin and iron.

Maillard Reaction

The Maillard reaction, the principles of which are discussed earlier in this article, can cause off colours particularly browning on canning of a wide variety of products.

The browning of navy beans in tomato sauce is primarily due to the formation of melanoidins through the Maillard reaction. Melanoidins are also partly responsible for the browning effect seen in canned apricots. Browning during canning of dark-fleshed fish, such as mackerel and tuna, is of little consequence, but in white fish such discoloration is a major problem and for this reason white fish is not routinely canned. Canning of milk can also lead to a brown tint, although cream is less affected.

Betalains

Betalains are water-soluble and split into two main groups, red-coloured betacyanins and yellow betaxanthins. The most important pigment in this group is betanin, the red pigment in beetroot which is often used as a natural colourant. Betanin is susceptible to oxi-

Table 2. The effect of heat processing on the major nutritional components

Nutrient	Effect
Water	Loss of total solids into canning liquor Dilution Dehydration
Proteins	Enzymic inactivation Loss of certain essential amino acids Loss of digestibility Improved digestibility
Carbohydrates	Starch gelatinization and increased digestibility No apparent change in content of carbohydrate
Dietary fibre	Generally no loss of physiological value
Lipids	Conversion of *cis* fatty acids to *trans* fatty acids by oxidation Loss of essential fatty acid activity
Water-soluble vitamins	Large losses of vitamins C and B_1 due to leaching and heat degradation Increased bioavailability of biotin and nicotinic acid as a result of enzyme inactivation
Fat-soluble vitamins	Mainly heat-stable Losses resulting from oxidation of lipids
Minerals	Losses resulting from leaching Possible increase in sodium and calcium levels by uptake from canning liquor

dation during canning which leads to a loss of colour, although this is often not noticeable because of the large amount present, and may also lead to brown discoloration.

Changes in Nutritional Properties of Foods

During the canning of food, both physical and chemical changes that are capable of affecting its nutritional status may occur. As well as damage to heat-labile nutrients, and physical loss of nutrients as a result of leaching, there are many reactions that occur on canning which affect the availability of nutrients within the foodstuff and, therefore, their usefulness to the body.

If comparing the nutritive value of canned foods with that of fresh foods, it is also important to consider any changes that occur during conventional preparation and cooking techniques (Table 2).

Moisture

The movement of water and solids during canning can cause very major changes in the nutritional status of the foodstuff. If the complete can contents are consumed, these changes can be largely disregarded, but when the canning liquor is discarded the effects of dilution, dehydration and loss of total solids must be taken into consideration. Dilution or dehydration will affect the relative proportions of other constituents in the food, while soluble nutrients can be leached into the liquor.

Proteins

Heating of proteins, as in canning, causes denaturation, rupturing of the hydrogen bonds and other noncovalent bonds, leading to changes in the conformation of the protein. The degree of denaturation depends on the level of heat treatment applied, but it can also be caused by oxidation and reaction with other food constituents, e.g. reducing sugars and lipid oxidation products. The total level of crude protein is generally unaffected by canning but both desirable and undesirable changes can occur in its nutritive quality and availability. Mild heating of proteins leads only to changes in tertiary structure which have little nutritional effect, although there is usually a loss in solubility. More severe heating, as in canning of vegetables, results in the Maillard reaction and the consequent loss in protein quality. These reactions occur mainly between lysine and sugars and cause a loss in availability of lysine, through cross-linking, with a loss of up to 40% observed on canning of potatoes. Canning of meat also leads to the reduction in availability of lysine and other essential sulphur-containing amino acids, and it may lead to a reduction in the digestibility of the meat.

The losses in protein availability that occur under normal canning conditions are, however, quite small and not nutritionally significant for most people in developed countries, as lysine is rarely the limiting amino acid in the diet. Canning may even lead to improved protein availability and digesitibility by denaturing antidigestive factors and by denaturing proteins. Some examples of advantageous effects of heat processing are mentioned below.

Heating of milk results in the proteins being precipitated by stomach acids as finely dispersed particles, making attack by digestive enzymes more effective than in raw milk. This can also enhance the formation of disulphide bonds, e.g. between β-lactoglobulin and κ-casein which leads to greater stability of the normally unstable β-lactoglobulin. The canning of legumes improves their digestibility, by unfolding of the major seed globulins, as well as increasing nutritional availability, especially of the sulphur-containing amino acids, by inactivation of trypsin inhibitors.

Quality Changes During Canning

Lipids

The nutritive value of the fat content of foods is not generally significantly altered during normal heat processing. Hydrolysis reactions that result in separaton of the fatty acids from the glycerol unit may occur, but this does not adversely affect the nutritional value of the fat as the resulting free fatty acids are available for digestion.

Saturated lipids are relatively stable, but unsaturated lipids are prone to oxidation when heated in the presence of oxygen or air. The exclusion of oxygen or use of antioxidants can be used to prevent the oxidation of lipids during canning, so that losses in the nutritional value of fats are unlikely to be significant. However, it is worth considering the effects of lipid oxidation, as any contact with oxygen during the history of the food can be sufficient for oxidation reactions to occur. *See* Antioxidants, Natural Antioxidants; Antioxidants, Synthetic Antioxidants

The major effect of lipid oxidation reactions is related to the flavour of food, but they can result in the conversion of *cis* fatty acids to *trans* fatty acids. The nutritional value in terms of energy is similar for the two fatty acid types, but the *trans* fatty acids do not generally possess essential fatty acid activity. The availability of the fat-soluble vitamins A, D and E, as well as vitamin C and folate, can also be reduced during lipid oxidation.

Carbohydrates

Carbohydrates have numerous characteristic properties, and the effects of canning are therefore varied. The levels of total and available carbohydrates have been found to be unaffected during canning of fruit and vegetables. In general, the effects of canning on carbohydrates are related not directly to their nutritional value but to their interaction with other food constituents and to the overall eating quality of the foodstuff. *See* Carbohydrates, Interactions with Other Food Components

On canning, reducing sugars can react with protein through the Maillard reaction, which causes loss in availability of certain amino acids. Other effects include increased bioavailability of iron through complexing with sugar molecules, and the breakdown of vaccinin, a natural sugar ester in cranberries, to produce benzoic acid which acts as a preservative.

Gelatinization of the starch granules improves the texture and, thereby, palatability of the food; it also aids digestibility of the food to the extent that many foods (e.g. potatoes, rice) are largely indigestible in the raw state.

The other constituent of carbohydrate in food is dietary fibre, which consists mainly of cellulose. Cellulose and other polysaccharides (i.e. hemicelluloses and pectins) are largely responsible for texture and structure of plant foods. *See* Dietary Fibre, Properties and Sources

Canning appears to have little effect on total dietary fibre levels, but the exact effects of canning on the various constituents of dietary fibre, and the effect of heat-induced fibre breakdown, are not fully known.

Minerals

Total mineral levels are not generally adversely affected by the canning process because they are relatively stable under conditions of heat, acid or alkali. However, minerals are susceptible to changes in bioavailability due to interactions with other food components. The bioavailability of iron can be enhanced during canning in the presence of vitamin C, or reducing sugars with which it forms available complexes. Oxalates, however, which occur naturally in many acidic plants, can inhibit calcium bioavailability. *See* Bioavailability of Nutrients; Minerals, Dietary Importance

The major changes that can occur in mineral levels on canning are caused by movement between the foodstuff and the canning liquor. Certain minerals, especially sodium and calcium, can be taken up by the food from the canning liquor; this can be seen especially during the canning of vegetables in brine. Minerals can also be leached out from the foodstuff into the canning liquor. Potassium is particularly prone to leaching, with losses of between 15% and 50% observed on canning of vegetables, while zinc, manganese and cobalt are also susceptible to leaching. *See* individual minerals

Storage of canned vegetables shows no further substantial changes in sodium or calcium levels, but slight further leaching of potassium and zinc does occur (Table 3).

Vitamins

Most vitamins are unstable under conditions of heat and are therefore susceptible to loss during the canning process. The fat-soluble vitamins are generally more stable than the water-soluble vitamins, but losses can occur during canning as a result of oxidation. Carotenoids are particularly prone to oxidation during heat processing, but this can be greatly reduced by the addition of antioxidants, e.g. vitamin C. *See* Vitamins, Overview

Losses of water-soluble vitamins during canning can be quite considerable, with vitamin C being the most labile. Vitamin C can be lost through the following processes: (1) oxidation, which can occur in the early stages of heat treatment before the ascorbic oxidase is inactivated; (2) chemical degradation, e.g. losses due to nonenzymatic browning reactions in fruit products with

Table 3. Mineral content (mg per 100 g, on a wet weight basis) in freshly cooked and canned cooked peas

Sample	Calcium	Sodium	Potassium	Zinc	Iron
Fresh	48	65	179	0·82	1·4
Zero time canned	47	320	152	1·0	1·4
Canned stored:					
3 months	40	315	79	0·72	1·3
6 months	31	—	82	0·44	0·9
9 months	28	295	84	0·53	1·5
12 months	—	280	108	0·55	1·2

high vitamin C levels; (3) through leaching into the canning liquor, which is generally the major cause of vitamin C loss in canned fruits and vegetables. The level of vitamin C remaining in canned vegetables has been shown to be as low as 20% of the vitamin C found in the fresh raw produce; however, vitamin C is lost during all stages of fresh storage, preparation, cooking or processing, and some canned vegetables have similar levels of vitamin C to the fresh product which had been stored prior to cooking. Thiamin is the most heat-sensitive of the B vitamins, especially under alkaline conditions. Thermal degradation of thiamin involves the cleavage of its methylene bridge, which gives rise to many volatile products. In the presence of reducing sugars, thiamin may take part in nonenzymatic browning reactions, and it also reacts with aldehydes in the presence of ascorbic acid. Thiamin can be lost through leaching, but it is less labile than vitamin C, and retention levels of between 60% and 90% are usual on canning. *See* Ascorbic Acid, Properties and Determination; Thiamin, Properties and Determination

Folic acid is lost on canning through heat degradation and oxidation, although it is stabilized in the presence of ascorbic acid, while pyridoxine can be lost through heat degradation and leaching. Losses of these two vitamins during canning of fruits and vegetables range between 30% and 80%. Losses on canning of meat can be very considerable, up to 90%. *See* Folic Acid, Properties and Determination; Vitamin B₆, Properties and Determination

Riboflavin and nicotinic acid are both relatively heat-stable, with minimal losses on canning of meat products; however, losses of between 20% and 50% have been found on storage of canned meats. Losses seen during the canning of fruits and vegetables, ranging from 25% to 70%, are mainly attributed to leaching. Nicotinic acid and riboflavin both show very high retention levels during milk processing, but riboflavin is lost from bottled milk as it is very sensitive to sunlight. *See* Niacin, Properties and Determination; Riboflavin, Properties and Determination

As can be seen, heat processing generally has a detrimental effect on most vitamin levels, but mild heating conditions can have a beneficial effect due to enzyme inactivation and the breakdown of binding agents which increases the bioavailability of certain vitamins, e.g. biotin and nicotinic acid. *See* Biotin, Properties and Determination

The canning of foods results in a wider choice of nutritious, good-quality foods available all year round in a convenient form for the consumer. When considering the quality of canned foods it is important to compare them with fresh or frozen foods at the point of consumption.

Many of the changes that occur in both sensory and nutritional aspects do so during any thermal process, whether it is conventional cooking, blanching or canning. For most foods the canning process replaces a conventional cooking process, and any mild reheating stage has no further significant effect on quality.

Losses in heat-labile nutrients such as vitamins can be significant. However, as canned products are usually produced from materials at optimum maturity and immediately after harvest, levels are often as high as the 'fresh' material purchased from the greengrocers and prepared in the home.

Bibliography

Bender AE (1978) *Food Processing and Nutrition*. London: Academic Press.

Hall MN, Edwards MC, Murphy MC and Pither RJ (1989) *A comparison of the composition of canned, frozen and fresh garden peas as consumed*. Technical Memorandum No. 553, Chipping Campden, UK: Campden Food and Drink Research Association.

Moyem T and Kvale O (eds) (1977) Physical, chemical and biological changes in food caused by thermal processing. Essex: Applied Science Publishers.

Priestley RJ (ed.) (1979) *Effects of Heating on Foodstuffs*. Essex: Elsevier Science Publishers.

Richardson T and Finley JW (eds) (1985) *Chemical Changes in Food during Processing*. Westport, Connecticut: AVI Publishing.

R. J. Pither
Campden Food and Drink Research Association, Chipping Campden, UK

Quality Changes During Canning

CARAMEL

Contents

Properties and Analysis

Home cooks used to burn sugar to obtain so-called caramel for flavouring food. Commercial caramel differs from the domestic product by its method of preparation and consequently in many of its properties. Several products called caramel are available commercially. Tables presented in this article summarize their physical and chemical properties and analytical problems are also discussed.

Definition of the Product

Caramel is a brown product originating from various sugars when they are heated either dry or in concentrated solutions and alone or with certain additives. It is designed as a food additive or ingredient for colouring and/or flavouring food.

In some countries the name 'caramel' is reserved for products manufactured from saccharides in the absence of nitrogen-containing compounds. Such products are used as flavouring ingredients. The products resulting from heating sugars with nitrogen-containing additives are called 'sugar colours' and they serve as colouring additives. *See* Colours, Properties and Determination of Natural Pigments; Flavour Compounds, Structures and Characteristics

Types and Standardization

The origin and properties of caramel are laid down in many producing countries. Also, the use of only a few, among many reported additives, is permitted in the manufacture of caramels. The World Health Organization and the Food and Agriculture Organization Joint Expert Committee on Food Additives distinguishes three general kinds of caramel: (1) caramel colour, plain (CP), (2) caramel colour, ammonia process or caustic (AC), and (3) caramel colour, ammonium sulphite process (SAC), depending on the additive used in their manufacture. Both the European Technical Caramel Association (EUTECA) and the International Technical Caramel Association (ITCA) have standardized the properties of four classes and 10 types of caramel (see Table 1).

4(5)-Methylimidazole in ammonia and ammonium sulphite caramel colours causes a special problem. This compound, which is formed from sugars and ammonia during manufacture of the caramel, is strongly neurotoxic. For this reason the daily intake of food containing ammonia caramel is controlled in some countries and in others ammonia caramel is banned.

Physical Properties

Caramel is polymeric in its character. Three main components of the plain type are called caramelan, caramelen and caramelin. Ammonia caramels additionally contain melanoidin, which is much darker in colour than the three other components mentioned above. Hence, ammonia caramels are the most intensively coloured.

Depending on their isoelectric points (pIs) caramels may be roughly divided into positive (pI 5·0–7·0), negative (pI 4·0–6·0) and spirit (pI < 3·0) types. The pI determines the possibility of application of caramels. The average molecular weight of compounds in caramels is between 5000 Da (electropositive caramels) and 10 000 Da (electronegative caramels). Other important properties are pH (see Table 1), aqueous solubility (should be completely soluble), specific gravity (usually 1·315 to 1·345), colour intensity (see Table 1) or tinctorial strength, hue index (called 'redness') as well as flavour and aroma. These last two organoleptic properties consist of two components: taste arising from the acidity (modifiable) and a taste contribution attributed to the nature of caramel (nonmodifiable).

Chemical Nature

The products of caramelization are distributed among volatile and nonvolatile fractions. The volatile fraction consists mainly of water, carbon monoxide, carbon dioxide, formaldehyde, acetaldehyde, methanol and ethanol. The composition of the low-molecular-weight portion of the nonvolatile fraction depends on the type of caramel. The plain caramel nonvolatile fraction

Table 1.   Classes of caramel colour according to ITCA/EUTECA

Class	Sort	Type	Colour intensity (ε_M at 610 nm)	EBC units ($\times 10^3$)	Dry residue (%)	4-Methylimidazole (mg kg^{-1})	Total nitrogen(%)	Total sulphur (%)	Ammonia nitrogen (%)	Sulphur dioxide (%)
I	Caramel colour, plain	CP-1	5–35	2–12	55–75	<25	<0·1	<0·1	<0·01	<0·005(<0·1)
		CP-2	40–80	15–25						
II	Caramel colour, caustic sulphite	CCS-1	40–80	15–25	62–82	<25	<0·1	0·15–2·5	<0·01	0·15
III	Caramel colour, ammonia	AC-1	60–90	16–24	55–75	<200	0·5–3·0	<0·3 (<0·7)	<0·5	<0·015(<0·02)
		AC-2	100–140	27–37·5			0·5–5·0			
		AC-3	150–200	40–54			1·5–6·5			
IV	Caramel colour, ammonium sulphite	SAC-1	35–70	8–16	55–75	0·1–1·3	0·3–2·0	0·3		0·08
		SAC-2	75–100	17·5–23		0·5–2·8	0·8–3·2 (<0·7)	0·5 (<0·5)		0·12 (<0·1)
		SAC-3	105–150	22·5–37		0·8–2·8	1·0–4·0	0·8		0·15
		SAC-4	210–270	40–52	47–57	2·0–4·0	1·0–5·0	1·5		0·28

The values in parentheses are FAO/WHO proposals dating from 1980. Permissible content (in mg kg^{-1}) of the heavy metals in caramel according to FAO/WHO standards are: total, 25; copper, 20; lead, 5; astatine, 3; mercury, 0·1. ε_M, Molar extinction coefficient; EBC, European Brewery Convention.

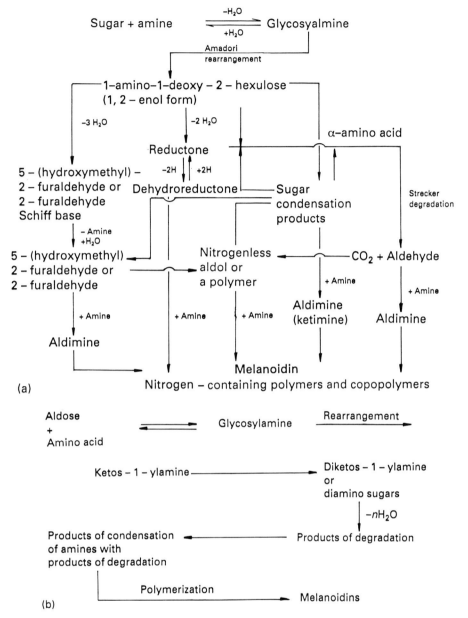

Fig. 1 Theoretical schemes for the formation of melanoidins according to (a) Hodge and (b) Reynolds.

contains the following saccharides: D-fructose, D-glucose, kojibiose, isomaltose, nigerose, sophorose, laminarabiose, maltose, gentobiose, cellobiose, isomaltotriose, panose and other oligosaccharides. There are also several carboxylic acids: formic acid and higher fatty acids, succinic, fumaric, pyruvic, levulinic and furancarboxylic acids. Oxaheterocycles are represented by 2-furaldehyde, 5-(hydroxymethyl)-2-furaldehyde, 2,3-dihydro-4-hydroxy-5-methylfuran-3-one, 2,3-dihydro-4-hydroxy-2-(hydroxymethyl)-5-methylfuran-3-one, bis(5,5-formylfurfuryl) ether and 2,3-dihydro-3,5-dihydroxy-6-methyl-4*H*-pyran-4-one. There are also various other aliphatic carbonyl compounds like glucoreductone (2-hydroxypropandial), pyruvaldehyde and α,β-unsaturated carbonyl compounds. A number of

other components which are products of reversion and polymerization remain uncharacterized. The low-molecular-weight fraction of caustic caramel contains about 50 components. Ammonia caramel contains in this fraction a certain amount of 4(5)-methylimidazole, 2-acetyl-4(5)-(1,2,3,4-tetrahydroxybutyl)imidazole and 3-hydroxy-6-methylpyridine, as well as at least 143 other components, including those mentioned above. *See* Carbohydrates, Classification and Properties; Fatty Acids, Properties; Fructose; Sucrose, Properties and Determination

The high-molecular-weight, nonvolatile fraction of plain caramels is composed of 1,6-anhydro-α-D-glucose, caramelan (formed in the reaction shown in eqn [1]), caramelen (resulting from the reaction shown in eqn [2]), caramelin (being the product of reaction shown in eqn [3]), structures of which remain unknown, and polymers composed of furan ring units.

$$6C_{12}H_{22}O_{11} \xrightarrow{-12H_2O} 6C_{12}H_{18}O_9 \qquad (1)$$

$$6C_{12}H_{22}O_{11} \xrightarrow{-18H_2O} 2C_{36}H_{48}O_{24} \qquad (2)$$

$$6C_{12}H_{22}O_{11} \xrightarrow{-27H_2O} 3C_{24}H_{26}O_{13} \qquad (3)$$

The interpretation of carbon-13 cross-polarized magic-angle sample spinning nuclear magnetic resonance (^{13}C CP/MAS NMR) spectra of plain caramels leads to the conclusion that there are 8–9% carbonyl and aldehyde carbon atoms, 7–7.7% carbon atoms in ester groups, 33–31% heterocyclic carbon atoms and 52.4–51.2% alkyl groups bonded to carbon atom and to oxygen. It may also be deduced that the furan system prevails among other heterocyclic systems present in caramel. *See* Spectroscopy, Nuclear Magnetic Resonance

Two consecutive steps may be distinguished in the formation of caramels without participation of either ammonia, ammonium sulphite, amines or amino acids and their salts, which may also be used as the catalysts. They are degradation reactions which lead to colourless or yellow compounds. First, water and carbon dioxide are evolved and furan derivatives are formed (2-furaldehyde from furanoses and 5-(hydroxymethyl)-2-furaldehyde from pyranoses). This step is a function of both temperature and time; atmospheric oxygen plays some role in the final stage. This is followed by the second step, polymerization and condensation reactions forming highly coloured compounds (caramelan, caramelen and caramelin as well as furan polymers).

In caramels manufactured with basic nitrogen-containing additives, melanoidins are the most important components. Their structure is unknown, but there is evidence that they have, at least in part, an amide structure. Moreover, they contain unpaired electrons, i.e. they have a free radical character. There is a great similarity between this product and humic acids resulting from the Maillard reaction. Two consistent schemes for the formation of melanoidins are proposed by Hodge (Fig. 1(a) and Reynolds (Fig. 1(b)). Both theories differ in the number of steps involved in the route from the preliminary reaction between sugar and amine to give glycosylamine and the final product – melanoidin. Recent studies have revealed that the possibility of the Strecker degradation as one of the processes involved should be rejected. *See* Browning, Nonenzymatic

Properties and Analysis

Table 2. Tests for particular types of caramel

Type of caramel[a]	Citric acid[b,c]	Alcohol[b,c]	Lassaigne
Spirit caramel			
I A	+	−	−
I B	−	−	−
I C	+	−	−
Non-ammonia caramel			
II	+	−	−
Beer caramel			
III A	−	±	+
III B	−	−	+
III C	−	+	+
Soft drink caramel			
IV A	−	+	+
IV B	−	+	+

[a] Consult also Tables 1 and 3 for classification of types.
[b] Formation of a precipitate.
[c] Solubility in citric acid–monosodium phosphate at pH 2.5.
[d] Solubility in 13:7 (v/v) ethanol–water.

Analysis of Caramels

The use of caramel is first of all limited by its type, which affects its use for a given food. For instance, a caramel may precipitate on contact with a product subjected to coloration, as a result of discharge of caramel micelles. The type and quality of caramel may easily be recognized by means of the citric acid, alcohol and Lassaigne tests (see Table 2). However, the complexity of caramel composition makes distinguishing between the different types difficult unless combined analytical methods are applied. These include chromatography of dilute solutions of caramel followed by thin-layer electrophoresis and size exclusion chromatography. Thus, full standardization of caramel may require many other determinations of chemical components as well as fractions, as shown in Table 3. This table presents several properties of certain types of caramel manufactured from sucrose. It is apparent that, for instance, two I CP-2 caramels listed therein differ from one another in the majority of their properties. It is a matter of discussion whether these findings will result in further attempts to standardize caramels within subtypes. These differences may also be considered as resulting from difficulties in the strict control of the caramelization process, which tends to be rather chimeric. *See* Chromatography, Principles; Electrophoresis

Determination of the pI may be carried out by means of electrophoresis, the flocculation test with tannin, ionic surface-active agents (an industrial approximate measure), the gelatin test and other more specific methods.

Table 3.   Analytical characteristics of some classes, sorts, types and subgroups of caramel colours

Properties	Type (carbohydrate, additive)						II (sucrose, sodium sulphite)
	I A (sucrose, sodium carbonate)			I B (sucrose, acid)			
	CP-2	CP-1	CP-2	CP-1	CP-1	CP-1	CCS
pH	3·7	3·1	3·1	3·6	3·9	3·5	3·0
Neutralization							
Nitric acid test	+	+	+	+	−	−	+
Alcohol test	−	−	−	−	−	−	−
Colour intensity (ε_{max})	65	32	71	29	38	29	100
Dry substance (%)	65·2	69·6	64·1	74·1	70·3	72·8	95·0
Ash (%)	0·55	1·16	0·47	0·09	0·38	0·06	0·07
Sodium (mg kg^{-1})	1825	2398	1856	126	1422	151	57
Sulphur dioxide (mg kg^{-1})	NF	NF	NF	NF	NF	NF	66
Sulphates in ash (%)	NF	NF	NF	NF	NF	NF	NF
Total nitrogen (%)	0·08	NF	NF	NF	NF	NF	NF
Basic nitrogen (mg kg^{-1})	NF	NF	NF	NF	NF	NF	
Formic acid (mg kg^{-1})	455	577	664	249	384	343	200
Glucose (%)	3·7	14·5	9·3	24·8	7·0	16·6	2·3
Fructose (%)	3·1	11·2	7·9	15·6	2·0	3·8	0·4
Sucrose (%)	0·6	NF	NF	NF	NF	0·8	NF
4-Methylimidazole (mg kg^{-1})	NF	NF	NF	NF	NF	NF	NF
'Glucoreductone' (%)	0·15	0·23	0·25	0·05	0·05	0·06	0·18
Gel permeation analysis							
Colour between R_{gp}	0·5–1·75	0·39–1·66	0·36–1·65	0·06–1·13	−0·02–10·7	−0·02–1·02	−0·05–1·39
Maxima at R_{gp}	0·98	0·91	0·91	0·35	0·32	0·32	0
	1·32	1·16	1·16	0·81	0·61	0·84	0·55
				0·96	0·86		1·09
Minima at R_{gp}	1·18	1·02	1·02	0·74, 0·87	0·56, 0·77	0·73	0·91

	III A (sucrose, ammonium carbonate)			III B (sucrose, ammonia)		
	AC 2	AC 3	AC 2	AC 1	AC 1	AC 2
pH	4·7	5·6	5·7	5·3	4·1	4·5
Neutralization		+	+	+	+	
Citric acid test	−	−	−	−	−	−
Alcohol test	−	+	+	−	−	−
Colour intensity (ε_{max})	108	194	113	79	86	99
Dry substance (%)	63·4	93·6	70·5	60·9	62·6	64·1
Ash (%)	0·30	0·58	0·27	0·36	0·45	0·38
Sodium (mg kg^{-1})	1198	1688	−	1265	1355	953
Sulphur dioxide (mg kg^{-1})	NF	NF	NF	NF	NF	NF
Sulphates in ash (%)	NF	NF	NF	NF	NF	NF
Total nitrogen (%)	4·73	6·7	2·5	4·70	4·95	4·45
Basic nitrogen (mg kg^{-1})	240	1690	NF	250	180	220
Formic acid (mg kg^{-1})	673	491	296	542	415	671
Glucose (%)	23·0	3·5	10·0	25·8	23·7	16·1
Fructose (%)	10·9	NF	8·0	10·7	8·9	5·1
Sucrose (%)	1·7	NF	NF	NF	5·4	3·1
4-Methylimidazole (mg kg^{-1})	128	119	51	118	151	47
'Glucoreductone' (%)	0·54	0·53	0·44	0·54	0·62	0·54
Gel permeation analysis						
Colour between R_{gp}	−0·99–1·66	−0·07–1·75	−0·09–1·69	0·41–1·80	0·39–1·73	0·54–1·61
Maxima at R_{gp}	0	0	0	0·84	0·91	0·97
	0·93	0·89	0·93	1·30	1·34	1·27
	1·23	1·18	1·23			
Minima at R_{gp}	0·07	0·25	0·09	1·02	1·04	1·11
	1·05	1·05	1·05			

(continued)

Table 3. (*continued*)

Properties	Type (carbohydrate, additive)		
	IV A (sucrose, ammonium sulphite)		
	SAC 2	SAC 3	SAC 2
pH	4·1	5·8	3·9
Neutralization		+	
Citric acid test	−	−	−
Alcohol test	+	+	+
Colour intensity (ε_{max})	78	123	98
Dry substance (%)	65·0	68·3	68·4
Ash (%)	1·80	2·18	1·96
Sodium (mg kg^{-1})	5230	5307	5540
Sulphur dioxide (mg kg^{-1})	369	337	234
Sulphates in ash (%)	49·6	67·1	54·5
Total nitrogen (%)	1·35	1·17	1·17
Basic nitrogen (mg kg^{-1})	260	150	280
Formic acid (mg kg^{-1})	277	438	393
Glucose (%)	28·8	31·4	28·5
Fructose (%)	3·8	NF	NF
Sucrose (%)	12·0	NF	NF
4-Methylimidazole (mg kg^{-1})	117	40	37
'Glucoreductone' (%)	0·07	0·09	0·09
Gel permeation analysis			
Colour between R_{gp}	−0·07–1·39	−0·04–1·34	−0·55–1·39
Maxima at R_{gp}	0	0	0
	0·30	0·27	0·27
	0·98	0·93	0·93
Minima at R_{gp}	0·09	0·07	0·09
	0·93	0·91	0·91

NF, not found; R_{gp}, retention factor on Sepharose C1-6B (calculated from retention volumes of caramel components relative to those of Blue Dextran and $NaHCO_3$).
Data abstracted from Hellwig E *et al.* (1981).

Table 4. Methods of detection of caramel in food

Method	Reagent	Appearance
Jaegerschmidt	Resorcinol + hydrochloric acid, ether or acetone	Red colour in ether Violet red colour in acetone
Amthor	Paraldydehyde + absolute alcohol	Brown precipitate after 24 h which reacts with phenylhydrazine hydrochloride to give a solid insoluble in hydrochloric acid but soluble in ammonia and alkali
Griessmeyer–Aubry	Ammonium sulphate in 96% ethanol	Yellow to brown colour
Lichthard	Tannin + sulphuric acid	Brown solid within 24 h
Fradiss	Dry 1-pentanol	A precipitate
Crampton–Simons	Floridin, Tonsil or Fuller's earth	Decoloration of aqueous or ethanol solutions in caramel followed by colorimetric determination of resulting colour
Straub	1% aqueous $SnCl_2$ + potassium acetate	Light yellow colour and precipitate
Nessler–Carles	Fresh egg white	Brown to orange colour
Ihl	Pyrogallic acid in hydrochloric acid	Dark red precipitate
Magalhaes	K_2SO_4 + cotton wool	Light orange colour on boiling for 10 min
Schenck	Phenol or 2-naphtol	Red brown colour immediately (phenol) or after 30 min (2-naphthol)

Isolation and separation of caramelan, caramelen and caramelin may be achieved by dialysis, electrofiltration through an ion exchange membrane or by determining solubilities in different solvents (84% aqueous ethanol, 1-propanol). Fractionation by gel filtration and adsorption on either charcoal or using ion exchangers are recommended mainly for elimination and separation of overall colouring matter from caramel. Anionic resins exhibit particular selectivity towards caramelan, which is adsorbed, leaving caramelen and caramelin in the unadsorbed state.

The determination of 4(5)-methylimidazole in ammonia caramel involves chromatographic techniques. Thus, extracts of caramels are developed on silica gel F_{254}-coated plates using a 4:1:1 ether–chloroform–methanol mixture (sodium nitrite with sulphanilic acid are used as a spray). Gas–liquid chromatography involves columns packed with 10% carbowax 20M with 25% potassium hydroxide on CPLA (80–100 mesh). *See* Chromatography, Gas Chromatography

There are several methods of detection of caramel in food. These are presented in Table 4. Furthermore, physical methods based on size exclusion chromatography and spectral measurements in the ultraviolet and visible region have recently been developed.

Bibliography

FAO Nutritional Meeting Report Series, No. 57. Geneva: Food and Agriculture Organization.
Greenshields RN and Macgillivray AW (1972) Caramel. 1. Browning reactions. *Process Biochemistry* 7(12): 11–13, 16.
Hellwig E, Gombocz E, Frischenschlager S and Petuely F (1981) Detection and identification of caramel color by gel permeation chromatography. *Deutsche Lebensmitteln Rundschau* 77: 165–174.
ITCA/EUTECA (1979) *ITCA/EUTECA Specifications for Caramel Color, 3rd Meeting of EUTECA Sub-Committee Specifications*, 4th May Paris: European Technical Caramel Association.
Tomasik P, Palasinski M and Wiejak S (1989) The thermal decomposition of carbohydrates. Part I. The decomposition of mono-, di, and oligosaccharides. *Advances in Carbohydrate Chemistry and Biochemistry* 47: 203–278.
Truhaut R, Vitte G and Lassale-Saint-Jean V (1962) Bibliographic study of caramel. *Bulletin de la Societe Pharmaceutique Bordeaux* 101: 97–120.
WHO (1977) *WHO Technical Report Series*, No. 617. Geneva: World Health Organization.

P. Tomasik
University of Zimbabwe, Harare, Zimbabwe

Methods of Manufacture

Commercial caramels, even if manufactured from the same materials, may have different properties depending on the additives used and the conditions of caramelization. Caramelization itself is a very chimeric process and the manufacture of caramel is sometimes considered to be an art. Ready made caramel is a rather unstable product and its storage is also a very important factor. The problems of production and storage of caramel are presented below.

Applications of Caramel

The classification of caramel into four classes results from the properties of the product and its intended food application. Thus, caramel of class I (CP-1 and CP-2) is designed as an additive to spirits, brandy, sweets, medicines, biscuits, pastries, aromas and spices. Caramel of class II (CSS-1) has very limited applications as it is used for special spirits as a flavouring rather than a colouring agent. Class III caramel (AC-1, AC-2 and AC-3) is used as brown colour for beer, malt liquor, bread, biscuits, pastries, soups, sauces, canned food, meat, tobacco and some spices. Finally, class IV caramel (SC-1 to SAC-4) is the colorant of cola-type beverages, soft drinks, vermouths and vinegar. The use of caramels for nonfood purposes is of marginal importance. The data published for 1986 set the world production at the level of 60000 tonnes: in the USA caramel of class IV was the only product manufactured to any significant extent (95% of overall production) whereas in the EEC the manufacture of both class IV (50%) and class III (45%) caramels was important (class I, 4%; class II, 1%) *See* Colours, Properties and Determination of Natural Pigments; Flavour Compounds, Structures and Characteristics

The isoelectric point and tinctorial strength are the most important criteria for selecting a class of caramel for a given purpose. However, flavour is also an important property. Incorrectly selected caramels can produce a haze in drinks and flocculation as well as nonuniform shades in finished products. Beer caramel (class III) has to withstand fermentation. The composition of caramel micelles, especially their calcium content, is another factor which can cause turbidity in some drinks finished with caramel. Caramel in brandy (0·2% v/v) accelerates its ageing. Aspartame in drinks is stabilized by the addition of caramel. Oriental cuisines commonly utilize caramel for colouring and flavouring soups, gravies and sauces, e.g. soy sauce (shoyu).

Sources for Manufacture

Some authors report that the quality of caramel depends, among other aspects, on its source. However, some authors express the opposite point of view, claiming that only parameters of caramelization (including catalysing additives) are responsible for the quality of the final product. Undoubtedly the presence of amino acids, proteins and hydroxy acids in materials used for caramelization contributes additional flavour and other specific organoleptic properties to the final product. As a matter of fact such additives have a catalysing role in the formation of the brown-coloured components of caramel. There is also some relationship between the content of D-glucose in the stock and firmness of caramel. D-Glucose decreases the hygroscopicity and maltose has practically no effect on it.

Sucrose as well as D-glucose and D-fructose, both resulting from its hydrolysis, are prime sources for the manufacture of caramel. Reducing sugars caramelize more readily than nonreducing sugars. The mode of preparation of sugar for caramelization has some influence on the caramelization process. Sugar from carbonation is better than that from sulphination as residual carbonates catalyse the caramelization better than sulphites. *See* Fructose; Sucrose, Properties and Determination

Other mono- and disaccharides have also been considered as sources of caramels, but they are only of theoretical importance. Molasses has attracted the attention of manufacturers as a relatively inexpensive source of caramel because of its brown components. A disadvantage in the the use of molasses is its high potassium content and the unfavourable viscosity of the resulting caramel. *See* Carbohydrates, Classification and Properties

Many reasons, among them economic and political, make sucrose, invert sugar and D-glucose rather unfavourable sources for the production of caramel. Oligo- and polysaccharides, which are hydrolysed by acids, bases or enzymes, provide a source of very stable caramels. Maize, cassave, sago and potato starch as well as starch waste may be employed. Starch syrups from enzymatic hydrolysis deliver caramels with a higher tendency towards crystallization due to their higher content of dextrins after acid hydrolysis. Microwave heating of starch in a sealed vessel causes its hydrolysis accompanied by caramelization of the hydrolysate. Nonconventional sources such as malt and soya bean carbohydrates have also been paid some attention as the sugar syrups derived from them contain 70–85% reducing sugars. *See* Starch, Sources and Processing

Additives and Catalysts of Caramelization

The caramelization of plain sugars produces flavouring rather than colouring caramels. Certain additives accelerate caramelization, influencing both flavour and tinctorial strength of caramel by being either reagents or catalysts. The use of the following additives has been published: acids – acetic, citric, phosphoric, sulphurous, sulphuric and carbonic acids; bases – ammonia as well as hydroxides of sodium, potassium and calcium; salts – carbonates, hydrogencarbonates, sulphates, sulphites or phosphates of ammonia, sodium, potassium and calcium. Alkaline additives catalyse caramelization of furanoses more efficiently than pyranoses. Some sodium compounds, mainly biogenic amino acids and their sodium, potassium, magnesium and calcium salts, taurine (2-aminoethanesulphonic acid) and sulphanilic acid, have also been tested. They may be of particular interest in view of the fact that the most effective catalyst, ammonia, produces caramel contaminated with the neurotoxin 4(5)-methylimidazole. Caramel sources as well as additives and catalysts are controlled by food laws of particular countries or economic unions. *See* Legislation, Additives

Apart from chemical catalysts the possibility of catalysis of caramelization by ultraviolet, microwave or γ radiation or ultrasound has also been studied with inconclusive results. In particular, ultraviolet and γ-radiation introduce competing reactions such as the free radical decomposition of carbohydrate to water and carbon dioxide and a number of lower carbonyl compounds (aldehydes, ketones, carboxylic acids). In the case of caramels with poor tinctorial strength (class I CP-1 and CP-2) attempts have been to increase their colouring ability by blending ready made caramels with certain additives. Among possible additives enhancing the tinctorial strength of caramels the following have been tested: magnesium and calcium hydroxides, calcium phosphate as well as oxides of magnesium, calcium, zinc and cobalt(II). Magnesium oxide appears to be a superior additive among those tested. Its application has, however, limited value. The increase of tinctorial strength of plain caramels has some limits because the most intensively coloured melanoids are absent. The effect of magnesium oxide seems to be due to modification of the micellar structure of plain caramel. This effect enables further dehydration of caramelan to the darker caramelen and caramelin. Apart from such procedures, ultrafiltration, centrifugation combined with size exclusion chromatography as well as ion exchange columns have been proposed as methods to increase the tinctorial strength of caramels. Thus far, these methods have not achieved any application on an industrial scale. *See* Chromatography, Principles

Preparation and Manufacture

The variability of the sources for caramelization causes a great deal of empiricism in this technology. Generally, the character of compounds constituting caramel

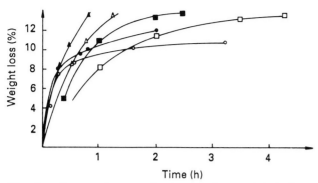

Fig. 1. Course of caramelization of glucose (circles), sucrose (triangles) and maltose (squares) in air (open symbols) and under nitrogen (solid symbols).

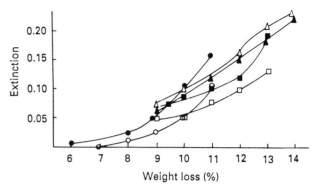

Fig. 2. Extinction of the absorption band at 35000 cm^{-1} in the ultraviolet/visible spectra of 0·1% aqueous solution of caramel from glucose (circles), sucrose (triangles) and maltose (squares). Open and solid symbols represent caramel prepared in air and under nitrogen, respectively.

depends on temperature of the process, its duration and the concentration of reactants. Increase in the colour of the product is proportional to the time of the process.

There are four aspects of thermolysis affecting caramelization and all of them have found practical industrial applications:

(1) Thermolysis of plain saccharides above their melting temperatures. This can be carried out under either normal, reduced or enhanced pressure. The last approach is usually employed when syrups from the hydrolysis of starch are caramelized. The initiation of the process readily takes place, after which the pressure may be released. The process is allowed to continue open to the atmosphere to develop all the colour, viscosity and desired organoleptic properties. The temperature range is between 180 and 250°C. Although it is commonly accepted that the contact of the reaction mixture with atmospheric oxygen does not play any role in the formation of caramel, one may see in Figs 1–4 that this is not so. Oxygen slows down the caramelization in later stages of the process. Its effect on the tinctorial strength of the final product is non-uniform and depends on the source. The elimination of nitrogen positively influences acid resistance and solubility of the final product.

(2) Thermolysis in the presence of catalyst. More recent procedures allow the temperature of caramelization to be reduced to 120–130°C. An increase of the temperature to above this range decreases the tinctorial strength of the caramel and develops an acid flavour.

(3) Thermolysis in the presence of either mineral acids or alkalis. These additives hydrolyse oligosaccharides which further caramelize. This process also requires lower temperature than these listed under (1). Increased pressures may also be used.

(4) Thermolysis with ammonia, ammonium salts, amino acids and their salts as well as proteins and

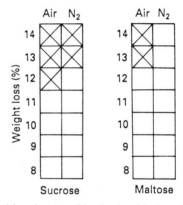

Fig. 3. Acid resistance (the hydrochloric acid test) of caramel from sucrose and maltose prepared in air and under nitrogen. Crossed squares denote flocculation of caramel.

polypeptides. Such caramels contain nitrogen heterocyclic components (imidazoles, pyroles, pyrazines and pyridines) which enrich the flavour and aroma of the final product.

Thermolysis should be carried out in entirely stainless steel equipment – kettles (open or pressurized), lines, storage tanks, fillers, agitators, valves and so on.

Careful control of the process as it proceeds is very important. The parameters of the caramelization have to be precisely adjusted for a given source and to obtain the desired properties of the final product. Caramels from sucrose, D-glucose and D-fructose with a distinct content of noncaramelized sugars have the best organoleptic quality. However, such caramels are quite hygroscopic and unstable. There are several techniques for the control of caramelization. One of

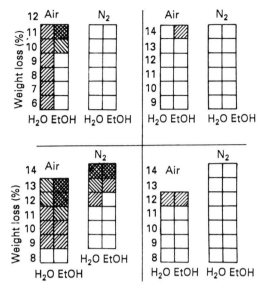

Fig. 4. Solubility in water and in 96% aqueous ethanol of caramel from various sugars made in air and under nitrogen: □, solution is transparent; ▨, traces of turbidity; ▧, solution is turbid; ▩, caramel is sparingly soluble.

the most recent developments is measuring the absorbance of free-flowing material in the near-infrared region. Lack of control of the process leads to loss of the micellar character of caramel and, in consequence precipitation occurs. For this reason the isoelectric point has to be adjusted. This must be done at the beginning of the caramelization as attempts to change the isoelectric point in the course of the process are quite complicated and frequently unsuccessful. The pH of caramels constitutes an important property. A high pH may indicate incomplete caramelization or the presence of alkali. Above pH 6·0, caramel is readily attacked by moulds and below pH 2·5 it quite easily resinifies.

The control of the viscosity of caramel is difficult. The rate of evolution of water (dehydration) significantly influences this property. The desired viscosity can be achieved by manipulation of the temperature and contact time with reagents.

Overburn caramel results from badly controlled temperature and from attempts to manufacture a highly coloured product. This may occur particularly in the manufacture of ammonia caramel. The control of the temperature is important throughout the whole period of production, including the final stage of killing heat, i.e. the fast cooling of a caramel to about 30°C.

The concentration and origin of the caramelized sources are of lesser importance. There is a relationship between the viscosity of caramel and its solubility. Less viscous caramels are usually more readily soluble and have more stable tinctorial strength, shelf life and retention of complete solubility. Such caramels are stored with the minimum of waste and effort.

For special use solid, dry caramels are manufactured. They are prepared by treating hot (120°C) viscous caramel with ammonium carbonate followed by adding sucrose and orthophosphoric acid, cooling to 100°C, and adding citric acid and sodium hydrogen carbonate. An alternative route involves addition of some cereal products, e.g. rye flour, and conditioning of the mass at 80–85°C at pH 3·5–5·5. Liquid caramel may also be thickened with a mixture of starch and dextrins. An extrusion of mono- and disaccharides at 150–300°C also leads to solid caramels.

Storage

Undesirable properties of caramel may appear even if the product has been properly manufactured. Caramels are not fully stable and caramelization slowly progresses on storage. Therefore, caramel should be stored at low temperatures. Caramelization on storage may be catalysed by metal ions. Hence tanks should be either plastic lined or made of stainless steel. These precautions slow down resinification of the product into an amorphous gel which becomes useless as either an additive or ingredient for food and drinks. The stability of caramel stored in ideal conditions is estimated to be about 5 years.

Bibliography

Greenshields RN (1973) Caramel. 2. Manufacture, composition and properties, *Process Biochemistry* 8(14): 17–20.
North RS (1973) Caramel versatile coloring. *Flavour Industry* 4(8): 337–338.
Smolnik MD (1987) Production and application of caramel from starch products. *Staerke* 39: 28–32.
Tomasik P, Palasinski M and Wiejak S (1989) The thermal decomposition of carbohydrates. Part I. The decomposition of mono-, di- and oligo-saccharides. *Advances in Carbohydrate Chemistry and Biochemistry* 47: 203–278.

P. Tomasik
University of Zimbabwe, Harare, Zimbabwe

CARBOHYDRATES

Contents

Classification and Properties

Structures of Sugars

'Carbohydrate', a term derived from the French '*hydrate de carbone*', and the similar German '*kohlenhydrate*', expresses the originally determined empirical formula of $C_x(H_2O)_y$. D-Glucose, the central metabolic sugar of most living organisms, was at first depicted as an open chain, then later and more accurately as a more stable hemiacetal in ring form (Haworth projection). It may also be shown in its most thermodynamically stable chair conformation. D-Glucose, a monosaccharide, has the empirical formula $C_6H_{12}O_6$, but the structural formula shows its aldehyde and polyhydroxyl functionality (Fig. 1). *See* Glucose, Function and Metabolism

When 2–10 monosaccharide units are linked together they form the class of oligosaccharides (from the Greek '*oligos*', meaning 'few'). When greater than 10 monosaccharide units are joined together they produce a polysaccharide (from the Greek '*polus*', meaning 'many'), although most polysaccharides have several hundred to several thousand monosaccharide residues.

Food monosaccharides are low-molecular-weight molecules containing five or six carbon atoms with the empirical formula $C_n(H_2O)_n$. Such monosaccharides readily form acetals. The carbonyl group can react with one of its own alcohol groups to form a hemiacetal. When C1 of D-glucose is involved in hemiacetal formation is has four different groups attached to it, and exists

in two forms called anomers. In the D-isomeric series to which natural glucose belongs, the α-D form has the oxygen of the anomeric carbon on the opposite side from C6 in the Haworth ring structure. β-D-Glucopyranose has the anomeric oxygen on the same side as C6. *See* Sugar Alcohols

Sugars differing in configuration at a chiral centre other than C1 are called epimers. D-Mannose is the C2 epimer of D-glucose, and D-galactose is the C4 epimer of D-glucose. *See* Galactose

Sugar rings are not flat as represented in the Haworth projections. Pyranoses may adopt different conformations, including chair and boat conformers (Fig. 2). Many hexoses occur mainly in the fairly rigid chair form, while fewer exist in the more flexible boat or twisted forms.

Monosaccharides occur naturally in only small amounts. D-Glucose is present in free form in a very small quantity in plants, but represents 0·8–1·0% of the carbohydrates in blood, where it is the main cellular energy source for humans and animals. D-Glucopyranosyl units, linked by α-1,4-D-linkages, comprise starches, and D-glucopyranosyl units also combine with other sugars in numerous other polysaccharides.

Disaccharides occurring in foods include sucrose (cane or beet sugar), maltose (corn sugar) and lactose (milk sugar). Disaccharides are not directly absorbed in the small intestine and are not nutritionally available to humans unless they are hydrolysed to monosaccharides. Oligosaccharides resistant to human enzymes, and

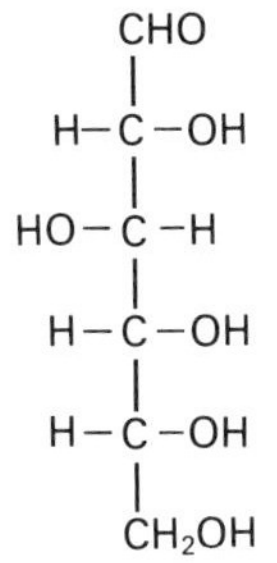

```
            CHO
             |
        H — C — OH
             |
       HO — C — H
             |
        H — C — OH
             |
        H — C — OH
             |
           CH₂OH
```

Fig. 1   Open chain representation of D-glucose.

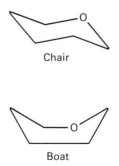

Chair

Boat

Fig. 2   Chair and boat conformation of the pyranose ring.

polysaccharides, pass through the digestive tract and may provide beneficial bulk (fibre). Oligosaccharides may be digested by microflora in the colon to give organic acids or gases that produce flatulence. Flatulence commonly results from ingestion of certain higher oligosaccharides, such as the trisaccharide raffinose and the tetrasaccharide stachyose, which are present in beans and other vegetables. *See* Dietary Fibre, Physiological Effects; Lactose; Malt, Malt Types and Products; Sucrose, Properties and Determination

Structures of Polysaccharides

Most polysaccharides have from 100 to several thousand sugar units. Some polysaccharides contain a single monomer monosaccharide (homoglycans). Cellulose and starch are homoglycans, yielding only D-glucose on hydrolysis. Xylan is a plant cell wall polymer solely composed of D-xylopyranosyl units. Some polysaccharides are linear chains and others are branched; some have single sugar unit branches on a main chain while others possess a more complex branch on branch, or bush-like, structure. *See* Cellulose; Starch, Functional Properties

Food polysaccharides include starch, cellulose, hemicellulose, pectic substances and the seed gums, exudate gums, seaweed gums, microbial gums and cellulose gums. Starch is the principal food reserve of plants and is isolated for commercial use from corn, wheat, rice, tapioca, arrowroot, potato and sago. Starch occurs in packets called granules, made up of starch molecules. Starch molecules are generally of two types, the linear amylose (an α-1,4-D-glucan) and a highly branched bush-like structure termed amylopectin (consisting of an α-1,4-D-glucan chain with α-1,6-D branch points). Most 'normal' starches contain three amylopectin molecules for every amylose molecule, but some starches (waxy starches) contain no amylose, while others (high-amylose starches) contain 50–80% amylose. When starch is heated in water the granules undergo an irreversible swelling known as gelatinization whereby they provide thickness and gel-forming ability. *See* Gums, Properties of Individual Gums; Hemicelluloses; Pectin, Food Uses

Starches may be modified to extend their properties for some food uses. Acid-modified starches are used in gum confectionery, starch ethers (such as hydroxyethyl starch) are used in salad dressings and pie fillings, and starch phosphate esters are useful because of their excellent freeze–thaw stability. Cross-linked starch is used in baby foods and fruit pie fillings as a thickener/stabilizer, and starch acetate esters are used in pie fillings because of the clarity and stability of their cooked pastes.

Cellulose is a β-1,4-D-glucan and is the principal

structural component of plant cell walls. Much of the texture of plant foods is due to cellulose, as well as the ligneous middle lamella pectic substances.

Hemicelluloses are present in plant cell walls and yield, on hydrolysis, an abundance of the five-carbon sugars L-arabinose and D-xylose (pentoses), along with D-glucuronic acid, and some deoxy sugars. D-Xylose-containing hemicelluloses (xylans) are common in foods, and those from wheat probably have an effect in baked goods where they promote water binding of the flour. They improve mixability of the bread dough, reduce mixing energy, aid incorporation of protein, increase loaf volume and decrease rate of staling.

Pectic substances occur with lignin in the middle lamella of plant cell walls and consist of the central pectin polymer composed of α-1,4-D-galactopyranosyluronic acid units as well as polymers composed mainly of D-galactosyl and L-arabinosyl units. The pectin D-galacturonic acid polymer occurs as the methyl ester, which loses some of its methyl groups as the plant matures or as the fruit ripens. Protopectin in immature fruits is highly esterified while pectin and pectinic acid have less esterification and pectic acid, the completely demethylated form, is found in overripe fruits. *See* Lignin; Ripening of Fruit

Commercial pectin is produced in three grades. High-methoxyl or rapid-set pectin contains 72–75% methoxyl groups and sets in 20–70 s at pH 3·0–3·1 at 0·3% pectin in 65% sugar. Slow-set pectin, having 62–68% methoxyl content, sets in 180–250 s. Medium-set pectins have methoxyl contents of 68–71%. Pectins are mainly used to produce jellies. Calcium ions combine with free carboxyl groups to cross-link pectin chains to induce gel formation, and are especially effective in medium- to low-methoxyl pectins. Calcium forms gels with low-methoxyl pectins without the need for sugar and are useful for making low-energy, dietetic jellies.

Many plant polysaccharides are soluble in water and find commercial uses in foods as thickeners or food modifiers. These are the industrial gums derived from seeds, plant exudates, seaweeds and gums produced by special fermentation or made by derivatization of cellulose.

Seed gums are principally the galactomannans from guar (*Cyamopsis tetragonolobus*) or from locust bean seeds (*Ceratonia siliqua*). Guar gum is composed of β-1,4-D-mannopyranosyl units with, on average, an α-D-galactopyranosyl unit linked (1,6) to every other main chain unit. In locust bean gum the single-unit side-chains are fewer and are linked to the main chain in a less regular order. Locust bean gum interacts in solution with carrageenan to give increased solution viscosity or even formation of a weak gel. *See* Gums, Nutritional Role of Guar Gum

Gum arabic is a plant exudate from the acacia tree. It is a large complex heteroglycan of up to 1 000 000 Da. It differs from other natural gums in being of high solubility, even producing solutions of 40% concentration, and has excellent ability to encapsulate flavour principles in dry beverage mixes.

Carrageenan, from the seaweed *Chondrus crispus*, is a mixture of several related galactans having one or two sulphate groups attached as half-esters to each sugar unit. Several molecular variations exist, designated κ, λ, μ, ι and ν. κ-Carrageenan forms strong gels in the presence of potassium cations. Carragenan has a particular affinity for protein and is used in chocolate milk to stabilize the protein and to suspend chocolate particles.

Alginate, another seaweed gum, is extracted from the giant kelp (*Macrocystis pyrifera*). Alginates contain D-mannopyranosyluronic acid and L-gulopyranosyluronic acid and the commercial polysaccharide is sold as the soluble sodium salt. Its solutions gel at room temperature in the presence of calcium ions. Alginates are used in ice cream, icings, glazes, pourable salad dressing and in beer for foam stabilization.

Of the microbially produced gums, dextran and xanthan are the most widely used. Dextran contains D-glucopyranosyl units linked 1,6, 1,3 and 1,4, and is used in confectioneries to inhibit sucrose crystallization and in ice cream to provide good mouth feel. *See* Dextran

Xanthan gum, a product of several *Xanthomonas* species, is basically a cellulose molecule substituted by a trisaccharide side-chain on every other D-glucopyranosyl unit. Xanthan is easily soluble in water and produces highly viscous, pseudoplastic dispersions at low concentrations. Xanthan enhances flavour release in certain foods, promotes cloud stabilization in orange juice, is used as a suspending–thickening agent in canned foods, and can be employed in milk-based instant puddings.

Derivatives of cellulose are also employed as food gums. If the amorphous region of cellulose is acid hydrolysed, the remaining material, known as microcrystalline cellulose, can be used as a nonmetabolizable bulking agent in many foods. Treatment of cellulose with chloroacetic acid under strongly alkaline conditions yields carboxymethylcellulose (CMC), which is mainly used as a viscosity builder in foods. It acts to thicken up pie fillings, custards and cheese spreads. It reduces ice crystal growth in frozen desserts, stabilizes emulsions in salad dressings, and provides bulk, body and mouth feel in dietetic foods.

Methylcellulose is prepared by heating cellulose with methyl chloride under strongly alkaline conditions. Methylcellulose, unlike most other gums, exhibits thermogelation, that is, it forms a gel when heated but returns to a normal flowable dispersion on cooling. Methylcellulose confers resistance to oil absorption in deep-fried foods, acts as a syneresis inhibitor, bulking agent, and provides texture and structure in certain foods. It acts as a thickener/stabilizer in salad dressings

and is used as an edible coating in a variety of food products.

Chemistry and Physical Properties of Sugars

Hydrolysis of food glycosides, including oligosaccharides and polysaccharides, is influenced by pH, temperature, anomeric configuration, and sugar ring size. Hydrolysis of carbohydrates is important in food processing and preservation and may cause undesirable changes in colour or, with polysaccharides, their inability to thicken or to form a strong gel. *See* Sugar, Handling of Sugar Beet and Sugar Cane

Glycosidic linkages are more readily cleaved in acidic media than in alkaline media, where they are fairly stable. The hydrolysis is believed to follow the mechanism shown in Fig. 3.

Increasing temperature greatly increases the rate of glycoside hydrolysis, as reflected by changes in the first-order rate constant. Also, anomers differ in hydrolysis rates, methyl β-D-glycosides generally being hydrolysed more rapidly than the α-D anomers.

In the 1970s, technology was developed to hydrolyse corn starch to D-glucose by using α-amylase followed by glucoamylase. The corn syrup so produced was then treated with isomerase, to produce an equilibrium mixture of 54% D-glucose and 42% D-fructose. This low-cost sweetener, known as high-fructose corn syrup (HFCS), has replaced 40–50% of the sucrose market in the USA and this percentage continues to increase. Composition and relative sweetness of typical industrial high-fructose corn syrups are shown in Table 1. *See* Fructose; Sweeteners – Intense

Mutarotation, the conversion of one anomer to another, is best illustrated polarimetrically by the equilibration of α- or β-D-glucose. β-D-Glucose in solution has an initial specific rotation of $[\alpha]_D + 18\cdot7°$, which increases in a few hours to $+53°$. α-D-Glucose

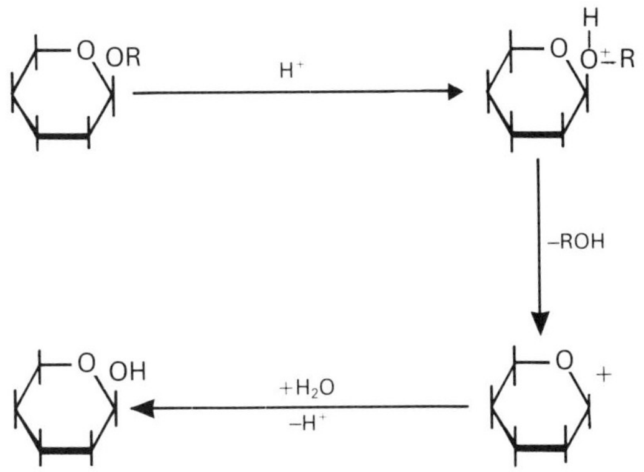

Fig. 3 Mechanism of acid-catalysed hydrolysis of alkyl pyranosides.

Table 1.   Percentage composition and sweetness of typical high-fructose corn syrups available commercially

Components	Type		
	Normal	55% fructose	90% fructose
D-Glucose	52	40	7
D-Fructose	42	55	90
Oligosaccharides	6	5	3
Relative sweetness[a]	100	105	140

[a] Sucrose=100.

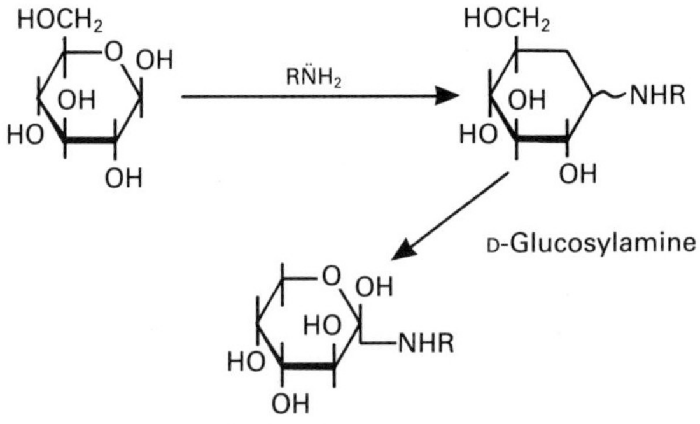

1-Amino-2-ketose
(Amadori product)

Fig. 5   Initial reactions of Maillard browning.

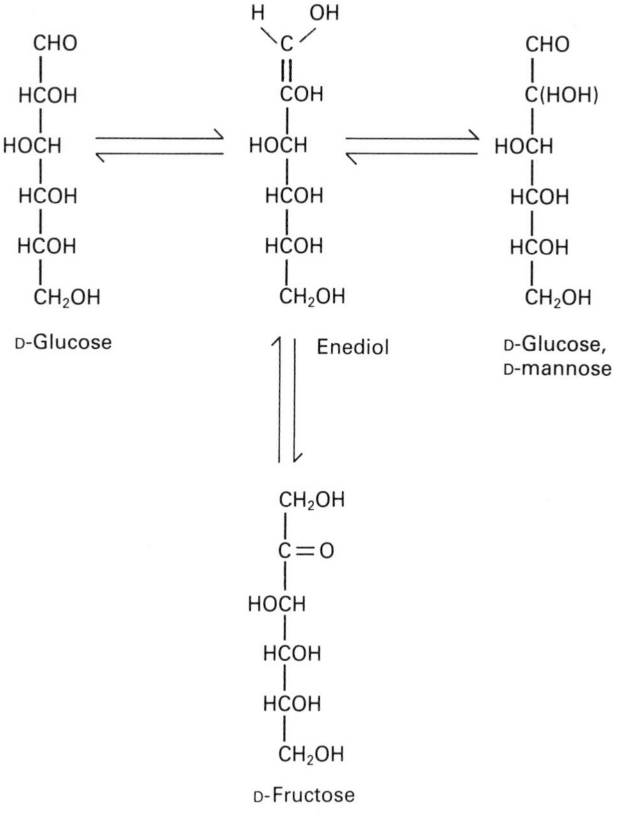

Fig. 4   Alkali-catalysed enolization of D-glucose.

initially has a specific rotation of $[\alpha]_D$ $+112°$, which decreases to $+53°$. The equilibrium corresponds to a composition of 36.2% α-D-glucose and 63.8% β-D-glucose. Acid or alkali serves as a catalyst, greatly increasing the rate of mutarotation.

Enolization, catalysed by alkali, occurs through the open-chair form to yield an enediol (Fig. 4). D-Glucose can undergo several reactions to yield a mixture of D-glucose, its C2 epimer D-mannose, and the ketose D-fructose.

Thermal degradation of sugars is an important reaction in foods, and is catalysed by acid or base.

Pentoses yield 2-furaldehyde as the principal dehydration product while hexoses yield 5-hydroxymethyl-2-furaldehyde (HMF) and other products such as 2-hydroxyacetylfuran and isomaltol. Some of these products are highly odiferous and may contribute desirable or undesirable flavours to foods.

Browning of foods is due to oxidative or nonoxidative reactions. Nonoxidative (nonenzymatic) browning is of great importance in many foods. It includes caramelization and the interaction of proteins or amines with carbohydrates. The latter reaction is known as the Maillard reaction. *See* Browning, Nonenzymatic

Thermal treatment of carbohydrates induces a complex group of reactions called caramelization. These reactions produce unsaturated rings and conjugated double bonds which absorb light and produce colour. Catalysts are frequently used to direct the reaction to specific types of caramel colours or flavours. Sucrose is normally used for preparing caramel colours and flavours. It is heated with acid or acidic ammonium salts to produce various products used in food. *See* Caramel, Properties and Analysis

Pyrolytic reactions produce unique unsaturated ring systems with unique tastes and fragrances. Maltol (3-hydroxy-2-methylpyran-4-one) and isomaltol (3-hydroxy-2-acetylfuran) contribute to the flavour of freshly baked bread. 2-*H*-Hydroxy-5-methylfuran-3-one has a cooked meat flavour and can be used as a flavour enhancer for various other flavours and sweeteners.

The other major type of nonenzymatic browning in foods is Maillard browning. The reactant requirements for Maillard browning are an amino-bearing compound (usually a protein), a reducing sugar and moisture. Reactions involved in the early steps of Maillard browning are shown in Fig. 5.

When an amino acid or part of a protein chain participates in the Maillard reaction the amino acid is made nutritionally unavailable. This is especially important for the essential amino acids, L-lysine being the most susceptible to the Maillard reaction.

Relatively mild conditions can cause loss of nutrients

Classification and Properties

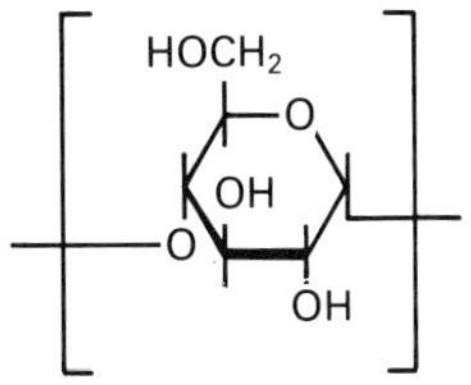

Fig. 6 D-Glucosyl residue of a polysaccharide, showing the potential sites for hydrogen-bonding interaction with water molecules.

Table 2. Sucrose in common foods (single analysis)

Food	Sucrose present (%)
Soft drink	8·8
Cracker	11·8
Ice cream	21·0
Hamburger	23·0
Ketchup	29·0
Cake	35·9
Nondairy creamer	65·0
Jelly	82·9

and, whenever foods containing protein and reducing sugars are heated, even at low temperatures for short time periods, losses of amino acids can occur. This degradation is especially pronounced for the essential amino acid L-lysine.

Control of the Maillard reaction is important not only because of contribution to flavour, odour and colour but because of possible toxicity of the products. Some authors have suggested that the 'premelanoidin' products of these reactions may be mutagenic. However, this area is still unsettled and more work needs to be conducted on the potential toxicity of Maillard products.

When Maillard browning is not desirable in foods, it may be limited by use of very low or very high water activities (a_w), low pH or low temperature. Browning can be reduced also by enzymatically altering one of the substrates, usually the sugar. For dried egg whites, this can be accomplished by adding D-glucose oxidase (prior to drying) to oxidize the D-glucose to D-gluconic acid. Sulphur dioxide or sulphites can also be used to inhibit browning.

Chemistry and Physical Properties of Polysaccharides

Most food polysaccharides are insoluble and nondigestible. Thus, cellulose and hemicellulose of plant cell walls are essentially nondigested. The same is true of water-soluble or water-dispersable polysaccharides in foods. Soluble polysaccharides serve various roles, such as providing thickening, viscosity, adhesiveness, gel-forming ability and sensory mouth feel.

Theoretically, polysaccharides should be water-soluble, since they are chains of glycosyl units composed of hexoses and pentoses. Each hydroxyl hydrogen or oxygen atom can potentially hydrogen bond to a water molecule (Fig. 6) and thus each chain sugar unit can be fully hydrated, inducing water solubility of the polymer. A polysaccharide will not be soluble in water when water access to all parts of the polymer does not occur. Purely linear polysaccharides like cellulose tend to associate or intermolecularly bond in an attempt at crystallization and exclude water to become water-soluble.

This interaction toward crystallization by soluble molecules of the same kind, with exclusion of water, is termed 'junction zone formation'. If additional molecules coalesce at the junction zone, the complex can become large enough that gravitation causes it to precipitate. If the junction zone does not enlarge and another junction zone, involving one of the original two molecules and a new molecule, forms elsewhere, a three-dimensional network, entrapping solvent water, is formed. This three-dimensional network is a gel. Gel strength, an important consideration in foods, depends largely on the strength of the junction zones that hold the gel together. Many degrees of gel strength and stability can be achieved by control of junction zones, and this ability is widely used in food science.

All water-soluble polysaccharides produce thickening because of their large molecular size. Viscosity depends on molecular size, shape and charge. Viscosity may be influenced by electrolytes, since they affect the conformation and size of the polymer. As a general rule, solutions of linear polysaccharides will be more viscous than solutions of branched polysaccharides of the same molecular weight. Since the main reason for using polysaccharide in foods is to provide viscosity, or gelling behaviour, linear polymers are generally more desirable.

Occurrence of Sugars and Polysaccharides in Foods

Carbohydrates constitute 75% of the dry weight of all land and marine plants, and are present in all plant parts consumed by humans. Since most of the metabolizable carbohydrate comes from sucrose or starch, plants high in these carbohydrates are more frequently consumed by humans. Nondigestible polysaccharides (fibre) are also consumed when plant material is eaten and the 'fibre' promotes healthy intestinal activity.

Sucrose is present in small quantities in most plants. Most dietary sucrose is derived from fabricated, processed foods containing sucrose isolated from sugar beets or sugar cane. The amount of sucrose in some commercial foods is shown in Table 2. Fruits and

Table 3. Free sugars in fruit (% fresh weight basis)

Fruit	Sucrose	D-Glucose	D-Fructose
Apple	3·78	1·17	6·04
Grape	2·25	6·86	7·84
Peach	6·92	0·91	1·18
Cherry	0·22	6·49	7·38
Strawberry	1·03	2·09	2·40

Table 4. Free sugars in vegetables (% fresh weight basis)

Vegetable[a]	Sucrose	D-Glucose	D-Fructose
Beet	6·11	0·18	0·16
Broccoli	0·42	0·73	0·67
Carrot	4·24	0·85	0·85
Cucumber	0·06	0·86	0·86
Onion	0·89	2·07	1·09
Spinach	0·06	0·09	0·04
Sweet corn	3·03	0·34	0·31
Tomato	0·01	1·12	1·34

[a] Layman's classification.

vegetables contain minor amounts of sucrose, as well as the monosaccharides D-glucose and D-fructose, as shown in Tables 3 and 4. *See* Fruits of Tropical Climates, Commercial and Dietary Importance; Fruits of Temperate Climates, Commercial and Dietary Importance; Vegetables of Temperate Climates, Commercial and Dietary Importance; Vegetables of Tropical Climates, Commercial and Dietary Importance

Cereals contain relatively small amounts of mono- and disaccharides, as most of the sugar transported to seeds is converted to starch. Starch is the major carbohydrate energy reserve of plants, being stored principally in seeds, roots and tubers. Starch dries easily at low relative humidities, regains softness on exposure to moisture and is rapidly hydrolysed to produce D-glucose for energy. *See* Cereals, Contribution to the Diet

Bibliography

Binkley RW (1988) *Modern Carbohydrate Chemistry*. New York: Marcel Dekker.

Birch GG and Green LF (eds) (1973) *Molecular Structure and Function of Food Carbohydrate*. New York: Wiley.

Capon B (1969) Mechanism in carbohydrate chemistry. *Chemical Reviews* 69: 407–498.

Guthrie RD (1974) *Introduction to Carbohydrate Chemistry*. Oxford: Clarendon Press.

Kennedy JF (ed.) (1988) *Carbohydrate Chemistry*. Oxford: Clarendon Press.

Shallenberger RS (1982) *Advanced Sugar Chemistry: Principles of Sugar Stereochemistry*. Westport, CT: AVI.

Whistler RL and Daniel JR (1985) *Carbohydrates, in Food Chemistry*, 2nd edn. New York: Marcel Dekker.

J.R. Daniel and R.L. Whistler
Purdue University, West Lafayette, USA

Interactions With Other Food Components

Interactions of Sugars with Other Food Components

An important function of sugars in food is their interaction with water. Low-molecular-weight carbohydrates such as D-glucose, D-fructose or sucrose lower the water vapour pressure as well as the water activity a_w. The ability to bind water is referred to as humectancy and affects the texture of food as well as its susceptibility to microbiological spoilage. For instance, it is the interaction of sugars and water that gives syrups their thick consistency and it is the relatively low a_w (0·65–0·75) of jellies, due to the interaction of sucrose and water, that lowers the ability of microorganisms to grow on the jelly surface. *See* Fructose; Sucrose, Properties and Determination; Water Activity, Principles and Measurement; Water Activity, Effect on Food Stability

Interactions of sugars and water is mainly due to hydrogen bonding ($ROH\cdots OH_2$) which decreases vapour pressure and a_w. This interaction also leads to a depression of the solution freezing point as seen in frozen desserts (freezing point −2 to −5°C) and to elevation of the solution boiling point as noted in the preparation of confectionery (see final cooking temperatures for various confectioneries in Table 1).

It is interesting to note that not all sugars have an equal affinity for moisture, as illustrated in Table 2.

Impure sugars or syrups absorb more water at a

Table 1. Final cooking temperatures for confectionery

Confectionery	Final cooking temperature (°C)
Fondant	114
Fudge	112
Panocha	112
Caramels	120
Peanut brittle	149
Marshmallows	116

Table 2. Percentage water absorbed by sugars

Sugar	Water (%) absorbed (60% relative humidity 1 h, 20°C)
D-Glucose	0·07
D-Fructose	0·28
Sucrose	0·04
Maltose, hydrate	5·05
Maltose, anhydrous	0·80
Lactose, hydrate	5·05
Lactose, anhydrous	0·54

Table 3. Percentage composition of high-fructose corn syrups

Components	Type		
	Normal	55% fructose	90% fructose
D-Glucose	52	40	7
D-Fructose	42	55	90
Oligosaccharides	6	5	3

higher rate than pure sugars. This is true even when the impurity is the anomeric form of the sugar. Impurities interfere with the orderly crystalline arrangement of molecules, making water absorption more likely.

Sugars, specifically glycosides, may also interact with acid in aqueous solution resulting in hydrolysis. Such hydrolysis is caused by common food acids such as citric acid (citrus juices), acetic acid (vinegar), and potassium acid tartrate (cream of tartar). The reaction involves the interaction of acid with the glycosidic linkage. Specifically, the glycosidic oxygen atom is protonated by a food acid and the aglycon is then displaced in a nucleophilic substitution (S_N2)-type reaction by water. The resulting sugar derivative loses a proton to regenerate the hydrogen ion catalyst.

Hydrolysis of sucrose is important in some foods but its major commercial importance lies in the production of high-fructose corn syrup (HFCS). Corn starch is initially hydrolysed to a mixture of D-glucose, maltose and dextrins. This 'normal' corn syrup is treated with an isomerase enzyme to convert about 42% of the D-glucose into D-fructose. Composition of some high-fructose corn syrups is shown in Table 3. *See* Dextrins; Malt, Malt Types and Products

Not all glycosides are equally susceptible to acid hydrolysis. Sucrose, in particular, is sensitive to acid hydrolysis where protonation of the sucrose glycosidic oxygen is followed by generation of D-glucose and a D-...osyl secondary carboxonium ion. The secondary carboxonium ion is very stable and has a low activation energy for its production. The result is that sucrose is quite labile to acid hydrolysis.

Sugars that are capable of forming open-chain isomers containing an aldehyde group are known as reducing sugars and can participate in a complex series of reactions with free amino-bearing compounds, called the Maillard reaction. This reaction is responsible for the desirable brown surface colour and some of the flavour of many food products, especially baked goods such as bread and biscuits. It is important, however, to know how to control this reaction because if it proceeds too far the product will have an undesirably dark colour and a strong, objectionable flavour. Also, products of the Maillard reaction containing essential amino acids may be nutritionally unavailable and some of the products generated by the Maillard reaction may be mutagenic. While dietary amino acid deficiencies are not likely to be a problem in developed countries where the population eats a varied diet, it may be of importance in developing countries where the diets tend to be predominantly (80–100%) grain based. This occurs because grains are already limiting in L-lysine even before any L-lysine degradation occurs. *See* Browning, Nonenzymatic

The minimum requirements for the Maillard reaction are a reducing sugar, an amino-bearing compound and moisture. The level of moisture can be very low as this reaction can occur in dried egg whites. This reaction in dried egg whites, though of historical importance, is now prevented by treating egg white (prior to drying) with the enzyme glucose oxidase. Such treatment converts D-glucose into nonreactive D-gluconic acid. This technique is employed in other foods as well, such as treatment of fish with a bacterium containing ribose oxidase activity, and represents one of the more recent methods for controlling Maillard browning. Other methods for controlling the browning reaction include maintaining a low moisture level (keeping the reactants insoluble), or by controlling pH to less than 6, which protonates the amino groups rendering them unreactive, or by use of sulphating agents such as sulphur dioxide to react with a furfural-type intermediate and interfere with the cascade of reactions leading to colour and aroma compounds.

Interactions of Polysaccharides and Other Food Components

Polysaccharides in foods interact with many other components, water being the most important. Polysaccharides are added to foods to produce thickened dispersions or gelled products. Formation of these specialized textures fundamentally involves control of a_w. Most food polysaccharides are effective at controlling a_w, exhibiting their characteristics at concentrations

Table 4. Qualitative effect of acid on polysaccharides in solution

Polymer	Susceptibility to acid hydrolysis
Gum arabic	+
Gum tragacanth	−
Guaran	−
Locust bean gum	−
Carrageenan	+
Alginate	−
Xanthan gum	−

of 1% (w/w) or less. Many foods benefit from the water-controlling, texture-building effects of polysaccharides, including frozen desserts, confectionery, salad dressings, puddings, gravies, cheese, pie fillings and a variety of dietetic foods.

Polysaccharides are high-molecular-weight compounds which can become hydrated to a greater or lesser extent on dispersion in aqueous media. Interactions between polysaccharide and water molecules are due to hydrogen bonding or ion–dipole attraction. In either case the large polymer molecule is surrounded by a layer of water (first hydration shell) and consequently can be dispersed in the bulk water of food. Hydrated polysaccharides are large molecules and are constantly 'bumping into one another'. This interaction, an internal fluid friction, gives rise to dispersion viscosity. If the interaction between the large polymers is more substantial, that is, if they interact and form a region where the two polymers are directly in contact (a junction zone), then a gel may be formed. Usually gel structures have a high water content (98–99%) and a low content of polysaccharide (1–2%).

Polysaccharides, including starch, cellulose, hemicellulose, pectin and plant gums, may interact with acids in foods and undergo hydrolysis. Typical food acids which may cause this include acetic acid (vinegar), citric acid (citrus juice) and potassium acid tartrate (cream of tartar). In most cases, hydrolysis is undesirable as it leads to loss of the polysaccharide's ability to gel or thicken the food in which it occurs. A qualitative indication of the effect of acid on polysaccharides is given in Table 4. *See* Cellulose; Gums, Properties of Individual Gums; Hemicelluloses; Pectin, Food Uses; Starch, Structure, Properties and Determination

Polysaccharides may also interact in important ways with ionic species in foods, especially cations. These interactions are of the ion–dipole type or Coulombic interactions. The effect may sometimes decrease the dispersion viscosity as in gum arabic, but more often increases viscosity and may even cause gel formation. Examples of these chemically set gels include low-methoxyl pectin, carrageenan and alginate gels.

While molecules of the same polysaccharides may interact with each other to build viscosity or form gels, it is also possible for polysaccharides of different types to interact with each other, largely through hydrogen bond interactions or ion–dipole interactions. For instance, carrageenan forms a gel in the presence of potassium salts but the gel is very brittle and undergoes extensive syneresis. However, addition of a small amount of locust bean gum modifies the carrageenan gel texture so that it is less brittle, more elastic and less prone to syneresis. Due to fine structural differences, polymers closely related to locust bean gum such as guaran do not interact with carrageenan.

Both guaran and locust bean gum interact with xanthan gum to produce increased dispersion viscosity. However, xanthan gum–locust bean gum combinations form thermally reversible gels when heated to greater than 54°C and then cooled. This behaviour indicates synergistic interaction between the two polymers.

Polysaccharides also interact with some proteins. Carboxymethylcellulose may be used to inhibit protein precipitation in fruit-flavoured milk drinks and carrageenan has been long used to stabilize casein against interaction with calcium ions. In breadmaking the interaction between the gluten protein and dough polysaccharides (starch, pentosans) are important in determining the quality of the product. Additionally, flour with inferior breadmaking properties, such as soft red winter wheat flour, may be improved by addition of polysaccharides such as xanthan gum and carrageenan. Sodium alginate (1%) has a beneficial interaction with soya protein in the preparation of soya bean grits used in making textured vegetable protein (TVP) products.

Interaction with Flavour Compounds

In many food systems, carbohydrates are important for retaining volatile flavour compounds. This is particularly true in processed foods where water has been removed by drying, as in the production of instant coffee. Effectively, the flavour compounds are replacing some of the water associated with the carbohydrate. Monosaccharide sugars are less effective in retaining compounds than disaccharides or polysaccharides. Schardinger dextrins, on account of their cyclic structures, form inclusion complexes with flavour compounds and other small molecules. These are particularly stable and lead to strong flavour retention. *See* Flavour Compounds, Structures and Characteristics

Gum arabic is an important polysaccharide in assisting flavour retention. It is able to form a film around flavour particles which reduces water absorption, loss by evaporation and chemical oxidation. Gum arabic–gelatin mixtures have been used for microencapsulation, which allows complete retention of flavour compounds prior to dissolution of the coating.

Interactions With Other Food Components

Table 5. Extent of starch gelatinization in baked products

Product	Loss of birefringence (%)
White bread	100
Cake doughnuts	98
Pie crust	50
Sweet biscuits	9

Changes During Processing

Most carbohydrates are susceptible to change during food processing, mainly from heat treatment. In many cases changes are due to a combination of heat and acid, or heat and amino acids. At temperatures above 100°C, starch and other polysaccharides are prone to some degree of thermal degradation. Even in cases where no degradation occurs, a decrease in viscosity is noted with an increase in temperature, as is normal for Newtonian fluids. More is known about changes in starch during processing than about other polysaccharides.

Most food uses of starch require cooking, either in the presence or absence of water. In the absence of water, thermal degradation, called dextrinization, occurs which results in lower paste viscosity when the product is subsequently cooked. When starch is heated in the presence of water it is gelatinized, that is, the granules irreversibly imbibe water to produce an extensive swelling. The extent of gelatinization, as measured by loss of birefringence, varies in different food products as shown in Table 5. *See* Starch, Functional Properties

Gelatinized starch, on cooling, undergoes retrogradation, an attempt at crystallization by the large, unwieldy starch molecules. This association of starch molecules or partial crystallization may lead to gel formation or to firming of the product, as in bread staling. Normal starches containing linear amylose molecules easily produce gels, but waxy starches have no amylose and do not form gels. In the case of normal starch, continued junction zone formation and enlargement eventually leads to changes in gel texture accompanied by syneresis. This phenomenon is especially noticeable in normal starch-containing products subjected to several freeze–thaw cycles. For this reason, starch-containing foods that are to be frozen are typically prepared with waxy starch which contains no amylose.

Bibliography

Blanshard JMV and Mitchell JR (eds) (1978) *Polysaccharides in Food.* Boston: Butterworths.
Lineback DR and Inglett GE (eds) (1981) *Food Carbohydrates.* Westport, CT: AVI.
Phillips GO, Wedlock DJ and Williams PA (eds) (1982) *Gums*
and Stabilizers for the Food Industry: Interactions of Hydrocolloids. Oxford: Pergamon Press.
Whistler RL and BeMiller JN (eds) (1973) *Industrial Gums.* New York: Academic Press.
Whistler RL and Daniel JR (1985) Carbohydrates. In: Fennema OR (ed.) *Food Chemistry*, 2nd edn. New York: Marcel Dekker.

J.R. Daniel and R.L. Whistler
Purdue University, West Lafayette, USA

Digestion, Absorption and Metabolism

The assimilation of dietary carbohydrate into the body is a complex process in four separate organs (salivary gland, stomach, small bowel, and colon) involving digestion, active and passive transport, and luminal fermentation with absorption of short-chain fatty acids (Fig. 1). Abnormalities in each of these organs or processes can lead to diminished assimilation of carbohydrates. *See* Fatty Acids, Metabolism

Digestion

The Effect of Food Sources and Processing

Starch is composed of a straight-chain polymer of glucose joined in α-1,4 linkages (amylose) and the branched glucopolymer amylopectin formed by α-1,6 linked chains at about every 25 glucose residues in the amylose polymer. Dietary fibre is the term used to describe substances (nearly all carbohydrates) in food that are not digested and absorbed in the small intestine. In the usual Western diet, starch provides about 50–60% of available carbohydrate, while disaccharides, largely sucrose (30%) and lactose (10%), comprise most of the rest. Content of starch, the major storage form of polysaccharide in plants, depends upon the type, part and age of the plant; thus actual dietary starch content may vary significantly from that reproduced in published tables. *See* Dietary Fibre, Properties and Sources; Starch, Structure, Properties and Determination

A high amylose content in starch is thought to reduce digestibility. Not only food source, but also food preparation can affect digestibility *in vivo*, although the relative importance of each factor is uncertain. In general, cooking and processing leads to more complete digestion. For example, wheat processing can affect starch digestion, and gluten has been suggested as the factor responsible for the variability. Starches and disaccharides are subject to digestion within the lumen of organs formed from the foregut and midgut, i.e.

674 Carbohydrates

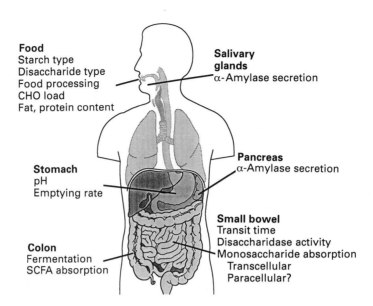

Fig. 1 Factors affecting carbohydrate assimilation.

mouth, stomach, and small intestine. Most of the over 200 plant polysaccharides comprising most of dietary fibre are digested by bacteria in the lumen of the nonruminant colon, derived from the hindgut. In the ruminant this digestion occurs in the forestomach.

Salivary and Gastric Hydrolysis

Salivary amylase is probably important in initiating starch digestion, depending upon the amount of time spent in chewing. Starch hydrolysis begins in random fashion on internal α-1,4 glucose bonds. As the reaction proceeds, hydrolysis becomes more and more selective, so that the final products of maltose and maltotriose are resistant to amylase action. Human salivary amylase is 94% identical with the predicted sequence of pancreatic amylase, and exists in both a glycosylated and nonglycosylated form. The physiological importance of the two forms is uncertain. Free salivary amylase is inactivated by the acid pH in the gastric lumen, but the presence of starch or its hydrolytic products can protect the enzyme from acid denaturation. In this way, some salivary amylase can reach the more neutral pH of the duodenal lumen.

In humans over one year of age the α-amylase activity in the duodenal lumen is fairly high. Before that age there is not much amylase activity in the lumen, because both salivary and pancreatic enzymes have not yet reached their normal rate of secretion. The protection of amylase by its hydrolytic products may be useful to the neonate, before amylase levels reach adult levels.

No other carbohydrases except for salivary amylase are present in gastric juice. Acid nonenzymic hydrolysis of some carbohydrates can occur, and presumably in the stomach, although the importance of this process is

probably small *in vivo*. The rate of gastric emptying is related to caloric load, and will be decreased by a large carbohydrate load. The purpose of this regulatory step is probably to limit the delivery of undigested food to the duodenum, avoiding overload of the capacity of the small intestinal lumen to hydrolyse all the carbohydrate.

Pancreatic Hydrolysis

α-Amylase is the only pancreatic enzyme active against carbohydrate substrates; in contrast, both lipid and protein substrates are attacked by more than one pancreatic enzyme. The presence of salivary amylase, however, provides a margin of safety needed for starch digestion. The pancreatic enzyme, like the salivary one, is active at neutral pH, and hydrolyses starch from internal α-1,4 bonds. In normal circumstances the bulk of dietary starch is hydrolysed in the lumen of the small intestine by the pancreatic enzyme.

There are multiple factors determining the completeness of starch digestion. Food processing (discussed above) is one factor. Altered intestinal transit is another such factor. Meal composition may affect variation in transit time from meal to meal. Fat and protein may influence the release of cholecystokinin and thus the release of amylase into the lumen. These nutrients may also delay gastric emptying, allowing more time for intraluminal digestion of starch. Amylase activity can be altered by intraluminal substances as well, including protein inhibitors that are found in certain plants. Although these inhibitors have been used in an attempt to limit the assimilation of carbohydrates in controlling obesity, their role in normal conditions is unclear. Dietary carbohydrate in the form of starch can increase α-amylase secretion in animals and in newborn humans

Digestion, Absorption and Metabolism

but oligosaccharides do not do so in humans. *See* Fats, Digestion, Absorption and Transport; Protein, Digestion and Absorption of Protein and Nitrogen Balance

The release of glucose from starch also elicits a hormonal response, not of cholecytokinin but of insulin. The amount of blood glucose rise (glycaemic response) varies among carbohydrate sources, depending upon the form and processing of the starch or carbohydrate, and upon the presence of dietary fibre. Meals containing fat increase secretion of gastric inhibitory polypeptide (GIP), whose major hormonal function appears to be the enhancement of glucose-mediated insulin release. Because of the variety of factors affecting the glycaemic response of carbohydrates in individual foods, it is not surprising that the causes of the differences in glycaemic response are poorly understood.

Intestinal (Membrane Surface) Digestion

The major products of intraluminal starch digestion by amylases are maltose, maltotriose, and α-limit dextrins, but not glucose, the only product that could be absorbed intact. α-Amylase cannot cleave the α-1,4 bonds near the α-1,6 branch points, and thus leaves about one third of the amylopectin undigested. These end products could act as inhibitors of further α-amylase activity, but are rapidly removed by hydrolysis by brush border enzymes. α-Amylase has been found to be attached by electrostatic charge to the brush border, an attachment once thought to confer a kinetic advantage to the hydrolysis of starch or to absorption of its products. Although an attractive hypothesis, evidence for its importance *in vivo* is lacking.

The major dietary disaccharides, sucrose and lactose, are also hydrolysed by brush border enzymes (Table 1). These enzymes are all large proteins (> 200 kDa), present either as heterodimers or as single subunits with transmembrane stalks and > 90% of their bulk extending into the lumen of the intestine. With the exception of trehalase, about which little is known, these enzymes are synthesized as large, single-peptide chains, and are modified by glycosylation and cleavage. Sucrase-isomaltase and glucoamylase are split into their final subunits on the external surface of the enterocyte, whereas lactase cleavage appears to occur both intracellularly (pig, human) and extracellularly (rat). The stalk segment of these proteins is cleaved by intraluminal pancreatic proteases which, in the case of lactase, additionally decrease the amount of active enzyme. The various processing steps in the synthesis of these proteins assume greater importance, because deficiency of sucrase-isomaltase and some of the relative deficiency of adult mammals for lactase can be explained by alterations in cellular processing.

The disaccharidases are responsible for the final steps in starch digestion, and for the entire digestion of disaccharides. This surface digestion is important because only monosaccharides can be absorbed from the intestinal lumen. Moreover, the activity of the disaccharidases may be rate limiting for absorption of the component sugars. This is clearly the case for lactase, which is limited in its tissue content in adult mammals. Glucoamylase hydrolysis of glucose oligomers may be rate limiting for glucose absorption when luminal α-amylase activity is scarce. The distribution of disaccharidases along the length of the gut is designed for efficient digeston, as the enzyme content rises in the duodenum, peaks in the jejunum, and declines in the ileum. Normally, carbohydrate digestion is nearly complete by midjejunum. Thus the ileal enzyme activity functions as a safety feature, provided that intestinal transit time is long enough for digestion to be completed.

Dietary factors can regulate brush border disaccharidase levels, as is the case for salivary or pancreatic amylases (Table 2). In rats, the high fasting levels of sucrase-isomaltase decline after eating because of rapid enzyme turnover mediated by pancreatic proteases. Other disaccharidases are also removed from the brush border surface by the action of pancreatic proteases. In pancreatic insufficiency the brush border content of disaccharidases is increased, perhaps to compensate for the decrease in pancreatic α-amylase activity. Although full levels of brush border enzymes are not yet present in the newborn, they may serve the same purpose in the face of low levels of pancreatic enzymes present at this age.

High dietary intake of sucrose or fructose in humans increases glucoamylase and sucrase-isomaltase activity, but not that of lactase. Lactose feeding does not appear to lead to a significant increase in lactase activity in humans; moreover, the absence of dietary lactose in patients with galactosaemia does not alter lactase activity. Fasting in rats leads to a decline in all disaccharidase activity except for lactase, which is preserved. During all these dietary or other experimental changes the alteration in disaccharidase activity appears to be due to changes in enzyme synthesis or in degradation. Enzyme activation does not seem to be a mechanism available for altering disaccharidase activity.

Lactase activity is high at birth in most mammals, and declines after the suckling period, reaching levels of about 10% of that at birth. Initiation of this process may be genetically determined, but can be altered by hormones and nutrients. The tissue content of mRNA (messenger ribonucleic acid) encoding lactase declines after suckling in most studies, while lactase synthesis is decreased, providing a likely mechanism for this striking adaptation. The correlation between the fall in lactase activity and the shortening of the lifespan of the

Table 1.   Mammalian carbohydrases used in dietary carbohydrate digestion

Enzyme	Size (kDa)			Specificity substrate	Bonds cleaved	K_m (mmol l^{-1})	Products
	Proprotein, nonglyco-sylated	Proprotein, glycosylated	Mature form				
α-Amylase (human)							
Salivary	a	a	55	Starch (Glu$_{n > 6}$)	Glc α-1,4 Glc	0·02^b	Maltose,
Pancreatic	a	a	60				maltotriose, α-limit dextrins
Glucoamylase							
Pig	200	225	245^c	Linear glucose	Glc α-1,4 Glc	1–4	Glucose
Rat	145		125 + 135	oligomers (Glc$_{n = 2-9}$)			
Sucrase-isomaltase (human)	210	217	231^d (145 + 151)	Sucrose, turanose	Glc α-1,2 Fru	20	Glucose, fructose,
				α-limit dextrins	Glc α-1,6 Glc	1–4	Glucose
Lactase-glycosyl ceramidase (human)	200	214	262^e (160)	Lactose, cellobiose β-glycosides with hydrophobic aglycon (e.g. phlorizin)	Glc β-1,4 Glc Glc β-1,4 Gal	18	Glucose, galactose, various aglycons
Trehalase							
Rabbit	?	?	75	Trehalose	Glc α-1,1 Glc	2–5	Glucose
Rat	?	?	94				

^{a} These enzymes are not synthesized as proproteins.
^{b} The K_m reported is for starch polymers of an average length.
^{c} Glucoamylase is a heterodimer, in which both fully processed peptides have similar activity.
^{d} Sucrase-isomaltase is a heterodimer containing a sucrase (145 kDa) and an isomaltase (151 kDa) subunit.
^{e} Lactase is converted to a single smaller peptide (160 kDa) containing both enzymatic activities.

Table 2.   Factors altering carbohydrase activity

Enzyme	Factor	Effect
α-Amylase	Starch feeding	Increased enzyme content
	Presence of hydrolytic products	Decreased degradation
	Prenatal development	Increased enzyme synthesis
Disaccharidases	End-product inhibition	Decreased activity
	Enzyme turnover (pancreatic enzymes)	Decreased enzyme content
	Pancreatic insufficiency	Increased enzyme content
Sucrase-isomaltase	Single meal feeding	Decreased enzyme content
	Sucrose, fructose feeding	Increased enzyme content
	Prenatal development	Increased enzyme content
Lactase	Postnatal development	Decreased enzyme content

enterocyte is very close, so much so that the two phenomena have been considered related. It seems possible that the decline in lactase activity after suckling may also involve post-transcriptional mechanisms.

In most mammals the α-glucosidases develop full activity after birth, a phenomenon under transcriptional control. But in the human both α- and β-glucosidase activity is well developed at birth. Premature infants have somewhat decreased lactase activity, but are usually not lactose intolerant, perhaps because enough activity is present, or because colonic digestion of lactose allows absorption of products from a more permeable colon. Some humans (mostly Caucasians) retain high levels of lactase activity after weaning, perhaps due to selection occasioned by herding and milking as a means of subsistence.

Colonic (Luminal) Digestion

Although carbohydrate digestion (and absorption) is very efficient, some dietary carbohydrate can escape digestion in the small intestine and can be delivered to the colon. Up to 70 g of carbohydrate (including the components of dietary fibre) may reach the colon each day in humans. This carbohydrate is fermented by colonic bacteria to short-chain fatty acids (largely acetate, propionate and butyrate), hydrogen gas and methane, as illustrated by the equation below estimating the overall fermentation reaction.

$$34 \cdot 5\ C_6H_2O_6 \rightarrow 48\ CH_3COOH + CH_3CH_2COOH +$$
$$5\ CH_3(CH_2)_2COOH + 23 \cdot 75\ CH_4 +$$
$$34 \cdot 25\ CO_2 + 10 \cdot 5\ H_2O$$

In ruminants these are produced in the forestomach, and in other mammals in the caecum and colon. Butyrate and caproate can be released by gastric lipase action on milk triacylglycerols, and may be nutritionally important in infants.

In the colon, bacteria produce both proteases and glycosidases to degrade mucins, presumably to support bacterial growth. Only certain species secrete the ABH-blood-group-degrading enzymes, which initiate hydrolysis of the carbohydrate moieties of mucins. Thus endogenous carbohydrates are important in perpetuating colonic bacterial cultures, which in turn are responsible for salvaging much of the nutrient value of unabsorbed dietary carbohydrate. *See* Colon, Structure and Function

Absorption and Metabolism

General Characteristics of the Mucosal Barrier

The absorption rate of a solute from the lumen of the intestine depends upon two factors: the concentration of the solute at the apical surface of the enterocyte, and the rate of transport either across the cell (transcellular) or between the cells (paracellular). The delivery of the solute to the cell surface is a function of the efficiency of luminal stirring. In humans the preepithelial diffusion barrier has been reported to produce a uniform thickness of unstirred water in excess of 600 μm, sufficiently large to be the rate-limiting step in absorption. Such an estimate is probably greatly exaggerated, and may have resulted from methodological problems: in the dog, using low concentrations of glucose and vigorous stirring, the unstirred layer is 40 μm. Nonetheless, diffusion through this barrier may still remain the rate-

limiting step for glucose, although the delay in traversing such a barrier should be brief. For passively absorbed compounds, such as high concentrations of glucose or fructose, such a diffusion barrier may represent a significant portion of the total resistance to absorption.

The major dietary monosaccharides (glucose, galactose and fructose) are all absorbed at rates that exceed those expected from passive diffusion. Saturable transport systems have been demonstrated for all three sugars. The intraluminal concentration of monosaccharides after a meal exceeds the observed K_m for monosaccharide transport (1–10 mmol l^{-1}), suggesting that much of postprandial sugar absorption occurs down a concentration gradient, and may not require active transport. Resistance to passive ion flow across the transcellular pathway varies from 1000 to 10 000 Ω cm^{-2}. The resistance of mammalian intestinal epithelium, however, is only 50–90 Ω cm^{-2}. Most (85%) of passive ion flow in the intestine appears to occur paracellularly, and most of that ($> 70\%$) is attributable to the crypt region. Although much of passive sugar transport seems to be carrier mediated, and thus transcellular, recent studies in small animals have suggested that paracellular transport may account for some sugar transport.

Brush Border Glucose Transport

The major systems involved in the uptake of glucose from the intestinal lumen are outlined in Table 3. Active hexose transport is driven by a sodium gradient, a system that has been localized to the apical brush border membrane. In the presence of sodium a membrane potential, as well as the sodium gradient itself, can drive glucose transport (electrogenic cotransport). It is this downhill electrochemical sodium gradient that drives the movement of glucose across the brush border. The stoichiometry for Na$^+$: glucose transport appears to be 1:1 for mammalian membranes, and 2:1 for chicken brush borders. This may represent differences in species or in experimental conditions.

Brush border membranes appear to contain at least two different types of Na$^+$-dependent glucose transporters; one with a $K_m < 50\ \mu$mol l^{-1}, and one with a K_m of 1–25 mmol l^{-1}, depending on the species. The high affinity system would be operating at concentrations even below that of serum glucose. Thus the low affinity system would appear to be operative at the high intraluminal postprandial concentrations. These systems appear to vary independently in conditions of fasting or feeding and during adaptation.

A nearly full-length cDNA (cyclic deoxyribonucleic acid) clone encoding the rabbit cotransporter has been identified and sequenced, yielding a 662 amino acid

Table 3.   Hexose transport pathways in the small intestine

Pathway	Membrane	Transporter	Size (kDa)	Na$^+$ dependent?	Substrate
Transcellular	Apical (brush border)	Na$^+$-glucose	73	Yes	D-Glucose, D-galactose, α-Methylglucoside
		Fructose	?	No	Fructose
	Basolateral	Glucose	57	No	D-Glucose, D-galactose D-Mannose
Paracellular	Basolateral	None	—	Yes[a]	Most monosaccharides

[a] Permeability altered by glucose absorption utilizing the Na$^+$-glucose apical cotransporter. Data limited to small mammals, mostly hamsters.

protein (predicted size 73 kDa) containing 11 membrane-spanning regions. Two hydrophilic segments are considered important in glucose binding. It would appear that the molecule may act as a gated pore, with glucose being translocated after a conformational change of the transporter, rather than being moved by a mobile carrier. The Na$^+$-glucose cotransporter has no detectable homology with the sodium-independent glucose transporters.

Basolateral Glucose Transporter

The concentration step for glucose transport is located at the brush border membrane; in contrast, glucose exit from the cell is mediated by facilitated diffusion by a Na$^+$-independent system shared by nonepithelial cells. In the steady state, the transport of sugars is coupled with electrical, chemical, and perhaps osmotic gradients across the basolateral membrane. These effects may trigger changes in the pump rate of Na$^+$ and K$^+$ movement across that membrane. The energy for this process derives from the action of Na$^+$,K$^+$-ATPase (adenosine 5′ triphosphatase). Na$^+$ can move into the cell to be extruded again, because of its availability at the basolateral membrane via the paracellular pathway.

The basolateral transporter appears to be similar to that in red blood cells. It facilitates exit of glucose and galactose. Similar facilitated diffusion of hexoses has been reported in the basolateral membranes of many tissues, including liver. A cDNA clone encoding this transporter in the intestine has been identified by using a cDNA probe encoding the liver transporter. The protein is a membrane protein with a predicted size of 57 kDa, and 12 hydrophobic transmembrane regions. After exit from the cell, glucose and galactose enter the portal vein, with very little metabolism within the enterocyte.

Fructose Transport

Fructose transport occurs by a Na$^+$-independent, carrier-mediated system. Absorption can occur against a concentration gradient, and presumably requires energy. This system has been localized to the brush border membrane by vesicle studies. Uptake of fructose was slower than that of glucose. After transport into the cell, fructose exits by diffusion across the basolateral membrane. Fructose does not appear to be a substrate for the basolateral Na$^+$-independent transporter. Whether or not a separate basolateral fructose transporter exists is not known. Fructose is more lipogenic than glucose, and causes elevations in triglycerides greater than that of other sugars. Unlike other hexoses, it is metabolized largely in the liver, but like glucose and galactose, very little fructose is metabolized in the intestinal cells.

Paracellular Absorption

In adult animals the ingestion and absorption of glucose far exceeds the rate of active, carrier-mediated transport, measured in anaesthetized animals *in vivo*, or *in vitro* cell preparations. The argument has been advanced that the difference must be accounted for by passive processes, primarily due to solvent drag. Activation of the Na$^+$-coupled transporter by glucose alters the zonula occludens at tight junctions, modifying the sieving properties of the epithelium. These phenomena occur at concentrations of glucose that saturate the transcellular pathway (< 25 mmol l^{-1}). Because glucose concentration after a meal may exceed 200 mmol l^{-1}, and because a more leaky paracellular pathway occurs at concentrations over 25 mmol l^{-1}, it is possible that some of the passive glucose absorption after a meal occurs paracellularly. This prediction is consistent with the observation that glucose uptake by the intestine continues to increase well past the point at which the transcellular pathway is saturated. To date, however, no direct evidence is available to verify and quantify the predictions of this interesting possibility.

In humans the difference between ingestion and active absorption rates is even greater than in animals. Minimum possible rates of glucose absorption in man have been measured as > 200 mmol per hour, or 10 times the estimated active transport capacity. The importance of passive glucose absorption depends upon which sets of data are used, ones which estimate the ingestion: active absorption ratio at 2 or at 10. Nonetheless, it seems apparent that some of the glucose absorbed after a meal probably crosses the apical brush border membrane passively. It is not yet clear whether all of this passively absorbed glucose passes transcellularly or whether some moves paracellularly. There is likely to be a species difference, and in normal humans with a relatively high intestinal resistance, the contribution of paracellular sugar transport will probably be small.

The possible importance of these potential paracellular pathways is emphasized by the observation made in disease states that passive sugar absorption is increased. A number of tests have been devised that compare disaccharide absorption (usually excluded) and monosaccharide absorption (usually absorbed), using poorly metabolized sugars (e.g. cellobiose and mannitol). The ratio of disaccharide to monosaccharide absorption may be an indirect measurement of the paracellular pathway. Employing such tests, increased paracellular absorption has been reported in patients with coeliac disease, Crohn's disease, food allergy, and dermatitis herpetiformis, among others.

Short-chain Fatty Acid Absorption

Short-chain fatty acids are the major nutrients produced by the process of bacterial fermentation. In ruminants (via the forestomach) and in herbivores (via coprophagy) they are delivered for absorption to the small intestine. In humans the fermentation products are produced and absorbed in the colon. The mucosa of both small and large intestine readily absorb unionized short-chain fatty acids. Protonation of these weak acids may occur in the lumen by hydration of carbon dioxide. Unlike hexoses in the small intestine, short-chain fatty acids are partly metabolized in the mucosal cells, and may be a major source of nutrition for colonic epithelial cells. Most of the short-chain fatty acids are metabolized intracellularly to carbon dioxide. In ruminants this metabolism accounts for 70–80% of their basal energy requirement. In mammals the contribution is smaller, but still considerable. Estimates of the contribution of short-chain fatty acid metabolism to the basal metabolic requirement vary from 1–2% in the pig, through 6–9% in humans, to 30–40% in the rabbit. The importance of this pathway in man increases in sugar malabsorption, when delivery of nonabsorbed sugar to the colon increases.

Bibliography

Alpers DH (1987) Digestion and absorption of carbohydrates and proteins. In: Johnson LR (ed) *Physiology of the Gastrointestinal Tract* 2nd edn, pp 1469–1487. York: Raven Press.

Bugaut M (1987) Occurrence, absorption, and metabolism of short chain fatty acids in the digestive tract of mammals. *Comparative Biochemistry and Physiology* 86B: 439–472.

Hallfrisch J (1990) Metabolic effects of dietary fructose. *FASEB Journal* 4: 2652–2660

Hopfer U (1987) Membrane transport mechanisms for hexoses and amino acids ikn the small intestine. In: Johnson LR (ed) *Physiology of the Gastrointestinal Tract* 2nd edn, pp 1499–1526. New York: Raven Press.

MacDonald I (1988) Carbohydrates. In: Shils ME and Young VR (eds) *Modern Nutrition in Health and Disease* 7th edn, pp 38–51. Philadelphia: Lea and Febiger.

Menzies I (1983) Transmucosal passage of inert molecules in health and disease. In: Skadhorge E and Heinfze K (eds) *Intestinal Absorption and Secretion*, pp 527–543. Baltimore: MTP Press.

Lloyd ML and Olsen WA (1991) Carbohydrate assimilation. In: Yamada T (ed) *Textbook of Gastroenterology* 1520–1529. Philadelphia: Lippincott.

Pappenheimer JR (1990) Paracellular intestinal absorption of glucose, creatinine, and mannitol in normal animals: relation to body size. *American Journal of Physiology* 259: G290–G299.

Semenza G and Aurrichio S (1989) Small-intestinal disaccharidases. In: Scriver CR et al. (eds) *The Metabolic Basis of Inherited Disease* 6th edn, pp 2975–2997. New York: McGraw-Hill.

D. H. Alpers
Washington University Medical School, St. Louis, Missouri, USA

Requirements and Dietary Importance

Dietary carbohydrates are the cheapest source of energy for metabolism by the body. They are cheap because they are produced by plants for energy metabolism and storage and consequently can be harvested by man in most temperate and humid climates. To produce a million calories for human consumption requires 0·08 ha for sucrose, 0·16 ha for potatoes, 0·4 ha for wheat and 6·88 ha for cattle. Thus a very important factor when considering requirement of dietary carbohydrate lies largely in economic necessity. Carbohydrates have long been the mainstay in world dietaries, with sucrose and starches being the major sources for human consumption. In regions where per capita incomes are low and the balance between food production and demand close, consumption of carbohydrates as cereals or starchy root vegetables largely meets the need for energy intake. In some underdeveloped countries carbohydrates supply up to 90% of the dietary energy consumed, and, of course, consumption at this level gives rise to concern about deficiencies of the other nutrients such as proteins, minerals and vitamins. In industrial countries dietary carbohydrates provide about half the daily energy intake.

Although the total carbohydrate intake may be similar between some developing and developed countries, the nature of the carbohydrates eaten and the proportion they contribute to the energy intake may not be similar. Carbohydrates from staple foods such as cereals and roots are composed mainly of starch and may represent 85% of the carbohydrate intake in developing countries but only 62% in affluent ones. The difference is largely made up by carbohydrates from fruit, sucrose, corn syrups (mainly in North America) and, to a lesser extent, lactose.

Surveys in the 1980s have shown that the consumption of sucrose is changing, tending to fall in the more developed countries while rising in the others, and it has been suggested that the saturation point occurs at about 160 g per day per person. In developing regions, starch consumption from cereals and roots seems to be related to income, rising when personal income rises. In developed regions, cereal consumption, and therefore starch intake, has fallen, especially in Japan and Eastern Europe, with little change in North America and Australia. These changes might also reflect income, for at higher income levels food choice is not limited to purchasing power and as income rises the proportion of energy derived from carbohydrate tends to fall.

Complex carbohydrates, like other insoluble components of the diet, have no taste, only 'mouth feel', but carbohydrates with a comparatively smaller molecular weight are soluble and stimulate the taste buds for sweetness. This property of sugars, and especially sucrose, makes them an organoleptic requirement for many, especially the young. It has been suggested that this property of the simple carbohydrates is useful in making palatable those foods which are nutritionally desirable but may not be so pleasant to consume. *See* Cereals, Contribution to the Diet; Sucrose, Dietary Importance

Metabolic Importance of Dietary Carbohydrate

The major carbohydrates that are found in the body tissues in humans are glycogen, glucose, fructose, galactose and lactose (in lactation).

Glycogen, the storage form of carbohydrate, is found in the liver and muscle. Before being released into the blood for transport to other regions of the body, it has to be hydrolysed to the monosaccharide, glucose. *See* Glycogen

Glucose is the common metabolic currency of carbohydrate in the body and all cells are able to metabolize glucose to carbon dioxide and water with the consequent release of energy. However, glucose it not only used as a readily available source of energy but it can also be converted to glycogen or to fat for storage. Although glucose can be utilized by all cells, it is only in a few organs that glucose is essential, and these include the brain and red cells of the blood. During pregnancy and growth, glucose is essential for the formation of cell constituents. *See* Glucose, Function and Metabolism

Fructose, which largely comes from the sucrose in the diet and also from honey, does not seem to have a specific role in the body and the only site of production of fructose in humans seems to be in the seminal vesicles, where it is made from glucose.

Galactose is, along with glucose, one of the monosaccharides in lactose; practically the only dietary source of galactose is milk. Galactose is synthesized from glucose in the lactating mammary gland. *See* Galactose

Metabolic Sources of Carbohydrate other than Dietary Carbohydrate

As glucose is essential to the biochemistry of the body it is not surprising that there are sources of glucose other than those in the diet. One of these is obviously liver or muscle glycogen but these stores of 'animal starch' are very limited. After 24 hours or so of complete starvation the stores are empty; yet, as long as water is supplied, a normal-weight person can survive complete starvation for 50–60 days, so alternative sources of glucose must exist.

Another source of glucose in the body is from the glycerol moiety of triglyceride. This part of the triglyceride molecule forms about 10% of its molecular weight, and when triglycerides are hydrolysed the released glycerol can be converted to glucose. Another source of glucose within the body is from the so-called glucogenic amino acids, which can be metabolized to glucose. *See* Triglycerides, Structures and Properties

Although dietary carbohydrates can be converted to fat in the body, fat cannot be converted to carbohydrate.

Metabolic Requirements for Dietary Carbohydrate

Apart from the fact that a diet with little or no carbohydrate would be most unpalatable, there is a metabolic need for dietary carbohydrate. Total deprivation of energy intake has been used in the treatment of obesity and this has provided the opportunity to study the effects of a zero intake of dietary carbohydrate. The effects of diets which are high in protein and fat and very low in carbohydrate have also been studied and the striking consequence of a low or zero carbohydrate intake is that the breakdown of fat in the body cannot go to completion. The final end product of fat metabolism is then a two-carbon chain remnant, existing in the blood as acetoacetic acid or β-hydroxy butyrate. The classical breath odour in this condition, known as 'ketosis', is due to acetone excretion by the lungs. Clinically, 'ketosis' occurs in uncontrolled diabetes mellitus and after 24 hours or more of dietary carbohydrate deprivation in otherwise healthy individuals. Thus carbohydrate is needed in order that the catabolism of fat can be completed to carbon dioxide and water. *See* Fats, Digestion, Absorption and Transport

There are two disadvantages of the ketotic state in an individual: (1) the judgement of such a person may be impaired and it could therefore be unwise to handle potentially dangerous machinery (e.g. a car) while ketotic; (2) the 'ketone bodies' excreted in the breath and urine contain utilizable energy and thus represent an energy loss to the body and diminishing body stores. Production of 'ketone bodies' in large quantities, as in uncontrolled diabetes mellitus, can lead to coma and death. Thus there is a need in all individuals for a minimal daily intake of carbohydrate that can supply the amount of glucose necessary to complete the breakdown of depot fat.

What is the minimum desirable intake of glucose or its equivalent? Under normal circumstances the adult brain needs about 140 g of glucose per day and the red blood cells need another 40 g per day. If diet contains no sugars or starch, about 130 g of glucose can be provided endogenously from the catabolism of protein and from the glycerol moiety of depot fat, thus leaving a shortfall of approximately 50 g per day to be obtained from the diet. It is therefore possible to state a minimum desirable intake of glucose or its equivalent for adults. After several days in the ketotic state the brain, a major consumer of glucose, adapts and can use, to some extent, the energy present in the 'ketone bodies', thus lessening the minimal daily requirement for dietary carbohydrate.

Metabolic 'Knock-on' Effects of Dietary Carbohydrate

All dietary carbohydrates have to be broken down to their constituent monosaccharides (glucose, fructose or galactose) before they can be absorbed from the intestine but only glucose stimulates the release of insulin, a hormone which not only accelerates the cellular uptake of glucose but also facilitates the uptake of amino acids. Insulin is, in general, an anabolic hormone, so that the glucose provided by the carbohydrate in the diet can have far-reaching effects on the metabolism of other dietary constituents, through its ability to bring about the release of insulin.

The amount of energy stored in the body as carbohydrate is minute when compared with that stored as fat or protein. The total quantity of carbohydrate in liver, muscle, kidney and other tissues, plus the glucose that circulates in the blood, amount to about 1800 kcal (7·56 MJ). However, it has been found that the carbohydrate stored in the skeletal muscle can be increased considerably by reducing the proportion of fat in the diet and replacing it with carbohydrate. This is of importance to those who compete in endurance sports and has led to the expression 'carbohydrate loading'.

Finally, there is what used to be called the 'protein sparing' effect of dietary carbohydrate. When the energy intake in the diet is below requirement, administration of carbohydrate (which raises insulin levels) reduces the breakdown of body protein, whereas dietary fat under comparable circumstances has a negligible effect on reducing protein breakdown. *See* Protein, Interactions and Reactions Involved in Food Processing

Bibliography

British Nutrition Foundation (1987) *Sugars and Syrups.* London: British Nutrition Foundation.
British Nutrition Foundation (1990) *Complex Carbohydrates in Foods.* London: Chapman and Hall.
Food and Agriculture Organization/World Health Organization (1980) Carbohydrates in human nutrition. *Food and Nutrition* Paper no. 15.

Ian Macdonald
University of London, London, UK

Metabolism of Sugars

There are only three sugars that are normally present within the body and these are the monosaccharides, glucose, fructose and galactose. Glucose is the prime carbohydrate in the body; fructose is consumed mainly with glucose as the disaccharide sucrose and plays a relatively minor role; galactose is associated with lactation and milk ingestion, and is, along with glucose, one of the monosaccharides of the lactose molecule. *See* Fructose; Galactose; Glucose, Function and Metabolism

Glucose

To produce energy the glucose molecule must enter a cell from the blood and there be converted to glucose 6-phosphate in the cytoplasm. This compound can then be metabolized in a number of ways, depending on the needs and versatility of the cell. It can (1) be broken down to pyruvic acid/lactic acid, (2) go down the

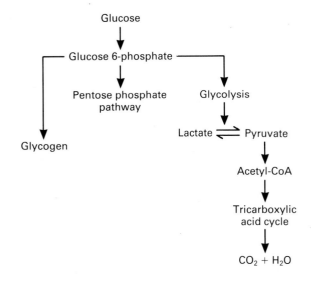

Fig. 1.   Metabolic options for glucose metabolism.

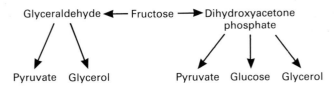

Fig. 2.   Metabolism of fructose.

pentose phosphate pathway, or (3) form glycogen (Fig. 1).

(1) The most important way by which energy is released from the glucose molecule is by the splitting of the molecule to form two molecules of pyruvic acid (glycolysis). This end product of glycolysis may then enter the tricarboxylic acid cycle inside the mitochondia of the cell and be broken down completely to carbon dioxide and water with the release of energy.

When quantities of pyruvic acid and hydrogen atoms become excessive, as in severe exercise, these two products inhibit glycolysis and react with each other to form lactic acid.

(2) The pentose phosphate pathway accounts for as much as 30% of the glucose metabolism in the liver and more than this in the fat cells. This pathway supplies reducing power for fat synthesis from carbohydrate sources.

(3) When glucose is not immediately required for energy, the extra glucose that continually enters the cells is stored as glycogen or converted to fat. Glucose is preferentially stored as glycogen and only when the cell approaches saturation with glycogen is the additional glucose then converted to fat. *See* Glycogen

Fructose

Fructose in the bloodstream is utilized about twice as fast as blood glucose; the liver and, to a lesser extent, the kidney and small intestine are the main sites of fructose metabolism. The utilization of fructose by other peripheral tissues seems to be negligible. The first step in the metabolism of fructose is the formation of fructose 1-phosphate which then splits to form two 3-carbon molecules, namely glyceraldehyde and dihydroxyace-

tone phosphate. As shown in Fig. 2, these trioses can form pyruvate, glycerol and, in the case of dihydroxyacetone phosphate, glucose.

Fructose is mainly converted to glucose and lactic acid, with perhaps up to 3% of the fructose being converted to triglycerides; ketone bodies; glycerol and sorbitol are minor end products.

Metabolism of Sugars in the Liver

Glucose

In the liver, glucose has no difficulty in crossing the cell wall; the main factors influencing the rate of entry are the concentration of glucose in the blood and the ability of the enzymes in the cell to dispose of the glucose. Much of the glucose that is absorbed from the intestine never reaches the peripheral circulation as it is taken up in the first pass through the liver.

The liver is also capable of releasing glucose into the blood, either as a result of the breakdown of glycogen or protein, or as a result of synthesis from glycerol. The balance of input and output of glucose by the liver is entirely controlled by hormones, acting via the enzymes within cells:

(1) Insulin, which is produced by the β cells of the pancreas, accelerates glycogen formation. In other cells in the body, insulin is solely concerned with the transfer of glucose into the cell, but in the liver insulin influences the synthesis of enzymes.
(2) Glucagon is produced by the α cells of the pancreas, and causes a rapid breakdown of liver glycogen.
(3) Adrenaline, like glucagon, stimulates the breakdown of glycogen but, unlike glucagon, it is able to do this in muscles as well; it does not stimulate insulin release.
(4) Glucocorticoids are produced by the adrenal gland. These hormones maintain and aid the formation of glycogen. *See* Hormones, Adrenal Hormones

Fructose

In man most of the fructose absorbed from the intestine is taken up by the liver, hence the low blood levels of fructose after its ingestion. Compared to glucose, fructose has a greater ability to form lactate but, unlike glucose, fructose administration leads to an increase in blood uric acid levels and, for this reason, has been used as a screening test for gout. Also in the liver, fructose is converted to the lipid triglyceride to a greater extent than is glucose; again unlike glucose, whether given orally or intravenously, fructose speeds up the metabolism of ethanol by the liver.

Sugars and Muscle

The muscle mass, because of its size and sheer need, plays a principal role in carbohydrate metabolism. The uptake of glucose by muscle cells is insulin sensitive but the metabolism of fructose in the cell is probably minimal and only the pyruvate and lactate formed from fructose in the liver would be of any support to the muscle cell.

Sugars and Depot Fat

The pioneering studies of Lawes and Gilbert in 1852 showed that dietary carbohydrate can be converted to depot fat, a fact known by most overweight people. Glucose and fructose are the two carbohydrates usually presented to the fat cell or adipocyte and the extent of their uptake into adipose tissue is closely controlled by hormones, the most influential of which is insulin. Part of the glucose taken up by the adipocyte is converted to glycerol but the main fate of the glucose is in the formation of fatty acids. Following a high carbohydrate diet there is an increase in both insulin levels and fatty acid synthesis from glucose. *See* Fatty Acids, Metabolism

Fructose can enter the adipocyte but its rate of transport is slow and only at high levels of fructose do significant levels enter the adipocyte.

Sugars and the Brain

The brain seems to be entirely dependent on glucose and oxygen, and a reduction in the supply of either will soon lead to irreversible damage. The brain removes a fixed amount of glucose per unit time irrespective of the blood concentration of glucose and its uptake is not dependent on insulin. There has been a suggestion that the insulin release following glucose ingestion increases the level of serotonin in the cerebral tissue and that this compound diminishes the sensation of pain and produces a feeling of wellbeing.

Sugars and the Metabolic Rate

The increase in metabolic rate after the ingestion of various sugars is greater after sucrose or a mixture of fructose and glucose than after glucose alone, suggesting that the body 'handles' fructose more efficiently than glucose.

Sugars and the Fetus and Neonate

As lipid does not cross the placenta to any great extent the fat present in the infant at birth must have been synthesized in the fetus from glucose or amino acid. Changes in the maternal blood glucose level are quickly reflected in the fetal blood.

In contrast to glucose, fructose cannot cross the placenta, although some animal species (not humans) can transform glucose to fructose in the placenta.

In the neonate the sole dietary source of carbohydrate is the lactose in milk but no specific role for lactose has been identified.

Factors Affecting the Metabolic Response to Dietary Sugars

Sex of the Consumer

The increase in blood triglycerides seen in men after a diet high in fructose is not seen in young women but is found in postmenopausal women. Although both sexes increase hepatic lipogenesis after fructose ingestion, it is possible that premenopausal women are able to remove the blood triglycerides more rapidly.

Type of Fat Accompanying the Carbohydrate

A synergistic effect of sucrose and animal fat on blood triglycerides has been shown, and the raised levels found after a diet high in sucrose are considerably reduced by polyunsaturated fat accompanying the sucrose.

Dietary Protein

The recovery of serum albumin after protein deficiency seems to be slower with sucrose in the diet than with starch, and the interplay of the metabolism of sugars and protein becomes more interesting when it is appreciated that the amino acids arginine and leucine stimulate the release of insulin. *See* Protein, Interactions and Reactions Involved in Food Processing

'Sensitivity' of the Consumer

The extent to which sugars are converted to lipids, especially triglycerides, seems to vary between individuals. Those persons whose level of triglycerides in fasted blood is high, and who may be more prone to coronary heart disease, have a greater increase in these triglycerides after consuming carbohydrates than persons with normal lipid levels.

Species

There are not only within-species differences in metabolic responses to sugars but also more marked differences between the species. For example, rats can absorb fructose from the intestine very rapidly and this will affect the metabolic handling of fructose when compared to humans.

Bibliography

Dickens F, Randle PJ and Whelan WJ (1968) *Carbohydrate Metabolism and its Disorders*, Vols 1–3. London: Academic Press.

Macdonald I and Vrana A (eds) (1986) Metabolic effects of dietary carbohydrates. *Progress in Biochemical Pharmacology* 21.

Reiser S and Hallfrisch J (1987) *Metabolic Effects of Dietary Fructose*. Boca Raton: CRC Press.

Sipple HL and McNutt KW (eds) (1974) *Sugars in Nutrition*. New York: Academic Press.

Ian Macdonald
University of London, London, UK

Determination

Food carbohydrates consist of a heterogeneous group of substances of widely differing physical and chemical properties. There are no simple methods by which they can all be determined at one time. The methods of choice (Table 1) depend on the reason for the analysis and the physical form and composition of the foodstuff. Legal requirements, quality control and dietary information are based on differing types of information and generally involve different analytical techniques. Rather outdated traditional methods are often used to comply with well-established legal requirements or long-standing practice. Accepted and recommended methods are regularly described by the International Standards Organization, Geneva, the International Commission

Table 1.   Analytical methods for food carbohydrates

Carbohydrate	Usual analytical methods	Comments
Common analyses		
Reducing sugars	Chemical	Mainly glucose and fructose
Sucrose	Chemical, physical, enzymatic	
Starch	Extractive, physical, enzymatic	Amylose and amylopectin rarely determined separately
Dietary fibre	Extractive	Includes the noncarbohydrate, lignin
Syrups	Physical, enzymatic, chromatography	Major constituents are glucose, fructose, sucrose or maltose
Less common analyses		
Glucose	Physical, enzymatic	
Fructose	Chemical, enzymatic	
Lactose	Enzymatic	
Dextrin	Physical, chromatography	Including maltose
Soluble fibre	Extractive, enzymatic	Mainly pectic substances and hemicelluloses
Insoluble fibre	Extractive, chemical	Mainly cellulose
Rare analyses		
Galactose	Enzymatic	
Maltose	Enzymatic, chromatography	
Raffinose	Enzymatic, chromatography	
Inulin	Enzymatic	
Glycogen	Enzymatic	
Sugar alcohols	Enzymatic, chromatography	Sorbitol and xylitol are examples
Algal polysaccharides	Chemical	Carrageenans, agar and alginates
Gluconic acid	Enzymatic	
Others	Enzymatic, chromatography	Other monosaccharides, oligosaccharides, gums, mucilages and additives

for Uniform Methods of Sugar Analysis, the *Official Journal of the European Communities* and the Association of Official Analytical Chemists, Washington, DC, USA. Some foodstuffs consist of carbohydrates in a state pure enough to enable immediate analysis without prior extraction or clean-up. Others are so heterogeneous that reproducible sampling is the major problem for the analyst. The value obtained for the carbohydrate will depend very much on the method of analysis chosen. Of all the methods currently in use, enzymatic analyses produce the most accurate data as they are specific for individual sugars. Such methods are gradually replacing many traditional procedures. One of the advantages of the use of enzymes, which is becoming increasingly important, is their use of safe reagents, particularly when compared with chemical analytical techniques. Other methods in common usage are non-specific and require some prior knowledge of the sample, obtained by past experience or from the literature, in order to give reliable and useful results. They have the advantage that a considerable amount of experience of these methods has accumulated over the years.

The reason for the analysis is often the primary determinant of the method chosen. Of secondary but significant importance is the cost in terms of trained personnel, assay time, capital equipment, reagents and waste disposal. Chromatography is chosen where several soluble carbohydrates are to be determined in the same sample. Where only the total reducing sugar or total carbohydrate is required, simpler chemical or physical methods may often be preferred.

Extraction and Clean-up

Many sugar-containing foodstuffs are already in a homogeneous liquid state (e.g. syrups) and do not require extraction. For other solid, solid–liquid, emulsified and multiphase materials, the sugars generally have to be extracted to produce an essentially clear and colourless solution. As the accuracy of the analytical results depends on the representative sampling of the starting material and the yield of the extractive process, these early stages are of prime importance. Material is carefully stored prior to assay to ensure that no changes in composition occur. Representative sampling can usually be guaranteed by the use of large, well-chosen samples. Solids are ground down and homogenized under conditions in which further metabolic changes, owing to enzyme action, are minimized. The process should be fast and efficient. Low-molecular-weight carbohydrates may be extracted with hot aqueous solutions or, to avoid coextracting the soluble polysaccharides, with 80% aqueous ethanol.

Methods for the clean-up of sugar extracts from foodstuffs depend not only on the nature of the

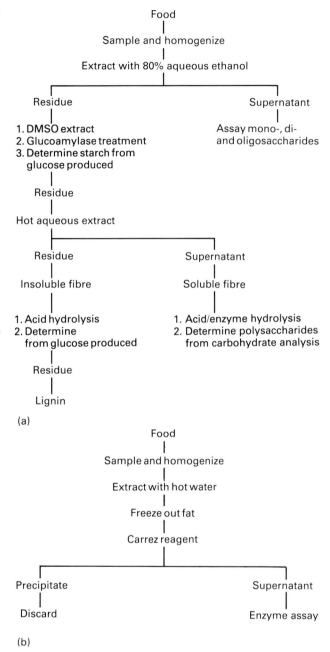

Fig. 1 Indicative outline of extraction and clean-up for (a) chemical analysis and (b) enzymatic analysis. DMSO, dimethyl sulphoxide.

foodstuff but also on the analytical methods which are to be employed (Fig. 1). As there are many methods for extraction and clean-up, the schemes shown are indicative only of the methods available. Solutions of low-molecular-weight carbohydrates are often deproteinized and clarified by coprecipitation with the zinc ferrocyanide precipitate formed by Carrez reagents (0·1 M sodium hydroxide added to an equal mixture of solutions I (0·085 M potassium ferrocyanide) and II (0·25 M zinc sulphate) until the pH is about 8). Alternatively, fat may be removed by freezing it out of the subsequent extracts or by back-extracting with nonpolar organic solvents. Protein can be specifically removed from solid material by the use of proteases. If necessary, solutions are decolourized with polyamide, gelatine or polyvinylpolypyrrolidone.

Extractive Methods

Polysaccharides are usually analysed as part of the extraction procedure. Starch is insoluble in hot aqueous ethanol and solubilized only with great difficulty by hot water. By preference, it is dissolved in hot acidified 80% aqueous dimethyl sulphoxide (DMSO) and quantified using the glucose produced from its subsequent acid or enzymatic hydrolysis (see later, eqn [6]) of the digest. Starch may also be determined gravimetrically after precipitation from solution by complexation with molecular iodine. The residue after starch hydrolysis contains the other food polysaccharides (Fig. 1a) as constituents of the various dietary fibre fractions (Table 1). Pectins are dissolved in hot water and quantified from the galacturonic acids produced on enzymatic hydrolysis. Hemicelluloses are determined by the analysis of acid hydrolysates after hot alkaline extraction. Soluble polysaccharides may be separated from each other by selective precipitation with salts or organic solvents. Residual cellulose, which is solubilized by treatment with concentrated sulphuric acid (12 M) is determined from the glucose produced by dilute acid hydrolysis. *See* Cellulose; Dietary Fibre, Determination; Hemicelluloses; Starch, Structure, Properties and Determination

Determination of the water content of pure syrups may be used to calculate the total carbohydrate content by difference. The weight loss on drying of concentrated syrups gives an approximate water content, the lack of accuracy being due to the fact that some of the water is very strongly bound, and conditions for its removal also cause the degradative dehydration of some carbohydrate compounds. A more accurate method is the Karl Fischer titration, in which the water is titrated against a solution of iodine and sulphur dioxide in anhydrous methanol.

The sucrose concentration of syrups is sometimes determined by isotope dilution.

Physical Methods

Physical methods are useful for the analysis of otherwise well-characterized sugar syrups. They are rapid, inexpensive and non-destructive but usually give inaccurate results for all but pure solutions. To determine the carbohydrate concentrations, published tables or empirical equations are often used, rather than the standard solutions used in chemical, enzymatic and chromatographic methods. Temperature has to be strictly controlled during these analyses.

Many carbohydrates are very soluble and produce concentrated solutions showing significantly higher densities and refractive indices than pure water. Determination of the specific gravity (ratio of the density of a solution compared to that of pure water at a defined temperature) or refractive index (ratio of the speed of light in a vacuum to its speed in the substance) allows the concentration of pure carbohydrate syrups to be established. Specific gravity is measured using a sugar hydrometer in the degassed solution at 20°C. The refractive index is measured using a sugar refractometer with thermostat and a yellow sodium light source. Sugar hydrometers and refractometers are calibrated directly in degrees Brix, which is equivalent to the percentage sucrose on a weight basis. As nonsugars have similar effects on density and refractive index, these methods may also be used to obtain an approximate measure of the total dry substance in less well-characterized syrups. The effects of concentration changes are slightly non-linear, a 10% increase in dry substance in solution producing an approximately 4% increase in density and 1% increase in refractive index.

The optical rotation of carbohydrate solutions also varies with the sugar concentration. The effect is a property of optically active substances and varies in magnitude and rotary direction with different carbohydrates. The optical rotation is determined on optically clear, or clarified, solutions with a polarimeter using yellow sodium light at 20°C. The change in optical rotation with concentration is slightly non-linear and temperature-dependent. Unknown mixtures of carbohydrates and solutions containing other optically active material (i.e. most biological molecules) cannot be analysed using this method. The α and β anomers of carbohydrates have different specific rotations (the angular rotation of plane-polarized light observed per unit concentration under specific conditions), necessitating the mutarotation (the equilibrium between the α and β forms of the reducing sugars) to equilibrium of solutions before analysis. As sucrose has a different specific rotation to that of invert syrups, the sucrose content of a complex mixture can be determined from the difference in optical rotation found before and after acid or enzymic inversion (eqn [5]). Other soluble di-, oligo- and polysaccharides may be determined in a similar manner. The specific rotation of glucose syrups varies in an almost linear manner with their dextrose equivalent (DE; the percentage hydrolysis of starch as measured by the reducing sugar produced), which allows the straightforward determination of the DE of pure starch hydrolysates. *See* Sucrose, Properties and Determination

Table 2. Important chemical methods of carbohydrate analysis

Carbohydrate group	Assay	Mechanism of action
Reducing sugars	Lane and Eynon titration	Reduction of alkaline cupric tartrate to cuprous oxide
	Luff–Schoorl method	Iodometric determination after the reduction of alkaline cupric citrate
	Dinitrosalicylic acid assay	Reduction of alkaline dinitrosalicylic acid to yield a green solution
	Ferricyanide assay	Reduction of alkaline ferricyanide to give Prussian Blue
Hexose (e.g. glucose)	Phenol sulphuric acid assay	Condensation of phenol with dehydrated hexoses to yield a yellow solution
	Iodometric titration	Oxidation by iodine to give aldonic acids
Ketose (e.g. fructose)	Phenol boric acid sulphuric acid assay	Condensation of phenol with dehydrated ketoses to yield a blue solution
Uronic acid	Carbazole assay	Condensation of carbazole with dehyrated uronic acids to yield a pink solution

Spectroscopic Methods

The infrared spectra of carbohydrates are complex and cannot easily be used to analyse mixtures of carbohydrates. However, Fourier transform infrared reflectance spectroscopy (FTIR) has been developed as a method for the analysis of the total carbohydrate content in complex mixtures, suspensions and solid foodstuffs. The major advantage of this method is that no sample preparation is necessary. *See* Spectroscopy, Near-infrared

Chemical Methods

Methods for the chemical analysis of carbohydrates depend on the chemical reactions of specific functional groups. They use inexpensive reagents and relatively straightforward protocols. The mechanisms of the analytical reactions are poorly characterized and optimum conditions have been determined empirically. Side-reactions always occur with varying importance dependent on the precise assay conditions and the type and concentration of the other components present. These analyses are reproducible, given reproducible assay conditions and analyte. However, they are generally inaccurate in that they show sample-dependent systematic errors. This is particularly relevant in the analysis of complex and poorly characterized foodstuffs. Different carbohydrates generally give different responses in all of these assays. With care, chemical methods can be used where absolute accuracy is not of the prime concern and in quality assurance with otherwise well-characterized samples. They are of similar sensitivity to enzymatic methods.

A carbohydrate analytical assay of great interest and importance in the food industry is the determination of reducing sugars (carbohydrates possessing a free alde-

hyde or ketone group) (Table 2). Such assays must be undertaken under strictly controlled conditions and both noncarbohydrate reducing agents (e.g. vitamin C) and molecular oxygen offer considerable interference. Since the 1920s, the commonly recommended procedure within the food industry has been the Lane and Eynon titration. The more recent constant-volume modification of this method involves the reduction of alkaline cupric tartrate, freshly prepared by mixing equal volumes of Fehling's solutions A (0·278 M copper sulphate) and B (1·226 M sodium potassium tartrate in 2·5 M sodium hydroxide), to cuprous oxide under very closely controlled conditions. The reaction is completed by boiling for a strictly controlled time, the steam generated preventing aerobic reoxidation. The reducing sugars are titrated until the colour of blue cupric tartrate is lost. Addition of the redox indicator, methylene blue, enables this end-point to be more precisely determined. The mixed Fehling's solution is precalibrated with a standard invert sugar solution. By preliminary testing of the approximate concentration of reducing sugar, it is ensured that the end-point is always reached at about the same final volume ($\pm 1\%$), so that the reagent concentrations remain closely controlled. The reaction is not stoichiometric, but reproducible results are obtained under these conditions. An empirical correction factor has to be applied if there is an excess of (nonreducing) sucrose present. The Luff–Schoorl method is another modification of the Lane and Eynon titration, whereby alkaline cupric citrate is reduced. It has been developed empirically to produce similar responses for glucose and fructose. Excess cupric ions left at the end of the reaction are reduced by excess iodide, and the iodine released is titrated against standard thiosulphate solution. This reaction is both nonstoichiometric and nonlinear, but adequate results are obtained by reference to standard tables. The reducing sugar assays can be applied to nonreducing carbohydrates if they are first hydrolysed to their constituent reducing sugars by acids or enzymes. Lactose, in mixtures with sucrose, glucose and fructose, may be determined after prior removal of the fermentable sugars with baker's yeast. *See* Lactose

Most of the other major chemical analytical methods (Table 2) involve the dehydration of the carbohydrates to furfuraldehyde or furancarboxylic acid derivatives, using hot concentrated sulphuric acid, followed by condensation with an organic reagent to produce coloured solutions. These assays can be made more or less specific by control of the precise conditions of dehydration and the careful selection of the condensing reagent. As the dehydration conditions are quite severe, oligomeric and polymeric carbohydrates also generally respond in these assays. *See* Spectroscopy, Visible Spectroscopy and Colorimetry

Enzymatic Methods

Enzymatic methods of analysis are applicable to a wide range of materials capable of acting as substrates, inhibitors or activators of enzymes. Such methods utilize the specificity of enzymes to pick out mainly biological substances from mixtures, and are ideally placed for the analysis of foodstuffs. If care is taken over the purity and specific activity (the enzymatic activity per unit weight of enzyme) of the enzyme(s), they are generally very reliable methods, of good sensitivity, accuracy, linearity and precision. Repeat experiments generally produce standard deviations of about 1–2% of the means. All currently accepted assays make use of end-point determinations where the analyte is the substrate of a single enzyme, or an enzymatic pathway. The quantification is determined on the basis of a change in colour or ultraviolet absorption between the material before and after it has totally reacted. Coupled enzymatic pathways are used in order to produce the change in absorption or to pull the reaction in the required direction. At least one of the enzymes, if there are more than one, is usually sufficiently specific so that only the required analyte gives a response. *See* Enzymes, Use in Analysis

Several carbohydrates may be determined in the same solution by timing the addition of the enzymes such that the absorption changes are noted sequentially. Interferences, owing to inhibitory effects, are rarely found in the enzymatic analysis of foodstuffs; antioxidants and preservatives do not interfere and heavy metal ions, which may inhibit enzymes, are not present at sufficient concentrations in routine analysis. As the analyses require the determination of absorption changes, practically clear and almost colourless solutions are required. This is generally achieved by coprecipitation of the coloured, suspended or emulsified material with Carrez reagent, as outlined in Fig. 1b.

Of all the enzymatic assays, that for glucose is the most important. This is not only because glucose is the most common single analyte, but also because it is often produced from other carbohydrates, in their assays, by hydrolysis. Analysis is by conversion of the glucose to 6-phosphogluconolactone with the concomitant conversion of the coenzyme NADP$^+$ (oxidized form of nicotinamide adenine dinucleotide phosphate) to its reduced form, NADPH, which absorbs light of wavelength 340 nm (eqns [1, 2]). Although hexokinase is not a very specific enzyme (Table 3), glucose-6-phosphate dehydrogenase is highly specific, making the coupled assay an excellent reference method specific solely for D-glucose.

$$\text{D-Glucose} + \text{ATP} \xrightarrow{\text{hexokinase}} \text{glucose 6-phosphate} + \text{ADP} \quad (1)$$

$$\text{Glucose 6-phosphate} + \text{NADP}^+ \xrightarrow{\text{Glucose-6-phosphate dehydrogenase}}$$
$$\text{6-phosphogluconolactone} + \text{NADPH} + \text{H}^+ \quad (2)$$

A similar assay can be applied to the determination of fructose, if the intermediate, fructose 6-phosphate, is converted to glucose 6-phosphate (eqns [3, 4] followed by [eqn 2]). Glucose can be determined in the same sample by delaying the addition of the phosphoglucose isomerase until all the glucose has reacted. Such assays are able to determine accurately as little as 0·002% glucose and fructose in 99·995% sucrose. If fructose alone is required, the last trace of glucose can be removed from solutions, by aerobic oxidation catalysed by glucose oxidase and catalase, prior to the fructose determinations. Mannose, produced by the hydrolysis of some thickening agents, may be determined similarly to fructose but with the addition of phosphomannose isomerase which converts the mannose 6-phosphate produced by hexokinase to fructose 6-phosphate. *See* Fructose

$$\text{D-Fructose} + \text{ATP} \xrightarrow{\text{hexokinase}} \text{fructose 6-phosphate} + \text{ADP} \quad (3)$$

$$\text{Fructose 6-phosphate} \xrightarrow{\text{Phosphoglucose isomerase}} \text{glucose 6-phosphate} \quad (4)$$

Sucrose can be determined by analysis of either the glucose or the fructose produced by hydrolysis (eqn [5]). Use of glucose is preferred as invertase produces fructose from other β-fructans; for example, raffinose produces fructose and melibiose. The presence of these β-fructans may be determined from the ratio of glucose to fructose.

$$\text{Sucrose} + \text{H}_2\text{O} \xrightarrow{\text{Invertase}} \text{D-fructose} + \text{D-glucose} \quad (5)$$

The difficulty with the determination of starch by enzymatic analysis concerns its poor solubility (Fig. 1a). It can be fully solubilized by hot acidic DMSO or by

Determination

Table 3. Sources and specificity of enzymes used in carbohydrate analysis

Enzyme[a]	Common name	Source	Specificity[b]
Oxidoreductases			
1.1.1.14	Sorbitol dehydrogenase	Sheep liver	Polyols
1.1.1.27	Lactate dehydrogenase	Pig muscle	L-Lactic acid
1.1.1.44	6-Phosphogluconate dehydrogenase	*Saccharomyces cerevisiae*	6-Phosphogluconate
1.1.1.48	β-Galactose dehydrogenase	*Pseudomonas fluorescens*	D-Galactose, L-arabinose
1.1.1.49	Glucose-6-phosphate dehydrogenase	*S. cerevisiae*	D-Glucose 6-phosphate
1.1.3.4	Glucose oxidase	*Aspergillus niger*	D-Glucose
1.6.4.3	Diaphorase	Pig heart	NADH
1.11.1.6	Catalase	Beef liver	Hydrogen peroxide
Kinases			
2.7.1.1	Hexokinase	*S. cerevisiae*	D-Hexoses
2.7.1.12	Gluconate kinase	*Escherichia coli*	D-Gluconic acid
Hydrolases			
3.2.1.3	Amyloglucosidase	*A. niger*	Internal α-linked D-glucose residues
3.2.1.20	α-Glucosidase	*S. cerevisiae*	Terminal α-linked D-glucose in dimers and trimers
3.2.1.22	α-Galactosidase	Green coffee beans	Terminal α-linked D-galactose in oligomers
3.2.1.23	β-Galactosidase	*E. coli*	Terminal β-linked D-galactose in dimers
3.2.1.26	Invertase	*S. cerevisiae*	Terminal β-linked D-fructose in oligomers
Isomerases			
5.3.1.8	Phosphomannose isomerase	*S. cerevisiae*	D-Mannose 6-phosphate
5.3.1.9	Phosphoglucose isomerase	*S. cerevisiae*	D-Glucose 6-phosphate

NADH, reduced form of nicotinamide adenine dinucleotide.
[a] Enzyme commission (EC) numbers.
[b] Specificity as shown in carbohydrate assays.

autoclaving its aqueous suspensions. When dissolved it is fully hydrolysed by amylogucosidase (eqn [6]), a hydrolytic enzyme specific for α-linked glucose oligomers and polymers. The glucose produced is analysed as above. The method is also applicable to glycogen, dextrins and maltose. α-Glucosidase is preferred to amyloglucosidase for the analysis of maltose and maltotriose as it does not hydrolyse higher dextrins (eqn [7]). Sucrose, being an α-glucoside as well as a β-fructoside, may also be determined using this latter assay (eqn [8]) by analysing the fructose produced.

$$\text{Starch} + (n-1)\,H_2O \xrightarrow{\text{Amyloglucosidase}} n\ \text{D-glucose} \quad (6)$$

$$\text{Maltose} + H_2O \xrightarrow{\text{α-Glucosidase}} 2\ \text{D-glucose} \quad (7)$$

$$\text{Sucrose} + H_2O \xrightarrow{\text{α-Glucosidase}} \text{D-fructose} + \text{D-glucose} \quad (8)$$

Lactose can be determined from the glucose or galactose produced by hydrolysis with β-galactosidase (eqns [9, 1 and 2 or 9 and 10], NADH also absorbing at 340 nm). Lactulose, produced in heated milk, may be similarly determined from the fructose produced (eqn [11], followed by eqns [3, 4, 2]). The α-linked galactose oligomers, raffinose, melibiose and stachyose (which produces two moles of galactose per mole), can be determined from the galactose produced by hydrolysis (eqns [12, 10]) with α-galactosidase. These galactosidases are anomer-specific, so that lactose does not interfere, even at high concentrations, in the assay of raffinose, nor raffinose in the assay of lactose. *See* Galactose

$$\text{Lactose} + H_2O \xrightarrow{\text{β-Galactosidase}} \text{D-Glucose} + \text{D-galactose} \quad (9)$$

$$\text{D-Galactose} + NAD^+ \xrightarrow{\text{β-Galactose dehydrogenase}} \text{galactonolactone} + NADH + H^+ \quad (10)$$

$$\text{Lactulose} + H_2O \xrightarrow{\text{β-Galactosidase}} \text{D-fructose} + \text{D-galactose} \quad (11)$$

$$\text{Raffinose} + H_2O \xrightarrow{\text{α-Galactosidase}} \text{D-galactose} + \text{sucrose} \quad (12)$$

Enzymes may be used in many other analyses. Thus inulin may be determined from the fructose it produces on mild perchloric acid hydrolysis. Sorbitol and xylitol are analysed following oxidation to fructose and xylulose respectively. This reaction, catalysed by NAD^+-dependent sorbitol dehydrogenase, is pulled to completion by the removal of the resultant NADH either by reaction with diaphorase and iodonitrotetrazolium chloride to produce the coloured formazan, or by pyruvate and lactate dehydrogenase, leaving the fructose to be determined as described earlier. Gluconic acid may be determined in an analogous manner to glucose but using the enzymes gluconate kinase and 6-phosphogluconate dehydrogenase.

Biosensors

Biosensors are analytical devices which convert biological responses directly to electrical signals. The biologically active material is often a oxidoreductase enzyme, bound at an electrode surface, which utilizes the redox electrons to produce the electrical response. Most of the early interest in these devices centred around clinical analysis, but they are now entering the food carbohydrate arena as sensors for glucose and sucrose. The primary enzyme used is glucose oxidase (eqn [13], Table 3). The sensor can be made responsive to other sugars by binding carbohydrate hydrolases (e.g. invertase) together with the glucose oxidase.

$$\text{D-Glucose} \xrightarrow{\text{Glucose oxidase}} \text{gluconolactone} + 2H^+ + 2e \qquad (13)$$

Chromatographic Methods

Chromatographic methods are used to separate carbohydrates. They give quantitative data where standards are available, and interference from other similarly behaved molecules is negligible. Positive confirmation of the identity of chromatographic peaks (e.g. by mass spectrometry) is rarely undertaken, reliance being placed on previous experience and the similarity to separately run standards. Thin-layer chromatography and paper chromatography are still used for the qualitative analysis of carbohydrates, particularly oligosaccharides (carbohydrate polymers containing from two to about ten residues). These methods have been considerably improved over the years, and can yield quantitative data. However, the most common methods of chromatographic analysis are gas chromatography (GC) and high-performance liquid chromatography (HPLC). *See* Chromatography, Principles; Chromatography, High-performance Liquid Chromatography; Chromatography, Gas Chromatography; Chromatography, Thin-layer Chromatography

Carbohydrate analysis using GC usually consists of the separation of the per-trimethylsilyl derivatives on packed-bed or highly efficient, fused-silica, wall-coated open tubular (WCOT) columns using nonpolar dimethyl silicone stationary liquid phase and a flame ionization detector. Separation results from the extractive distillation of the volatile derivatives.

A wide variety of columns may be used for HPLC but columns containing calcium (Ca^{2+})- or silver (Ag^+)-loaded cation exchangers, at moderately high temperatures, or amino-bonded silica operating at around ambient temperature have recently become most popular. The metal-loaded cation exchangers act primarily by size exclusion, elution being roughly in order of decreasing molecular weight. Amino-bonded silica columns use an acetonitrile–water mobile phase and separate mainly by partition between the acetonitrile-rich mobile phase and the water-enriched stationary phase. Detection is usually by means of changes in refractive index, although mass detectors, which utilize the light-scattering of particles left after solvent evaporation and detect all nonvolatile materials, are becoming more popular. Solutions for HPLC must be free of salts, amino acids and proteins as these interfere with detection and the chromatographic separation. The extra clean-up this necessitates is often achieved by solid-phase extraction using syringe-operated cartridge mini-columns and guard columns (small HPLC columns used primarily to protect the main HPLC column but also often used to remove low levels of contaminants).

The choice between GC and HPLC depends on the carbohydrates present and the purpose of the analysis. The latter method is generally preferred for the analysis of simple monosaccharide mixtures and for oligosaccharide analysis and purification, whereas GC can be used on very complex monosaccharide mixtures and to avoid the much more extensive clean-up needed for HPLC. As GC requires the time-consuming and error-prone preparation of volatile derivatives of the carbohydrates for the analysis, higher-molecular-weight molecules should be analysed by HPLC. There is generally sufficient material available to the food analyst that the 100-fold greater sensitivity of GC over HPLC is of no importance. In practice, HPLC is becoming the method of choice, particularly as more efficient and selective columns become available.

Bibliography

Anonymous (1989) *Methods of Biochemical Analysis and Food Analysis.* Mannheim, FRG: Boehringer Mannheim GmbH.

Ball GFM (1990) The application of HPLC to the determination of low molecular weight sugars and polyhydric alcohols in foods: a review. *Food Chemistry* 35: 117–152.

Birch GG (ed.) (1985) *Analysis of Food Carbohydrate.* Essex: Elsevier Science Publishers.

Chaplin MF and Bucke C (1990) *Enzyme Technology.* Cambridge: Cambridge University Press.

Chaplin MF and Kennedy JF (eds) (1986) *Carbohydrate Analysis. A Practical Approach.* Oxford: IRL Press.

Kirk RS and Sawyer R (1991) *Pearson's Composition and Analysis of Foods* 9th edn. Essex: Longman Scientific and Technical.

Determination

Schneider F (ed.) (1979) *Sugar Analysis. ICUMSA Methods.* Norwich: The International Commission for Uniform Methods of Sugar Analysis.

Southgate DAT (1991) *Determination of Food Carbohydrates* 2nd edn. Essex: Elsevier Science Publishers.

M. F. Chaplin
South Bank Polytechnic, London, UK

Sensory Properties

Sweetness of Sugars in Relation to Structure

The first sensory response expected of low-molecular-weight carbohydrates is sweetness. More than 100 substances are sweet and chemically identified as sugars, or nutritive carbohydrate sweeteners. Many other unrelated substances of diverse molecular geometry elicit the sweet taste, including some aliphatic and aromatic organic compounds, amino acids and certain inorganic salts. However, the sensory properties of foods that are influenced by carbohydrates extend far beyond sweetness. Flavours, in addition to the sweet taste, develop from browning reaction products. Colour is another sensory property developed with browning reactions. Textural attributes are influenced in numerous ways: the low-molecular-weight carbohydrates contribute body or viscosity or interact with other components, including the high-molecular-weight carbohydrates, to influence sensory properties of food products; and the starches and gums contribute thickening and gel structure alone and by interactions with each other to alter other mechanical and geometrical textural characteristics. *See* Sensory Evaluation, Appearance; Sensory Evaluation, Texture; Sensory Evaluation, Taste

Stereochemical Similarities of Sweet Compounds

AH–B Groups

Sweet-tasting compounds have a common structural feature identified as the geometric separation of the two electronegative atoms, A and B. The hydrogen atoms link covalently to A, thereby creating a proton-donating AH component, while B maintains the role of the proton or hydrogen bond acceptor, as shown in Fig. 1. The AH–B system of a stimulating compound combines reversibly by intermolecular hydrogen bonding with a commensurate AH–B system on a proteinaceous receptor molecule of the tongue. The perception of a sweet taste occurs if the distance between A and B is between 0.25 and 0.4 nm.

The primary AH–B system of the common sugars is the α-glycol grouping, the portion farthest from the reactive, anomeric centre; for example, the 3,4α-glycol system of glucopyranose structures is responsible for its sweet taste. The glycol group is found in any of four steric positions: gauche, staggered, anticlinal, and eclipsed (Fig. 2). When glycol pairs are in the gauche or staggered position, hydroxyl groups are equidistant and the centre of the oxygen orbitals are close enough (0.286 nm) for sweetness to occur.

Anticlinal hydroxyl groups are too far apart (> 0.4 nm) to bond intermolecularly to receptor AH,B sites. Strong intramolecular hydrogen bonding occurs when the α-glycol group is eclipsed, decreasing the number of glycol units available to elicit the sweet taste, so that those compounds do not taste sweet. The decrease of sugar sweetness is especially true if the primary AH unit is involved. However, in the case of sugar alcohols, such as maltitol and lactitol, intramolecular hydrogen bonding between AH and B promotes sweetness in comparison to maltose and lactose, respectively. *See* Lactose; Malt, Malt Types and Products; Sugar Alcohols

Hydrophobic Site

In some carbohydrates and the potent sweeteners, a third hydrophobic bonding site probably functions. Apparently, the bipartite AH–B interaction between stimuli and receptor provides sweetness, but the tripartite interaction governs the intensity of response and temporal differences. This hydrophobic site is located sterically at the same position with respect to AH and B, about 0.35 nm from A and 0.55 nm from B if a tripartite AH–B–X interaction is to occur between stimuli and receptor. This component is not a lock-and-key mechanism, but a directing, aligning, or entrapping influence

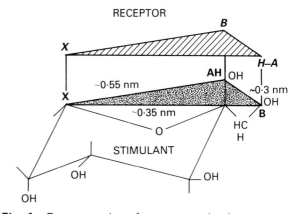

Fig. 1 Representation of sweetness stimulant–receptor interaction showing the location of AH–B–X units on a sugar (β–D–fructopyranose) for the stimulant template and its relationship to the template for the corresponding receptor site.

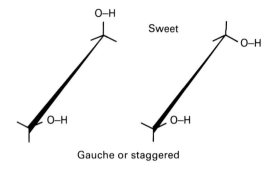

Sweet

Gauche or staggered

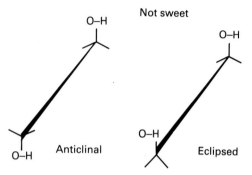

Not sweet

Anticlinal   Eclipsed

Fig. 2 Conformation of glycol units for sweet and not sweet sugars. (Reprinted by permission from Shallenberger RS and Acree TE (1967) Molecular theory of sweet taste. *Nature* 216: 480; Copyright ©1967 Macmillan Magazines Ltd.)

as the stimulus molecule approaches the receptor site. *See* Sweeteners – Intense

In the chlorosugars the chlorine atoms probably increase the lipophilicity and improve the access to the sweetener receptors. Chlorosubstituents at the 4, 1′, and 6 positions of sucralose induce sweetness; two or more chlorosubstituents on the sugar have synergistic effects. Not all molecules with apparent AH–B–X 'glucophores' are sweet; additional structural characteristics relevant to the elicitation of sweetness include hydrogen bonding in aqueous solutions, chiral centres, and deoxy, methylene and methyl groups. Factors that seem to depress sweetness include ring oxygens, glycosidic oxygens, ether linkages at secondary positions, and methyl ethers.

Bitter Components

Many derivatives and some unmodified sugars have a bitter, as well as a sweet, component. The anomeric carbon, anomeric hydroxyl groups and the ring oxygen atom of some carbohydrates elicit bitterness, but have no role in the sweetness response. The bitter/sweet molecules polarize on the taste receptors so that the hydrophilic end of the molecule interacts with a sweet receptor and the hydrophobic end with a bitter receptor, rather than some molecules orienting themselves on sweet receptors and some orienting on bitter receptors.

Receptor Sites for Sweet Substances

Several hypothetical receptor sites on the tongue and in the oral cavity have been proposed, but the nature of the receptor for sweet compounds remains unclear. The sweet response involves a chemical stimulation of a heterogeneous population of electrically charged taste cells, but responses vary among species, individuals, and cells. The receptor sites for sugars are not identical from one taste bud to the next, and different receptor sites exist on the same taste bud. Apparently, several receptor sites of variable but low specificity cooperate in the sweet taste chemoreception. The various sweeteners do not trigger each of the mechanisms in the same proportions. It is supposed that sugars cannot persist at the receptor site because they lack the lipophilic bonding site. Hence, once the appropriate number of receptor sites are occupied by sugars, the remaining sugar molecules are diffused away from the site.

Temperature can influence the nature of the sweet response. An increase in temperature causes an increase in sucrose sweetness intensity but a decrease in persistence of sugar sweetness. Increasing the temperature has no effect on the binding to the receptor site, but temperature apparently affects the approach of the stimulus molecules to the receptor site. The optimum temperature for the detection of sweetness is near the temperature of the tongue, since electrophysical responses are maximal at this point. Acuity to all tastes is minimized if the food is very hot or cold. Temperature of the stimuli not only affects the sensitivity of the taste receptors, but also can affect the conformation and configuration of the sweetener. Heat can break the intramolecular hydrogen bonds, freeing more hydroxyl groups to participate in the AH–B system. *See* Sucrose, Properties and Determination

Intensity of Sweetness

Sweetness generally decreases with the molecular weight of a sugar, although the reason is unknown. Perhaps only one sugar residue in each oligosaccharide binds to the taste bud, or only that part of the sugar is responsible for eliciting a sweet response. Lack of sweetness in certain compounds is caused by steric interference of one or both of the axial hydroxyl groups, thus preventing binding to the taste bud protein.

Relative sweetness, defined as the 'ratio of concentration of substances matching in sweetness', is a common means of characterizing the sweet sensation. Sucrose is the reference for rating the sweetness of other compounds (Table 1).

Synergistic effects are inferred when the sweetness of the mixture is greater than the sum of the components, a well-known phenomena in psychophysics and flavour

Table 1. Relative sweetness of sugars

Bulk solids	
Fructose	1·2–1·7
Glucose	0·7–0·8
Invert sugar	1·0
Isomalt (Palatinit®)	0·5–0·6
Lactitol	0·3
Lactose	0·2–0·4
Maltose	0·4–0·5
Mannitol	0·4–0·7
Mannose	0·6
Sorbitol	0·5–0·6
Xylitol	0·9–1·2
Xylose	0·7
Bulk syrups	
Corn syrup, unmixed, acid-converted	
30 DE	0·3–0·35
36 DE	0·35–0·4
42 DE	0·45–0·5
54 DE	0·5–0·55
62 DE	0·6–0·7
High-fructose corn syrup	
42%	0·9–1·0
55%	1·0–1·1
90%	1·2–1·6
Hydrogenated glucose syrup (Lycasin®)	0·4–0·75
Chloroderivatives of sucrose (sucralose)	5–2000
Stevioside	300

[a] Sucrose=1·0. Sweetness is a subjective measurement dependent upon many external factors, including concentration, temperature, pH, structural configuration, and degree of hydrolysis.
DE, dextrose equivalent.

research. Synergism can result from solute–solute, solute–water and solute–receptor interactions. Some sugars react synergistically but the effect with any given sugar is not universal. Fructose, for example, shares a synergistic relationship with saccharin and glucose but not necessarily with other carbohydrate sweeteners. Synergism between the sugars and several of the high-potency sweeteners is common. *See* Fructose

Intensity of sweetness also relates to concentration, but this relationship is not always linear. The concentration effect results, in part, from the saturation of taste cell receptors. If all receptors are activated or satiated, the presentation of more sweetener to the receptor site will not produce a noticeable difference in response.

Concentration increases can negate or alter intensity differences or induce unpleasantness. Relative sweetness of sucrose, fructose, glucose, and starch hydrolysis products increases with an increase in concentration, but the relative sweetness of sucralose, a potent sweetener, decreases with increases in concentration at the high concentrations. Whether the sweetener is in solution or in its crystalline form, the age of the test medium, and the degree to which the sugar has mutarotated are

further factors influencing relative sweetness. *See* Starch, Functional Properties

Temporal Effects and the Sweetness Response

Onset time and duration of sweetness can influence the acceptability of a sweetener. Consumers detect sucrose sweetness within 1 s and that sweetness lasts about 30 s. Any sweetening agent that has a delayed initial sweetness or a sharp or prolonged sweetness sensation will probably taste unusual to many people. A localized concentration of stimulus molecules at the receptor site is believed to govern the persistence or duration of sweetness. The lipophilic site could be responsible for directing potent sweeteners into localized concentrations (or 'queques') at a nonspecific area of the cell membrane and account for persistence of sweetness. Thus the physical length of the queque determines the duration of sweetness by how long the receptor is supplied with stimuli.

Synergism of Sugars with Other Food Components

Interaction of Components and Effects on Sweetness

The following factors influence and modify perception of sweetness from sugars: the presence and concentration of other tastes, sweeteners and flavours; the structural matrix, whether a solid, liquid or gas; viscosity and solvent polarity of the medium; temperature of processing, storage and preparation, and the microbes and enzymes present. Typically, sweet compounds are embedded in a complex matrix with bitter, sour and salty tastes and the flavour nuances of other ingredients. The 'taste modifiers' alter sweetness quality, increase or reduce intensity, or mask aftertaste, probably by exerting a physical or chemical effect on the stimulus rather than the taste receptor. Sensory acuity to carbohydrate sweetness diminishes in the presence of other tastes, but the degree of suppression depends on the nature of the secondary agent, the concentration, and the intensity of taste.

Sweetness seems to be enhanced at low ($<0·4\%$) sodium chloride concentrations but perceived sweetness declines if the concentration of salt is high. Sweetness of sucrose, fructose, and glucose is affected differently by various acids and the relative concentrations of each of the components. Fruit flavourings alter sweetness perception of aqueous systems, generally enhancing the sweetness of the carbohydrate sweetener. The sugar decrease the perception of bitterness in foods and beverages.

Relative initial and maximum sweetness of sugars in food products differs from that in model systems.

Thickened stimuli generally are perceived to be less sweet than those in thinner mediums with equal concentrations of the sugars. Texture and physical properties of a food affect its taste because texture partially controls the amount and the rate at which the taste compound reaches the taste buds. Thresholds for the four basic tastes are higher in food products than in aqueous solutions. Sweetness perception is maximal when there is little or no interference from physical behaviour of the taste medium. Viscous and oil solvents exhibit an interfering behaviour which raises the threshold and minimizes the perceived sweetness intensity.

Sugar–Protein Interactions

Flavours and colours of foods are altered by nonenzymatic browning of carbohydrates. Thermal decomposition of simple and complex carbohydrates usually occurs in combination with inorganic or organic catalysts and results in caramelization, the key pathway for the formation of flavours associated with molasses, maple syrup, and caramel flavourings and colourings. The carbonyl-amine reaction involves a thermally induced interaction between an amino acid and a reducing sugar. Many pathways and reaction schemes follow ring opening and enolization of the sugars and their interactions with nitrogenous amino groups. The unique colour and flavour compounds produced in roasted coffee, nuts, meats, chocolate, maple syrup, and bakery products result, in large part, from the carbonyl-amine reaction. Products of the carbonyl-amine reaction and interactions of the caramelization and carbonyl-amine reactions include pyrroles, pyridines, imidazoles, pyrazines, furfurals, furanones, oxazoles, and thiazoles; and they can form numerous brown to black polymers. Maltol and isomaltol, with their fragrant, caramel-like aromas, enhance both the flavour and sweetness of many foods. In foods cooked by microwaves and in extruded foods, the time, temperature and moisture conditions result in a lack of flavour and colour because only low levels of the browning reaction products are formed. Strecker degradation and the fragmentation of carbonyl-amines are well-defined pathways that can also result in many off-flavour compounds in foods. During the final stages of the Strecker degradation reaction, formaldhydes and pyrazines evolve from amino ketone fragments of the reducing sugar. Food processors should optimize desirable caramel-type aromas but must minimize the burnt, bitter and acrid notes that can be produced. *See* Browning, Nonenzymatic

Sugar Interactions and Textural Changes in Foods

Sweeteners, such as maltodextrins and low-dextrose-equivalent (DE) corn syrups, impart the desired degree of body, cohesiveness, or chewiness to table syrups, fruit beverages, confectionery products, fruit bars, ice cream, sherbet and other frozen desserts. Viscosities of most carbohydrate sweeteners in solution are similar except for glucose syrups. A large percentage of high-molecular-weight polysaccharides increases the relative viscosity of glucose syrups. Consequently, these syrups impart more cohesiveness, body and adhesiveness to a food system than other types of sweeteners. Viscosity of carbohydrate-sweetened solutions is also governed by solute concentration and temperature. With an increased temperature, molecular motion is increased, reducing the friction among the molecules and resulting in a decreased resistance to flow.

Low-DE syrups are viscous and increase the chewiness of products such as caramels and cookies (biscuits) more than an equal concentration of a higher-conversion, lower-viscosity syrup. The low-viscosity syrups decrease the viscosity of a candy mass of a given sucrose composition by decreasing air retention. The candy is brittle and good flavour release in the mouth is promoted. *See* Biscuits, Cookies and Crackers, Methods of Manufacture

The sharp crystalline edges of sugars contribute to the aerated nature of chemically leavened bakery products by helping to disperse the lipid portion of a batter in the initial creaming stages of multi-stage mixed batters and doughs. This creaming of the shortening allows the formation of many air cells, thus increasing the volume and tenderness. Sugars further tenderize bakery products by controlling starch hydration and by dispersing protein and starch molecules. Starch and protein molecules are separated by the sugars, as well as by lipids, and are prevented from forming a continuous mass. The structure remains flexible and pliable enough to allow for maximum expansion during leavening and before thermal setting. Excessive sugar can increase the fluidity of the batter, increase the coagulation temperature of the egg proteins, and increase the temperature at which starch gelatinization occurs to the extent that the structure is too weak to support its weight. The batter rises before thermal set, but then collapses. *See* Cakes, Nature of Cakes

Regulating the amount and type of sugar controls cookie spread. Increasing the amount of sugar with a given amount of water generates more solution than is available with water alone. Small crystals increase cookie spread because fine crystals dissolve more readily, gelatinization and thermal set times are delayed, the dough is more fluid, the cookie spreads farther before the structure sets, and it is crisper. When cookies contain high levels of sucrose, a hard, sweet cookie with 'snap', or a crispness and crunch, results after cooling as the sugar syrup recrystallizes to form an amorphous glass. Molasses, honey, glucose syrups, and high-fructose corn syrup inhibit crystallization and give softer cookies that are chewy rather than crisp.

Sensory Properties of Polysaccharides in Relation to Structure

Polysaccharides affect the sensory properties, particularly the texture, of food products by retarding the flow as well as modifying gelling characteristics. Nonstructured, amorphous regions of polysaccharides are highly hydratable, and bind large quantities of water. In contrast, areas that contain a large portion of straight-chained crystalline regions, such as retrograded starch gels, exclude water. Most natural and synthetic hydrocolloids, or gums, display pseudoplastic flow properties, i.e. the viscosity of the solution decreases as the shear rate increases. With high shear rates, viscosity decreases because the particles are oriented parallel to the shear field. In general terms, viscosity also decreases as temperature increases.

Sensory Properties and Rheological Character

The predominant sensory property of many gum solutions is slimy; a thick, mouth-coating material which is difficult to swallow. Dispersions that approach Newtonian flow behaviour are associated with a high degree of sliminess, and gums in solution that depart considerably from Newtonian flow and have a high degree of shear-thinning are less slimy in the mouth. Other sensory attributes used to describe gum solutions are adhesive, starchy, gummy, astringent, slippery, and oily. 'Starchy' is a flavour related to an undercooked product, but the other parameters are related to mouth-feel and mechanical textural properties. Blandness is normally the desired flavour quality for carbohydrate thickeners in food products.

Pseudoplastic behaviour is associated with a less slimy mouth-feel because the viscosity of the fluid decreases at the shear rate encountered in the mouth (approximately $50\,s^{-1}$). High-viscosity seed and exudate gums – guar, tragacanth, and locust bean – are more pseudoplastic than alginates and cellulose ethers, while gum arabic has a very low viscosity and nearly Newtonian flow properties up to a concentration of at least 40%. Dispersions of microcrystalline cellulose, a synthetic gum, show both thixotropic and plastic behaviour. The behaviour that dominates depends upon concentration and shear history. Starches can be modified to alter their consistency; cross-linking contributes short, stringless consistency in waxy and tapioca starches. The unmodified starches will have a stringy, cohesive consistency. High levels of highly cross-linked waxy cornstarch (cornflour) will increase chewiness in a product. *See* Gums, Properties of Individual Gums; Gums, Nutritional Role of Guar Gum

Gel Properties

Several polysaccharides provide partial gel structure in some food products and total structure in others. High-

methoxyl pectins in fruit jellies, low-methoxyl pectins for dietetic gels, starches in puddings, agar in meat products, carrageenan for kosher fruit gels and milk puddings and alginate in pie fillings, reformed vegetables, fruits and meat chunks are all examples in which the carbohydrates provide either total or partial gel structure.

Gels can be brittle, rigid, springy, firm, soft, spreadable, cutable, rubbery, smooth, or grainy depending upon the degree of interactions of the polymers and the concentration. Gelation balances polymer–polymer and polymer–solvent interactions to form a tertiary network or matrix; a gel is an intermediate state between a solution and a precipitate. Enhanced interactions among polymer molecules result as their solubility decreases and generally lead to firm, rubbery, springy, rigid gels. Gels tend to become more brittle as concentration increases, but faster rates of setting and decreased uniformity of matrices also result in increased brittleness. Crisp or crunchy mouth-feel for snack foods is obtained with high amylose of slightly degraded waxy pregels that expand to tender structures with heating and drying. Rubbery structures are obtained with thin boiling corn starch in the presence of high concentrations of sugars. In other instances, substances influence the rigidity or strength by (1) competing with water for the binding loci, such as sugar softening a starch gel, (2) competing with the solid phase for the liquid, as sugar does in high methoxyl pectin gels, (3) altering the pH, as acids do in pectin systems, (4) interacting chemically with either or both phases, as calcium ions forming cross-bridges with alginates or low-methoxyl pectins, and (5) altering the charge distribution on the polymer molecules.

Relationship of Gel Strength to Interactive Forces

The type and strength of the crystalline junction zones in polysaccharide gel networks govern the strength, elasticity, and flow behaviour of the gel. If the junction zone is short and chains are not held together strongly, the polysaccharide molecules will separate under physical pressure or with slight increases in temperature. One or more polysaccharides can be involved in the junction zone; the zones can involve multiple helices or aggregates of ordered ribbons. Agar forms one of the strongest gels known via bundles of associated double helices, and the gels remain stable at temperatures of 30–85°C. Helical junction zones are also involved in carrageenan and furcelleran gels. Low-methoxyl pectins, with less than 50% esterification, can form stable gels using divalent ions, such as calcium, to form cross-links. Alginate gelation occurs at room temperature in the presence of calcium or other di- or trivalent ions, or in the absence of ions at pH 3 or less. Gellan, in the presence of ions, gels similarly to alginate but gives brittleness, elasticity and cohesiveness that are similar to those of agar gels, except that gellan gels are more firm. In the case of carrageenans, ions are immobilized at the junction zones, although the primary gelation mechanism is believed to be hydrogen bonding. κ-Carrageenans form firm gels with potassium, but not with sodium ions, and ι-carrageenan is calcium sensitive. Both κ- and ι-carrageenans form a gel; however, λ fractions are strongly anionic, do not complex readily with cations, and do not gel.

Polysaccharides with carbonyl groups also do not gel easily because of electrical repulsion between approaching chain segments. High-methoxyl pectin (55–80% esterification) forms strong gels only if (1) the pH is adjusted to 2·0–3·5 to prevent charge repulsion and ionization of the carboxylate groups and (2) a dehydrating material is used to increase the intermolecular interactions by hydrogen bonding among the polymers. A synergism between alginates and pectins for gel formation occurs if the system is first acidified in order to reduce electrostatic repulsion and permit molecular association.

Molecular Configuration and Gel Character

Branched molecules do not form strong junction zones; thus they do not form strong, elastic gels. Studies on cross-linking mechanisms of mixed gels (agarose, carrageenans or xanthan plus galactomannans such as guar or locust bean) suggest an ordered binding between extended ribbon conformations of smooth sites (unbranched areas) on the galactomannan chains and double helices of the agarose or carrageenan. In the case of the xanthan gum, the unstructured smooth regions of the mannan and the xanthan are involved in the junction zone of thermally reversible gels.

Concentration Effects

Gel strength in simple gel systems, such as alginate or pectin gels, and in the more complex starch gel is strongly concentration-dependent. For a given polymer type, a critical concentration, specific for any given polymer–solvent pair, is required. Polysaccharide solutions generally form gels at relatively low concentrations of gelling material, and firm gels can be prepared from a few types of gums, such as pectins, at levels of 1% or lower. Other colloidal gelling agents require a concentration of as much as 10%. A higher polymer concentration is probably needed in some systems to allow close association of molecules for aggregate formation at low temperatures where less opportunity exists for intermolecular interaction. An aggregated-type gel structure requires higher particle concentrations than a polymer network. Overall strength of starch gels depends upon

the residual swollen gelatinized granules to reinforce the strength of the amylose gel matrix. Soft jelly gums can be obtained with high-amylose starches. The retrogradation of amylose is controlled to give textures ranging from a short, clean bite to a long, somewhat chewy bite in products such as gum drops, orange slices, and gummy bears. Thin boiling starches obtained by acid treatment to produce short chains in the amylopectin portion are used with high concentrations of starch and sugar for the manufacture of firm, rubbery gum candies (sweets).

In polysaccharide gels, crystalline junction zones can also occur to such a degree with time that retrogradation and corresponding syneresis occurs. Increased polyguluronate junction zones in alginate gels result in rigid, brittle gels with high syneresis, whereas few junction zones produce an elastic gel with less tendency to synerese. In general, syneresis is promoted by increases in temperature and ionic strength of the dispersing medium. Syneresis resulting from compression can give a feeling of juiciness in the mouth.

Synergism of Polysaccharides with Other Food Components

Gel Structures

Mixed gels and filled or composite gels are utilized to obtain specific textural properties in food products. The texture is dependent on the relative proportions of each component and the overall concentration. Locust bean gum and κ-carrageenan form brittle, slightly elastic gels, whereas xanthan gum and κ-carrageenan or low-methoxyl pectin and ι-carrageenan form soft, cohesive gels. Low levels of gellan gum can give similar gel characteristics as high levels of κ-carrageenan with locust bean gum. Myoglobin and bovine serum albumin are proteins that promote low-methoxyl pectin gelation, but they inhibit formation of alginate gels. Each of the gelling agents can contribute to the gel formation in mixed gels, or one of the agents can be considered nonactive, modifying the characteristics but not interacting to form a gel network. For example, agar forms microgels in the gelatin matrix of an agar–gelatin mixed gel.

Flavour Carrying and Encapsulation

Carbohydrates can enrobe, absorb and retain flavour volatiles during processing, and this has important implications in food systems. Gum arabic, guar gum, modified starches, and maltodextrins, as well as sucrose and lactose, are commonly used for encapsulation by spray-drying or extrusion processes. Inclusion complexing is used for encapsulation by the β-cyclodextrins. *See* Flavour Compounds, Production Methods

Bibliography

Birch GG (1976) Structural relationships of sugars to taste. *CRC Critical Reviews in Food Science and Nutrition* 9: 57.
Birch GG (1980) Theory of sweetness. In: Koivistoinen P and Hyvönen L (eds) *Carbohydrate Sweeteners in Foods and Nutrition*, pp 61–75. New York: Academic Press.
Koivistoinen P and Hyvönen L (eds) (1980) *Carbohydrate Sweeteners in Foods and Nutrition*. New York: Academic Press.
Lineback DR and Inglett GE (eds) (1982) *Food Carbohydrates*. Westport, Connecticut: AVI Publishing.
Morris VJ (1986) Gelation of polysaccharides. In: Mitchell JR and Ledward DA (eds) *Functional Properties of Food Macromolecules*, pp 121–170. New York: Elsevier Science Publishers.
Oakenfull D (1987) Gelling agents. *CRC Critical Reviews in Food Science and Nutrition* 26 (1): 1.
Reineccius GA (1989) Flavor encapsulation. *Food Reviews International* 5(2): 147–176.
Shallenberger RS (1977) Chemical clues to the perception of sweetness. In: Birch G, Brennan J and Parker K (eds) *Sensory Properties of Foods*, pp 167–283. Essex: Elsevier Science Publishers.
Waller GR and Feather MS (1983) *The Maillard Reaction in Foods and Nutrition*. ACS Symposium Series 215. Washington, DC: American Chemical Society.

Carole S. Setser
Kansas State University, Manhattan, USA

CARBOXYLIC ACIDS

See Acids

CARCINOGENS

Contents

Carcinogenic Substances in Food

Risk to Humans

Cancer is, after cardiovascular disease, the most important cause of nonaccidental mortality in industrialized countries. Furthermore, in certain Third World countries, cancer of the liver is the single most important cause of death in individuals aged 20–35 years. Whereas current estimates suggest that smoking-related cancers may account for 30% of all cancer deaths in the USA, with a range of between 25% and 40%, diet is considered to be an equally important risk factor. The best estimate of the proportion of cancer deaths associated with diet is 35%; however, the range of 10–70% indicates the uncertainty inherent in the epidemiological data. *See* Cancer, Epidemiology; Liver, Nutritional Management of Liver and Biliary Disorders; Smoking, Diet and Health

It is now accepted that cancer development is a complex, multistep process, making the identification of specific stages and causes difficult. Nonetheless, epidemiological data, the study of familial associated cancers and experimental work in animals suggest that damage to the genetic material may be an important event in cancer development. Carcinogens that react with deoxyribonucleic acid (DNA), and are active in various short-term tests (see later), are said to be genotoxic carcinogens, and many have been implicated in the initial stages of carcinogenesis. In experimental systems, these chemicals act rapidly and their effect is only slowly reversible. Numerous other carcinogenic chemicals do not react with DNA and show no activity in short-term tests. These are described as nongenotoxic carcinogens and appear to act through epigenetic mechanisms. Many cause the disease to progress by their action on previously initiated cells, and are described as promoters.

Both macro- and microcomponents of the diet may contribute to the development of cancer. In experimental animals it has been clearly shown that dietary levels of fat, protein and carbohydrate (the macronutrients) may greatly modify the incidence of cancer. In man the association is less clear, although there is compelling circumstantial evidence relating the intake of fat, both in quality and quantity, to the incidence of cancer at certain defined sites, such as the colon and mammary gland. The microcomponents include both man-made and natural compounds, either added deliberately or incorporated through unintentional contamination. In addition, storage practices or cooking processes may result in the production of potentially carcinogenic agents. *See* Breast Cancer and Diet; Colon, Cancer of the Colon

Diversity of Dietary Carcinogens and Levels in the Diet

While the human epidemiological data on dietary carcinogens are sparse, a carcinogenic effect has been described in animals for a variety of compounds that occur, or may occur, in the diet of humans. The main sources of dietary carcinogens are as follows:

1. Food additives.
2. Contaminants: migration from packaging materials; pesticides and herbicides; animal drug residues.
3. Naturally occurring carcinogens: natural components; mycotoxin contaminants – aflatoxin B_1, ochratoxin A.
4. From preparation, preservation or cooking.

It must be emphasized that the identity of these groupings is based largely on data from experimental animals, and any attempt to partition the relative risks from these sources is based on hazard assessment from animal data. The role of bulk components of the diet in such risk assessment is poorly understood, as is the role of certain protective factors. For example, the observed decrease in gastric cancer in Western countries may be a result of an increase in the intake of vitamins C and E, which may act to prevent the formation of gastric carcinogens, or as a result of a reduction in the levels of carcinogens in the diet resulting from improvements in food storage methods. *See* Ascorbic Acid, Physiology; Cancer, Diet in Cancer Prevention; Cancer, Diet in Cancer Treatment; Oesophageal Cancer; Tocopherols, Physiology

Most carcinogens identified in diet are those that generally show genotoxic activity and have been recognized as carcinogens in animal experiments. These are a numerous, diverse group of chemicals and are widely distributed. Their concentration in food is usually measured in mg per kg, or parts per million (ppm), or in μg per kg, or parts per billion (ppb). For example, the carcinogen N-methyl-N-formyl hydrazide is found in mushrooms at 500 ppm, mixed hydrazines in *Agaricus bisporus* at 400 ppm, psoralens in parsnips at 40 ppm and in celery at 1 ppm, and pyrrolizidine alkaloids in plants at 100–6000 ppm. Nitrosamines have been reported in cooked meats at levels of up to 5 ppb, while polycyclic aromatic hydrocarbons have been reported at levels of 1–200 ppb, depending on the type of food and method of cooking. In addition, pyrolysis products of various amino acids, such as Trp-P-1, Trp-P-2, Glu-P-1 and Glu-P-2, have been described at levels of 10–50 ppb in food. *See* Nitrosamines; Polycyclic Aromatic Hydrocarbons

Another group of carcinogens to which particular attention has been directed are the mycotoxins, of which the most extensively investigated has been aflatoxin B_1. Contamination with aflatoxin results from the presence in food of certain strains of *Aspergillus flavus*. In the tropics, peanuts and peanut products are often contaminated with aflatoxins, and levels as high as 15 600 μg per kg have been reported. Such contamination would lead to overt hepatotoxicity, while contamination with aflatoxin B_1 at lower levels of between 2 and 200 μg per kg may play an important role in the development of liver cancer. Infection with hepatitis B virus may also be an important contributory factor in aflatoxin-induced liver cancer. Infection with hepatitis B virus may also be an important contributory factor in aflatoxin-induced liver cancer. At present, the evidence does not allow a complete assessment of the importance of the various risk factors. *See* Mycotoxins, Occurrence and Determination

Attempts to categorize carcinogenic risks from food exposure are complicated by the variety of materials present, the uncertainty of individual exposure, and the various additive and protective factors that may exist. Recent assessments have suggested that the traditional food components contribute the bulk of the effect (41–98%). In contrast, contamination with pesticides and animal drugs may account for between 0·02% and 0·81% of the foodborne risk. Food preparation and contamination with mycotoxins may also account for relatively small risks of 0·01% and 0·0001%, respectively, in developed countries. However, in the case of food preparation, this risk may be comparable to that attributed to traditional foods under some circumstances.

Biochemical Metabolism and Transformation of Carcinogens

Many of the carcinogens that have been described undergo extensive transformation within the body. Such metabolic changes are frequently essential for the acquisition of carcinogenic activity. Oxidation reactions are of paramount importance in this process and are mediated

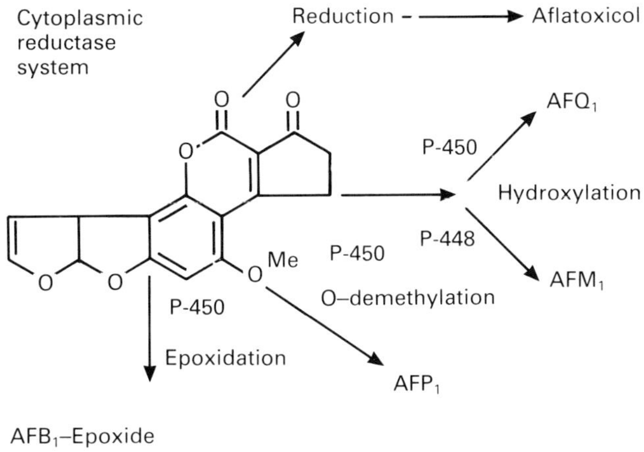

Fig. 1 The metabolism of aflatoxin B$_1$.

principally through the cytochrome P-450 family of mixed-function oxidase enzymes. In addition, flavine-dependent enzymes, the prostaglandin endoperoxide synthetase system, and other peroxidases may also be involved. The primary oxidative product of such metabolism may be further metabolized by reaction with, for example, sulphate or glutathione (phase II reactions) which may result in detoxification. In some instances, however, phase II reactions may lead to the carcinogenic moiety. Examples of the two mechanisms are given by N-nitrosodimethylamine (NDMA) and 2-acetylaminofluorene (2-AAF). Nitrosodimethylamine is oxidized by the P-450 monooxygenase enzymes to hydroxymethyl-methylnitrosamine. This is unstable and decomposes to formaldehyde and nitrosomethylamine. It is presumed that the latter yields nitrogen and methyl carbonium ion, the proximate methylating agent through breakdown of the unstable intermediate methyl diazonium hydroxide. 2-Acetylaminofluorene undergoes N-hydroxylation to yield a compound which is more carcinogenic than the parent compound. However, this compound, N-hydroxy-2-AAF, is not itself the active agent; conjugation with sulphate or acyl groups, mediated by sulphotransferases and acetyltransferases, respectively, leads to a highly reactive intermediate group, the breakdown of which results in the production of arylamidonium ions which may react with DNA or other cellular targets.

The metabolism of these agents is complex and the overall result (activation or detoxification) is often dependent on a number of competing pathways. This can be illustrated with reference to aflatoxin B$_1$, the metabolism of which is shown in Fig. 1. In these processes the epoxidation pathway is considered to be the primary activation step and the balance between the various primary steps, together with various conjugation reactions along with the stability of the DNA adducts (see later) may determine the relative effectiveness of aflatoxin B$_1$ as a carcinogen in different species.

Interaction of Carcinogens with Macromolecules and other Cellular Constituents

The metabolic pathways described above give rise to reactive molecular species that may readily interact with a variety of cellular molecules having nucleophilic sites. Thus the methylcarbonium ions, resulting from the metabolism of NDMA, methylate both proteins and nucleic acids. In this regard interaction with DNA is considered the primary event for agents which initiate carcinogenicity. Fifteen different sites susceptible to attack by alkylating agents have been identified, relative reaction rates being dependent on the nucleophilic strength of the reaction site, the reactivity of the electrophilic agent, and steric factors. For simple alkylating agents promutagenic adducts are formed by reaction with the oxygen atom at position 6 (O^6) of guanine, O^2 and O^4 of thymidine and O^2 of cytosine. *See* Gene Expression and Nutrition

The production of DNA adducts, however, is only the first stage of the process leading to neoplasia, and different adducts show different probabilities of causing particular genotoxic events. For example, the adduct formed at the N^7 position of guanine is not associated with a high rate of point mutation, whereas there is a high frequency of point mutation following formation of O^6-methylguanine.

The major DNA adduct of aflatoxin is 2,3-dihydro-3-hydroxy-(N^7-guanyl)aflatoxin B$_1$ (AFB$_1$-N^7-GUA). Binding is linear over a wide dose range, but it is dependent on both activation and detoxification pathways. Thus ethoxyquin administration markedly reduces aflatoxin binding to DNA by activating a competing pathway which leads to binding with glutathione. The considerable species differences in susceptibility to aflatoxin-induced carcinogenicity have been correlated with differences in activation and covalent binding of this compound.

It is now generally accepted that a cancer cell has to have some heritable defect to pass on to its progeny. This is most easily conceived as resulting from alteration in DNA. However, chemical carcinogens may react with a variety of cellular macromolecules, including proteins and RNA. Indeed, metabolites of the carcinogen AAF bind to a cytosolic protein, designated h$_2$ protein; this protein is not present in the cells of tumours produced by AAF, and the discovery of this fact led to the protein deletion hypothesis of carcinogenesis. In addition, binding to histones and to chromatin-associated proteins has also been described. As these proteins are important in the control of gene expression, alteration may lead to disturbance in cellular function. Binding to RNA has also been described: for example, a high degree of methylation occurs following the administration of nitrosamines. Adduct formation may interfere with codon–anticodon recognition, which may affect base-pairing during translation.

The biological consequence of interaction with DNA depends on the nature and site of the interaction, and three major effects may result. With polycyclic hydrocarbons, insertion of the planar molecule between the bases of DNA may lead to distortion of the helix and to a frame-shift mutation. Alkylations can result in the insertion of other inappropriate bases at the alkylated site, resulting in base transition. Some adducts lead to reduced stability of the bond between the purine base and deoxyribose, which may then undergo cleavage by DNA glycosylase and result in an apurinic site.

Clearly, DNA damage of the type described above could result in heritable defects in the cells, initiating the process of carcinogenesis. However, many compounds that do not react with DNA and are not genotoxic agents will, when given to animals, produce tumours. Little is known of the mechanism by which many of these compounds cause cancer. For example, there are a number of chemicals that produce tumours in the kidney in the male rat only. Among these compounds are unleaded gasoline, decalin, 1,4-dichlorobenzene and D-limonene. Tumours are preceded by a nephropathy which is characterized by the accumulation of α_2-microglobulin. The latter is a low-molecular-weight protein which is synthesized in the liver of male rats. A number of metabolic products have been shown to bind to this protein. This reduces the rate of proteolytic hydrolysis of the protein, resulting in accumulation at the site of its catabolism, the kidney. Accumulation of the proteins is associated with cytolysis and resultant compensatory hyperplasia. This chronic hyperplastic response eventually progresses to tumour development in some animals.

Other organs in which carcinogenicity is not associated with a primary genotoxic mechanism include the thyroid, the forestomach of the rodent, and the liver. One common feature of these forms of carcinogenesis, as in the kidney model, seems to be chronic hyperplasia.

Considerable impetus has been given in recent years to the recognition of oncogenes in carcinogenesis. These genes, which may play an important role in normal cell function, were first identified because they were present in transforming retroviruses. Single point mutations in a number of these oncogenes have been found in tumours from both animals and man. Under certain experimental conditions, insertion of oncogene DNA in fibroblast cells grown in culture may result in transformation of the cells. Such a mechanism is an attractive pathway for carcinogenesis as a result of chemically induced mutations. However, such point mutations are not always acquired at the time of first exposure to the carcinogen; thus they may not constitute the primary event. Other genes may play a suppressor function in cancer development and may be of equal, if not greater importance, in cancer development.

There is still considerable doubt as to which are the significant rate-limiting steps in cancer development, particularly with regard to the relative importance of the initiation and the promotional phase. Even for cigarette smoking, an accepted cause of human cancer, it is by no means certain whether mutation *per se* is the most important event. Although cigarette smoke contains a large number of potential genotoxic (initiating) agents, the shape of the dose–response curve, especially when cessation of smoking is considered, suggests that the promotional stage may be the most important determining factor in the development of cancer.

Carcinogens in the Food Chain: Levels in the Diet

The number of 'natural' carcinogens in food, or that result from food preparation, is high. For example, dietary estimates of the intake of nitrosamines in the USA range between 1 and 10 μg per day. Furthermore, Bruce Ames and his colleagues have drawn attention to the inappropriate, in his view, preoccupation with synthetic as opposed to naturally occurring carcinogens. Many compounds such as formaldehyde are present in most commonly used foods while a whole variety of polycyclic hydrocarbons may be produced in the cooking process. The consumption of these 'naturally' occurring carcinogens is difficult, if not impossible, to control and it therefore seems likely that exposure to such chemicals will remain inevitable. Whether a further concerted effort to restrict such exposure would be beneficial therefore seems questionable. Caloric restriction has been shown to reduce tumour incidence in rodents. In addition, the National Academy of Sciences in the USA has indicated that the observed differences in cancer incidence between human populations may be associated with bulk components of the diet and that modification of dietary practices may reduce the incidence of cancer in the USA by approximately one third. This risk is not associated with specific carcinogen contamination but with the possible promotional characteristics of one or other of the major constituents. *See* Cancer, Diet in Cancer Treatment

Monitoring and Control of Hazards

The complex mixture of chemicals that constitute food, together with the uncertainty of the specific role of the various components in the diet, has made monitoring and control of specific items difficult. However, control of potential carcinogens in food can be considered in terms of specific items: bulk components of food; minor natural components; specific additives; components that arise through food preparation; contaminants, either natural or man-made.

As previously indicated, there has been considerable discussion on the relationship between the minor and major components of food and human disease patterns. The realization that animal carcinogens, as identified by standard animal bioassay, are widely distributed in the general environment, including food, has made control by total elimination impossible. *See* Diseases, Diseases of Affluence

A degree of control has been attempted in certain areas, particularly contaminants and additives. This has been achieved through the establishment of no-effect-levels (NEL) in animal experiments, followed by the setting of an allowable daily intake (ADI) through some arbitrary extrapolaton. This extrapolation may take into consideration other properties of the chemical concerned, particularly genotoxic potential. For geno-toxic carcinogens, a maximum risk of 10^{-6} cancers in a lifetime may be taken as an acceptable risk, and exposure estimates extrapolated from animal data. For nongenotoxic agents a safety factor of a hundred may be used for the carcinogenic effect, based on the association of carcinogenicity with some other feature of the compound's activity such as toxicity. It must be said that there is little scientific evidence to support either of these approaches, as even for the best documented cases the mechanism of the carcinogenic effect is poorly understood.

In practice, carcinogens or potential carcinogens, as determined by various short-term tests, are dealt with in a hierarchical way, depending on their source. In other words, they are classified either as natural components of food, e.g. solanine in potatoes or hydrazines in mushrooms, as specific contaminants resulting from agricultural or manufacturing processes, or as specific food additives. *See* Food Additives, Safety; Pesticides and Herbicides, Toxicology

The major problem in all these discussions is how a carcinogen is identified. Clearly, the most appropriate model for humans is the human being. Epidemiological data involving both prospective and retrospective studies, and using case controls in certain investigations, may be used. These techniques have limited applications to diet-associated carcinogenesis and have proved most useful in identifying specific carcinogens in the work place or as therapeutic agents. The problem in investigating diet relates to its complexity, the difficulty in identifying specific components, and the sensitivity of the epidemiological methods themselves. Such methods have indicated the relative importance of 'life style' factors in carcinogenesis: in particular, associations have been made between lack of dietary fibre and colon cancer, between fresh fruit and vegetables and stomach

cancer, and between excess dietary fat and colon and breast cancer. However, it would seem unlikely that epidemiological data will be able to link specific chemical carcinogens in food with a carcinogenic effect. These chemicals are likely to be present at low levels, to express a 'weak' carcinogenic effect and if producing any detrimental health effects, these will be below the sensitivity threshold of current epidemiological methods. It is generally assumed that the most potent carcinogens will be readily identified, but that the weaker carcinogens will be the most important in human cancer and will be the most difficult to identify.

At present, carcinogenic or potential carcinogenic effect is identified through animal bioassays or short-term tests for mutagenesis, of which the Ames test has been predominant. Analytical methods have improved greatly over the last decade such that carcinogens can be detected at levels of parts per billion, or even parts per trillion. This has meant that even in food that is considered wholly safe, low levels of 'carcinogens' may be detected; perhaps no food material is totally free of such materials. *See* Mutagens

Most of the activity aimed at controlling carcinogens in food has been directed at preventing additions to this natural background, through the application of laws governing the adulteration of food, the first of which were enacted in the mid-nineteenth century in the UK. The current UK legislation is the 1990 Food Safety Act, governing the nature and quality of food and its nutritive value. This Act, like its forerunner, the 1955 Food and Drugs Act, requires that the constituents of food should not be injurious to health. Thus, while there is no specific requirement for carcinogenicity testing in the current act, consideration is given to all available data, including the result of mutagenicity tests and long-term tests in animals. These data are considered by the Food Additives and Contaminants Committee and, if satisfactory, a regulation may be proposed and drafted, allowing the addition of the specific additive to the Permitted List of Food Additives. *See* Legislation, International Standards

The position in the USA up to 1958 was similar to that in the UK. Food was considered adulterated if injury could arise from its use. Legislation was based on traditional food, added substances and unavoidably added substances (contaminants). For added substances, the food was adulterated if the added substance could render the food injurious to health; for unavoidably added substances, a balance was applied between the essential nature of the food material and the degree of contamination. These strictures applied to both carcinogenic and noncarcinogenic toxicants. In 1958 a change in emphasis was introduced through the Food Additives Amendment. This established a licensing scheme for substances deliberately added to foods or for food substances that could migrate into food, but excluded

Carcinogenic Substances in Food

materials that were generally, through usage, regarded as safe (GRAS). For licensing purposes, the material has to be shown to be 'safe' for its intended use. *See* Legislation, Contaminants and Adulterants

In 1958 the Delaney Clause was enacted; this required that if there was evidence of carcinogenicity the material should be prohibited from food usage. Improved analytical techniques, as already indicated, have shown that foods from various sources contain both unintentionally added and natural carcinogens, such as polynuclear aromatic hydrocarbons and nitrosamines, and no form of regulation could control these materials. The bulk components of food may themselves play an important role in the promotional phase of carcinogenesis. These factors have meant that the exclusion of all potentially carcinogenic additives under the Delaney Clause has given way to the concept of 'safe' tolerance, and that 'safe levels' may be set by appropriate, conservative risk assessment in which an 'insignificant life time risk' of 10^{-6} is considered acceptable.

Bibliography

Ames BN, Durston WE, Yamasaki E and Lee FO (1973) Carcinogens are mutagens: a simple test system combining liver homogenates for activation and bacteria for detection. *Proceedings of the National Academy of Sciences of the USA* 70: 2281–2285.

Anderson D (1988) Genetic toxicology. In: Anderson D and Conning DM (eds) *Experimental Toxicology: The Basic Issues*, pp 242–286. London: Royal Society of Chemistry.

Ashby J and Tennant RW (1991) Definitive relationships among chemical structures, carcinogenicity and mutagenicity for 301 chemical tested by the US NCI/NTP. *Mutation Research* 257: 229–306.

Douglas JF (1984) *Carcinogenesis and Mutagenesis Testing*. Clifton, New Jersey: Humana Press.

Grasso P (1988) Testing for carcinogenicity. In: Anderson D and Conning DM (eds) *Experimental Toxicology: The Basic Issues*, pp 309–334. London: Royal Society of Chemistry.

Milman HA and Weisburger EK (eds) (1986) *Handbook of Carcinogen Testing*. Path Ridge, New Jersey: Noyes Publications.

Scheuplein RJ (1990) Perspectives on toxicological risk – an example: food borne carcinogenic risk. In: Clayson DB, Munro IC, Shubik P and Swenberg JA (eds) *Progress in Predictive Toxicology*, pp 365–372. Amsterdam: Elsevier Science Publishers.

Tennant RW, Margolin BH, Shelby MD *et al.* (1987) Prediction of chemical carcinogenicity in rodents from *in vitro* genetic toxicity assays. *Science* 236: 933–941.

J. G. Evans, J. C. Phillips and D. Anderson
BIBRA Toxicology International, Carshalton, UK

Carcinogenicity Tests

Carcinogenesis Bioassay (Animal studies)

As the mechanism of carcinogenesis in both humans and animals is poorly understood, no mechanistically based,

short-term predictive test has been entirely successful. The most acceptable procedure for cancer prediction is still the exposure of animals to the test material for a considerable period of their lives. The assumption of such tests is that animals will behave in essentially the same way as humans to carcinogen exposure, i.e. the mechanism of tumour induction will be similar in both animals and humans.

The procedures for carcinogenicity bioassays are set out in specific guidelines, both national and international. Although there is a general level of conformity, there are differences related to national requirement and to the nature and use of the test material. Thus the guidelines for testing industrial chemicals, pharmaceuticals and agrochemicals may differ. It is only in the USA that specific guidelines refer to food additives. *See* Food Additives, Safety

The standard basis of most guidelines is that the test material be fed to two suitable species for a considerable proportion of their natural lifespan. For mice this is usually between 18 months and 2 years, and for rats between 2 years and 30 months. In some cases the animals may be kept until a certain proportion in one or other of the treatment groups has died or has been killed in a moribund state. Tests are essentially of two types: the first, used widely under the National Toxicology Program (NTP) in the USA, is designed to examine the ability of the test material to induce cancer in the species used; the second type is aimed at determining the cancer incidence in respect of dose – a classical dose–response study. The latter requires several treatment groups, each containing a large number of animals. In general, therefore, it is a test for carcinogenic potential that is usually carried out. Because of their small size and relatively short life expectancy, the rat and mouse are the species of choice, although the hamster is occasionally used. Other larger species, such as dogs and primates, are more difficult to house, and their long lifespan makes their use impractical. In the USA, inbred strains of animals are widely used (the F344 rat and the B6C3F$_1$ hybrid mouse), although out-bred strains are commonly used in Europe.

In order to maximize the chance of detecting a carcinogenic effect, the administered compound is usually given at a relatively high dose. This dose may be the maximum tolerated dose (MTD) and is determined from a series of acute, subacute and subchronic studies. The maximum tolerated dose may be defined in a number of different ways; the most commonly used is the highest dose that, when given to the animals under the conditions of the bioassay, does not significantly alter the animals' survival. In practice, the MTD is often set at the dose that in subchronic studies produces, at most, a 10% reduction in bodyweight gain.

As well as the highest dose set at the MTD, a lower dose or doses may be used. Commonly, there may be three treated groups and one or two appropriate control groups. If only a single additional dose group is used, this is usually set at half the MTD. As a minimum, 50 animals are allocated at random to each of the experimental groups. For carcinogenic potential of food components, the test substance is usually given in the diet; occasionally, application may be in the drinking water or by gavage.

Following administration for the required time, the animals are killed and tissues fixed for histological examination. This may involve approximately 30–40 different tissues, with multiple samples taken from major organs such as the liver, lung, kidney and gastrointestinal tract. All these tissues may be examined histologically from all groups or only from the top-dose and control groups, with only target organs and any other gross abnormalities being examined from the lower-dose groups. A classification of both neoplastic and non-neoplastic lesions is made and a summary table prepared.

The procedures of these bioassays are conducted under rigorous conditions, defined by the Code of Good Laboratory Practice (GLP). Compliance with the principles of GLP is confirmed by independent study auditors, the so-called quality assurance (QA) function. The purpose of GLP is to ensure that the conduct of such studies is satisfactory with regard to (1) resources, which includes personnel, the adequacy of the facility and equipment, chemicals and management, and (2) processes, including study design, study conduct, documentation and QA.

In practice, this means that the test article should be properly defined, stored and prepared for administration and that appropriate staff should be available at the critical phases of the study. The animals' clinical state should be monitored appropriately during course of the study, and the animals killed at the right time, or if found dead or killed *in extremis*, appropriate steps should be taken for tissue preservation and examination. At the end of the study a proper necropsy should be performed, and appropriate tissues selected, weighed if necessary, and preserved for subsequent processing. All tissues, as defined by the protocol, should be examined by the pathologist. The essence of GLP is that these essential stages are defined and correct records kept.

The analysis of a carcinogenicity bioassay is aimed at determining whether the administration of the test article has resulted in an increase in the incidence of tumours at one or more sites. In order to accomplish this analysis, two major confounding factors may have to be taken into consideration. The first is the effect of differences in mortality rates between the control and treated groups and the second is the effect of differences in food intake and its consequence on bodyweight. Both factors can substantially alter the tumour pattern

observed in different groups. Early deaths may prevent the animals reaching tumour-bearing age, and reduced food intake and the associated reduction in bodyweight may result in a considerable reduction in tumour incidence.

Statistical analysis of the data is usually based on the assumption that different tumour types in the same organ, or tumours in different organs, are independent events and can be treated individually. In some cases the numbers of benign and malignant tumours may be combined for statistical analysis: whether or not this is appropriate should be determined by the pathologist following discussion with a statistician and toxicologist.

Survival rates are generally determined by the product-limit procedure of Kaplan–Meier and may be shown in graphical form. An analysis of dose-related trend may be given, whereas the determination of tumour incidence is generally based on an analysis of the numbers of site-specific tumours compared with the number of animals in which that site was examined. As a minimum, a direct pairwise comparison using Fisher's exact test and an analysis of dose–response using the Cochran–Armitage linear trend test is made. In addition, some form of time–adjusted analysis or life table methods may be used. The latter are complicated by non-tumour-induced intercurrent mortality and so proposals have been made to distinguish between tumours that caused the early death of the animals (fatal tumours) and those that do not (incidental tumours). The latter are tumours that were found at the time of necropsy only because the animal died from a non-tumour-related disease. The identification of the precise cause of death may be difficult and some authorities have advocated the practice of making two analyses, one in which all tumours of the type of interest are considered 'fatal' and the other in which the tumours are considered 'incidental'. In the former case the denominator is considered to be all animals at risk, while in the latter the denominator is all animals that died during the time interval of interest.

Irrespective of the statistical methods used, the bioassay itself is not particularly sensitive. Indeed, even when there are no tumours of the type of interest in the control group, at least 10% of the animals in the treated group must bear tumours for the number to be statistically significant. If tumours occur at the site of interest in the control group, then a bioassay would not efficiently detect an increased risk of 10%. This lack of sensitivity must be considered in the context of the often stated human risk factor of 10^{-6}.

The interpretation of the results of a bioassay are complex but most authorities work to the 'weight of evidence' principle. This evidence is taken in the light of the 'adequacy' of the bioassay, which is dependent on some of the factors previously discussed. Strong evidence for carcinogenicity would be increased malignant tumour incidence in two species, with tumours at multiple sites and also showing a clear dose–response relationship. Rare or unusual tumours at a site would be given added weight. Equivocal evidence may result from a statistically marginal result; the effect may only be seen in one species and be associated with species-specific toxicity, or there may only be an increase in commonly occurring benign tumours. Sometimes, problems associated with such findings may be clarified by further mechanistic studies or by reference to historical data. Unequivocally negative data are taken as no evidence of carcinogenicity in two species in adequate bioassays. When the data from bioassays are considered in human risk assessment, other factors must clearly also be taken into consideration. These may include evidence of genotoxicity and data on metabolism and potential human exposure. Furthermore, a measure of risk at doses substantially below the bioassay dose may be needed. This may require an extrapolation using mathematical models. As yet no general agreement as to the most appropriate of these methods has been determined, and the calculated risk given by different methods may vary considerably. Thus the final assessment may be made on quite pragmatic grounds, in which the experience and expertise of a number of individuals are drawn on to reach a consensus opinion.

Tests with DNA

There are various tests which measure damage to DNA. These include assays for detecting gene mutation, damage to chromosomes or damage to the whole genome. Tests for chromosome damage detect breakages (clastogenicity) or numerical changes. Sister chromatid exchanges can also be detected in chromosomes. Damage to the whole genome can be measured in DNA repair assays. Most of these assays can be performed *in vitro* and *in vivo* in both somatic and germ cells.

Gene mutation can be measured in microbial assays using bacteria (such as *Salmonella typhimurium* and *Escherichia coli*), yeasts (*Saccharomyces cerevisiae* and *Schizosaccharomyces pombe*) or mammalian cells in culture; the most frequently used cells include Chinese hamster ovary (CHO), Chinese hamster lung (V79) and mouse lymphoma (L5178Y) cells. The microbial assay which is most well validated and universally used is the so-called Ames test, using *Salmonella typhimurium* as the test organism. The advantages of using bacteria to detect mutagenic potential are counterbalanced, however, by the inability of these cells to activate metabolically many classes of unreactive, but nevertheless mutagenic chemicals. The Ames test overcomes this deficiency by incorporating an exogenous metabolizing system into the assay. This is known as the S-9 mix and is the supernatant fraction derived from the liver of rats treated with a wide-spectrum enzyme inducer. The liver homogenate is spun at 9000 g and supplemented with appropriate cofactors. *See* Mutagens

The essential feature of the Ames test is the reversion of a mutant form of the test organism requiring histidine for growth (auxotrophy) to a wild type form which does not (prototrophy) on exposure to a mutagen. There are various tester strains which can detect either base-pair or frame-shift mutations; strains TA1535 and TA100 detect the former and TA1537, TA1538, TA97 and TA98 the latter. The bacterium has a 'leaky' coat, which allows large chemical molecules to enter and renders it nonpathogenic. The bacteria lack a DNA repair system and strains TA97, TA98 and TA100 contain a plasmid which confers resistance to ampicillin and increased sensitivity to mutagens. Other strains (e.g. TA102 and TA104) have been more recently developed to detect chemicals which operate through oxygen radical involvement.

The mammalian cell lines are used to detect mutations at different loci. Mutation results in resistance to the toxic effects of various nucleic acid base analogues, such as 6-thioguanine and trifluorothymidine, due to loss of hypoxanthine guanine phosphoribosyl transferase (HPRT) and thymidine kinase (TK) enzyme activity, respectively.

Gene mutation assays *in vivo* include the spot test and the specific locus assay. In the spot test, pregnant female animals are exposed to the test chemical, and spots of changed colour occur in the coat of the offspring as a result of mutation. In the specific locus assay, animal strains with recessive markers are mated. When mutation occurs, coat colour changes are seen in the F_1 offspring.

Chromosome damage is generally measured *in vitro* in cell lines such as those derived from Chinese hamster ovary (CHO) cells or fibroblasts (CHL) and in human peripheral blood lymphocytes. The former have a lower number of chromosomes ($n = 22$) than the human ($n = 46$) and consequently are easier to evaluate.

Human lymphocytes can also be used to monitor populations for exposure to mutagenic agents. Peripheral blood is taken from an exposed individual and chromosome preparations are made in the same way as for cell lines. However, lymphocytes are essentially resting cells which have to be stimulated into cell division by the addition of a mitogen. Metaphase preparations of treated cells are examined for chromosome aberrations, which include chromosome and chromatid gaps and breaks, rings, fragments, dicentrics, translocations and inversions.

Chromosome damage can also be detected via *in vivo* assays in, for example, rodent bone marrow cells after chemical exposure, either directly using metaphase analysis or indirectly by assaying micronuclei. These are formed when the main nucleus is extruded from the mature erythrocyte and a fragment or whole chromosome is left behind.

An *in vivo* assay measuring unscheduled DNA synthesis (UDS) in rat liver or gut is recommended by most regulatory authorities if there is a positive response in any *in vitro* assay and a negative response in an *in vivo* cytogenetics assay. In the UDS assay, scheduled DNA synthesis is arrested by treatment with hydroxyurea, and unscheduled DNA synthesis is assessed by measuring incorporation of a radiolabelled precursor. This is usually carried out using autoradiographic methods, and is shown as an increase in silver grains in the cell nucleus by comparison with the cytoplasm.

Sister chromatid exchanges can also be scored in chromosomes. These are exchanges of regions of chromatid arms and are increased after exposure to mutagens. They are visualized for microscopic examination by differential staining following treatment with bromodeoxyuridine, which is incorporated into DNA in place of thymidine and stains more heavily. A variety of other *in vivo* assays can be used to measure chromosome damage in germ cells. These include the dominant lethal assay in which treated males are mated to virgin females on consecutive weeks over the 8 weeks of the spermatogenic cycle in mice (10 weeks in rats). This allows sensitivity of the various stages of maturation of germ cells to be determined. The transmission of damaged chromosomes can be measured in the heritable translocation assay, either by cytogenetic examination of germ cells or by mating studies. In mating studies, a chromosomal translocation results in sterile or partially sterile males.

The last two decades have seen extensive efforts to evaluate short-term tests for their suitability for predicting carcinogenic potential. The early validation studies suggested good predictability, with correct identification of over 90% of carcinogens (high sensitivity) and over 90% of noncarcinogens (high specificity). In a more recent evaluation, rodent carcinogenicity and short-term test data for 73 compounds were compared and a somewhat lower figure (60%) was obtained. However, when carcinogens known to react by nongenotoxic mechanisms (e.g. hormones or peroxisome proliferators) were excluded, the predictability was improved to approximately 80%. This suggests that short-term tests are suitable for detecting those carcinogens which act by a genotoxic mechanism. Logically, this is precisely what would be expected since the tests are designed to detect DNA damage (i.e. genotoxicity).

Although many regulatory authorities have guidelines for carcinogenicity evaluation which include short-term tests, all still require animal studies as the ultimate test for carcinogenicity. Some expert bodies, such as The International Agency for Research in Cancer, use short-term tests as an adjunct to animal carcinogenicity studies in their evaluation process, giving added weighting to an animal carcinogen that is also positive in short-term tests in their assessment of its likely human hazard.

Since foods are an extremely diverse mixture of chemicals, the complexity of which may be altered by the various processing methods used, and by the use of additives, the determination of their potential mutagenicity or carcinogenicity is difficult. Assessment of food additives is relatively straightforward since they can be tested directly in short-term tests. Similarly, some food constituents and contaminants such as aflatoxin B_1 and some compounds formed by processing, notably polycyclic aromatic hydrocarbons and nitrosamines, can be chemically identified and similarly tested. However, most foodstuffs cannot be evaluated so easily since the macromolecular constituents render them unsuitable for incorporation into short-term test systems. One possible approach is to digest and/or solvent-extract the foodstuff and investigate the activity of the various extracts (acidic, basic and neutral). When foods are tested *in vivo* in short-term tests (e.g. bone marrow assay), it may be difficult to use dose levels above the normal levels encountered in the diet. Thus no margin of safety can be identified, whereas for additives and contaminants dose levels in excess of those encountered in the diet can be tested, allowing the determination of appropriate safety factors. In addition, confounding factors may alter the response of foods in these tests (e.g. the presence of histidine could interfere with the end-point of the Ames test). *See* Nitrosamines; Polycyclic Aromatic Hydrocarbons

It must be emphasized that short-term tests are used not only as predictors of carcinogenic potential, but in their own right for predicting potential human mutagenicity. Some regulatory authorities, such as the UK Department of Health, use them in this way.

Nutrition and Cancer

Geographic epidemiological data show considerable differences in the pattern of cancer between different populations. In a number of instances these differences have been related to the nature of the diet. In particular, cancers of the colon, breast and pancreas have been correlated with a high intake of fat. However, detailed case control and follow-up studies do not show such a clear-cut association. For colorectal cancer and cancer of the breast, the evidence is often inconsistent and does not suggest a *direct* association. Nonetheless, a consistent association between breast cancer and dietary fat is seen, and in the case of large bowel cancer the association is stronger for the intake of saturated rather than unsaturated fats. *See* Breast Cancer and Diet; Cancer, Epidemiology; Colon, Cancer of the Colon

One problem with all the data is the difficulty in determining the exact component of the diet that may be important in a particular disease. This may be made through recall with estimates of past dietary habits or through contemporary dietary surveys such as the British National Food Study. Furthermore, estimates of fat intake may be made using a surrogate measure such as the intake of meat, but such data do not give details of the type and quantity of different fats ingested. *See* Dietary Surveys, Measurement of Food Intake

Variation in one component of the diet is frequently associated with changes in other components, so that several associations may be made in terms of diet and cancer incidence. An inverse relationship between vitamin A and selenium intake has been described, although the results of epidemiological studies are often inconsistent. It is clear from both human observation and experimental data that total caloric intake is an important risk factor, irrespective of source. However, the analysis of total caloric intake is complex as intake is related to physical activity as well as other social factors. Obesity has also been suggested as a risk factor for certain forms of cancer. Other data suggest that obesity *per se* may not be the prime determining factor and that lean body mass may be more important. At a number of sites, such as the lung, gastrointestinal tract and breast, other confounding factors are often difficult to eliminate entirely. Thus alcohol intake at quite moderate levels has been associated with an increased risk for breast cancer which is at least as great as that associated with dietary differences. *See* Retinol, Physiology; Selenium, Physiology

Experimental data from laboratory animals, particularly mice, has shown a clear relationship between food intake (caloric intake) and the incidence of spontaneous tumours. Thus the total tumour burden may be reduced from 40–50% to less than 10% by reducing food intake by approximately 20%. The reduction in tumours occurs primarily at four sites: the lung, the lymphoreticular system, mammary gland and liver. However, recent data also suggest a reduction in tumours at other sites. *See* Cancer, Diet in Cancer Prevention

Considerable experimental evidence does exist to show that dietary manipulation may also affect the development of tumours induced by genotoxic agents in various model systems. These data show that both total caloric intake and specific components may be important. For example, caloric restriction can markedly inhibit the development of benzo(a)pyrene-induced skin tumours, while corn oil or sunflower oil, when given at 20–30% by weight in the diet, increases significantly the incidence of dimethylbenzanthracene- or N-methyl-N-nitrosourea-induced mammary tumours in rats. The most effective oils in these models are rich in ω_6-polyunsaturated fatty acids, whilst oils rich in ω_3-polyunsaturated fatty acids are not effective. However, linoleic acid at 4.4% of the diet is most effective at increasing mammary tumours. As in human studies, these data are confounded by difficulty in distinguishing the effect of oils from caloric differences resulting from dietary manipulation, and the effect of age-specific sensitivity to such alterations. Furthermore, a balance may be set between lean body mass and obesity which may result in conflicting results. *See* Essential Fatty Acids, Physiology

The mechanism through which nutritional factors affect cancer incidence is poorly understood. A direct mechanistic relationship between fat intake and the generation of free radicals has been suggested. However, current research indicates that a more insidious effect may be through the possible contribution of diet on cell proliferation in a wide variety of organs. This may be controlled through an effect on the endocrine system, the production of growth factors, and the expression of various oncogenes. Data in the literature show that dietary restriction alters the level of a variety of hormones, growth factors and oncogenes, and the balance of such alteration indicates a reduced growth stimulation.

Thus it is clear that the relationship between human cancer incidence and diet is complex, and much more research is needed to identify specific dietary factors responsible for human cancer and for protecting against endogenous and exogenous carcinogens.

Bibliography

Ames BN, Durston WE, Yamasaki E and Lee FO (1973) Carcinogens are mutagens: a simple test system combining liver homogenates for activation and bacteria for detection. *Proceedings of the National Academy of Sciences of the USA* 70: 2281–2285.

Anderson D (1988) Genetic toxicology. In: Anderson D and Conning DM (eds) *Experimental Toxicology: The Basic Issues*, pp 242–286. London: Royal Society of Chemistry.

Ashby J and Tennant RW (1991) Definitive relationships among chemical structures, carcinogenicity and mutagenicity for 301 chemical tested by the US NCI/NTP. *Mutation Resarch* 257: 229–306.

Douglas JF (1984) *Carcinogenesis and Mutagenesis Testing*. Clifton, New Jersey: Humana Press.

Grasso P (1988) Testing for carcinogenicity. In: Anderson D and Conning DM (eds) *Experimental Toxicology: The Basic Issues*, pp 309–334. London: Royal Society of Chemistry.

Milman HA and Weisburger EK (eds) (1986) *Handbook of Carcinogen Testing*. Path Ridge, New Jersey: Noyes Publications.

Scheuplein RJ (1990) Perspectives on toxicological risk – an example: food borne carcinogenic risk. In: Clayson DB, Munro IC, Shubik P and Swenberg JA (eds) *Progress in Predictive Toxicology*, pp 365–372. Amsterdam: Elsevier Science Publishers.

Tennant RW, Margolin BH, Shelby MD *et al.* (1987) Prediction of chemical carcinogenicity in rodents from *in vitro* genetic toxicity assays. *Science* 236: 933–941.

J. G. Evans, J. C. Phillips and D. Anderson
BIBRA Toxicology International, Carshalton, UK

Carcinogenicity Tests

CAROTENOIDS

Contents

Properties and Determination

Structures and Occurrence in Foods

Among the naturally occurring pigments, carotenoids are notable for their wide distribution, diversity and varied functions. In nature more than 100 million tonnes of these compounds are produced annually. The latest compilation consists of 563 carotenoids that have been isolated and characterized. This remarkable number includes the enormous variety of carotenoids in algae, bacteria and fungi. In foods the number is much more restricted, nonetheless the carotenoid composition can be complex.

Food carotenoids are generally C_{40} tetraterpenoids formed from eight isoprenoid units joined so that the arrangement is reversed at the centre; the two central methyl groups are separated by six carbon atoms and the others by five (Fig. 1). The distinctive feature of carotenoids, responsible for their special properties and functions, is a series of conjugated double bonds. The basic skeleton may be modified in many ways, such as cyclization, hydrogenation, dehydrogenation, insertion of oxygen in various forms and chain shortening, resulting in an immense array of structures.

These compounds are traditionally referred to by trivial names. A semisystematic nomenclature, conveying structural information, has been devised by the Commission on Biochemical Nomenclature. The molecule is considered in two halves and the carotenoid is named as a derivative of the parent carotene. Greek letters describe its end-groups, and conventional prefixes and suffixes indicate change of hydrogenation and the presence of substituent groups. The semisystematic names are given in parentheses in the figures; those of other carotenoids will be cited with the trivial names when first mentioned. Thereafter only the more well-known trivial names will be used.

Hydrocarbon carotenoids (e.g. β-carotene, lycopene) are known as carotenes; oxygenated derivatives are called xanthophylls. The oxygen functions most commonly encountered are hydroxyl (as in β-cryptoxanthin), oxo (as in echinenone), epoxy (as in violaxanthin) and aldehyde (as in β-citraurin). Carotenoids may be acyclic (e.g. ζ-carotene, lycopene), monocyclic (e.g. γ-carotene) or bicyclic (e.g. α- and β-carotene). Cyclization is limited to the formation of a six-membered (occasionally five-membered) ring at one or both ends of the molecule.

In nature carotenoids exist primarily in the more stable all-*trans* form, but *cis* isomers do occur. The first C_{40} compound in the biosynthetic pathway has the 15-*cis* configuration. Small amounts of *cis* isomers of other carotenoids have been increasingly reported. Naturally occurring poly-*cis* isomers have been isolated, such as prolycopene (7Z,9Z,7′Z,9′Z-lycopene) in the tangerine tomato. The stem name carotene implies a *trans* configuration at all double bonds. The *cis* form is indicated by citing the double bond which has this configuration either as *cis* or (Z).

Although masked by chlorophylls, carotenoids are found universally in the chloroplasts of green tissues. Leaves of all species studied revealed the presence of the same major carotenoids: β-carotene, lutein, violaxanthin and neoxanthin. Small amounts of α-carotene, α-[(3R,6′R)-β,ε-caroten-3-ol] or β-cryptoxanthin, zeaxanthin, antheraxanthin ((3S,5R,6S,3′R)-5,6-epoxy-5,6-dihydro-β,β-carotene-3,3-diol) and lutein-5,6-epoxide ((3S,5R,6S,3′R,6′R)-5,6-epoxy-5,6-dihydro-β,ε-carotene-3,3′-diol) may also be found. The xanthophylls are unesterified and relative ratios of the individual compounds are fairly constant, but the absolute concentrations vary considerably. *See* Chlorophyll

In fruits carotenoids are usually located in chromoplasts and the hydroxycarotenoids are mostly esterified with fatty acids. The composition varies dramatically from fruit to fruit, but eight major patterns can be discerned: (1) insignificant levels of carotenoids; (2) small amounts generally of chloroplast carotenoids (e.g. grape); (3) considerable amounts of lycopene (e.g. tomato, watermelon, red-fleshed guava and papaya); (4) predominance of β-carotene and/or β-cryptoxanthin (e.g. mango, peach, loquat); (5) large amounts of epoxides (e.g. carambola); (6) preponderance of unusual or species-specific carotenoids (e.g. red pepper); (7) substantial amounts of poly-*cis*-carotenoids (e.g. tangerine tomato); (8) significant levels of apocarotenoids (carotenoids with a shortened carbon skeleton) (e.g. citrus species). Some merging of these patterns can be seen in many fruits.

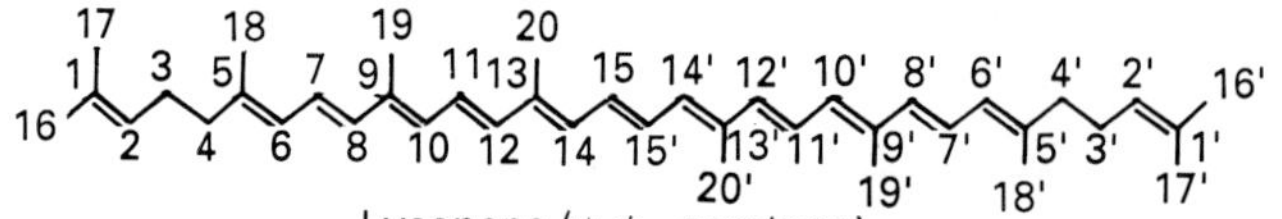

Lycopene (ψ,ψ - carotene)

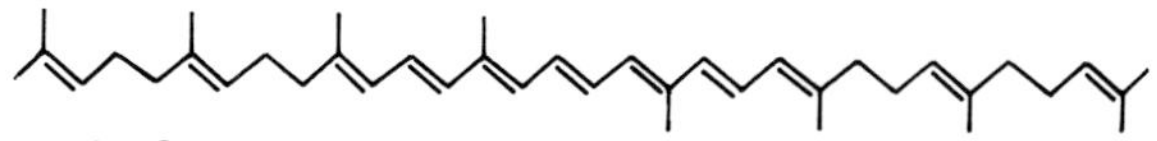

ζ - Carotene (7, 8, 7', 8' - tetrahydro - ψ,ψ - carotene)

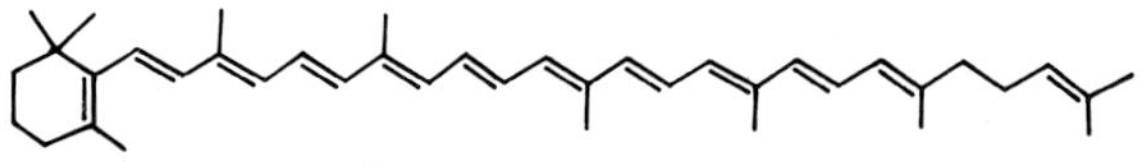

γ - Carotene (β,ψ - carotene)

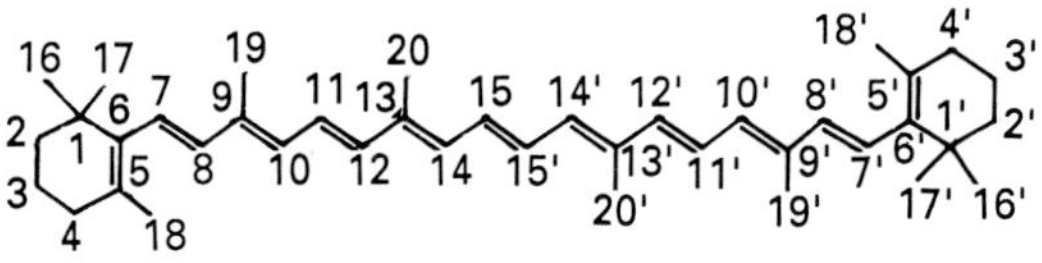

β - Carotene (β, β - carotene)

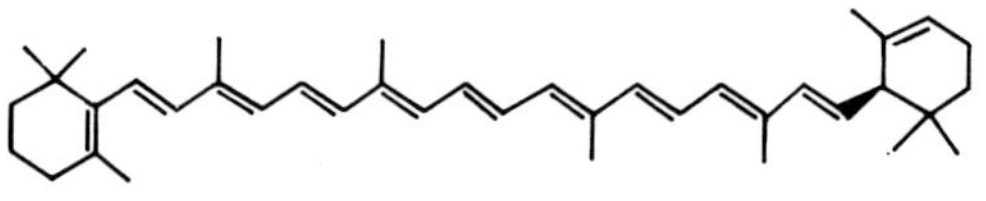

α - Carotene ((6'*R*) - β,ε - carotene)

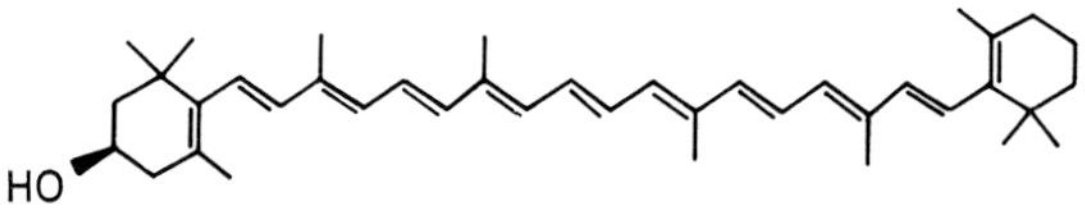

β - Cryptoxanthin ((3*R*) - β,β - caroten - 3 ol)

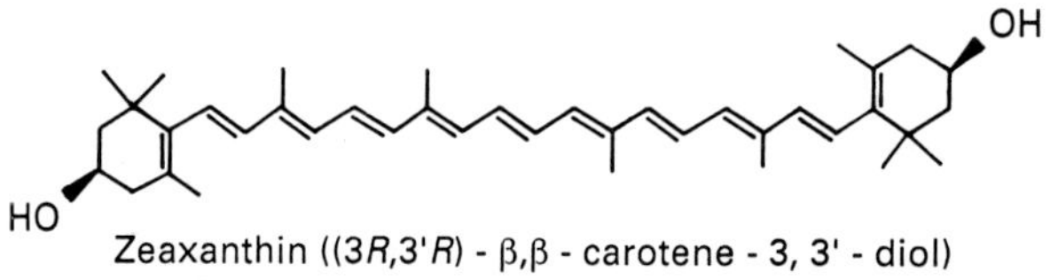

Zeaxanthin ((3*R*,3'*R*) - β,β - carotene - 3, 3' - diol)

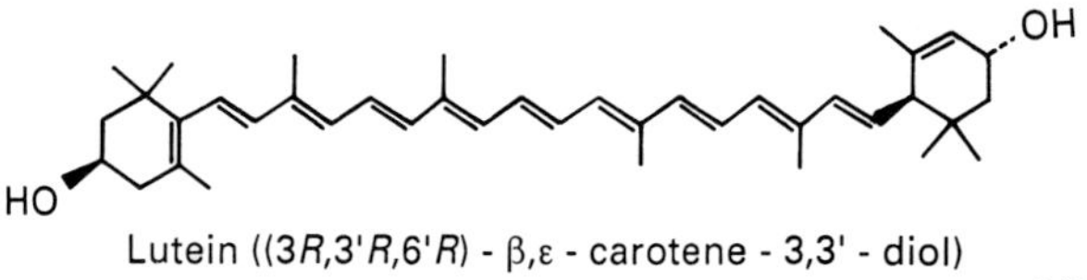

Lutein ((3*R*,3'*R*,6'*R*) - β,ε - carotene - 3,3' - diol)

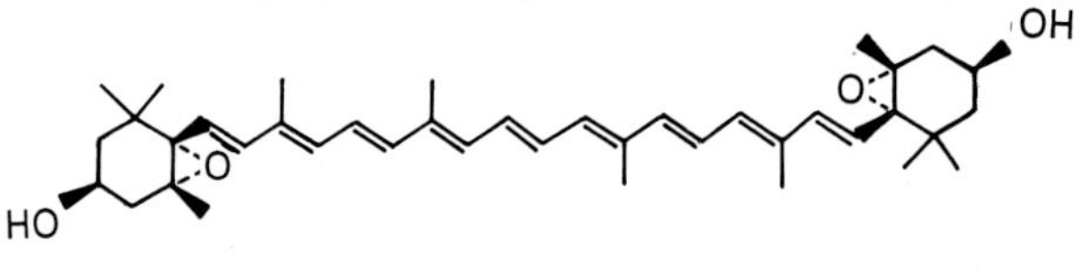

Violaxanthin ((3*S*,5*R*,6*S*,3'*S*,5'*R*,6'*S*) - 5,6,5',6' - diepoxy - 5,6,5',6' - tetrahydro - β,β - carotene - 3,3' - diol)

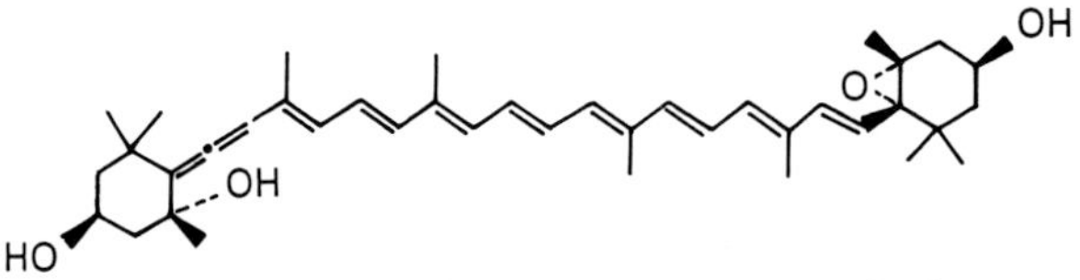

Neoxanthin ((3*S*,5*R*,6*R*,3'*S*,5'*R*,6'*S*) - 5',6' - epoxy - 6,7 - didehydro - 5,6,5',6' - tetrahydro - β,β carotene - 3,5,3' - triol)

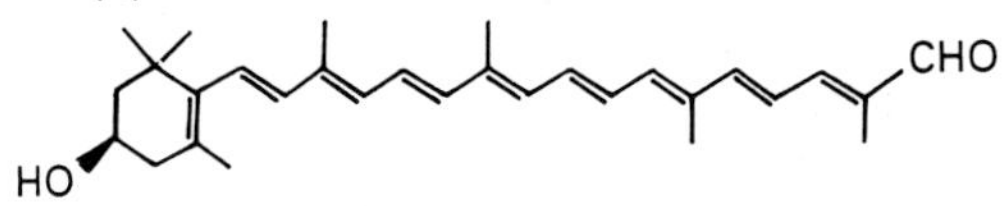

β - Citraurin ((3*R*) - 3 - hydroxy - 8' - apo - β - caroten - 8' - al)

Fig. 1. Structures of common carotenoids in foods of plant origin.

Properties and Determination

Table 1. Carotenoid distribution in some foods

Food	Total carotenoid content (μg per g fresh food)	Major carotenoids	Other carotenoids
Carrot	14–122	β-Carotene α-Carotene	ζ-Carotene, γ-carotene, δ-carotene, lycopene, lutein, neurosporene, β-zeacarotene
Egg yolk	∼16	Lutein Zeaxanthin	Isolutein, β-cryptoxanthin, β-carotene, α-carotene, neoxanthin, ζ-carotene
Guava (pink-fleshed)	57–70	Lycopene	β-Carotene, ζ-carotene, γ-carotene, zeinoxanthin, 5,6,5′,6′-diepoxy-β-carotene, unidentified 5,8-furanoid triol
Loquat	16–27	β-Cryptoxanthin β-Carotene	γ-Carotene, lutein, violaxanthin, neoxanthin, 5,6-monoepoxy-β-cryptoxanthin, phytofluene, mutatochrome, ζ-carotene, luteoxanthin
Mango	13–154	β-Carotene	Violaxanthin, luteoxanthin, mutatoxanthin, α-cryptoxanthin, mutatochrome, ζ-carotene, auroxanthin, phytoene, phytofluene, antheraxanthin
Milk	5–10	β-Carotene	α-Carotene, γ-carotene, β-cryptoxanthin, lycopene, lutein, zeaxanthin
Tomato	90–190	Lycopene	Phytoene, phytofluene, β-carotene, ζ-carotene, γ-carotene, neurosporene

Semisystematic names: neurosporene (7,8-dihydro-ψ,ψ-carotene); δ-carotene ((6R)-ε,ψ-carotene); β-zeacarotene (7′,8′-dihydro-β,ψ-carotene); isolutein ((3S,5R,6S,3′S,6′R)-5,6-epoxy-5,6-dihydro-β,ε-carotene-3,3′-diol); zeinoxanthin ((3R,6′R)-β,ε-caroten-3-ol); 5,6,5′,6′-diepoxy-β-carotene (5,6,5′,6′-diepoxy-5,6,5′,6′-tetrahydro-β,β-carotene); 5,6-monoepoxy-β-cryptoxanthin (5,6-epoxy-5,6-dihydro-β,β-caroten-3-ol); 5,6,5′,6′-diepoxy-β-cryptoxanthin (5,6,5′,6′-diepoxy-5,6,5′,6′-tetrahydro-β,β-caroten-3-ol); mutatochrome (5,8-epoxy-5,8-dihydro-β,β-carotene); luteoxanthin (5,6,5′,8′-diepoxy-5,6,5′,8′-tetrahydro-β,β-carotene-3,3′-diol); auroxanthin (5,8,5′,8′-diepoxy-5,8,5′,8′-tetrahydro-β,β-carotene-3,3-diol); phytoene (7,8,11,12,7′,8′,11′,12′-octahydro-ψ,ψ-carotene); phytofluene (7,8,11,12,7′,8′,-hexahydro-ψ,ψ-carotene).

In the few carotenogenic roots (e.g. carrot, sweet potato), the carotenes are preponderant. In maize (seed) the xanthophylls predominate.

Since plants are able to synthesize carotenoids *de novo*, their composition is enriched by the presence of minor or trace amounts of biosynthetic precursors along with derivatives of the main components (Table 1). Compositional variations occur as a consequence of varietal differences, climatic conditions, agricultural variables, stage of maturity, harvesting and postharvest handling, conditions during storage and transportation.

Carotenoids are not as widely distributed in animal foods and the total content is much less. In animals, ingested carotenoids are selectively or unselectively absorbed, converted to vitamin A, deposited as such or slightly altered before tissue storage to form carotenoids typical of animal species (Fig. 2). Astaxanthin is the major carotenoid in most crustaceans, either free, esterified or as carotenoproteins (complexes in which carotenoid molecules are bound to proteins in stoichiometric proportions). β-Carotene, echinenone and canthaxanthin are the other pigments usually encountered. When found in fish, carotenoids are located in the skin and flesh. The xanthophylls predominate over the carotenes; astaxanthin is the most common, followed by lutein (dominant in freshwater fishes) and tunaxanthin (ε,ε-carotene-3,3′-diol) (characteristic of marine fishes).

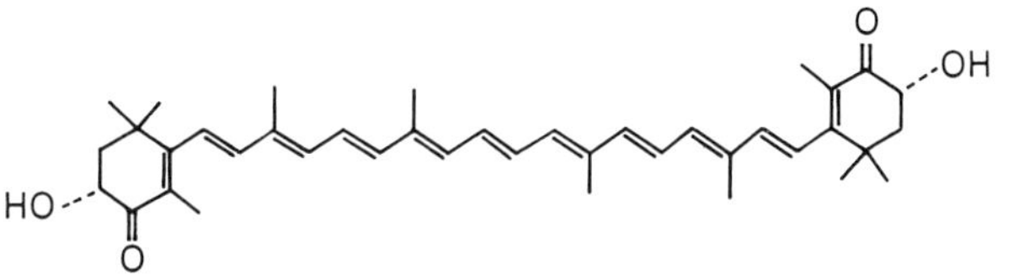

Astaxanthin (3, 3′ - dihydroxy - β, β - carotene - 4, 4′ - dione)

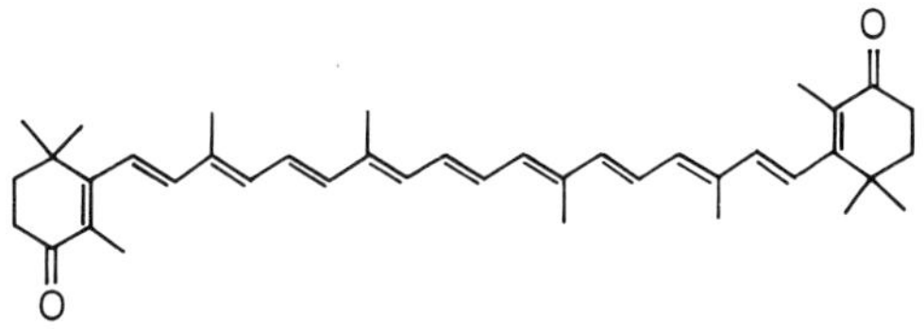

Canthaxanthin (β, β - carotene - 4, 4′ - dione)

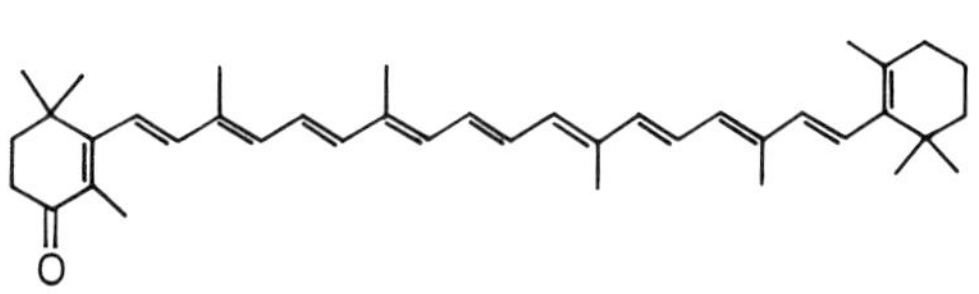

Echinenone (β, β - caroten - 4 - one)

Fig. 2. Some carotenoids typical of foods of animal origin. Astaxanthin occurs as a mixture of the (3S,3′S), (3R,3′R) and (3R,3′S) forms.

Avian species preferentially accumulate certain xanthophylls which provide the colour of eggs, body skin and fat. Diet-derived β-carotene predominates in milk.

Properties and Determination

Physical and Colour Properties

The extensive conjugated double-bond system constitutes the light-absorbing chromophore that gives carotenoids their attractive colours and provides the visible absorption spectrum which serves as the basis for their identification and quantitation. The structure–spectrum relationship has been extensively described; a few examples will be cited, referring to carotenoids dissolved in petroleum ether. The most unsaturated acyclic carotenoid lycopene, with 11 conjugated double bonds, is red and absorbs at the longest wavelengths (λ_{max} at 446, 472, 505 nm). At least seven such bonds are needed for a carotenoid to have perceptible colour. Thus, ζ-carotene is light yellow and its spectrum resembles that of lycopene in shape, with three well-defined peaks, but at much lower wavelengths (378, 400, 425 nm). The two carotenoids which precede ζ-carotene in the desaturation biosynthetic pathway, phytoene (three conjugated double bonds) and phytofluene (five conjugated double bonds), are colourless and absorb maximally at 276, 286, and 297 nm, and 331, 347 and 367 nm, respectively. Cyclization results in steric hindrance between the methyl groups at C5 and the polyene chain, taking the π electrons of the ring double bond out of plane with those of the chain. Consequently, a hypsochromic shift, hypochromic effect and loss of fine structure are observed. Thus, β-carotene, although possessing the same number of bonds as lycopene, is yellow-orange and has λ_{max} at 448 and 475, with a mere inflection at 425 nm. γ-Carotene is red-orange and exhibits a spectrum intermediate between those of lycopene and β-carotene. The double bond in the α-ionone ring of α-carotene is out of conjugation, thus it is light yellow and the absorption maxima are slightly more defined and at slightly lower wavelengths (422, 444, 473 nm) compared to β-carotene. Conjugated carbonyl groups cause a bathochromic shift and loss of fine structure to the extent that the three-maxima spectrum is replaced by a broad curve, asymmetrical with a maximum at 456 nm and a shoulder at 482 nm for echinenone (orange) and symmetrical with the maximum at 463 nm for canthaxanthin (red-orange). Hydroxyl substituents result in virtually no change in colour and absorption spectrum. Thus, lutein resembles α-carotene; β-cryptoxanthin and zeaxanthin are similar to β-carotene in these properties. Cis isomerization of one of the chromophore's bonds causes a slight loss in colour, hypsochromic shift and hypochromic effect, accompanied by the appearance of a new 'cis' peak in the ultraviolet region. The 5,6-mono- and 5,6,5',6'-diepoxides, having lost one and two ring double bonds, respectively. absorb maximally at wavelengths some 3 and 7 nm lower and are lighter than the parent compound. On transformation to the 5,8-furanoid form, two double bonds (one ring, one chain) are lost. Thus, the maxima of the 5,8-mono- and 5,8,5',8'-diepoxide are 20–25 and 50 nm lower, respectively, than those of the parent compound. Solvent effects are pronounced; the λ_{max} are higher relative to petroleum ether by 0–2 nm in methanol and ethanol, 1–3 nm in diethyl ether, 2–4 nm in acetone, 12–16 nm in chloroform and 14–20 nm in benzene. The absorbance ($A_{1\,cm}^{1\%}$) of a carotenoid also varies markedly with the solvent.

The intensity and hues of plant foods depend on which carotenoids are present and their concentrations, as well as their localization in the plastids. In animals, complexation of carotenoids with proteins can extend the colour to green, purple, blue or black. A well-known example is the blue carotenoprotein crustacyanin of the lobster carapace, an astaxanthin complex. On denaturation of the protein (e.g. heating), astaxanthin is released and its vivid red colour ensues.

Carotenoids are liposoluble and dissolve in fat solvents such as acetone, alcohol, ethyl ether and hexane. Xanthophylls are more polar but still insoluble in water; they dissolve more readily in methanol and ethanol. In plants and animals, carotenoids occur in solutions in fat depots, in colloidal dispersion in lipid media, or combined with protein in the aqueous phase.

Chemical Properties

The highly unsaturated carotenoid molecule is prone to isomerization and oxidation. Heat treatment, light and acids promote trans–cis isomerization. Oxidative degradation is stimulated by light, enzymes, metals and co-oxidation with lipid hydroperoxides. Carotenoids apparently have different susceptibilities, ζ-carotene, lutein and violaxanthin being cited as more labile. In studies involving β-carotene, the initial site of attack appears to be the terminal double bond, forming the 5,6-mono- and 5,6,5',6'-diepoxide, both of which undergo acid-catalysed conversion to the 5,8-mono- and 5,8,5',8'-diepoxide. Subsequent fragmentation yields a series of low-molecular-weight compounds similar to those obtained in fatty acid oxidation. *See* Oxidation of Food Components

There is increasing evidence that carotenoids can function directly as antioxidants. The primary mechanism of action appears to be their ability to quench singlet oxygen and interact with radical species, formed enzymatically or chemically. Quenching characteristics seem to be maximal with those having nine or more double bonds; the carotenoid molecule is destroyed in the process. At elevated oxygen pressures, however, carotenoids are reported to act as pro-oxidants. *See* Antioxidants, Natural Antioxidants

Xanthophylls undergo specific group reactions which serve as simple chemical tests in the determination of the structure. For example, primary and secondary hydroxyl groups are acetylated by acetic anhydride in

Properties and Determination

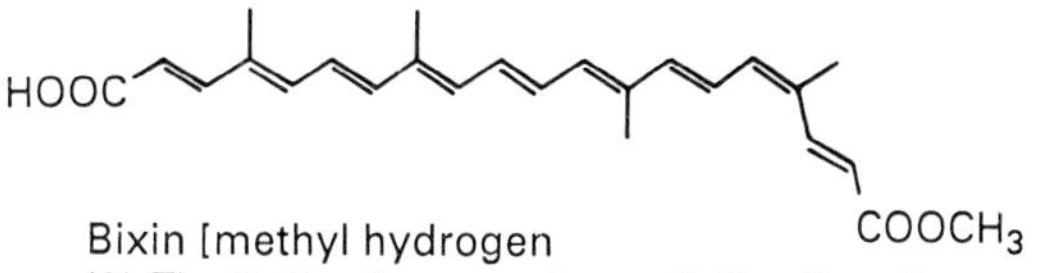

Bixin [methyl hydrogen
(9' Z) - 6, 6' - diapocarotene - 6, 6' - dioate]

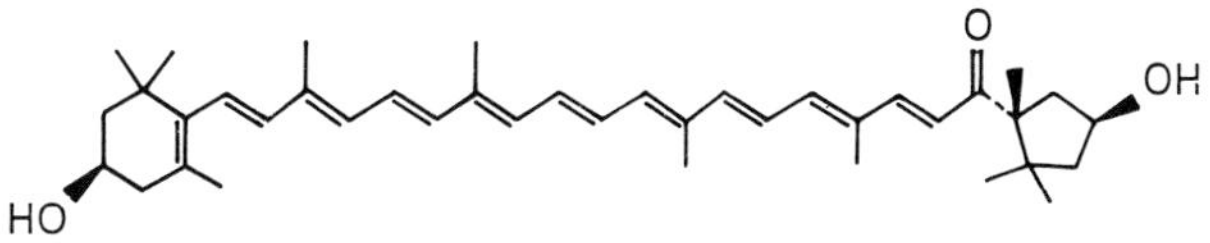

Capsanthin ((3R, 3'S, 5'R) - 3, 3' - dihydroxy - β, κ - caroten - 6' - one)

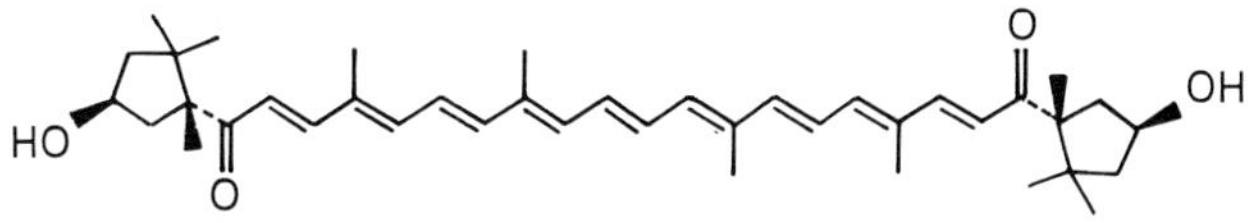

Capsorubin ((3S, 5R, 3'S, 5'R) - 3, 3' - dihydroxy - κ, κ - carotene - 6, 6' - dione)

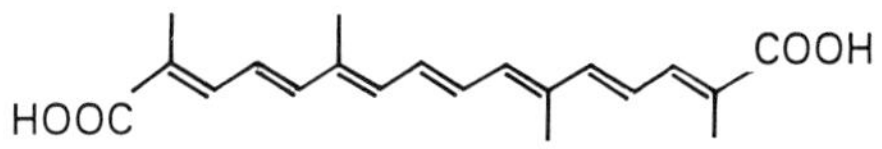

Crocetin (8, 8' - diapocarotene - 8, 8' - dioic acid)

Fig. 3. Principal carotenoids of natural extracts used as food colorants.

pyridine. Allylic hydroxyls, isolated or allylic to the chromophore are methylated with acidified methanol. In both reactions, a positive response is shown by an increase in thin-layer chromatography (TLC) R_F values, the extent of which depends on the number of hydroxyl substituents. Epoxy groups in the 5,6- or 5,6,5',6'-positions are easily detected by their conversion to the furanoid derivatives as described above. Oxo carotenoids undergo reduction with reducing agents such as $LiAlH_4$ or $NaBH_4$, manifested by the appearance of the three-peak spectra of the resulting hydroxycarotenoids. On the other hand, allylic hydroxyl groups are oxidized to the corresponding ketones by ρ-chloranil. Treatment with acidified chloroform results in the elimination of allylic hydroxyl groups as water, extending the chromophore and thus resulting in a bathochromic spectral shift. *See* Chromatography, Thin-layer Chromatography

Use as Food Colorants

Carotenoids as colorants find their way into food products by direct addition or indirectly through an animal's feed. Commercial formulations are of two types: natural extracts and synthetic nature-identical carotenoids. *See* Colours, Properties and Determination of Natural Pigments

Annatto, paprika, palm oil and tomato extracts, and saffron have been used for generations. Annatto is a series of red colouring preparations all based on the extracts of *Bixa orellana* seeds where the pigments are concentrated in the thin seed coat. Bixin (Fig. 3) is the main component of oil-soluble formulations and its saponification product, norbixin, the major colouring matter of water-soluble products. Oleoresin of paprika is the oil extract of *Capsicum annum*, which imparts a pinkish-yellow to crimson-red colour to foods, the main pigments being capsanthin and capsorubin. Saffron consists of the dried stigma of *Croccus sativus*, and is used as a spice and yellow colouring agent. It contains mainly crocin, the digentiobioside of crocetin. Lutein-containing marigold petals have been commercialized for poultry feed and a recent trend is to use β-carotene-rich algae as commercial sources of carotenoids.

The first carotenoid prepared by chemical synthesis, β-carotene, was introduced commercially by Roche in 1954. It was followed by β-apo-8'-carotenal in 1960, β-apo-8'-carotenoic acid ethyl ester in 1962 and canthaxanthin in 1964. In 1968 BASF introduced citranaxanthin and in 1984 Roche launched (3RS, 3'RS)-astaxanthin as feed additives. Crystalline carotenoids suffer from problems which render their commercialization in this form impractical: instability, insolubility in water and limited solubility in fats and oils. To satisfy the needs of the food industry, special application forms have been developed. Oil suspensions are the major marketable forms for colouring fat-based foods. For water-based foods, emulsions or colloidal preparations are available.

Advantages cited for carotenoids as food colorants are: natural connotation; high tinctural potency; unaffected by reducing conditions; non corrosive; good stability in the pH range of most food products; provitamin activity of some. Their disadvantages are: limited colour range; more expensive than azo dyes; sensitive to oxidative degradation.

Stability on Processing and Storage

Naturally present or added carotenoids are subject to isomerization and oxidation during food processing and storage, the practical consequence being loss of colour and biological activity and formation of volatile compounds that confer desirable or undesirable aromas to some foods. Oxidation, the major cause of degradation, depends on: the amount of oxygen; the carotenoids present and their physical state; water activity; presence of antioxidants (e.g. tocopherols and ascorbic acid); exposure to light; presence of metals, enzymes and peroxides; severity of the treatment (i.e. destruction of the ultrastructure that protects the carotenoids, increase of surface area, duration and temperature of heat treatment); packaging material; storage conditions. *See* Ascorbic Acid, Properties and Determination; Tocopherols, Properties and Determination

Reports on carotenoid retention appear conflicting, some claiming no loss or increase in carotenoid content and others showing considerable reductions. Some caution must be taken in interpreting the data since the divergence may be due to analytical factors. Calculations may not account for weight losses due to leaching of soluble solids (e.g. during blanching), giving erroneously high results for the processed products. Also, extraction of the carotenoids may be more effective in the processed products as compared to the raw material where solvent penetration may be difficult. On the other hand, care must be taken so as not to attribute carotenoid losses during analysis to processing effects.

Notwithstanding the diverging results, blanching, retorting and freezing are widely considered to have little effect on carotenoids and stability is good to excellent in frozen and heat-sterilized foods throughout the normal shelf life. Oxygen content is minimized by hot packing, vacuum packing, and oxygen scavenging with ascorbic acid. Heat does cause isomerization of *trans*-carotenoids to *cis* forms. Stability in dehydrated and powdered fruits and vegetables is generally poor, unless the product has been carefully processed and placed in a hermetically sealed, inert atmosphere for storage. A considerable portion of the carotenoids may be destroyed or removed by milling and processing of seeds and grains. Crude oil, such as palm oil, may contain significant levels of carotenoids, which are degraded on refining. *See* Freezing, Structural and Flavour Changes; Heat Treatment, Chemical and Microbiological Changes; Vegetable Oils, Refining

Analysis

With carotenoids two distinct analytical activities are conducted: elucidation of the structure of unknown carotenoids and determination of composition. Although they often overlap, there are nuances which are evident. In the former the major concern is to obtain the pure and unaltered carotenoid; the criteria of purity are rigorous, but quantitative losses are tolerated. In the latter, the purity requirement is not as strict, but complete extraction, efficient separation, conclusive identification and accurate quantitation are necessary. In both cases stringent precautions are essential, such as: (1) use of fresh samples and purified solvents; (2) short analysis time; (3) protection from oxygen (e.g. use of nitrogen gas), light (working under subdued light) and acids.

The general scheme for structure elucidation consists of extraction, saponification, partition, chromatography and rechromatography (open column chromatography, TLC, high-performance liquid chromatography (HPLC)), crystallization, check of purity, recrystallization and characterization by ultraviolet–visible, nuclear magnetic resonance (NMR) and mass spectroscopy (MS) techniques, chemical reactions and circular dichroism (CD). HPLC has greatly improved and facilitated carotenoid purification. Considerable amounts of NMR and MS data and also CD properties (to deduce absolute configurations) have been published. *See* Chromatography, High-performance Liquid Chromatography; Chromatography, Thin-layer Chromatography; Mass Spectrometry, Principles and Instrumentation; Spectroscopy, Nuclear Magnetic Resonance

Quantitative analysis has been approached differently, depending on the objective of the analyst. As a measure of colour, index of maturity (colour development) or processing parameter (loss of colour), it may simply involve extraction, spectrometric measurement and calculation of the total content, using the $A_{1\,cm}^{1\%}$ of β-carotene or that of the principal carotenoid. Not showing the qualitative pattern, the information obtained is limited. It is also inadequate for assessing vitamin A activity because of the presence of large amounts of vitamin A-inactive carotenoids in many foods. Thus, some methods include partial open column (gravity-flow) chromatography to separate the 'carotene' fraction. Depending on the adsorbent used and the extent of the separation, however, this fraction also contains less active and inactive carotenoids, which are quantified as β-carotene, or excludes active xanthophylls. Chromatography should be carried out further to separate the nonprovitamin carotenoids from the provitamins, which must be separated from each other and quantified individually. The vitamin A value can then be calculated, taking into account the different activities. *See* Retinol, Properties and Determination

The importance of the complete carotenoid composition, first recognized in efforts to understand the biosynthesis, has been reinforced by recent findings attributing to carotenoids roles other than and independent of the provitamin A activity (e.g. cancer inhibition). The analysis involves extraction, partition to petroleum ether or hexane (necessary for open column chromatography, optional for HPLC), saponification (needed for some samples), concentration in a rotary evaporator, chromatographic separation (open column chromatography or HPLC), confirmation of identity and quantitation.

The extraction procedure should be adapted to the sample under investigation. It is usually accomplished with mechanical tissue disruption, using a water-miscible organic solvent such as acetone, methanol or ethanol. Dried samples can be extracted with petroleum ether or ethyl ether, but more efficient extraction is achieved by moistening the sample with water and proceeding in the usual way.

Saponification is effective in removing chlorophylls and unwanted lipids and in hydrolysing carotenol esters (to simplify the separation). It must be avoided whenever possible, however, because artifact formation and quantitative losses may occur, depending on the conditions used.

The classical technique for separating carotenoids is open column chromatography. MgO:Hyflosupercel and neutral alumina are the preferred adsorbents. Fractions are eluted successively with solvents of increasing polarity (e.g. increasing concentration of diethyl ether or acetone in hexane or petroleum ether) and quantified spectrophotometrically. Reproducibility and efficiency of separation depend heavily on the analyst's skill and experience.

HPLC offers several advantages: high separation efficiency, reproducibility, sensitivity, inert conditions and speed. Most methods employ reversed-phase C_{18} columns and both nonaqueous and aqueous solvent systems have been used. Isocratic operation is preferred for provitamin A determination and gradient elution for complete carotenoid analysis. Quantitation is still problematic, however, considering that: (1) carotenoids absorb maximally at different wavelengths; (2) their absorption coefficients differ; (3) solvent effects are substantial. Thus, quantitative data based on peak area percentages can only be taken as rough estimates of the relative ratios, especially when detection is set at a single wavelength. A diode array detector will allow monitoring at different wavelengths but will not solve the other problems. Use of solvent mixtures isocratically or with gradient elution not only influence the quantitation but may also mislead the identification, since published spectral data refer to pure solvents. External or internal calibration is needed to determine the absolute concentrations. Both techniques, however, require standard solutions of the different carotenoids and only two or three are available commercially and are of varying purity. Unavailability and instability of carotenoid standards particularly affect external calibration which requires constant use of these standards. On the other hand, an ideal commercial internal standard has not been found. It is probably for this reason that most HPLC papers report only qualitative data or quantitation of major carotenoids.

Identification of the carotenoids should not be based solely on chromatographic data. Routine confirmation of the identity of well-known carotenoids can be achieved by electronic absorption spectra, corroborated by chemical reactions and the chromatographic behaviour. Otherwise, MS and/or NMR spectroscopy are required.

Bibliography

Bauernfeind JC (ed) (1981) *Carotenoids as Colorants and Vitamin A Precursors*. New York: Academic Press.

Britton G (1985) General carotenoid methods. *Methods in Enzymology* 111: 113–149.

Davies BH (1976) Carotenoids. In: Goodwin TW (ed.) *Chemistry and Biochemistry of Plant Pigments*, 2nd edn, pp 38–165. London: Academic Press.

Goodwin TW (1980) *The Biochemistry of the Carotenoids*, 2nd edn, vol. 1, London: Chapman and Hall.

Goodwin TW and Britton G (1988) Distribution and analysis of carotenoids. In: Goodwin TW (ed.) *Plant Pigments*, pp 61–132. London: Academic Press.

Gross J (1987) *Pigments in Fruits*, London: Academic Press.

Isler O (ed) (1971) *Carotenoids*, Basel: Birkhauser.

Krinsky NI, Mathews-Roth MM and Taylor RF (eds) (1990) *Carotenoids: Chemistry and Biology*, New York: Plenum Press.

Pfander H (ed) (1987) *Key to Carotenoids*, 2nd edn. Basel: Birkhauser.

Rodriguez-Amaya DB (1989) Critical review of provitamin A determination in plant foods. *Journal of Micronutrient Analysis* 5: 191–225.

D. B. Rodriguez-Amaya
Universidade Estadual de Campinas, Campinas SP, Brasil

Physiology

Absorption and Bioavailability of Carotenoids

There is considerable species variability in efficiency of absorption and in metabolism of carotenoids. Humans are apparently unusual in efficiently absorbing, transporting and storing both carotenes and xanthophylls. Although the rat and the chick have been used as experimental models for human carotenoid metabolism, recent work recommends the ferret as a better animal model. Some fish and birds absorb xanthophylls particularly well, and use them as pigments.

Intestinal absorption of carotenoids requires the presence of bile acids, as for absorption of other lipids; human subjects with impaired bile flow (biliary atresia) show low levels of liver carotenoids compared with normal subjects. The presence of other dietary lipid promotes intestinal micelle formation and carotenoid absorption. Animal feeding studies have shown that the biological matrix of food carotenoids affects absorption of dietary carotenoids, and dietary β-carotene in plant tissues has lower bioavailability than β-carotene in oil solution. Hence the plant source and method of preparation of feeds affect the bioavailability of β-carotene; processes which break down the biological matrix (e.g. grinding, mild cooking) improve carotenoid absorption.

Unequivocal estimation of the extent of absorption of dietary carotenoids is very difficult because of the ubiquitous presence of carotenoids in the diet, the slow absorption kinetics of carotenoids, the partial metabolism of carotenoids, and considerable apparent individual variation in extent of absorption and metabolism. However, it has been shown with an unmetabolized carotenoid analogue (ethyl β-apo8′carotenoate) in human studies that at least 40% of a moderate oral dose (100 μmol) was circulating in blood at about 16 h after dosing (Zeng, Furr and Olson, unpublished observations); since this peak concentration is due to the competing processes of intestinal absorption and redistribution from plasma to other tissues, absorption of dietary carotenoids may be quite efficient in the normal human, contrary to common belief.

In humans given approximately equal amounts of all-trans-β-carotene or a cis-β-carotene preparation, more all-trans-β-carotene was found in the blood, suggesting that (1) cis-β-carotene was not absorbed as efficiently, or (2) cis-β-carotene is preferentially metabolized to vitamin A, or (3) there was significant cis-to-trans isomerization in the human.

Transport, Distribution and Storage of Carotenoids

As with other lipids, freshly absorbed carotenoids are transported in the lymph via chylomicra. It is believed that the carotenoids, as with other lipid components of the chylomicron remnants, are taken up by the liver, and then released into the blood stream as components of very-low-density lipoproteins (VLDLs). The VLDLs

are taken up by extrahepatic tissues, their components processed into low-density lipoproteins (LDLs), and eventually into high-density lipoproteins (HDLs). Early studies showed that in human plasma the hydrocarbon carotenoids β-carotene and lycopene are predominantly associated with LDL (75%) and HDL (25%); the xanthophyll lutein is approximately equally distributed between HDL and LDL. The predominant human serum carotenoids, in studies in the USA, are β-carotene, α-carotene, lycopene, β-cryptoxanthin, lutein and zeaxanthin, also the colourless carotenoids phytoene and phytofluene; serum carotenoid profiles and concentrations are highly dependent on dietary intake. It is estimated that serum carotenoids represent about 1% of total body carotenoids in the human. *See* Lipoproteins

Adipose tissue (80–85% of total body carotenoids) and liver (8–12%) are the major sites of carotenoid deposition in humans when total mass of tissue carotenoid is considered. Typical total human carotenoid levels of 100–150 mg are reported from autopsy analyses. Human adipose carotenoid profiles are similar to those of serum. Reported values for total human liver carotenoids range between 0 and 97 μg per g of liver (i.e. $0–0.18$ μmol g^{-1}; total carotenoids were expressed as β-carotene in older studies), and include lutein, lycopene, α-carotene and β-carotene. Other tissues that are known to contain high concentrations of carotenoids include adrenals (20 μg (37 nmol) per g of tissue, mostly as β-carotene) and human macular pigment (containing predominantly the xanthophylls lutein and zeaxanthin). It has been suggested that organs with high numbers of LDL receptors and high rates of LDL uptake show higher tissue levels of carotenoids.

Carotenoid–protein interactions have been studied in plants, bacteria, and marine invertebrates. In these species the strength of specific protein–carotenoid binding depends, not surprisingly, on carotenoid structure. Distinctive interactions between a binding protein and its carotenoid ligand are evident by the spectral changes of the carotenoid on binding; these spectral changes may reflect physiological functions as well as producing colour polymorphism among species.

Retinol Equivalents of Different Carotenoids

Of the more than 600 known carotenoids, only about 60 have been reported to be precursors of vitamin A. In order to serve as a precursor of vitamin A, a carotenoid must have at least one unsubstituted β-ionone ring (2,6,6-trimethyl-1-cyclohexen-1-yl) with a polyene side-chain of at least 11 carbon atoms. Thus α-carotene (with one β-ionone ring) has half the biological activity of β-carotene, and canthaxanthin (with keto substitutions on both rings) has no provitamin A activity. Absolute vitamin A activity, however, depends on a number of other factors, not all of which are well understood. In general, it seems that efficiency of conversion of carotenoids to vitamin A depends on vitamin A status; high intakes of preformed vitamin A result in poor efficiency of conversion to vitamin A, perhaps owing to metabolic control of the cleavage enzyme(s). Frank vitamin A deficiency is also associated with impaired conversion efficiency, perhaps because of damaged intestinal epithelial function in vitamin A inadequacy. Vitamin A deficiency disease is more rapidly cured by providing preformed vitamin A than by providing dietary carotenoids because conversion of β-carotene to vitamin A is impaired in vitamin A deficiency. Excessive vitamin E intake seems to impair carotenoid cleavage (or interferes with intestinal absorption); vitamin E deficiency decreases vitamin A formation, perhaps because adequate vitamin E is needed to protect carotenoids and vitamin A from oxidation. Conversion efficiency of β-carotene and other carotenoids to vitamin A is also decreased at high carotenoid intakes, perhaps as a result of either impaired intestinal absorption or metabolic control of the cleavage enzyme(s). Protein deficiency impairs cleavage, suggesting that protein malnutrition in humans exacerbates vitamin A deficiency. *See* Retinol, Physiology

Common dietary sources of provitamin A carotenoids are carrots, yellow squash, dark-green leafy vegetables, yellow maize, tomatoes, papaya, and oranges. Cereal grains and white maize contain little or no provitamin A. Red palm oil is one of the richest sources of provitamin A carotenoids, containing approximately 0·5 mg α- and β-carotene per ml; as little as 7 ml palm oil per d may provide adequate vitamin A for the preschool child. On a global basis, β-carotene is the most important vitamin A precursor, both because of its greater provitamin A activity and because of its wide distribution in plant products. However, other provitamin A carotenoids, such as α-carotene and β-cryptoxanthin and β-apocarotenals, can be nutritionally important sources of vitamin A from particular foods (Table 1). Other carotenoids, such as lycopene (which has no β-ionone rings) and the dihydroxycarotenoids lutein and zeaxanthin (which are substituted on both ionone rings), may be major carotenoids in particular foods and may have other important physiological functions, but have no provitamin A activity.

Estimation of provitamin A content of foods from food composition tables is problematic: carotenoid composition of raw fruits and vegetables varies with species, growth conditions, and mode of storage. Furthermore older tables often express total carotenoids as 'β-carotene', ignoring the different provitamin A activity of different carotenoids. Biological activity of carotenoids in foodstuffs may differ from the analysed content because of mode of preparation, binding of carotenoids within the foodstuff, and the nature of the meal (presence or absence of fat).

Although central cleavage of 1 mol of β-carotene should, in theory, yield 2 mol of vitamin A, such a high yield is not found reproducibly in feeding studies. Instead, the biological activity of β-carotene compared with that of vitamin A seems to be in a range of 2:1 to 12:1 (weight of β-carotene:weight of vitamin A); in most domestic animals and in humans, the ratio is 4:1 to 10:1 (mean 7:1). Currently a conversion ratio of 6 μg β-carotene to 1 μg vitamin A alcohol (approximately 3 mol β-carotene to 1 mol vitamin A) is generally accepted for humans and domestic animals, although this value clearly depends on other nutritional factors (as discussed above). Other provitamin A carotenoids are considered to have half this activity (12 μg carotenoid is equal to 1 μg retinol). Table 2 compares different methods of expressing vitamin A values.

Enzymatic Conversion to Vitamin A

By comparison of the structure of β-carotene with that of vitamin A, it would appear that β-carotene could be cleaved in its centre (between the 15 and 15′ carbon atoms) to give two molecules of vitamin A per molecule of carotenoid. Such a mechanism was first proposed by Karrer. However, in addition ot this central (symmetric) cleavage, a random (asymmetric) cleavage has been proposed. Glover first suggested that asymmetric cleavage of the symmetric β-carotene molecule could be followed by stepwise shortening to vitamin A. In support of this hypothesis, small amounts of labelled β-apo8′-, β-apo10′, and β-apo12′carotenal (and their alcohols and acids) have been found in rat tissues after feeding radioactive β-carotene. These apo-carotenals can be formed by chemical reaction of oxidizing agents (hydrogen peroxide, potassium permanganate) with β-carotene *in vitro*, and they are found in small amounts in plants. However, no enzymatic asymmetric cleavage activity has been demonstrated *in vitro*. On the other hand, *in vitro* experiments using partially purified intestinal homogenates (from rat, rabbit, or guinea pig) have demonstrated symmetric cleavage of β-carotene, with retinal (vitamin A aldehyde) as the only detectable product. This enzymatic activity requires the presence of oxygen, and has been named '15,15′β-carotenoid dioxygenase' (EC 1.13.11.21). This enzymatic activity has been demonstrated in intestine, liver, kidney, and several other tissues *in vitro*.

The 'random-cleavage' hypothesis is supported by the experimental observation that 1 mol of dietary β-carotene never has more biological activity than 1 mol of vitamin A (not 2 mol as predicted by the 'central-cleavage' hypothesis) in animal studies. However, this

Table 1. Vitamin A activity of common carotenoids relative to β-carotene

Carotenoid	Activity (%)	Occurrence (partial list)
β-Carotene	100	Green plants, vegetables, carrots, yellow sweet potatoes, squash, tomatoes, red and yellow fruits
α-Carotene	50–54	Green plants, carrots, squash, maize, green peppers
γ-Carotene	42–50	Carrots, sweet potatoes, maize, tomatoes, algae, some fruits
β-Carotene 5′,6′monoepoxide	21	Plants, potatoes, red peppers
β-Carotene 5,6,5′,6′diepoxide	Active?	Plants
β-Carotene 5′,8′monofuranoxide (mutatochrome, citroxanthin, flavacin)	50	Orange peel, red peppers, tomatoes, sweet potatoes, cranberries
4-Keto-β-carotene (4-oxo-β-carotene, echinenone, aphanin, myxoxanthin)	44–54	Algae, sea urchins, *Daphnia*, *Hydra*, red sponges, brine shrimp, crustaceans
3-Keto-β-carotene (3-oxo-β-carotene)	52	
3-Hydroxy-β-carotene (β-cryptoxanthin)	50–60	Yellow maize, green peppers, lichens, persimmons, papayas, lemons, oranges
4-Hydroxy-β-carotene (isocryptoxanthin)	48	Brine shrimp
3,4-Dehydro3′hydroxy-β-carotene (anhydrolutein, deoxylutein)	Active, *c.* 10	Alfalfa meal, acidulated soya bean soapstock
3-Hydroxy-4-keto-β-carotene (hydroxyechinenone)	Probably active	Algae, bacteria, flowers
β-Apo2′carotenal	Active	Citrus fruit
β-Apo8′carotenal	36–72	Citrus fruit, green plants
β-Apo10′carotenal	Active	Citrus fruit, green plants, alfalfa meal
β-Apo12′carotenal	120	Alfalfa meal
β-Apo8′carotenoic acid	Active	Maize, animal tissue
β-Apo8′carotenoic acid ethyl ester	25, 78	
Lycopene	Inactive	Tomatoes, carrots, green peppers, pink citrus fruit
3,3′Dihydroxy-β-carotene (zeaxanthin)	Inactive	Spinach, paprika, yellow maize, green peppers, fruits
3,3′Dihdroxy-α-carotene (lutein)	Inactive	Green leaves, yellow maize, potatoes, spinach, green peppers, carrots, tomatoes, fruits
3,3′Dihydroxy-4,4′diketo-β-carotene (astaxanthin)	Inactive	Oranges, crustaceans, lobster, fish, algae, *Daphnia*, trout, salmon
4,4′Diketo-β-carotene (canthaxanthin, aphanicin)	Inactive	Mushrooms, trout, *Daphnia*, *Hydra*, microorganisms, algae, crustaceans, brine shrimp
Capsanthin	Inactive	Red peppers, paprika
Capsorubrin	Inactive	Red peppers, paprika
Bixin	Inactive	Annatto seeds

Adapted and shortened from Bauernfeind JC, Adams CR and Marusich WL (1981) Carotenes and vitamin A precursors in animal feed. In: Bauernfeind JC (ed.) *Carotenoids as Colorants and Vitamin A Precursors*, pp 563–743. New York: Academic Press.

effect might be explained by inefficiencies of absorption and enzymatic cleavage. The 'random-cleavage' mechanism requires the step-wise shortening of longer-chain apocarotenoids to vitamin A; β oxidation (in analogy to fatty acid metabolism) has been proposed, but such a mechanism would produce retinoic acid instead of retinal or retinol, and there is strong evidence against biological reduction of retinoic acid to the other forms of vitamin A. The random-cleavage mechanism has in its favour that small amounts of apocarotenoids have been found in animal tissues. However, shorter aporetinoid fragments (fewer than 20 carbon atoms), required as remnants of asymmetric cleavage, have not been isolated and identified. β-Apocarotenoids have provitamin A activity in animal experiments (a necessary condition for the random-cleavage hypothesis), but can

be cleaved to retinal by intestinal homogenates *in vitro* under conditions used to assay the 15,15′dioxygenase enzymatic activity (central cleavage). β-Carotene is not a source of vitamin A in the cat, and it has been reported that 15,15′dioxygenase activity is not present in cat intestine, consistent with the central-cleavage hypothesis. Hence there is no definitive answer at this time as to the mechanism used *in vivo*, or, if both are used in the animal, which predominates. Considering the importance of carotenoids as precursors of vitamin A in higher animals, this remains an important question in carotenoid metabolism.

It seems that some fish and birds can also convert the xanthophylls, astaxanthin, canthaxanthin and isozeaxanthin, to vitamin A; some freshwater fish can convert lutein to 3,4-didehydroretinol (vitamin A$_2$). Ketocarote-

Table 2. Conversion factors for estimating vitamin A value from carotenoid composition

	Conversion factors and formulae
1 retinol equivalent (RE)[a]	$= 1\ \mu g$ all-*trans*-retinol
	$= 6\ \mu g$ all-*trans*-β-carotene
	$= 12\ \mu g$ other provitamin A carotenoids
	$= 3\cdot33$ iu vitamin A
	$= 10$ iu provitamin A carotenoids
1 International Unit of vitamin A (iu$_A$)	$= 0\cdot3\ \mu g$ all-*trans*-retinol
	$= 0\cdot3$ RE
	$= 3$ iu$_C$ carotene
	$= 1\cdot8\ \mu g$ all-*trans*-β-carotene
	$= 3\cdot6\ \mu g$ other provitamin A carotenoids
1 International Unit of provitamin A carotenoids (iu$_C$)	$= 0\cdot6\ \mu g$ all-*trans*-β-carotene
	$= 0\cdot1$ RE $= 0\cdot1\ \mu g$ all-*trans*-retinol
	$= 0\cdot33$ iu$_A$
	$= 1\cdot2\ \mu g$ other provitamin A carotenoids
Retinol and β-carotene given in μg	RE $= \mu g$ retinol $+ (\mu g\ \beta\text{-carotene}/6)$
Retinol and β-carotene given in iu	RE $= (\text{iu retinol}/3\cdot33) + (\text{iu }\beta\text{-carotene}/10)$
β-Carotene and other provitamin A carotenoids given in μg	RE $= (\mu g\ \beta\text{-carotene}/6) + (\mu g$ other provitamin A carotenoids/12)

[a] Note that 1 RE $= 1\cdot15\ \mu g$ retinyl acetate (M_r 328) $= 1\cdot83\ \mu g$ retinyl palmitate (M_r 524), i.e. molar equivalence.
Adapted from Olson JA (1987) Recommended dietary intakes (RDI) of vitamin A in humans: appendix. *American Journal of Clinical Nutrition* 45: 704–716.

noids can be reduced to the corresponding alcohols and esterified with long-chain fatty acids.

Toxicity of Carotenoids

There is virtually no toxicity resulting from high intakes of carotenoids, in marked contrast to vitamin A. Excessive human ingestion of β-carotene can cause high serum carotenoid levels and yellowing of light-coloured skin, but such overconsumption is very unusual, and no harmful physiological effect from even such high intakes of β-carotene have been reported. The effects disappear when high carotenoid intakes cease. Ingestion of large amounts of carotenoids does not give rise to hypervitaminosis A, probably because of decreased efficiency of conversion of carotenoids to vitamin A at high intakes. Tetratogenicity caused by carotenoids has never been suggested. β-Carotene supplementation in humans does not produce elevated serum triacylglycerols or cholesterol. *See* Hypovitaminosis A

The only carotenoid which has been associated with adverse effects is canthaxanthin (4,4′diketo-β-carotene which has been used in treatment of patients with erythropoietic protoporphyria and related skin disorders. High daily doses (50–100 mg) have resulted in canthaxanthin retinopathy (crystalline deposits in the retina leading to impaired night vision); the effect is slowly reversible on cessation of intake. Pharmacological doses of canthaxanthin have depressed liver accumu-

lation of dietary vitamin A in rats. Human ingestion of large amounts of canthaxanthin gives a yellowish colouration to light-coloured skin; this is the basis of some 'skin tanning' pills.

Therapeutic Role of Carotenoids

In addition to the important roles of some carotenoids as vitamin A precursors, there is evidence that carotenoids can quench singlet oxygen and can serve as radical-trapping antioxidants; it has also been suggested that carotenoids may have a role (apart from a provitamin A function) in enhancing immune function in animals. Singlet-oxygen trapping and antioxidant functions are exhibited *in vitro* by carotenoids which have no provitamin A activity (such as lycopene and astaxanthin) as well as by provitamin A carotenoids. *See* Antioxidants, Role of Antioxidant Nutrients in Defence Systems

Both β-carotene and canthaxanthin have been used in large-dose regimens to ameliorate photosensitivity associated with erythropoietic protoporphyria (a genetic disease of porphyrin metabolism). β-Carotene also prevents photosensitivity caused by quinidine ingestion, but not photosensitivity to ultraviolet (UV) light, although it has been reported that human serum carotenoid levels decrease after repeated exposure to UV light.

Epidemiological evidence strongly suggests a role for

carotenoids in human cancer prevention, although some studies may be confounded by other factors. The strongest evidence is for a protective effect of carotenoids against lung cancer; tomato products (which provide lycopene) may be more effective than carrots and squash (sources of β-carotene). Protective effects of carotenoids against laryngeal cancer, gastric cancer, invasive bladder cancer and cervical dysplasia and cervical cancer have also been suggested; these effects are not shown by vitamin A, suggesting a direct role of carotenoids. Neither carotenoids nor vitamin A protect against cancers of the oesophagus or gastrointestinal tract, breast, head, or neck. A variety of cancers in animal models are prevented or delayed by carotenoids, including skin tumours and mammary tumours. In studies in cells in culture, carotenoids can prevent malignant transformation, sister chromatid exchange, and mutagenic effects in bacterial systems. *See* Cancer, Diet in Cancer Prevention

A recent report suggests that coronary heart disease may be reduced in populations consuming higher quantities of carotenoid-containing foods. *See* Coronary Heart Disease, Antioxidant Status

Carotenoids have been found to enhance both specific and nonspecific immune functions, including proliferation of T and B lymphocytes, induction of specific effector cells capable of killing tumour cells and increased production of tumour necrosis factor, and secretion of factors required for communication between cells (prostaglandins and leucotrienes). It has been suggested that the mechanism(s) may involve quenching singlet oxygen and trapping free radicals (generated by neutrophils to kill invading cells), or maintaining cell membrane fluidity (important for func-tion of membrane receptors and for release of immuno-modulating factors). Again, some of the immunological functions of carotenoids seem to be independent of any provitamin A activity, although retinoids are also important in immune function. Elucidation of these biochemical effects of carotenoids, and explanation of the conversion of carotenoids to vitamin A, remain central issues in the study of carotenoid metabolism. *See* Immunity and Nutrition

Bibliography

Bauernfeind JC (ed.) (1981) *Carotenoids as Colorants and Vitamin A Precursors*. New York: Academic Press.
Bendich A and Olson JA (1989) Biological actions of carotenoids. *FASEB Journal* 3: 1927–1932.
Isler O (ed.) (1971) *The Carotenoids*. Basel: Birkhauser Verlag.
Glover J and Redfearn ER (1954) The mechanism of the transformation of β-carotene into vitamin A in vivo. *Biochemical Journal* 58: xv.
Karrer P, Morf R and Schopp K (1931) Zur Kenntnis des Vitamin-A aus Fischtrannen II. *Helvetica Chimica Acta* 14: 1431–1436.
Krinsky NI, Mathews-Roth MM and Taylor RF (eds) (1990) *Carotenoids: Chemistry and Biology*. New York: Plenum Press.
Mathews-Roth MM (1991) Recent progress in the medical applications of carotenoids. *Pure and Applied Chemistry* 63(1): 147–156.
Pfander H (1987) *Key to Carotenoids* 2nd edn. Basel: Birkhauser Verlag.
Straub O (1976) *Key to Carotenoids: List of Natural Carotenoids*. Basel: Birkhauser Verlag.

Harold C. Furr
University of Connecticut, Storrs, USA

CASEIN AND CASEINATES

Contents

Methods of Manufacture

The commercial production of casein, the principal protein in cow's milk, has occurred for most of the twentieth century. During the period to 1960, the major proportion of casein was used in technical (or nonfood) applications. More recently, however, there has been a significant change from technical to edible uses for casein products and this has been reflected in the introduction of requirements for pasteurization of milk intended for casein manufacture (*c.* 1970) and the greater number of specifications for microbial quality and freedom from impurities. At the present time, the major producers of casein include the EEC (Denmark, France, Germany, the Irish Republic and the Netherlands), New Zealand and Poland, and world production is of the order of 220 000–250 000 tonnes. This article describes the manufacture of the main casein products. *See* Pasteurization, Principles

General

The proteins that exist in milk can be broadly divided into two groups, viz. casein and whey proteins. Caseins may be considered as those proteins that are precipitated when unheated (raw) milk is acidified to pH 4·6 (the isoelectric point of casein) whereas whey proteins remain in solution. Commercial casein is a mixture of several different caseins, e.g. α_{s1}-, β- and κ-casein, and may sometimes be referred to as whole casein. As a phosphoprotein, casein belongs to a relatively rare class of proteins. It contains 0·7–0·9% phosphorus, covalently bound to the casein by a serine ester linkage. Casein exists in milk in combination with calcium, inorganic phosphate and citrate as a colloidal suspension of complex 'micelles' and accounts for 2·6–2·9% by weight of whole milk. *See* Whey and Whey Powders, Production and Uses; Whey and Whey Powders, Protein Concentrates and Fractions; Whey and Whey Powders, Fermentation of Whey

Manufacture of Casein

Casein may be precipitated from skim milk to produce several products such as acid casein, rennet casein and coprecipitate. All these products are insoluble in water after precipitation. However, addition of alkali to acid casein yields water-soluble caseinate.

Acid Casein

Acidification

When milk (pH 6·6) is acidified, the calcium and inorganic phosphate are removed from the casein micelles, the net charge on the micelles decreases and the micelles become less and less stable until the casein precipitates. Complete precipitation of the casein occurs at the isoelectric point, pH 4·6. Acidification of the milk may be carried out by one of the following processes:

(1) Inoculation of milk with lactic acid-producing bacteria such as *Lactococcus lactis* subspecies *lactis* or *cremoris*. These bacteria, commonly known as 'starters', convert some of the lactose in the milk to lactic acid during the period of incubation (about 16–18 h). This method of manufacture is the most common one employed in New Zealand (see Fig. 1).
(2) Direct addition of dilute acid to skim milk. Hydro-

chloric acid, sulphuric acid, phosphoric acid or lactic acid (and, occasionally, other organic acids) may be used for this purpose. The most common method of producing acid casein in countries other than New Zealand is by means of hydrochloric acid precipitation. *See* Lactic Acid Bacteria

Cooking/Acidulation

In the manufacture of acid casein, acidification of the milk is followed, or occasionally preceded, by heating of the mixture. Heating promotes agglomeration of the casein curd particles which subsequently shrink ('syneresis') to expel whey. At the same time, the curd becomes firmer and is able to withstand the mechanical processing that follows. Heating of the acidified milk is sometimes termed 'cooking' and may be carried out, usually in the temperature range 45–55°C, by:

(1) injection of steam into the pipeline carrying the acidified milk;
(2) indirect heating by means of a heat exchanger; or
(3) a combination of both—preheating through a heat exchanger with steam injection to complete the heating process (e.g. see Fig. 1).

In each case, the cooked curd and whey are held in a 'cooking pipe' for a period of about 10–20 s before they emerge into an 'acidulation' vat. The curd and whey may remain here for a period varying from 30 s to about 15 min, during which time the curd is gently agitated in the whey until equilibrium between the calcium in the curd and whey is attained.

Alternative processes may employ a 'syneresis tube' in which the cooked curd and whey are held in a large-diameter tube for a period of several minutes (also undergoing 'acidulation' or equilibration).

Dewheying and Washing

Following acidulation, the curd and whey are transferred by pump or discharged by gravity to a dewheying screen above the first washing vat. The whey is removed and the curd falls into the vat. Alternatively, the curd and whey may be more completely separated using a horizontal solid-bowl centrifuge (decanter) or a casein-dewatering press before the curd is transferred to the first wash. A combination of screening and decanter dewheying can be used to reduce the hydraulic load on the decanter. The purpose of washing is to remove whey (containing mainly lactose) from the curd so that the casein produced is relatively pure. It is normal practice to wash the curd several times in water. The temperature of the wash water may be varied, depending upon particular requirements. Casein is usually subjected to

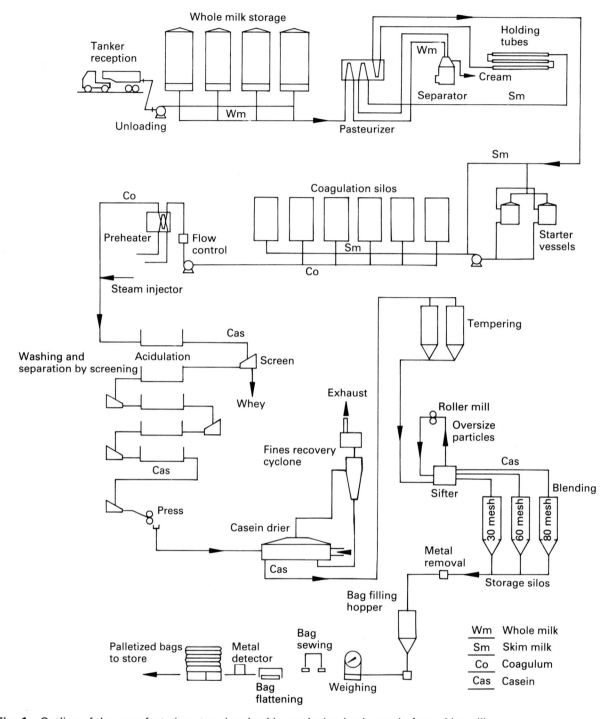

Fig. 1   Outline of the manufacturing steps involved in producing lactic casein from skim milk.

multiple washes and these are operated in a counter flow to the direction of the curd, with the purest curd meeting the cleanest water.

Dewatering

After washing, the curd is mechanically 'dewatered' to remove excess water before drying. As drying is a relatively expensive operation, it is obviously worthwhile to remove as much water as possible from the curd before transferring the casein to the drier. The texture of the curd is affected by temperature; as the temperature of the wash water is increased, the curd releases more water during dewatering but becomes firm and more plastic and is consequently harder to mince and dry. Therefore, it is necessary to regulate carefully the temperature of the last wash to optimize the conflicting

Table 1. Typical composition and properties of casein products

Component	Acid casein	Rennet casein	Sodium caseinate (spray dried)
Component	*Amount per 100 g*		
Moisture (g)	11·5	11·5	4·5
Fat (g)	1·1	0·4	1·0
Protein (g) (nitrogen × 6·38)	86·2	81·3	92·0
Ash (g)	1·8	8·2	3·6
Lactose (g)	0·1	0·1	0·1
	Amount per 1 kg		
Copper (mg)	2	2	2
Lead (mg)	<1	<1	<1
Iron (mg)	5–20	5	5–10
Physical properties			
Colour	Creamy white	Creamy white	White
Flavour	Bland, clean	Bland, clean	Bland, clean
Solubility in water	Insoluble	Insoluble	Soluble

requirements of minimum water content and maximum friability of the curd.

Equipment for dewatering casein curd consists of roller or belt presses, decanters and screen-bowl centrifuges. The roller press, used for many years, is designed to reduce the moisture content of curd to about 55%. The belt press will do a similar duty. Solid-bowl decanters or screen-bowl centrifuges are capable of reducing the moisture content of acid casein curd to about 52%.

Drying

Drying of casein curd is most commonly carried out using horizontal vibrating fluid-bed driers. These driers have two or more perforated stainless steel decks (see Fig. 1). The combined effect of vibration of the decks and the flow of hot air (typical temperature range 75–115°C) up through the holes in the decks causes the casein curd to become fluidized and materially helps in the removal of moisture from the particles. Most of the water is removed during the early stages of drying of the casein as it is evaporated from the surface of the particle. The later stages of drying require the transfer of moisture from the centre to the surface of the particle, and this is a much slower process.

Pneumatic-conveying ring driers and attrition driers are also used for drying casein. These employ in-line milling and tend to produce finer casein products than those dried in fluid-bed driers. *See* Drying, Spray Drying

Cooling, Tempering, Grinding, Sifting, Blending, Bagging

Casein that is produced using fluid-bed driers is warm and soft and unsuitable for grinding immediately in some mills such as roller mills. The casein consequently may be cooled and then transferred to 'tempering' bins where equilibration of moisture can occur in and between all the particles during a period of 8–24 h.

The casein may then be ground and sieved, using multideck, gyrating screens, into various particle sizes, usually < 600 μm. Very fine casein (e.g. < 150 μm) is generally produced using pin mills.

Following blending of the ground casein, it is packed into multiwall bags equipped with plastic liners and stored. A typical composition of acid casein is shown in Table 1.

Rennet Casein

Action of Chymosin

Casein may also be precipitated from milk by the action of a proteolytic enzyme, such as chymosin, which is present in calf rennet. Chymosin (and other enzymes from animal and microbial sources that cause milk to clot) splits off a portion of the κ-casein (referred to as glycomacropeptide or GMP) from the micelle. As a result, the micelle is no longer stabilized in the presence of calcium ions and the destabilized casein subsequently forms a three-dimensional clot. This process is essential in the production of most types of cheese. *See* Cheeses, Chemistry of Curd Manufacture

Methods of Manufacture

Clotting of Milk

Pasteurized skim milk at a temperature of 29°C (or lower) is mixed with calf rennet (or other milk-clotting enzyme) in the approximate ratio (by volume) of 1:7500 rennet to milk. Clotting usually occurs from 20 to 40 min after addition of rennet to the milk. If lower setting temperatures are used, renneting times must be correspondingly increased. It is also possible to reduce the quantity of rennet added under these conditions and consequently allow a longer time for the renneting action to occur.

Cooking

The usual technique for the cooking of rennet casein involves the injection of steam into a cooking line of clotted milk pumped from a vat. However, the vat cooking technique (similar to that used in cheesemaking) is also practised in some countries. The cooking temperature employed in making rennet casein usually varies from about 50 to 60°C.

Dewheying, washing, dewatering and drying of curd then proceed in a manner similar to that described for acid casein, and the dried casein is also treated as outlined previously.

Where indirect cooking of rennet casein is employed, a tubular heat exchanger may be used to cook the curd and whey to a temperature similar to that used in the 'direct cook' (steam injection) process. Other processing steps are similar to those described above and no acidulation step occurs after cooking of the rennet casein.

A typical composition of rennet casein is shown in Table 1.

Coprecipitates

Coprecipitates are combinations of casein and whey proteins that are precipitated together from heated milk. When milk is heated to temperatures greater than 70°C, some of the whey proteins are heat denatured and may interact with some of the caseins. When a casein precipitant (such as acid or calcium chloride) is added to the heated milk, the casein and whey proteins coprecipitate together. Depending upon the pH of precipitation (which may vary from 6·6 to 4·5), the coprecipitate will contain different quantities of calcium ('high-calcium' at pH 6·6 to 'low-calcium' at pH 4·5). As whey proteins have a higher nutritional value than casein, coprecipitates also have an enhanced nutritional value compared with casein. The yield of coprecipitate from skim milk is usually 5–20% greater than that of casein. *See* Calcium, Physiology

Caseinates

Caseinates are produced by the neutralization of acid casein with alkali. All caseinates are substantially water-soluble and are typically prepared as a solution of about 20% solids prior to spray drying. Roller-dried caseinates may be prepared from more concentrated solutions. It is also possible to prepare granular, partly soluble or semidispersible forms of caseinate in which the casein and alkali have only been partly reacted. Sodium caseinate is the most common form of this class of product and is prepared by mixing a solution of sodium hydroxide, bicarbonate or carbonate with acid casein curd or dry acid casein that has been suspended in water. It dissolves completely in water to produce a viscous, sticky, straw-coloured solution.

Calcium caseinate, on the other hand, produces a thin, opaque, white colloidal dispersion in water, similar in appearance to milk. Other caseinates, such as those of potassium and ammonium, are similar in general properties to sodium caseinate. Magnesium caseinate has properties that are intermediate between those of sodium and calcium caseinates. Relatively insignificant commercial quantities of these products are, however, manufactured at the present time.

A typical composition of sodium caseinate is shown in Table 1. Acid (low-calcium) coprecipitates can be dissolved in alkali in a similar manner to that used for acid casein. Both rennet casein and high-calcium coprecipitate (precipitated at a pH of 6 or greater) are usually rendered soluble by means of complex phosphates, such as sodium tripolyphosphate, to produce translucent solutions with viscosities somewhat higher than that of the corresponding caseinates.

In the great majority of applications, in both edible and technical (nonfood) uses, casein must first be made soluble before it can be employed in its final application. Although some users will convert the casein to caseinate themselves, others tend to purchase the caseinate directly from the producer. For applications, refer to the next article.

Bibliography

Australian Society of Dairy Technology (1972) *Casein Manual*. Victoria: Australian Society of Dairy Technology, Parkville.

Farrell Jr, HM (1988) Physical equilibria: proteins. In: Wong NP, Jenness R, Keeney M and Marth EH (eds) *Fundamentals of Dairy Chemistry*, 3rd edn, pp 461–510. New York: Van Nostrand Reinhold.

Muller LL (1971) Manufacture and uses of casein and co-precipitates: a review. *Dairy Science Abstracts* 33: 659–674.

Muller LL (1982) Manufacture of casein, caseinates and co-precipitates. In: Fox PF (ed.) *Developments in Dairy Chemistry*, vol. 1. *Proteins*, pp 315–337. London: Applied Science.

Southward CR (1985) Manufacture and applications of edible

casein products. 1. Manufacture and properties. *New Zealand Journal of Dairy Science and Technology* 20: 79–101.

Southward CR (1986) Utilization of milk components: casein. In: Robinson RK (ed.) *Modern Dairy Technology*, vol. 1. *Advances in Milk Processing*, pp 317–368. London: Elsevier.

Southward CR and Walker NJ (1980) The manufacture and industrial use of casein. *New Zealand Journal of Dairy Science and Technology* 15: 201–217.

Spellacy JR (1953) *Casein, Dried and Condensed Whey*. San Francisco: Lithotype Process

Whitney RMcL (1988) Proteins of milk. In: Wong NP, Jenness R, Keeney M and Marth EH (eds) *Fundamentals of Dairy Chemistry*, 3rd edn, pp 81–169. New York: Van Nostrand Reinhold.

C.R. Southward
New Zealand Dairy Research Institute, Palmerston North, New Zealand

Uses in the Food Industry*

Although casein, as it exists in milk, has been consumed as 'food' for thousands of years, the extracted form of casein had very little application in foods prior to 1960. Instead, from early in the twentieth century, and in some cases before then, it was used as an adhesive in wood glues and paper coating, and in paints, fibres, plastics and leather finishing. The introduction of coffee whiteners and whipped toppings, in particular, by the food industry in the USA during the 1960s played a significant part in the establishment of casein products in foods. These two product groups were based on vegetable fat and contained casein in a water-soluble form (usually sodium caseinate), together with carbohydrate, emulsifiers and stabilizers. They were promoted as 'nondairy' foods (as casein was *derived* from milk, it was not considered to be a dairy product). Nondairy coffee whiteners and whipped toppings were thus presented as alternatives to the traditional dairy products of milk, cream and whipping cream, and offered advantages of lower price (because the raw materials from which they were made were cheaper than the domestic milk solids they were replacing), convenience and shelf stability (several of the products were sold in powder form). Other non-dairy products followed, many of them containing casein, e.g. so-called imitation milks, imitation cheese and salad dressings. Food supplements and dietary products were also produced and a number of these were based on casein. A variety of such products is shown in Plate 12. This article reviews the use and function of casein products in food.

The colour plate section for this article appears between p. 556 and p. 557.

General

The main applications of casein products in foods, together with their functions in such foods, are shown in Table 1. As a high-quality protein, casein can provide nutrition in foods but this is often not the main reason for its use. It is frequently incorporated into food products for its ability to impart so-called 'functional' properties of whipping, foaming, fat emulsification, water binding and thickening. Consequently, casein can have a significant effect on the texture or consistency of a food.

Animal and Pet Foods

Extensive nutritional feeding trials for ruminants were undertaken in the late 1960s and 1970s to determine the effect – on milk production and wool growth respectively – of feeding 'protected' casein to cows and to sheep. The casein was protected by reaction with formaldehyde, which prevented it from being broken down by the rumen microflora. It was able to pass undigested to the abomasum where the acidic conditions were able to promote digestion of the casein. These studies were also extended to determine how the feeding

Table 1. Use and function of casein products in foods

Application	Principal functions
Animal and pet foods	Nutrition, binder for moisture and fat
Bakery products	Nutrition, texture, water binding
Beverages, including soups	Emulsifier, stabilizer, nutrition
Coffee whiteners and creamers	Resistance to feathering, emulsifier
Confectionery	Nutrition, texture
Cultured products	Stabilizer, emulsifier, consistency, nutrition
Extruded snack foods	Texture
High-fat powders and shortenings	Emulsifier, whipping
Ice cream, mousse and desserts	Whipping, foaming, emulsifier
Imitation cheese and other cheeselike products	Texture, emulsifier
Infant foods	Nutrition
Instant breakfasts and dietary preparations	Nutrition
Meat products	Emulsifier, water binding
Pasta	Nutrition, texture
Pharmaceuticals	Nutrition, therapeutic
Spreads	Texture, stabilizer
Whipped toppings	Stabilizer, emulsifier

of polyunsaturated oils, encapsulated in formalin-treated caseins, to ruminants affects the quantity of polyunsaturated fat in meat and milk.

Casein (generally in the form of sodium caseinate) may be used as a nutritional supplement in pet foods and calf milk replacers, and it has also been reported as an ingredient in fish food.

Bakery Applications and Extruded Snack Foods

The water-binding properties of casein (as well as nutrition) are important in bakery applications where this product may be used. Soluble forms of casein (such as caseinates) tend to bind too much water and may make the food too sticky or 'doughy'. Accordingly, insoluble or partly soluble casein products are used more often, because these have less water binding than the fully soluble caseinates. Some bakery products that have been made with casein include doughnuts, biscuits, waffles, cake mixes and bread. The purposes of using casein products in extruded (high-protein) snack foods are to produce the required texture and for nutritional fortification. *See* Cakes, Methods of Manufacture

Beverages

Imitation Milks

In the USA, so-called 'filled milk', which contains vegetable fat and skim milk solids, has been sold for many years. In the late 1960s and 1970s a new class of milk – 'imitation milk' – appeared on the market. This contained vegetable fat and various other ingredients, including protein as sodium or potassium caseinate or from soy beans, and a carbohydrate source such as corn syrup solids. Artificial milks were also reported in the UK and the USSR. The lower cost of the ingredients and the absence of lactose (for which some people show intolerance) were no doubt significant factors in the establishment of such products. However, concerns were voiced over the generally lower nutritional quality (e.g. lack of vitamins and minerals and, sometimes, lower protein content) and often poorer flavour compared with 'normal' cows' milk. Casein products have also been used to fortify fresh milk, though this has occurred in Europe rather than in North America. *See* Milk, Dietary Importance; Recombined and Filled Milks

Cream Liqueurs

Casein, in the form of sodium caseinate, has found application recently in cream liqueurs, especially in the UK and the Irish Republic, where they have been, apparently, one of the fastest growing markets for cream. Other ingredients include sugar, alcohol and trisodium citrate. In this application, the sodium caseinate acts mainly as an emulsifier. *See* Liqueurs, Cream Liqueurs

Soups

When casein products are used in soups, their purpose may be for nutrition (e.g. as calcium caseinate) or for increasing the consistency or viscosity of the mixture (possibly in the form of sodium caseinate). Occasionally, hydrolysates of casein products may be used in soups and gravies for flavour enhancement.

Coffee Whiteners and Creamers

As shown in Table 1, the main functions of casein (as sodium caseinate) in coffee whiteners are to provide emulsification and to promote resistance to 'feathering'. It has been claimed that sodium caseinate (or other protein) also imparts body, provides some whitening (though this is mainly due to the fat) and improves flavour. Although both liquid and dry (powdered) coffee whiteners have been produced, the most popular by far appear to be the latter because, as mentioned in the introduction to this article, they have the advantages of being shelf stable and convenient to use. In addition, the low price of the major ingredients (vegetable fat and carbohydrate, usually as corn syrup solids) compared with that of milk solids makes coffee whitener an attractive alternative to milk or cream.

Confectionery

Casein products are used much less in confectionery than are other milk products (e.g. skim milk powder, whole milk powder and sweetened condensed milk). Nevertheless, their use has been described in toffees, caramels and fudges, where they can form a firm, chewy body, and in marshmallow and nougat to produce heat-stable whips and foams. Casein products have also been used to produce high-protein chocolate snacks and confectionery sticks or bars.

Cultured Products

In the manufacture of yoghurt, casein products have been incorporated for protein enrichment, and improvement in consistency and stability; they give less syneresis than standard yoghurt products. *See* Yoghurt, The Product and its Manufacture

Imitation sour cream products have been produced from vegetable fat, sodium caseinate and other ingredients. The purposes of adding sodium caseinate to these are to act as a stabilizer, to increase the consistency and to emulsify the fat – functions that sodium caseinate performs in mayonnaise as well. Although some publications have claimed nutritional fortification as a reason for incorporating casein products in cultured milk products, this does not seem to be as significant as the 'functional' properties mentioned earlier.

High-fat Powders and Shortenings

Sodium caseinate has been used to encapsulate and emulsify the fat in powders with a very high (> 70%) fat content. Such powders, which remain relatively free-flowing at high temperatures and are not usually greasy, can be used as shortening in baking or cooking. Whipping fats and whipping creams (fat content 30–65%) have been produced successfully for use as base products in instant desserts and whipped toppings. *See* Fats, Uses in the Food Industry

Ice Cream, Mousse and Desserts

The incorporation of casein products in ice cream has not been commercially extensive, generally because of various legal restrictions. Several ice-cream substitutes, however, did appear in the USA in the 1960s (e.g. 'Mellorine') and some of these products had casein (usually as sodium caseinate) incorporated in their formulations. Sodium caseinate functions in ice cream and frozen desserts as a stabilizer, improves the whipping properties of the mix and imparts 'body'. Other properties of sodium caseinate that are important in these products include emulsification, foam stability and film formation.

Imitation Cheese and other Cheeselike Products

Although casein has been used as an extender and texture modifier in processed cheese, and even to increase the yield of cheese from cheese milk (e.g. in Europe), probably the most significant use of casein in cheese products has been in the production of so-called 'imitation' or synthetic cheese. This product, similar in properties to processed cheese, is made from water, casein (e.g. acid casein, rennet casein, or sodium or calcium caseinate), vegetable fat, stabilizers and emulsifiers. The food industry in the USA was first to develop imitation cheese, in the early 1970s, and the quantity produced grew to a maximum of about 5% of the total

cheese sales in the USA. It found its application as a cheaper alternative to natural cheese, particularly in fast-food outlets, in frozen pizza and hamburgers, for instance. The main function of the casein product in this use is to provide the required body and texture, with emulsification of fat, as well as the melting properties of the finished cheese in pizza. Although the use of imitation cheese in the UK and Japan has been mentioned, its main area of commercial significance is in the USA. *See* Cheeses, Processed Cheese

Infant Foods

The use of casein products in infant foods is not widespread. Many infants are fed on cows' milk preparations, which contain a much higher ratio of casein to whey protein than is found in human milk. Therefore the aim is generally to reduce the ratio of casein to whey protein, e.g. by adding whey powder. *See* Infant Foods, Milk Formulas

A number of specialized infant feeding preparations have, however, been developed from casein hydrolysates. Thus Lofenalac® (manufactured by Mead Johnson), which is a casein hydrolysate from which 95% of the phenylalanine has been removed, has been used in feeding infants suffering from phenylketonuria. Several hypoallergenic formulas are available commercially, and these may be employed in treating infants who show allergy to whole-milk protein.

Casein products may be used in some circumstances for nutritional fortification of beverages and foods for infants and children.

Instant Breakfasts and Dietary Preparations

So-called instant breakfast formulations were introduced to the US market in the 1960s and 1970s, and subsequently spread to other countries. These usually consisted of skim milk powder, sucrose, sodium caseinate, vitamins and minerals, and were sold in different flavours. They were intended to be mixed with milk (one sachet per glass) to provide a 'fast breakfast' with adequate nutrition. *See* Breakfast – Role in the Diet

As a high-quality protein (casein has been used as a reference protein for many years in trials to determine the nutritional quality of proteins by testing for PER, or protein efficiency ratio), casein is used in many nutritional and dietary products that are sold in pharmacies, health food shops and even in supermarkets. These preparations may be for people who are, or have been, ill or debilitated, or even for those wishing to improve their sporting prowess. Studies in the last-named area (in sports medicine) have claimed improved performance from weightlifters and swimmers who had included a milk protein supplement in their diet during training.

Meat Products

Comminuted Meats

The reason for using casein products (usually as sodium caseinate) in comminuted meat products such as sausages and mincemeat is to emulsify fat, bind water and generally improve consistency. Sometimes, milk protein may be added for nutritional purposes. The use of casein in meat products is strictly controlled by legislation in most countries and the quantity that may be added is generally less than 5% of the weight of the meat. One estimate suggests that the potential world market for the use of high-protein milk products in processed meats is about 100 000 t. *See* Meat, Sausages and Comminuted Products

Textured Protein

Meat analogues (with a texture resembling the fibrous nature of meat muscle) have been prepared from casein, either using a spinning technique (similar to methods used for producing textile fibres in the 1930s, in which a protein solution is forced through spinnerets into a coagulating bath) or by production of chewy, meatlike gels. The general disadvantage of using casein in this form is that when the fibres are heated in a moist environment they tend to melt together and lose the individual fibrous structure – which is why casein readily forms a smooth plastic or molten mass in the production of (processed) cheese or casein plastic for buttons.

Pasta

Where casein is used in pasta products, it is mainly to enhance their nutritional quality because the high lysine content of the casein complements the low lysine- and high sulphur-containing amino acids of wheat and other vegetable proteins present in such products. In some cases, casein plays an important part in forming a suitable texture matrix for the pasta product. Thus casein products have been reportedly used in macaroni, spaghetti, rice and noodles. *See* Pasta and Macaroni, Methods of Manufacture

Pharmaceuticals

Various casein preparations have been used in a range of pharmaceutical applications. These include casein hydrolysates for intravenous nutrition in intestinal disorders, veterinary medicine and disorders involving protein metabolism. Some preparations of casein have been used for feeding patients following surgery, as a therapeutic agent in dressing wounds, in cosmetics, in toothpaste for inhibition of dental caries, and in hair shampoos. The potential for producing specific drugs, such as opiates, from casein has been described, and other extracts from casein have been claimed as being suitable for treatment of arthrosis (pain in a joint) and gastric ulcers, for enhancement of calcium and iron absorption, and to augment immunity.

Spreads

With the concerns about the effects of consumption of fats and cholesterol on coronary heart disease, which have been given considerable publicity, particularly in the West, since the 1960s, there has tended to be a decline in the consumption of 'standard' butter and margarine (the so-called 'yellow fats'), especially in Europe. Lower fat spreads have been introduced to complement or replace the traditional fats and, in some of these products, casein (usually in the form of sodium caseinate) has been used to stabilize the water phase and to improve the texture of the product. In addition, casein has been used in some (processed) cheese spreads, presumably for similar (functional) reasons.

Whipped Toppings

As described in the introduction to this article, whipped toppings which contained vegetable fat, water and sodium caseinate (together with other ingredients) appeared in the USA in the 1960s as specific competitors for whipping cream. In this application, sodium caseinate is used in forming a film to trap aerating gases. It also functions in fat encapsulation, as a bodying agent and as a stabilizer. Such products are now manufactured in other countries, including the UK, Italy, Israel and Japan.

Conclusion

In the majority of the applications described above, where casein is used to provide a specific functional or physical effect, it is incorporated in the food in relatively small quantities, i.e. generally below 10% by weight of the product. Unlike other dairy products, such as milk and milk powder, butter and cheese, it is not consumed as a food *per se*. However, when it is used for nutrition, it may indeed represent a significant proportion of the total weight of the food. In pharmaceutical and medical applications, there are some indications that derivatives of casein may be important therapeutic agents in the future.

Uses in the Food Industry

Bibliography

Centre National du Commerce Extérieur (1970) *The United States Market for Edible Caseins and Caseinates*. Paris: Centre National du Commerce Extérieur.

Lim DM (1980) *Functional Properties of Milk Proteins with Particular Reference to Confectionery Products*, Scientific and Technical Survey No. RA120. Leatherhead, Surrey: British Food Manufacturing Industries Research Association.

Manson W (1980) The use of milk and milk constituents in pharmaceutical preparations. *Factors Affecting the Yields and Contents of Milk Constituents of Commercial Importance*. International Dairy Federation Bulletin, Document 125, pp 60–65. Brussels: International Dairy Federation.

Muller LL (1971) Manufacture and uses of casein and co-precipitate, *Dairy Science Abstracts* 33: 659–674.

Schuette HA (1939) Alimentary and medicinal uses of casein. In: Sutermeister E and Browne FL (eds) *Casein and Its Industrial Applications*, pp 366–390. New York: Reinhold Publishing Corporation.

Southward CR (1986) Utilisation of milk components: casein. In: Robinson RK (ed) *Modern Dairy Technology*, vol. 1, pp 317–368. London: Elsevier Applied Science Publishers.

Southward CR (1989) Uses of casein and caseinates. In: Fox PF (ed), *Developments in Dairy Chemistry*, vol. 4, pp 173–244. London: Elsevier Applied Science Publishers.

Southward CR and Walker NJ (1982) Casein, caseinates and milk protein co-precipitates In: Wolff IA (ed), *CRC Handbook of Processing and Utilization in Agriculture*, vol. I, pp 445–552. Boca Raton, Florida: CRC Press.

Webb BH (1970) Miscellaneous products. In: Webb BH and Whittier EO (eds) *Byproducts from Milk*, pp 285–330. Westport, Connecticut: AVI Publishing.

C.R. Southward
New Zealand Dairy Research Institute, Palmerston North, New Zealand

CASHEW NUTS AND CASHEW APPLES*

The cashew is one of the two costliest nuts marketed in quantity worldwide. Formerly second to the macadamia nut in retail value, it is now more expensive because of short supply. Few people in the Northern Hemisphere question why the cashew nut is never sold in the shell as peanuts, pecans, walnuts and almonds often are. There is a good reason for this. The cashew, by nature, is much more complex than other nuts and a technical explanation of its processing is required.

Description

The cashew tree, *Anacardium occidentale*, of the family Anacardiaceae, is short-trunked, up to 13 m high and normally with a very broad crown, although it is often stunted and bushy on coasts. There is an enormous, very old, wild cashew tree in Natal, Brazil, that covers 0·75 ha and is a great tourist attraction. Its leathery, evergreen leaves are clustered at the branch tips. The small, yellow-and-red flowers are borne in open sprays. The true fruit of the tree is the kidney-shaped, hard-shelled nut that is at first green, later turning an ashy brown; it grows to 3 cm or more in length and develops at the tip of a fleshy stalk. As the 'nut' matures, the stalk inflates to form a showy, pear-shaped, smooth-skinned, succulent, juicy pseudofruit (false fruit), which is bright-red, orange, yellow, or two-tone; usually viewed, and utilized, as a fruit (Fig. 1). The weight of the expanded pseudofruit causes the nut to fall to the ground at its peak of maturity. A caustic oil in the honeycomblike cells within the double-layered shell of the 'nut' protects it from being destroyed by foragers that feed on the 'apple'. However, the oil seriously complicates the processing of the 'nut' and extraction of its kernel for food use.

Origin and Distribution

The cashew tree is native from southern Mexico to Peru, Brazil, and the West Indies. Wild stands extend along the coast of Brazil from Pará to Rio de Janeiro, and the nut and apple have always been of importance to the indigenous people. The cashew was one of the first tropical American fruit trees to be introduced by early Portuguese and Spanish voyagers into the tropics of the Old World. In the sixteenth century the Portuguese planted it, especially on the west coast of India and the east coast of Mozambique, in order to halt soil erosion and, in time, it formed extensive forests.

The tree soon became commonly cultivated and naturalized at low altitudes in East, Central and West Africa, Southeast Asia, Ceylon, Malaysia, the Philippines, Mauritius and the Seychelles. In addition, it has been planted around villages in most of the Pacific Islands including Hawaii, and is occasionally grown in dooryards in southern Florida.

---

* The colour plate section for this article appears between p. 556 and p. 557.

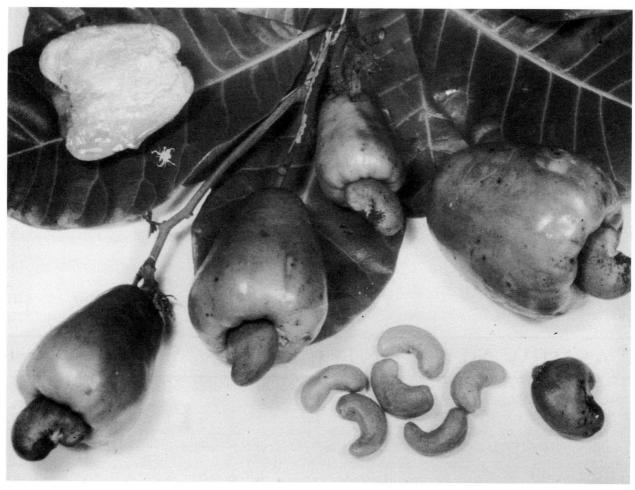

Fig. 1 The cashew nut, shaped like a boxing glove, develops at the tip of a fleshy, juicy, fruitlike stalk (peduncle), called 'cashew apple', which enlarges as the nut matures, becomes red, orange, yellow, or two-tone, and is eaten raw or preserved.

The name 'cashew' is derived from the Brazilian *acaju*, usually abbreviated to *caju*. In the Orinoco region, the tree is known as *pauji*. In all the Spanish-speaking countries of Latin America and the Caribbean area, the common name is *marañon*, except in Venezuela where it is called *merey*. In French it is *cajou* or *acajou*.

Climate and Soil

The tree requires a tropical or subtropical climate. It is highly sensitive to frost when young, but later is able to withstand brief cold spells. It is well adapted to sandy soil, intolerant of heavy clay, and is drought and salt tolerant, succeeding on land too poor for most other crops. It thrives from sea level to an altitude of 1000 m.

Commercial Development

India pioneered the domestication and commercialization of the cashew and, for a long time, augmented her

supply by importing raw nuts from Mozambique. The 1950s saw large-scale planting of cashew trees in Africa, India and Brazil. In northeastern Brazil there was first a private plantation of about 1500 ha. Then, in 1957, a programme was begun to plant a million trees in the State of Ceará, the Government supplying the seeds and a bonus for each tree set out in plots of 100 or more. From 1957 to 1972, a company in Pacajus set out 2000 ha. Another surge of government-stimulated plantings totalled nearly 136 000 ha by 1972, mostly in Ceará. Later, 18 000 ha were developed in Rio Grande do Norte. By 1986, more than 40 000 ha of cashew had been added in reforestation programmes in Ceará, Piaui, Rio Grande do Norte, and Bahia.

There have been sporadic attempts to develop cashew industries in Venezuela, Colombia, Peru, Guatemala, Belize and Jamaica. Some have been moderately successful. The primary problem is that cashew trees are still mainly grown from seed and there is great variation in yield, and great variability in the form and size of the nuts from seedling trees (Fig. 2). The nuts may range

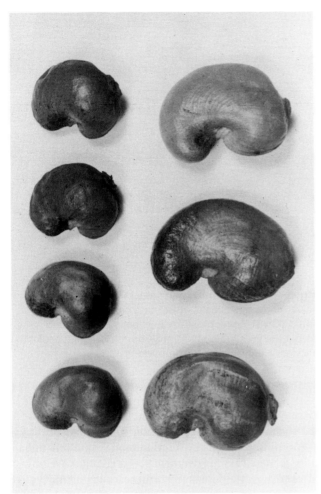

Fig. 2 Cashew nuts range from 2·5 to 5 cm in length and this variability, together with the odd shape, contributes to the difficulties of opening them mechanically. They are never sold in the shell.

from 3 to 32 g in weight and the apples (mostly orange or yellow) from 15 to 650 g. Trees bearing small nuts tend to produce heavily, while trees with large nuts and apples are less productive and may bear in alternate years.

Much research in Mozambique and India has been devoted to techniques of vegetative propagation (by cuttings, grafting, budding, or air layering) to achieve uniformity, but it is still not widely practised, mainly because of the costs involved. India has accomplished much in rejuvenation of old groves by top-working beheaded, unproductive, trees. Side-veneer grafting has been recommended in Venezuela. In Trinidad and India air-layered trees have poor form and tend to blow over in the wind. Once a method of propagation has been adopted, there must be a search for the best types to be grown. An experimental planting of grafted trees was initiated in Ceará but did not prosper because of a prolonged drought. In 1980, a selected clone of a 'dwarf' cashew was grafted onto *Anacardium microcarpum* and

the 40 trees set out fruited early and were highly drought-resistant. This trial encouraged experiments with other rootstocks and selection of high-quality clones, but low yields have caused such work to languish. There are still no commercial orchards of selected, vegetatively propagated trees.

Varieties

Generally, named varieties have been distinguished merely by colour and size of the apple; as, the 'Vermelho' (yellow) and 'Amarello Gigante' (large yellow) of Brazil, and the 'Marañon Amarillo' (yellow) and 'Marañon Rosado' (red) of Colombia. Natural hybrids in Colombia have been named 'La Gigante (huge) del Rio Magdelena', 'La Larga (long) de Nazareth', and 'La Pequeña (small) del Meta'. Usually the nut and apple are larger in the yellow forms than in the red, and the apple is less astringent. One name pertaining not to the apple but to the nut is the 'Jumbo' grown by the late Edward B Smith, Crescent Estate, Trinidad, who has supplied air layers to people from South America wishing to establish this large-seeded type in their countries.

In evaluating cashew trees, preference should be given to a cashew tree of slender, compact form because the cashew needs light to flower and fruit and bears only on its outer circumference. The interior of a broad-spreading tree is devoid of foliage and fruit. Likewise, if cashew trees are planted too close together, the branches that overlap or shade each other will be nonbearing and may die back. From an experimental plantation of compact trees, the grower should select those that produce a high yield of large nuts and multiply them vegetatively, rather than increasing labour costs by simply planting more and more seedling trees with yields varying from 5 to 100 kg per tree. There is variation also in the colour of the young leaves of cashew trees. On some, the new shoots at the branch tips are purplish-red, on others, more or less yellow. The yellow leaves are heavily attacked by leaf-eating insects while the red, being richer in phenolic compounds, are naturally insect-resistant.

Diseases and Pests

In humid atmospheres and in seasons of excessive rainfall, cashew trees are subject to attack by the fungus *Colletotrichum gloeosporioides*, which causes anthracnose, a disease affecting the foliage, especially young shoots, the twigs, flowers, the apple, and the developing nut. A parasitic fungus, *Oidium anarcardii*, appears on the leaves, shoots and flowers when there are periods of alternating sun and rain. They become coated with a powdery white substance and this is followed by blackening, shrivelling and shedding. The nut may be ruined by the fungus, *Nematospora* sp., which invades it through minute perforations caused by sucking insects. A large wasp sucks the juice from immature apples, causing them to shrivel and blacken while the nut is still green. Yellow, red-banded thrips (*Selenothrips rubrocinctus* Giard) often infest the foliage. Cashew apples are commonly eaten by birds, bats, monkeys and squirrels.

Harvesting and Drying

Harvesting of cashew nuts is extremely labour-intensive. The entire crop does not ripen at one time, and harvesting may extend over a period of 40 to 75 days. The nuts ideally should be allowed to fall (with the apple attached) when perfectly mature. Some people unwisely shake the branches to bring them down or knock them off with a pole. This results in slightly immature nuts of high moisture content being mixed with partly dried mature nuts and makes it impossible to assure uniform drying, thereby adversely affecting all subsequent steps in processing. In Brazil, cashews are plucked from the tree only if perfect apples are desired for dessert use. If allowed to fall, the apple will remain in good condition on the ground for 2–3 days. If it is not to be utilized, it is twisted off and left on the ground for cattle or pigs to consume. If it is wanted for preserving, it is salvaged and transported to a packing plant. The nuts are conveyed separately to be spread out in the sun and dried, with constant raking, and then stored if they are not to be immediately shelled. Thoroughly dried nuts can be stored for 1 or 2 years.

Processing

In Latin America and the West Indies there have been crude pre-cracking practices such as boiling the nuts in steel barrels, simply drying them in the sun for 2 or 3 days, or sweating them in cement bins for several months. There was much loss because many nuts were found to be infested with insects or fungi on opening. In some cases the nuts were cut open by machete wielders with their hands wrapped in layers of plastic. The half-kernels were then picked out and sent to local clubs or bars, but these nuts were too contaminated with the cashew nut shell liquid (CNSL) to be fit for consumption (Fig. 3).

Sanitary processing of cashews in the past was best performed in India by roasting the nuts in shallow pans over open fires to expel the caustic CNSL, some of which was caught in jars below for various local uses. Then they rubbed the nuts with sand or ashes before hand-shelling, at which the Indian female workers were especially adept. But the fumes from the roasting were

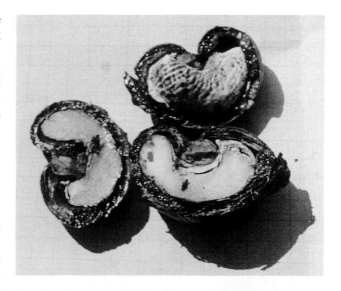

Fig. 3   Cut open with a machete, these cashew nut halves show the caustic, glistening cashew nut shell liquid (CNSL) which is usually expelled by roasting before the nuts are opened, the kernel extracted, peeled, and reroasted before consumption.

extremely irritating to eyes, nose, throat and skin, and the shellers frequently had to dip their hands in lime, ash, or linseed or castor oil to minimize skin inflammation. A merciful improvement was a change to roasting in rotating cylinders over furnaces with chimneys to carry off the toxic fumes. The next advance, brought about by Mortimer Harvey, of New Jersey, who had investigated the chemistry and potential industrial uses of the shell oil, was a method of heating the nuts in baths of the oil kept at 188–194°C. This method resulted in greater recovery of higher quality oil.

Semimechanized shelling was initiated in Brazil in 1946. Dried raw nuts were first steamed to moisten the shells and then fed into a device, operated by hand and footpedal simultaneously, which cut the shell into two halves, leaving the kernel whole or cut in half. Facing the cutter, a seated operator pries the kernel loose from the cut shells if it adheres. This system is still used in Ceará for shelling very large nuts.

When East African countries achieved independence from colonial governments, they wanted to cease exporting their raw cashews to India in order to gain more revenue by processing the nuts themselves. A simple, raw-cashew opening-machine was invented by a mining engineer in Tanzania in 1960. The operator protected his hands with barrier cream. There followed the development of complete factory installations of cashew-shelling equipment in Italy, France and Germany. Mozambique obtained its first full-scale factory in 1964 and 2 years later set a world record in cashew production; most of the crop went to India for shelling, the rest (26 000 t) of the locally shelled kernels were exported to the USA, West Germany and South Africa.

The various systems of cracking by pressure, centrifugal cracking, and cutting or sawing were evaluated by the Tropical Products Institute of London (now the Natural Products Institute), and the Sturtevants Engineering Company began producing and exporting the centrifugal shelling equipment in 1970. This system is now used by Brazil Oiticica, and modified versions are used in northeastern Brazil. An Italian factory installation of a series of machines, designed by the Instituto Agronomico per l'Oltremare, involves 15 steps. The dried nuts are cleaned, roughly sorted according to size, wetted for several days to the desired moisture content, roasted in CNSL, centrifuged to eliminate any oil residue, cooled, and mechanically calibrated to separate eight sizes. The nuts are then machine cut, and the shell separated from the kernel and removed by pneumatic tubes for use as a fuel. The kernels are dried for 48 h in the sun or in ovens until the testa wrinkles and is removed mechanically. The kernels are rehumidified to resist breaking; they are then sorted into wholes and pieces. Lastly, kernels that still having clinging testa must be hand-peeled. Japanese processors freeze the nuts instead of roasting them before shelling.

However, none of these or other factory systems have given ideal results, mainly because of the variability of the raw material. There is a great need for a portable, simple cashew sheller that can take dehydrated, raw nuts of any size, splitting them without contamination of the kernel. The shells would be sent to facilities for total extraction of the oil for industrial purposes, and the split kernels of 'Jumbo' cashews should not be inferior to whole kernels from smaller nuts. Such shelling has been achieved experimentally with explosive decompression, but further refinement of the method is needed.

The latest development in India is a cashew kernel drier, electronically controlled, with timer and alarm to avoid scorching, and adjustable dampers for air-inflow; the drier turns out higher quality kernels in 60–90 min.

Economic Status

In the past, the cashew ranked as India's second dollar earner. After mechanization, India found that the total crop of her cashew plantations could not keep her big factories busy, the productivity of the trees having declined after they reached 35 years of age. In Kerala, the leading growing area, cashew orchards have been cut down and replaced by more profitable rubber plantations. From 1980 to 1987, the World Bank assisted India in a Cashew Development Project to improve old plantations and establish new ones. In 1990, adverse weather conditions in India and other major cashew areas seriously affected the supply of cashews for export.

Indian production was reduced by 20–25%, causing a sharp increase in prices. Nevertheless, the demand for cashew kernels has increased, especially with the opening of markets in Eastern Europe. In 1989, world export of cashew kernels from India, Brazil, Mozambique, Kenya, Tanzania, and other areas, amounted to 90 000 t. If horticultural improvement could be brought up to the level of cashew engineering, this figure could be doubled or tripled, and cashews would be less expensive and more widely enjoyed.

Inspection, Grading and Packing

Before export, cashew kernels go through rigid inspection systems, are classified according to grade – Wholes, Butts, Splits, Large and Small pieces and Baby Bits, also White, Scorched and Dessert – and are carefully vacuum packed in 11·3 kg-capacity metal containers, two to a crate. They are then held in cold storage at temperatures below 9°C. For retail sale, cashew kernels are usually reroasted in olive, peanut or other oil, an adhesive and salt are applied and the kernels are packed in glass jars or cans. In recent years, many are dry roasted without salt. High grades have a minimum of split or broken kernels. Lower grades are utilized mainly by the bakery or confectionery industries. They are familiar ingredients in cookies, chocolate bars and other products, and are made into cashew butter.

Cashew Apple

Because of the difficulty of cracking cashew nuts, many Latin Americans have habitually discarded the nut and consumed the 'cashew apple' or, in Spanish, *manzana del marañon*, large heaps of which are seen on native markets at the height of the season. As it is fibrous, the apple is massaged and the juice is squeezed into the mouth as a thirst-quencher, especially out in the countryside. Inferior types that are still astringent when ripe are eaten with salt so that they will not irritate the throat. In the kitchen, cashew apples may be sliced and stewed or used to make juice, fruit soup, jam, jelly, paste, or chutney. The best cashew apples are preserved whole in syrup in glass jars. The less perfect are candied – cooked thoroughly in heavy syrup until well wrinkled, and then dried and sometimes rolled in granulated sugar. This is an excellent product resembling candied figs but it is, of course, seedless.

In India, the Central Food Technological Research Institute at Mysore has found that the astringency and acidity of cashew apple juice, due to 35% tannin content and 3% of an oily substance, can be eliminated by pressure steaming for 5–15 min and thorough washing. Then the juice is mechanically extracted. In the

Table 1. Food value of Cashew nuts, oil roasted and dry roasted

Nutrients and units[a]	Mean amount per kg, edible portion	
	Oil roasted	Dry roasted
Proximate		
Water (g)	39·1	17·0
Food energy (kcal)	5760	5740
(kJ)	24 090	24 020
Protein (N × 5·30) (g)	161·5	153·1
Total lipid (fat) (g)	482·1	463·5
Carbohydrate, total (g)	285·2	326·9
Fibre (g)	12·7	7·0
Ash (g)	32·1	39·5
Minerals (mg)		
Calcium	410	450
Iron	41·0	60·0
Magnesium	2550	2600
Phosphorus	4260	4900
Potassium	5300	5650
Sodium[b]	170	160
Zinc	47·5	56·0
Copper	21·7	22·2
Manganese	8·07	—
Vitamins[c]		
Ascorbic acid (mg)	0·0	0·0
Thiamin (mg)	4·24	2·00
Riboflavin (mg)	1·75	2·00
Niacin (mg)	18·00	14·00
Pantothenic acid (mg)	11·90	12·17
Vitamin B_6 (mg)	2·50	2·56
Folacin (μg)	677·0	692·0
Vitamin B_{12} (μg)	0	0
Vitamin A (RE)	0	0
(iu)	0	0
Lipids (g)		
Fatty acids		
Saturated, total	95·26	91·57
4:0	—	—
6:0	—	—
8:0	1·37	1·32
10:0	1·37	1·32
12:0	8·16	7·84
14:0	3·61	3·47
16:0	45·26	43·51
18:0	30·91	29·72
Monounsaturated, total	284·15	273·17
16:1	3·31	3·18
18:1	278·86	268·08
20:1	1·44	1·39
22:1	—	—

Continued

Table 1. *Continued.*

Nutrients and units[a]	Mean amount per kg, edible portion	
	Oil roasted	Dry roasted
Lipids (g)		
Fatty acids		
Polyunsaturated, total	81·52	78·36
18:2	79·68	76·60
18:3	1·67	1·61
18:4	—	—
20:4	—	—
20:5	—	—
22:5	—	—
22:6	0	—
Cholesterol	—	0
Phytosterols	—	1·58
Amino acids (g)		
Tryptophan	2·50	2·37
Threonine	6·25	5·92
Isoleucine	7·71	7·31
Leucine	13·56	12·85
Lysine	8·62	8·17
Methionine	2·89	2·74
Cystine	2·99	2·83
Phenylalanine	8·35	7·91
Tyrosine	5·18	4·91
Valine	10·97	10·40
Arginine	18·37	17·41
Histidine	4·20	3·99
Alanine	7·40	7·02
Aspartic acid	15·87	15·05
Glutamic acid	38·24	36·24
Glycine	8·47	8·03
Proline	7·28	6·90
Serine	8·96	8·49

[a] 28 g=approximately 14 large, 18 medium, or 26 small kernels.
[b] Value based on data for product without added salt. Oil-roasted product with added salt contains 626 mg sodium per 100 g, dry-roasted contains 640 mg of sodium per 100 g.
[c] α-Tocopherol=0·57 mg per 100 g of dry-roasted product.
McCarthy MA and Matthews RH (1984) *Composition of Foods: Nut and Seed Products (Raw, Processed, Prepared)*. Agriculture Handbook No. 8–12. US Department of Agriculture.
One retinol equivalent (RE)=6 μg beta-carotene or 10 international units (iu) vitamin A activity from beta-carotene

Philippines, the Bureau of Plant Industry, Manila, designed a cashew-apple-crushing machine for this purpose. To free the juice of some other undesirable elements, casein, gelatin, pectin or lime juice may be added before straining or centrifuging. After the addition of sugar and citric acid to arrive at 15° Brix and 4% acidity, the juice is boiled for 1 min and then bottled or canned, alone or with other fruit juices.

In Brazil, it is estimated that less than 10% of the total cashew apple crop is processed, though the juice is

Table 2. Food value of cashew apple, raw caju, *Anacardium occidentale* L.

Nutrients and units	Mean amount per kg, edible portion
Nutrients and minerals (g)	
Food energy (kcal)	460·0
Moisture	871·0
Proteins	8·0
Lipids	2·0
Glycides	116·0
Fibre	15·0
Ash	3·0
Calcium	0·04
Phosphorus	0·18
Iron	0·01
Vitamins (mg)	
Retinol	0·40
Vitamin B$_1$	0·30
Vitamin B$_2$	0·30
Niacin	4·0
Ascorbic acid	2190·0

Anonymous (1981) *Tabelas de Composição de Alimentos, Estudo Nacional da Despesa Familiar – Endef.* Rio de Janeiro: Secretaria de Planejamento da Presidência da República Funacao Instituto Brasileiro de Geografia e Estatística.

locally popular and, with suspended pulp or clear, it is pasteurized, preservatives are added, and it is bottled and exported. The unclarified juice may be concentrated and bottled as nectar, or made available as frozen concentrate. Cashew apple juice is also made into vinegar. In Cuba, Costa Rica and the Philippines, and formerly in Brazil, it has been fermented into wine. Cashew apple brandy is subject to government control in East Africa and Goa. In the late nineteenth century, in Mozambique, the cashew was denounced as a source of vice and ruin because of the highly intoxicating liquor distilled from the apple. Cultivation of the tree was banned for a while; later a tax was imposed on plantations as a possible deterrent.

Food Value of Cashew Nut and Cashew Apple

See Tables 1 and 2. *See* individual nutrients.

Cashew Nut Shell Liquid

This toxic oil is highly heat- and friction-resistant and is valuable for many industrial uses. When it was first used in aircraft paint-stripping products, mechanics suffered skin reactions. Mortimer Harvey promptly patented processes of detoxification and its uses have multiplied. It has been standard material for automobile clutch facings and brake linings and in insulation for electrical tools. It is incorporated into marine paints, water-resistant plywood, resins utilized in laminating, varnishes, floor tiles, cold-setting cements, moulding powders for plastics, and many other products. In addition, the testa, which is removed from cashew kernels, has a high level of condensed tannin (as much as 25%) and the extract has been used for tanning leather.

Bibliography

Agnoloni M and Guiliani F (1977) *Cashew Cultivation.* Florence, Italy: Instituto Agronomico per l'Oltremare, Ministry of Foreign Affairs.
Cashew Export Promotion Council of India (1990) World Bank assisted cashew development scheme. *Indian Cashew Journal* 10 (3): 18–20.
Khan MM, Hegde M, Mallik B, Hiremath IG, Hanamashetti SI, Madhava Rao VN and Krishnamurthy K (1987) Rejuvenation of old cashew trees by top-working. *Indian Cashew Journal* 17 (3): 9–25.
Morton JF (1967) Marañon! Necesidad urgente de un programa para la seleccion de variedades. *La Hacienda* 62 (9): 38–43.
Morton JF and Venning FD (1972) Avoid failures and losses in the cultivation of the cashew. *Economic Botany* 26 (3): 245–254.
Ohler JG (1979) *Cashew.* Communication 71. Amsterdam: Department of Agricultural Research, Koninklijk Instituut voor de Tropen.
Santos Lima V de PM (ed.) (1988) *A cultura do cajueiro no Nordeste do Brasil.* Fortaleza, Brazil: Banco do Nordeste do Brasil.
Wilson RJ (1975) *The Market for Cashew-Nut Kernels and Cashew-Nut Liquid.* London: Tropical Products Institute.

Julia F. Morton.
University of Miami, Florida, USA

CASSAVA

Contents

The Nature of the Tuber[*]

The cassava plant is a highly efficient producer of carbohydrate, mainly in the form of starch. It is the fourth most important source of calories in the human diet in tropical regions of the world, and is consumed in a wide variety of forms. This article will review the origin and current distribution of the crop, the anatomy of the edible root and its chemical composition. Special emphasis will be placed on the starch component of the root and on the presence of cyanide-containing glucosides.

Cassava Production

Crop Distribution

Cassava originated in the Americas, although the exact centre of origin is disputed: northern Brazil, northern Colombia/Venezuela, Paraguay and southern Mexico have been suggested. The crop was widely grown in the Amazon basin by 2000 BC, and remains a traditional staple of many tribal groups. Cassava was taken by Spanish and Portuguese traders to Africa, India and Southeast Asia in the sixteenth and seventeenth centuries, but did not become widespread in Africa until the late nineteenth century. It is currently cultivated in almost all tropical and subtropical countries, the major producers being Thailand, Indonesia, India, Brazil, Zaire and Nigeria. Total world production in 1989 reached 149×10^6 t, of which Americas, Africa and Asia counted for 22%, 42% and 36% respectively.

Cassava has found acceptance over a diverse range of agricultural and food systems due to its tolerance of poor soil and harsh climatic conditions. Yields in excess of 10 t per ha per year are achieved with minimal inputs under conditions of acid soils (pH < 4), low rainfall (< 1000 mm per year) and nutrient deficiency. Cassava has thus gained a reputation as a food security and famine reserve crop, and as such has become especially important to small farmers living in marginal areas of the tropics. In addition, the efficiency of carbohydrate production, due to cassava's unique combination of C_3 and C_4 photosynthetic pathways, has promoted its agroindustrial use in the last 30 years, especially in Thailand, Indonesia and southern Brazil, for starch extraction and as a component of dried animal feed.

This short daylength, perennial crop can be grown from 30°N to 30°S latitude, and up to an altitude of 2000 m at the equator, where the mean annual temperature is at least 17°C in the high-altitude tropics, or 20°C in lowland areas. Established plants can withstand over 6 months of drought, but cannot tolerate prolonged flooding or saline conditions. In the humid lowland tropics, roots can be harvested after 6–7 months' growth. This increases to 18 months at higher altitudes, and 2 years in the subtropics. Propagation is by woody stem pieces called stakes. When grown in high fertility soils with good agronomic practices, up to 50 t per ha can be produced in 12 months. On a worldwide basis, the crops most frequently interplanted with cassava are maize, cowpea, sorghums and millets.

Traditional varieties tend to be of restricted agroecological range, having been selected by small farmers over many years. Many countries have introduced new varieties over the last decade, especially Thailand, Indonesia, Colombia and Nigeria. Varietal improvement has focused on yield, adaptation to environmental and biotic stresses, and recently on root quality.

The Morphology and Anatomy of the Storage Root

The cassava root is anatomically a true root, not a tuberous root. The root cannot serve for vegetative propagation. Root size and shape depend on variety and environmental conditions. Variability in size within a variety is greater than that found in other root crops. Cassava roots are generally from 15–100 cm long and 3–15 cm wide. They are cylindrical, conical or oval, with a coffee, pink or cream-coloured peel which is covered by a thin brown bark. The parenchyma is generally white, cream or yellow. Plants produce 5–10 roots weighing 0·5–2·5 kg each.

The root is composed of three distinct tissues: bark (periderm), peel and parenchyma. The parenchyma is the edible portion of the fresh root, and comprises

[*] The colour plate section for this article appears between p. 556 and p. 557.

approximately 85% of total weight. The parenchyma consists of xylem vessels radially distributed in a matrix of starch-containing cells. A central fibrous vascular bundle becomes progressively larger as the roots mature. Other fibrous bundles may develop throughout the root. The peel layer comprises sclerenchyma, cortical parenchyma and phloem, and consistutes 12% of root weight, with the periderm layer comprising another 2%.

Harvesting, Root Deterioration and Storage

Harvesting

The cassava root has no fixed period of optimum maturity: the woody plant is perennial, and starch deposition will continue for many years in most ecosystems. Harvest time is therefore determined by a combination of factors relating to yield, quality (starch content, etc.), the farmer's need to clear the field, climatic factors and market prices. Climate affects starch content, fresh root eating quality, and hence market acceptability. Roots left beyond their optimum time for the fresh market are often used for animal feed or industrial processing at a later date, giving the farmer great flexibility of harvest time.

Harvesting is almost entirely manual. Although mechanical harvesters have been developed in Brazil, Venezuela, Nigeria, and Cuba, use of these is limited and occurs primarily in southern Brazil. In most countries, cassava is planted in small plots, often on sloping terrain unsuited to mechanical operations. Manual harvesting represents one of the major production costs, along with weeding, often accounting for 30% of total cost. Ease of harvesting depends on variety, soil type and moisture content. The aerial part of the plant is frequently removed before harvesting. At harvest, roots destined for the fresh market are sorted, based on size, into commercial and noncommercial classes. For industrial processing, all roots are collected.

Deterioration

Freshly harvested cassava roots have the shortest post-harvest life of any of the major staple food crops. Roots become inedible within 24–72 h after harvest due to a rapid physiological deterioration process. This deterioration is a major constraint for industrial processing of the fresh roots, and for marketing them to distant urban centres. Deterioration is due to the rapid, *de novo*, post-harvest synthesis of simple phenolic compounds (catechins, coumarins, leucoanthocyanins) which polymerize to form blue, brown and black pigments (condensed tannins). The accumulation of the

coumarin, scopoletin, is especially rapid, reaching 80 mg per kg (dry weight) in 24 h. Scopoletin has intense blue fluorescence in UV light and can be confused with aflatoxins B_1 and B_2, which also have blue fluorescence and similar R_f values under some chromatographic systems: many reports of aflatoxins in fresh and processed cassava should therefore be treated with caution. *See* Mycotoxins, Occurrence and Determination; Phenolic Compounds

Rapid physiological deterioration is an oxidative process. Tissue dehydration, especially at sites of root mechanical damage encourages the rapid onset of this phenomenon. Care at harvest to reduce mechanical damage is beneficial. Tissue discoloration is initiated at damage sites, and rapidly spreads through the entire root, starting in the vascular system, but later spreading to parenchymal cells. Within 3 days after harvest, a ring of discoloured tissues arranged around the outer portion of the parenchyma (Plate 14) typically appears. In advanced cases, dehydrated, brown-white parenchyma tissues result. *See* Oxidation of Food Components

A secondary deterioration can follow physiological or primary deterioration 5–7 days after harvest. This is due to microbial infection of mechanically damaged tissues, and results in the same tissue discoloration with vascular streaks spreading from the infected tissues. Generalized rotting and fermentation of tissues follow.

Storage

Conditions of high temperature (30°C) and high relative humidity (85%) favour the rapid wound healing of mechanically damaged tissues (curing). Under these conditions, the physiological processes described above are localized in the vicinity of the wound itself. The cured tissues represent a barrier to further oxygen entry, thus preventing the oxidative reactions which lead to formation of condensed tannins. Encouragement of this curing process is the basis for several simple storage methods for fresh cassava.

Traditionally, cassava roots are preserved in the fresh state by reburying them in soil or moist sand. Field clamps, using straw and roots in layers below a soil-covered mound, with adequate ventilation, were developed in the 1970s. Packing roots in boxes with moist sawdust, coconut fibre or other locally available materials has also been successful. More recently, packing roots in polyethylene bags (with or without perforations) and protecting against microbial deterioration with a Thiabendazole-based fungicide of low toxicity, has been developed as a simple and effective storage technology. Treated cassava packed in 3–5 kg bags is now commercially available in Colombia and Paraguay. With all these storage methods, root quality is maintained for 2–3 weeks. Beyond this time, starch break-

Table 1. Constituents of cassava root parenchyma and peel

Constituent	Percentage of dry weight	
	Parenchyma	Peel
Dry matter (%, fresh wt.)	23–44	15–34
Starch	70–91	44–59
Total sugars	1·3–5·3	5·2–7·1
Crude fibre	3·0–5·0	5·0–15·0
Ash	1·0–2·5	2·8–4·2
Protein	1·0–6·0	7·0–14·0
Fat	0·3–1·5	1·5–2·8

Table 2. Vitamin, mineral and cyanide constituents of cassava root parenchyma and peel

Constituent	Milligrams per kilogram dry weight	
	Parenchyma	Peel
Total cyanide	30–1350	60—550
Calcium	480–920	—
Phosphorus	770–150	—
Potassium	6000–10 000	—
Iron	5–25	—
Vitamin A	0–70	—
Vitamin C	380–900	—

down to free sugars gives roots an unacceptable sweet taste. *See* Fungicides; Storage Stability, Mechanisms of Degradation

For export markets, paraffin-coating of fresh roots provides an artificial barrier to oxygen entry and hence to deterioration. Costa Rica and the Dominican Republic export paraffin-coated roots to the USA and Europe. Peeled, frozen cassava pieces are also exported from these and other countries.

No economically viable method for fresh root storage at the plant level prior to industrial processing is available. Fresh roots should be processed within 2 days of harvest to ensure acceptable quality and yield: starch extracted from deteriorated roots is light brown in colour, of poor functional quality, and the starch yield decreases by 10% for each day beyond the initial 2 days of storage. Excellent links between processing plant and cassava producers are essential to avoid deliveries of roots of unacceptable quality. The lack of a large-scale storage method for fresh cassava limits processing-plant operations to cassava harvest periods. However, in many areas, cassava can be harvested year round, especially if irrigation is available. If necessary, fresh roots can be chipped and sun-dried: the dried chips can be used for starch extraction at a later date, although starch yield and quality is lower.

Chemical Composition of the Cassava Root

The chemical composition of cassava roots is shown in Tables 1 and 2. The composition of peel and parenchyma is different: the peel has more protein, fibre, sugars and cyanide than the parenchyma, and less dry matter and starch. A wide range of values is reported in the literature for each root component. Reports of whole-root dry-matter contents vary from 20% to 40%, and between 70% and 90% of dry matter is composed of starch, with average values between 80% and 85%. Total carbohydrates, including starch, free sugars and

other cellulose or hemicellulose components, together make up over 90% of parenchyma dry weight. Protein content is uniformly low (below 2% on a fresh weight basis), as are fats and ash content. Fibre contents are more variable, and increase with plant age. Great variation in total cyanide content is also found, with parenchyma values of 30–100 mg per kg common for low-cyanide cultivars destined for direct consumption, compared with 1350 mg per kg in bitter varieties used for processing. *See* Carbohydrates, Classification and Properties; Starch, Sources and Processing

Variation in chemical composition is found between cassava varieties, and also within varieties at different plant ages, and is due to changing environmental and biotic stress factors. For example, parenchyma dry-matter content may decrease from 35% to 28% after a period of drought followed by the onset of rainfall. Under these conditions, starch is rapidly hydrolysed to free sugars, especialy sucrose, which are used by the plant to initiate regrowth of foliage. These large fluctuations in root quality over relatively short periods must be taken into account in planning harvesting times, both for direct consumption and for processing. *See* Starch, Modified Starches

Cyanide in Cassava Roots

All known *Manihot* species contain cyanide. In cassava, cyanide is synthesized in the leaf and transported to the roots, where it is partitioned between peel and parenchyma. Some 85% of the cyanide occurs as cyanoglucosides, mainly linamarin. Linamarin is broken down by the enzyme linamarase, also found in cassava tissues. In intact roots, the compartmentalization of linamarase in cell walls and linamarin in cell vacuoles prevents the formation of free cyanide. On processing, the disruption of tissues ensures that the enzyme comes into contact with its substrate, resulting in rapid production of free cyanide via an unstable cyanhydrin intermediary.

The Nature of the Tuber

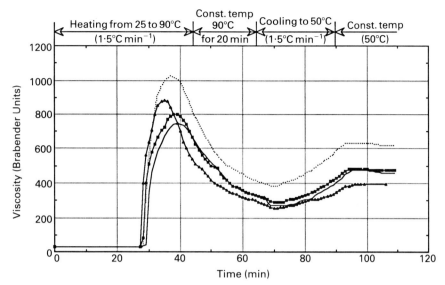

Fig. 1   Brabender viscoamylograms of starch from four cassava varieties (4% w/v paste). ──── CMC-40; ─■─ CM 523-7; ········ MCol 8; ─▲─ MCol 1684. Source: CIAT (International Centre for Tropical Agriculture), Cali, Columbia.

Cassava varieties differ in their total cyanide content, and although variation in content is continuous, two distinct types can be discerned in many regions of the world: low- and high-cyanide varieties. Low-cyanide varieties are often called sweet, although confusion with elevated free sugar contents in some conditions may occur. These are grown for fresh consumption, or for simple processing. High-cyanide varieties are called bitter, although the phenolic compounds involved in root physiological deterioration can also produce a bitter taste. These are invariably grown for processing, especially for farinha in Brazil and gari in Africa. It is interesting that low cyanide varieties are rarely used for processing: the reasons for preference for high-cyanide varieties is unclear. Contrary to anecdotal evidence, high-cyanide varieties do not yield more than low-cyanide ones. There is some evidence that cyanide may protect against rodent pests and robbery, and also that there may be a link between end-product quality (e.g. farinha texture) and cyanide content.

Cyanide is concentrated in the root peel, especially in low-cyanide varieties where peel:root ratios of 40:1 are found. In high-cyanide varieties ratios of 1·6:1 are common. The use of whole or peeled roots for processing may therefore result in great differences in end-product cyanide content. In root parenchyma tissues, free cyanide – hydrogen cyanide (HCN) plus cyanhydrin – normally accounts for 15% of total cyanide; the remainder is bound as linamarin or lotaustralin. All cassava varieties characterized to date contain cyanide. Projects involving genetic manipulation are currently under way to reduce the toxicity problems of cassava, though regulation of cyanide synthesis and increasing the activity of linamarase.

Starch

Cassava starch has many food and industrial uses, which are linked to its functional properties. Although the basic properties of this starch are known, much research is required to complete our knowledge, especially as regards varietal differences in composition and functional properties. Cassava starch granules are round with a truncated end and a well-defined hilum. Granule size is between 5 and 35 μm. The starch has an A-type X-ray diffraction pattern, usually characteristic of cereals, and not the B type found in other root and tuber starches. The C-type spectrum, intermediate between A and B types, has also been reported. The nonglucosidic fraction of cassava starch is very low: protein and lipid content is below 0·2%. There is thus no formation of an amylose complex with lipids in native starch. Amylose contents of 8–28% have been reported, but most values lie within the range of 16–18%. *See* Starch, Structure, Properties and Determination

Fig. 1 shows Brabender amylographs of starch from four cassava varieties. Although significant varietal variation is present, all curves follow the same general pattern, and are similar to all high-amylopectin starches. The starch gelatinizes at relatively low temperatures. Initial and final gelatinization occurs at 60°C and 80°C, respectively. Peak viscosity is high and is reached rapidly, within 2 min. At high temperatures starch viscosity decreases greatly. Viscosity increases again on cooling (setback), and then remains stable. Cassava starch has a low retrogradation tendency (i.e. viscosity is stable over time following the cooling episode), and produces a very stable and clear gel. The swelling power of the starch is also very high: 100 g dry starch will absorb 120 g water at 100°C. At this temperature, over 50% of the starch is soluble. *See* Starch, Functional Properties

Bibliography

Bradbury JH and Holloway WD (1988) Chemistry of tropical root crops: significance for nutrition and agriculture in the Pacific. *Australian Center for International Agricultural Research Monograph* No. 6.

Cock JH (1985) *Cassava: New Potential for a Neglected Crop.* Boulder, Colorado: Westview Press.

Cooke RD and Coursey DG (1981) Cassava: a major cyanide containing food crop. In: Conn E, Knowles EJ, Vennesland B, Westley E and Wissung F (eds) *Cyanide in Biology*, p 193. New York: Academic Press.

Kay DE (revised by Gooding EGB) (1987) *Crop and Product Digest No. 2-Root Crops* 2nd edn. London: Natural Resources Institute XV.

Rickard JE and Coursey DG (1981) Cassava storage. Part 1: storage of fresh cassava roots. *Tropical Science* 23: 1–32.

Wheatley CC and Best R (1991) How can traditional forms of nutrition be maintained in urban centers: the case of cassava. *Entwicklung & Landlicher Raum* 1: 13–16.

C. C. Wheatley
International Centre for Tropical Agriculture (CIAT), Cali, Colombia
G. Chuzel
Centre d'Etudes et de Expérimentation du Machinisme Agricole Tropical, Montpellier, France

Use as a Raw Material

The fresh cassava root is an important staple in many rural areas of the tropics, especially in sub-Saharan Africa where it is the principal carbohydrate source for 40% of the population. More recently, the crop has been used as a raw material for food and other industries. This article will briefly review the wide range of products made from cassava roots and then focus on four of the most important products.

Use as a Staple Food

The fresh, peeled root is commonly boiled for 15–30 min, either alone or with other ingredients in a soup. Raw or boiled root pieces can also be fried. Boiled cassava should have a soft, floury texture, but is sometimes hard and glassy, leading to rejection by consumers. The causes of glassy texture are unknown. Bitter taste is frequently due to residual cyanide remaining after boiling, although the phenolic compounds involved in physiological deterioration can also produce a bitter taste. Cultivars with low cyanide content in the

parenchyma are invariably used for fresh consumption. Consumption per capita of fresh cassava may reach very high levels (e.g. 405 kg per year in Zaire, and over 200 kg per year in rural areas of Paraguay). A variety of foods made with grated or mashed, boiled cassava are prepared at the household level. Examples of other staple foods based on cassava are gari in Nigeria and farinha in Brazil. These processed products will be considered in the next section. *See* Phenolic Compounds

Cassava leaves form an important part of the diet in Zaire and other African countries, and are of minor importance in Southeast Asia. In Zaire, cassava leaves comprise nearly 70% by weight of all vegetables consumed. They are normally chopped and boiled, a process which greatly reduces the level of residual cyanide.

Cyanide Toxicity and Processing

Tissue disruption (chipping, grating or fermentation) is effective in bringing linamarase into contact with the linamarin substrate, thereby liberating hydrogen cyanide (HCN). Processes such as sun-drying of large root pieces or boiling are less effective. Toxicity problems may result when poorly processed cassava products are consumed. Acute cyanide toxicity appears when more than 30 mg is consumed over a 24 h period. The body's natural thiocyanate detoxification mechanism requires a good supply of sulphur-containing amino acids: a protein-deficient diet in combination with cyanide consumption can therefore result in health problems. In addition, thiocyanate interferes with iodine uptake by the thyroid gland, leading to goitre and, in extreme cases, cretinism. Epidemic spastic paraparesis has been reported on several occasions in Africa since 1981, affecting a total of 5000–10 000 people with leg paralysis. The exact metabolic processes involved are unknown, but each outbreak was clearly associated with famine-induced consumption of poorly processed cassava and a lack of protein in the diet. *See* Thyroid Diseases

The toxicity of processed cassava products is due to the residual linamarin and cyanhydrin remaining after the action of linamarase ceases. Once consumed, linamarin reaching the gut may be broken down by microbial enzymes or by ingested linamarase. This process is incomplete, since linamarin can also be detected in the urine. The percentage of linamarin which may be degraded in the gut has received little research attention; however, individual sensitivity to cyanide toxicity seems to vary with nutritional status. Adequate cassava processing (grating, fermentation, slow sun-drying), combined with sufficient dietary protein, is necessary for populations at risk in order to take advantage of the food security offered by cultivating high-cyanide cassava varieties. The use of cassava varieties low in cyanide also has potential.

Overview of Cassava Processing

Processing of cassava has several objectives: to produce a more stable product, capable of being stored in tropical environments for extended periods with no decrease in quality or deterioration; to reduce the content of cyanide to innocuous levels; to reduce bulk and hence lower transport costs; to diversify the food and other uses of cassava, leading to market expansion; and to provide food and other industries with a low-cost raw material for further processing.

Cassava roots may be processed whole, after removal of the peel, or after washing, a process which also removes most of the outer barky layer. The roots can then be grated, chipped or sliced. Grated roots may be pressed to remove excess water, and then toasted to produce the flour called farinha, or a flat bread called cassabe. These are staple foods in several Latin American and Caribbean countries. If a fermentation stage is included, using peeled roots, the product is gari, a staple in West Africa. Alternatively, starch can be extracted from the grated roots, and can either be dried directly, or fermented to produce a modified starch (sour starch). Cassava chips are usually sun-dried to produce a dried chip (gaplek) which is used for human consumption in Indonesia, and for animal consumption in Latin America. Larger root pieces are sun-dried in Africa. *See* Starch, Sources and Processing

A high-quality cassava flour can be produced from washed or peeled roots, chipped and sun-dried on trays or artificially dried to avoid microbial contamination. This flour can replace wheat and other imported flours in tropical countries. In Africa, pieces of cassava roots are fermented and dried to produce a flour called lafun. In Indonesia, root pieces are fermented using an innoculum of *Amylomyces* and *Endomycopsis*, to produce a moist product called tape. In Africa, whole roots are retted, grated and boiled to produce a fermented dough called chickwangwe or fu-fu.

A great diversity of products are prepared from cassava roots in rustic, small-scale facilities, using traditional methods. Over the last decades, medium-scale processing of these traditional products has developed on all continents. This had led to the design of more efficient processing equipment, and to improvements and standardization of quality. In recent years large-scale operations for starch and farinha have been developed to supply urban and export markets, especially in Brazil, Thailand and Indonesia. *See* Traditional Food Technology

Important Products

Gari

Gari, a fermented, cooked and dehydrated cassava meal, is widely consumed in West Africa. It is a stable, ready-to-use foodstuff, well-suited to urban markets. Gari consumption is increasing even in countries where it is not a traditional food. Gari is principally consumed in the main meal with vegetable sauces and meat. It can also be eaten as a snack soaked in cold water or milk, with roasted peanuts or coconut. Gari contributes up to 60% of the total calorie intake in West Africa, where an average of 150 g per person per day is consumed. Gari is mainly produced on a small scale and marketed by women; it provides an important source of income in many rural areas. Although many process improvements have been designed, diffusion of equipment has been slow and patchy, so that today most of the gari consumed is still manufactured using the traditional process.

In traditional preparation of gari (Fig. 1), the roots are hand-peeled, then grated into a pulp, often using a roughly perforated iron sheet. This pulp or mash is placed in hessian sacks, under heavy weights (logs, rocks) to squeeze out excess water. The mash is left to drain for 1–6 days, during which natural fermentation occurs. The pressed cake is shredded by hand and then rubbed through a woven palm-frond sieve to remove fibre and large lumps. This sieved mash is toasted (garified) in clay or iron vessels over a wood fire until the starch gelatinizes and the moisture content is reduced to 10–15%. The mash must be stirred constantly to avoid sticking or burning. Palm oil may be added to facilitate this operation, and imparts a yellow colour to the final product.

Great variability exists in consumer perception of gari quality, and it is difficult to establish optimum values for the different quality parameters. However, in general, consumers prefer a crisp, fine-grained, slightly sour product with good swelling power in water, and a lightly toasted colour. Although all the processing steps are important in determining end-product quality, some of them are only mechanical (peeling, grating, sieving, dewatering), while others involve some physical and chemical modifications which improve digestibility and reduce cyanide toxicity (fermentation, garification). The fermentation step is crucial to the development of the characteristic aroma and sour flavour of gari, imparted mainly by lactic acid bacteria, which produce lactic acid and volatiles such as aldehydes, diacetyl esters and ethanol. Fermentation also helps to detoxify the mash, while grating allows linamarase to come into contact with cyanoglucoside substrates. During fermentation, free HCN is released. The pH falls from 6·8 to 4·5 after 24 h of fermentation. Because the cyanohydrin interme-

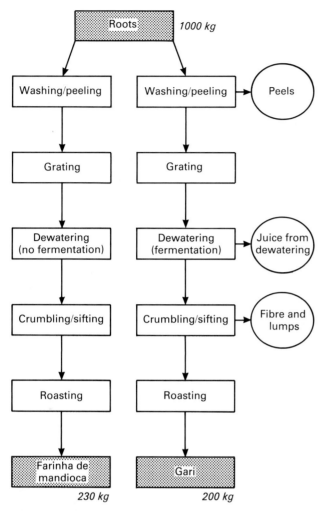

Fig. 1 Flow diagram of the traditional processes for production of gari (West Africa) and farinha de mandioca (Brazil).

diary is quite stable in acidic conditions and linamarase activity is also reduced, less free cyanide is produced and cyanhydrins accumulate in the fermented mash. Cyanide detoxification of the mash occurs in three ways: enzymic hydrolysis of cyanoglucosides, solubilization of cyanide in the water lost during dewatering, and volatilization of free cyanide during garification, at temperatures over 26°C. The combination of these is not enough to completely remove all cyanide from the end product: total cyanide contents of 15–33 mg per kg, with 5–25 mg per kg of free cyanide, have been reported. *See* Lactic Acid Bacteria

The garification step is essential to obtain good quality gari, for which 60–80% of starch should be gelatinized. This also improves starch digestibility. The starch is not completely gelatinized during garification because of the low initial moisture content of the dewatered mash (50–55%) and the temperatures used (60–85°C). Gelatinization proceeds until moisture content is reduced to about 40%, after which only drying

occurs. The efficiency of manual stirring during garification is an additional variable affecting final quality.

Farinha

Farinha de mandioca is a major dietary staple in Brazil, especially in the northeast region of the country where per capita consumption is over 40 kg per year or 1881 J (450 cal) per person per day. This represents 25% of total calories consumed – more than rice and wheat combined. In Brazil as a whole, farinha contributes an average of 752 J (180 cal) per person per day to the diet. Farinha is a traditional cassava product and is still the major source of dietary energy for many of the indigenous peoples of the Amazon basin; one study of the Colombian Vaupes region found that cassava provided over 80% of dietary calories, and that farinha was the major product consumed.

The process for the production of farinha is similar to that of gari (Fig. 1). It is probable that gari is an adaptation of farinha to African tastes, which occurred when cassava was introduced from Brazil to Africa. Unlike gari, however, typical farinha preparation does not include a fermentation step. The operation proceeds directly from grating through pressing and sieving to toasting. Another difference is the use of washed but unpeeled roots. The end product is thus a cream/yellow-coloured meal with no fermented taste. The final moisture content is the same as in gari, but the residual cyanide content is lower (10 mg per kg). Since no fermentation occurs, acid conditions do not develop and the cyanhydrin intermediate rapidly breaks down to free cyanide.

Farinha is an integral ingredient in many traditional dishes. Mixed with beans, farinha provides a thicker texture. Farinha is also consumed with meats. Consumption decreased markedly between 1960 and 1980, as government subsidies on wheat reduced the competitiveness of farinha. However, over the last few years, elimination of wheat subsidies has resulted in an increase in the attractiveness of farinha. As a storable, rapidly prepared and well-accepted food, farinha integrates easily into urban food habits.

Considerable applied research has resulted in the design, testing, commercial construction and use of efficient medium- and large-scale farinha production facilities in Brazil. Plants with a capacity of 50–200 t of cassava roots per day are in operation. Alongside this, many thousands of small-scale traditional 'casas de farinha' exist, especially in the northeast, providing employment over vast areas of this region, the poorest in Brazil. Over 460 000 such plants exist, often run as communal operations at the village level. The range of scales of operation, and the regional differences in cassava varieties and in the process itself, result in large

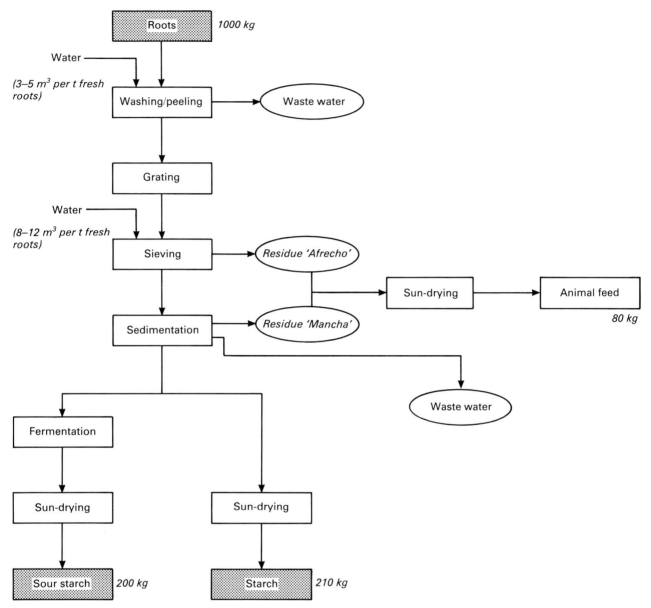

Fig. 2 Flow diagram of the process for production of fermented (sour) and nonfermented (sweet, native) cassava starch.

variations in end-product quality. Variation in quality and its effect on consumption patterns needs more study. Research aimed at improvement and standardization of quality has yet to produce results.

Starch

Although cassava is an efficient starch producer, only 5% of total starch traded worldwide is from cassava, representing about $0.8-1.0 \times 10^6$ t per year. The main industrial-scale producers of cassava starch are Brazil, China and Indonesia for national use, and Thailand, mainly for export. National use of cassava starch is now increasing in Southeast Asia, especially as a feedstock for derived products for the food industry. In addition to the large-scale industries, many small-scale starch extraction plants operate in South and Southeast Asia and in Latin America. Here, cassava starch is used in the local food industry to make a wide range of traditional food products (tapioca or sago in India; krupuk in Indonesia; chipa in Paraguay). In Brazil and Colombia, moist starch is fermented before drying, and a naturally modified starch is obtained which has functional properties distinct from those of native cassava starch. This is used in several traditional breads (pandebono, pan de queijo, biscoicho).

Cassava roots are washed and peeled; sometimes only the outer bark is removed, and then grated to release starch granules (Fig. 2). The starch is extracted under running water, and separated from the fibre and other root components by screening. Solid starch is separated from the starch/water slurry by sedimentation or centrifugation. The resultant starch is dried to a final moisture content of 12–14%. Sun-drying in small-scale operations and flash-drying in large-scale plants are typical. To obtain sour, fermented starch, the sedimented starch is left in tanks for 20–30 days before drying. While a small-scale extraction plant may process only 2–10 t of cassava per day, large-scale operations in Brazil and Thailand can handle 200 t per day. Starch extraction rates are usually 18–22% for small-scale plants and 20–25% in larger operations, depending on process efficiency and initial root starch content. In small-scale plants, operations are manual or semimechanized, resulting in less efficient starch extraction: in Columbia, 45% of the starch contained in the roots is lost in the waste water from the process, or remains in the peel and fibre byproduct, which is dried and used for animal feed. Waste water from processing plants can present severe environmental contamination problems, due to significant concentrations of starch and cyanide. Simple water treatment systems are available and are being implemented in several countries.

In India, Brazil, and Malaysia, partially dried native cassava starch is used to make tapioca or sago: the still moist starch is globulated on a vibrating surface, then the resulting small spheres are steamed or baked to gelatinize the surface layers of starch. The end product, tapioca pearls, is used to make a variety of desserts. In Indonesia and Malaysia, the native starch is mixed with water, fish or prawn flavouring and colouring. This dough is steamed, then sun-dried to make krupuk, or prawn crackers. When fried, these expand to several times their original size. They are a major snack food in Java and elsewhere in the region.

Fermented or sour starch has excellent expansion power; thus the volume of a dough containing this starch increases greatly during baking. Although many factors affect the expansion power of sour starch, including environmental conditions, cassava variety and water quality, the major factor is fermentation. During fermentation, amylolytic organisms produce reducing sugars which are immediately consumed by lactic acid bacteria to produce organic acids (lactic, propionic, butyric, acetic etc.) and carbon dioxide (CO_2). High lactic acid content in sour starch correlates with good expansion power and a good-quality final baked product. The action of the amylolytic enzymes and the acidification of the fermentation medium (pH 3·2) result in a lower viscosity, improved ease of baking and reduced gelling ability of sour starch compared to native cassava starch. During baking of doughs containing sour starch, the moisture content loss (from 50% to 8–12%) together with volatilization of lactic acid and CO_2 result in the increased expansion power and

reduced gelling ability, giving the end product its characteristic texture.

Flour

In several regions of Africa and in Indonesia, cassava roots are chopped into pieces, sun-dried and then pounded into a coarse meal or flour. This flour serves as a base for the production of many dishes at the household level. More recently, in Thailand, sun-dried cassava chips have been produced on a large scale, over 6×10^6 t per year, for export to Europe as an animal feed. The chips are ground to a meal, which is then converted under steam and pressure to hard pellets. Dried cassava for animal feed is now expanding rapidly in Latin America as an alternative to imported grains for internal use. Potential also exists to produce high-quality cassava flour to replace imported wheat flour in bakery and other products in many tropical countries. One such programme in Brazil was halted during the 1970s by wheat flour subsidies which made it impossible for cassava flour to compete. With many countries now removing subsidies, an opportunity for cassava flour is reemerging. In Brazil, food industry use of cassava flour is increasing again.

The process for the production of high-quality cassava flour requires the use of cleaned roots with the bark removed. Peel removal is optional. Roots are chipped and sun-dried on trays or artificially dried (60°C for 8–10 h) to obtain a hygienic product. The dried chips, with 12% moisture content, can be reduced in size (premilled) sufficiently to permit them to enter into standard wheat flour roller mills. Conversion rates in excess of 90% can be obtained in this way, compared with 72% for wheat grains. If roots are not peeled before chipping and drying, the peel and fibre fractions can be removed efficiently during the milling and grading process. A conversion rate of 3:1 is possible with cassava flour, compared to 4·5–5:1 for starch. The approximate composition of the flour is as follows: moisture 12%; carbohydrate 75%; protein 3%; fibre 5%; and lipids 2%. Total cyanide content should be below 50 mg per kg.

Industry trials with cassava flour in Colombia have recently demonstrated that some specific attributes of the flour are especially suited to certain products. A 40–50% substitution of cassava for wheat flour produced biscuits with superior texture and colour compared to 100% wheat flour controls. In Indonesia, a wide range of bakery products are being manufactured from cassava flour for internal consumption and export. The quality advantages apparent for cassava flour, combined with its competitive price in countries where wheat flour is not subsidized, could permit an expansion in the use of this product over the coming decades. *See* Flour, Analysis of Wheat Flours; Flour, Dietary Importance; Flour, Roller Milling Operations

Bibliography

Balagopalan C, Padmaja G, Nanda SK and Moorthy SN (1988) *Cassava in Food, Feed and Industry*. Boca Raton, Florida: CRC Press.

Campbell-Plat G (1987) *Fermented Foods of the World*. London: Butterworth.

Cereda MP (1987) Tecnología e qualidade do polvilho azedo (Technology and quality of sour starch). *Informe Agropecuario Belo Horizonte* 13: 145.

Chuzel G and Griffon D (1989) Le gari. In: Bourgeois CM and Larpent JP (eds) *Microbiologie Alimentaire*, pp 175–188. Paris: Technique et Documentation, Lavoisier.

Lancaster PA, Ingram JS, Lim MY and Coursey DG (1982) Traditional cassava based food: survey of processing techniques. *Economic Botany* 36: 12–45.

Muchnik J and Vinck D (1984) *La Transformation du Manioc: Technologies Autochtones*. Paris: Presses Universitaires de France.

Onyekwere OO, Akminrele IA, Koleojo OA and Heys G (1989) Industrialisation of gari fermentation. In: Steinkraus KH (ed.) *Industrialisation of Indigenous Fermented Foods*, pp 363–408. New York: Marcel Dekker.

Rosling H (1988) *Cassava Toxicity and Food Security: a Report for UNICEF African Household Food Security Programme*. Uppsala, Sweden: International Child Health Unit, University Hospital.

Wheatley CC and Best R (1991) How can traditional forms of nutrition be maintained in urban centers: the case of cassava. *Entwicklung Landlicher Raum*. 1: 13–16.

C. C. Wheatley
International Centre for Tropical Agriculture (CIAT), Cali, Colombia
G. Chuzel
Centre d'Etudes et d'Expérimentation du Machinisme Agricole Tropical, Montpellier, France